Frontiers in Cognitive Neuroscience

Frontiers in Cognitive Neuroscience

edited by Stephen M. Kosslyn and Richard A. Andersen

A Bradford Book

The MIT Press
Cambridge, Massachusetts
London, England

First MIT Press paperback edition, 1995

This book was printed and bound in the United States of America.

Library of Congress Cataloging-in-Publication Data

Frontiers in cognitive neuroscience/edited by
Stephen M. Kosslyn and Richard A. Andersen.
p. cm.
"A Bradford book."
Includes bibliographical references and index.
ISBN 0-262-11163-2 (HB), 0-262-61110-4 (PB)
1. Cognitive neuroscience. I. Kosslyn, Stephen Michael, 1948– . II. Andersen, Richard A.
QP360.5.C64 1992
153—dc20 91-36146
CIP

Contents

Reasoning

Language

General Introduction
Stephen M. Kosslyn and Richard A. Andersen

It has sometimes been said that "the mind is what the brain does." Cognitive neuroscience is built on this assumption, and its goal is to understand how brain function gives rise to mental activities such as perception, memory, and language. To understand the excitement surrounding the emergence of cognitive neuroscience, we must see how it arose from the confluence of several fields.

Cognitive neuroscience rests in part on the idea that different parts of the brain do different things—an idea with a checkered history. To understand the cognitive neuroscience approach, and why the time is finally ripe for this enterprise, we will consider first its historical roots and then turn to the factors that led to its recent emergence.

Historical Roots

Although philosophers have always been interested in the mind, it was not until the nineteenth century that scientists began to consider in earnest how mental activity arises from the brain. The major issue was whether the brain functions as a single, integrated whole (as the "globalists" believed) or as a collection of distinct organs, each responsible for a separate ability (as the "localizationists" believed). This central debate involved several lines of research during this period. Three examples are the phrenologists' view of localization of mental abilities, Pierre Flourens's and Gustav Theodor Fritsch and Edvard Hitzig's rather different conclusions based on experiments in animals, and Paul Broca's clinical findings of very specific deficits following brain lesions in humans.

The phrenologists, led by Franz Joseph Gall and J. G. Spurzheim, developed a "faculty psychology," which claimed that different regions of the brain implement distinct mental faculties, a not-so-unreasonable hypothesis. They also claimed, unfortunately, that more accomplished abilities are carried out by larger regions of the brain and that larger regions of the brain in turn create larger bumps on the skull. Neither assumption proved correct. Moreover, phrenologists characterized these faculties using rather arbitrary categories of human behavior and experience, which led them to assume that faculties such as sublimity, secretiveness, and parental love are carried out by distinct regions of the brain. This also proved to be off the mark.

Although phrenology was deeply flawed, it also produced some important concepts. For example, the phrenologists were the first to emphasize the importance of the surface of the brain, the cortex; previous theorists focused on the interior of the brain (typically concentrating on the role of the ventricles). In addition, phrenologists stressed that the brain is not a single, undifferentiated system, which also turns out to be correct.

Perhaps the most serious shortcoming of the phrenologists was that they were not really scientists; they did not put their ideas to rigorous empirical test. Instead, they felt bumpy skulls and made claims about the owners' personalities and mental abilities without trying carefully to validate their claims. Although phrenology was a pseudoscience, it did develop a clear set of ideas that could be treated as hypotheses by working scientists, who took up the challenge. These early researchers focused on the claim that mental abilities are localized to specific brain sites, rather than on the ancillary conceptions of what the abilities are and how to assess them. In these studies physiologists examined the effects of lesions or stimulation of different brain areas on the behavior of animals.

Pierre Flourens (1794–1867) is usually cited as one of the first physiologists to spearhead an attack against the localizationist view by using animal experiments. Flourens performed ablation studies on birds, removing only selected parts of their brains and then observing their behavior after they recovered. He claimed that the birds recovered, regardless of where the brain was cut, and regained the same set of abilities. These findings led Flourens to argue that the brain works as an integrated whole and that specific abilities are not localized to particular sites.

In retrospect, Flourens's research was flawed in several critical respects. First, his behavioral tests were crude. These methods were so insensitive that Flourens probably would not have noted selective deficits even if they were present. Indeed, modern researchers now report selective effects of damaging specific locations of birds' brains (e.g., Nottebohm 1981). Second, one must wonder about the precision of his surgery; it seems likely that his lesions often produced widespread damage, and so they may not have selectively affected specific neural structures.

Moreover, other scientists did produce evidence for the localization of function. Perhaps the best example is the research of Fritsch and Hitzig (1870), who delivered electrical stimuli to the cerebral cortex of dogs. Fritsch and Hitzig discovered that shocking specific locations of the cortex caused certain muscles to twitch. These results supported the idea that at least some functions are localized to distinct sites in the brain.

The third facet of the debate took place at about the same time that the animal experiments were underway. In contrast, however, this aspect of the debate focused on clinical phenomena. This third set of researchers were primarily physicians, who observed selective behavioral deficits when their patients suffered brain damage. Although others predated him, Broca's 1863 report probably had the most impact on the debate.

Broca described a patient who had suffered a stroke. A stroke occurs when blood is cut off from part of the brain, which causes those cells to die. This patient had a severe language deficit following his stroke; indeed, after the stroke all he could say was "tan." Broca examined the patient's brain immediately after he died and found that the stroke had damaged the posterior part of the left frontal lobe. Broca reported a second case with similar damage later that year. After seeing a number of such cases, Broca inferred that language depended on specific folds in the cortex, specifically the left posterior portion of the third frontal convolution.

The localizationist view received even stronger support when, in 1874, Carl Wernicke reported that a different language deficit occurred when a different part of the brain was damaged. His patient had damage to the left superior temporal gyrus and had trouble not in producing language—as had Broca's patients—but rather in comprehending language.

It was not long before others reported a wide variety of behavioral deficits that were correlated with damage to different brain sites. These reports led to the "era of the diagram makers." These investigators constructed diagrams that specified the locations of various brain sites for specific behaviors and described how these sites are anatomically connected. These early diagrams were often based on superficial analyses of the behavioral deficits and on the suspected localization of the damage. Thus, it was not surprising that many viewed them with skepticism.

At about the same time that these clinical findings were being reported on the Continent, the British neurologist John Hughlings Jackson offered a more sophisticated view (which in some ways was similar to Wernicke's views), suggesting that multiple brain areas contribute to complex brain processes. Although Jackson discovered that damage to the right cerebral hemisphere impairs visual perception more than damage to the left hemisphere, he rejected the idea that such a complex cognitive function can be carried out solely in one particular location of the brain. Rather, Jackson found that particular functions were never completely lost after a stroke; in fact, in some contexts patients could often exhibit abilities that were impaired or absent in other contexts. For example, it is not uncommon to find patients who cannot touch their lips with their tongue when asked to do so, but have no trouble performing this act to remove a crumb. Indeed, some patients cannot say specific words, such as "no," unless they are emotionally agitated. These sorts of observations led Jackson to claim that multiple regions of the brain are involved in carrying out complex functions such as perception, action, and language (see Taylor 1932).

The Twentieth Century

Remarkably, this debate continued into the twentieth century, in spite of the rather strong data for localization of function that existed in the experimental and clinical literature. The turn of the century marked the Golden Age of neuroanatomy. Santiago Ramón y Cajal, a Spanish neuroanatomist, using a stain developed by his contemporary (and competitor) Camillo Golgi, documented the immense complexity and anatomical specificity of the brain during the last part of the previous century and the early part of this century. Of particular interest is Cajal's theory that the brain is made up of individual elements, neurons. This idea was in contrast to the views of Golgi, who believed that the neural plexus was a continuous structure, a syncytium. Another insight of Cajal's was that nerve cells are unipolar, collecting information in the dendrites and sending it out along the axon. These basic ideas are some of the building blocks that began a century of progress in our understanding of brain function.

At the turn of the century, the famous German neuroanatomist Korbinian Brodmann used a stain originally developed by Franz Nissl (which stains the endoplasmic reticulum in the cytoplasm of cells) to study differential staining in the cortex. He used cytoarchitecture, the variation in appearance of various cortical areas due to different packing densities and cell morphologies, to distinguish roughly 50 areas. A large number of cytoarchitectural studies emerged in the period following Brodmann, including those by the Vogts, von Economo, von Bonin and Bailey, and Walker, which further divided the cortex into many cortical areas. Some of the most obvious divisions have remained, such as the border dividing Brodmann's area 17 (striate cortex) from Brodmann's area 18. Many other divisions have not remained; for instance it is now known that area 18 contains several different visual areas. Although perhaps a majority of the subdivisions recognized by the cytoarchitectonic studies have not stood the test of time, the paper by Merzenich and colleagues in this collection is a small victory for Brodmann. Areas 3a, 3b, 1, and 2 of Brodmann had been lumped in subsequent years by physiologists into one somatosensory area, SI. Merzenich and colleagues showed that there are, in fact, at least three representations of the body surface within SI, which correspond to Brodmann areas. Another more recently exploited technique involves staining the myelin sheaths that surround the axons of nerve cells; the use of myeloarchitecture has proved valuable in distinguishing area MT, the visual motion area whose function is described in the papers by Allman, Miezin, and McGuinness and by Movshon, Adelson, Gizzi, and Newsome in this collection.

The discovery in the earlier part of this century that the brain has a complex physical structure seemed to many to be strong support for the localizationist view. Some researchers felt at that time (circa 1930), however, that differences in appearance did not necessarily imply differences in function, and others questioned whether these structural differences existed at all. In particular, an influential psychologist, Karl Lashley, and his colleagues not only challenged many of the claims about the physical variations within the cortex (Lashley and Clark 1946), but also performed Flourens-like experiments on rats and reported similar findings. These findings were consistent with two principles Lashley (1929) used to explain the effects of brain damage on behavior. The principle of *mass action* stated that the brain operates as a single, integrated system, and the principle of *equipotentiality* stated that all portions of the brain have equal abilities. Taken together, these principles imply that the sheer amount of the brain that is damaged determines the behavioral deficit, not which particular parts are damaged.

Although Lashley's experiments were methodologically superior to those of Flourens, they were still crude by contemporary standards—and in fact failed to reveal selective deficits that have since been reported. Fortunately this brief regression was followed by an explosion of important discoveries regarding functional specialization in the cortex, and Lashley's influence was mitigated.

An important step forward in neurophysiological research occurred in the late 1930s when Woolsey, Bard, Rose, and their colleagues began novel experiments in which they mapped the evoked activity for sensory stimuli by placing wick electrodes on the surface of the cortex of animals. They mapped two auditory areas, AI and AII, and two somatosensory areas, SI and SII. As mentioned above, it was later found that SI contains several distinct areas, and their area AII contains three areas. Based on their recordings from visual cortex, they also proposed two areas; although there is a certain symmetry to their initial studies, it is now appreciated that there are at least 30 visual areas in the monkey cortex.

The surface electrodes used by these investigators recorded the composite activity of many thousands of nerve cells. With the advent of single-cell recording, using very fine wires insulated except at their tips, John Allman and Jon Kaas (reviewed in Woolsey 1981) began to map the visual cortex in new-world monkeys. They found one representation of visual space in the primary (striate) visual cortex, a fact that had been known for many years based on scotomas (blind spots) experienced by humans with brain lesions and the surface electrode technique with animals. When they continued to move into visual cortex outside of the primary visual cortex, however, they found several more representations of visual space, corresponding to several other visual fields. At this time Semir Zeki began tracing connections between the primary visual cortex and the extrastriate cortex and found that there were projections to several areas. This work is reviewed in Zeki's paper in this collection. Zeki also made the seminal finding that cells in area MT (V5) preferred moving visual stimuli, and cells in area V4 were selective for color. These important experiments laid the foundation for an exciting two decades of discovery, providing evidence for separate processing streams within the visual cortex. Much of this work is summarized in the papers by DeYoe and Van Essen, Livingstone and Hubel, and Schiller and Logothetis in this volume. At the same time a similar set of investigations was discovering multiple areas in the auditory cortex (reviewed by Brugge and Reale) and in the somatosensory cortex (Merzenich, Kaas, Sur, and Lin).

These empirical studies have led to a simple, elegant solution to the globalist/localizationist controversy. The brain is precisely organized, more so than any of the early researchers ever imagined. For instance, there is a small subdivision of the medial superior temporal area, about 3 mm in diameter, which in every monkey contains receptive fields that are selective for patterns of motion, such as rotation or expansion, occurring anywhere in their large visual fields. Similarly, circuits that perform specific transformations of the sensory input are found in striate cortex (Bolz, Gilbert, and Wiesel 1989). The mistake of the early localizationists is that they tried to map behaviors and perceptions into single locations in the cortex. Any particular behavior or percept is produced by many areas, located in various parts of the brain. Thus, the key to resolving the debate is to realize that complex functions such as perception, memory, reasoning, and movement are accomplished by a host of underlying processes, each of which confers only a single facet of the ability. These processes are relatively simple and mechanical; they do not "think" but rather reflexively perform a specific operation when provided with appropriate input. It is these simple, underlying processes that are carried out in a single region of the brain. Indeed, the abilities themselves typically can be accomplished in numerous different ways, which involve different combinations of processes. An example of this new synthesis can be gleaned from the readings in the section on attention, which include discussions of how the behavior of attending invokes the activity of many cortical areas (for example, Crick; Moran and Desimone; Richmond and Sato; Wurtz, Goldberg, and Robinson). Mesulam points out in his article, however, that lesions in humans to different attention-related brain structures produce different types of attentional deficits, leading him to suggest that the attention system is represented by a distributed network with its different nodes accomplishing different aspects of the process.

Any given complex ability, then, is not accomplished by a single part of the brain. So in this sense, the globalists were right. The kinds of functions posited by the phrenologists are not localized to a single brain region. However, simple processes that are recruited to exercise such abilities are localized. So in this sense, the localizationists were right (for further discussion, see Kosslyn and Koenig 1992; Luria 1980; Squire 1987).

Thus the stage was set for cognitive neuroscience: Two central questions emerged from the efforts of previous researchers. First, what are the simple, underlying processes that are carried out by the brain? And second, how do these processes work together to produce "mental" abilities? Both questions led to a new way of conceptualizing brain function.

The Emergence of Cognitive Neuroscience

Cognitive neuroscience arose when researchers conceived of brain function from a new perspective. This perspective grew out of a confluence of discoveries and ideas in three older disciplines, namely neuroscience (specifically neuroanatomy and neurophysiology), experimental psychology, and computer science. Although there are many modern precursors to the field (e.g., see Grossberg 1987; McCulloch and Pitts 1943), cognitive neuroscience probably did not truly come into its own until the late 1970s.

One foundation of cognitive neuroscience emerged in large part from the work of David Hubel and Torsten Wiesel at the Harvard Medical School and Vernon Mountcastle at Johns Hopkins University. These researchers led the way in helping us to understand how specific neural events could give rise to perception. They not only began to characterize elementary processes that are carried out by individual neurons but also discovered key facts about how the brain is organized. They found that some neurons are tuned for specific types of stimuli, that neurons are organized into "columns" with an orderly internal structure, and that these columns are interconnected in orderly ways. By combining neurophysiology (the study of dynamic properties of brain cells) and neuroanatomy (the study of the structure of the brain), these researchers and their contemporaries made great strides in showing how specific neural processes might be neurally integrated to produce sensory percepts.

Another important advance in neuroscience came with the melding of psychophysics with neurophysiology. Psychophysics is not the product of a deranged physicist but rather the study of the limits and parameters of human perception and ability. It represents an early branch of experimental psychology whose roots are the work of some of the great psychologists of the nineteenth century, and it has undergone a recent rebirth since the advent of computers, which enable highly precise stimulus control and response measurement. Psychophysical results tell us what the neural machine can do—its specifications, if you will—and give neurophysiologists clues about what to look for when deciphering brain mechanisms. An example is the study of depth perception. Bela Julesz, then at Bell Labs, and Gerald Westheimer, at the University of California at Berkeley, studied the abilities of humans to see depth from stereopsis. Their findings, and a unique stimulus developed by Julesz (the random-dot stereogram) enabled physiologists such as Gian Poggio, at the Johns Hopkins Medical School, to search for and find the neural substrate of this perceptual process in the monkey visual cortex.

An important technical advance in neuroscience was the advent of recording the activity of single nerve cells in behaving animals. This technique was first exploited in a systematic fashion by Edward Evarts at NIH. Evarts studied the motor cortex, which can only be appreciated when an animal can make voluntary movements. Soon after Evart's initial studies, David Robinson and his colleagues at the Johns Hopkins Medical School began using this technique to study the control of eye movements in monkeys. The eye movement system is a much simpler system than the limb movement system and as a result has proved to be an important model system for the study of motor control. Emilio Bizzi and his colleagues at the Massachusetts Institute of Technology further advanced this field by studying the coordination of combined eye and head movements.

Another foundation of cognitive neuroscience grew out of experimental psychology. Although there were a vast number of important contributors, three played a special role. Saul Sternberg, at the University of Pennsylvania, developed a ground-breaking technique for characterizing individual mental operations. Sternberg (1969) showed that some tasks are accomplished by a series of discrete processing stages and developed a method for characterizing the individual stages. Each stage was understood in terms of information that is stored and operated on in specific ways. Although his method has since proven less straightforward than originally conceived (because many tasks are not performed by a series of discrete serial operations), Sternberg's work helped to focus experimental psychologists on the problem of measuring individual processes that underlie complex abilities. One consequence of this analysis was the development of many sensitive behavioral tasks, which subsequently have allowed researchers in cognitive neuroscience to assess the effects of brain damage and to correlate local brain activity with specific types of information processing.

Another key contributor was Michael Posner, at the University of Oregon. Posner developed tasks that assess relatively simple aspects of information processing (e.g., see the paper reprinted in this volume), and developed conceptual foundations for the study of attention and related abilities. Like Sternberg, Posner developed ways of testing individual components of information processing, but his ideas were not tied to specific models of sequential processing. His elegantly simple tasks and sophisticated ideas have subsequently played a major role in the study of effects of brain damage on behavior and in the use of brain-scanning techniques to study the localization of cognitive function.

Much research in experimental psychology stressed the discrete nature of cognitive operations. This point of view was nicely counterbalanced by the work of Roger N. Shepard, at Stanford University. Shepard used behavioral data to demonstrate that the brain performs "analog" operations, such as mentally rotating or folding objects in visual mental images. For example, he and his colleagues found that subjects required progressively more time to imagine an object rotating through greater arcs or being folded more times (see Shepard and Cooper 1982). This work also demonstrated that there must be internal representations of images in the brain and challenged many researchers to gain an understanding of the properties of different kinds of internal representations. One of the papers in this collection has taken up this challenge. Georgopoulos and his colleagues report what appears to be a neural correlate of a mental rotation of a planned movement.

The idea that behavior can be understood in terms of operations on internal representations led many experimental psychologists into cognitive science. Cognitive science likens the mind to a computer program, which has led researchers to try to characterize the representations and operations carried out by the mind. This new brand of experimental psychology has played a special role in the development of cognitive neuroscience, emphasizing the structural organization of information processing.

Another important development in experimental psychology was the widespread realization that behavioral data alone are not sufficient to characterize mental processes. John Anderson (1978) proved that any set of behavioral data could always be explained by more than a single theory and suggested that neurophysiological constraints would help to ameliorate this problem. This approach led some experimental psychologists to look more seriously at the neural substrate of behavior.

The third foundation of cognitive neuroscience was provided by developments in computer science—in particular in the subdiscipline of artificial intelligence (AI). The reconciliation of the globalist/localizationist debate led researchers to expect relatively simple processes to be localized in specific regions of the brain; however, researchers in neuroscience characterized brain function largely on the basis of common sense. For example, if a single cell in the visual cortex responded vigorously to an oriented line segment, it might be construed as an "oriented-line detector." Unfortunately, many neurons respond in complex ways to stimuli, and common sense falters when trying to characterize their function.

Computer science provided a new, more powerful way to think about brain function. From the start, researchers in AI were confronted with the problem of characterizing elementary processes. Their goal is to build machines that behave "intelligently," and they typically build such machines by programming hierarchies of processes. That is, they compose complex functions out of sets of simpler ones. Indeed, Herbert Simon, one of the founders of AI, argued that all complex devices should be built in this way (Simon 1981).

The simple processes in AI programs execute individual *computations*. The concept of a "computation" is closely related to the concept of a mapping; a computation systematically maps an input to an output. Moreover, both the input and the output convey information, and the relation between the two can be characterized in terms of a (mathematical) function. Computations transform inputs to produce appropriate outputs.

Because a computation describes a type of mapping, this concept could be applied equally easily to a computer or to a brain—as the early researchers in cybernetics, who focused on analog computing systems, concluded. Indeed, John von Neumann (1958), Norbert Wiener (1948), Warren McCulloch and Walter Pitts (1943), and others regarded neural processes as performing computations.

Many researchers adopted this conceptualization of brain function after learning about the work of one man, the late David Marr of the Massachusetts Institute of Technology. At the time, Marr's work was uniquely interdisciplinary and was particularly important because it provided the first rigorous examples of cognitive neuroscience theories (Kosslyn and Maljkovic 1990). A classic example of Marr's approach is the paper by Marr and Nishihara in this volume. Marr borrowed from the work of the experimental psychologist J. J. Gibson and emphasized the importance of careful analyses of the visual input to understand the "problems" that must be solved by a vision system with abilities like ours. Marr went a step beyond his predecessors by showing how such observations could be used to analyze what computations are necessary to produce specific behaviors. And Marr did even more than this: His analyses were informed by facts about neurophysiology and neuroanatomy.

Marr stressed the idea that neural computation can be understood at multiple levels of analysis. Philosophers of science observed long ago that a single phenomenon can be examined at multiple levels of analysis (e.g., Putnam 1973; see also chapter 8 of Churchland 1986). When considering psychology, philosophers such as Jerry Fodor (1968) distinguished between a functional and physical level; the functional level ascribed roles and purposes to brain events, and the physical level characterized the electrical and chemical characteristics of those events.

Marr took these earlier analyses several steps further. He posited a hierarchy of levels that is rooted in the idea that the brain computes. He divided the functional level into two levels, one that characterizes *what* is computed and another that characterizes *how* the computation is accomplished (i.e., the algorithm), and he showed how these levels related to the lowest one, the level of the implementation. The theories of the computation and the algorithm are cast in the vocabulary of computation, referring to data structures and processes that operate on them, whereas the theory of the implementation is cast in the vocabularies of biology and biophysics, referring to properties of neurons and their physical interactions.

Marr's analysis held enormous appeal. Part of this appeal came from the idea that we could understand cognitive function by reason alone. If we could divine the correct theory of what had to be computed to solve a specific problem, we were most of the way there. Unfortunately, this has not turned out to be the case. The distinction between the levels of the algorithm and the implementation is not clear-cut. Indeed, if one is trying to understand brain function, then theories of computations and algorithms are necessarily descriptions of neural activity. Hence, properties of neurons cannot help but bear on these theories. It is clear that the structure of the brain (its neuroanatomy) and its dynamic properties (its neurophysiology) provide hints as to what the brain is doing. Marr himself noted the receptive field properties of different types of neurons and used this information to constrain his theory.

The interdependence of the levels has been driven home by the rise of "neural network" modeling since Marr's death (e.g., Grossberg 1987; Rumelhart and McClelland 1986). These models conflate all three levels. The functional properties of these models, several of which are described in articles we have reprinted here, are intended to mirror those of the underlying neural substrate.

Thus it became clear to many that research in brain function required a combination of complementary approaches, and the idea of a new field of research was born. The term "Cognitive Neuroscience" was coined in 1970 by Michael S. Gazzaniga, presently at the University of California, Davis. This field has since evolved as new technologies became available and the field became more interdisciplinary (Kosslyn and Koenig 1992), as we discuss in the following section.

The Cognitive Neuroscience Approach

The three foundations of cognitive neuroscience—neuroscience, experimental psychology, and computer science—have melded into a new discipline. The cognitive neuroscience approach can be schematized by a triangle. At the top of the triangle is behavior, and at its lower vertices are neuroscience and computation.

Consider first the top vertex. Our goal is to understand the regularities in how a system (vision, memory, etc.) behaves. Thus the behavioral sciences play a critical role in cognitive neuroscience; cognitive psychology, linguistics, psychophysics, and related disciplines provide detailed descriptions of what the brain does. Not all of the information produced by researchers in these fields is equally useful for cognitive neuroscientists, however; because our goal is to understand how the brain produces behavior, we need descriptions of behavior that can be related relatively directly to underlying neural mechanisms. Many sorts of behavior reflect complex interactions among many mechanisms. Unfortunately, there is no way to know in advance which regularities in behavior will mesh neatly with distinct properties of the brain and which regularities will reflect complex interactions among numerous properties. In general, however, behavioral studies that are designed to bear on issues about the brain seem more likely to alert us to relevant behavioral phenomena than studies that ignore such issues.

In cognitive neuroscience, explanations of behavioral regularities hinge on a confluence of facts and concepts about the brain and computation, which we schematize at the lower two vertices of the triangle. Our goal is to understand how a machine with the physical properties of the brain can produce specific behaviors when given specific inputs. Neuroscience, then, is the second vertex of our triangle; it provides information about the neuroanatomy and neurophysiology of the brain. Anatomical facts are often critically important because they specify the information flow within the brain, which places strong constraints on what a given part of the brain can do. And neurophysiological findings provide hints about how the brain represents and processes information.

Neuroscience has undergone a split; the part of this field that is concerned with behavior is now closely allied with cognitive neuroscience, and the other part has focused on the brain for its own sake. Even this second branch of the field, however, is beginning to feed into cognitive neuroscience. For example, the powerful methods of molecular biology are now being applied in studies of the neurochemical bases of brain function. In the future, we will understand brain function at multiple levels of analysis, ranging from the activity of circuits to the activity of genes that produce the neurotransmitters that are essential in making circuits work. The section on memory in this volume provides good examples of how cognitive functions are being approached from many levels. Memory is beginning to be understood from the levels of the transmitter, synapses and receptors (Bliss and Lømo), the function of neural circuits (Ambros-Ingerson, Granger, and Lynch; Barto and Jordan; Funahashi, Bruce, and Goldman-Rakic; Fuster and Jervey; Gluck and Thompson; Gnadt and Andersen; Hawkins and Kandel; Miyashita and Chang), and the behavior of the whole organism (Corkin; Mishkin; Schacter; Shimamura et al.; Squire).

Computer science is the third vertex of our triangle; it has given us not only the idea of computational analyses but also the possibility of computer models. As noted earlier, computational analyses lead to a theory of how input can be converted to output by a mechanism; such analyses are based on careful considerations about what kinds of input/output transformation would be necessary to produce a specific kind of behavior. However, in cognitive neuroscience we are not interested in any physical system that could perform computations and produce behavior. Rather, we are interested in one particular system, namely, the brain. Hence, computational analyses must be informed by neuroanatomy and neurophysiology.

The brain is very complex, as are the ways in which even relatively simple organisms can behave. Thus after computational analyses have led us to hypothesize specific computations, we often need *computer models* to discover the implications of these hypotheses. A computer model is a program that is designed to mimic a dynamic system. The program plays the same role as that played by a model aircraft in a wind tunnel when a new airplane is being designed. By observing the way the model behaves, researchers generate accounts for the way the actual object or system behaves and generate predictions about how it should behave in novel circumstances.

In cognitive neuroscience, models of neural networks allow researchers to discover how specific types of inputs can be mapped to specific types of outputs. The recent advent of neural network computer models has led to an explosion in modeling complex neural circuits; some of these models can produce remarkably brainlike behaviors and sometimes can offer insight into the underlying processes that produce these behaviors. Indeed, as is illustrated in several of the papers in this volume (Kosslyn et al.; Lehky and Sejnowski; Zipser and Andersen), the network models themselves can be analyzed after they "learn" to perform the mapping, providing the researcher with insights into what aspects of the input were used to achieve the mapping. These network models have also helped us to understand how individual nerve cells can show a very broad selectivity but the network as a whole can be very precise (see Kosslyn et al., this volume).

Finally, we must note that the invention of more powerful computers has in turn engendered advances in medical technologies, which have had a large impact on the study of human brain function. Thanks to CT and MRI scans, clinicians now know exactly where brain damage is located when they evaluate cognitive functions and deficits of their patients following brain injury. Moreover, new brain scanning techniques allow researchers to observe which specific regions of the brain are active while human subjects perform specific tasks. Some of these methods (such as positron emission tomography (PET) and magnetoencephalography (MEG)) are illustrated in articles we have reprinted in this book (Kaufman and Williamson; Petersen et al.; Roland and Friberg).

We have schematized the interactions among these fields with a triangle because each pair of considerations may cross-fertilize. For example, discoveries about behavior can lead researchers to make discoveries about the brain; for instance, the existence of "illusory contours" (visible edges that do not actually exist) allowed researchers to study where in the brain such contours are provided (von der Heydt et al., this volume). And such discoveries can provide direct hints as to how to build a computational system that behaves as we do—one goal of AI. Similarly, the concepts and facts schematized at both bottom vertices can lead researchers to discover more about how the system behaves; for example Lowe's (1987a, 1987b) computational ideas about visual encoding led Biederman (1987) to perform a series of experiments on the properties of human perception. The finding that the visual system constructs surfaces from sparse data and that it deals with motion transparency through early segmentation of surfaces led to new computer algorithms for analyzing structure-from-motion that are much more powerful than previous algorithms (Andersen et al. 1991).

In short, cognitive neuroscience involves an interplay between three different kinds of concepts and findings. No discipline or approach is paramount; they all lean on each other. Furthermore, no single type of theory or analysis necessarily precedes the others; we need not begin with a particular behavior in mind in order to discover something interesting about the brain that ultimately helps to explain behavior. The field necessarily involves a dynamic interplay between three kinds of information.

Although it is difficult to categorize all scientific investigations in a field, for purposes of clarity we will attempt to distinguish cognitive neuroscience from computational neuroscience, cognitive science, and some areas of research within the field of neuropsychology. Of course, there is a great deal of overlap between these fields and cognitive neuroscience. First, cognitive neuroscience and *computational neuroscience* differ in the kinds of questions that are asked and the kinds of answers that are sought. Computational neuroscience focuses on specific problems, such as stereopsis or motion detection, from a relatively abstract perspective and typically seeks an answer at the level of what Marr called the algorithm. The approach tends to focus more on the mathematical solution of a problem than on the detailed brain mechanisms or behavioral correlates involved.

Second, cognitive neuroscience also differs from *cognitive science* in its style of investigation. Cognitive neuroscientists ask questions about how the brain produces behavior; that is why "neuroscience" is the noun. In contrast, cognitive science focuses on function per se, with little specific regard for the brain. A cognitive neuroscientist attempts to characterize the functions of neurons or networks of neurons, whereas a cognitive scientist does not.

Third, cognitive neuroscience differs from some research avenues in contemporary *neuropsychology*. Contemporary neuropsychology has split into three major groups. (1) Clinical neuropsychologists are interested primarily in diagnosing the effects of brain damage so that effective rehabilitation programs can be designed. To the extent that these clinicians perform research, it tends to be descriptive (documenting patterns of deficits) and often does not rely on rigorous formal experimentation or theorizing. (2) Another part of neuropsychology evolved into *cognitive neuropsychology* (which is exemplified by articles published in the journal of the same name). These researchers attempt to characterize mental function in its own right, typically by studying the effects of brain damage on behavior; however, they are not as interested in characterizing what is contributed by specific parts of the brain. Thus cognitive neuropsychologists ask the questions similar to those of cognitive scientists, with little concern about the exact implementation of functions by neural structures. Cognitive neuropsychologists differ from cognitive scientists in two ways: they try to characterize mental function by observing selective behavioral deficits following brain damage, and they rely less heavily on computational approaches. (3) Finally, the third wing of neuropsychology represents a major force in the field of cognitive neuroscience. These researchers have adopted neuroanatomical, neurophysiological, and computational perspectives in order to understand how the brain gives rise to mental activity. Several examples of this approach are the articles by Coltheart and colleagues, Corkin, Farah, Gazzaniga and colleagues, Geschwind, Levine, Marshall and Newcombe, McCarthy and Warrington, Milner and Petrides, Mishkin, Schacter, Shimamura and colleagues, and Squire, in this volume.

Structure of the Book

Cognitive neuroscience is inherently interdisciplinary. It draws on concepts, findings, and methods from fields that focus on behavior, neuroscience, and computation; the brain is regarded as a living machine that produces behavior. One of the exciting aspects of this field is that anyone entering it will find something new. But this variety is also one of its drawbacks. It is often difficult to come into an area and discover the relevant literature, let alone determine which papers are of most importance. The purpose of this book is to make it easier for researchers and students to enter cognitive neuroscience by pulling together many of the key articles that form the foundations of the field.

A survey of the papers included in this volume will show that the field of cognitive neuroscience continues to approach many of the traditional questions in psychology and neuroscience, reshaping and refining them as the field evolves. The book begins with key articles in the cognitive neuroscience of vision. Because vision has been such an active area, we divided this part into two sections, one that focuses on the nature of distinct "streams" of visual processing and one that focuses on the ways in which neurons code information. We next present articles on other sensory modalities, specifically audition and somatosensory processing. We then present a set of articles on attention. Research on this higher cognitive function has enjoyed success in part because of the ability of researchers to define the problem and develop inventive behavioral tasks. We then turn to memory; this part is also relatively long, and it has been divided into a section on the mechanisms used to store new information and another section on the nature of distinct memory systems. We close with a part on higher cortical functions, which we organize into a section on reasoning and a section on language.

Although the field is very young, we were surprised by the large number of first-rate articles that have already been published. Thus we had some difficult choices to make, given the limited space available. Some of our choices were influenced by our observation that the advent of neural network computer models has sometimes had an unfortunate consequence: Some researchers have tended to focus on the requirements of simply building a system that produces a behavior and have not exploited hints from the brain or heeded its warnings. Mindful of this shortcoming, we have focused in this volume on reprinting papers that bear directly on how the brain functions. "Neuroscience" is, after all, the noun. We have chosen papers that examine specific aspects of behavior, either explicitly or implicitly, and that cast their findings in a way that provides direct constraints on computational theories. A minority of papers actually present computational models, in part because such models have only recently been brought to bear on many issues in the field. But all of the papers in this volume provide the foundations for further research in cognitive neuroscience, and it is our goal that this volume will allow more researchers to join us in the enterprise.

We hope that the reader will come away with an appreciation not only of the complexities but also of the excitement that is generated when a new field evolves—one that is ready and willing to incorporate technical advances and use them to attack one of our final frontiers.

References

Allman, J. M., J. F. Baker, W. T. Newsome, and S. E. Petersen. 1981. Visual topography and function: Cortical visual areas in the owl monkey. In *Cortical Sensory Organization.* Vol. 2, *Multiple Visual Areas,* ed. C. N. Woolsey, 171–186. Clifton, NJ: Humana Press.

Andersen, R. A., R. J. Snowden, S. Treue, and M. Graziano. 1991. Hierarchical processing of motion in the visual cortex of monkey. *Cold Spring Harbor Symposia on Quantitative Biology* 55: 741–748.

Anderson, J. R. 1978. Arguments concerning representations for mental imagery. *Psychological Review* 85: 249–277.

Biederman, I. 1987. Recognition-by-components: A theory of human image understanding. *Psychological Review* 94: 115–147.

Bolz, J., C. D. Gilbert, and T. N. Wiesel. 1989. Pharmacological analysis of cortical circuitry. *Trends in Neurosciences* 12: 292–296.

Broca, P. 1863. Localisations des fonctions cérébrales.—Siège du langage articule. *Bulletins de la sociéte d'anthropologie* 4: 200–204.

Brodmann, K. 1909. *Vergleichende Lokalisationlehre der Grosshirnrinde in Ihren Prinzipien Dargestellt auf Grund des Zellenbaues.* Leipzig: A. J. Barth.

Churchland, P. S. 1986. *Neurophilosophy: Toward a Unified Science of the Mind-Brain.* Cambridge, MA: MIT Press.

Flourens, P. 1824. *Recherches expérimentales sur les propriétés et les fonctions du système nerveux dans les animaux vertébrès.* Paris: Crevot.

Fodor, J. A. 1968. *Psychological Explanation: An Introduction to the Philosphy of Psychology.* New York: Random House.

Fritsch, G. T., and G. Hitzig. 1870. Uber die elektrische Erregbarkeit des Grosshirns. *Archiv für Anatomie, Physiologie und Wissenschaftliche Medizin* 37: 300–332.

Gall, F. J. 1812. *Anatomie et physiologie du système nerveux en général, et du cerveau en particulier.* Paris: Schoell.

Grossberg, S., ed. 1987. *The Adaptive Brain.* New York: North-Holland.

Kosslyn, S. M., and O. Koenig. 1992. *Wet Mind: The New Cognitive Neuroscience.* New York: Free Press.

Kosslyn, S. M., and V. Maljkovic. 1990. Marr's metatheory revisited. *Concepts in Neuroscience* 1: 239–251.

Lashley, K. S. 1929. *Brain Mechanisms and Intelligence.* Chicago: University of Chicago Press.

Lashley, K. S., and G. Clark. 1946. The cytoarchitecture of the cerebral cortex of Ateles. *Journal of Comparative Neurology* 82: 233–306.

Lowe, D. G. 1987a. Three-dimensional object recognition from single two-dimensional images. *Artificial Intelligence* 31: 355–395.

Lowe, D. G. 1987b. The viewpoint consistency constraint. *International Journal of Computer Vision* 1: 57–72.

Luria, A. R. 1973. *The Working Brain.* London: Allen Lane.

Luria, A. R. 1980. *Higher Cortical Functions in Man.* New York: Basic Books.

McCulloch, W. S., and W. Pitts. 1943. A logical calculus of the ideas imminent in nervous activity. *Bulletin of Mathematical Biophysics* 5: 115–133.

Marr, D. 1982. *Vision: A Computational Investigation into the Human Representation and Processing of Visual Information.* San Francisco: W. H. Freeman.

Marr, D., and H. K. Nishihara. 1978. Visual information processing: Artificial intelligence and the sensorium of sight. *Technology Review* 81: 2–23.

Marr, D., and T. Poggio. 1976. Cooperative computation of stereo disparity. *Science* 194: 283–287.

Nottebohm, F. 1981. Laterality, seasons and space governing the learning of a motor skill. *Trends in Neurosciences* 4/5: 104–106.

Penfield, W., and P. Perot. 1963. The brain's record of auditory and visual experience. *Brain* 86: 595–697.

Posner, M. I. 1978. *Chronometric Explorations of Mind.* Hillsdale, NJ: Erlbaum.

Putnam, H. 1973. Reductionism and the nature of psychology. *Cognition* 2: 131–146.

Ramón y Cajal, S. 1888. Estructura del cerebelo. *Gac. med. Catalana* 11: 449–457.

Ramón y Cajal, S. 1911. *Histologie du système nerveux de l'homme et des vertébrés.* Paris: Maloine.

Rumelhart, D. E., and J. L. McClelland, eds. 1986. *Parallel Distributed Processing.* Vol. 1. Cambridge, MA: MIT Press.

Shepard, R. N., and L. R. Cooper. 1982. *Mental Images and their Transformations.* Cambridge, MA: MIT Press.

Simon, H. A. 1981. *The Sciences of the Artificial.* Cambridge, MA: MIT Press.

Squire, L. R. 1987. *Memory and Brain.* New York: Oxford University Press.

Sternberg, S. 1969. The discovery of processing stages: Extensions of Donders' method. *Acta Psychologia* 30: 276–315.

Taylor, J. 1932. *Selected Writings of John Hughlings Jackson.* London: Hodder and Stoughton.

von Neumann, J. 1958. *The Computer and the Brain.* New Haven, CT: Yale University Press.

Walsh, K. W. 1978. *Neuropsychology: A Clinical Approach.* New York: Churchill Livingstone.

Wernicke, C. 1874. *Der Aphasische Symptomenkomplex.* Breslau: Cohn & Weigert.

Wiener, N. 1948. *Cybernetics.* New York: Wiley.

I
Vision

Introduction to Part I

The visual system is the best understood of the sensory systems in primates. Advances have been made rapidly in this system for at least four reasons. First, we have a good animal model of vision; in most cases monkey and human visual functions appear to be remarkably similar. Second, a large number of researchers work on vision, far surpassing the number working in any of the other areas of neuroscience. Perhaps this intense interest in vision is due to the highly visual character of our experiences and thoughts. Indeed, the highly visual nature of primates is reflected in estimates that over half of the neocortex of macaque monkeys is devoted to largely visual and visual-motor functions (Felleman and Van Essen 1991). Third, progress has also been rapid thanks to a strong foundation in visual psychophysics; the results of careful behavioral studies of our visual abilities have accumulated over the last century and are now being applied to both neurophysiological and computational investigations. And fourth, work in computer vision and image analysis has helped us to understand the problems inherent in analyzing the visual world. We see so effortlessly that we often do not appreciate how complex visual processing is; the visual system is bombarded with an enormous amount of information, which can be understood only if certain constraints about the structure of the world are used to construct a mental representation of the environment.

In the last few years the most rapid developments in vision research have centered on two areas, functional subdivision within the visual pathway and the neural representation of specific types of information. The first section of this part contains some of the seminal papers that document the existence of distinct functional streams for the processing of color, motion, depth, and form. The second section contains articles that report key findings about how patterns of neural activity represent specific sorts of information. Not surprisingly, modeling the activity of populations of neurons has been important in helping researchers to understand the nature of these representations. What is learned in both of these areas will no doubt also be useful in understanding the organizing and representational principles of other neural systems.

Processing Streams

To understand a complex system, we often use a strategy of divide-and-conquer—breaking the system into separate components and studying each individually. Fortunately for neuroscientists, the visual system has been found to be highly modular and is amenable to this form of analysis. The first paper in this section reviews seminal studies by Zeki, who in the late 1960s and early 1970s found several independent projections from the striate cortex (also known as the primary visual cortex, area 17, or area V1) to separate areas within the extrastriate cortex. He reasoned that it is unlikely that the same information is sent to these different extrastriate areas and attempted to elucidate what sorts of information might be sent to the different target areas. He found that area V4 contains large numbers of cells that are influenced by color stimuli, whereas area V5 (also known as MT) largely contains cells that are responsive to moving stimuli. These experiments were performed on old-world monkeys, and similar evidence for multiple and functionally distinct cortical areas in new-world monkeys was also being obtained at that time by Allman and Kaas.

Anatomists have also documented two general projection systems from the striate cortex into the extrastriate cortex. One system progresses ventrally from the occipital lobe to the inferotemporal cortex, whereas the other system projects dorsally from the occipital lobe to the posterior parietal cortex. The article by Mishkin, Ungerleider, and Macko advances the idea that the ventral pathway is specialized for the perception of object recognition, whereas the dorsal pathway is specialized for the perception of spatial location. These two pathways are often referred to as the "what" and "where" systems, respectively.

The distinction between the "what" and "where" pathways was made largely on the basis of behavioral deficits that occurred following lesions to the ventral and dorsal extrastriate cortex. Anatomical and detailed functional mapping experiments indicated that there are many complex interconnections between cortical areas that belong to these two pathways; indeed, separate parallel streams can be traced that begin at the much earlier level of the retinal ganglion cells. The articles by Livingstone and Hubel, DeYoe and Van Essen, and Schiller and Logothetis are concerned with how these different anatomical pathways might carry out different aspects of visual perception. Livingstone and Hubel and DeYoe and Van Essen review evidence for two processing streams coming from the retina, one passing through the magnocellular division of the lateral geniculate and one through the parvocellular division. They show that neurons in different cortical subdivisions respond selectively to color, orientation, and motion, as well as other stimulus properties. These results indicate that there are three distinct channels in areas V1 and V2—two that receive input primarily from the parvocellular system and one that receives input from the magnocellular system. Whereas Livingstone and Hubel stress the independence of the pathways, DeYoe and Van Essen emphasize the redundancy within pathways and interactions among pathways. DeYoe and Van Essen suggest that many visual percepts cannot be attributed to events in a single stream but rather result from activity in numerous pathways and cortical areas.

Schiller and Logothetis review experiments in which the magno or parvo channels were selectively removed by lesioning the magnocellular and parvocellular divisions of the lateral geniculate nucleus. The results lead them to propose that the magno system should be conceptualized as the "broad band system," which is not selective for color and extends vision into the higher temporal frequencies, and the parvo system should be conceptualized as the "color opponent system"; however, besides being specialized for color, the color opponent system extends vision into the higher spatial frequencies. Furthermore, lesions to areas MT and V4 have relatively small effects on perceptual thresholds for specific visual capacities, which leads Schiller and Logothetis to conclude that these two pathways are only partially segregated in the extrastriate visual cortex.

An interesting question that arises from the finding that different attributes of visual experience are processed in different brain structures is, How is it all put back together? For example, if one sees a red bouncing ball, how are the color, motion, and shape properly joined? Gray, König, Engel, and Singer report a discovery that may hint at a mechanism for conjoining separate representations; they find that neurons in the cat's visual cortex oscillate at a particular frequency and that these oscillations are synchronized in relatively distant parts of the cortex. It is possible that this oscillation is a "signature" that serves to bind separate patterns of activity so that they can be paired properly during later processing.

The final two papers in this section report behavioral results from human subjects. Cavanagh provides psychophysical evidence that stimulus properties are processed simultaneously in separate systems. His behavioral results also suggest that these systems are not entirely segregated, although they do make distinct contributions to information processing.

Finally, Levine summarizes compelling evidence that the human brain includes a ventral and dorsal pathway. He shows that stroke patients exhibit deficits that parallel those found in monkeys who have had one or the other pathway disrupted; human deficits in recognizing objects tend to arise following lesions to the occipital-temporal area, whereas deficits in registering location or other spatial properties tend to arise following lesions to the parietal lobe.

Representation

One of the most direct ways to understand neural representations is to examine the receptive field characteristics of single neurons. In the first section, we see that lower levels of the visual system extract information about color, contrast, motion, and disparity. In a ground-breaking paper that begins this second section, Gross, Rocha-Miranda, and Bender examine the receptive field properties of cells in the inferotemporal cortex, a higher-level area that is important for visual discrimination learning and object recognition. They find very large receptive fields in this area, which—unlike most other visual cortical areas—generally includes the ipsilateral as well as the contralateral visual field. They note that these large receptive fields allow input to be processed when it falls in a wide range of positions on the retina. In addition, they also find that some neurons respond selectively to visual stimuli, including monkey and human hands. In later papers they and others report cells that are selective for faces. These findings have shaped our view that the inferotemporal cortex is important for object recognition and have stimulated other researchers to search for the mechanisms that produce this selectivity.

Turning to the dorsal pathway, Motter and Mountcastle document detailed properties of the receptive field properties of neurons in the posterior parietal cortex. These cells sometimes respond to stimuli only if they are presented away from the point of fixation. These results are in striking contrast to those reported by Gross et al. in the inferotemporal cortex; these neurons typically respond most vigorously to stimuli when their images fall on the fovea. Motter and Mountcastle also find parietal cells that have an opponent vector organization, with cells preferring motion either toward or away from the point of fixation. They propose that this complex organization of motion selectivity may serve to analyze visual motion during locomotion or may alert the animal to the sudden movement of an object in the receptive field.

A neuron's receptive field is generally defined by the area of space over which a stimulus will increase or decrease its activity. However, there are extensive interconnections between cortical neurons both within and between visual areas, hence it is reasonable to suspect that stimuli presented outside the "classical" receptive field of a neuron might influence its response to a stimulus presented within the receptive field. Thus it is of interest that Allman, Miezin, and McGuinness find that many direction selective MT neurons are suppressed if motion in the same direction is simultaneously present outside their receptive fields. Allman et al. point out that such a local-global antagonism would be useful for perceptual functions such as figure-ground segregation and depth from motion parallax.

In another innovative paper that shook the traditional view of neuronal receptive fields, von der Heydt, Peterhans, and Baumgartner report "non-classical" receptive fields in area V2. They find that "illusory contours" produce a neural response when they fall within the receptive field, just as if a luminance gradient were actually within the receptive field. In this case physical stimuli outside the receptive field actually produce activity, whereas stimuli outside the receptive field only modulate the response of MT neurons to a stimulus within the receptive field. Illusory contours are useful in forming perceptions of continuous contours when parts of the contour are occluded, and these results suggest that some neural "interpolating" is in fact performed.

Receptive fields become progressively larger in areas that are farther up the visual pathways. This progression makes sense if "later" areas perform progressively more abstract processing, which is not tied to particular places in the visual field. A classic example of this hierarchical scheme comes from the study of Movshon, Adelson, Gizzi, and Newsome. Neurons in V1 that respond to motion sample too small a region of space to distinguish the true direction of motion. Many of these cells project to area MT, and Movshon and his colleagues show that some MT neurons can code the true direction of a two-dimensional pattern by combining information from groups of V1 neurons. These experiments show for the first time how small pieces of a picture, existing at a low level in the nervous system, can be brought together at a higher level to code a more general feature of a stimulus—in this case, its direction of motion.

In recent years computational and theoretical studies have provided additional insights about the neural representations that underlie vision. The papers by Marr and Nishihara, Lehky and Sejnowski, Zipser and Andersen, and Kosslyn, Chabris, Marsolek, and Koenig are good examples of this approach. These papers all underline the fact that information is coded by populations of neurons. Most studies that examine the activity of single cells tap into single points in an extremely complicated and distributed information-processing system. The use of mathematical techniques enables investigators to understand these complicated systems when intuition and common sense fall short in the face of this complexity. Having quantitative models also can directly verify or rule out qualitative ideas. Combining computational investigations with neurophysiological and psychophysical experiments is a new and very powerful approach, which is likely to become standard in the near future.

Marr and Nishihara stress that information-processing systems must be understood at several levels of analysis, and they outline several problems in vision that they have approached from their highest, "computational" level. This level is concerned with abstract solutions to problems in perception and does not address how the brain's "wetware" actually solves these problems. The papers by Lehky and Sejnowski, Zipser and Andersen, and Kosslyn et al. use neural network computer simulation models to understand how the brain might go about solving problems in vision. This approach integrates the abstract computation performed by the network with the algorithm for carrying out the computation.

Lehky and Sejnowski's results should give pause to researchers who use the activity of single neurons to draw inferences about the function of an area. They train a neural network to extract information about three-dimensional curvature from shading. The units at an intermediate stage in the network develop receptive fields that respond selectively to edges or bars; these receptive fields are similar to those found in the primary visual cortex. These results show that similar receptive fields could process either edges or shape from shading, and only an appreciation of the functional properties of the entire network could distinguish between these possibilities.

Zipser and Andersen examine how visual space is represented in the activity of populations of neurons in one region of posterior parietal cortex. This study was the first of its kind, using neural network techniques to explain data from single-cell recording experiments. Andersen and his colleagues had previously determined that visual and eye position signals are combined in area 7a of the posterior parietal cortex and had speculated that this information is used to code the location of targets relative to the head (in so-called head-centered coordinates). Zipser and Andersen train their network model to localize positions in head-centered coordinates, given only eye and retinal position signals like those found converging on the posterior parietal cortex. During training, the network spontaneously becomes organized so that some of its units have activity that is very similar to that of cells in the posterior parietal cortex that receive eye and retinal position inputs. The individual units of the model contain a limited amount of information about the location of a target, and the activity of several different units is required to specify location unambiguously. This model provides insight into the form of a distributed representation that is not intuitively apparent at the level of individual neurons.

Kosslyn et al. study representations of spatial relations, which presumably are computed in the parietal lobes. They provide an explanation for earlier findings that the brain represents spatial relations in two ways: as categories (such as "above/below," "on/off," "left/right") or in terms of precise distances. They show that networks that receive their input from lower-level units with relatively large receptive fields compute metric distance better than networks that receive their input from lower-level units with relatively small receptive fields; this computation makes use of "coarse coding," in which responses of units with overlapping receptive fields combine to specify location precisely. In contrast, networks that receive their input from lower-level units with relatively small, less overlapping receptive fields compute a categorical spatial relation better than networks that receive their input from lower-level units with relatively large receptive fields. There is some evidence that the left cerebral hemisphere operates preferentially on outputs from lower-level neurons with relatively small receptive fields, whereas the right hemisphere operates preferentially on outputs from lower-level neurons with relatively large receptive fields. Hence, these models suggest one possible mechanism underlying some aspects of the cerebral lateralization of visual function.

Reference

Felleman, D. J., and D. C. Van Essen. 1991. Distributed hierarchical processing in the primate cerebral cortex. *Cerebral Cortex* 1: 1–47.

1

S. M. Zeki

The functional organization of projections from striate to prestriate visual cortex in the rhesus monkey

1976. *Cold Spring Harbor Symposia on Quantitative Biology* 40: 591–600

It is now well established that two of the major functions of the primary visual cortex (area 17) in the rhesus monkey are to bring the input of the two eyes together and to analyze the visual fields in detail for retinal contour (Hubel and Wiesel 1968). If one were to study the distribution of the efferent cortical projections from area 17, one might well suppose that another one of its major functions might be to segregate out the information coming over the retinogeniculo cortical pathways and parcel this information out to different cortical areas for further analysis. Powerful evidence for such a supposition would be available if it could be shown that the distinct cortical areas to which the primary visual cortex projects have different populations of functional cell types. In a sense, this question is related to another question that has long excited the interest of neurologists: To what extent is there a division of labor within the visual cortex for handling information relating to different aspects of the visual environment? Although the evidence available is far from complete and certainly does not allow us to reach definitive conclusions, our understanding of the anatomical connections of the areas receiving direct inputs from area 17 has increased considerably over the past few years. Hand in hand with this has come an increased knowledge of the functional properties of the cells in these different areas, and this evidence has tended to suggest, but by no means proves, that there is indeed a concentration of different cell types in the different cortical areas and that, consequently, these different cortical areas may be specialized to handle different types of visual information.

PARALLEL AND INDEPENDENT EFFERENT OUTPUTS FROM AREA 17

Area 17 is surrounded by a wide cortical zone, commonly known as the prestriate cortex. There are no obvious cytoarchitectonic subdivisions within this prestriate cortex, but it has been customary since the time of Brodmann (1905) to subdivide it into two cytoarchitectonic fields, 18 and 19 (Fig. 1). Area 17 (VI) has five independent and parallel projections to the cytoarchitectonic area 18 (Fig. 2). The first of these is to V2, the second to V3, and the third to the cortex of the posterior bank of the superior temporal sulcus. Finally, there are projections, mainly, but not exclusively, from the region of foveal representation in area 17 to two further areas, V4 and V4a[1] (Cragg 1969; Zeki 1969, 1971a) (see Figs. 1 and 2). As yet, we have no information concerning the laminar origins in area 17 of these different cortical output systems, and it is possible, and even likely, that different laminae in area 17 contribute differently to these efferent systems. But it would be difficult to suppose that the information carried out from area 17 in these distinct anatomical pathways is the same information. One way of studying this problem further, perhaps the simplest and most direct, is to record the responses of single cells or groups of cells in these cortical recipient zones, compare the responses of cells in one area with those in another, and determine whether there are any recognizable differences.

Recordings from Single Cells in Separate Prestriate Areas

The overall differences in the different prestriate areas can be illustrated by looking at a long penetration that starts through V2, crosses the lunate sulcus, passes through V4 and white matter, and finally terminates in the cortex of the posterior bank of the superior temporal sulcus (Fig. 3). In this way, the electrode passes through three of the five areas that receive direct inputs from area 17. In this particular penetration, all the cells illustrated in area V2 were binocularly driven complex cells with a well-defined orientational preference. However, such cells, which form the "ordinary cells of area 18" (Hubel and Wiesel 1970), constitute only about one-half of the population of cells in V2. There is, in addition, a heavy concentration of another type of cell, not found in area 17, which responds optimally when the visual stimulus falls on slightly disparate points in the two retinas (Hubel and Wiesel 1970). Other types of cells, including color-coded cells (S. M. Zeki, unpubl.), have also been found in V2, but these appear to be in a minority. One may conclude that among the functions emphasized in V2 is the analysis of the visual fields for binocular disparity.

[1] Areas V2 and V3, as defined anatomically by degeneration methods, have also been called 18 and 19, but these are not to be confused with the cytoarchitectonic 18 and 19 of Brodmann (1905). However, to avoid confusion, in this paper we shall simply speak of areas V2 and V3, although it should be understood that these terms are interchangeable with 18 and 19, as defined by degeneration techniques (Zeki 1969).

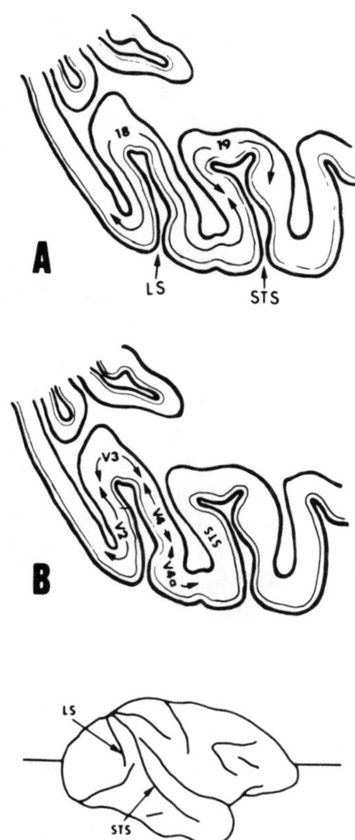

Figure 1. Tracings of horizontal sections taken through the brain of a rhesus monkey at the level indicated to show (*A*) the extent of area 18 as defined cytoarchitectonically by Brodmann (1905) and (*B*) the different anatomical zones within the cytoarchitectonic area 18 receiving direct inputs from the primary visual cortex (area 17). Only the posterior part of the brain is shown in these horizontal tracings. LS, lunate sulcus; STS, superior temporal sulcus.

As the electrode crosses the lunate sulcus, the picture changes dramatically. Here the cells become much more difficult to drive, and the number of frustrating experiments increases. And here, too, in a successful penetration, the type of cell encountered changes, with a relatively large number of cells responding to stimuli of specific wavelengths. In this particular penetration (Fig. 3), all the cells illustrated were excited by blue light, or blue-green light, but, as we shall see below, there are several varieties of color-coded cells in V4.

Returning once again to the penetration illustrated in Figure 3, one notes another striking change in the properties of the neurons as the electrode hits the cortex of the posterior bank of the superior temporal sulcus. In this particular penetration, all the cells illustrated were of the directionally selective type, responding to motion in the appropriate direction irrespective of the form or orientation of the stimulus or its color. It is characteristic of the cells of this area that they are almost all responsive to movement, and a large majority are of the directionally selective type (Zeki 1974a), as opposed to the cells of area 17 in which directional selectivity is not nearly so prominent a feature (Hubel and Wiesel 1968). There are several subvarieties of such directionally selective cells: e.g., complex and hypercomplex cells, cells responding preferentially to small spots moved in the appropriate direction, and cells responding to motion in the appropriate direction regardless of the shape of the stimulus. There are also pandirectional cells, capable of responding to motion in any direction within the receptive field. We studied many, though not all, of the cells in this area that we have recorded from for wavelength preferences. In general, the cells appeared to respond autonomously regardless of wavelength, and once the appropriate stimulus was found, it seemed to make little difference what color the stimulus was.

Such cells would be well situated to analyze motion in all directions in the frontoparallel plane. But to analyze motion towards or away from the animal, a different type of cell would be needed. To date, we have found two major types of cells capable of signaling motion towards or away from the animal, both of which are located in the cortex of the posterior bank of the superior temporal sulcus (Zeki 1974b). In one type, also found in cat area 18 by Pettigrew (1973), the cells respond differently to stimulation of the two eyes (Fig. 4). A cell might

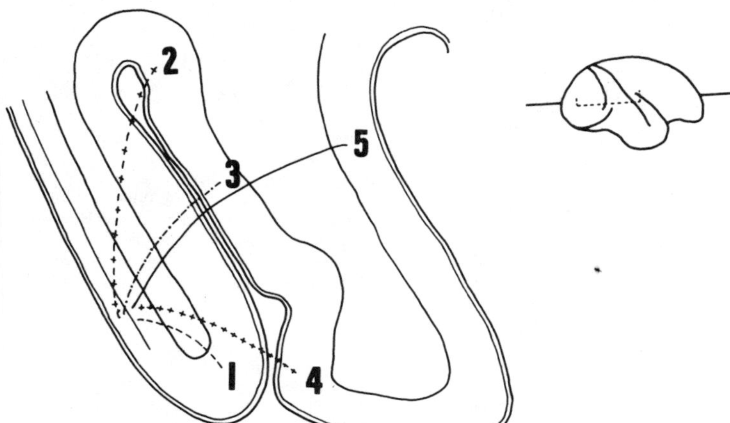

Figure 2. Tracings of a horizontal section through the brain of a rhesus monkey to show, diagrammatically, the five independent and parallel projections from area 17 (continuous line in the cortex) to the prestriate cortex. Exact topographic relations are not indicated in this figure. For further details, see text.

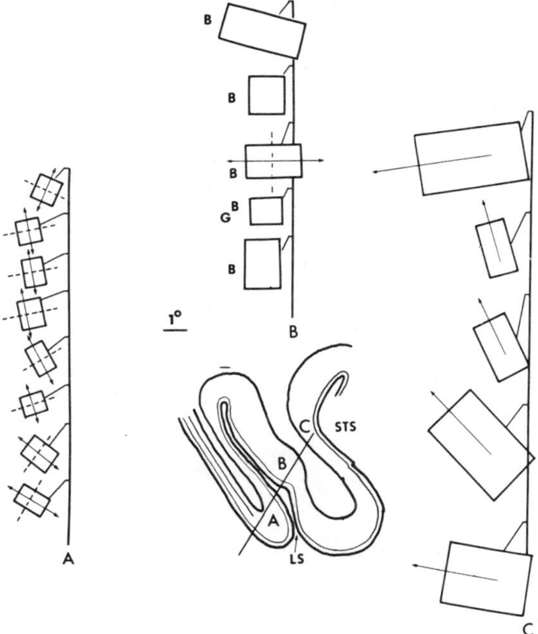

Figure 3. Diagrammatic reconstruction of a long penetration through the prestriate cortex of a rhesus monkey. The electrode entered the cortex through V2. For each cell, the receptive field position is separately indicated with reference to the fovea, which is indicated by the intersection of the short horizontal lines with the long, common vertical lines. Interrupted lines within the receptive field indicate the orientational preference of the cells. Where there is no such line, the cell had no orientational preference. The first cells recorded from (*A*, to left of figure) were in V2; they were all binocularly driven, orientation-selective cells, without any color preference. As the electrode crossed the lunate sulcus and hit V4 (*B*, in the center of figure), the cells recorded from were color-coded. In this penetration, all the cells, except cell 4, responded exclusively to blue light. Cell 4 had a wider spectral sensitivity, responding to green light as well (see text). The cells were binocularly driven. In the cortex of the posterior bank of the superior temporal sulcus, the character of the cells changed once again (*C*, to right of figure). The cells recorded from in this part of the penetration were binocularly driven, directionally selective cells for which the form, orientation or color of the stimulus were not relevant. Arrows indicate the preferred direction of motion of the stimulus.

B, blue; G, green; LS, lunate sulcus; STS, superior temporal sulcus.

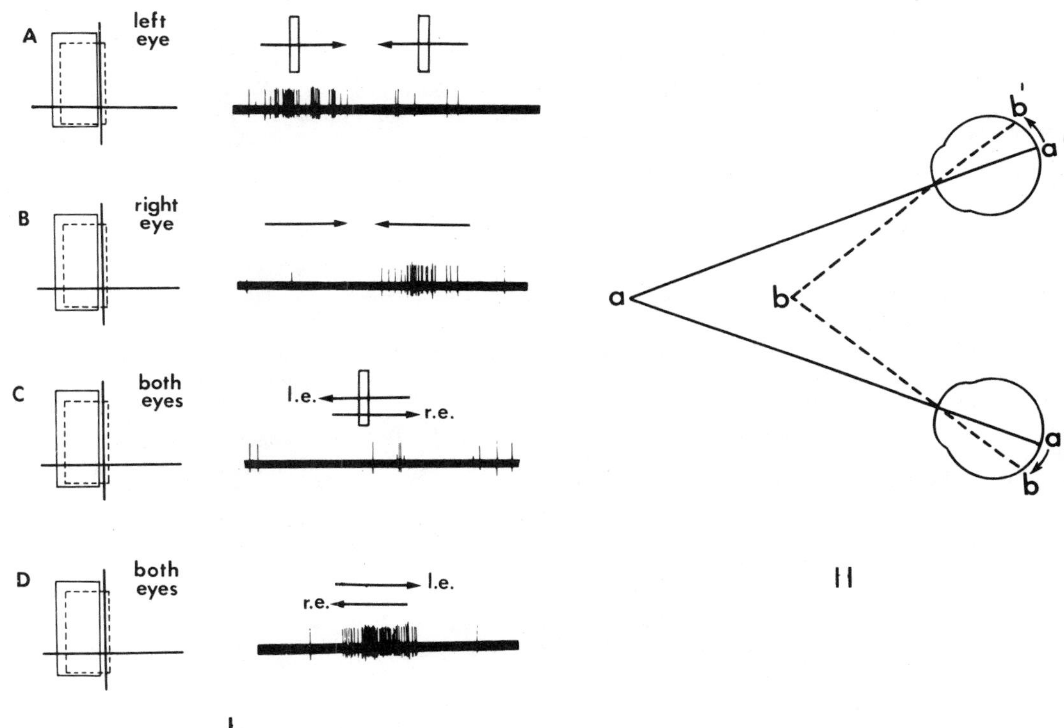

Figure 4. (*I*) The response of a cell in the cortex of the posterior bank of the superior temporal sulcus to stimulation of the two eyes. The receptive field for the right eye is marked by the interrupted rectangle, that for the left eye by the solid rectangle. (*A*) Stimulation of the left eye by a slit of light moved in the direction marked by the arrow; (*B*) the same as in *A* but for the right eye. (*C*) The response to simultaneous movement in the null direction for each eye. (*D*) The response to simultaneous movement of a slit of light in the preferred direction for each eye. Duration of each trace is 5 s. Left eye, l.e.; right eye, r.e. In *II* it is shown that when a point a, having its image at a and a′, is displaced to b, having its image at b and b′, the displacement is in opposite directions in each eye. For purposes of illustration, the distances on the retina are exaggerated in this figure. (Reprinted, with permission, from Zeki 1974a,b.)

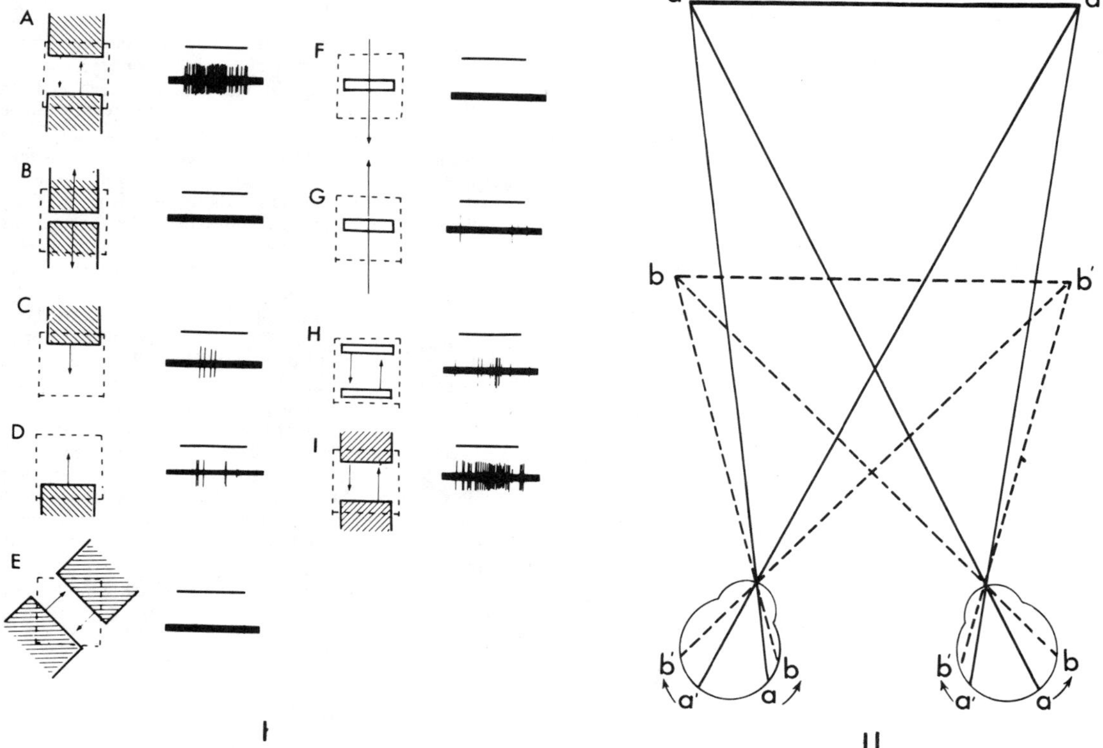

Figure 5. (*I*) The response of a binocularly driven, opposed movement complex cell in the cortex of the superior temporal sulcus to stimulation of the right eye. The cell gave a powerful response (*A*) when two dark edges were moved towards each other within the receptive field. Movement of the two edges away from each other (*B*) was ineffective, as was the movement of single, appropriately oriented edges or slits (*C, D, F, G*) or of two appropriately oriented slits moved in the appropriate direction. Orientation was critical (*E*). The size of the receptive field was 5°×5° and was located in the lower, contralateral quadrant. Duration of each sweep was 4 s. (*II*) A diagram to show that when a large bar, aa′, is moved to bb′, the image will move in opposite directions in each eye. (Reprinted, with permission, from Zeki 1974b.)

respond to motion from 3 o'clock to 9 o'clock for the right eye and from 9 o'clock to 3 o'clock for the left eye, thereby signaling motion towards the animal together with the changing disparity. The power of each of the two eyes to drive such a cell is not always equivalent, and for some of these changing disparity cells one eye may be more potent than the other in eliciting a response—presumably this mechanism aids in detecting motion towards the animal from the side.

Another type of cell capable of signaling motion towards or away from the animal is the opposed movement complex cell (Fig. 5). These cells, which may be driven either monocularly or binocularly, respond to two edges moving towards or away from each other, the orientation of the two edges being very critical. However when such a cell is driven monocularly, there is an ambiguity in the information that it may signal (Fig. 6); it could equally well signal information about an object at a fixed plane increasing

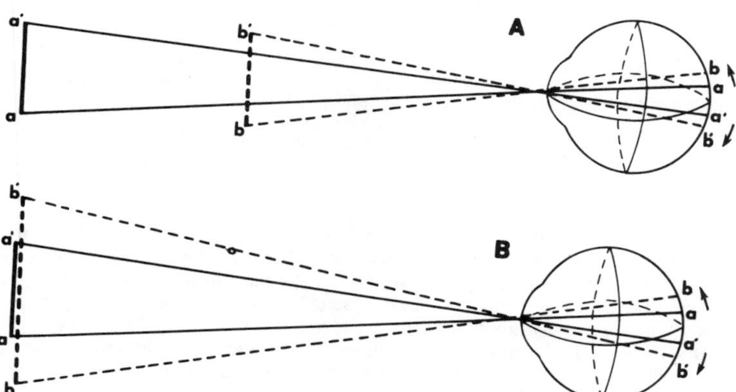

Figure 6. Diagram to show that when a bar, aa′, viewed monocularly, is displaced to bb′, its image will move in opposite directions in each eye (*A*), and that the same motion across the retina will occur if instead of moving towards the eye, aa′ becomes enlarged to bb′ (*B*). (Reprinted, with permission, from Zeki 1974b.)

or decreasing in size. It is not known how the nervous system is able to differentiate between these two types of information.

Recordings from V4

Color-coded cells are in a minority in area 17 (Hubel and Wiesel 1968), and most of the color-coded cells to be found in area 17 are concentrated in the region of foveal representation (Dow and Gouras 1973). In contrast in V4, around 80% of the cells that we have successfully driven have been color-coded, and there are several categories of color-coded cells to be found in this area. One type, perhaps the simplest, responds to stimulation of a small part of the visual field with light of one wavelength, for example, red. In this case, there is no response to white light, even if it is more intense, or to other colors when radiometrically equated (Fig. 7). The cell illustrated in Figure 7 responded specifically to a red slit at a given orientation. But for many color-coded cells, orientation was not critical, nor was the direction of motion of the stimulus, and merely illuminating the receptive field with light of a particular color gave a powerful response. Although the absence of a response to white light immediately suggests that there is an opponent color input to such a cell, it is not always possible to obtain an off response to stimulation with other colors or inhibit the (frequently low) spontaneous discharge of the cell by stimulating the receptive field with light of other colors. For other cells, however, it is possible to study the opponent response. Such a cell might, for example, have a receptive field which is excitatory red on-center and inhibitory green off-center. Switching on the green light leads to a very striking suppression of the firing rate and switching it off causes a powerful off response.

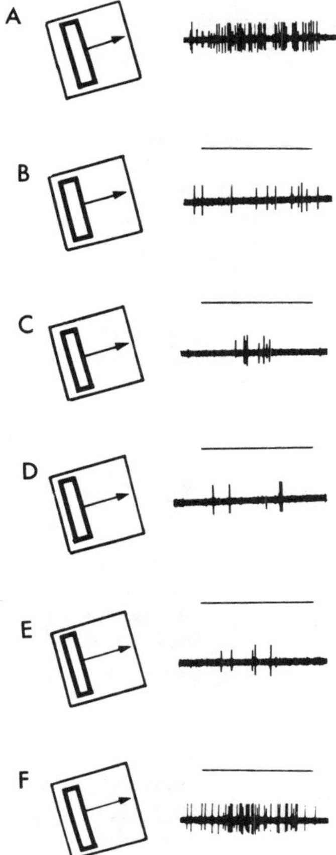

Figure 7. Responses of a group of cells in the V4 area of a rhesus monkey to stimulation with slits of monochromatic light (*A*, 640 nm; *D*, 520 nm; *E*, 480 nm; *F*, 640 nm) and to slits of white light at different intensities (*B*, *C*). The monochromatic lights were generated by interposing an interference filter in the light path. The cells were binocularly driven, but only the responses to stimulation of the contralateral eye are shown. The receptive field was located in the lower contralateral quadrant and was 2.5°×4° in size. Each sweep was about 3 s.

Another type of cell behaves somewhat differently with regard to center and surround. Such a cell might, for example, be red on-center, giving a vigorous response when the stimulus is moved within the receptive field. However, invading the surround with red light might abolish the firing of the cell altogether. When such cells are orientation-selective, they are of the color-coded, "hypercomplex" type (Hubel and Wiesel 1968). When orientation is not critical, these cells show a remarkable similarity to the cells of the lateral geniculate nucleus (Wiesel and Hubel 1966), except that they are far more exigent in their requirements for specific wavelengths and are binocularly driven.

A cell in V4 can be even more exigent in the distribution of spectral sensitivity within its receptive field. Instead of the two spectral contributions being concentrated in one part of the receptive field, or the one spectral contribution in adjacent parts, the receptive field may be subdivided into antagonistic regions, with the regions having different, and opponent, color properties (see Fig. 3 in Zeki 1973). One color (e.g., green) may excite the center, and the opponent color (e.g., red) may have an inhibitory influence when flashed in the surround. Such cells may have various other distinctive features. The excitatory center may be completely enveloped by the opponent surround, or the opponent surround may be identifiable only around limited regions of the center. Where the excitatory center is surrounded on only two sides by antagonistic areas, these areas need not be equivalent in size. Finally, both the center and the surround may respond to the appropriate wavelength independently of contour, or contour may be critical for the center but not for the opponent color surround.

For another type of cell, the successive contrast cell, the most powerful response is obtained when the receptive field is flooded with light of a particular color and then changed to its opponent color. For example, the cell might respond to a change from green to red but not green to white, or red to green, or to green off, or to white on and white off.

The preceding gives a summary of the types of color-coded cells encountered in V4. Looking next at the spectral sensitivities of such cells, it is found that they vary from one cell to the next. Some "red cells," for example, respond over a range of 50 nm (from 670–620 nm), with a very sharp cut off at 600 nm. With such cells, it was usually not possible to elicit a response using other colors or white light at the highest intensities available. A "blue-green" cell may have a slightly wider spectral sensitivity, responding to light coming through interference filters between 560 nm and 480 nm. On the other hand, the spectral sensitivity of a "blue cell" may be narrower, the cell responding over a range of 40 nm. But cells with sharper spectral sensitivities have also been found. There are, for example, cells responding at 440 and 460 nm, in that end of the spectrum commonly known as violet. The cells give a powerful response at these wavelengths but respond weakly, if at all, to red or to blue. The violet cell (Fig. 8) is remarkable not only for displaying a sharp spectral curve, but also for having other specific attributes, namely, responding to a violet bar at a specific orientation.

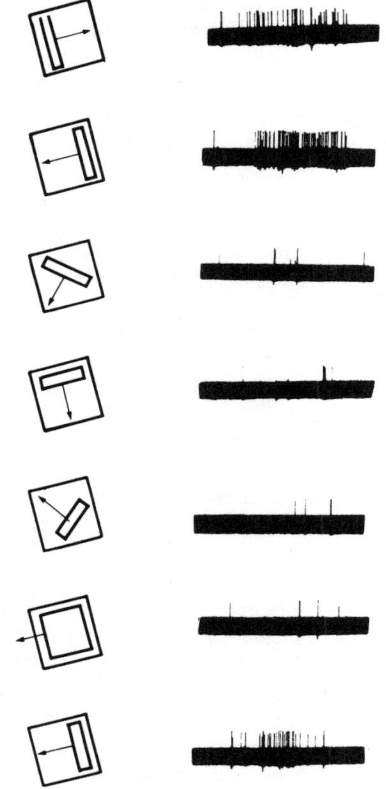

Figure 8. Responses of a binocularly driven, color-coded cell in the cortex of the V4 area of a rhesus monkey. The cell responded selectively to a violet bar (440–460 nm) at the appropriate orientation. Stimulation of the contralateral eye. The receptive field was located in the lower contralateral quadrant and was 3°×2°. Each sweep was 3 s.

We have also encountered color-coded cells responding to the extraspectral color magenta, or purple. The cell responded both to blue or to red but gave its optimal response to a superimposition of red and blue—an extraspectral color. It was fortunate that some of these cells had a high enough background activity for us to determine that green did provide an opponent input to these cells.

Color-coding in Cortical Areas Surrounding V4

The V4 area, as we have defined it elsewhere (Zeki 1971a), is flanked medially by V3 and laterally by V4a. We were naturally interested in exploring these two areas, especially the latter since it has an anatomical input closely similar to that of V4 (Zeki 1971a), to see whether there was any color-coding in either area.

Responses of cells in area V3. Area V3 lies immediately medial to V4. One is not always able to draw the boundary between V3 and V4 accurately in a Nissl-stained section. We were anxious to be secure in the knowledge that we were recording from area V3. The simplest way around this awkward problem was to section the corpus callosum several days prior to recording. The first area of degeneration in the anterior bank of the lunate sulcus defines the anterior boundary of area V3 (Cragg 1969; Zeki 1969, 1970). Electrode tracks within this area of degeneration or more medial to it were therefore accepted as being in area V3. In the 128 cells we have recorded from in area V3, we could not find any convincing example of color-coded cells. Complex cells formed the major segment of the population, followed by hypercomplex cells (Fig. 9). Cells were not studied for retinal disparity. Of course, the sampling was small, and a more extensive investigation may well show color-coded cells. Nevertheless, it seems clear that cells coded for color cannot be present in great concentrations in area V3.

Responses of cells in V4a. The cells of area V4a, lying lateral to V4 (Zeki 1971a), were difficult to drive, and many cells either habituated rapidly or had high spontaneous discharges, making their study difficult. Nevertheless, it was clear that these were visual cells, and it was only our own limitations that prevented us from driving them adequately. In addition to these vaguely driven cells, we succeeded in adequately driving 293 cells in this area, and the results are intriguing because many different varieties of cells may be found here. Complex cells, hypercomplex cells, cells having antagonistic surrounds but no orientational preference, pandirectional cells, cells responding to changes in intensity and color-coded cells were all encountered. Frequently, these different types of cells would all occur in the same penetration (Fig. 10), or a penetration would yield only one type of cell, for example, cells with orientational preferences (Fig. 11). Given the great variety of specific responses we have seen in this area, it is not clear what the

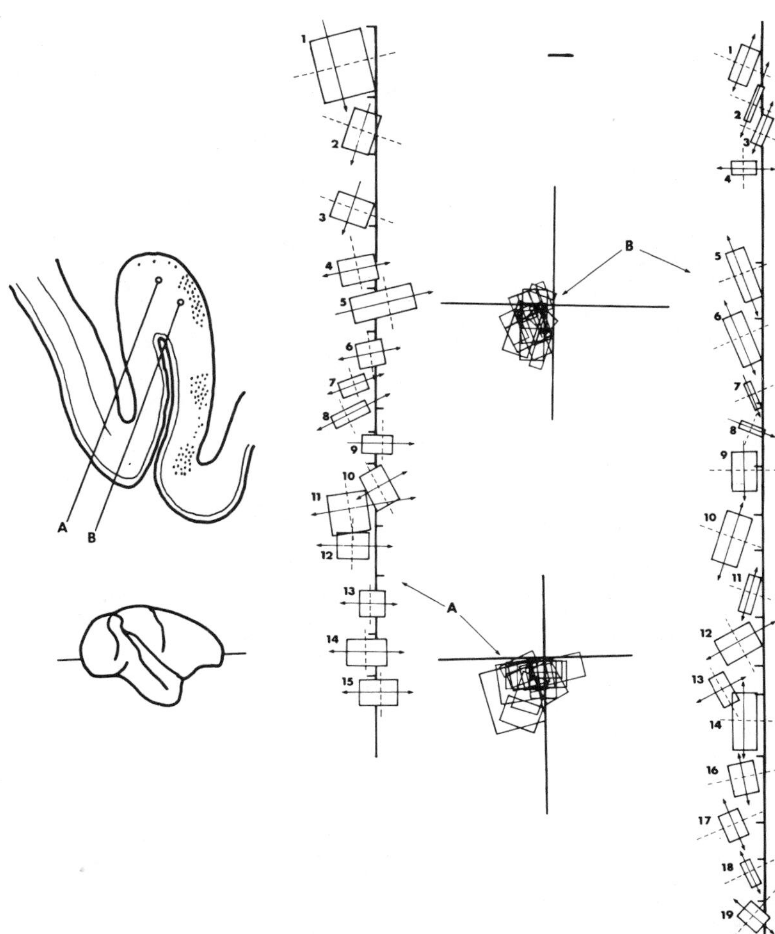

Figure 9. Reconstructions of penetrations through the depth and anterior bank of the lunate sulcus in a rhesus monkey at the level indicated. The dots in the cortex represent the degeneration following sectioning of the corpus callosum, and the most medial patch of degeneration (where the recordings were made) represents the anterior boundary of V3. Clearly the recordings were from V3. Conventions as in Figure 3. None of the 34 cells in the two penetrations was color-specific. The scale is 1°.

function of this area may be. It certainly contains types of cells found in other cortical areas. From the point of view of color-coding, something on the order of 25% of the cells recorded from in this area have been color-specific, but there did not appear to be any striking differences between the color-coded cells of this area and the color-coded cells of V4. Despite having recorded from 293 cells in this cortical area, we are still uncertain of its status.

Differentiation between the Areas of the Prestriate Cortex

In summary, then, as one explores the five separate prestriate areas that receive a direct input from area 17, differences begin to appear. The cortex of the posterior bank of the superior temporal sulcus contains, on the whole, cells that are quite different from the cells of V2. The cells of V2 are, on the whole, different from the cells of V4 or V4a. If one were to judge globally, one would certainly be justified, at least based on the present evidence, in concluding that the analysis of different aspects of the visual environment may be emphasized in these different areas. However, the distinction is not all that clear cut. There are, for example, similarities in the color-coded cells of V4 and V4a. There are complex cells in V2 as well as in V4a. Although in the minority, there are color-coded cells in V2, and some of these have remarkable properties. By the same token, although also in the minority, there are non–color-coded cells in V4. It is not clear why there should be this duplication, if indeed it is a duplication. It is possible that these recurring cells may have different attributes in different areas and that we have simply not discovered them.

Convergent and Divergent Connections between Visual Cortical Areas

The existence of divergent connections from area 17 to the different prestriate areas—an obvious anatomical step for parceling out different types of information to different cortical areas—does not preclude the existence of convergent connections within each system. The anatomical evidence is that both strategies are simultaneously employed. An obvious example is the cortex of the posterior bank of the superior temporal sulcus. Although this zone receives one of the divergent outputs from area 17, the input to it from area

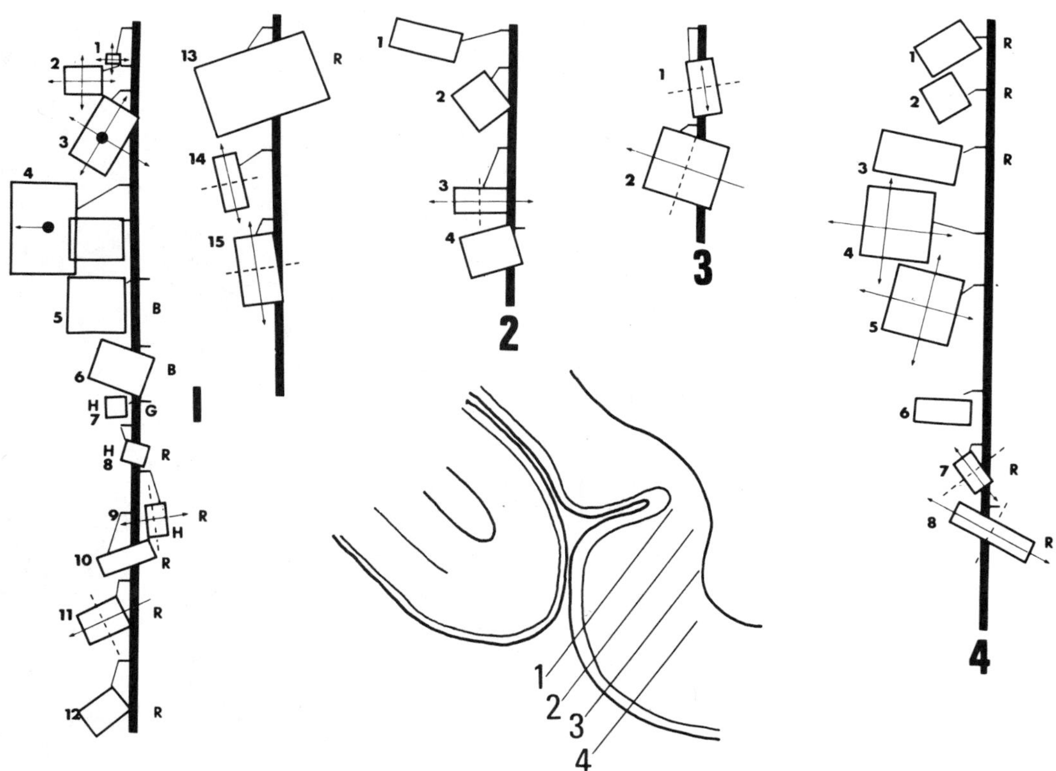

Figure 10. Reconstruction of four penetrations through the cortex of V4a in a rhesus monkey. In the center is a tracing of a horizontal section to show the positions of the electrode tracks. Conventions as in previous reconstructions. Black spots indicate that the cells preferred movement of a spot in the direction marked. Where only arrows are shown, the cells responded to movement in the appropriate direction irrespective of the shape or orientation of the stimulus. B, blue; G, green; R, red. H indicates that to obtain a response, the surround of the receptive field must not be invaded. Where both an H and an interrupted line are indicated, the cell was of the hypercomplex variety. Cell 9, for example, was a color-coded, hypercomplex cell. Where nothing is indicated within the receptive field, the cell responded to all orientations and all directions of motion, as well as to all colors. Note the wide variety of cells encountered in V4a.

17 is highly convergent (Zeki 1971b). Moreover, the input to this visual cortical area from area 17 is convergent with the input to this same cortical field from V2. Thus after making a small electrolytic lesion in V2 and injecting tritiated leucine into area 17, one finds degenerating fibers and autoradiographic grains in the same part of the cortex of the posterior bank of the superior temporal sulcus (Fig. 12). Thus one may speculate, for example, that the properties of most of the cells of the superior temporal sulcus are built up by an input from area 17, and that the opposed movement complex cells, with the changing disparity that they are able to signal, are built up by an input from V2. This would be a logical and economical strategy for the cortex to use. Instead of sending multiple inputs to V2 for the analysis of fixed disparities and another set of inputs to the cortex of the posterior bank of the superior temporal sulcus for the analysis of changing disparities, one need only build up fixed disparity cells in V2 by a direct input from area 17 and then build up changing disparity cells in the cortex of the superior temporal sulcus by a direct input from V2. There is, of course, no evidence that this is necessarily the case; one could equally argue that all the properties of the cells of the superior temporal sulcus are built up by an input from area 17. The point is that the anatomical pathways are there, and it is not altogether implausible that such a strategy, or one similar to it, is used. Also, V4 receives an input from V2 and V3, in addition to the input from foveal 17 (although we do not know whether the two sets of inputs overlap), and it is possible that both the striate and prestriate inputs to V4 take part in building up the properties of the cells in this cortical field.

When one considers that there is a multiplicity of distinct anatomical areas within the visual cortex of the monkey (Zeki 1969, 1971a,b, 1972) and that each one of these areas may have convergent inputs from one or from several antecedent areas and divergent outputs to more central cortical areas as well, then the possibilities for generating an endless variety of new cell types for analyzing in detail the many aspects of the visual environment become almost limitless.

Acknowledgment

This work was supported by the Science Research Council.

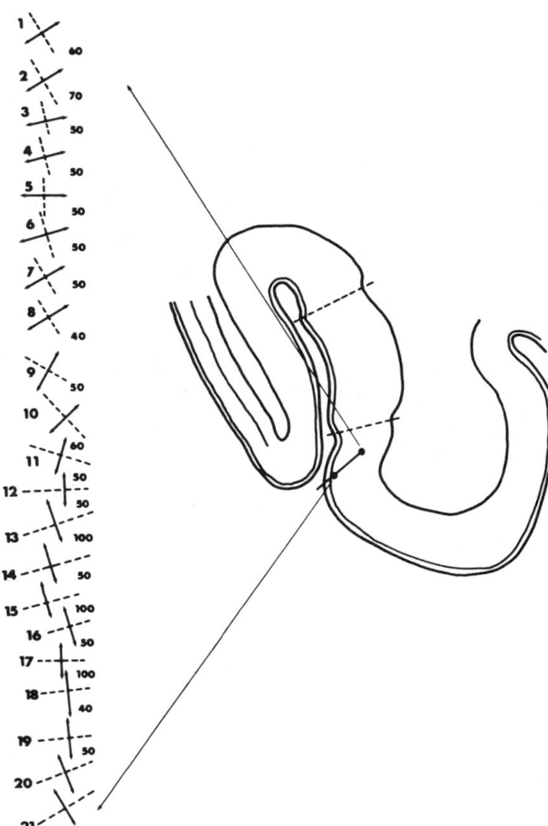

Figure 11. Reconstruction of a penetration through the cortex of area V4a of a rhesus monkey. To the left are shown the orientational preferences of the successive cells (dashed lines) and their preferred directions of motion (arrows). Numbers to the left of the column indicate the number of the cell; numbers to the right, the distances, in microns, between the cells. On the right in the figure is a tracing of a horizontal section to show the electrode track. The two small dots mark the positions of lesions made at the beginning and end of the track. All the cells in this penetration responded to the appropriate orientation regardless of wavelength. The dashed lines in the cortex indicate the limits of V4.

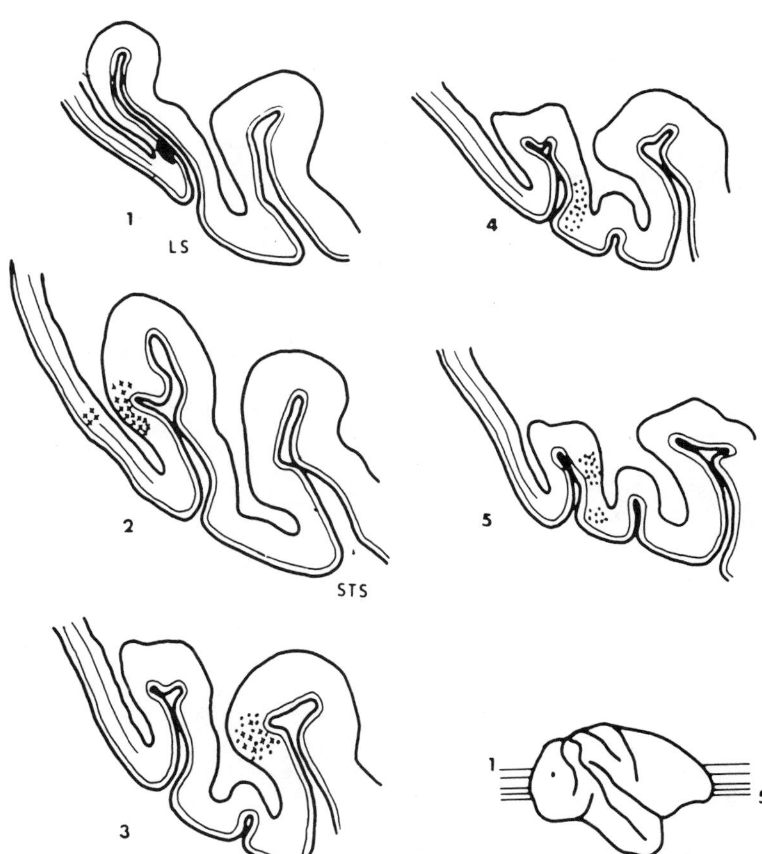

Figure 12. Tracings of horizontal sections through an experimental brain in which a small electrolytic lesion (black area in 1) was made in V2 and tritiated leucine was injected into area 17 (position marked by the four crosses in 2). The dots indicate the distribution of the degeneration following the lesion, and the crosses indicate the distribution of the autoradiographic grains following the injection of labeled leucine. Note that in the posterior bank of the superior temporal sulcus (3), the autoradiographic grains and the degeneration appear in the same region of the same section, showing that fibers from area 17 and from V2 converge on the same part of the cortex of the posterior bank of the superior temporal sulcus. LS, lunate sulcus; STS, superior temporal sulcus.

REFERENCES

BRODMANN, K. 1905. Beitrage zur histologischen Lokalisation der Groshirnrinde. *J. Psychol. Neurol.* (Leipzig) **4:**176.

CRAGG, B. G. 1969. The topography of the afferent projections in the circumstriate visual cortex (C.V.C.) of the monkey studied by the Nauta method. *Vision Res.* **9:**733.

DOW, B. M. and P. GOURAS. 1973. Color and spatial specificity of single units in rhesus monkey foveal striate cortex. *J. Neurophysiol.* **36:**79.

HUBEL, D. H. and T. N. WIESEL. 1968. Receptive fields and functional architecture of monkey striate cortex. *J. Physiol.* **195:**215.

———. 1970. Cells sensitive to binocular depth in area 18 of the macaque monkey cortex. *Nature* **225:**41.

PETTIGREW, J. D. 1973. Binocular neurones which signal change of disparity in area 18 of cat visual cortex. *Nature* **241:**123.

WIESEL, T. N. and D. H. HUBEL. 1966. Spatial and chromatic interactions in the lateral geniculate body of the rhesus monkey. *J. Neurophysiol.* **29:**1115.

ZEKI, S. M. 1969. Representation of central visual fields in prestriate cortex of monkey. *Brain Res.* **14:**271.

———. 1970. Interhemispheric connections of prestriate cortex in monkey. *Brain Res.* **19:**63.

———. 1971a. Cortical projections from two prestriate areas in the monkey. *Brain Res.* **34:**19.

———. 1971b. Convergent input from the striate cortex (area 17) to the cortex of the superior temporal sulcus in the rhesus monkey. *Brain Res.* **28:**338.

———. 1972. Comparison of the cortical degeneration in the visual regions of the temporal lobe of the monkey following section of the anterior commissure and the splenium. *J. Comp. Neurol.* **148:**167.

———. 1973. Color coding in rhesus monkey prestriate cortex. *Brain Res.* **53:**422.

———. 1974a. Functional organization of a visual area in the posterior bank of the superior temporal sulcus of the rhesus monkey. *J. Physiol.* **236:**549.

———. 1974b. Cells responding to changing image size and disparity in the cortex of the rhesus monkey. *J. Physiol.* **242:**827.

2

M. Mishkin, L. G. Ungerleider, and K. A. Macko

Object vision and spatial vision: Two cortical pathways

1983. *Trends in Neurosciences* 6: 414–417

Evidence is reviewed indicating that striate cortex in the monkey is the source of two multisynaptic corticocortical pathways. One courses ventrally, interconnecting the striate, prestriate, and inferior temporal areas, and enables the visual identification of objects. The other runs dorsally, interconnecting the striate, prestriate, and inferior parietal areas, and allows instead the visual location of objects. How the information carried in these two separate pathways is reintegrated has become an important question for future research.

Thirty-five years ago Lashley concluded that visual mechanisms do not extend beyond the striate cortex. He was led to this view after finding that 'None of the lesions in the prestriate region of the monkey has produced symptoms resembling object agnosia as described in man ... Uncomplicated destruction of major portions of the prestriate region ... has not been found to produce any disturbances in sensory or perceptual organization'[14].

We now know, of course, that Lashley's conclusion was wrong. Tissue essential for vision extends far beyond striate cortex to include not only the prestriate region of the occipital lobe but also large portions of the temporal and parietal lobes. Neurobehavioral studies since Lashley's[3,6,20–23,28], together with converging evidence from physiological[1,6,10,24,30,44] and anatomical studies[5,31,39,41–43], indicate that these extrastriate regions contain numerous visual areas that can be distinguished both structurally and functionally. Moreover, recent work from our own laboratory[40] suggests that these multiple visual areas are organized hierarchically into two separate cortical visual pathways, one specialized for 'object' vision, the other for 'spatial' vision.

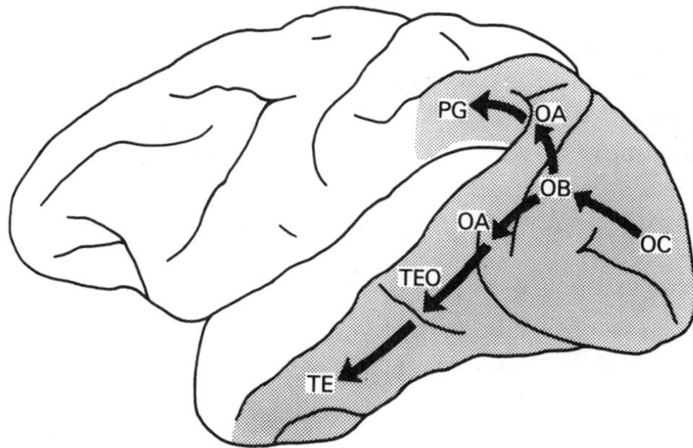

Figure 1. Lateral view of the left hemisphere of a rhesus monkey. The shaded area defines the cortical visual tissue in the occipital, temporal and parietal lobes. Arrows schematize two cortical visual pathways, each beginning in primary visual cortex (area OC), diverging within prestriate cortex (areas OB and OA), and then coursing either ventrally into the inferior temporal cortex (areas TEO and TE) or dorsally into the inferior parietal cortex (area PG). Both cortical visual pathways are crucial for higher visual function, the ventral pathway for object vision and the dorsal pathway for spatial vision.

Two Pathways

The two cortical visual pathways are schematized in Fig. 1. One of them consists of a multisynaptic occipitotemporal projection system that follows the course of the inferior longitudinal fasciculus. This pathway, which interconnects the striate, prestriate, and inferior temporal areas, is crucial for the visual identification of objects[21]. Subsequent links of the occipitotemporal pathway with limbic structures in the temporal lobe[36] and with ventral portions of the frontal lobe[13] may make possible the cognitive association of visual objects with other events, such as emotions and motor acts.

The other pathway consists of a multisynaptic occipitoparietal projection system that follows the course of the superior longitudinal fasciculus. This pathway, which interconnects the striate, prestriate, and inferior parietal areas, is critical for the visual location of objects[40]. Subsequent links of the occipitoparietal pathway with dorsal limbic[26] and dorsal frontal cortex[13,26] may enable the cognitive construction of spatial maps, as well as the visual guidance of motor acts[8] that were initially triggered by activity in the ventral pathway. In contrast to the ventral pathway, which remains modality-specific throughout its course, the later stations in the dorsal pathway appear to receive convergent input from other modalities and so may constitute polysensory areas[10,32].

The notion that separate neural systems mediate object and spatial vision is not new[11,25]. In previous formulations, however, these two types of visual perception were attributed to the geniculostriate and tectofugal systems, respectively, rather than to separate cortical pathways diverging from a common striate origin. The shift to the present view is in keeping with the cumulative evidence that, in primates at least, all forms of visual perception, as distinguished from visuomotor functions, are more heavily dependent on the geniculostriate than on the tectofugal system.

Object Vision

The anterior part of inferior temporal cortex, or area TE in Bonin and Bailey's terminology[2], is the last exclusively visual area in the pathway that begins in the striate cortex, or area OC, and continues through the prestriate and posterior temporal areas, OB, OA and TEO (Fig. 1). This ventrally directed chain of cortical visual areas appears to extract stimulus-quality information from the retinal input to the striate cortex[20], processing it for the purpose of identifying the visual stimulus and ultimately assigning it some meaning through the mediation of area TE's connections with the limbic and frontal-lobe systems[12]. According to this view, the analysis of the physical properties of a visual object (such as its size, color, texture and shape) is performed in the multiple subdivisions of the prestriate–posterior temporal complex[44] and may even be completed within this tissue. Such a proposal gains support from the striking loss in pattern-discrimination ability that follows damage to the posterior temporal area[20]. But the synthesis of all the physical properties of the particular object into a unique configuration appears to entail the funnelling of the outputs from the prestriate–posterior temporal region into area TE[21]. This postulated integration of the coded visual properties of an object within area TE would make TE especially well suited to serve not only as the highest-order area for the visual perception of objects but also as the storehouse for their central representations and, hence, for their later recognition.

That area TE is important for the retention of some form of visual experience has been suspected for decades[18]. Numerous behavioral studies[6] have demonstrated that bilateral removal of inferior temporal cortex in monkeys yields marked impairment both in the retention of visual discrimination habits acquired prior to surgery and in the postoperative acquisition of new ones. This impairment, which is exclusively visual, appears in the absence of any sensory loss and thus has long been considered a higher-order, or 'visuopsychic', dysfunction.

But that the impairment is in fact a visual retention disorder was demonstrated only later when it was found that area TE lesions impair performance on visual tests that tax memory even more than they do on visual tests that tax perceptual ability[3]. Now, having examined the ability of monkeys with TE lesions simply to remember the visual appearance of newly presented objects, we have uncovered what is perhaps the most dramatic impairment of all[21]. After just a few days of training, normal monkeys shown an object only once will demonstrate that they recognize that object when it is presented several minutes later (Fig. 2A). Thus, somewhere in the visual system the single presentation of a complex stimulus leaves a trace against which a subsequently presented stimulus can be matched. If it does match, i.e. if the original neural trace is reactivated, there is immediate recognition, as demonstrated by the monkey's highly accurate performance. The area in which the neural trace appears to be preferentially established is area TE, since lesions here—but not lesions elsewhere in the cortical visual system—nearly abolish the monkey's ability to perform the recognition task. Apparently, area TE contains the traces laid down by previous viewing of stimuli, and these serve as stored central representations against which incoming stimuli are constantly being

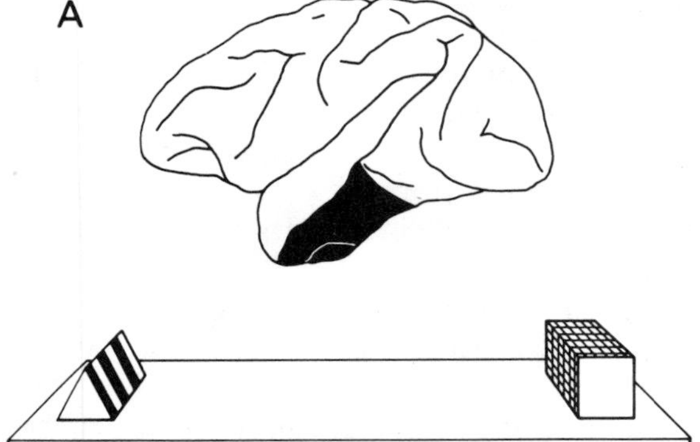

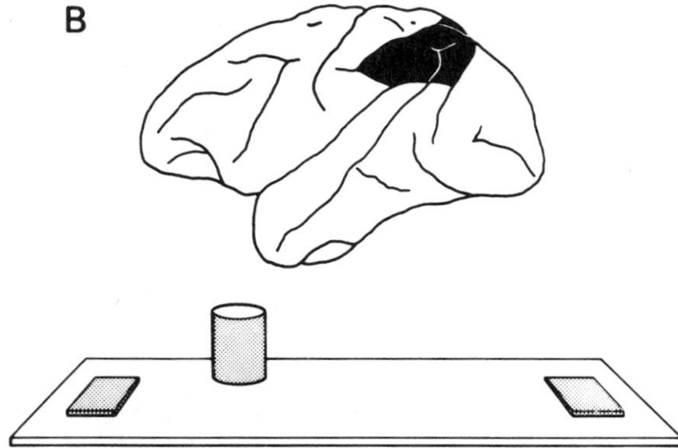

Figure 2. Behavioral tasks sensitive to cortical visual lesions in monkeys. **(A)** Object discrimination. Bilateral removal of area TE in inferior temporal cortex produces severe impairment on object discrimination. A simple version of such a discrimination is a one-trial object-recognition task based on the principle of non-matching to sample, in which monkeys are first familiarized with one object of a pair in a central location (familiarization trial not shown) and are then rewarded in the choice test for selecting the unfamiliar object. **(B)** Landmark discrimination. Bilateral removal of posterior parietal cortex produces severe impairment on landmark discrimination. On this task, monkeys are rewarded for choosing the covered foodwell closer to a tall cylinder, the 'landmark', which is positioned randomly from trial to trial closer to the left cover or closer to the right cover, the two covers being otherwise identical.

compared. In the process, old central representations may either decay, be renewed, or even be refined, while new representations are added to the store.

It is significant that by virtue of the extremely large visual receptive fields of inferior temporal neurons[6] this area seems to provide the neural basis for the phenomenon of stimulus equivalence across retinal translation[7]; i.e. the ability to recognize a stimulus as the same, regardless of its position in the visual field. But a necessary consequence of this mechanism for stimulus equivalence is that within the occipitotemporal pathway itself there is a loss of information about the visual location of the objects being identified.

Spatial Vision

The neural mechanism that enables the visual location of objects also entails the transmission of information from striate through prestriate cortex; however, the prestriate route in this case, as well as the rest of the pathway for spatial vision, appears to be quite separate from the pathway for object vision (Fig. 1). Evidence in support of this dichotomy of cortical visual pathways has come from our studies of posterior parietal cortex.

In the initial study of the series, Pohl[28] demonstrated a dissociation of visual deficits after inferior temporal and posterior parietal lesions. That is, whereas the temporal but not the parietal lesion produced severe impairment on an object-discrimination learning task, just the reverse was found on tests in which the monkey had to learn to choose a response location on the basis of its proximity to a visual 'landmark' (Fig. 2B). These results provided compelling evidence that 'the inferior temporal cortex participates mainly in the acts of noticing and remembering an object's qualities, not its position in space. Conversely, the posterior parietal cortex seems to be concerned with the perception of the spatial relations among objects, and not their intrinsic qualities'[20].

The effective lesions in Pohl's study were large, since they included not only inferior parietal cortex, or area PG, but also dorsal prestriate tissue within area OA. To test for the possibility of a further localization of function within this region, additional experiments were performed with more restricted lesions[22]. The results, however, failed to reveal any evidence of a cortical focus serving spatial vision; rather, the severity of impairment on the landmark task was found to depend on the amount of tissue included in the lesion, completely independent of the lesion site. Since damage to the same region, no matter how extensive, failed to produce any impairment in the acquisition of a visual pattern discrimination, it appears that the entire posterior parietal region, including dorsal OA cortex, participates selectively in the processing of visuospatial as distinguished from visual object-quality information.

Our findings support the accumulating neurobiological evidence that parietal area PG, rather than being a purely tactual association area as was once thought, is a polysensory area to which both the visual and tactual modalities contribute[10,24,30]. The findings are thus consistent with the proposal[33] that area PG serves a supramodal spatial ability that subsumes both the macrospace of vision and the microspace encompassed by the hand. According to this proposal, visuospatial and tactual discrimination deficits, as well as the inaccuracies in reaching that also follow inferior parietal damage, are different reflections of a single, supramodal disorder in spatial perception.

Polysensory area PG is presumed to depend for its visual input on the modality-specific prestriate area OA, which appears to serve visual spatial functions selectively. Such a hierarchical model for spatial perception suggests, in turn, that the source of the critical visual input for the entire dorsal prestriate–parietal region is, again, the striate cortex. The alternative possibility, namely, that the source of the critical input is the superior colliculus, found no support in a study of the effects of tectal lesions on performance of the landmark task; even complete bilateral destruction of the superior colliculus failed to produce a reliable loss in retention. We therefore examined the contribution of striate inputs to the visuospatial functions of posterior parietal cortex[23], using a disconnection technique analogous to the one used originally to examine the contribution of striate inputs to the object-vision functions of inferior temporal cortex[19]. Our results suggested that the posterior parietal cortex, like the inferior temporal, is totally dependent on striate input for its participation in vision; but unlike the inferior temporal, the posterior parietal cortex does not seem to receive a heavy visual input via the corpus callosum. It therefore appears that each posterior parietal area may be organized largely as a substrate for contralateral spatial function, which could account in part for the symptom of contralateral spatial neglect that has so often been reported after unilateral parietal injury in man[4,9,17].

A second difference in the organization of visual inputs to posterior parietal and inferior temporal cortex was uncovered in an experiment that compared the effects of selective removals of striate cortex[23]. In this experiment, monkeys received bilateral lesions of the striate areas representing either central vision (lateral striate) or peripheral vision (medial striate). The results indicated that while inputs from central vision are the more important ones for the object-recognition functions of inferior temporal cortex, inputs from central and peripheral vision are equally important for the visuospatial functions of posterior parietal cortex.

In summary, interactions with striate cortex are critical for the parietal just as they are for the temporal area, but the striate inputs to these two cortical targets are organized differently: relative to inferior temporal cortex, posterior parietal cortex receives a greater contribution from inputs representing both the contralateral and the peripheral visual fields. These differences, which are seen also in the visual receptive field topography of inferior temporal vs. posterior parietal neurons[6,30], presumably reflect differences in the sensory processing required for object vs. spatial vision.

Metabolic and Anatomical Mapping

The evidence from our behavioral work demonstrates that the neural mechanisms underlying object and spatial vision depend on the relay of information from striate cortex through prestriate cortex to targets in inferior temporal and inferior parietal areas, respectively. We have now mapped the full extent of both cortical visual pathways combined, using the 2-[^{14}C]-deoxyglucose method[15]. By comparing a blinded and a seeing hemisphere in the same monkey we have found that the entire visual system can be outlined on the basis of differential hemispheric glucose utilization during visual stimulation. Reduced glucose utilization in the blind as compared with the seeing hemisphere was seen cortically throughout the entire expanse of striate and prestriate cortex (areas OC, OB and OA), inferior temporal cortex as far forward as the temporal pole (areas TEO and TE), and the posterior part of the inferior parietal lobule (area PG). These results, which are in remarkably close agreement with our neurobehaviorally derived model of the two cortical visual pathways, have allowed us to delineate the exact limits of the entire system[16] (Fig. 1).

To trace the flow of visual information within each system we undertook a series of studies using autoradiographic and degeneration tracing techniques. Our goal in these anatomical investigations was to identify the multiple visual areas within the prestriate cortex, explore their organization, and map their projections forward into both the temporal and parietal lobes.

The findings indicated that the striate cortex is indeed the source of two major cortical projection systems. The first system begins with the known striate projection to the second visual area, V2[31,35,42,43]. We found that V2 in turn projects to areas V3 and V4[38]. These three prestriate areas are arranged in adjacent 'belts' that nearly surround the striate cortex, and, like striate cortex, each belt contains a topographic representation of the visual field. Area V2 corresponds to prestriate area OB, while V3 and V4 are both contained within prestriate area OA, exclusive of its dorsal part. Area V4 in turn projects to both areas TEO and TE in the inferior temporal cortex[5].

The second major system begins with both striate and V2 projections to visual area MT[31,35,39,41–43], which is located in the caudal portion of the superior temporal sulcus, mainly within dorsolateral OA. Area MT in turn projects to four additional areas in the upper superior temporal and the intraparietal sulci[37]. Although the total extents of these four areas are not yet completely established, the more anterior one in the intraparietal sulcus clearly falls within area PG. Thus, one major system of projections out of striate cortex is directed ventrally into the temporal lobe, while a second is directed dorsally into the parietal lobe. Furthermore, the divergence between these two systems appears to begin almost immediately after striate cortex, i.e. in its initial projections.

The two multisynaptic projection systems that we have traced provide not only the anatomical substrate for our two functionally defined visual pathways but also a partial solution to the puzzle that was presented at the outset, namely, why extensive removals of prestriate cortex in monkeys have repeatedly failed to yield the expected losses in either object or spatial vision[14,29,40]. If prestriate cortex constitutes an essential relay in both a striate–temporal and a striate–parietal pathway, then damage to this relay should yield effects at least as severe as damage to both its target areas. Yet such dramatic effects have not been found. The reason appears to be that no prestriate lesion to date has produced a total visual disconnection of the temporal and parietal lobes, since all removals have spared varying extents of prestriate tissue that could continue to relay visual information. Comparison with our anatomical maps indicates that the portions of prestriate cortex that have consistently escaped damage are those parts of both the belt areas and the MT-related areas that represent the peripheral visual fields. Thus, just as we had found from sparing in striate cortex, sparing of peripheral-field representations in prestriate cortex will protect both object and spatial vision from serious losses.

Objects in Spatial Locations

A major question posed by the present analysis is how object information and spatial information, initially carried together in the geniculostriate projections but then analysed separately in the two cortical visual pathways, are eventually reintegrated. As already noted, both pathways have further connections to the limbic system and the frontal lobe, and each of these target areas therefore constitutes a potential site of convergence and synthesis for object and spatial information. This theoretical possibility has not yet been sufficiently tested. Preliminary work does indicate, however, that one such site of reintegration may be the hippocampal formation and that one of its functions may be to enable the rapid memorization of the particular locations occupied by particular objects[27,34]. Further application of this concept of reintegration to research on the limbic system and the frontal lobe could throw new light on some old questions of local cerebral function.

Reading List

1. Allman, J. M., Baker, J. F., Newsome, W. T. and Petersen, S . E. (1981) in *Cortical Sensory Organization, Vol. 2: Multiple Visual Areas* (Woolsey, C. N., ed.), pp. 171–185, Humana Press, Clifton, NJ.

2. Bonin, G. von and Bailey, P. (1947) *The Neocortex of Macaca Mulatta*, The University of Illinois Press, Urbana, IL.

3. Cowey, A. and Gross, C. G. (1970) *Exp. Brain Res.* 11, 128–144.

4. Denny-Brown, D. and Chambers, R. A. (1958) *Res. Publ. Assoc. Res. Nerv. Ment. Dis.* 36, 35–117.

5. Desimone, R., Fleming, J. and Gross, C. G. (1980) *Brain Res.* 184, 41–55.

6. Gross, C. G. (1973) in *Handbook of Sensory Physiology VII/3* (Jung, R., ed.), pp. 451–482, Springer-Verlag, Berlin.

7. Gross, C. G. and Mishkin, M. (1979) in *Lateralization in the Nervous System* (Harnad, S., Doty, R. W., Goldstein, L., Jaynes, J. and Krauthamer, G., eds), pp. 109–122, Academic Press, New York.

8. Haaxma, R. and Kuypers, H. G. J. M. (1975) *Brain* 98, 239–260.

9. Heilman, K. M. and Watson, R. T. (1977) in *Advances in Neurology, Vol. 18* (Weinstein, E. A. and Friedland, R. P., eds), pp. 93–106, Raven Press, New York.

10. Hyvärinen, J. (1981) *Brain Res.* 206, 287–303.

11. Ingle, D., Schneider, G. E., Trevarthan, G. B. and Held, R. (1967) *Psychol. Forsch.* 31, 42–348.

12. Jones, B. and Mishkin, M. (1972) *Exp. Neurol.* 36, 352–377.

13. Kuypers, H. G. J. M., Szwarcbart, M. K., Mishkin, M. and Rosvold, H. E. (1965) *Exp. Neurol.* 11, 245–262.

14. Lashley, K. S. (1948) *Genet. Psychol Monogr.* 37, 107–166.

15. Macko, K. A., Jarvis, C. D., Kennedy, C., Miyaoka, M., Shinohara, M., Sokoloff, L. and Mishkin, M. (1982) *Science* 218, 394–397.

16. Macko, K. A., Kennedy, C., Sokoloff, L. and Mishkin, M. (1981) *Soc. Neurosci. Abstr.* 7, 832.

17. Mesulam, M.-M. (1981) *Ann. Neurol.* 10, 309–325.

18. Mishkin, M. (1954) *J. Comp. Physiol. Psychol.* 47, 187–193.

19. Mishkin, M. (1966) in *Frontiers of Physiological Psychology* (Russell, R., ed.), pp. 93–119, Academic Press, New York.

20. Mishkin, M. (1972) in *Brain and Human Behavior* (Karczmar, A. G. and Eccles, J. C., eds). pp. 187–208, Springer-Verlag, Berlin.

21. Mishkin, M. (1982) *Philos. Trans. R. Soc. London, Ser. B* 298, 85–95.

22. Mishkin, M., Lewis, M. E. and Ungerleider, L. G. (1982) *Behav. Brain Res.* 6, 41–55.

23. Mishkin, M. and Ungerleider, L. G. (1982) *Behav. Brain Res.* 6, 57–77.

24. Mountcastle, V. B., Lynch, J. C., Georgopoulos, A., Sakata, H. and Acuna, C. (1975) *J. Neurophysiol.* 38, 871–908.

25. Newcombe, F. and Russell, W. R. (1969) *J. Neurol. Neurosurg. Psychiatry* 32, 73–81.

26. Pandya, D. N. and Kuypers, H. G. J. M. (1968) *Brain Res.* 13, 13–36.

27. Parkinson, J. K. and Mishkin, M. (1982) *Soc. Neurosci. Abstr.* 8, 23.

28. Pohl, W. (1973) *J. Comp. Physiol. Psychol.* 82, 227–239.

29. Pribram, K. H., Spinelli, D. N. and Reitz, S. L. (1969) *Brain* 92, 301–312.

30. Robinson, D. L., Goldberg, M. E. and Stanton, G. B. (1978) *J. Neurophysiol* 41, 910–932.

31. Rockland, K. S. and Pandya, D. N. (1981) *Brain Res.* 212, 249–270.

32. Seltzer, B. and Pandya, D. N. (1980) *Brain Res.* 192, 339–351.

33. Semmes, J. (1967) in *Symposium on Oral Sensation and Perception* (Bosma J. G., ed.), pp. 137–148, Thomas, Springfield, IL.

34. Smith, M. L. and Milner, B. (1981) *Neuropsychologia* 19, 781–793.

35. Tigges, J., Tigges, M., Anschel, S., Cross, N. A., Letbetter, W. D. and McBride, R. L. (1981) *J. Comp. Neurol.* 202, 539–560.

36. Turner, B. H., Mishkin, M. and Knapp, M. (1980) *J. Comp. Neurol.* 191, 515–543.

37. Ungerleider, L. G., Desimone, R. and Mishkin, M. (1982) *Soc. Neurosci. Abstr.* 8, 680.

38. Ungerleider, L. G., Gattass, R., Sousa, A. P. B. and Miskkin, M. (1983) *Soc. Neurosci. Abstr.* 9.

39. Ungerleider. L G. and Mishkin. M. (1979) *J. Comp. Neurol.* 188, 347–366.

40. Ungerleider, L. G. and Mishkin, M. (1982) in *Analysis of Visual Behavior* (Ingle, D. J., Goodale, M. A. and Mansfield, R. J. W., eds), pp. 549–586, The MIT Press, Cambridge, MA.

41. Van Essen, D. C., Maunsell, J. H. R. and Bixby, J. L. (1981) *J. Comp. Neurol.* 199, 293–326.

42. Weller, R. E. and Kaas, J. H. (1981) in *Cortical Sensory Organization, Vol. 2: Multiple Visual Areas* (Woolsey, C. N., ed.), pp. 121–155, Humana Press, Clifton, NJ.

43. Zeki, S. M. (1969) *Brain Res.* 14, 271–291.

44. Zeki, S. M. (1978) *Nature (London)* 274, 423–428.

3

M. Livingstone and D. Hubel

Segregation of form, color, movement, and depth: Anatomy, physiology, and perception

1988. *Science* 240: 740–749

Anatomical and physiological observations in monkeys indicate that the primate visual system consists of several separate and independent subdivisions that analyze different aspects of the same retinal image: cells in cortical visual areas 1 and 2 and higher visual areas are segregated into three interdigitating subdivisions that differ in their selectivity for color, stereopsis, movement, and orientation. The pathways selective for form and color seem to be derived mainly from the parvocellular geniculate subdivisions, the depth- and movement-selective components from the magnocellular. At lower levels, in the retina and in the geniculate, cells in these two subdivisions differ in their color selectivity, contrast sensitivity, temporal properties, and spatial resolution. These major differences in the properties of cells at lower levels in each of the subdivisions led to the prediction that different visual functions, such as color, depth, movement, and form perception, should exhibit corresponding differences. Human perceptual experiments are remarkably consistent with these predictions. Moreover, perceptual experiments can be designed to ask which subdivisions of the system are responsible for particular visual abilities, such as figure/ground discrimination or perception of depth from perspective or relative movement—functions that might be difficult to deduce from single-cell response properties.

PEOPLE WITH NORMAL COLOR VISION WILL PROBABLY FIND the left illustration in Fig. 1 less clear and three-dimensional than the one on the right. But it springs forth if you look at it through a blue filter, such as a piece of colored glass or cellophane. In the left version the gray and yellow are equally bright, or luminant, for the average person, whereas the right version has luminance-contrast information. The ability to infer distance and three-dimensional shape from a two-dimensional image is an example of a visual function that can use luminance but not color differences. Depth from perspective and color perception are thus aspects of vision that seem to be handled by entirely separate channels in our nervous system.

Even though intuition suggests that our vision can plausibly be subdivided into several components—color, depth, movement, form, and texture perception—our perception of any scene usually seems well unified. Despite this apparent wholeness, studies of anatomy, physiology, and human perception are converging toward the conclusion that our visual system is subdivided into several separate parts whose functions are quite distinct. In this article we summarize some of these anatomical, physiological, and human-perceptual observations.

Physiological and Anatomical Studies

Occasionally people with strokes suffer surprisingly specific visual losses—for example, loss of color discrimination without impairment of form perception, loss of motion perception without loss of color or form perception, or loss of face recognition without loss of the ability to recognize most other categories of objects or loss of color or depth perception (*1*). Such selectivity seems to indicate that the visual pathway is functionally subdivided at a fairly gross level.

Anatomical and physiological studies in monkeys also support this idea of functional divergence within the visual pathway. They reveal major anatomical subdivisions at the earliest peripheral stages in the visual system as well as segregation of function at the highest known cortical stages, but until recently there was little information about corresponding subdivisions in the intermediate levels, the first and second cortical visual areas.

Subdivisions at early stages in the visual pathway. It has been known for a century that the nerve fibers leaving the eyes diverge to provide input both to the lateral geniculate bodies and to the superior colliculi. The colliculus seems to be relatively more important in lower mammals than it is in primates, in which its main role is probably orientation toward targets of interest; here we will be

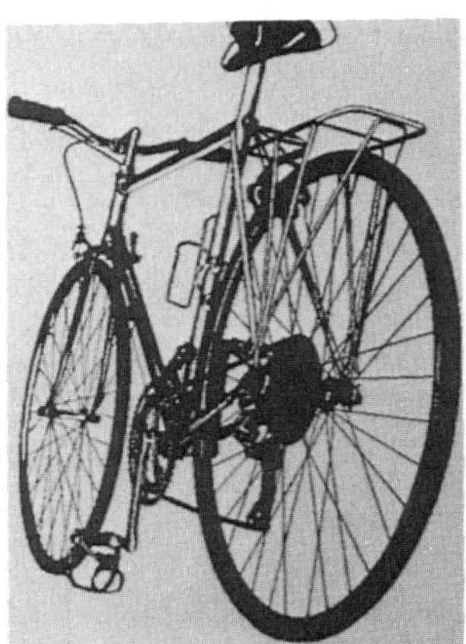

Fig. 1. The same image at equiluminance (left) and non-equiluminance (right). Depth from perspective, spatial organization, and figure/ground segregation are diminished in the equiluminant version. To convince yourself that the left version does indeed contain the same information as the other, look at it through a piece of blue cellophane or glass. These two colors may not be close enough to your equiluminance point to be effective. Changing the light source may help.

The authors are members of the faculty, Department of Neurobiology, Harvard Medical School, Boston, MA 02115.

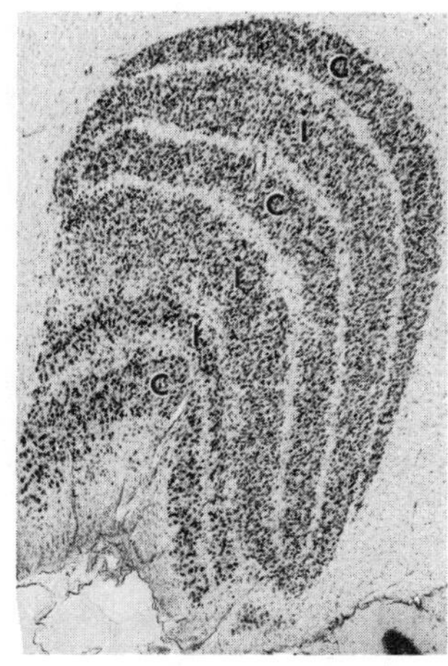

Fig. 2. The primate lateral geniculate body. This six-layered structure is the first stage in the visual system after the retina, and it consists of two distinct subdivisions, the ventral two magnocellular layers and the dorsal four parvocellular layers. The two eyes project to different layers in the interdigitating fashion shown: c indicates layers that are innervated by the contralateral eye; i indicates layers with input from the ipsilateral eye.

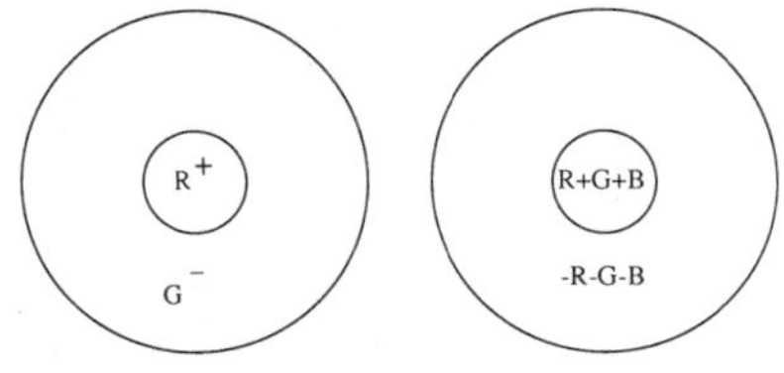

Fig. 3. Receptive fields for (**left**) typical color-opponent parvocellular geniculate neuron, excited over a small region by red light and inhibited over a larger region by green light and (**right**) typical broadband magnocellular neuron, excited by all wavelengths in the center and inhibited by all wavelengths in its surround.

concerned exclusively with the geniculo-cortical part of the visual system, which seems to be directly concerned with visual perception (*2*)—what we think of as seeing.

The primate lateral geniculate body is a six-layered structure, with two obviously different subdivisions: the four dorsal, small-cell (parvocellular) layers and the two ventral, large-cell (magnocellular) layers; these two subdivisions differ both anatomically and physiologically. In 1920 Minkowski (*3*) discovered that each eye projects to three of the six layers in the peculiar alternating fashion shown in Fig. 2: each half-retina is mapped three times onto one geniculate body, twice to the parvocellular layers and once to the magnocellular, and all six topographic maps of the visual field are in precise register (*4*).

The four parvocellular layers seem to be very similar, if not identical, anatomically and physiologically. But the magno- and parvocellular divisions are profoundly different, implying a major split in the visual pathway. This division is most obvious, and was first recognized, in the geniculate, but it does not originate there; the two geniculate subdivisions receive input from two intermixed but anatomically distinct types of retinal ganglion cells: type A cells are larger and project to the magnocellular division, and the smaller type B cells project to the parvocellular division (*5*). These two subdivisions of the visual pathway, which we will refer to as magno and parvo, are distinguishable both anatomically and physiologically. Whether this duality in the visual path arises even earlier, at the bipolar or horizontal cells in the retina, is not known. We can at least be reasonably certain that the two components must both derive their inputs from the same rods and cones and that the marked differences in response properties must therefore depend on the way the photoreceptor inputs are combined.

Though they differ significantly in their response characteristics, the magno and parvo systems do share some basic physiological properties. Their receptive fields (the regions of retina over which their impulse activity can be influenced) are all circularly symmetrical, and about 90% show center-surround opponency (*6, 7*); some cells are excited (impulse rate speeded up) by illumination of a small retinal region and inhibited (impulse rate slowed down) by illumination of a larger surrounding region, whereas others are the reverse, inhibited from the center and excited from the surround. Because of the antagonism between center and surround, large uniform spots produce feeble responses or none. This center-surround arrangement is found also at earlier levels, starting with the retinal bipolar cells. Clearly these cells are wired up so as to convert the information from the photoreceptors into information about spatial discontinuities in light patterns. This should not be surprising, since we ourselves are very poor in judging overall levels of illumination, as anyone who tries doing photography without a light meter well knows—we are lucky if we can come within an *f* stop (a factor of 2) of the right exposure. On the other hand we can detect a spot that is as little as a few percent brighter or darker than its immediate surround.

The magno and parvo divisions nevertheless differ physiologically in four major ways—color, acuity, speed, and contrast sensitivity (*7–10*).

Color. About 90% of the cells in the parvocellular layers of the geniculate are strikingly sensitive to differences in wavelength, whereas cells in the magnocellular layers are not. The three types of cones in the primate retina have broad, overlapping spectral sensitivities and can be loosely termed red-, green-, and blue-sensitive, to indicate that their peak sensitivities are in the long-, middle-, and short-wavelength regions of the spectrum. Parvo cells are wavelength selective because they combine these cone inputs so as in effect to subtract them (Fig. 3, left). A typical parvo cell may, for example, receive excitatory inputs to its receptive field center from red cones only, and inhibitory inputs to its receptive field surround from green cones only. Such a cell will be excited by long wavelengths (reds), inhibited by short wavelengths (blues and greens), and be unresponsive to some intermediate wavelength (yellow). Besides such red–on center, green–off surround cells, most of the other possibilities also occur, most commonly red cones antagonized by green, and blue versus the sum of red and green (that is, yellow). In contrast to the color selectivity of most parvo cells, magno cells (and also the remaining 10% of the parvo cells) sum the inputs of the three cone types, so that the spectral sensitivity curves are broad, and the response to a change in illumination is of the same type, either on or off, at all wavelengths (Fig. 3, right) (*11*). The magno system is thus in effect color-blind: as in black-and-white photography, two different colors, such as red and green, at some relative brightness will be indistinguishable.

Acuity. The second difference between magno and parvo cells is the size of their field centers. For both systems the average size of the receptive field center increases with distance from the fovea, consistent with the differences in acuity between foveal and peripheral vision. Yet at any given eccentricity, magno cells have larger receptive field centers than parvo cells, by a factor of 2 or 3.

Speed. Magno cells respond faster and more transiently than parvo cells. This sensitivity to the temporal aspects of a visual stimulus suggests that the magno system may play a special role in detecting movement. Many cells at higher levels in this pathway are selective for direction of movement.

Contrast. Shapley *et al.* (*10*) found that magno cells are much more sensitive than parvo cells to low-contrast stimuli. Both begin to respond when the center and surround brightnesses differ by only 1 or 2%, but with increasing contrast magno responses increase rapidly and level off at about 10 to 15% contrast, whereas parvo responses increase more slowly, and saturate at far higher contrasts.

These four major differences between the two subdivisions, in color, acuity, quickness, and contrast sensitivity, imply that they contribute to different aspects of vision. Exactly what aspects have become clearer recently, with new anatomical techniques that have made it possible to follow these subdivisions farther into the central nervous system and to correlate them with the response selectivity of cells at later stages in each subdivision for more abstract stimulus features.

Continuation of the magno and parvo subdivisions in visual area 1. The segregation of the two pathways is perpetuated in the primary visual cortex (*12*) (Fig. 4). Cells in the magnocellular geniculate layers project to layer 4Cα, which projects in turn to layer 4B, which then projects to visual area 2 and to cortical area MT. Parvo cells project to layer 4Cβ, and from there the connections go to layers 2 and 3, and from there to visual area 2. The parvocellular division splits to form an additional subdivision in the upper layers of visual area 1. The first evidence for this further subdivision came in 1978 when Wong-Riley (*13*) stained visual area 1 for the mitochondrial enzyme cytochrome oxidase and saw alternating regions of light and dark staining. The dark regions are round or oval in sections cut parallel to the surface; they are most prominent in the upper layers (2 and 3) but are also faintly visible in layers 5 and 6. They turned out to represent pillar-like structures about 0.2 mm in diameter, spaced 0.5 mm apart (*14*). We term these structures blobs because of their three-dimensional shape. Blobs are found only in the primary visual cortex; they occur in all primates that have been looked at, and in the prosimian *Galago*, but have not been found in other prosimians or any lower mammals (*15*).

Since layers 2 and 3 receive most of their inputs from parvo-recipient layer 4Cβ, both the blobs and the interblobs could be considered continuations of the parvo subdivision. Nevertheless the blobs should probably be thought of as a separate subdivision, because they have somewhat different inputs and very different response properties from the interblobs (*16–18*). The visual response properties of cells in the blobs suggest that they may also receive magnocellular input (*17, 18*).

Thus by the output stage of visual area 1 the magno system remains segregated, and the parvo system seems to have split into two branches. All three subdivisions, magno→4Cα→4B, parvo→4Cβ→interblob, and parvo(+magno?)→4Cβ→blob, then project to visual area 2.

These anatomically defined subdivisions in the primary visual cortex differ from each other in the kinds of visual information they carry (*18*), as in earlier stages.

In the magno pathway, cells in layer 4B are orientation selective; that is, they respond best to lines of a particular orientation, and most of them also show selectivity for the direction of movement (*18, 19*)—for example, a cell preferring horizontal lines may respond when an edge is moved upward but not when it moves downward. Like magnocellular geniculate cells, cells in 4B lack color selectivity.

In the interblobs, most, perhaps all, cells are also orientation selective. Unlike cells in layer 4B, most are not direction selective; 10 to 20% are end-stopped, responding to short but not long line or edge stimuli. The receptive fields are small, and the optimum line thickness is similar to the optimum spot size of cells in the geniculate parvocellular layers at the same eccentricity. This system may therefore be responsible for high-resolution form perception. Although anatomical evidence indicates that the interblob system receives its major input from the color-coded parvocellular geniculate layers, most of the interblob cells are not explicitly color-coded: they show no color opponency and respond well to achromatic luminance contrast borders. Nevertheless, many of them respond to an appropriately oriented color-contrast edge regardless of the colors forming the edge or the relative brightness of the two colors. Similarly, they usually respond to lines or borders of any brightness contrast (light-on-dark or dark-on-light), even though the antecedent geniculate cells are either on-center or off-center but not both. This suggests that much of the color-coded parvocellular input is pooled in such a way that color contrast can be used to identify borders but that the information about the colors (including black versus white) forming the border is lost (*20*).

Blob cells are not orientation selective but are either color or brightness selective. The blob system thus seems to carry information complementary to the information carried by the interblob system. The brightness-selective (non–color-coded or broadband) blob cells have larger receptive field centers than the broadband geniculate cells but are otherwise similar—they are either excited or inhibited by small spots of light, and they respond less well to large spots, indicating surround inhibition. These broadband blob cells could receive input from either the magnocellular geniculate cells or from the broadband parvo cells, but the physiological properties of many of them would be more consistent with input from the magno system (*17, 18*). We assume that the color-opponent blob cells receive input from the color-opponent parvocellular geniculate cells,

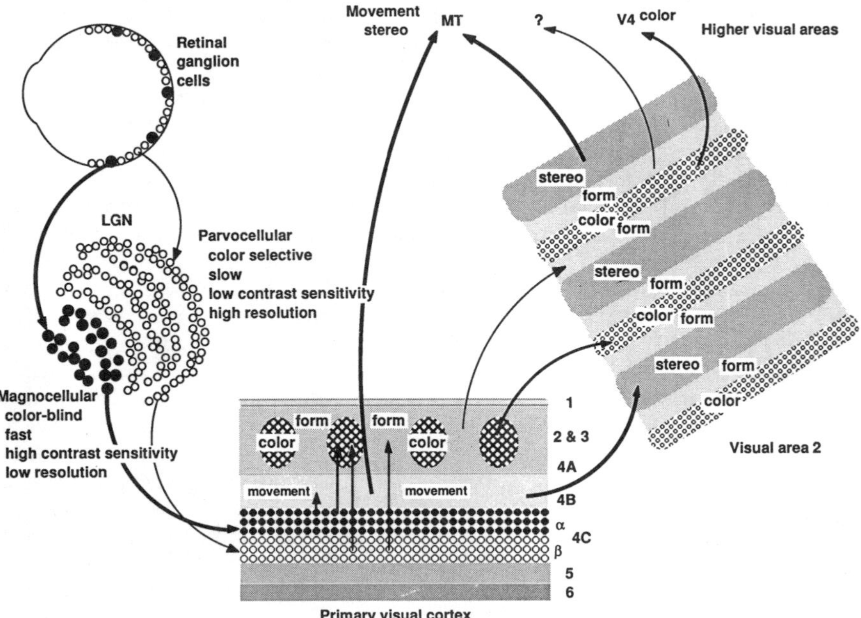

Fig. 4. Diagram of the functional segregation of the primate visual system. MT, middle temporal lobe; V4, visual area 4; LGN, lateral geniculate body.

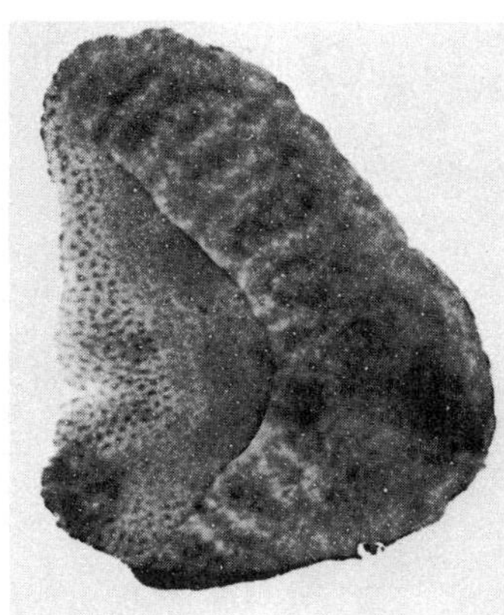

Fig. 5. Section parallel to the surface through visual areas 1 and 2 of a squirrel monkey, stained for cytochrome oxidase. Visual area 1 is on the left; the blobs appear as small round dots. In Visual area 2 the cytochrome-oxidase stain reveals a pattern of alternating thin, thick, and pale stripes.

though they differ from them in that their receptive field centers are larger and their color coding is doubly opponent—they give opposite responses to different parts of the spectrum in the center (say, on to red and off to green), and both types of center response are reduced when the spot is made larger.

The blob and interblob systems thus work in entirely different and complementary ways. Blob cells are explicitly color-coded, excited by colors in one region of the spectrum and inhibited by others, and not selective for stimulus orientation. Interblob cells are selective for stimulus orientation but mostly are not color selective, responding to a line or edge of the correct orientation regardless of its color. The strategy of carrying orientation information in a system that mostly pools color information and color-contrast information in a separate system that does not carry orientation information is probably more efficient than having single cells selective for both the orientation and color of a border. Nevertheless, as emphasized earlier, although most of the interblob cells are not overtly color selective, they probably receive their inputs from explicitly color-coded parvocellular geniculate cells and are most likely not color-blind in the sense that the cells in the magno system probably are. Most interblob cells, even though they lose the information about the colors that form a border or the sign of the contrast of the border, should respond to color-contrast borders in which the two colors are equally bright; such borders would be invisible to magno cells.

Visual area 2. The main target of visual area 1 is visual area 2 (Brodmann's area 18), which shows an equally intriguing pattern when stained for cytochrome oxidase (Fig. 5) (*16, 21*). Instead of small round dots, tangential sections show a pattern of stripes, much coarser than the blobs of visual area 1; these alternately dark and light stripes are several millimeters wide and run perpendicular to the border between visual areas 1 and 2, probably extending over the entire 8- to 10-mm width of visual area 2. The dark stripes are themselves of two types, thick and thin. The regularity of this pattern of thick, thin, and pale stripes varies from animal to animal and is clearer in New World monkeys than in Old World ones, at least partly because in Old World monkeys visual area 2 is buried in the lunate sulcus. Given three histologically defined regions in visual area 2 and the fact that visual area 1 has three kinds of subdivisions that project to other cortical areas, it was natural to ask if they were related. And indeed, from tracer injections into the three kinds of stripes in visual area 2, we found that the blobs are reciprocally connected to the thin stripes, the interblob regions to the pale stripes, and layer 4B to the thick stripes (Fig. 4) (*18, 22*).

The next step was to record from cells in visual area 2, to learn whether the three subdivisions carry different types of visual information. We did indeed find marked differences, which were consistent with the properties of cells in the antecedent subdivisions of visual area 1 (*18, 23*).

Cells in the thin stripes showed no orientation selectivity, and over half were color-coded, just as we had found in the blobs. As in the blobs, most of the color-coded cells were doubly opponent, with two antagonistic inputs to their centers, and surround antagonism for both of these center inputs. About half of the thin-stripe cells, both broadband and color opponent, exhibited an additional property not seen in the blob cells: the receptive field centers were bigger, yet optimum spot sizes were about the same. A typical cell might respond best, say, to a 0.5° diameter spot, give no response at all to 2° or 4° spots (indicating surround antagonism), and yet respond actively to the 0.5° spot anywhere within an area about 4° in diameter. These cells can be broadband or color opponent. Several years ago Baizer, Robinson, and Dow (*24*) described this kind of broadband cell, which they called "spot cells," in visual area 2.

Cells in the pale stripes are orientation selective but not direction selective. At least half of them are end-stopped; this represents a dramatic increase in the proportion of end-stopping over what is seen in visual area 1. We have argued that end-stopping, like center-surround antagonism, is an efficient way of encoding information about shape (*23*). Like cells in the interblobs, pale-stripe cells are not explicitly color-coded, and we expect that they would respond to color-contrast borders at all relative brightnesses, though we have not yet tested this.

In the thick stripes the great majority of cells likewise show orientation selectivity, but are seldom end-stopped. The most consistent response selectivity we see in the thick stripes is for stereoscopic depth—most cells respond poorly to stimulation of either eye alone but vigorously when both eyes are stimulated together, and for most cells the responses are extremely sensitive to variations in the relative horizontal positions of the stimuli in the two eyes (retinal disparity). Poggio and Fischer (*25*) had seen similar disparity-tuned cells in visual area 1 in alert monkeys, predominantly in layer 4B, the layer that projects to the thick stripes of visual area 2. In the thick stripes we find the same three basic

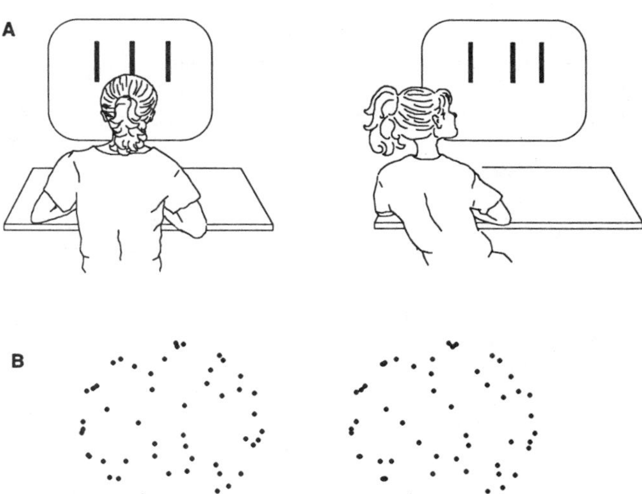

Fig. 6. (**A**) Loss of depth from parallax at equiluminance. The position of the middle bar is made to vary with the observer's head position. In this case, the center bar appears to lie in front of the reference bars, except when the bars are made equiluminant with the background. (**B**) Two frames of a movie in which the movement of dots generates the sensation of a three-dimensional object. The dots appear to lie on the surface of a sphere (which you can see by stereo-viewing these two frames). All sensation of depth is lost when the dots are equiluminant with the background.

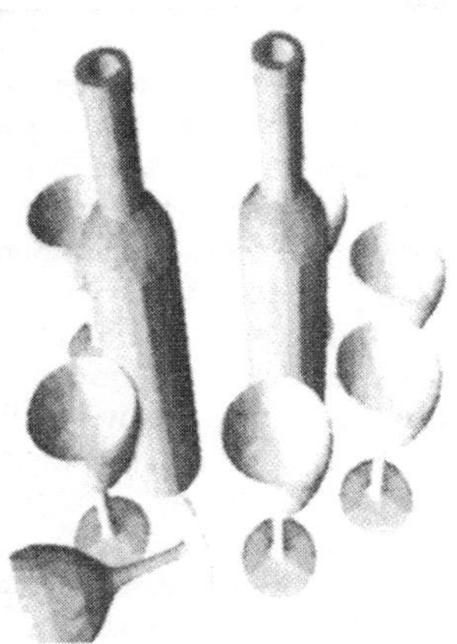
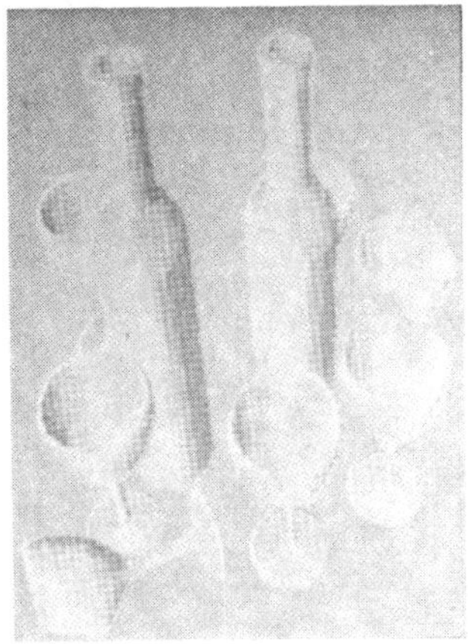
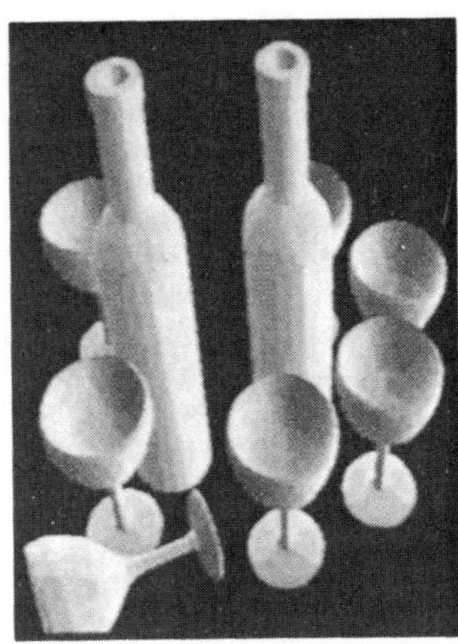

Fig. 7. Computer-generated images in which shape is generated by shading. In the middle image the two colors are equiluminant, and the three-dimensional shape is harder to discern than in the other two images, which have luminance-contrast.

classes of cells described by Poggio and Fischer—cells selective for near stimuli, far stimuli, or stimuli falling on exactly corresponding retinal points. Like cells in the pale stripes, these cells show no color selectivity; moreover, we would predict that these cells would be like their magnocellular predecessors and would not respond to color-contrast borders when the colors are equally bright, though we have not yet tested responses to equiluminant color-contrast borders either in layer 4B of visual area 1 or in the thick stripes of visual area 2.

Other studies (*26, 27*) have not reported such a clean segregation of cells with different physiological properties in visual area 2, or as clear a correlation of physiological subtypes with the three types of stripes. How clear the functional segregation is in visual area 2 remains to be resolved, but we suspect that these differences are due to choice of classification criteria (*23*).

Higher visual areas. Meanwhile, explorations of visual areas beyond 1 and 2 are helping close the gap between the functions suggested by electrophysiological studies and what clinical observations imply about the segregation of various functions in the human visual system. The response properties of cells at levels beyond visual area 2 suggest that the segregation of functions begun at the earliest levels is perpetuated at the highest levels so far studied. Indeed, the segregation seems to become more and more pronounced at each successive level, so that subdivisions that are interdigitated in visual areas 1 and 2 become segregated into entirely separate areas at still higher levels. One higher visual area in the middle temporal lobe, MT, seems to be specialized for the analysis of movement and stereoscopic depth (*28*). It receives input not only from layer 4B in visual area 1 (*29*), which is also rich in directionality and disparity selectivity, but also from the thick stripes in visual area 2 (*26, 30*), which, as already described, contain many cells selective for binocular disparity (*23*). Another higher visual area, visual area 4, has been reported to contain a preponderance of color-selective cells (*31*), but just how specialized visual area 4 is for color is still unclear since many of the cells show some selectivity for orientation. Visual area 4 receives input from the color-coded thin stripes in visual area 2 and possibly from the pale stripes (*26, 30, 32*). The notion that there is a higher visual area devoted largely to the processing of color information is consistent with the clinical observation that patients with strokes in the posterior inferior occipital lobe (perhaps in a region homologous to visual area 4) can lose color perception without impairment of form or movement perception.

There are strong suggestions that these channels remain segregated through still higher levels in the brain (*33*). From lesion studies Pohl (*34*) and Ungerleider and Mishkin (*35*) have defined two functionally distinct divisions of visual association areas: the temporal-occipital region, necessary for learning to identify objects by their appearance, and the parieto-occipital region, needed for tasks involving the positions of objects, a distinction they refer to as "where" versus "what." Visual area 4 preferentially projects to the temporal division and MT primarily to parietal cortex (*36*). Thus the temporal visual areas may represent the continuation of the parvo system, and the parietal areas the continuation of the magno pathway. There can be little doubt that in the next few years work on the dozen or so areas north of the striate cortex will greatly enhance our understanding of vision in general.

Human Perception

Despite many gaps, the picture beginning to emerge from the anatomical and electrophysiological studies summarized above is that the segregation begun in the eye gives rise to separate and independent parallel pathways. At early levels, where there are two major subdivisions, the cells in these two subdivisions exhibit at least four basic differences—color selectivity, speed, acuity, and contrast sensitivity. At higher stages the continuations of these pathways are selective for quite different aspects of vision (form, color, movement, and stereopsis), thus generating the counterintuitive prediction that different kinds of visual tasks should differ in their color, temporal, acuity, and contrast characteristics. To test this prediction, we asked whether the differences seen in the geniculate can be detected in conscious human visual perception by comparing the color, temporal, spatial, and contrast sensitivities of different visual functions. Many of these questions, not surprisingly, have already been asked, and the answers are wonderfully consistent with the anatomy and physiology. For several decades psychologists have accumulated evidence for two channels in human vision, one chromatic and the other achromatic, by showing that different tasks can have very different sensitivities to color and brightness contrast. Given what we know now about the electrophysiology and the anatomy of the subdivisions of the primate visual system, we can begin to try to correlate the perceptual observations with these subdivisions (*37*). Though at higher cortical levels there seem to be three subdivisions, possibly with some mixing of magno and parvo inputs to the blob system, the most important distinction is probably between the magno system (magno→4Cα→4B→MT) and the parvo-derived subdivisions (parvo→4Cβ→interblobs→pale stripes→ visual area 4?) and [parvo(+magno?)→4Cβ→blobs→thin stripes→visual area 4]. In our discussion of human perception we will, therefore, stress the distinctions between functions that seem to

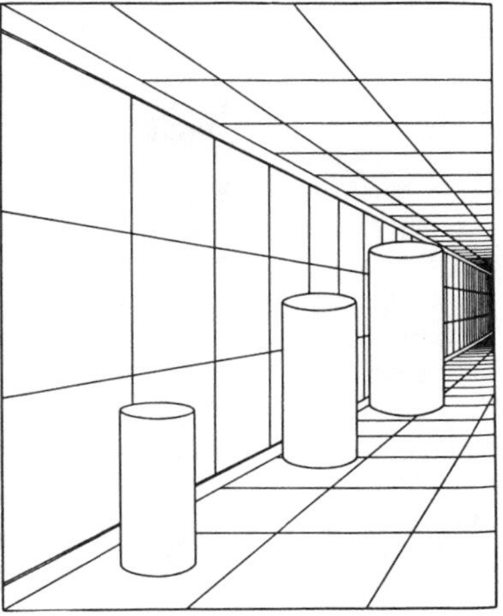

Fig. 8. Gibson's corridor illusion. [From (*47*) with permission, copyright 1950, Houghton Mifflin] At equiluminance the image no longer appears to recede into the distance, and the cylinders all appear to be the same size, as indeed they actually are.

be carried exclusively by the magno system and those that seem to be carried by the parvo-derived pathways.

From the fact that the magno system is color-blind and is faster than the parvo system, we can predict that discrimination of color and discrimination of brightness should have different temporal properties. This is indeed so: in 1923 Ives (*38*) showed that people can follow brightness alternations at much faster rates than pure color alternations.

The high incidence of movement and direction selectivity in MT suggests that this area may be particularly concerned with movement perception. Because anatomically MT receives its major inputs from layer 4B of the primary visual cortex and from the thick stripes of visual area 2, both part of the magno pathway, one would predict that human movement perception should somehow reflect magno characteristics: color blindness, quickness, high contrast sensitivity, and low acuity. Perceptual experiments indicate that movement perception does indeed have these characteristics. First, it is impaired for patterns made up of equiluminant colors: Cavanagh, Tyler, and Favreau (*39*) found that if they generated moving red and green sinewave stripes, "the perceived velocity of equiluminous gratings is substantially slowed . . . the gratings often appear to stop even though their bars are clearly resolved . . . the motion is appreciated only because it is occasionally noticed that the bars are at some new position" (*39*, p. 897; *40*). Second, movement perception is impaired at high spatial frequencies, consistent with the lower acuity of the magno system. Campbell and Maffei (*41*) viewed slowly rotating gratings and found a loss of motion perception at the highest resolvable frequencies, "At a spatial frequency of 16 and 32 cycles/deg a strange phenomenon was experienced, the grating was perceived as rotating extremely slowly and most of the time it actually appeared stationary. Of course, the subject could call upon his memory and deduce that the grating must be moving for he was aware that some seconds before the grating had been at a particular 'clock-face position.' Even with this additional information that the grating must be rotating the illusion of 'stopped motion' persisted" (*41*, p. 714). What is most surprising about the perception of both the equiluminant stripes and the very fine stripes is that even though the sensation of movement is entirely, or almost entirely, lost, the stripes themselves are still clearly visible—they are clear enough that changes in their position can be seen, even though they do not seem to be moving. Last, movement can be vividly perceived with very rapidly alternating or very low contrast images (*37*, *41*). Thus, as summarized in Table 1, the properties of human movement perception are remarkably consistent with the properties of the magno system.

Finding cells in the thick stripes of visual area 2 and in MT that are tuned to retinal disparity suggests that the magno system is also involved in stereoscopic depth perception. Consistent with this, Lu and Fender (*42*) found that subjects could not see depth in equiluminant color-contrast random-dot stereograms even though the dots making up the stereogram remained perfectly clear (*43*). This finding has been disputed, but we found that differences in results can arise from variations in subjects' equiluminance points with eccentricity, which make it difficult to achieve equiluminance across the visual field. Like movement perception, stereopsis fails for stereograms containing only high, but resolvable, spatial frequencies, but it is not diminished for rapidly alternating or very low contrast stereograms (*37*) (Table 1).

Deduction of further magno or parvo functions from perceptual tests. Since the functions that electrophysiological studies had suggested should be carried by the magno system did indeed show all four distinguishing characteristics of that system, we decided to ask whether other visual functions, ones not predicted by single-cell response properties, might also manifest some or all of these properties.

If a particular magno cell sums red and green inputs, there will be a red : green ratio at which the red and green will be equally effective in stimulating the cell. This need not imply that every magno cell has the same ratio of red to green inputs and therefore necessarily the same equiluminance point. Nevertheless, the fact that movement and stereopsis fail at equiluminance implies that, for a given observer, the null ratio must be very similar for the majority of his cells responsible for that function. Krüger (*44*) found that of 33 magnocellular geniculate cells studied in two monkeys, 75% were unresponsive to a moving color-contrast border at a particular relative brightness—a brightness ratio that was very close to a human observer's equiluminant point. Thus not only do individual cells in the magno system seem to be color-blind, but the properties of stereopsis and movement perception indicate that the magno system as a whole is color-blind. [There is, however, currently some disagreement about whether the magno system is inactive at equiluminance (*45*).] People with the most common forms of color

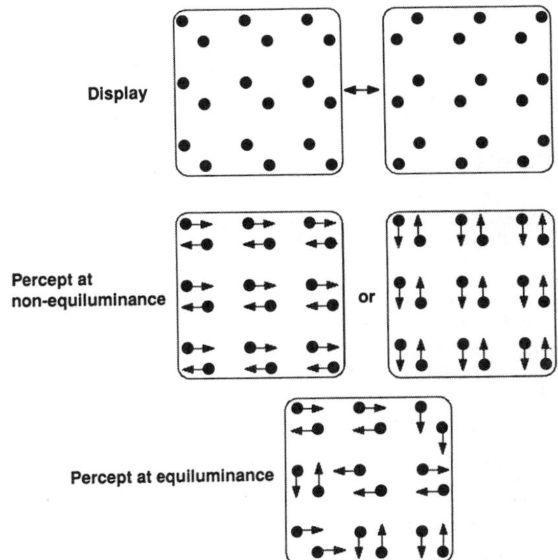

Fig. 9. Linking by movement is lost at equiluminance. All nine of the ambiguous motion squares appear to move in synchrony, even though any one seen alone could be seen moving either horizontally or vertically. This linking disappears at equiluminance, and the dots move every which way.

blindness, due to the lack of one of the three cone pigments, are not nearly as color-blind as the magno system appears to be. They still have two cone types to compare, and so they confuse only a small fraction of possible color pairs and can differentiate most color pairs at all relative brightnesses.

Since both motion perception and stereoscopic depth perception are lost at equiluminance, we suspected that the ability to use relative motion as a depth cue might also be lost. Relative motion is a very powerful depth cue: when an observer moves his head back and forth or moves around in his environment, the relative motion of objects provides information about their distance. In the experiment shown in Fig. 6A, the position of the middle bar was coupled to head movement, and the middle bar appeared to be either behind or in front of the reference bars, depending on whether its movement was the same as, or contrary to, the head movement. When the bars were made equiluminant with the background, all sensation of depth disappeared (*37*).

Relative movement of different parts of a three-dimensional object is also a powerful depth cue. Figure 6B shows two frames of a movie in which random dots move, some to the right and some to the left, as if they were pasted on a rotating spherical surface. The movie gives a powerful sensation of a rotating spherical surface—unless the dots are equiluminant with the background, and then all sensation of depth is lost (*37*), and the dots seem to dance aimlessly. Thus depth from motion, both from viewer parallax and from object motion, seems also to depend on luminance contrast and could well be a function of the magno system. Consistent with this idea, we could see depth from motion at very low levels of luminance contrast (*37*).

The retinal image is of course two-dimensional, and to capture the three-dimensional relationships of objects the visual systems uses many kinds of cues besides stereopsis and relative motion—perspective, gradients of texture, shading, occlusion, and relative position in the image. We wondered whether the sensation of depth from any of these other cues might also exhibit magno characteristics. It seemed especially likely that the ability to perceive depth from shading might be carried by an achromatic system, because shading is almost by definition purely luminance-contrast information; that is, under natural lighting conditions a shaded region of an object has the same hue as the unshaded parts, simply darker. But in biology just because something could, or seemingly even should, be done in a certain way does not mean that it will be. Nevertheless, Cavanagh and Leclerc (*46*) found that the perception of three-dimensional shape from shading indeed depends solely on luminance contrast. That is, in order to produce a sensation of depth and three-dimensionality, shadows can be any hue as long as they are darker than unshaded regions of the same surface. Many artists seem to have been aware of this; for example, in some of the self-portraits of Van Gogh and Matisse the shadows on their faces are green or blue, but they still convey a normally shaped face. Black-and-white photographs of these paintings (taken with film that has approximately the same spectral sensitivity as humans) confirm that the shadows are actually darker than the unshaded parts. The converse can be seen in Fig. 7; here the green shadows do not convey a sensation of depth and shape when they are the same brightness as the blue but do when they are darker (when the blue is darker, the blue parts are interpreted as shadowed).

Perspective was well known to artists by the time of the Renaissance and is a powerful indicator of depth. Converging lines or gradients of texture are automatically interpreted by the visual system as indicating increasing distance from the observer; thus the image in Fig. 8 (*47*) looks like a corridor receding into the distance despite the conflicting information from other depth cues, the absence of stereopsis or relative motion, which tells us we are looking at a flat surface. The perception of depth from perspective probably underlies many illusions: the two cylinders in Fig. 8 are the same size (and they each cover the same area on your retina), but are perceived by most people as being unequal.

We found that when images with strong perspective are rendered in equiluminant colors instead of black and white, the depth

Table 1. Summary of the correlations between human psychophysical results and the physiological properties of the three subdivisions of the primate geniculo-cortical visual system. A check indicates that the psychophysical results are consistent with the physiology, and a blank indicates that such an experiment has not been done.

Magno System

Physiology	Color selectivity	Contrast sensitivity	Temporal resolution	Spatial resolution
	no	high	fast	low
Human perception				
Movement perception				
Movement detection	√	√	√	√
Apparent movement	√	√	√	√
Depth cues				
Stereopsis	√	√	√	√
Interocular rivalry	√			√
Parallax	√			
Depth from motion	√	√		
Shading	√	√		
Contour lines	√			√
Occlusion	√			
Perspective	√	√	√	
Linking properties				
Linking by movement	√	√		
Linking by collinearity (illusory borders)	√	√	√	√
Figure/ground discrimination	√			

Parvo System

Parvo → Interblob pathway

Physiology	Color selectivity	Contrast sensitivity	Temporal resolution	Spatial resolution
	yes	low	slow	high
Human perception				
Shape discrimination				
Orientation discrimination	√	√	√	√
Shape discrimination	√	√	√	√

Parvo+(Magno?) → Blob pathway

Physiology	Color selectivity	Contrast sensitivity	Temporal resolution	Spatial resolution
	yes	high	slow	low
Human perception				
Color perception				
Color determination	√		√	√
Flicker photometry	√		√	

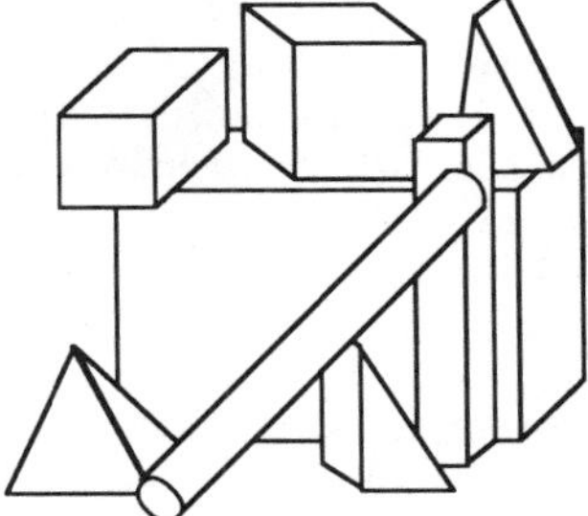

Fig. 10. Linking by collinearity. It is clear which edges are part of the same object, even when occluded by another object. At equiluminance this linking disappears, and it looks like a jumble of lines instead of a pile of blocks. After (*49*).

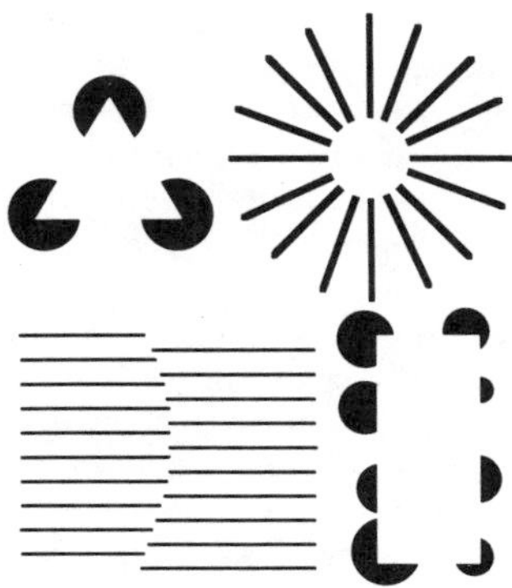

Fig. 11. Illusory borders, which disappear at equiluminance. Redrawn from (*52*).

sensation is lost or greatly diminished (*37*). Illusions of size are likewise lost at equiluminance—the cylinders in Fig. 8 are then all correctly perceived as being the same size. As with movement and stereopsis, the most startling aspect of this phenomenon is that even though the sensation of depth and the illusory distortions due to inappropriate scale all disappear at equiluminance, the lines defining the perspective and the individual elements in the image are nevertheless still clearly visible. This seems to us to rule out high-level, cognitive explanations for depth from perspective and the illusions of perspective; if you see depth because you merely know that converging lines mean increasing distance, you should be able to perceive the depth from the converging lines at equiluminance. Thus at a relatively low level in the visual system some simple interactions must initiate the automatic interpretation of a two-dimensional image into three-dimensional information; moreover, these operations seem to be performed only in the achromatic magno system, not in the parvo system.

Why should the depth and movement functions described above all be carried by the magno system and not by the parvo system? We at first assumed that it was because they might all be performed best by a system with the special characteristics of the magno system. But later we wondered if these various functions might be more related than they seemed at first—whether they could all be parts of a more global function. We were struck by the similarity between the list of functions we had ascribed to the magno system and the Gestalt psychologists' list of features used to discriminate objects from each other and from the background—figure/ground discrimination (*48*). Most scenes contain a huge amount of visual information, information about light intensity and color at every point on the retina and the presence and orientation of discontinuities in the light pattern. The Gestalt psychologists recognized that one important step in making sense of an image must be to correlate related pieces of visual information; that is, to decide whether a series of light/dark discontinuities forms a single edge, whether adjacent edges belong to the same object, whether two parts of an occluded edge are related, and so on. They determined that several kinds of cues are used in this way and to organize the visual elements in a scene into discrete objects, to distinguish them from each other and from the background. Barlow (*49*) has called these "linking features" because they are used to link or join related elements. These linking features include: common movement (objects move against a stationary background; contours moving in the same direction and velocity are likely to belong to the same object, even if they are different in orientation or not contiguous); common depth (contours at different distances from the observer are unlikely to belong to the same object); collinearity (if a straight or continuously curved contour is interrupted by being occluded by another object, it is still seen as a single contour); and common color or lightness. The results described below suggest, however, that only luminance contrast, and not color differences, is used to link parts together.

Ramachandran and Anstis (*50*) discovered a powerful example of linking by movement. If two dots on a diagonal are alternated with two other dots, in mirror-image positions, an observer sees apparent movement, which can be either horizontal or vertical. The direction of the observed alternating movement is completely ambiguous; observers usually see one direction for a few seconds, and then flip to the other. With a display of several such ambiguous-motion squares in an array (Fig. 9) all the squares are perceived as moving in the same direction, like Rockettes, either all horizontally or all vertically (even though any one of them viewed alone is equally likely to be perceived as moving in either direction), and when one flips its apparent direction of movement, they all flip. When the dots are made equiluminant with the background the synchrony breaks down and they all seem to move independently (*37*).

Linking by collinearity (Fig. 10) also breaks down when the lines are equiluminant with the background; the figure then just looks like a jumble of lines instead of a pile of blocks. Linking by collinearity is seen in the phenomenon of illusory contours (*51, 52*), figures that produce a vivid perception of an edge in the absence of any real discontinuity (Fig. 11). When these figures are drawn in equiluminant colors, the illusory borders disappear, even though the elements defining them (the pacmen, the spokes, the lines, or the circles) remain perfectly visible. Because the perception of illusory borders also manifests fast temporal resolution, high contrast sensitivity, and low spatial resolution, we suspect that it too may represent a magno function. Illusory borders have been called "cognitive contours" because of the suggestion that the perception of the border is due to a high-level deduction that there must be an object occluding a partially visible figure (*53*). We suspect that this is not the case because the illusory borders disappear at equiluminance, even though the real parts of the figure are still perfectly visible.

Fifty years ago the Gestalt psychologists observed that figure/ground discrimination and the ability to organize the elements in a scene decrease at equiluminance. Equiluminant figures have been described as "jazzy," "unstable," "jelly-like," or "disorganized" (*43, 54*). Koffka (*55*) pointed out that luminance differences are strikingly more important than color differences for figure/ground segregation: "Thus two greys which look very similar will give a perfectly stable organization if one is used for the figure and the other for the ground, whereas a deeply saturated blue and a grey of the same luminosity which look very different indeed will produce practically no such organization" (*54*, p. 127). Edgar Rubin's popular demonstration of the problem of figure/ground discrimination is the vase/faces (Fig. 12). At non-equiluminance the percept is bistable, so that one sees either the faces or the vase, but usually not both at the same time. At equiluminance the two percepts reverse rapidly, and one can occasionally see both the vase and the faces simultaneously. The distinction between figure and ground thus gets weaker or even disappears entirely.

Color contrast versus color bleeding. At any point in the visual field, cells in the blobs have receptive field centers that are two to four

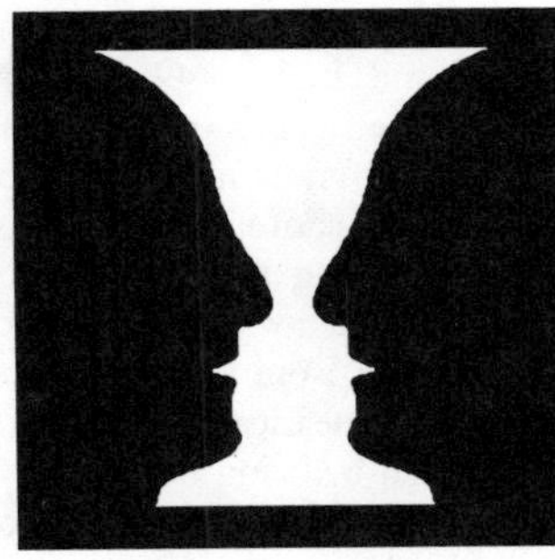

Fig. 12. Rubin's demonstration of figure/ground discrimination [after (*48*)]. In a luminance-contrast image like this you see either the vase or the faces but not both. At equiluminance you can see both simultaneously, or they alternate very rapidly.

times larger than those in the interblobs (*18*). Since only the blobs seem to retain information about the sign of color contrast, we suspect that they are responsible for the perception of the actual colors of objects, as opposed to the ability to use color or luminance contrast to perceive the borders of objects. This implies that color perception should have lower spatial resolution than form perception. This difference in spatial resolution may explain a phenomenon of color perception described by Chevreul (*56*) in 1839 and by von Bezold (*57*) in 1876, the phenomenon of bleeding. The way two adjacent colors can affect each other depends on their geometrical arrangement. When two large regions of color abut, their apparent colors and lightnesses repel each other, each making the other look more like its complement, a phenomenon consistent with the center/surround antagonism in the blob system. For example, a gray spot surrounded by red will look slightly greenish, and the same gray surrounded by green will appear slightly reddish; surrounding the gray by white will make it appear dark, and surrounding it by black will make it seem lighter. This is called simultaneous contrast and can be seen in Fig. 13. Two colors can have exactly the opposite effect on each other if their geometrical arrangement is such that one forms a very fine pattern, such as fine stripes or dots, with the other as a background. In the lower half of Fig. 13, the mortar seems to bleed into the surrounding gray; the white mortar makes the gray look lighter, and the black mortar makes the same gray look darker. We suspect that bleeding occurs when a pattern is too fine to be resolved by the low acuity color system but not too fine for the higher-resolution form system. Thus you see a pattern, but the colors do not seem to conform to the pattern. We think that the interblob system and the magno system can both define shape, and we cannot predict whether one or the other is more important in defining the borders to which the color is assigned. Some observations, however, suggest that the magno system can influence the spreading of color: color bleeding can be contained by illusory borders or by borders defined only by stereopsis; also, stationary patches of color can seem to move with moving luminance-contrast stimuli (*58*).

Of course a pattern can be too fine to be seen by either system, as in the microscopic dots used in magazine illustrations. In this case the individual dots cannot be seen, and the colors simply blend. Many artists of the Impressionist period were aware of the way the colors in a resolvable pattern can bleed; they often made dots or dabs of paint large enough to be seen, but small enough that their colors blended (*59*). The television industry takes advantage of these differences in spatial resolution by broadcasting the color part of the image at a lower resolution than the black and white part, thus reducing the amount of information to be carried.

Why should the visual system be subdivided? Electrophysiological studies suggest that the magno system is responsible for carrying information about movement and depth. We extended our ideas about the possible functions of the magno system with perceptual studies and concluded that the magno system may have a more global function of interpreting spatial organization. Magno functions may include deciding which visual elements, such as edges and discontinuities, belong to and define individual objects in the scene, as well as determining the overall three-dimensional organization of the scene and the positions of objects in space and movements of objects.

If the magno system covers such a broad range of functions, then what is the function of the tenfold more massive parvo system? The color selectivity of the parvo system should enable us to see borders using color information alone and thus borders that might be camouflaged to the color-blind magno system. But defeating camouflage may be only a small part of what the parvo system is specialized for. Experiments with fading of low contrast images (*37*) indicate that the magno system is not capable of sustained scrutiny, since images that can be seen by only the magno system disappear after a few seconds of voluntary fixation. Thus while the magno system is sensitive primarily to moving objects and carries information about the overall organization of the visual world, the parvo system seems to be important for analyzing the scene in much greater and more leisurely detail. These postulated functions would be consistent with the evolutionary relation of the two systems: the magno system seems to be more primitive than the parvo system (*60*) and is possibly homologous to the entire visual system of nonprimate mammals. If so, it should not be surprising that the magno system is capable of what seem to be the essential functions of vision for an animal that uses vision to navigate in its environment, catch prey, and avoid predators. The parvo system, which is well developed only in primates, seems to have added the ability to scrutinize in much more detail the shape, color, and surface properties of objects, creating the possibility of assigning multiple visual attributes to a single object and correlating its parts. Indeed, if the magno system needs to use the various visual attributes of an object in order to link its parts together, this could preclude its being able to analyze the attributes independently. It thus seems reasonable to us that the parvo→ →temporal lobe system might be especially suited for visual identification and association.

Is the existence of separate pathways an accident of evolution or a useful design principle? Segregating the processing of different types of information into separate pathways might facilitate the interactions between cells carrying the same type of information. It might also allow each system to develop functions particularly suited to its specialization. If the parvo system did evolve after the magno system, by duplication of previously existing structures, it should not be surprising to find some redundancy in the properties of the two systems. Indeed, both seem to carry information about orienta-

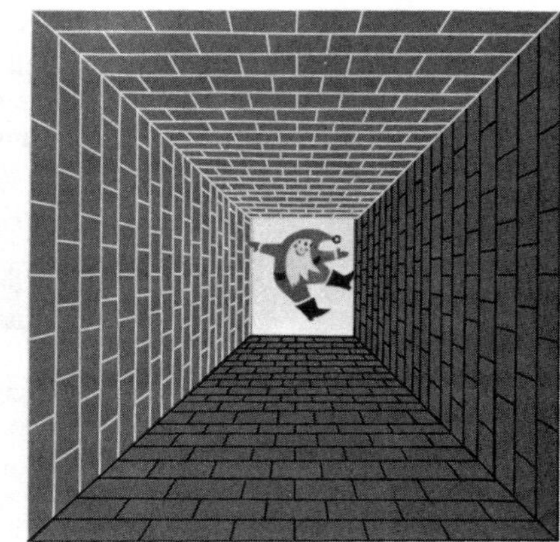

Fig. 13. Simultaneous contrast versus bleeding. This phenomenon is shown for black and white, but it is also true for colors. When a spot is surrounded by another color or brightness, the apparent color of the spot tends toward the opposite, or complement, of the surround. The exact opposite happens when one color forms a fine pattern on the other; then the colors bleed.

tion, and perceptual experiments indicate that both systems can be used to determine shape.

We have summarized the anatomical, physiological, and psychological evidence for segregation of function in the primate visual system. By comparing our own perceptual abilities with the electrophysiological properties of neurons in different subdivisions of the visual system, we may be able to deduce functions of particular visual areas, functions that might not have been obvious from electrophysiological observations alone. We can now go back to physiological experiments to test some of the ideas raised by the perceptual experiments.

REFERENCES AND NOTES

1. H. Lissauer, *Arch. Psychiatr. Nervenkr.* **21**, 22 (1890); J. Bodamer, *ibid.* **179**, 6 (1947); A. R. Damasio, T. Yamada, H. Damasio, J. Corbett, J. McKee, *Neurology* **30**, 1064 (1980); A. L. Pearlman, J. Birch, J. C. Meadows, *Ann. Neurol.* **5**, 253 (1979); D. Verrey, *Arch. Ophthalmol. (Paris)* **8**, 289 (1888); R. Balint, *Monatsschr. Psychiatr. Neurol.* **25**, 51 (1909); J. Zihl, D. Von Cramon, N. Mai, *Brain* **106**, 313 (1983). Cortical loss of color perception and loss of face recognition usually occur together, but each can occur independently.
2. H. Munk, *Centralbl. Prakt. Augenheilk.* **3**, 255 (1879).
3. M. Minkowski, *Arch. Neurol. Psychiatr.* **6**, 201 (1920).
4. W. E. Le Gros Clark and G. G. Penman, *Proc. R. Soc. Lond. Ser. B* **114**, 291 (1934); S. Brody, *Proc. Kon. Ned. Akad. Wet.* **37**, 724 (1934); J. G. Malpeli and F. H. Baker, *J. Comp. Neurol.* **161**, 569 (1975).
5. A. G. Leventhal, R. W. Rodieck, B. Dreher, *Science* **213**, 1139 (1981).
6. S. W. Kuffler, *J. Neurophysiol.* **16**, 37 (1953).
7. T. N. Wiesel and D. H. Hubel *ibid.* **29**, 1115 (1966); P. H. Schiller and J. G. Malpeli, *ibid.* **41**, 788 (1978).
8. R. L. De Valois, E. Abramov, G. H. Jacobs, *J. Opt. Soc. Am.* **56**, 966 (1966); R. L. De Valois, D. M. Snodderly, Jr., E. W. Yund, N. K. Hepler, *Sens. Process.* **1**, 244 (1977); A. M. Derrington, J. Krauskopf, P. Lennie, *J. Physiol. (London)* **357**, 241 (1984); E. Kaplan and R. M. Shapley, *ibid.* **330**, 125 (1982); *Proc. Natl. Acad. Sci. U.S.A.* **83**, 2755 (1986); B. Dreher, Y. Fukada, R. W. Rodieck, *J. Physiol. (London)* **258**, 433 (1976); T. P. Hicks, B. B. Lee, T. R. Vidyasagar, *ibid.* **337**, 183 (1983); P. Gouras, *ibid.* **199**, 533 (1968); *ibid.* **204**, 407 (1969); F. deMonasterio and P. Gouras, *ibid.* **251**, 167 (1975).
9. A. M. Derrington and P. Lennie, *J. Physiol. (London)* **357**, 219 (1984).
10. R. Shapley, E. Kaplan, R. Soodak, *Nature (London)* **292**, 543 (1981).
11. The magno system clearly combines the inputs from the red and the green cones, but the contribution from the blue cones is so small that it is not clear whether the magno system receives any input at all from the blue cones. Also, magno cells are not completely broadband, in that their receptive field surrounds are often weighted toward the red (*7*).
12. D. H. Hubel and T. N. Wiesel, *J. Comp. Neurol.* **146**, 421 (1972); J. S. Lund, *ibid.* **147**, 455 (1973); ——— and R. G. Boothe, *ibid.* **159**, 305 (1975).
13. M. Wong-Riley, personal communication.
14. A. E. Hendrickson, S. P. Hunt, and J.-Y. Wu, *Nature (London)* **292**, 605 (1981); J. C. Horton and D. H. Hubel, *ibid.*, p. 762.
15. J. C. Horton, *Philos. Trans. R. Soc. London* **304**, 199 (1984); E. McGuinness, C. MacDonald, M. Sereno, J. Allman, *Soc. Neurosci. Abstr.* **12**, 130 (1986).
16. M. S. Livingstone and D. H. Hubel, *Proc. Natl. Acad. Sci. U.S.A.* **79**, 6098 (1982).
17. C. R. Michael, *Soc. Neurosci. Abstr.* **13**, 2 (1987); D. Fitzpatrick, K. Itoh, I. T. Diamond, *J. Neurosci.* **3**, 673 (1983); R. B. H. Tootell, S. L. Hamilton, E. Switkes, R. L. De Valois, *Invest. Ophthalmol. Visual Sci.* (suppl.) **26**, 8 (1985).
18. M. S. Livingstone and D. H. Hubel, *J. Neurosci.* **4**, 2830 (1984).
19. B. Dow, *J. Neurophysiol.* **37**, 927 (1974).
20. P. Gouras and J. Krüger, *ibid.* **42**, 850 (1979).
21. R. B. H. Tootell *et al.*, *Science* **220**, 737 (1983).
22. M. S. Livingstone and D. H. Hubel, *J. Neurosci.* **7**, 3371 (1987).
23. D. H. Hubel and M. S. Livingstone, *ibid.*, p. 3378.
24. J. S. Baizer, D. L. Robinson, B. M. Dow, *J. Neurophysiol.* **40**, 1024 (1977).
25. G. F. Poggio and B. Fischer, *ibid.*, p. 1392; G. F. Poggio, in *Dynamic Aspects of Neocortical Functions* G. M. Edelman, W. E. Gall, W. M. Cowan, Eds. (Wiley, New York, 1984), pp. 631–632.
26. E. A. DeYoe and D. C. Van Essen, *Nature (London)* **317**, 58 (1985).
27. A. Burkhalter and D. C. Van Essen, *J. Neurosci.* **6**, 2327 (1986).
28. R. Dubner and S. M. Zeki, *Brain Res.* **35**, 528 (1971); J. H. R. Maunsell and D. C. Van Essen, *J. Neurophysiol.* **49**, 1148 (1983).
29. J. S. Lund, R. D. Lund, A. E. Hendrickson, A. H. Bunt, A. F. Fuchs, *J. Comp. Neurol.* **164**, 287 (1975); W. B. Spatz, *Brain Res* **92**, 450 (1975); L. G. Ungerlieder and M. Mishkin, *J. Comp. Neurol.* **188**, 347 (1979).
30. S. Shipp and S. Zeki, *Nature (London)* **315**, 322 (1985).
31. S. Zeki, *ibid.* **284**, 412 (1980).
32. References (*26*) and (*30*) are in agreement that the thick stripes project to MT and that the thin stripes project to visual area **4**, but only (*26*) reports that the pale stripes project to visual area 4.
33. For a review, J. H. R. Maunsell, *Matters of Intelligence*, L. M. Vaina, Ed. (Kluwer Academic, Norwell, MA, 1987), pp. 59–87.
34. W. Pohl, *J. Comp. Physiol. Psychol.* **82**, 227 (1973).
35. L. G. Ungerleider and M. Mishkin, in *Analysis of Visual Behavior*, D. J. Ingle, M. A. Goodale, R. J. W. Mansfield, Eds. (MIT Press, Cambridge, MA, 1982), pp. 549–586.
36. K. S. Rockland and D. N. Pandya, *Brain Res.* **179**, 3 (1979); R. Desimone, J. Fleming, C. G. Gross, *ibid.* **184**, 41 (1980); J. H. R. Maunsell and D. C. Van Essen, *J. Neurosci.* **3**, 2563 (1983).
37. M. S. Livingstone and D. H. Hubel, *J. Neurosci.* 7, 3416 (1987).
38. H. E. Ives, *J. Opt. Soc. Am. Rev. Sci. Instr.* 7, 363 (1923).
39. P. Cavanagh, C. W. Tyler, O. E. Favreau, *J. Opt. Soc. Am.* **8**, 893 (1984).
40. We found (*37*) that apparent movement as well as real movement disappeared at equiluminance. This result is controversial, but we suspect that different findings may be due to difficulties in achieving equiluminance across the visual field.
41. F. W. Campbell and L. Maffei, *Vision Res.* **21**, 713 (1981).
42. C. Lu and D. H. Fender, *Invest. Ophthalmol.* **11**, 482 (1972).
43. R. L. Gregory, *Perception* **6**, 113 (1977).
44. J. Krüger, *Exp. Brain Res.* **30**, 297 (1979).
45. Derrington and Lennie (*9*) have reported that magnocellular neurons are less responsive than parvocellular neurons at equiluminance, but are not unresponsive. P. H. Schiller and C. L. Colby [*Vision Res.* **23**, 1631 (1983)] and A. C. Hurlbert, N. K. Logothetis, E. R. Charles, and P. H. Schiller [*Soc. Neurosci. Abstr.* **13**, **204** (1987)] have reported that cells in the parvo system, not the magno system, become unresponsive at equiluminance. This issue clearly remains to be resolved and is discussed in (*37*).
46. P. Cavanagh and Y. Leclerc, *Invest. Ophthalmol. Visual Sci.* (suppl.) **26**, 282 (1985).
47. J. J. Gibson, *The Perception of the Visual World*, L. Carmichael, Ed. (Houghton Mifflin, Boston, 1950).
48. E. Rubin, *Synsoplevede Figurer* (Glydendalska, Copenhagen, 1915).
49. H. B. Barlow, *Proc. R. Soc. London* **212**, 1 (1981).
50. V. S. Ramachandran and S. A. Anstis, *Perception* **14**, 135 (1985).
51. F. Schumann, *Z. Psychol.* **23**, 1 (1900).
52. G. Kanizsa, *Riv. Psicologia* **49**, 7 (1955).
53. R. L. Gregory, *Nature (London)* **238**, 51 (1972).
54. S. Liebmann, *Psychol. Forsch.* **9**, 300 (1926).
55. K. Koffka, *Principles of Gestalt Psychology* (Harcourt Brace, New York, 1935).
56. M. E. Chevreul, *De la Loi du Contraste Simultané des Couleurs* (Pitios-Levrault, Paris, 1839).
57. W. von Bezold, *The Theory of Color*, S. R. Koehler, Transl. (Prang, Boston, 1876).
58. H. F. J. M. van Tuijl, *Acta Psychol.* **39**, 441 (1975); K. Nakayama and S. Shimojo, personal communication; V. S. Ramachandran, *Nature (London)* **328**, 645 (1987).
59. M. S. Livingstone, *Sci. Am.* **258**, 78 (January 1988).
60. R. W. Guillery, *Prog. Brain Res.* **51**, 403 (1979); S. M. Sherman, *Prog. Psychobiol. Physiol. Psychol.* **2**, 233 (1985).

4

E. A. DeYoe and D. C. Van Essen

Concurrent processing streams in monkey visual cortex

1988. *Trends in Neurosciences* 11: 219–226

The concept of multiple processing streams has emerged as a major theme in many studies of the primate visual system. However, the perception of basic attributes such as color, form, depth, and movement cannot be mapped onto different neuronal pathways as a set of simple, one-to-one relationships. Rather, we suggest that many aspects of perception involve significant overlap across a number of paths and cortical areas. Anatomical divergences and convergences that have been reported among processing streams may be related to the multiplicity of strategies for deriving perceptual attributes from the low-level cues provided by retinal images.

E. A. DeYoe and D. C. Van Essen are at the Division of Biology 216–76, California Institute of Technology, Pasadena, CA 91125, USA.

Several lines of anatomical, physiological, and behavioral evidence suggest that a small number of processing streams originate within retina, continue within the lateral geniculate nucleus, and further differentiate within striate and extrastriate visual cortex[1–6]. To understand the functional significance of this architecture, it is essential to know what types of information are carried in each stream and also how that information is used in perception and the control of behavior. A popular notion in recent years has been that each stream emphasizes the analysis of a particular type of low-level sensory cue, which in turn contributes to a single aspect of perception. For example, it has been suggested[4,7] that the perception of movement is mediated by a pathway that includes the middle temporal visual area (MT), whose cells respond selectively to motion in the retinal image. Similarly, it has been hypothesized that the analysis of wavelength and hence the perception of color are mediated by a pathway including visual area V4[8–10]. Analogous proposals link the analysis of contour orientation to the perception of form and the analysis of binocular disparity to the perception of depth. Thus, in its extreme form, this line of reasoning links each sensory cue to a single aspect of perception and assigns the analysis to a single processing stream (one cue: one stream: one percept).

In the first part of this article, we argue for a broader conceptual framework, centered around the proposition that each low-level sensory cue typically provides a basis for perceiving not one, but several distinct attributes of objects in the external world. Conversely, most attributes can be inferred concurrently from several sensory cues rather than just one. For example, image motion cues can engender perceptions of three-dimensional shape as well as movement *per se*. Additional cues, including geometric perspective, binocular disparity, and shading can reinforce and enrich the perception of shape over that attainable from motion cues alone. Accordingly, there is a specific yet manifold relationship between low-level cues and high-level aspects of perception. In contrast to a strict parallelism of processing streams, this leads us to expect redundant representation of sensory cues in different anatomical streams and to expect divergence and convergence of streams at successive stages of processing. In the second part of this article, we use this framework as a perspective for reviewing the anatomical connections and physiological characterization of different compartments and streams in visual cortex, which in several respects are more closely intertwined than has generally been appreciated.

Our analysis complements and extends the proposition that cortical processing streams reflect a basic dichotomy between two general tasks of perception: object identification on the one hand and the analysis of spatial relationships on the other (i.e. 'what' vs. 'where'). In broad terms, these two tasks have been associated with anatomically distinct streams leading to temporal and parietal visual cortex, respectively[5,11,12]. Our emphasis here is first to analyse the spectrum of subtasks associated with object identification and spatial relationships and second, to outline the complexity of the linkages between particular subtasks and the low-level cues on which they are based.

Information flow in early visual processing

Images, cues, and attributes

Vision is a process for making inferences about the three-dimensional (3-D) structure and composition of the external physical world, based upon information contained in two-dimensional (2-D) retinal images[13]. The net result is a seemingly unified visual percept, yet the process itself is inherently multifaceted. This is evident from the multiplicity of physical parameters needed to describe retinal images; from the multiplicity of low-level cues that contribute to perceptions;

Retinal images	Sensory cues	Inferred attributes
		(1) **3-D Form** Shape Size Rigidity
Intensity = f(position - x, y; wavelength; time; eye - r, l)	**Primary** Luminance Spectral **Feature-based** Contrast 2-D Velocity Disparity 2-D Orientation	(2) **Surface properties** Color (brightness, hue, saturation) Visual texture Specular reflectance Transparency (shadows, highlights) (3) **3-D Spatial relationships** Relative positions (X, Y, distance-Z) 3-D Orientation in space
		(4) **3-D Movement** Trajectory Rotation

Fig. 1. *Representations of visual information at levels associated with retinal images (left), sensory cues (center), and attributes inferred about the physical world (right). Sensory cues listed here are a subset of the possible distinct types of low level information that can be derived from the images. Feature-based cues are derived in turn from the primary cues. Attribute groups (3) and (4) are meant to include the problem of determining the observer's position and motion as well. Inferences about the nature and direction of illumination should also be accounted for.*

and from the multiplicity of attributes that we can discriminate and ultimately use to describe what we see (Fig. 1). At each level of description, information has been parcelled into several distinct types, and the nature of the parcellation is quite different from one level to the next. Our immediate goal is to discuss the divergence and convergence of information flow that is associated with these transformations. To this end, it will be helpful to state more explicitly what we mean by the terms 'cue' and 'attribute' and to indicate how they may be related to the neural representation of information at different stages of the visual pathway.

Any retinal image can be completely and explicitly described as an intensity distribution that is a function of five physical parameters (Fig. 1, left): retinal position (two dimensions), wavelength, time, and eye (right or left). In the conversion of images into neural signals by the mosaic of retinal photoreceptors, much information is lost at the outset. For example, the exact spectral composition of the image is inevitably obscured by having only three cone types with broad spectral sensitivities; nonetheless, the information that is retained obviously suffices to yield a robust capacity for hue discrimination and color perception.

By combining inputs from groups of photoreceptors in various ways, cells at later stages become selective for particular spatial, temporal, and/or chromatic aspects of a restricted portion of the retinal image. Hence, the neural representation of visual information is in general quite different from the description of images in terms of physical parameters. To assist the discussion of early and intermediate neural representations, we will use the term 'sensory cue' to signify a particular type of information that is (1) present in the images, (2) can be extracted by local processing, and (3) contributes to perception or visually guided behavior.

Initially, each location in an image can be described in terms of two primary cues: luminance, which reflects the aggregate level of photoreceptor activation; and spectral composition, which reflects the differential activation of the different cone types (Fig. 1, center). Any perceptible inhomogeneity in the spatial or temporal distribution of luminance or spectral cues can be regarded as a primitive 'feature'. From these features other cues can be derived, such as spatial contrast (light/dark or spectral), 2-D retinal velocity, binocular disparity, and 2-D orientation. In principle, an unlimited variety of cues can be described, and these can be arranged hierarchically insofar as higher-order cues can be described as combinations of low-order cues. We focus here on a representative set of low-level cues that can profitably be compared to neuronal selectivities that have been studied in various cortical areas. In a more fundamental sense, the choice of cues that are most appropriate in discussing early visual processing is not arbitrary. Rather, it should reflect types of information that are richly represented in natural visual scenes, and descriptions that are matched to the specific informational needs of various higher-level processes.

Once extracted, sensory cues can be used to infer many different properties of the external world. We will refer to the internal representations of these properties as 'perceived attributes'. We emphasize that they are a product of neural processing within the visual pathway. Attributes typically represent good approximations to the physical properties of natural objects, but under some circumstances they may deviate markedly from physical reality, as in many visual illusions. The notion of attributes provides a basis for parcellation of visual information that differs from sensory cues and physical image parameters. Attributes are more closely related to perception and behavior, since visual information is now divided into categories useful in identifying objects and determining their positions or motions in space.

In order to give an intuitive feel to our discussion of attributes, it is useful to consider the following specific (albeit whimsical) example. Suppose that an observer is standing in a room, say at a cocktail party, viewing a balloon drifting near the ceiling. In a broad sense, the visual system has the task of informing the observer about what the object is, where it is located, and where it is going. These general attributes may be further subdivided and naturally grouped into four psychophysically distinct sets which are listed at the right side of Fig. 1. Intuitively, one perceives the shape, color, rotation, and other attributes of the balloon as qualitatively different properties. In a more rigorous sense, these categories can be studied psychophysically using various tests in which an observer is asked to identify objects that are matched for one attribute. For example, given a cluster of different balloons, the observer can be asked to identify those matching in color. Matches will be easily found despite wide differences in other attributes such as shape, size, location, and motion. Such tests of equivalence can reveal how an attribute, as an internal representation, is related to the actual properties of external objects.

In Fig. 1, the first set of attributes pertains to 3-D form: the shape, size, and rigidity of the balloon. These geometrical attributes reflect the spatial extent and arrangement of an object's parts to one another. The second set of attributes pertains to intrinsic surface properties: the balloon's color, texture, shininess, and degree of transparency. These involve inferences about the reflectance and transmittance properties of surface materials. Taken together, the first two groups provide information especially useful in identifying, recognizing and discriminating among objects. In contrast, attributes of the third and fourth groups are primarily involved in determining the locations of objects. The third set concerns static spatial relationships, such as a balloon's 3-D orientation (e.g. tilted back) and its 3-D location relative to the observer (e.g. close by and head-high) and to the rest of the room (e.g. above the table). Finally, the fourth set pertains to motions, including internal rotations (e.g. spinning) and the 3-D trajectory of an object relative to the observer and the rest of the room (e.g. drifting away toward the window).

Direct and concealed contributions of cues

Attributes depend on cues in several ways, some less obvious than others. We say there is a *direct* linkage if the quality of the attribute depends on the particular value of a cue, rather than just its presence. For example, if a balloon reflects longer wavelength light than its neighbors, it will appear more red; hence spectral composition contributes directly to perceived color. Similarly, if a stereogram contains crossed rather than uncrossed disparities, the corresponding regions will appear closer rather than more distant, signifying that disparity contributes directly to depth perception. In addition to these obvious and well-known relationships, there can be hidden linkages between cues and attributes that are also very important but not as widely appreciated. We say that the contribution of a cue is *concealed* if it aids perception in only an indirect way. For example, a pattern whose movement is incoherent or ambiguous when seen in black and white (luminance cues only) can, under certain conditions, produce an unambiguous percept of motion after addition of appropriate spectral cues[14]. To give an intuitive grasp, this finding can be transposed to our hypothetical cluster of balloons, where one would expect an impression of coherent motion to emerge if all the red balloons happened to have a common velocity. The particular color (red) would help in generating the percept of coherence even though it obviously is irrelevant to knowing the direction and speed of motion. In analogous fashion, orientation cues can also make a concealed contribution to movement perception[14]. Another example has been demonstrated in stereopsis, where spectral cues can permit fusion and depth perception in a random-dot stereogram that otherwise appears diplopic[15].

Another way in which the role of a cue may be concealed is through the generation of contours that are not distinguishable by luminance differences, but rather by discontinuities in spectral, disparity, or motion cues. For instance, an isoluminant border, delineated only by spectral contrast (e.g. green stripes on a red balloon), may yield contours contributing to shape perception. Only positions of the discontinuity are needed to describe the contour; the values of the cues (red vs. green, etc.) are largely irrelevant to the subsequent process of inferring shape. However, it is important to note that the discrimination of motion, depth and 3-D shape are all markedly impaired when viewing isoluminant patterns[3,16,17], suggesting that isoluminant contours are mainly useful in two-dimensional aspects of shape perception.

The manifold linkage of cues and attributes

We now turn to a more systematic consideration of how various cues do or do not contribute to different perceived attributes. In general, the inference of a particular attribute (e.g. red, round, falling) depends more heavily on some cues than others. Each pairing between a cue and an attribute to which it contributes can be regarded as a 'computational strategy'. Fig. 2 graphically enumerates a number of computational strategies linking the different sensory cues to five of the perceptual attributes listed in Fig. 1. The simplest case is that of color perception, in which the attributes of hue, brightness, and saturation are inferred mainly from luminance and spectral contrast cues (Fig. 2, blue lines); other cues are largely irrelevant. The actual computations used to infer surface color are complex, involving integration of luminance and chromatic cues across boundaries and over the entire image in order to compensate for the spectral composition of the source of illumination[19]. However, our goal here is simply to enumerate the computational strategies (linkages) without specifying in detail the particular computations involved.

In contrast to color, the attributes of shape, distance, and motion trajectory each can be partially or completely inferred from one or more of three feature-based cues by using any of several computational strategies. For instance, 2-D retinal velocity cues (Fig. 2, orange lines) can help in inferring shape (structure from motion), distance from the observer or other objects (motion parallax), and overall 3-D trajectory (2-D to 3-D motion transformation, which includes optical flow and looming). In each case, the particular velocities are important, signifying that the contribution of the cue is a direct one as described above. Likewise, disparity and orientation (contour) cues can each contribute directly to inferences about shape, distance, and 3-D trajectory using the processing strategies denoted by red and green lines in the figure. In addition, shape can be inferred partly from luminance contrasts involved in shading.

A similar analysis can be applied to visual texture. In general, texture is a complex attribute that pertains to the overall spatial pattern of markings on a surface. The basis for perceiving texture can arise not only from contrast and 2-D orientation, but also from velocity cues (as in a rippling surface) and possibly from disparity cues (but see Ref. 30). Each of these cues can be associated with basic elements of textures known as textons[20].

Complementary strategies and the interactions among cues

Thus far, we have stressed the independence of computational strategies, insofar as a single cue operating in isolation (often contrived) can elicit a well-defined percept. A notable example is the random-dot stereogram, which can yield robust perceptions of 3-D shapes dependent exclusively on binocular disparity cues[15]. However, multiple cues acting in concert can help to specify the uniqueness or strengthen the robustness of the percept. For example, the well-known Necker cube, when projected as a 2-D image, has two equally plausible interpretations that alternate as competing percepts, but the addition of disparity cues can bias the outcome to favor a single percept. In a broader sense, the information contained in 2-D retinal images is fundamentally inadequate for an unambiguous reconstruction of the external world. In other words, the computational problem is severely 'ill-posed'[31]. In order to reduce the inherent ambiguity, it is necessary to impose additional constraints and assumptions – for example, that images arise mainly from piecewise continuous surfaces[13]. The coordinated use of multiple computational strategies may reduce the need for such constraints and help to insure the most plausible interpretation of images[32].

In summary, Fig. 2 makes it clear that the relationship between cues and attributes is rarely one-to-one. Rather, there is a manifold relationship in which each sensory cue can be used in multiple ways to contribute to inferences about colors, textures, shapes, distances, and trajectories. From this perspective, vision clearly involves concurrent processing of different cues with both divergence (one cue contributing to multiple attributes) and convergence (multiple cues contributing to a single attribute). To the extent that different attributes are processed separately in the brain, this leads to the expectation

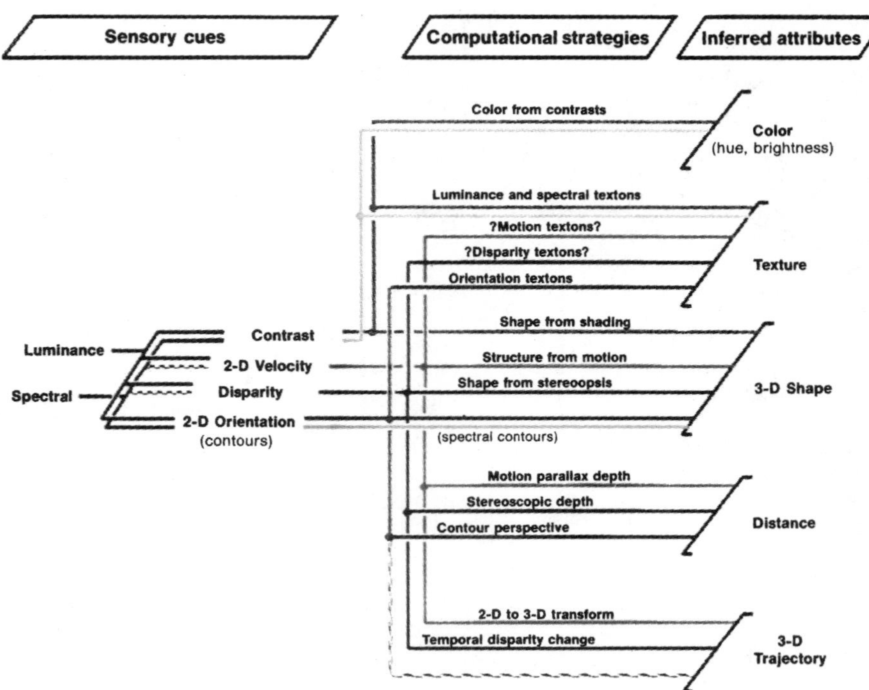

Fig. 2. *Schematic diagram of possible associations between sensory cues and various attributes of the visual scene. Only a subset of all possible cues and attributes are illustrated here. Note that 'color' refers here to brightness as well as hue. Dashed lines indicate concealed contributions of spectral cues (red dashed lines) or orientation cues (green dashed line) (see text). Although 2-D orientation cues are linked to 3-D shape by a line marked 'spectral contours', the actual contribution may be limited to the perception of 2-D shape. Question marks signify uncertainty about the sufficiency of motion and disparity cues in contributing to the perception of surface texture. Informative references relevant to each computational strategy are as follows: color from contrasts[18,19]; textons[20,21]; shape from shading[22,23]; structure from motion[24]; form from stereopsis[15,25]; form from contours[26,27]; 2-D form (but little else) from chromatic contours[3]; motion parallex depth[24]; stereoscopic depth[15,25]; contour perspective[26,27]; 2-D to 3-D motion transform (includes flow field and looming strategies)[28,29]; temporal sequence of disparity[29].*

that different neuronal selectivities will be represented redundantly in pathways that sometimes run in parallel but that can also split or join together. In the next section, we evaluate the degree to which such organizational principles are reflected in the anatomy and physiology of primate visual cortex.

Anatomical and physiological evidence for concurrent processing streams

Anatomy

Parallel anatomical pathways in the primate visual system begin within the retina, where there are two major classes of ganglion cells, large (magnocellular) and small (parvocellular) neurons, that project to the lateral geniculate nucleus (LGN)[33]. Within cortical areas V1 and V2, a tripartite organizational pattern emerges that is closely related to the pattern of lamination and to the tangential distribution of staining for cytochrome oxidase (CO). In V1, these three compartments include layer 4B plus a tangentially organized array of CO-rich 'blobs' separated by CO-sparse 'interblobs'[34–39]. In V2, there is a coarser array of irregular, stripe-like regions (most apparent in layers 3–5), which run roughly orthogonal to the V1/V2 border. These can be subdivided into alternating thick (wide) stripes and thin (narrow) stripes, both rich in CO, which are separated by CO-sparse interstripes[1,34,40].

Fig. 3 shows a hierarchical scheme that represents the major interrelationships among the various compartments in the LGN, V1, and several extrastriate visual areas. The lines linking the various boxes represent prominent anatomical connections, which are known in most cases to be reciprocal (bi-directional); line styles reflect robustness or consistency of projections (see legend). Many of these pathways are multiple-neuron sequences involving additional layers that have been omitted from the diagram for clarity. The icons within each box represent physiological selectivities revealed by single unit recordings, as discussed below.

Based on the connections among the different compartments illustrated schematically in Fig. 3, we distinguish three major processing streams[35,41–44]. The M (magno) stream, dominated by magnocellular LGN inputs, includes several substreams linking layer 4B of V1, the CO thick stripes of V2, and areas V3 and MT. The outputs of the M stream are distributed from MT and V3 mainly to visual areas in posterior parietal cortex[6,12,45]. The P–I (parvo–interblob) stream, dominated by parvocellular LGN inputs, includes the interblobs of V1 and the interstripes of V2. The P–B (parvo–blob) stream includes the blobs of V1 and the thin stripes of V2. It receives indirect inputs from the parvocellular LGN and direct inputs from 'interlaminar' and 'S-layer' neurons of the LGN, at least in the squirrel monkey[46–48]. Both the P–I and P–B streams project heavily to area V4[42,44], and there is anatomical[49] and physiological evidence[50] suggesting that the streams remain distinct within V4. The outputs of these streams project most heavily via V4 to subdivisions of inferotemporal cortex[6].

There are several types of cross-connection between streams. Explicitly noted in Fig. 3 are examples of divergence of outputs (from V3 to both V4 and MT; from V4 to both parietal and inferotemporal cortex[51]), as well as convergence of inputs (a variable projection to MT from thin stripes as well as thick stripes of V2[42]), and lateral connections (between layer 4B and superficial layers in V1[35], between thin stripes and thick stripes in V2[39] and between V4 and MT[6]).

In squirrel monkeys, the output from V2 to MT apparently arises primarily from CO thin stripes[52], which in the macaque contribute only a small and variable projection to MT[42]. This is surprising insofar as the organization of connections from V1 to V2 appears to be similar in the two species[39]. Since the pattern of connections among higher cortical areas is poorly understood in squirrel monkeys, the functional significance of these species variations is unclear.

Physiology

Major physiological differences between processing streams are evident in the retina and LGN, in conjunction with the pronounced anatomical differentiation there. In particular, magnocellular neurons are notable for their high contrast sensitivity, transient responses, and lack of overt wavelength selectivity; parvocellular neurons differ in having lower contrast sensitivity, sustained responses, and pronounced wavelength selectivity[53,54]. Within visual cortex, many additional receptive field properties are generated that involve selectivity for the feature-based sensory cues noted in Figs 1 and 2. The prevalence of different selectivities in each area and compartment is portrayed schematically by the different icons in Fig. 3 and more quantitatively in Table I (see table legend for references). These include selectivity for stimulus direction (pointing hand), contour orientation (angle icons), wavelength (rainbow icons), and binocular disparity (spectacles).

It is evident from this figure and from the summary data provided in Table I that the overall distribution of receptive field properties bears a systematic relationship to the three major anatomical streams (P–B, P–I, and M). For example, wavelength selectivity is prevalent in the P–B stream, whereas direction selectivity is most common in the M stream. However, rather than a one cue:one stream allocation, each type of selectivity occurs in more than one stream, and two of the streams are associated with multiple types of selectivity. In a general sense, the divergence of connections, resulting in multiple, pathways and redundant cue selectivities, as well as the subsequent convergence of pathways, is reminiscent of the key organizational features of Fig. 2. Based on the sensory cues represented within each stream, and the known specializations of inferotemporal and parietal cortex, we can now begin to consider which computational strategies the different streams are likely to support.

The P–B stream

The P–B stream is the simplest to discuss, as it is mainly associated with a high incidence of wavelength selectivity typically combined with a preference for low spatial frequency stimuli[1,39,42,62,63]. Other types of selectivity, as measured with current techniques, have been reported to be low or absent. Referring to Fig. 2 (blue lines), we see that the selective representation of spectral cues suggests a natural link between the P–B stream and the computational strategy for inferring hue from spectral (and luminance) contrast cues, as has been suggested by others[1,3,10,38,39]. There is no direct evidence linking this stream to other aspects of color perception, including saturation and brightness, or with the perception of luminance or spectral cue-based textures. However, blobs and thin stripes are prominent in bushbabies and owl monkeys, both nocturnal primates with poor color vision, which strongly suggests that the P–B stream is involved in more than just hue discrimination[34,64].

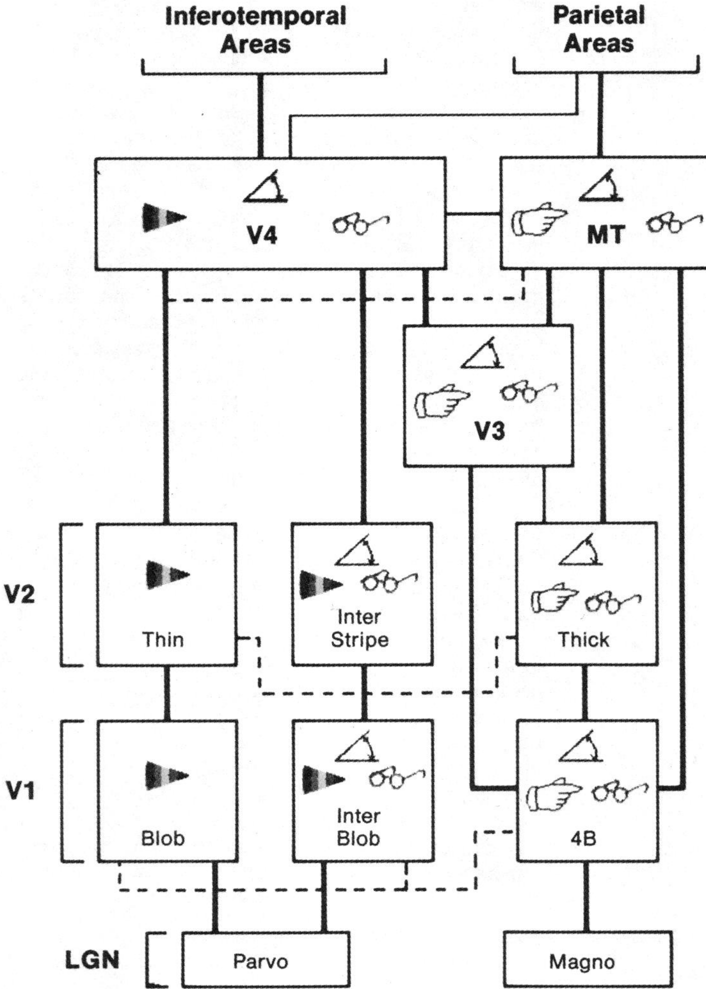

Fig. 3. *Schematic diagram of anatomical connections and neuronal selectivities of early visual areas in the macaque monkey. LGN = lateral geniculate nucleus (parvocellular and magnocellular divisions). Divisions of V1 and V2: blob = cytochrome oxidase blob regions; interblob = cytochrome oxidase–poor regions surrounding the blobs; 4B = lamina 4B; thin = thin (narrow) cytochrome oxidase strips; interstripe = cytochrome oxidase–poor regions between the thin and thick strips; thick = thick (wide) cytochrome oxidase strips; V3 = visual area 3; V4 = visual area(s) 4; MT = middle temporal area. Areas V2, V3, V4, MT have connections to other areas not explicitly represented here. Area V3 may also receive projections from V2 interstripes or thin stripes[79]. Heavy lines indicate robust primary connections, and thin lines indicate weaker, more variable connections. Dotted lines represent observed connections that require additional verification.* **Icons**: *rainbow = tuned and/or opponent wavelength selectivity (incidence at least 40%); angle symbol = orientation selectivity (incidence at least 20%); spectacles = binocular disparity selectivity and/or strong binocular interactions (V2) (incidence at least 20%); pointing hand = direction of motion selectivity (incidence at least 20%).*

The P–I stream

Physiological properties of the P–I stream overlap those of the M stream in selectivity for orientation and disparity, but wavelength selectivity is more prevalent and direction selectivity less so (though not entirely absent). Many individual cells in V1, including some specifically in the interblob portions, show joint selectivity for multiple cues such as orientation and wavelength[47,59,65,66]. Whether this is also true of V2 interstripes is less clear, since there are discrepancies in the reported incidence of any type of wavelength selectivity in the interstripes[1,42].

The P–I stream is a major source of orientation and probably also disparity information reaching inferotemporal cortex (by way of V4) from the high-spatial resolution parvocellular neurons of the retina. Referring again to Fig. 2 (green and red lines), contour-orientation and disparity cues can contribute to a variety of attributes. Since lesion studies have implicated inferotemporal cortex in shape and pattern recognition[5,11], this stream is likely to be involved in strategies deriving 3-D shape from luminance contours and perhaps from stereoscopic cues as well. The P–I stream might also provide texture information for use in other object recognition processes associated with inferotemporal cortex. It is less clear whether the P–I stream is involved in other computational strategies, such as the perception of distance from stereo cues and orientation (perspective) cues, the outputs of which should presumably be directed mainly to parietal cortex because of its involvement in the analysis of spatial relationships (see below).

It is intriguing to speculate on the possible significance of wavelength selective cells in the P–I pathway, particularly since many such cells are known to be concurrently orientation selective. We suggest that the activity of these cells may involve the operation of spectral contrast as a concealed cue, rather than as a direct cue (see above). Consider, for example, the information signalled by a cell selective for both long wavelengths and vertical orientations. Suppose that by virtue of its higher-order connections, this cell is associated only with the strategy for computing shape from contours. Its output, then, would be used to signal the presence of a contour at or near a vertical orientation. Although the cell would not contribute to color perception *per se*, its wavelength selectivity could be important in eliciting a vigorous response when the contour is based more on spectral differences (e.g. red–green) contrast, than on luminance differences. Many cells selective for both wavelength and orientation in V1 do indeed respond well to isoluminant color-contrast borders[65,66]. The possibility that different pathways subserve the direct and concealed contributions of spectral cues is supported by observations on achromatopsic patients, who are unable to perceive colors as a result of a bilateral cortical lesion. At least some of these individuals are able to indentify the shapes of 'hidden' figures in pseudoisochromatic (Ishihara) patterns despite their failure to perceive any color difference[9,67].

The M stream

The M stream has often been linked to motion analysis, in large part because of the high incidence of direction selectivity reported for area MT and also for layer 4B of V1[1,4,6,57,68]. Recent work has buttressed this hypothesis by showing that lesions of MT produced by ibotenic acid injections cause deficits in pursuit eye movements and in discriminating directions of motion[69]. In addition, some direction selective neurons in MT show a more complex form of motion analysis that closely parallels perception. When presented with stimuli consisting of two superimposed sinusoidal gratings that are drifting in different directions, these cells respond preferentially to an intermediate direction that corresponds to the 'pattern' direction perceived by human observers[70]. All these findings are commensurate with a role for MT in analysing the trajectories of objects. However, processing in the M stream may be more complex in two important ways. First, as already noted in Fig. 2 (orange lines), velocity cues can be used to support a variety of perceptual attributes in addition to the perception of object motion *per se*. In accordance with this, lesions of MT also cause deficits in discriminating the three-dimensional shape of moving dot patterns, suggesting an additional role for this stream in structure-from-motion computations[71]. The second complexity is the prevalence in the M stream of selectivity for other cues besides velocity, namely disparity and orientation. Such properties may be related to strategies for inferring 3-D trajectories[14,68], but they also suggest a plausible role for the M stream in other tasks (Fig. 2, red and green lines). One such candidate is the estimation of relative distances through a number of different strategies, including contour perspective, stereoscopic depth, and motion parallax.

Since numerous strategies, especially those based on velocity cues, may be associated predominantly with area MT and the M stream, it is interesting to consider the distribution of their various outputs with regard to cortical areas concerned with the analysis of spatial relationships versus object recognition. For example, it seems appropriate that the M stream projects heavily into the parietal lobe, so that information about object trajectories and distances can

TABLE I. Neuronal selectivities of visual areas in the macaque[a]

P–B stream		P–I stream		M stream
	V4			**MT**
	WVL 50			WVL 0
	DIR 5		**V3**	DIR 85
	ORI 50		WVL 15	ORI 75
	DIS 40		DIR 40	DIS 70
			ORI 70	
			DIS 40	
V2 thin		**V2 inter**		**V2 thick**
WVL 85		WVL 65(−)		WVL 15
DIR 5		DIR 0		DIR 20
ORI 20(−)		ORI 20		ORI 50
DIS 30(−)		DIS 20		DIS 70
	V1			
V1 blob	**Blob+inter**	**V1 inter**		**V1 4B**
WVL 65	WVL 45	WVL 40		WVL 10
DIR−	DIR 10	DIR −		DIR 50
ORI−	ORI 70	ORI++		ORI 85
DIS?	DIS++	DIS++		DIS+

[a]Numbers indicate percentages of cells selective for wavelength (WVL), direction of motion (DIR), orientation (ORI), or disparity (or having strong binocular interactions) (DIS). P–B = parvo–blob; P–I = parvo–interblob; M stream = magnocellular-dominated streams. Qualitative estimates of selectivity: little or none (−), moderate incidence (+), high incidence (++), not tested (?). Estimates in parentheses indicate notable discrepancies between quantitative and qualitative measurements. Many early studies of V1 did not distinguish between blob and inter-blob regions, so data from those studies are presented under 'V1 Blob+inter'. Values are best estimates compiled from a variety of studies that did not always provide similar percentages for the same regions. Fig. 3 is a schematic attempt to reconcile these differences to the best of our knowledge. Interested readers should consult Refs 41, 45, 55 for V4, V3, and MT; Refs 1, 42, 44 and 56 for V2; and Refs 39, 57–61 for V1.

subserve mechanisms concerned with spatial relationships (and changes in them). In contrast, 3-D shape information presumably should converge in the temporal lobe for use in object recognition. To the extent that the strategy of structure-from-motion is part of the M stream, its outputs would then need to be distributed to temporal as well as parietal areas. This could occur via the pathway between MT and V4 or via other possible routes. However, there is no direct evidence bearing on this hypothesis, and it remains a reasonable alternative that both parietal and temporal lobes could be involved with shape analysis but associated with different computational strategies (e.g. structure-from-motion versus shape-from-contours).

Because neurons at various stages of the M stream generally lack substantial wavelength selectivity, it is tempting to presume that this stream is in effect 'color-blind'. However, there is evidence from recent neurophysiological and 2-deoxyglucose experiments that isoluminant spectral borders can be effective in driving many neurons of the M stream, including the magnocellular LGN layers[72], the thick stripes of V2[62], and area MT (Saito, H., pers. commun.). This is consistent with our earlier suggestion that spectral cues can contribute in a concealed fashion to certain aspects of motion perception.

Our discussion of the M stream has emphasized area MT because of the intensive scrutiny it has recently received, and because at least three parallel paths originating in layer 4B of V1 converge there. Though not evident in Fig. 3, each of these converging paths has its own distinctive characteristics. The thick stripes of V2, for example, have a lower incidence of direction selectivity than MT (20–25%, which is nonetheless higher than in the rest of V2), and are more distinctive for their disparity selectivity (including many 'binocular only' neurons)[1,42,56]. V3 has an intermediate incidence of direction selectivity (40%) and even a significant incidence of wavelength selectivity[41]. An open question is why these areas all project to MT. An attractive hypothesis is that different computational strategies are associated with each input to MT. By converging there, they may cooperate to (1) establish cue-invariant representations of trajectory[73] and distance, and (2) enhance the accuracy of motion perception compared to that attainable using only a single computational strategy.

Interactions among streams

Though we have stressed the concurrent nature of processing in these three streams, it is important to recognize that they may interact significantly. For example, a stationary isoluminant red square on a green background will appear to move along with an overlying pattern of drifting black dots[74]. One interpretation is that the dots generate a motion percept via the M pathway that is linked to the color percept generated via the P–B pathway. Any of several cross-connections shown in Fig. 3 could form the basis of such an inter-stream link. In a similar vein, it has been suggested that the perceptual filling-in of contour-bounded regions with color and texture is a separate process, computationally distinct from boundary segmentation[75]. Plausibly, this might reflect interactions between the P–B and P–I streams or even among all three streams, since boundaries and textures can be derived from a variety of cues.

For all the complexities brought forth in this article, we have nonetheless presented an oversimplified view of several potentially significant aspects of cortical organization. First, the compartments within V1 and V2 (blobs and stripes) have been described as though they were entirely discrete, whereas their borders may in reality be genuinely fuzzy. Second, although we have emphasized the anatomical and physiological characteristics in common within each area and compartment, each one is inhomogeneous in ways that may prove to be very significant. Third, the physiological properties of cells were treated as though a given type of selectivity is either present or absent, e.g. that a cell either is or is not orientation selective. In reality, such properties often are distributed along a continuum, from highly selective to non-selective. High selectivity at least indicates that reliable information about a particular cue is available, but it does not reveal the way in which the information is actually used. Finally, there is no fundamental reason that any of the particular computational strategies listed in Fig. 2 must be restricted to a single neural pathway. Psychophysical evidence, for example, indicates that the perception of motion involves two underlying processes (short range and long range) each having different characteristics[76], and perhaps involving different pathways or different stages of processing.

Concluding remarks

Through the conceptual framework and analysis presented here, we have attempted to integrate and reconcile several different notions about concurrent processing in primate visual cortex. We have emphasized the manifold relationships between sensory cues and perceived attributes, and we have suggested that the connectional patterns and physiological specializations of cortical pathways are likely to reflect the complexity of those relationships. In the face of such complexity, it would serve accuracy and clarity if hypotheses about the functional contributions of particular streams were framed in terms of specific computational strategies that link a particular cue with a particular attribute. Of the 15 specific computational strategies identified in Fig. 2 (which itself is far from an exhaustive listing), only a few can at present be strongly linked to a particular processing stream – a notable example being the proposed involvement of the P–B stream in mediating color perception from spectral contrast cues. The prospects for obtaining a more thorough charting of these relationships are good, particularly in view of recent refinements in techniques for chemically lesioning restricted cortical regions[69] or restricted types of neurons[77,78]. However, one should not anticipate that the typical outcome will be a simple one-to-one relationship between a particular stream and a particular computational strategy. Rather, it seems likely that some strategies will be handled in parallel by more than one stream or will involve significant crossover between streams.

As our ability to understand and model neural function grows, it will become increasingly important to deal with the detailed subtleties and heterogeneous characteristics of cells at each processing stage. This should not be a disconcerting prospect, however, for

Acknowledgements
We thank many of our colleagues for valuable discussions and criticisms of the manuscript. Work in this laboratory was supported by NIH grant EY 02091, ONR contract N00014-85K-0068, the Del Webb Foundation, and by NIH training grant T32NS07251-01 to E.A.D.

the mechanisms underlying the extraordinary flexibility and well-intergrated capacities of the visual system must surely operate under a richly complex set of rules.

Selected references

1 Hubel, D. H. and Livingstone, M. S. (1987) *J. Neurosci.* 7, 3378–3415
2 Lennie, P. (1980) *Vision Res.* 20, 561–594
3 Livingstone, M. S. and Hubel, D. H. (1987) *J. Neurosci.* 7, 3416–3468
4 Maunsell, J. H. R. and Newsome, W. T. (1987) *Annu. Rev. Neurosci.* 10, 363–401
4 Ungerleider, L. G. and Mishkin, M. (1982) in *Analysis of Visual Behavior* (Ingle, D. J., Goodale, M. A. and Mansfield, R. J. W., eds), pp. 549–586, MIT Press
6 Van Essen, D. C. and Maunsell, J. H. R. (1983) *Trends Neurosci.* 6, 370–375
7 Zihl, J., Von Cramon, D. and Mai, N. (1983) *Brain* 106, 313–340
8 Damasio, A., Yamada, T., Damasio, H., Corbett, J. and McKee, J. (1980) *Neurology* 30, 1064–1071
9 Pearlman, A. L., Birch, J. and Meadows, J. C. (1979) *Ann. Neurol.* 5, 253–261
10 Zeki, S. (1980) *Nature* 284, 412–418
11 Mishkin, M., Ungerleider, L. G. and Macko, K. A. (1983) *Trends Neurosci.* 6, 414–417
12 Ungerleider, L. G. and Desimone, R. (1986) *J. Comp. Neurol.* 248, 190–222
13 Marr, D. (1982) *Vision* W. H. Freeman
14 Gorea, A. and Papathomas, T. V. (1987) AT&T Bell Laboratories Technical Memorandum 11223–87TM
15 Julesz, B. (1971) *Foundations of Cyclopean Perception*, University of Chicago Press
16 Anstis, S. and Cavanagh, P. (1983) in *Colour Vision*, (Mollon, J. D. and Sharpe, L. T., eds), pp. 155–166, Academic Press
17 Lu, C. and Fender, D. H. (1972) *Invest. Ophthalmol. Visual Sci.* 11, 482–489
18 Hurlbert, A. (1986) *J. Opt. Soc. Am.* 3, 1684–1693
19 Land, E. H. (1983) *Proc. Natl Acad. Sci. USA* 80, 5163–5169
20 Julesz, B. (1984) *Trends Neurosci.* 7, 41–45
21 Julesz, B. and Bergen, J. R. (1983) *Bell Sys. Tech. J.* 62, 1619–1645
22 Ikeuchi, K. and Horn, B. K. P. (1981) *Artif. Intell.* 17, 141–184
23 Lehky, S. R. and Sejnowski, T. J. (1987) *Soc. Neurosci. Abstr.* 13, 1451
24 Ullman, S. (1983) in *Human and Machine Vision* (Beck, J., Hope, B. and Rosenfeld, A., eds), pp. 459–480, Academic Press
25 Poggio, G. and Poggio, T. (1984) *Annu. Rev. Neurosci.* 7, 379–412
26 Barrow, H. G. and Tenenbaum, J. M. (1981) *Artif. Intell.* 17, 75–116
27 Stevens, K. A. (1981) *Artif. Intell.* 17, 47–74
28 Hildreth, E. C. and Koch, C. (1987) *Annu. Rev. Neurosci.* 10, 477–533
29 Regan, D. and Beverly, K. I. (1979) *Vision Res.* 19, 1331–1342
30 Nothdurft, H. C. (1985) *Perception* 14, 527–537
31 Poggio, T., Torre, V. and Koch, C. (1985) *Nature* 317, 314–319
32 Poggio, T. (1985) Working Paper No. 285, Artificial Intelligence Lab, MIT
33 Perry, V. H., Oehler, R. and Cowey, A. (1984) *Neuroscience* 12, 1101–1123
34 Allman, J. (1987) in *Neurobiology of Neocortex* (Dahlem Konferenzen), John Wiley & Sons (in press)
35 Blasdel, G. G., Lund, J. S. and Fitzpatrick, D. (1985) *J. Neurosci.* 5, 3350–3369
36 Carroll, E. W. and Wong-Riley, M. (1984) *J. Comp. Neurol.* 222, 1–17
37 Hendrickson, A. E. (1985) *Trends Neurosci.* 8, 406–410
38 Horton, J. C. (1984) *Philos, Trans. R. Soc. London Ser. B* 304, 199–253
39 Livingstone, M. S. and Hubel, D. H. (1984) *J. Neurosci.* 4, 309–356
40 Tootell, R. B. H., Silverman, M. S., DeValois, R. L. and Jacobs, G. H. (1983) *Science* 220, 737–739
41 Fellemen, D. F. and Van Essen, D. C. (1987) *J. Neurophysiol.* 57, 889–920
42 DeYoe, E. A. and Van Essen, D. C. (1985) *Nature* 317, 58–61
43 Livingstone, M. S. and Hubel, D. H. (1987) *J. Neurosci.* 7, 3371–3377
44 Shipp, S. and Zeki, S. (1985) *Nature* 315, 322–324
45 Maunsell, J. H. R. and Van Essen, D. C. (1983) *J. Neurosci.* 3, 2563–2586
46 Fitzpatrick, D., Itoh, K. and Diamond, I. T. (1983) *J. Neurosci.* 3, 637–702
47 Michael, C. R. (1987) *Soc. Neurosci. Abstr.* 13, 2
48 Weber, J. T., Huerta, M. F., Kaas, J. H. and Harting, J. K. (1983) *J. Comp. Neurol.* 213, 135–145
49 DeYoe, E. A., Felleman, D. J., Knierim, J. J., Olavarria, J. and Van Essen, D. C. *Invest. Ophthalmol. Visual Sci.* (Suppl.) (in press)
50 Zeki, S. (1983) *Proc. R. Soc. London Ser. B* 217, 449–470
51 Felleman, D. J. and Van Essen, D. C. (1983) *Soc. Neurosci. Abstr.* 9, 153
52 Krubitzer, L. A. and Kaas, J. H. (1987) *Soc. Neurosci. Abstr.* 13, 3
53 Schiller, P. H. and Malpeli, J. G. (1978) *J. Neurophysiol.* 41, 788–796
54 Shapley, R., Kaplan, E. and Soodak, R. (1981) *Nature* 292, 543–545
55 Desimone, R. and Schein, S. J. (1987) *J. Neurophysiol.* 57, 835–868
56 Hubel, D. H. and Livingstone, M. S. (1985) *Nature* 315, 325–327
57 Dow, B. M. (1974) *J. Neurophysiol.* 37, 927–946
58 Gouras, P. (1974) *J. Physiol (London)* 238, 583–602
59 Michael, C. R. (1985) *Vision Res.* 25, 415–423
60 Poggio, G. F. (1984) in *Dynamic Aspects of Neocortical Function*, (Edelman, G., Cowan, W. M. and Gall, E., eds), pp. 613–635, John Wiley & Sons
61 Schiller, P. H., Finlay, B. L. and Volman, S. F. (1976) *J. Neurophysiol.* 39, 1320–1333
62 Tootell, R. B. H. and Hamilton, S. L. *J. Neurosci.* (in press)
63 Tootell, R. B. H., Silverman, M. S., Hamilton, S. L., Switkes, E. and DeValois, R. L. *J. Neurosci.* (in press)
64 Tootell, R. B., Hamilton, S. L. and Silverman, M. S. (1985) *J. Neurosci.* 5, 2786–2800
65 Gouras, P. and Kruger, J. (1979) *J. Neurophysiol.* 42, 850–860
66 Thorell, L. G., DeValois, R. L. and Albrecht, D. G. (1984) *Vision Res.* 24, 751–769
67 Mollon, J. D., Newcombe, F., Polden, P. G. and Ratcliff, G. (1979) in *Colour Vision Deficiencies* (Verriest, G., ed.), pp. 130–135, Adam Hilger
68 Albright, T. D. (1984) *J. Neurophysiol.* 52, 1106–1130
69 Newsome, W. T., Wurtz, R. H., Dursteler, M. R. and Mikami, A. (1985) *J. Neurosci.* 5, 825–840
70 Movshon, J. A., Adelson, E. H., Gizzi, M. S. and Newsome, W. T. (1985) in *Pattern Recognition Mechanisms*, (Chagas, C., Gattass, R. and Cross, C., eds), pp. 117–151, Springer-Verlag
71 Siegel, R. M. and Andersen, R. A. (1986) *Soc. Neurosci. Abstr.* 12, 1183
72 Hurlbert, A. C., Logothetis, N. K., Charles, E. R. and Schiller, P. H. (1987) *Soc. Neurosci. Abstr.* 13, 204
73 Albright, T. D. (1987) *Soc. Neurosci. Abstr.* 13, 1626
74 Ramachandran, V. S. (1987) *Nature* 328, 645–647
75 Grossberg, S. and Mingolla, E. (1985) *Psychol. Rev.* 92, 173–211
76 Braddick, O. J. (1974) *Vision Res.* 14, 519–527
77 Merrigan, W. H. and Eskin, T. A. (1986) *Vision Res.* 26, 1751–1761
78 Schiller, P. (1984) *Vision Res.* 24, 923–932
79 Felleman, D. J., DeYoe, E. A., Knierim, J. J., Olavarria, J. and Van Essen, D. C. *Invest. Ophthalmol. Vis. Sci.* (Suppl.) (in press)

5

P. H. Schiller and N. K. Logothetis

The color-opponent and broad-band channels of the primate visual system

1990. *Trends in Neurosciences* 13: 392–398

Peter H. Schiller and Nikos K. Logothetis are at the Department of Brain and Cognitive Sciences, Massachusetts Institute of Technology, Cambridge, MA 02139, USA.

Physiological, anatomical and psychophysical studies have identified several parallel channels of information processing in the primate visual system. Two of these, the color-opponent and the broad-band channels, originate in the retina and remain in part segregated through several higher cortical stations. To improve understanding of their function, recent studies have examined the visual capacities of monkeys following selective disruption of these channels. Color vision, fine- but not coarse-form vision and stereopsis are severely impaired in the absence of the color-opponent channel, whereas motion and flicker perception are impaired at high but not low temporal frequencies in the absence of the broad-band channel. The results suggest that the color-opponent channel extends the range of vision in the spatial and wavelength domains, and that the broad-band channel extends it in the temporal domain. Lesion studies also indicate that these channels must reach higher cortical centers through extrastriate regions other than just area V4 and the middle temporal area, and that the analysis performed by these two regions cannot be uniquely identified with specific visual capacities.

Physiological and anatomical studies have distinguished several distinct classes of retinal ganglion cells in the mammalian retina, each of which appears to be involved in the analysis of a different aspect of the visual scene[1]. Since the various ganglion cell classes carry out their analyses concurrently and show considerable specificity in their central connections, they are generally conceived of as parallel information-processing channels[2–5]. Clarifying the role of these channels in perception has become a central quest in vision research. During the past few years significant advances have been made in our understanding of two major channels in the primate, the color-opponent and broad-band channels. Here we consider the various hypotheses, the controversies and the evidence regarding their function.

Physiological characteristics

The characteristics of the color-opponent and broad-band channels were first delineated in single-cell recording experiments[6–10]. The retinal ganglion cells of both classes have a concentric, antagonistic center–surround organization as depicted in Fig. 1. The receptive field center region of most color-opponent cells is believed to receive input from only one cone type, whereas the input to the center of each broad-band cell is from all three of the cone types found in Old World monkeys[6,8,9,11]; contrary to the earlier belief that the surround of the color-opponent cells obtains its input from a different set of cones than does the center (for example, center input from red cones and surround input from green cones), recent studies of horizontal cell connectivity suggest that the receptive field surround of both cell types may receive undifferentiated input from all cones[12,13]. The receptive field of the color-opponent cells is small, the cells respond in a sustained fashion to visual stimulation, and their axons have medium conduction velocity. By contrast, the broad-band cells have much larger receptive fields, are more sensitive to small changes in luminance, respond transiently, and have rapidly conducting axons[10,14]. Morphological studies have established that the shape and size of the dendritic arbors of the retinal ganglion cells, as viewed head-on in retinal whole mounts, correspond to the shape and size of their receptive field centers; color-opponent cells have small arbors as well as small, β-type cell bodies and the broad-band cells have large arbors and α-type cell bodies[15,17]. Figure 1 shows some of the basic differences between the two cell types.

Examination of the central connections of these two systems revealed that they project to different laminae of the lateral geniculate nucleus of the thalamus: the color-opponent cells, which comprise about 90% of the neurons of the geniculostriate system, terminate in the four parvocellular layers of the lateral geniculate nucleus; the broad-band cells on the other hand terminate in its two magnocellular layers[16–19]. Since the characteristics of these two systems are not really described adequately by the terms 'color-opponent' and 'broad-band', some investigators prefer to call them the P (for parvocellular) and M (for magnocellular) channels, terms that are not entirely satisfactory either since the mode of action of the channels is defined by retinal and not by lateral geniculate nucleus circuitry; therefore, we retain the original terms.

Based on the analysis of the receptive field properties of single cells at various levels of the visual system it was proposed that the color-opponent channel plays a central role in color vision and in the perception of high spatial frequency patterns[20], whereas the broad-band system, referred to by some investigators as the luminance channel, plays an important role in the perception of motion[20], in the perception of low-contrast stimuli and in night vision when only the rod receptors are active[21].

Psychophysical studies

In the attempt to obtain additional lines of evidence regarding the functions of these two systems, one of the more provocative ideas advanced recently is that their role in vision can be determined in psychophysical experiments in which information based on luminance contrast is eliminated and only differences in wavelength are available for contour detection. Under such 'isoluminant' conditions a number of perceptual functions are compromised[22,23], a loss ascribed to the presumed unresponsiveness of the broad-band system in the absence of luminance cues[20]. The results of isoluminance experiments led to the suggestion that the 'color-blind' broad-band system mediates motion perception, the ability to determine the spatiotemporal relationship of objects and depth perception, while the color-opponent system mediates color and form perception[3,20]. Perceptions produced by the broad-band system might therefore be caricatured as three-dimensional black and white movies and those of the color-opponent system as two-dimensional color films of limited contrast.

The rationale of the isoluminance experiments, however, has been challenged on several grounds. (1) Visual functions that are believed to be processed by the color-opponent system, such as fine-pattern and texture perception, are also compromised at isoluminance[24]. (2) The cells of the broad-band system are not rendered silent by isoluminant conditions at the level of the retina[25], the lateral geniculate nucleus[24,26] or the middle temporal visual area[27], which receives a heavy projection from the broad-band system[28,29]. (3) The color-opponent system responds selectively to both luminance and color contrast; thus in the absence of luminance information the discharge characteristics of this system are also altered; it is noteworthy that the 15–20% of the parvocellular lateral geniculate nucleus cells that lack sharply defined color-opponency become especially unresponsive under isoluminant conditions[24,26]. (4) It has been shown that color information can be effectively used by the visual system in the absence of luminance cues for the perception of form, motion and depth[24,30–34]. (5) Some of the perceptual capacities compromised by isoluminance are also compromised by low levels of achromatic contrast. For example, the illusory slowing down of red/green drifting sinusoidal gratings under isoluminant conditions, attributed to the inactivation of the broad-band system[3,20], also occurs with low-contrast achromatic luminance gratings[35,36] to which the broad-band system is believed to be considerably more responsive than the color-opponent system.

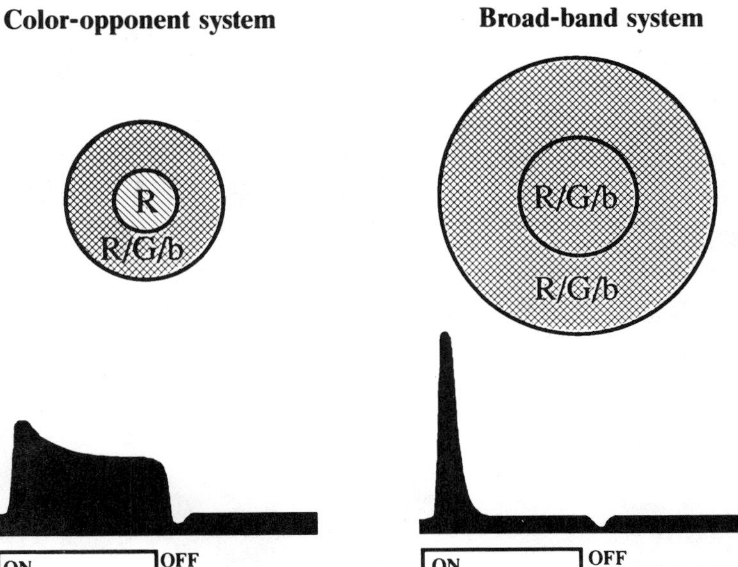

Fig. 1. *The major differences in the characteristics of the color-opponent and broad-band cells of the trichromatic primate. The color-opponent cells have small receptive fields and their center typically receives input from just one cone type; the surround input, according to recent work, may comprise input from all cone types. The color-opponent cells respond in a sustained fashion to light stimulation confined to the center of their receptive fields as indicated in the schematized cumulative-response histogram. The broad-band cells have large receptive fields; they receive undifferentiated input from all cone types in both the center and the surround regions of their receptive fields. The light-evoked responses of the broad-band cells are transient. R, G and b indicate different cone type inputs. The blue cones are indicated with a lower case 'b' because only one out of ten cones is blue in the monkey retina.*

Lesion experiments

As a result of these problems with isoluminance experiments, and the limitations inherent in single-cell recording studies, it became desirable to turn to different, perhaps more direct methods to assess the roles of the color-opponent and broad-band channels in vision. To do so, investigators have recently devised ways to block selectively each of the channels in rhesus monkeys, whose visual system is remarkably similar to that of humans, and then to test their visual functions. Two methods are at present in use. The first, introduced by William Merigan[37], attempts to block the color-opponent system selectively by repeated systemic administrations of acrylamide, a toxin that has been shown to destroy visual neurons with fine axons, thereby acting preferentially on the color-opponent retinal ganglion cells. The second approach, used in our experiments[38,39], involves the creation of small lesions in either the parvocellular or the magnocellular portions of the lateral geniculate nucleus by first taking electrophysiological recordings to establish the layers and visual field representations to be lesioned, and subsequently injecting minute quantities of the neurotoxin ibotenic acid[38,39]. To confine the stimuli to the lesioned or intact portions of the visual field, each trial is initiated by having the animal fixate a central fixation spot; this is verified by eye-movement recordings. A number of different visual capacities is assessed, using either a detection or a discrimination paradigm, which include the perception of color, form, brightness, depth, flicker and motion. In the detection paradigm, following fixation, a single target appears in one of several locations and the animal has to make a saccadic eye movement to it to be rewarded with a drop of apple juice. In the discrimination paradigm, several stimuli appear, one of which is different from the others (in either color, form, brightness, or depth); choice is indicated by making a direct saccade to the stimulus that is different. Figure 2 provides examples for some of the tasks used in these experiments. Since the rhesus monkeys used in this work willingly perform several thousand trials per day and readily master all of the visual tasks, reliable psychophysical functions can be generated.

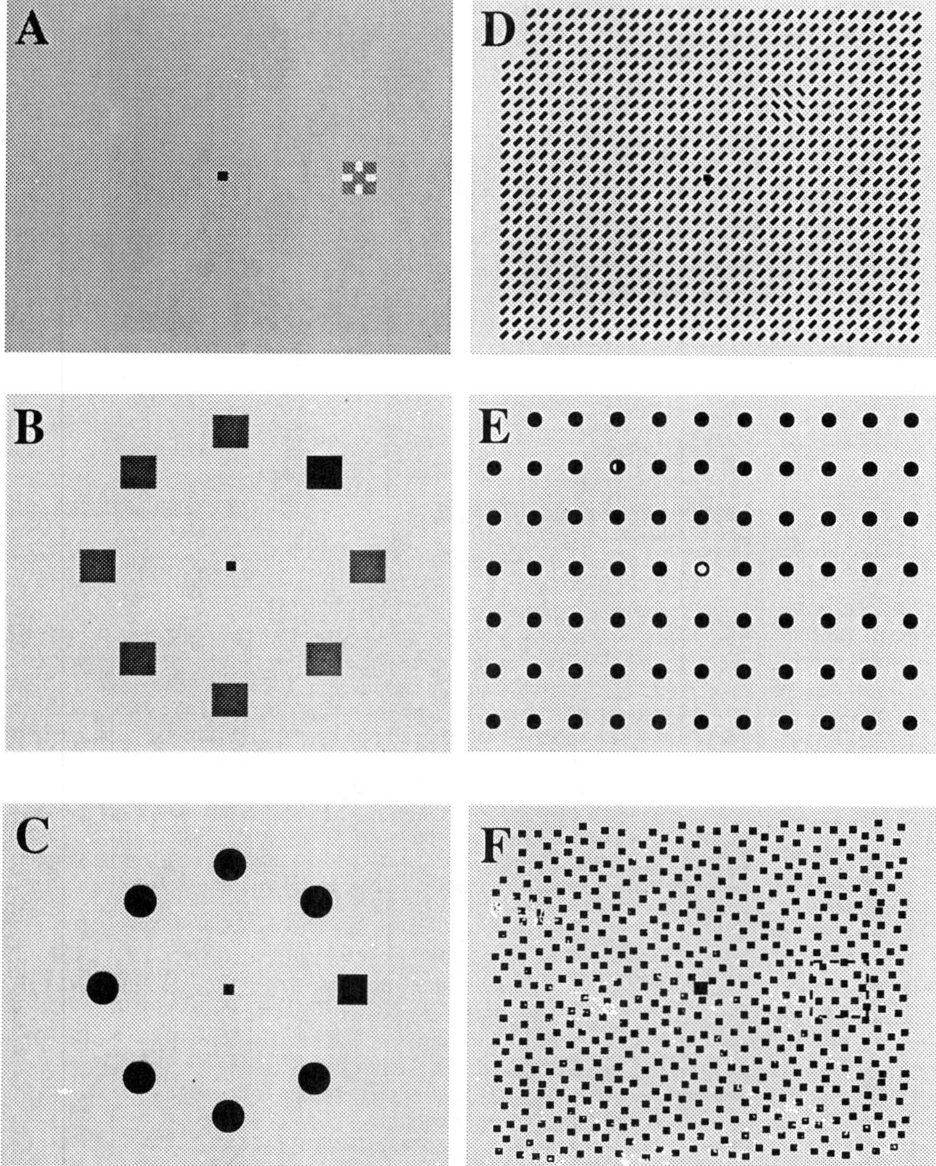

Fig. 2. *Examples of the tasks used.* **(A)** *Detection task for contrast sensitivity: the position of the checkerboard target, its spatial frequency and contrast are varied randomly from trial to trial. Each trial begins with the appearance of the central fixation spot. After the animal has directed its gaze to this spot as assessed by eye-movement recordings and a computer system, the checkerboard target appears. To be rewarded a saccade has to be made to it.* **(B)** *Brightness discrimination: one of the eight stimuli, the target, is brighter or darker than the others; the position of the target stimulus and its luminance are varied randomly by trial. To be rewarded the animal has to make a direct saccade to the target.* **(C)** *Shape discrimination: the target is the square.* **(D)** *Texture discrimination: the target is the square area within which the diagonal lines have the opposite slant.* **(E)** *Flicker perception: an array of LEDs is shown. Following fixation of the central LED, one of the LEDs flickers as indicated by the half-filled circle. This is the target to which the animal has to make a saccade to be rewarded.* **(F)** *Motion detection: in a small region of this dot array, as indicated by the hatched square area, the dots are set in motion. To be rewarded the animal has to make a saccade to this location. Not shown in this figure are pattern-discrimination and stereo-detection tasks. For pattern discrimination high-contrast checkerboard patterns were used and the target stimulus had a different spatial frequency to the seven other stimuli. They were presented in a manner similar to that shown in (B) and (C). For stereopsis, random-dot stereograms were used, and a small square appeared in depth by having the dots within this area displaced horizontally for one of the two stereograms; the stereograms were viewed through a stereoscope.*

The major results obtained in lesion experiments[37–40] are outlined in Table I. The first two columns show the magnitude of deficits following lesions of the parvocellular and magnocellular layers of the lateral geniculate nucleus. These are detailed below.

Color vision. When color vision is tested by having monkeys discriminate stimuli only on the basis of color differences, parvocellular lesions are shown to lead to severe deficits: animals can no longer discern color differences at all. However, when a single, low spatial frequency color stimulus appears on an isoluminant background, they have no difficulty detecting it. The various color stimuli in these experiments are set to be isoluminant with each other, or their relative luminances are randomly varied to eliminate any brightness information. The isoluminant point is determined in separate experiments in which the luminance ratio of two colors is systematically varied in various discrimination tasks to derive the ratio at which perception is maximally affected. These experiments establish then that parvocellular lesions abolish the capacity for discriminating color differences (to ascribe color values to various wavelength compositions) but do not interfere with the capacity to 'see' stimuli on the basis of wavelength differences. Magnocellular lesions have no effect on color discrimination.

Form vision. At high spatial frequencies all three kinds of form vision studied, pattern, texture and shape (see Fig. 2C and D for examples of shape and texture discrimination), are severely compromised following lesions of the parvocellular layers of the lateral geniculate nucleus. The deficits are considerably less pronounced with low spatial frequency stimuli. Magnocellular lesions have no discernible effect on any of these tasks.

Brightness perception. Neither lesion causes deficits in the detection or the discrimination of low spatial frequency stimuli on the basis of luminance differences alone (see Fig. 2B for brightness discrimination task). This is true for both photopic vision subserved by the cones and for scotopic or night vision, subserved by the rods. Thus it appears that luminance information at low spatial frequencies can be processed by both the color-opponent and the broad-band systems. These findings also suggest that the broad-band channel cannot be conceived of as a unique luminance channel.

Luminance contrast sensitivity. One of the most efficient and informative ways to describe spatial visual capacity is to generate contrast sensitivity functions. These can be obtained by systematically assessing visual sensitivity for various contrasts and spatial frequencies. This is typically done using sinusoidal gratings, but similar results can also be obtained with checkerboard patterns of various spatial frequencies and contrasts (see Fig. 2A for one example). In Fig. 3 an array of such checkerboard patterns is shown on the left and sinusoidal gratings on the right; for each figure, contrast is decreased uniformly on the vertical axis from the bottom up and spatial frequency is increased from left to right. By fixating above or below the figure the contrast sensitivity function of the reader can readily be observed. At high spatial frequencies only the highest contrasts are visible. Perception is best at intermediate frequencies. William Merigan has studied luminance contrast sensitivity extensively using sinusoidal gratings following parvocellular and magnocellular lesions[37,40]. We obtained quite similar results with checkerboard patterns. What these experiments show is that parvocellular lesions cause pronounced deficits in contrast sensitivity at high spatial frequencies, but produce only small deficits at low spatial frequencies. Surprisingly, there are only minor or no deficits in contrast sensitivity following magnocellular lesions in spite of the fact that the cells of the broad-band system have been shown to be more sensitive than those of the parvocellular system[14,26,41].

Stereoscopic depth perception. Studying stereopsis with random-dot stereograms of various spatial frequencies and degrees of disparity shows that lesions to the parvocellular layers of the lateral geniculate nucleus produce major deficits in fine but not coarse static stereopsis; no deficits are obtained with magnocellular lesions. These findings dispute the claim that stereopsis is processed exclusively by the broad-band system as has been proposed by Livingstone and Hubel[3,20].

Motion and flicker perception. The major deficits that arise following lesions of the broad-band system fall into the temporal domain. Most dramatically affected is the perception of flicker and motion, especially at low contrasts (see Fig. 2E and F for testing procedures). Magnocellular lesions produce significant deficits in the detection of both monochromatic and heterochromatic flicker at high frequencies indicating that the temporal limits of flicker perception are set by the broad-band system. These and the color vision results fit with the observation that in the course of increasing red/green flicker rate, human observers experience three perceptions: at low rates the stimulus is seen as alternating between red and green; as the rate is increased, the colors fuse and a yellow flickering stimulus is perceived; at high rates the sensation of flicker is lost and a steadily illuminated yellow stimulus is seen. The presumption is that the color sensations are mediated by the color-opponent system and rapid flicker by the broad-band system. It should be emphasized that while deficits in motion and flicker following magnocellular lesions are pronounced, neither of these capacities is eliminated; at low temporal frequencies and high contrasts the deficits are small, suggesting that the color-opponent system can make a significant contribution to the temporal aspects of perception[37–40].

The results of studies using lesions to the lateral geniculate nucleus lead to the conclusion that the color-opponent system is crucial for color discrimination and is essential for form and depth perception at high but not at low spatial frequencies. The broad-band system plays an important role in motion and flicker perception; however, the color-opponent system can process these capacities at high contrasts and low temporal rates. Both systems can process brightness, shape and stereo information at low spatial frequencies. Thus, while some of the perceptual losses caused by lesions to the

TABLE I. Deficit magnitude following PLGN, MLGN, V4 and MT lesions

Function		PLGN	MLGN	V4	MT
Color vision		Severe	–	Moderate	–
Texture perception		Severe	–	Mild	–
Pattern perception		Severe	–	Moderate	–
Shape perception:	fine	Severe	–	Mild	–
	coarse	Mild	–	–	–
Brightness perception		–	–	–	–
Coarse scotopic vision		–	–	–	–
Contrast sensitivity:	fine	Severe	–	Mild	Mild
	coarse	Mild	–	–	Mild
Stereopsis:	fine	Severe	–	–	–
	coarse	Pronounced	–	–	–
Motion perception		–	Moderate	–	Moderate
Flicker perception		–	Severe	–	Pronounced

Abbreviations: MLGN, magnocellular layer of the lateral geniculate nucleus; MT, middle temporal area; PLGN, parvocellular layer of the lateral geniculate nucleus. Dashes indicate no deficit.

lateral geniculate nucleus are profound, it is important to note that except for color discrimination, the deficits for the various visual capacities are not all or none but are graded: at low spatial and temporal frequencies, high contrasts and low disparities, perceptual losses are generally small. Deficits become pronounced as spatial and temporal frequencies are increased and/or contrast and disparities are decreased. It should also be noted that in no case did a deficit in any one of the visual functions we studied occur both after a parvocellular and after a magnocellular lesion, i.e. the deficits incurred by these two types of lesions seem mutually exclusive (see Table I). This suggests that no visual capacity studied in our experiments is produced by integrative action between the two systems.

Central connections

One of the most exciting discoveries relating to the organization of the visual system made during the past few decades has been the discrimination of numerous visual areas in the occipital, parietal and temporal lobes[42]. There has been extensive speculation as to why there are so many areas, and one of the central claims that has emerged is that each of them is involved in the analysis of a different aspect of visual perception[43,44]. Thus, it has been argued that area V4 is involved in color vision and that the middle temporal area (MT) is involved in motion perception. It has also been found that the color-opponent and broad-band systems show considerable specificity in their projection to the various extrastriate areas[28,29,45,46]. One appealing hypothesis, which integrates these and related findings, is that there are two major information-processing streams in the visual cortex, one, dominated by the color-opponent channel, that projects from the striate cortex to the temporal lobe via area V4 and the other, dominated by the broad-band channel, that projects to the parietal lobe via area MT[47].

There are a number of problems with these ideas. (1) In V1 there is evidence of partial convergence between the color-opponent and broad-band systems[45,48–50]; thus, it has been shown that a significant number of single cells receive convergent input from the two systems[49] and that both the cytochrome oxidase-stained 'blob' regions and the 'interblob' regions receive projections from both channels[51]. (2) Several of the extrastriate areas are not homogeneous. Instead, they show a modular organization[2,4]. For example, in area V2, which lies adjacent to area V1, cytochrome oxidase staining disclosed the existence of three kinds of regions that receive selective connections from the blob and interblob regions of V1 and hence had been thought to process different kinds of information. However, the receptive field properties of single cells in these regions do not appear to be quite as distinct from each other as would be expected on the basis of a strict segregation of function[52]. (3) Although there is strong evidence that the direction-specific cells of area MT are devoted to the analysis of various aspects of motion perception, current work on area V4 suggests that this area is far more complex than originally thought. In addition to specificity for color, many single cells in this area are orientation- and direction-selective[53], and studies in alert monkeys reveal that such factors as attention and stimulus relevance for the successful execution of a behavioral task can significantly modulate the responses of many cells[54–56]. (4) While there is compelling evidence to the effect that the input to area MT is dominated by the broad-band channel[57], area V4 appears to receive extensive projections from both systems (Maunsell, J. H. R., pers. commun.). (5) Extrastriate areas interconnect profusely. Thus area MT and parietal cortex have been shown to make reciprocal connections with the temporal lobe[4].

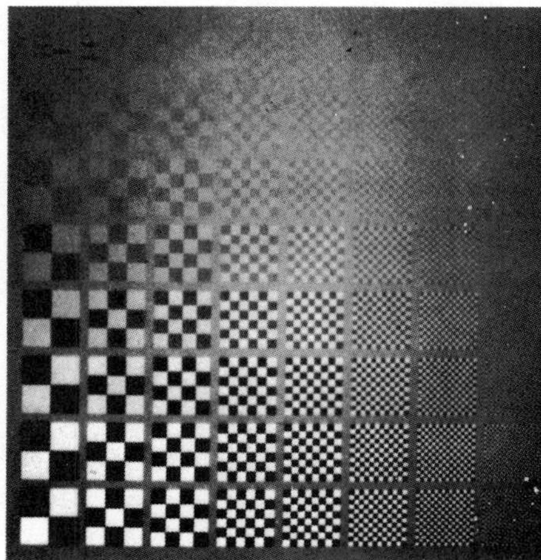

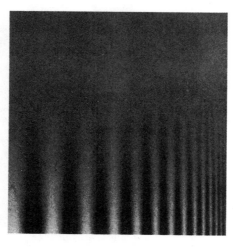

Fig. 3. *Stimulus configuration demonstrating visual sensitivity for various spatial frequencies. Checkerboard patterns are shown on the left and sinusoidal gratings on the right. Contrast is varied uniformly on the Y-axis and spatial frequency on the X-axis. By fixating above or below the figure or by moving it to a greater distance, it can be seen that perceptual abilities fall off notably at both high and low spatial frequencies with the sinusoidal gratings. The fall-off at low spatial frequencies is less evident with the checkerboard patterns because the low frequencies, due to the relatively well-defined edges, contain significant high spatial frequency components.*

Lesion studies also raise several questions about the idea that various extrastriate areas receive selective connections from the color-opponent and broad-band systems and play a unique role in analysing specific visual functions: area V4 lesions produce losses in both color and pattern vision as well as in the learning of new perceptual tasks[58–60]. The color deficits are much less pronounced than those obtained with lesions to the parvocellular layer of the lateral geniculate nucleus[59,60]. For example, following parvocellular lesions, monkeys cannot discriminate yellow from isoluminant red, blue or green. Following V4 lesions, however, they have no problem with this task. Deficits can be demonstrated, though, for subtle differences in hue; thus, difficulties occur when yellow has to be discriminated from orange-yellow or orange, but even this deficit declines with practice. Therefore, it must be that other cortical areas can contribute to color vision. Lesions of area MT produce deficits in motion and flicker perception and in visually guided pursuit eye movements[61,62]. Recovery has been reported over time. Lesions of the magnocellular layer of the lateral geniculate nucleus produce greater deficits and show less recovery[63]. Most notable in our experiments was the fact that neither lesions to area V4 nor to area MT produced deleterious effects on stereoscopic depth perception. This was the case not only for static but also for dynamic stereopsis. However, slight deficits in static stereopsis following V4 lesions have been reported by Cowey[64]. Summary comparisons for deficit magnitude for various visual capacities following parvocellular, magnocellular, V4 and MT lesions appear in Table I. The conclusions to be drawn from these comparisons are that (1) areas V4 and MT are not unique in processing color, form, motion and stereopsis, and (2) they are not the sole gateways to the temporal and parietal lobes for the color-opponent and broad-band systems as also indicated by recent anatomical and physiological studies[2,4]. These conclusions suggest that there must be other ways of passing the information to higher cortical regions, either through interactions between the two major pathways or through yet undiscovered regions and connections. The possibility remains that stereopsis can be processed by *either* channel independently. Studies using paired V4 and MT lesions, yet to be done, will test this alternative.

How do these considerations fit with data obtained from human clinical studies? It has been shown that following damage to areas tentatively associated with V4, deficits arise in the characterization of color stimuli[65,66] but not in color contrast sensitivity[66]; following damage to areas considered to include MT, deficits have been noted in motion perception[67]. These results support the idea that various brain regions in the occipital cortex have considerable functional specificity in spite of the fact that the input to them from the color-opponent and broad-band channels is not fully segregated. Such specificity is likely to be created, therefore, by intracortical circuitry. However, the inferences made from human data about the functions of V4 and MT must be tempered since the location of these areas in the human brain, as generally acknowledged, has not yet been pinpointed, and infarcts or other forms of brain damage are seldom if ever confined entirely to a single specific extrastriate region and typically involve damage not only to gray matter but also to underlying white matter[67]

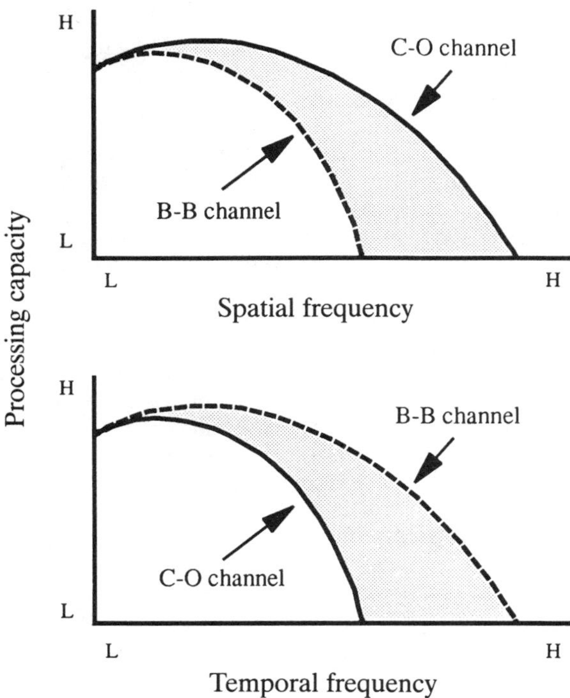

Fig. 4. *Schematic showing processing capacity for the color-opponent and broad-band channels along spatial and temporal frequency axes. In the spatial frequency domain, the ability of the broad-band system to process information falls off more rapidly with increasing spatial frequencies than does that of the color-opponent system. In the frequency domain the opposite is the case: the broad-band system can process information to higher temporal frequencies than the color-opponent system. Further insights into the functions of these two channels could be gained in psychophysical experiments by testing subjects within the shaded areas of the figure. The Y-axis shows information processing capacity where H stands for high and L for low. On the X-axis, L and H stand for low and high spatial or temporal frequencies.*

Evolutionary considerations

What general statement can be made about why the color-opponent and broad-band channels have evolved? In pondering this question it may be profitable to turn, as an analogy, to another system, the receptors of the retina, which were identified by Schultze[68] in 1866 to be dual in nature. He correctly hypothesized that the cones subserve day vision and the rods night vision. The hypothesis suggests that the evolution of rods and cones extended the range of vision in the domain of light intensity. In a similar vein, we propose that the evolution of the color-opponent and the broad-band channels also extended the range of vision, with the former extending it in the domain of wavelength and spatial frequency and the latter in the domain of temporal frequency as shown in Fig. 4. Why should there be more than one system? Probably because of conflicting requirements. Conflicting, because for high-resolution vision one needs small windows to the world, small receptive fields that is, that are available in relatively large numbers. One also needs cells that respond in a sustained fashion to optimize the extraction of static spatial information during each brief period of maintained gaze, the duration of which in diurnal primates is typically 200–500 ms followed by a rapid saccadic eye movement to another part of the visual scene to repeat the process. In addition, for color vision one needs spatially segregated input from different cone types. The small degree of convergence of receptors in this system and the sustained responses it gives, limit sensitivity and temporal resolution. High temporal frequency selectivity, and the concomitant sensitivity required for it, need large receptive fields with non-specific convergence of receptors and with transient responses. What is consequently given up in the broad-band system is the processing of color and of pattern at high spatial frequencies.

In summary, we propose that the color-opponent and broad-band channels form two separate but overlapping systems that extend visual capacities in the spatial, wavelength and temporal domains. Their segregation at higher cortical levels is only partial, and for the analysis of several visual capacities their signals are funneled.

Acknowledgements
We thank Eliot R. Charles and Kyoungmin Lee for their participation in the research reported here from our laboratory, which was supported in part by NIH grant EY00676.

Selected references

1 Schiller, P. H. (1986) *Vision Res.* 26, 1351–1386
2 DeYoe, E. A. and Van Essen, D. C. (1988) *Trends Neurosci.* 11, 219–226
3 Livingstone, M. S. and Hubel, D. H. (1988) *Science* 240, 740–749
4 Zeki, S. and Shipp, S. (1988) *Nature* 335, 311–317
5 Martin, K. A. C. (1988) *Trends Neurosci.* 11, 380–387
6 Wiesel, T. N. and Hubel, D. H. (1966) *J. Neurophysiol.* 29, 1115–1156
7 De Valois, R. L. and Jacobs, G. H. (1968) *Science* 162, 533–540
8 Gouras, P. (1968) *J. Physiol. (London)* 199, 533–547
9 De Monasterio, F. M. and Gouras, P. (1975) *J. Physiol. (London)* 251, 167–195
10 Schiller, P. H. and Malpeli, J. G. (1978) *J. Neurophysiol.* 41, 788–797
11 Derrington, A. M., Krauskopf, J. and Lennie, P. (1984) *J. Physiol. (London)* 357, 241–265
12 Roehrenbeck, J., Waessle, H. and Boycott, B. B. (1989) *Eur. J. Neurosci.* 1, 407–420
13 Waessle, H., Boycott, B. B. and Roehrenbeck, J. (1989) *Eur. J. Neurosci.* 1, 421–435
14 Shapley, R. M., Kaplan, E. and Soodak, R. (1985) *Nature* 292, 543–545
15 Boycott, B. B. and Waessle, H. (1974) *J. Physiol. (London)* 240, 397–419
16 Leventhal, A. G., Rodieck, R. W. and Dreher, B. (1981) *Science* 213, 1139–1142
17 Perry, V. H., Oehler, R. and Cowey, A. (1984) *Neuroscience* 12, 1101–1123
18 Dreher, B., Fukada, Y. and Rodieck, R. W. (1976) *J. Physiol. (London)* 258, 433–452
19 Schiller, P. H. and Malpeli, J. G. (1978) *J. Neurophysiol.* 41, 788–797
20 Livingstone, M. S. and Hubel, D. H. (1987) *J. Neurosci.* 7, 3416–3468
21 Purpura, K., Kaplan, E. and Shapley, R. M. (1988) *Proc. Natl Acad. Sci. USA* 85, 4534–4537
22 Lu, C. and Fender, D. H. (1972) *Invest. Ophthalmol.* 11, 482–490
23 Ramachandran, V. S. and Gregory, R. L. (1978) *Nature* 275, 55
24 Logothetis, N. K., Schiller, P. H., Charles, E. R. and Hurlbert, A. C. (1989) *Science* 247, 214–217
25 Lee, B. B., Martin, P. R. and Valberg, A. (1989) *J. Neurosci.* 9, 1433–1442
26 Schiller, P. H. and Colby, C. L. (1983) *Vision Res.* 23, 1631–1641
27 Saito, H., Tanaka, K., Isono, H., Yasuda, M. and Mikami, A. (1989) *Exp. Brain Res.* 75, 1–14
28 DeYoe, E. A. and Van Essen, D. C. (1985) *Nature* 317, 58–61
29 Shipp, S. and Zeki, S. (1985) *Nature* 315, 322–325
30 Cavanagh, P. and Favreau, O. E. (1985) *Vision Res.* 25, 1595–1601
31 Cavanagh, P., Boeglin, J. and Favreau, O. E. (1985) *Perception* 14, 151–162
32 Cavanagh, P. and Anstis, S. M. (1986) *Invest. Ophthalmol. Visual Sci. Suppl.* 27, 291
33 Comerford, J. P. (1974) *Vision Res.* 14, 975–982
34 de Weert, C. M. M. (1979) *Vision Res.* 19, 555–564
35 Campbell, F. W. and Maffei, L. (1981) *Vision Res.* 21, 713–721
36 Thompson, P. (1982) *Vision Res.* 22, 377–380
37 Merigan, W. H. (1989) *J. Neurosci.* 9, 776–783
38 Schiller, P. H., Logothetis, N. K. and Charles, E. R. (1989) *Nature* 343, 68–70
39 Schiller, P. H., Logothetis, N. K. and Charles, E. R. *Visual Neurosci.* (in press)
40 Merigan, W. H. (1989) *Soc. Neurosci. Abstr.* 15, 1256
41 Kaplan, E. and Shapley, R. M. (1986) *Proc. Natl Acad. Sci. USA* 83, 2755–2757
42 van Essen, D. C. (1985) in *Cerebral Cortex, Vol. 3* (Peters, A. and Jones, E. G., eds), pp. 259–329, Plenum Press
43 Cowey, A. (1979) *Q. J. Exp. Psychol.* 31, 1–17
44 Zeki, S. M. (1980) *Nature* 284, 412–418
45 Lund, J. S. and Boothe, R. G. (1975) *J. Comp. Neurol.* 159, 305–334
46 Livingstone, M. S. and Hubel, D. H. (1984) *J. Neurosci.* 4, 2830–2835
47 Ungerleider, L. G. and Mishkin, M. (1982) in *Analysis of Visual Behavior* (Ingle, D. J., Goodale, M. A. and Mansfield, R. J. W., eds), pp. 549–586, MIT Press
48 Fitzpatrick, D., Lund, J. S. and Blasdel, G. G. (1985) *J. Neurosci.* 5, 3329–3349
49 Malpeli, J. G., Schiller, P. H. and Colby, C. L. (1981) *J. Neurophysiol.* 46, 1102–1119
50 Ts'o, D. and Gilbert, C. (1988) *J. Neurosci.* 8, 1712–1727
51 Casagrande, V. (1990) *Invest. Ophthalmol. Visual Sci. Suppl.* 31, 396
52 Levitt, J. B. and Movshon, A. (1990) *Invest. Ophthalmol. Visual Sci. Suppl.* 31, 89
53 Desimone, R. and Schein, S. J. (1987) *J. Neurophysiol.* 57, 835–868
54 Moran, J. and Desimone, R. (1985) *Science* 229, 782–784
55 Henny, P. E., Maunsell, J. H. R. and Schiller, P. H. (1988) *Exp. Brain Res.* 69, 245–259
56 Maunsell, J. H. R., Nealy, T. A., Sclar, G. and DePriest, D. D. (1989) in *Neural Mechanisms of Visual Perception* (Lam, D. and Gilbert, C., eds), pp. 223–235, Portfolio
57 Maunsell, J. H. R., DePriest, D. D. and Nealy, T. A. (1989) *Invest. Ophthalmol. Visual Sci. Suppl.* 30, 427
58 Schiller, P. H., Logothetis, N. K. and Charles, E. R. (1989) *Invest. Ophthalmol. Visual Sci. Suppl.* 30, 323
59 Dean, P. (1979) *Exp. Brain Res.* 35, 69–83
60 Heywood, C. A. and Cowey, A. (1987) *J. Neurosci.* 7, 2601–2617
61 Duersteller, M. R., Wurtz, R. H. and Newsome, W. T. (1987) *J. Neurophysiol.* 57, 1262–1287
62 Newsome, W. T., Wurtz, R. H., Duersteller, M. R. and Mikami, A. (1985) *J. Neurosci.* 5, 825–840
63 Schiller, P. H., Logothetis, N. K. and Charles, E. R. (1988) *Soc. Neurosci. Abstr.* 14, 456
64 Cowey, A. (1985) in *Brain Mechanisms and Spatial Vision* (Ingle, D. J., Jeannerod, M. and Lee D. N., eds), pp. 259–278, Martinus Nijhoff
65 Damasio, A., Yamada, T., Damasio, H., Corbett, J. and McKee, J. (1980) *Neurology* 30, 1064–1071
66 Victor, J. D., Maiese, K., Shapley, R., Sidtis, J. and Gazzaniga, M. S. (1989) *Clin. Vision Sci.* 4, 183
67 Zihl, J., Von Cramon, D. and Mai, N. (1983) *Brain* 106, 313–340
68 Schultze, M. (1866) *Arch. Mikr. Anat. Entwicklungsmech.* 2, 175–286

6

C. M. Gray, P. König, A. K. Engel, and W. Singer

Oscillatory responses in cat visual cortex exhibit inter-columnar synchronization which reflects global stimulus properties

1989. *Nature* 338: 334–337

A FUNDAMENTAL step in visual pattern recognition is the establishment of relations between spatially separate features. Recently, we have shown that neurons in the cat visual cortex have oscillatory responses in the range 40–60 Hz (refs 1, 2) which occur in synchrony for cells in a functional column and are tightly correlated with a local oscillatory field potential. This led us to hypothesize that the synchronization of oscillatory responses of spatially distributed, feature selective cells might be a way to establish relations between features in different parts of the visual field[2,3]. In support of this hypothesis, we demonstrate here that neurons in spatially separate columns can synchronize their oscillatory responses. The synchronization has, on average, no phase difference, depends on the spatial separation and the orientation preference of the cells and is influenced by global stimulus properties.

We recorded multi-unit responses to appropriately oriented moving light bars simultaneously from 5 to 7 spatially separate sites in cortical area 17 of 13 adult cats. To determine the temporal relationship of the firing patterns recorded at two sites, we computed both the auto- and cross-correlation functions of the spike trains[4,5]. For 132 of 199 recording sites, the auto-correlation function of the responses was periodic, indicating that the neuronal responses were oscillatory. To establish an objective criterion for the occurrence of oscillatory responses, we fitted a damped sine wave (Gabor function) to the auto-correlograms. Responses were considered to be oscillatory when the fitted function had at least three peaks and when the amplitude of the sinusoidal modulation was significantly different from zero ($P < 0.05$) and exceeded 10% of the amplitude of the cross-correlogram recomputed after shuffling the trial sequence by one stimulus period. The frequency of these oscillatory responses ranged from 40 to 60 Hz (mean, 50 ± 6 Hz), was similar for different recording sites in the same animal and depended only slightly on stimulus configuration (orientation, direction)[2]. Of these 132 recordings, we selected 99 pairs in which oscillatory responses occurred simultaneously at two sites, and used these in cross-correlation analysis. Applying the same criteria used for auto-correlograms, 51 of the cross-correlograms had a significant correlation between the oscillatory responses.

Figure 1 illustrates a typical case in which neuronal responses were oscillatory and synchronized across spatially separate columns. Responses were recorded from five closely spaced sites near the representation of the area centralis of the retina. The receptive fields were overlapping but had different orientation preferences at adjacent sites. Stimulation with a light bar of 112° orientation evoked vigorous responses at sites 1, 3 and 5 but not at sites 2 and 4. As indicated by the periodic modulations of both auto- and cross-correlation functions, these responses were oscillatory and the oscillations were tightly correlated with zero phase difference. Changing the orientation of the stimulus to 22°, to maximize activation of the units at sites 2 and 4 produced synchronized oscillatory responses at these sites (data not shown). In all cases the correlations were abolished in the shuffled cross-correlogram[4-11].

When the recording sites had a larger spatial separation (>2 mm) the receptive fields were non-overlapping and could be stimulated independently. This enabled us to activate the units at each site even if their preferred orientations differed and to determine more precisely if the extent of correlations depended on the similarity of orientation preferences. Figure 2 illustrates the typical case where oscillatory responses in remote columns were synchronized if their orientation preferences were similar but showed no fixed phase relationship when the orientation preferences differed.

TABLE 1 Correlated oscillatory neuronal responses in area 17 as a function of spatial separation of recording sites and angular difference in preferred stimulus orientation

Angular difference of preferred orientation	Spatial separation	
	0.4–2.0 mm (overlapping fields)	2.0–7.0 mm (non-overlapping fields)
0–22°	90% (28/31)	54% (7/13)
45°	73% (8/11)	0% (0/8)
67–90°	44% (7/16)	25% (1/4)

Data were taken from a total of 99 cross-correlograms in which simultaneous oscillatory responses were recorded from two electrodes in area 17. Correlograms computed for responses at sites separated by 8–12 mm ($n = 16$) were excluded. The correlograms were classified into six categories based on the difference in orientation preference of the neurons at the two recording sites and whether or not the receptive fields were overlapping. The results are presented as the percentage of recordings showing oscillatory correlations. The numbers in parentheses correspond to the number of oscillatory correlations and the total number of response pairs analysed for that category, respectively. The correlograms which showed no periodic modulation (48 out of 99) showed either a single peak centred around a 0 ms time delay ($n = 11$) or a flat distribution ($n = 37$).

In two individuals we recorded at two sites separated by 7 mm in which the receptive fields were non-overlapping, had the same orientation preference and were aligned colinearly. This enabled us to co-activate the units at both recording sites with a single long light bar, as well as with two short, independently moving stimuli (Fig. 3). In both cases, the stimuli evoked oscillatory responses at each site. When the short light bars were moved in opposite directions over the two receptive fields, the respective responses showed no phase locking. When the two stimuli were moved in the same direction, however, the oscillations became weakly synchronized and this synchronization was markedly enhanced in each case when the responses were evoked with a single long light bar that co-stimulated the two receptive fields. This suggests that synchronization depends on global features of the stimuli such as coherent motion and continuity, which are not reflected by the local responses alone.

The probability for the occurrence of phase locking depended both on the distance between recording sites and on the angular difference between preferred stimulus orientations (Table 1). There was no phase locking of the oscillatory responses when the electrodes were separated by 7-12 mm ($n = 16$). At intermediate distances of 2-7 mm, when the receptive fields of the recorded neurons were non-overlapping, phase locking occurred mainly between neuronal groups with similar orientation preferences. The same trend was observed for more closely spaced neurons (0.4-2.0 mm), which had overlapping receptive fields but in these cases phase locking was also observed for cells with different orientation preferences. Phase locking of oscillatory responses typically occurred with a phase difference of 0 ms (32 out of 51) and the phase difference rarely exceeded ±3 ms.

Our auto-correlation data confirm that the responses of a large fraction of cortical neurons are oscillatory and that these oscillations are synchronous for cells that are close enough together to be recorded with a single electrode[1,2]. Thus, we could take advantage of multi-unit recordings for the cross-correlation analysis, considerably increasing the number of events per unit time and allowing us to confine the analysis to short epochs. Correlations between the firing probabilities of neurons in the visual cortex have been described previously[6-12] and shown to be dependent on orientation preference[6,9] but only one study has provided evidence for oscillatory correlograms[11]. This rela-

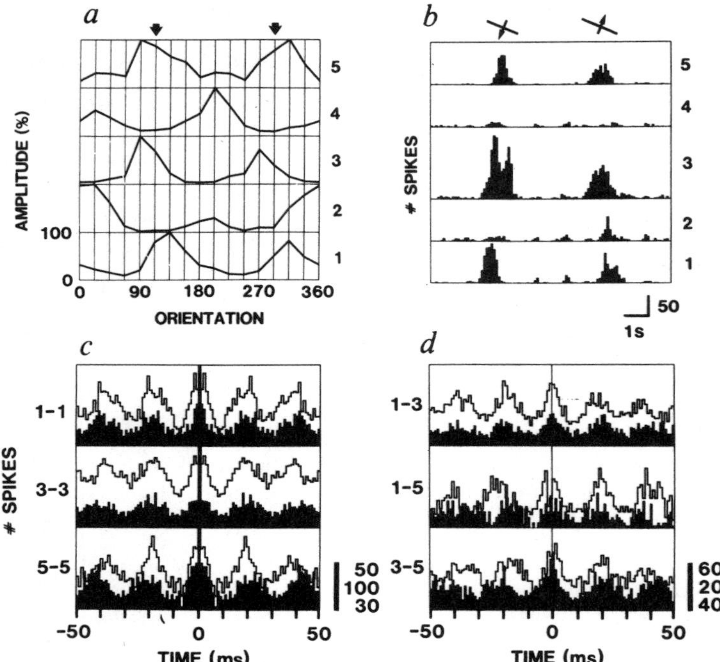

FIG. 1 Orientation-specific intercolumnar synchronization of oscillatory neuronal responses in area 17 of an adult cat. *a*, Normalized orientation tuning curves of the neuronal responses recorded from five electrodes spaced 400 μm apart and centred on the representation of the area centralis. Response amplitudes (ordinate) to stimuli of different orientations (abscissa) are expressed as a percentage of the maximum response for each electrode. The arrows indicate the stimulus orientation (112°) at which the responses were recorded in *b*, *c* and *d*. *b*, Post-stimulus time histograms recorded simultaneously from the same five electrodes at an orientation of 112°. Note the small difference in the latencies of the responses indicating overlapping but slightly offset receptive field locations. *c*, Auto-correlograms of the responses recorded at sites 1 (1–1), 3 (3–3) and 5 (5–5). *d*, Cross-correlograms computed for the three possible combinations (1–3, 1–5, 3–5) between responses recorded on electrodes 1, 3 and 5. Correlograms computed for the first direction of stimulus movement are displayed with unfilled bars with the exception of comparison 1–5 in *d*.

METHODS. Adult cats were prepared for acute physiological recordings from the visual cortex using standard procedures[2]. Anaesthesia was induced with a short acting anaesthetic (hexobarbital, 15 mg per kg or ketamine, 15 mg per kg) and then supplemented with a mixture of 30% O_2, 70% N_2O and 0.1–0.3% halothane. Multi-unit activity was recorded from an array of 4–6 closely spaced (300–500 μm) platinum–iridium electrodes (25 μm tip diameter) and an additional single electrode that was moved independently. The array was inserted in the vicinity of the representation of the area centralis. The single electrode was positioned anteriorly and advanced down the medial bank of area 17. All receptive field locations were within 15° of the area centralis. Spikes exceeding a threshold of twice the noise level were detected with a window discriminator and digitized with a resolution of 1 ms. All recordings used binocular stimulation after the receptive fields for the two eyes had been aligned using prisms. When neurons recorded from different electrodes had overlapping receptive fields but differing orientation preferences, we used a stimulus orientation that evoked a response at each site of at least half the maximal amplitude. Responses that did not meet this criterion and that did not overlap in time were excluded from the analysis. In the case of non-overlapping receptive fields we applied two independently controllable stimuli. For each trial the stimuli were moved across the receptive fields, at the preferred velocity, in both directions of movement perpendicular to the axis of orientation. Each trial lasted for 10 s and was repeated 10 times.

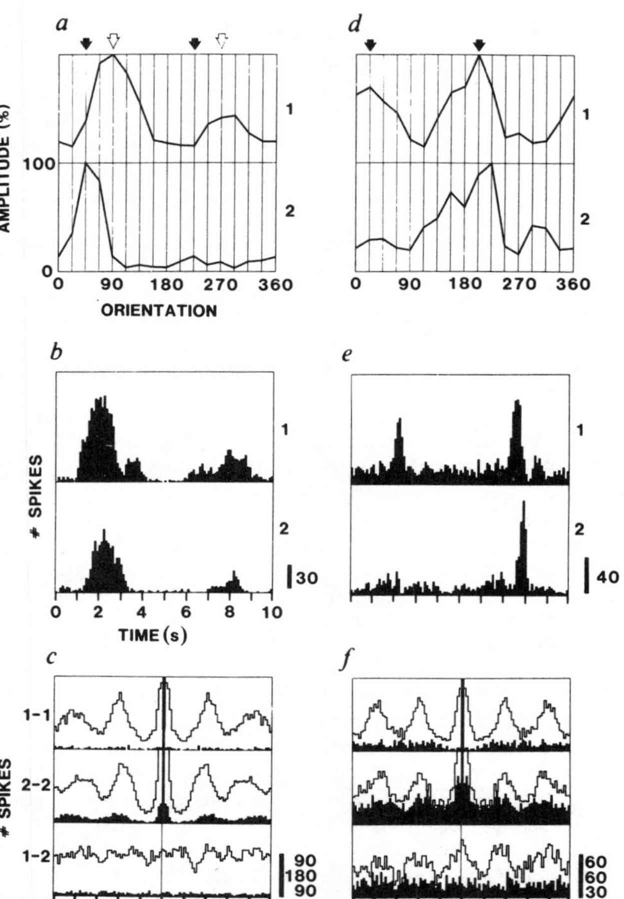

FIG. 2 Long-range inter-columnar synchronization of oscillatory responses depends on the similarity of orientation preference. *a*, Orientation tuning curves of multi-unit responses recorded at two sites (1 and 2) separated by 6 mm in area 17. The neurons had non-overlapping receptive fields and a clear difference in orientation preference of 45° (open and closed arrows). *b*, Post-stimulus time histograms of the responses recorded to stimulation of each receptive field at its own respective optimal orientation (open and closed arrows in *a*). *c*, Auto- (1–1, 2–2) and cross-correlograms (1–2) computed from the neuronal responses recorded from both electrodes revealed that oscillatory responses occurred at both sites but were not correlated. Unfilled bars are for the first direction of stimulus movement. *d*, Orientation tuning curves of multi-unit responses recorded from the same animal at two different cortical sites (1 and 2), separated by 7 mm. The neuronal responses at each site had similar orientation and directional preferences. *e*, Post-stimulus time-histograms of the activity recorded at each site in response to their optimal stimulus orientation of 22° (arrows in *d*). *f*, Auto- (1–1, 2–2) and cross-correlograms (1–2) computed from the neuronal responses recorded on the two electrodes demonstrate oscillatory responses at both sites which were correlated with zero phase difference. Unfilled bars are for the second direction of stimulus movement.

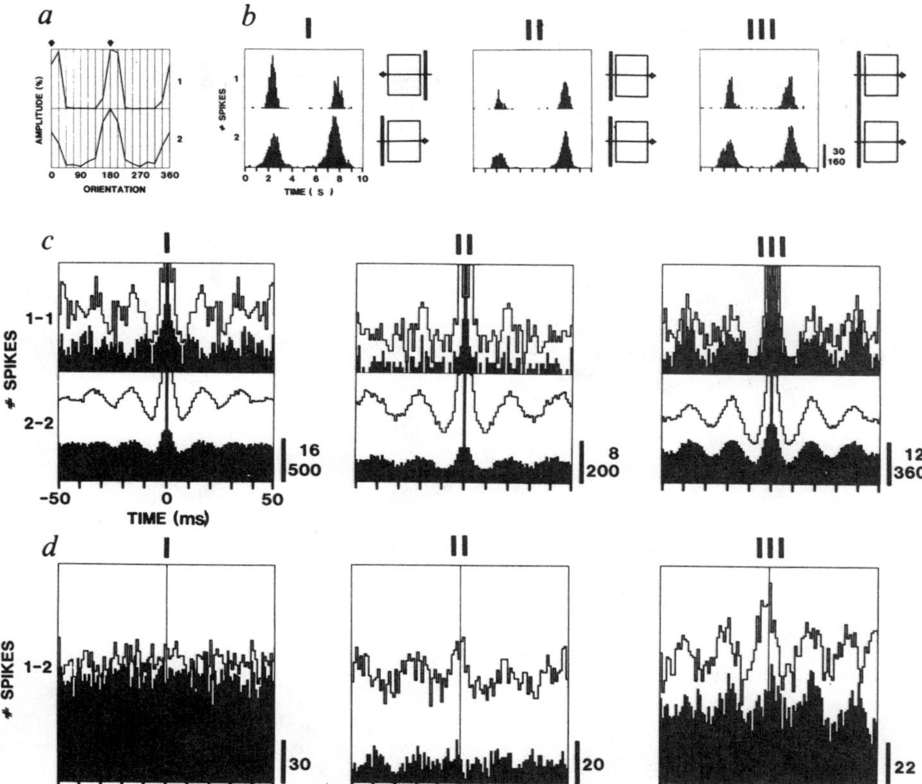

FIG. 3 Long-range oscillatory correlations reflect global stimulus properties. *a*, Orientation tuning curves of neuronal responses recorded from two electrodes (1, 2) separated by 7 mm show a preference for vertical light bars (0 and 180°) at both recording sites. *b*, Post-stimulus time-histograms of the neuronal responses recorded at each site for each of three different stimulus conditions: (I) two light bars moved in opposite directions; (II) two light bars moved in the same direction; and (III) one long light bar moved across both receptive fields. A schematic diagram of the receptive field locations and the stimulus configuration used is displayed to the right of each post-stimulus time histogram. *c*, *d*, Auto-correlograms (*c*, 1–1, 2–2) and cross-correlograms (*d*, 1–2) computed for the neuronal responses at both sites (1 and 2 in *a* and *b*) for each of the three stimulus conditions (I, II, III) displayed in *b*. For each pair of correlograms except the two displayed in *c* (I, 1–1) and *d* (I) the second direction of stimulus movement is shown with unfilled bars.

tive lack of evidence for oscillatory responses in the cortex has several possible explanations. First, only a fraction of cortical neurons have oscillatory responses[2]; second, averaging procedures mask the oscillations because they are not phase-locked to the stimulus[2]; and third, previous studies may have excluded oscillatory activity because cross-correlograms of rhythmic responses were interpreted as misleading[6,12].

The system of tangential intracortical connections[13-19], or the reciprocal projections from other cortical areas[20] may provide the anatomical substrate for the synchronization of oscillatory responses between remote columns. Common input from subcortical structures can be excluded because collaterals of geniculate afferents do not span sufficiently large distances and do not have oscillatory responses in this frequency range[1,2].

We propose that the synchronization of oscillatory responses in spatially separate regions of the cortex may be used to establish a transient relationship between common but spatially distributed features of a pattern[21]. Our data show that synchronization is sensitive to global features of stimuli such as continuity, similarity of orientation and coherency of motion. Synchronization may therefore serve as a mechanism for the extraction and representation of global and coherent features of a pattern. Such processes are crucial for the analysis of visual scenes and figure-ground segregation[3,22-26]. Synchronization of oscillatory responses may however also have a more general function in cortical processing because it is a powerful mechanism for establishing cell assemblies that are characterized by the phase and the frequency of their coherent oscillations. □

1. Gray, C. M. & Singer, W. *Soc. Neurosci. Abstr.* **404,** 3 (1987).
2. Gray, C. M. & Singer, W. *Proc. natn. Acad. Sci. U.S.A.* (in the press).
3. von der Malsburg, C. & Singer, W. in *Neurobiology of Neocortex (Proceedings of the Dahlem Conference)* 69–99 (eds Rakiç, P. & Singer, W.) (Wiley, Chichester, 1988).
4. Perkel, D. H., Gerstein, G. L. & Moore, G. P. *Biophys. J.* **7,** 391–418 (1967).
5. Perkel, D. H., Gerstein, G. L. & Moore, G. P. *Biophys. J.* **7,** 419–440 (1967).
6. Tso, D., Gilbert, C. D. & Wiesel, T. N. *J. Neurosci.* **6,** 1160–1170 (1986).
7. Toyama, K., Kimura, M. & Tanaka, K. *J. Neurophys.* **46,** 191–201 (1981).
8. Toyama, K., Kimura, M. & Tanaka, K. *J. Neurophys.* **46,** 202–213 (1981).
9. Michalski, A., Gerstein, G. L., Czarkowska, J. & Tarnecki, R. *Expl Brain Res.* **51,** 97–107 (1983).
10. Aiple, F. & Krüger, J. *Expl Brain Res.* **72,** 141–149 (1988).
11. Krüger, J. *Rev. Physiol. Biochem. Pharmac.* **98,** 177–233 (1983).
12. Hata, Y., Tsumoto, T., Sato, H., Hagihara, K. & Tamura, H. *Nature* **335,** 815–817 (1988).
13. Creutzfeldt, O. D., Garey, L. J., Kuroda, R. & Wolff, J.-R. *Expl Brain Res.* **27,** 419–440 (1977).
14. Gilbert, C. D. & Wiesel, T. N. *Nature* **280,** 120–125 (1979).
15. Rockland, K. S. & Lund, J. *Science* **215,** 1532–1534 (1982).
16. Mitchison, G. & Crick, F. *Proc. natn. Acad. Sci. U.S.A.* **79,** 3661–3665 (1982).
17. Gilbert, C. D. & Wiesel, T. N. *J. Neurosci.* **3,** 1116–1133 (1983).
18. Martin, K. A. C. & Whitteridge, D. *J. Physiol.* **353,** 463–504 (1984).
19. Kisvarday, Z. F. *et al. Expl Brain Res.* **64,** 541–552 (1986).
20. Montero, V. M. *Brain Behav. Evol.* **18,** 194–218 (1981).
21. Barlow, H. B. *Proc. R. Soc.* **B212,** 1–34 (1981).
22. Marr, D. & Poggio, T. *Science* **194,** 283–287 (1976).
23. Julesz, B. *Nature* **290,** 91–97 (1981).
24. Ballard, D. H., Hinton, G. E. & Sejnowski, T. J. *Nature* **306,** 21–26 (1983).
25. von der Malsburg, C. & Schneider, W. *Biol. Cybern* **54,** 29–40 (1986).
26. Nelson, J. I. in *Models of the Visual Cortex* (eds Rose, D. & Dobson, V. G.) 108–122 (Wiley, Chichester, 1985).
27. Gray, C. M. & Singer, W. *Eur. J. Neurosci.* Suppl. 1, 86.4 (1988).
28. Singer, W., Gray, C. M., Engel, A. & König, P. *Soc. Neurosci. Abstr.* **14,** 362.13 (1988).

ACKNOWLEDGEMENTS. The results presented in this study were presented previously in abstract form (refs 27, 28).

7

P. Cavanagh

Multiple analyses of orientation in the visual system

1989. In *Neural Mechanisms of Visual Perception*, edited by D. M.-K. Lam and C. Gilbert. Houston: Gulf Publishing Co.

We have examined aftereffects and illusions using images defined by five different visual attributes: luminance, color, texture, motion, and binocular disparity. Our results suggest that, for all five attributes, the initial representation of two-dimensional shape involves information about local size and orientation and that in many cases, these size and orientation codes are analyzed independently for individual attributes. Why should these two-dimensional size and orientation analyses be duplicated for several attributes? First, multiple analyses increase reliability. In particular, color and texture borders are more reliably linked to object borders than is luminance (luminance contours are often confounded by shadow borders). Second, using similar codes for each attribute allows a standardized image description that facilitates the subsequent integration of the separate images.

Why are the low-level codes specifically size and orientation? Again reliability may be the reason. Early contour extraction is significantly more accurate when based on local size and orientation information, and the ultimate role of these codes may be to develop a contour representation of the image. On the other hand, difficulties in classifying different types of image contours suggest that the initial memory access should not be based on explicit contour representations but on representations that are invariant to size and orientation. These also depend on the early extraction of size and orientation information. The functionally independent pathways that are demonstrated in the experiments reported here do not appear to do much more than extract two-dimensional representations. It seems very unlikely that such an early stage in visual processing would involve all the visual cortices up to and including areas MT and V4. It is proposed that these cortices are the beginnings of a different set of pathways that are not specific to stimulus attributes.

Introduction

The goal of vision is to inform us both of the identity of objects in view and their spatial positions. Research in several fields has recently indicated that the initial information concerning the scene may be analyzed as several separate images, each involving a particular visual attribute such as texture, color, or motion. Each of these separate images conveys a message about the value of the attribute in question, indicating whether a particular position is, say, red or green. Some of these images also provide three-dimensional information such depth from binocular disparity or surface slants from local gradients of motion or texture. Although the analysis of these attribute-specific images likely involves specialized processes, all of the images convey a message about the two-dimensional shape of regions, and all of these may represent two-dimensional shape in a similar manner. These two-dimensional shape descriptions can then be used to infer three-dimensional object structure through cues such as occlusion, perspective, contour junctions, and the change of shape over time (structure from motion). The extraction of a two-dimensional description of the retinal image is a major step in visual analysis and the purpose of this paper is to examine the nature and degree of independence of the analyses of two-dimensional shape for different visual attributes.

Physiological studies have given clear evidence of multiple analyses at early levels in vision. An image can be considered a superposition of several surface attributes such as color, texture, and luminance and in the first area of visual cortex, V1, cells respond to many of these attributes conjointly: orientation, size, color, direction of motion, binocular disparity. We could imagine processes that operate on this combined image in order to segment regions defined by various attributes but that does not seem to be the case. Cowey[1] and Barlow[2] have argued that local interactions are an integral part of the low-level processes that the visual system applies to these attributes and that for reasons of simplicity and economy (length of axons), the visual system has opted to analyze different attributes in physically separate areas. There is physiological evidence that relative motion and color are analyzed by specialized cortical areas[3,4] and therefore that the stimulus information defined only by color or only by motion will follow separate pathways through these areas. Visual deficits following brain lesions in human patients have shown independent losses of vision for motion,[5] color,[6] and luminance,[7] indicating some physical separation in the cortical representations or projections for these attributes. Although the existence of multiple representations in extrastriate cortex is widely accepted, the routing of information through these areas and the stimulus and/or response attributes processed by each are not yet clearly established.[8]

The work described in this paper examines the functional pathways of information by using perceptual tasks in normal humans. We have studied five stimulus attributes (Figure 1): color, luminance, texture, binocular disparity, and relative motion. Undoubtedly, the actual pathways are considerably more tortuous than those shown in Figure 1, but this simplified schematic can serve as a useful point of departure for research. To construct images defined by a single attribute, texture for example, we start with a black and white figure and replace the black areas with one texture and the white areas with a different texture having the same

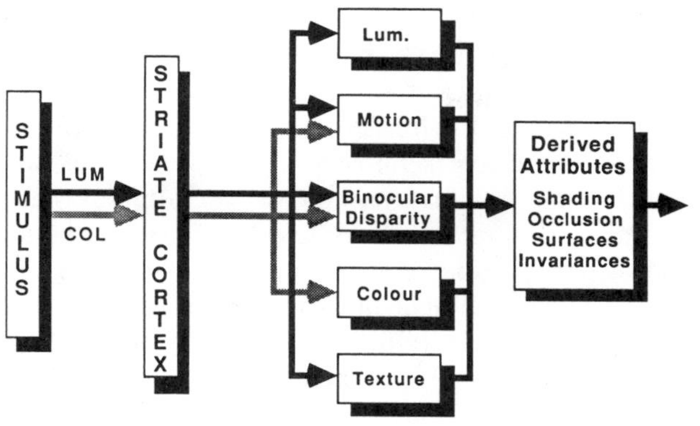

Figure 1. Perceptual pathways in the visual system. Luminance, motion, binocular disparity, color, and texture are stimulus surface qualities that may receive independent analyses. Each of these analyses generates a two-dimensional representation of the attribute, contributing to an overall representation of stimulus shape. These independent representations may be followed by one or more high-level representations that reintegrate information from all attributes and from which are drawn inferences of shading, occlusion, and surfaces inferences.

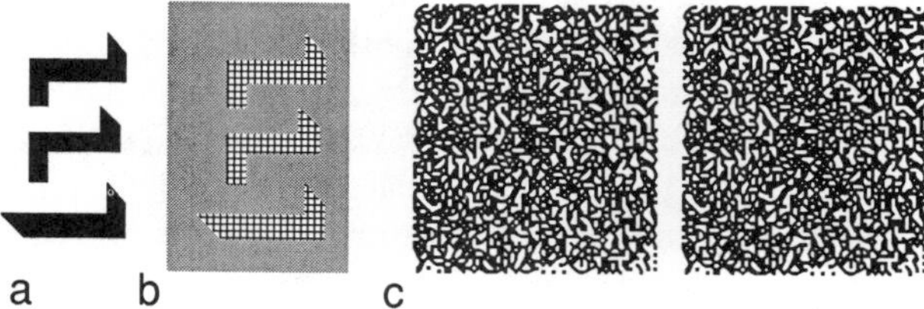

Figure 2. Representations of a shadowed, block letter E defined by (a) luminance, (b) texture, and (c) binocular disparity (the left and right hand panels must be fused).

mean luminance. Figure 2 demonstrates this attribute replacement for texture and binocular disparity. Using images defined by individual attributes, we have been able to demonstrate psychophysically that there are independent analyses of several attributes.[9–12] Whether or not analyses that are functionally independent are also physically separate is a question best answered with physiological methods. In fact, since several studies have shown that analysis of different attributes can be compartmentalized within one visual cortex (for example, processing of chromatic properties in the cytochrome oxidase blob areas of V1 and achromatic properties in interblob regions),[13,14] functional independence may imply either physical separation in local compartments or in separate cortices.

Whatever the routing of information through various stages of early analysis, the separate descriptions must at some point be recombined, and this raises interesting questions concerning the extent of the independent analysis, the cooperation across attributes, and the resolution of conflicts. Bulthoff and Mallot[15] and Sperling and Dosher[16] have described situations

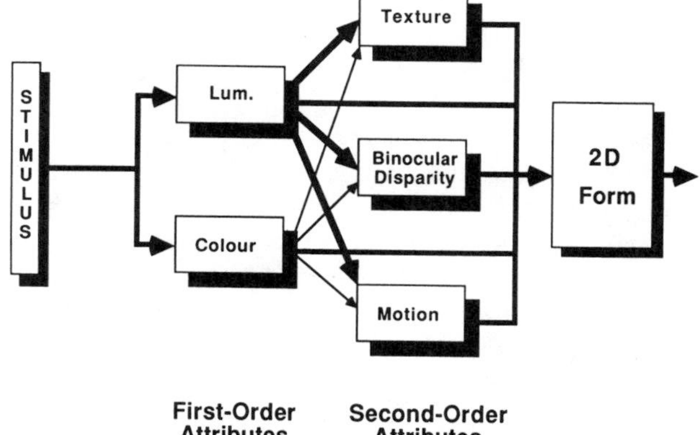

Figure 3. Texture, binocular disparity, and motion are second-order attributes of patterns defined by luminance or color. Color makes a weaker contribution to these second-order attributes than does luminance.

of conflict between various cues in establishing three-dimensional shape. Gregory[17] has proposed that luminance is the primary attribute in determining contour location and that other attributes simply fill out to the luminance-defined border. He calls this border locking and claims that the luminance information is the master map and that the others are adjusted into register with it. Our work[9–11,18–22] gives no evidence of special primacy or privilege for luminance information other than the extra resolution it affords. We feel that the determination of object borders involves much more interattribute cooperation. In fact, the redundancy offered by the independent analysis of separate attributes may be the most important advantage of separate analyses.

What follows this initial two-dimensional analysis of visual attributes? Are rudimentary object descriptions built up from these two-dimensional images of individual attributes at an early level in vision? The object-based approaches of Marr[23] and Biederman[24] suggest that they are. Work that we have just begun[25,26] takes a quite different approach, suggesting that object parts and boundaries should not be explicitly identified at such an early stage and that matching of raw two-dimensional views may be the most effective way to make the initial memory contact. I will not describe the nature of object representations here but concentrate rather on the nature of the multiple representations in early vision.

Inputs

Although Figure 1 places all the five attributes we have considered at the same level, the different attributes, in fact, become explicitly represented at different stages in the visual system. As shown schematically in Figure 3, luminance and color are the initial attributes that represent the image, and these are followed by binocular disparity, motion, and texture, each of which emerges as a property of contours defined by the first two.

Since there is an area specialized for the analysis of color (V4, 3) it is often assumed that color information does not contribute to the pathways involved in the analysis of motion and binocular disparity. However, color does contribute to motion[27–30] and to binocular disparity.[31,32] Our most recent studies[30,33] suggest that the contribution of color to motion passes through the opponent-color (parvocellular) pathway from the retina to the striate cortex rather than “leaking” into the non-opponent (magnocellular) pathway that carries the luminance contribution to motion.[8] These separate routes for color and luminance then converge to form a common motion pathway and a common site for motion aftereffects.[29] Although color does contribute to the second-order attributes as shown in Figure 3, its contribution is much weaker than that of luminance.

Shape Primitives

The two-dimensional shape of a stimulus is coded on a global level by the spatial arrangement of image information in each pathway. To segment image areas defined by a particular attribute, the visual system must be able to distinguish one region from another which it can do very well by simply coding the value of the attribute (say, color) at each point in a retinotopic map. In the case of luminance, however, it has been demonstrated that the visual system goes beyond this simple coding and extracts local structure (shape primitives) directly with cells that are selective to orientation and size[34] and perhaps curvature.[35] The visual system may use similar shape primitives (receptive-field structures) for all attributes or may have some specialized encoding for particular attributes, for example, extracting local orientation and size for luminance and but only coding values point by point for other attributes. The shape primitives available for each attribute limit, and in a way, identify the algorithms the visual system can use to represent shapes. For example, position-, size-, and orientation-invariant descriptions that could form the basis for memory and recognition operations[36,37] require size and orientation coding at an early level.

Physiological studies have identified receptive-field structures at several stages in the visual system. In the retina and lateral geniculate, for example, information is coded by antagonistic center and surround organization and these contribute, in the striate cortex, to the formation of orientation- and size-selective cells.[34] Cells in area V4 appear to have both oriented and nonoriented receptive fields selective for color[3] while many cells in area MT,[38] although directionally selective, do not appear to be orientation-selective, at least not for the orientation of a moving bar. Whether or not they are selective for the orientation of bars defined by relative motion has not been determined. Cells in area V1 and V2 that respond to random-dot stereograms do not appear to be selective for the orientation of bars presented as random-dot stereograms.[39] Although this catalogue of receptive-field structures is extensive, it is not sufficient to identify the coding dimensions ultimately available for all of the attributes we are studying. We have, therefore, developed a series of psychophysical tests to identify coding primitives for these attributes.

Aftereffects

Size[40] and tilt aftereffects[41] have been used to infer the existence of size and orientation coding dimensions and we have examined these aftereffects for each attribute. We have already demonstrated size aftereffects for color stimuli.[9] Elsner[42] has demonstrated orientation specificity for color stimuli using a tilt aftereffect, and Tyler[43] has reported tilt and spatial frequency aftereffects for random-dot stereograms.

With Patrick Flanagan and Olga Favreau, I have examined the tilt aftereffect paradigm to determine whether there are orientation-tuned detectors specialized for luminance, color, texture, relative motion, and binocular disparity. We use a standard induction and test procedure for all the candidate pathways: observers are exposed to the adapting stimulus for 8.0 seconds and then to the test for 0.3 seconds in a repeating cycle. The stimuli are square-wave gratings of 0.5 cycles per degree presented in an 8° square display. The adapting stimuli are tilted 15° off vertical. When the test is present, they match the apparent tilt of the test by adjusting a comparison stimulus presented in an unadapted region of the visual field. We recently compared tilt aftereffects for all five attributes (Figure 4) and found that they were all of similar strength.[12,44]

This result may imply either that each attribute undergoes a separate but similar orientation analysis or that a single orientation analysis operates on a higher image that recombines the images from the separate attributes in some manner. In order to distinguish between these two possibilities, we have used an opposing adaptation technique where we induce opposite aftereffects for two attributes simultaneously. Observers alternately adapt to, for example, texture gratings tilting to the left of vertical and luminance gratings tilting to the right (Figure 5). Three observers participated in these experiments. Following adaptation, vertical test gratings appear tilted to the right if they are defined by texture but tilted to the left if defined by luminance. These independent tilt aftereffects demon-

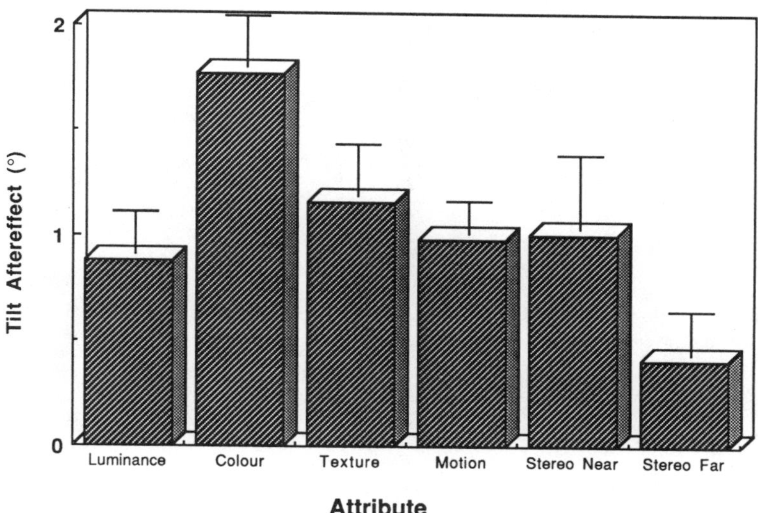

Figure 4. Tilt aftereffects as a function of the attribute defining the bars of the adapting and test gratings. Vertical handles show standard errors (+1.0 S.E.).

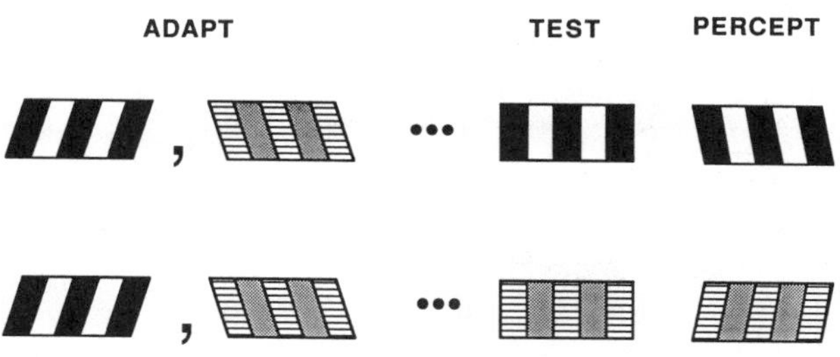

Figure 5. Opposing aftereffects paradigm. Observers alternated adaptation between a luminance-defined grating tilted one way and a texture-defined grating tilted the other way. Vertical tests defined by luminance appeared tilted the opposite direction from the luminance-defined adapting gratings and vertical tests defined by texture appeared tilted the opposite direction from the texture-defined adapting grating.

strate that similar analyses of orientation must be occurring in parallel for texture and luminance. In addition, we have been able to show independent aftereffects for color and texture, and color and luminance (Figure 6). In fact, we have found[10] independent analyses of orientation for a luminance pathway and two chromatic pathways, one red-green and the other aligned with the short-wavelength cone axis (tritanopic confusion line). Since orientation analysis does not emerge until the first cortical visual area, this represents evidence of the use of cardinal color axes[45] at the cortical level.

In contrast to these independent tilt aftereffects, we find no independence in the opposed adaptation paradigm whenever one of the tilted gratings is defined by either motion or binocular disparity (Figure 7). In this case, the observed tilt on the motion or binocular disparity-defined test grating is in the same direction as that seen on the other test (luminance-, color-, or texture-defined). This may imply that the adaptation effects of motion or binocular disparity-defined stimuli are simply overwhelmed by the stronger stimuli. If this were the case, then pitting motion-defined stimuli against binocular disparity-defined stimuli should involve equal adaptation strengths, and the independent aftereffects should reappear. Figure 8 shows that this is not the case. When motion-defined stimuli and binocular disparity-defined stimuli are opposed, there is little or no aftereffect in either direction. These results suggest that there is no independently adaptable orientation analysis for motion-defined or binocular disparity-defined stimuli. The tilt aftereffects seen in the original experiment following adaptation for motion-defined or binocular disparity-defined stimuli presented alone (Figure 4) must have been based in a higher-level representation, common to all the attributes, that also represented orientation explicitly and was adaptable. For size aftereffects, we have demonstrated independent size aftereffects for color and luminance[9] and we shall shortly begin to test for independence with other attributes.

Illusions

Two illusions, horizontal-vertical illusion and tilt illusion (Zöllner), were tested with composite figures (Figure 9). Figure 10 gives an example of the horizontal-vertical illusion presented as a composite figure with the horizontal bar defined by texture and the vertical bar defined by binocular disparity (the two images in the figure must be fused to produce the stereoscopic effect). Composite figures like that of Figure 10 allow us to test the level at which illusions occur. An illusion

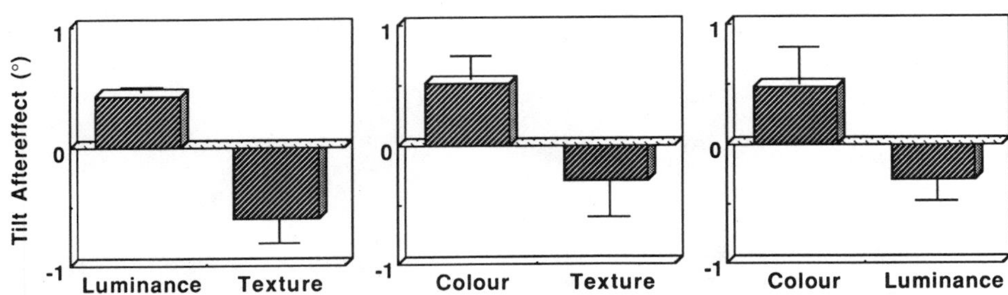

Figure 6. Tilt aftereffects measured in opposing adaptation conditions for luminance versus texture, color versus texture, and color versus luminance. Vertical handles show standard errors (+1.0 S.E.).

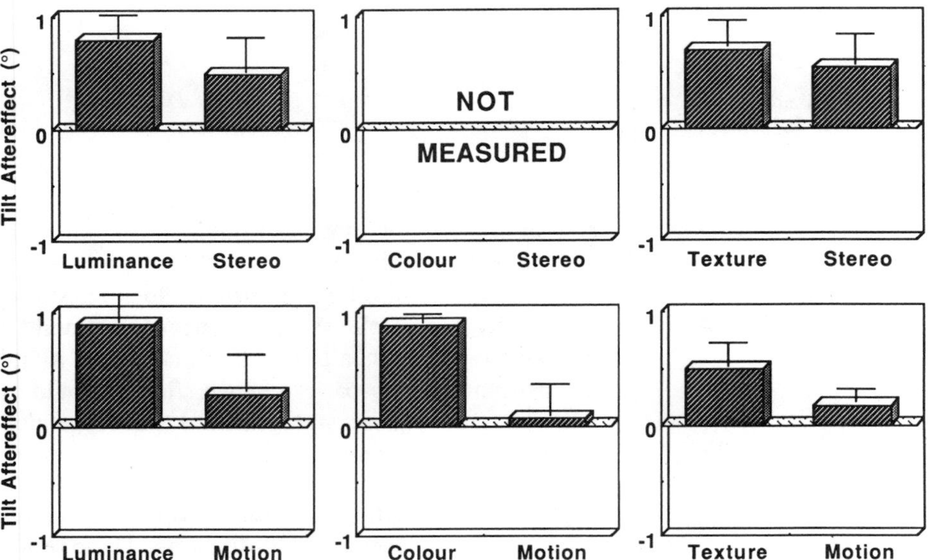

Figure 7. Tilt aftereffects measured in opposing adaptation conditions for stereo versus luminance and texture, and for motion versus luminance, color, and texture. The condition of stereo versus color could not be measured because red-green anaglyphs were used to present the random-dot stereograms and the color stimuli could not be seen properly through the filter glasses. Vertical handles show standard errors (+1.0 S.E.).

that remains undiminished in a composite figure must involve processes that operate on a combined image. An illusion whose strength is reduced in a composite figure must involve processes that operate independently on individual attributes.

With two exceptions (color and stereo could not be combined because red-green anaglyphs were used to present the random dot stereograms, and the color stimuli could not be seen properly through the filter glasses), all possible combinations of the five attributes were used in these figures producing 23 different versions: five "within" figures with both the inducing and the test portion of the illusion figure defined by the same attribute and 18 "between" figures with the two components defined by different attributes. The display subtended 10° of visual angle and, for the horizontal-vertical illusion, observers adjusted the length of the horizontal bar until it appeared to equal that of the vertical bar. Four observers participated. The results are shown in Figure 11. The values shown for the "between" results for each attribute are the average of results involving that particular attribute in all its combinations with the four others. The strength of the horizontal-vertical illusion was very similar for all the attributes whether both lines were defined by the same attribute (within) or by different attributes (between).

For the Zöllner illusion, a small dot was placed 2° from the end of the central shaft of the Zöllner figure. Observers adjusted the position of this dot until they felt that it was colinear with the apparent direction of the central shaft. Four observers participated. Other than the change in the illusion figure, the conditions used were the same as those in the horizontal-vertical tests described above. The results are shown in Figure 12. The strength of the illusion was similar for all attributes in the "within" conditions and similar, as

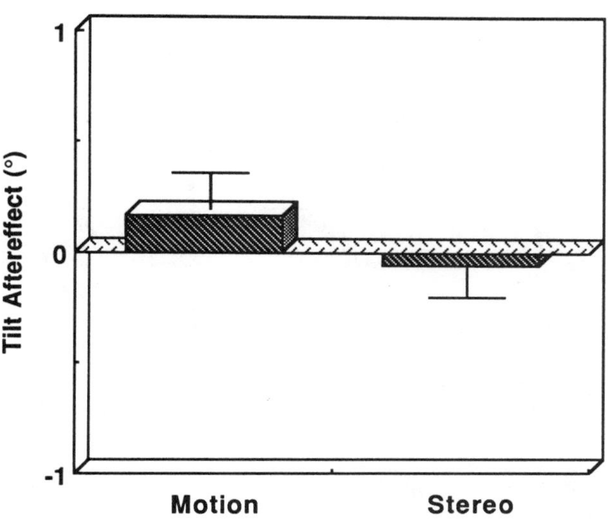

Figure 8. Tilt aftereffects measured in opposing adaptation conditions for motion versus stereo. Vertical handles show standard errors (+1.0 S.E.).

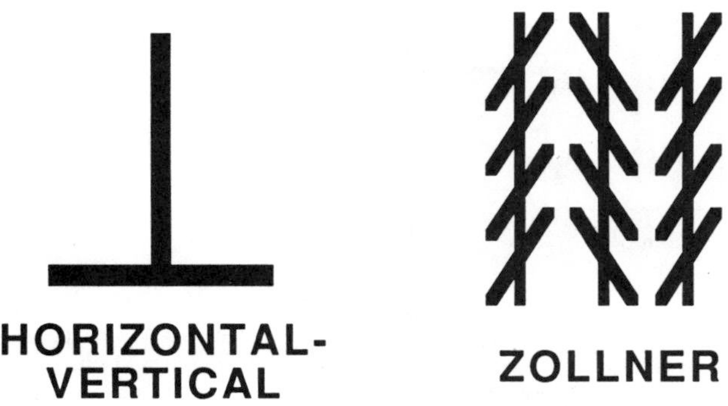

Figure 9. Two illusions, horizontal-vertical and Zöllner, used to test effects in composite figures.

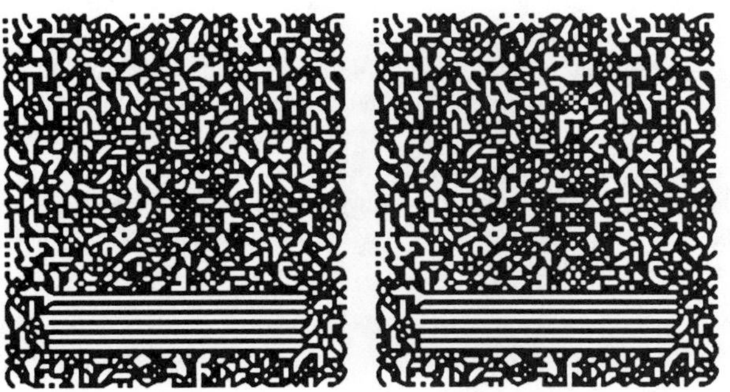

Figure 10. Horizontal-vertical illusion presented as a composite figure. The two images must be fused to see the vertical bar defined by stereo. The horizontal bar is defined by texture.

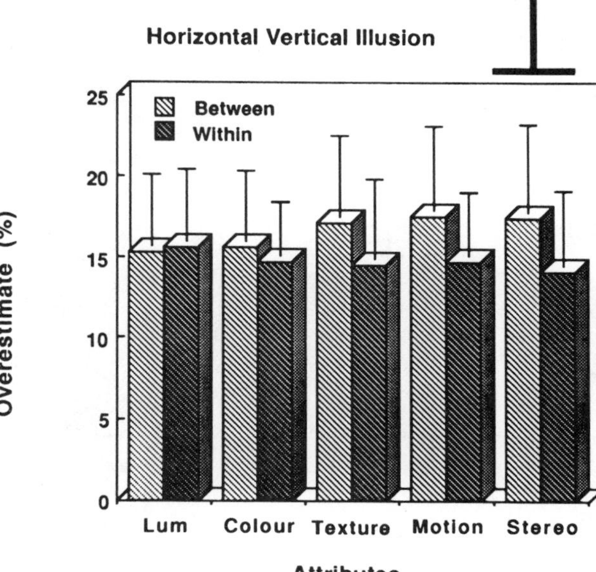

Figure 11. Horizontal-vertical illusion as a function of stimulus attribute and whether the attribute was used to defined both bars ("within" condition: dark striped columns) or only one of them ("between" condition: light striped columns), the other being defined by a different attribute. The vertical axis shows the percent lengthening of the horizontal bar required for it to appear equal in length to the vertical bar. Vertical handles show standard errors (+1.0 S.E.).

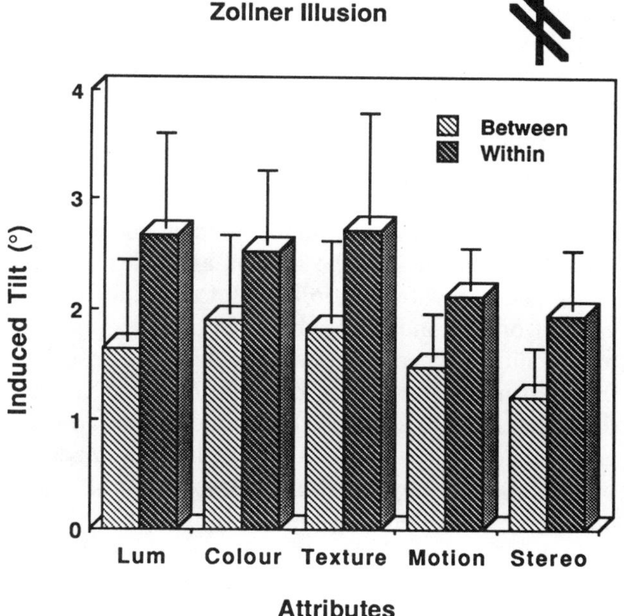

Figure 12. Zöllner illusion as a function of stimulus attribute and whether the attribute was used to define both the central shaft and the inducing bars ("within" condition: dark striped columns) or only one of them ("between" condition: light striped columns), while the other was defined by a different attribute. The vertical axis shows the apparent angular tilt of the central shaft. Vertical handles show standard errors (+1.0 S.E.).

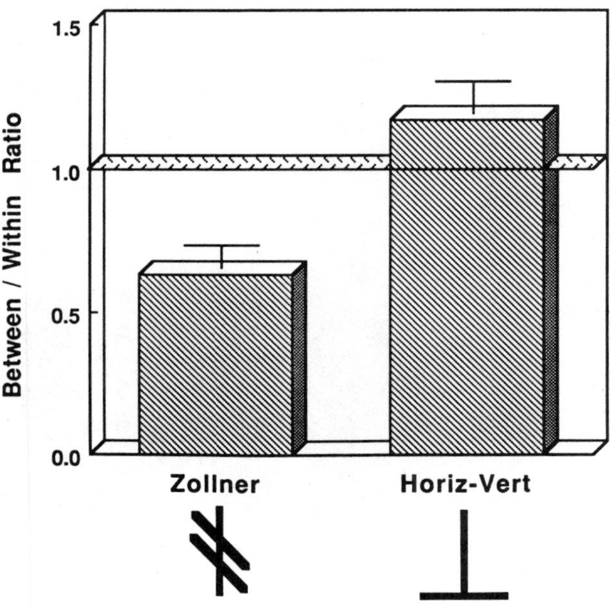

Figure 13. Illusion strength for "between" conditions divided by that for "within" conditions as a function of illusion. Vertical handles show standard errors (+1.0 S.E.).

well, across attributes in the "between" conditions. However, the illusion strength was uniformly smaller in the "between" conditions than in the "within" conditions.

A "between-within" ratio was computed by dividing the average illusion strength for all "between" figures by the average strength for all "within" figures (Figure 13). A value of 1.0 for this ratio indicates that processes responsible for the illusion could access a combined shape representation while a value less than 1.0 indicates that the processes responsible must, at least in part, be located in the individual pathways so that the integrated figure was unavailable to them and so could not trigger the illusion. The horizontal-vertical illusion had a between-within ratio that did not differ significantly from 1.0, indicating that the processes underlying the illusions access an integrated image. Processes involved in spatial scaling of horizontal and vertical dimensions might be expected to operate on an integrated image since they must deal with scenes made up of objects defined by an arbitrary assortment of attributes. For the Zöllner illusion, on the other hand, the ratio was significantly less than 1.0, implying that the orientation coding underlying this tilt illusion must be occurring independently in each pathway to some extent: a composite figure would, therefore, produce less illusion than one defined by a single attribute (Figure 14). The ratio was, nevertheless, also greater than zero indicating that there is some interpathway interaction for orientation coding or alternately some orientation coding in a common high-level representation.

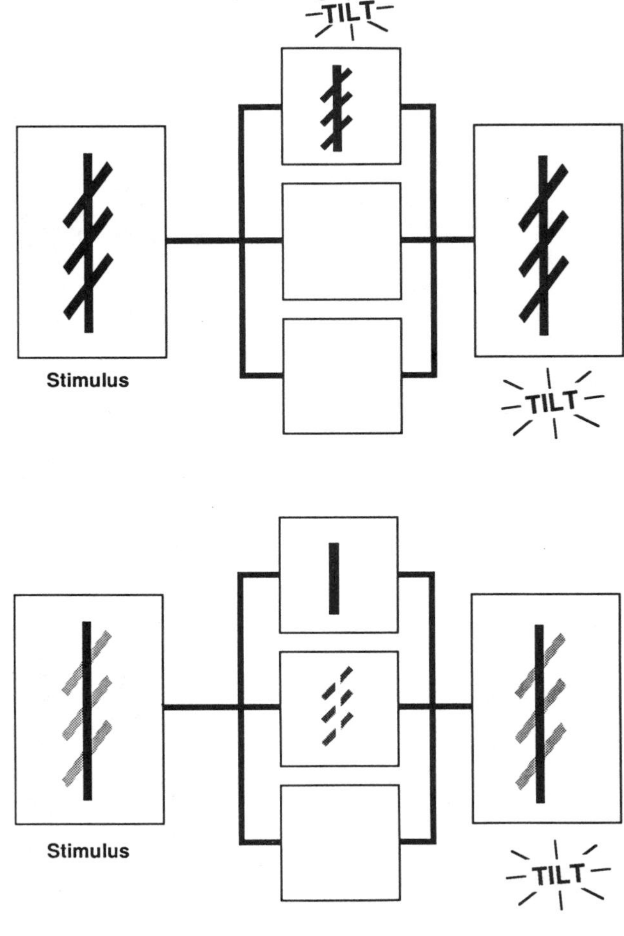

Figure 14. Schematic representation of the difference in tilt illusion for a figure with shaft and inducing bars both defined by the same attribute (top) and the same figure with the shaft defined by one attribute and the inducing bars defined by another (bottom). On the top in the "within" condition, a tilt illusion is generated by orientation analyses both in the independent pathways depicted in the center and the common representation at the right. The two effects combine to produce a total effect greater than either alone. On the bottom in the "between" condition, a tilt illusion is generated by orientation analyses only in the common representation at the right. The inducing bars and the central shaft are represented in separate independent pathways and so no interaction can take place to produce a tilt illusion at this level. The final result in the "within" condition is therefore larger than in the "between" condition.

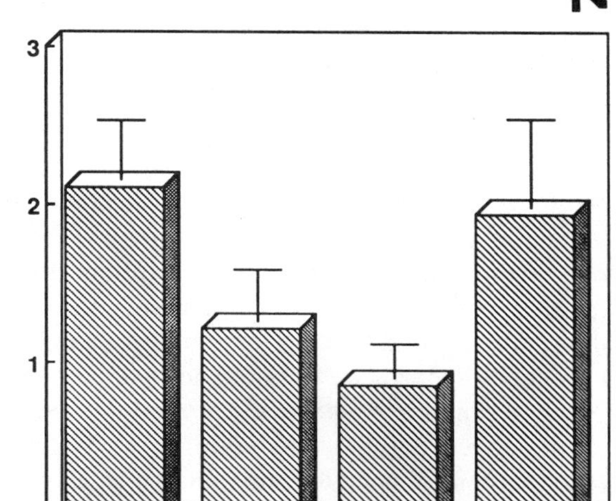

Figure 15. Zöllner illusion as a function of the stimulus attribute defining the central shaft and that defining the inducing bars for the attributes stereo and motion only. The vertical axis shows the apparent angular tilt of the central shaft. Motion-motion and stereo-stereo are "within" conditions while motion-stereo and stereo-motion are "between" conditions. Vertical handles show standard errors (+1.0 S.E.).

The previous experiments on tilt aftereffects had indicated that stimuli defined by motion or binocular disparity did not produce independent tilt aftereffects. For purposes of comparison, the results of the tilt illusion for figures involving motion and binocular disparity are shown in Figure 15. The data show a drop in illusion strength for Zöllner figures composed of both motion and binocular disparity-defined bars compared to those composed of only motion-defined bars or only binocular disparity-defined bars. The tilt illusion data suggests that there is independent analysis of orientation for motion binocular disparity pathways, at least to the same extent as for the other pathways. The results from the tilt aftereffect study indicate that the orientation analysis, although it occurs, may not involve adaptable mechanisms. Both studies do suggest the role of an orientation analysis that operates on a common representation.

Discussion

These results raise several intriguing questions: why there are several analyses, why they seem similar and why they involve, in particular, size and orientation. Since our work here is not yet complete, the answers are speculative and offer interesting directions for further research.

Why Are There Several Analyses?

It is clear that if at least one analysis of shape, say based on luminance, is useful, more may be significantly better. Many surfaces are distinguished from their surrounds not only by luminance differences but also by texture and color so that shape analyses for additional features would improve the segmentation of the surfaces in the scene. In fact, it is easy to argue that luminance, the favored attribute in most shape analysis programs in computer vision, is a problematic choice because many luminance edges in the scene are irrelevant shadow borders. Color and texture differences are much more reliably linked to object boundaries than are luminance edges.

Why Are They Similar?

We have established that there is independent orientation analysis for several attributes and independent size analysis for at least two. We have not yet established that the analysis of each attribute is similar in every respect but one very important reason for the degree of similarity that we have found may be the exchange of image information between analyses. If an integrated higher-level image is to be formed, it is useful to have all lower-level images defined in a standard format. Size and orientation coding may therefore be part of an internal standard for image exchange in the visual system.

If the shape codes for all the attributes are similar, we would expect that processes that depend on two-dimensional shape should be effective on a given two-dimensional shape no matter what attribute is used to define it. For example, we should be able to interpret an ellipse as a tilted circle whether the ellipse is defined by color (red on green of equal luminance), by a random-dot stereogram or by luminance (black on white). Phenomena that depend on information other than shape or that depend on a particular encoding of two-dimensional shape may be preserved for stimuli defined by some attributes but lost for others.

In 1971, Julesz[46] reported that shapes defined by random-dot stereograms produced classical visual illusions, identifiable letters and various other perceptual phenomena. In extending Julesz's approach to additional attributes, we have found that all three-dimensional shape inferences involving objects defined by explicit contours work for all attributes.[18,19,21,22,47] These results are directly opposed to the claims of Livingstone and Hubel[14] that monocular depth cues are ineffective unless luminance defines the stimulus contours. Our studies clearly show that this is not the case, and we attribute their failures to find three-dimensional depth to the fine detail in their images, detail that is critical to the interpretation of their figures. In their stimuli, this fine detail can only be resolved across the entire image if luminance is present and both the stimulus and the depth are lost at equiluminance.

Not all three-dimensional inferences are possible for every attribute, however. Stimuli involving implicit object borders appear to require luminance. For example, shadows and subjective contours both can be perceived with stimuli defined by luminance but both fail to be perceived for the same stimuli when defined by other attributes (for example, Figure 3) even when the object is in motion.[47] The luminance pathway is essential for shadows and subjective contours and the essential information that is derived in the luminance pathway may be the polarity of contrast across the borders.[19,48]

Why Size and Orientation?

There are two possible answers for the popularity of these two image codes. The first is that local size and orientation information significantly improves the detection of contours in the image. These multi-scale approaches[49] to contour identification are the initial stages of contour labeling involved in recognition-by-component models. Contours are extracted and object parts, whether generalized cylinders[23] or geons,[24] are identified from these contours using simple image constraints. These early representations then index memory to retrieve object identity and other useful information for completing the three-dimensional model. Memory representations are assumed to be object-centered in that arbitrary views of the object can be matched to the memory prototype.

The second possibility is that size and orientation codes are an intermediate step in obtaining size- and orientation-invariant shape descriptions. Fourier-Mellin transforms[50] and Fourier-log polar-Fourier transforms[36,37] are representatives of this class of transform. The coincidence between the size and orientation representation which is an intermediate step in these transforms and that seen in local regions of striate cortex, and revealed by the aftereffects that we have studied, may simply be a coincidence. But it may be an indication that the visual system uses a transform of this type.

Cortical Areas

It has been proposed that the existence of separate cortical areas specialized for different visual attributes allows for a more economical analysis of each. Although each of these areas may perform some specialized tasks such as color constancy or contour polarity, the results of the experiments reported here suggest that, other than these specialized analyses, the independent analysis of visual attributes may involve only the extraction of two-dimensional shape. The cortical areas that have been proposed as the sites for these independent analyses include all those up to MT and V4.[3] These independent representations would involve a very large proportion of visual cortex in what is only a preliminary step in vision. It may be that the functionally independent analyses that we have demonstrated in our experiments occur before these regions and involve perhaps only compartmentalized representations rather than physically separate ones. Orientation tuning for disparity- and direction-selective units is seen as early as the striate cortex. However, in our oriented gratings presented as random-dot stereograms or random-dot kinematograms, these striate units must respond to the orientation of individual, luminance-defined elements and not to the orientation of the alternating broad strips of random dots which are at different depths (stereogram) or moving in different directions (kinematogram) and which all have the same mean luminance. Some of the orientation effects we measure must therefore be based in extrastriate cortices although not necessarily as far along as V4 or MT. Area MT and V4 might then be candidates for a new set of pathways that are not specific to stimulus attributes. V4 might be the site of a common two-dimensional shape representation that combines information from all visual attributes. Note that if this were the case, V4 cells would not necessarily respond to motion, for example, but to the shapes defined by motion differences between regions; it would not necessarily respond to stereo but to the shapes of regions defined by stereo. Specifically, some cells in V4 ought to show tuning for the orientation of contours that are defined by any feature—color, luminance, texture, motion, or disparity—as if these cells performed an OR function on the outputs of lower-level, orientation-tuned units. Conversely, area MT might respond to motion of shapes no matter how they are defined.

Acknowledgments

This research was supported by NSERC grants A8606 to Patrick Cavanagh and A8333 to Olga Eizner Favreau and by the Ministère d'Education du Québec.

References

1. A. Cowey, *Q. J. Exp. Psych.* **31**, 1 (1979).

2. H. B. Barlow, *Vision Res.* **26**, 81 (1986).

3. S. M. Zeki, *Nature (London)*, **274**, 423 (1978).

4. D. C. van Essen, in *Cerebral Cortex Vol. III*, A. Peters and E. G. Jones, Eds., (Plenum Publishing, New York, 1985), p. 259.

5. J. Zihl, *Brain* **106**, 313 (1983).

6. A. Damasio *et al., Neurology* **30**, 1064 (1980).

7. J. Rovamo, L. Hyvarinen, and R. Hari, *Doc. Ophthal. Proc. Series* **33**, 457 (1982).

8. J. H. R. Maunsell and W. T. Newsome, *Ann. Rev. Neurosci.* **10**, 363 (1987).

9. O. E. Favreau and P. Cavanagh, *Science* **212**, 831 (1981).

10. P. Flanagan, P. Cavanagh, and O. E. Favreau, *Optics News*, **13**, 161 (1987).

11. P. Flanagan, P. Cavanagh, and O. E. Favreau, *Invest. Ophthalmol. Vis. Sci. Suppl.* **29**, 327 (1988).

12. P. Cavanagh, paper presented to the Symposium on New Insights on Visual Cortex, Rochester, June 1988.

13. M. S. Livingstone and D. H. Hubel, *J. Neurosci.* **4**, 309 (1984).

14. M. S. Livingstone and D. H. Hubel, *J. Neurosci.* **7**, 3416 (1987).

15. H. H. Bülthoff and H. A. Mallot, *Invest. Ophthalmol. Vis. Sci. Suppl.* **29**, 40 (1988).

16. G. Sperling and B. Dosher, *Vision Res.*, **26**, 973 (1986).

17. R. L. Gregory, *Proc. R . Soc. London*, **B204**, 467 (1979).

18. P. Cavanagh, *J. Opt. Soc. Am.* **A2**, P51 (1985b).

19. P. Cavanagh, *Bull. Psychonomics Soc.* **23**, 273 (1985c).

20. P. Cavanagh, *Bull. Psychonomics Soc.* **24**, 291 (1986).

21. P. Cavanagh, *Computer Vision, Graphics and Image Processing*, **37**, 171 (1987).

22. P. Cavanagh, in *Computational Processes in Human Vision: An Interdisciplinary Perspective*, Zenon Pylyshyn, Ed. (Ablex, Norwood, N.J., 1987), p. 254.

23. D. Marr, *Vision* (Freeman, San Francisco, 1982).

24. I. Biederman, *Psych. Rev.* **84**, 115 (1987).

25. P. Cavanagh, S. Peters, and M. von Grünau, paper presented to the annual meeting of the European Conference on Visual Perception, Bristol, August 1988.

26. P. Cavanagh and M. von Grünau, paper presented ARVO, Sarasota, May 1989.

27. P. Cavanagh, J. Boeglin, and O. E. Favreau, *Perception* **14**, 151 (1989).

28. P. Cavanagh, C. W. Tyler, and O. E. Favreau, *J. Opt. Soc. Am.* **1**, 893 (1984).

29. P. Cavanagh and O. E. Favreau, *Vision Res.* **25**, 1595 (1985).

30. P. Cavanagh and S. M. Anstis, *Invest. Ophthalmol. Vis. Sci. Suppl.* **27**, 291 (1986).

31. C. M. M. de Weert and K. J. Sadza, in *Colour vision: Psychophysics and physiology*, J. D. Mollon and L. T. Sharpe, Eds. (Academic Press, London, 1983), pp. 553–562.

32. D. L. Grinberg and D. R. Williams, *Vision Res.* **25**, 531 (1985).

33. P. Cavanagh, *Invest. Ophthalmol. Visual Sci. Suppl.* **29**, 196 (1988).

34. D. H. Hubel and T. N. Wiesel, *J. Physiol.*, **195**, 215 (1968).

35. A. Dobbins, S. W. Zucker, and M. S. Cynader, *Nature (London)* **322**, 196 (1987).

36. P. Cavanagh, in *Figural Synthesis*, P. C. Dodwell and T. Caelli, Eds. (Lawrence Erlbaum Associates, Hillsdale, N.J., 1984), pp. 185–218.

37. P. Cavanagh, in *Models of the Visual Cortex*, D. Rose and V. G. Dobson, Eds. (John Wiley & Sons, London, 1985), pp. 85–95.

38. J. A. Movshon *et al.*, in *Pattern Recognition Mechanisms*, C. Chagas, R. Gattass, and C. Gross, Eds. (Springer Verlag, Berlin, 1986), pp. 117–151.

39. G. F. Poggio *et al.*, *Vision Res.* **25**, 397 (1985).

40. C. Blakemore and P. Sutton, *Science* **166**, 245 (1969).

41. F. W. Campbell and L. Maffei, *Vision Res.* **11**, 833 (1971).

42. A. Elsner, *Perception and Psychophysics* **24**, 451 (1978).

43. C. W. Tyler, *Perception* **4**, 187 (1975).

44. P. Cavanagh, M. Arguin, and P. Flanagan, paper presented to the annual meeting of the English Pychological Association, Oxford, July 1987.

45. J. Krauskopf, D. R. Williams, and D. W. Healy, *Vision Res.* **22**, 1123 (1982).

46. B. Julesz, *Foundations of Cyclopean Perception* (University of Chicago Press, Chicago, 1971).

47. P. Cavanagh and V. S. Ramachandran, paper presented to the annual meeting or the Canadian Psychology Association, Montreal, June 1988.

48. P. Cavanagh, and Y. Leclerc, *J. Exp. Psychol. [Hum. Percept.]*, 3 (1988).

49. A. P. Witkin, *Proceedings of the 8th International Joint Conference on Artificial Intelligence* **2**, 1019 (1983).

50. D. Casasent and D. Psaltis, *Applied Optics* **15**, 1793 (1976).

8

D. N. Levine

Visual agnosia in monkey and in man

1982. In *Analysis of Visual Behavior*, edited by D. J. Ingle, M. A. Goodale, and R. J. W. Mansfield. Cambridge, MA: MIT Press

In recent years, there have been few attempts to relate disorders of visual recognition in man to visual disturbances resulting from circumscribed cerebral ablations in animals. Early workers (see Lissauer 1890) had no hesitation in attempting to relate their observations in patients to experimental results. Indeed, the term *Seelenblindheit* (psychic blindness) that was used to describe the syndrome known today as associative visual agnosia was taken directly from Munk's (1881) description of the behavior of dogs after bilateral occipital lesions. In the ensuing decades, however, the laboratory and the clinic drifted apart in the study of cerebral disturbances of vision. Perhaps part of the reason for this drift lay with Lissauer himself. In choosing to give a psychological explanation for his well-defined syndrome he opened the door to a controversy that continues to this day among clinicians as to the psychological nature of visual agnosia. Whether "perception" can be intact but have no "meaning" has been the focus of this controversy and has diverted attention from the study of the comparative anatomy and comparative behavior of the syndrome.

Geschwind (1965) discussed "agnosias" in animals and in man, and pointed out that one cannot understand visual agnosias in man without considering the specialization of the left hemisphere for speech and the effects of disconnecting the nonverbal right hemisphere from the speaking left. He concluded that "visual agnosias" in monkey and in man had entirely different anatomical and psychological substrates. "Visual agnosia" in the monkey was conceived as a disconnection of the calcarine cortex from the "limbic" regions anatomically and as the loss of visual-visceral (olfactory, gustatory) associations psychologically. Visual agnosia in man was conceived as a disconnection of the calcarine cortex from the angular gyrus of the dominant hemisphere anatomically and as loss of visual-language associations psychologically.

The purpose of this chapter is to reexamine the degree to which the syndromes of visual agnosia in man parallel the syndromes of impaired visual discrimination in the monkey. Given Geschwind's cogent arguments, it would be unwise to expect complete correspondence, because the monkey lacks speech and its underlying lateralized cerebral substrate. Nevertheless, I will attempt to show that there are remarkable parallels both in behavioral abnormalities and in pathological anatomy between the visual agnosias in monkey and in man. In both primates, similar impairments in visual discrimination result from interruption of an interconnected system of neurons in striate cortex, visual association cortex, and inferior temporal neocortex. In both man and monkey, these syndromes can be distinguished from those involving other cerebral areas. The appearance of hemispheric specialization in man results in a greater variety of visual-discrimination deficits than are seen in the monkey, but this greater variety can be seen as a differentiation in man of a common behavioral and anatomical pathology that is shared with the monkey.

The Anatomic Basis of Impaired Visual Discrimination in the Monkey

Munk (1881) performed bilateral occipital ablations in dogs. The animals appeared to see in that they walked about without colliding with obstacles. But they did not otherwise behave discriminatively toward visual stimuli, no longer taking food, no longer cringing from fire, and remaining indifferent to the sight of their master though responding to his voice.

Brown and Schafer (1888) were the first to produce a similar picture in the primate. After removal of both temporal lobes, a rhesus monkey oriented its body and limbs properly to visually presented objects, but appeared tame, allowing itself to be handled. It approached and investigated by feeling, tasting, and smelling all sorts of objects, animate or inanimate, edible or inedible. This syndrome was largely forgotten until the experiments of Klüver and Bucy (1937, 1939) confirmed that after bilateral temporal lobectomy monkeys were tame, compulsively examined every visual object in the environment ("hypermetamorphosis"), and tended to chew, lick, or sniff all such objects (oral tendencies). In addition, the monkeys would often eat meat, which a normal monkey will not do, and displayed excessive indiscriminate (auto-, hetero-, and homo-) sexual behavior. Although visual acuity appeared intact, as did orientation of the body and limbs to visual objects, these monkeys had great difficulty (but eventual success) in learning to discriminate visually a circle from a square and also in retaining such discriminations that had been learned before the operation.

Numerous studies followed in an attempt to delimit more precisely the lesions necessary to produce the syndrome. Early studies (Blum et al. 1950; Chow 1951, 1952) demonstrated that impaired acquisition and retention of visual discriminations resulted from lesions involving only neocortex of temporal lobe. Shortly thereafter, studies with less extensive lesions demonstrated that ablation of the neocortex of the inferior temporal lobe, coinciding roughly with von Bonin and Bailey's (1947) area TE, would produce the visual-discrimination deficits, but that lesions of superior temporal gyrus (Mishkin and Pribram 1954), hippocampus, and amygdala (Mishkin 1954) or of temporal pole, anterior insula, and orbital frontal cortex (Pribram and Bagshaw 1953) would not. The inferotemporal lesions, while producing defects in acquiring and retaining visual discriminations, did not as a rule produce the other manifestations of the "Klüver-Bucy syndrome"—the tameness, hypermetamorphosis, oral tendencies, and changes in dietary habits or sexual behavior.

Once it was shown that lesions of inferior temporal neocortex (TE) were crucial in producing impaired acquisition and retention of visual discrimination, further studies attempted to determine which anatomical connections to this area were necessary for adequate function of this region. It seemed possible, on the one hand, that cortico-cortical connections (striate cortex → visual association cortex → inferotemporal cortex) were important; on the other hand, cortico-subcortical relays (striate cortex → pulvinar → inferotemporal cortex) or extrageniculostriate pathways (retina → superior colliculus → pulvinar → inferotemporal cortex) might be crucial. Mishkin (1966) demonstrated the importance of cortico-cortical connections. He ablated inferotemporal cortex in one hemisphere and striate cortex in the other. The monkeys were somewhat impaired in retaining visual discriminations but could be retrained. He then sectioned the corpus callosum, destroying the only remaining cortico-cortical connection between striate and inferotemporal cortex. Severe impairment in retention of visual discriminations ensued. Thus Mishkin demonstrated the importance of striate-inferotemporal connections, both ipsilateral and crossed (via corpus callosum) in ensuring adequate visual discrimination performance in the monkey.

Mishkin's results heightened a paradox that had existed for almost two decades. Modern studies employing the Nauta technique (Kuypers et al. 1965; Jones and Powell 1970) have confirmed earlier conclusions, based on strychnine neuronography, that striate cortex projects to inferotemporal cortex not directly but through visual-association cortex. Thus, if cortico-cortical pathways from striate to inferotemporal regions were necessary for intact visual discrimination, impairment should result from lesions of visual-association cortex as well. Yet earlier investigators (Lashley 1948; Chow 1951, 1952; Evarts 1952) had ablated extensive areas of visual-association cortex in the monkey without producing impairment in the acquisition of visual form discriminations. This failure had prompted either of two alternative conclusions: that cortico-subcortical loops were more important than cortico-cortical connections and capable of maintaining normal visual discrimination when cortico-cortical connections were interrupted (Pribram 1960); or that cortico-cortical paths were indeed important, but that association cortex was equipotential and highly redundant, so that even small areas remaining after large ablations could subserve the acquisition of simple visual discriminations (Lashley 1948). Though experiments such as Mishkin's demonstrated the insufficiency of cortico-subcortical pathways alone, only recently has sufficient anatomic information about the organization of visual-association cortex become available to offer an alternative to Lashley's conclusion.

Investigations (Iwai and Mishkin 1968; Cowey and Gross 1970) taking advantage of new information about the anatomic organization of visual-association cortex have contributed to the resolution of the above paradox. This anatomic information was derived from studies employing the Nauta technique and its variations to trace fiber pathways after focal occipital ablations (Myers 1965a; Kuypers et al. 1965; Zeki 1969, 1970, 1971a, b) and from studies employing microelectrodes to map visual areas by determining receptive fields of single neurons (Allman and Kaas 1971, 1974a, b, 1975, 1976). These studies have demonstrated that visual-association cortex is not a mass of equivalent neurons in which visual information is represented diffusely. Instead, it appears to consist of numerous, geographically distinct representations of the visual fields with complex interconnections.

A detailed review of the results of these still-incomplete studies is beyond the scope of this article (see Allman 1977). Of importance to us is that these studies consistently demonstrate that the representation of the fovea in striate cortex projects to specific, restricted areas of visual-association cortex. The densest projections are to the immediately anterior cortex on the ventrolateral convexity of the occipitotemporal region (figure 1). This "foveal prestriate" cortex (Cowey and Gross 1970) appears to correspond to the representations of foveal information in several electrophysiologically mapped visual areas, including Allman and Kaas's V2, DL, and MT (Allman 1977).

When Iwai and Mishkin (1968) and Cowey and Gross (1970) made small bilateral lesions restricted to the foveal prestriate area (much smaller than the extensive lesions of previous investigators), their monkeys were impaired in learning visual form discriminations even more than animals with the usual, more anterior inferotemporal (TE) lesions. These investigators pointed out that all of their predecessors had spared part or all of the foveal prestriate region in their ablations for fear of damage to the underlying visual radiations.

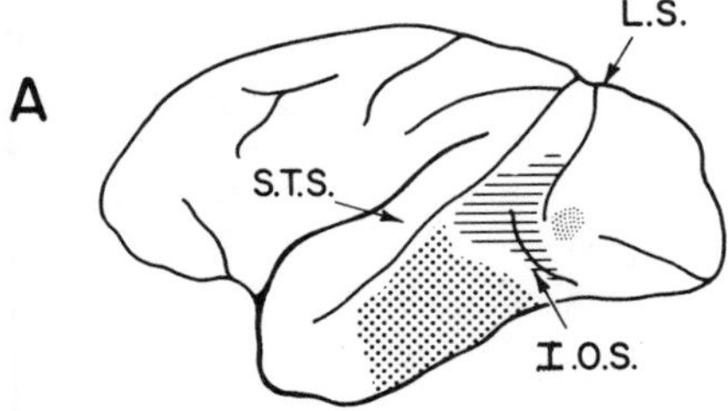

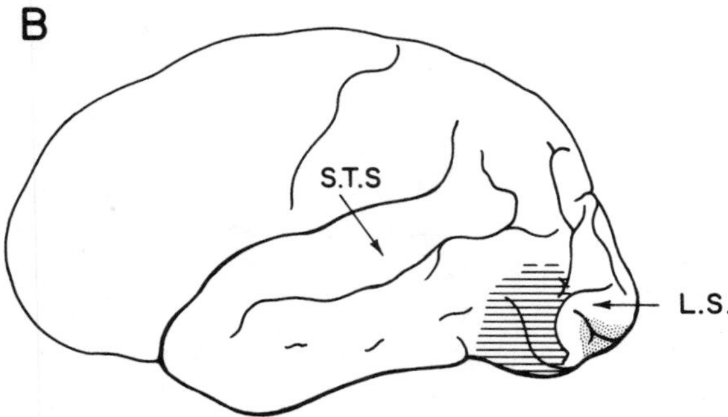

Figure 1. (A) The foveal prestriate (horizontal lines) and inferotemporal regions (coarse dots) in the rhesus monkey, as demonstrated by Zeki. (B) The site of lesions resulting in human visual agnosia according to Nielsen (horizontal lines). L.S.: lunate sulcus. I.O.S.: inferior occipital sulcus. S.T.S.: superior temporal sulcus. Fine dots represent anterior extent of foveal representation in striate cortex.

Thus the paradox of the apparent dispensability of the visual association areas despite the proven importance of cortico-cortical connections was solved. The solution was that some areas of association cortex were more important than others with respect to the acquisition of visual form discrimination. The area of foveal representation was crucial; when it was destroyed, performance was impaired.

Thus, a coherent anatomic basis for understanding impaired visual form discrimination in the monkey has begun to emerge. At the cortical level, an interconnected system consisting of the portions of striate, prestriate, and inferotemporal cortex representing central vision is necessary for intact visual form discrimination. This interconnected system, if intact in *either* cerebral hemisphere, will allow visual discrimination learning. Even after certain bihemispheral lesions of this system (e.g., striate cortex in one hemisphere and inferotemporal cortex on the other), discrimination may be relatively preserved because posterior callosal fibers may suffice to interconnect remaining foveal striate, prestriate, and inferotemporal regions. The crossed connections, however, do not appear as strong as the intrahemispheric ones (Myers 1965b; Mishkin 1972).

Although the necessity of the above interconnected cortical system for normal visual discrimination is now clear, a role for the pulvinar in visual discrimination cannot be dismissed on the basis of the experiments to date. As previously indicated, the pulvinar might relay information either from superior colliculus or from striate cortex to the prestriate and inferotemporal regions. Early studies (Chow 1954; Rosvold et al. 1958) demonstrated that bilateral pulvinar ablations did not produce impairment in acquisition of visual discriminations, suggesting that these routes were relatively unimportant. However, modern anatomical studies have confirmed earlier work establishing the anatomic specificity of the different subdivisions of the monkey pulvinar. In the squirrel monkey (Mathers 1971), as in the macaque (Chow 1950), it is the inferior nucleus of the pulvinar that projects to the foveal prestriate region of occipital cortex. Also, it is only the inferior pulvinar in the squirrel monkey that receives projections from the superficial layers of the superior colliculus (Mathers 1971). Allman et al. (1972) have mapped a representation of the contralateral visual half-field in this region. Thus, a clear-cut route from superior colliculus to foveal prestriate cortex exists via the inferior nucleus of the pulvinar. The existence of striate cortex → pulvinar connections is disputed. Siqueira and Franks (1974), using both Marchi and Nauta techniques, found no such projections in the macaque, whereas Campos-Ortega et al. (1970) found projections from striate cortex to inferior pulvinar. Thus, if a route to inferotemporal cortex from striate cortex via pulvinar exists, it too is probably via the inferior nucleus.

If one now reviews the studies of the effects of pulvinar lesions on visual discrimination learning, it is clear that in no case has there been bilateral destruction of all or even of a substantial portion of the inferior nucleus. In Chow's studies, the published reconstructions of the lesions demonstrate this to be the case. In the work of Rosvold et al., pulvinar lesions were produced by mistake when lesions of superior colliculus were intended, and it was the medial, not the inferior, pulvinar that was affected. Thus, it is possible that appropriately placed lesions, bilaterally destroying nucleus pulvinaris inferior, will produce impairment in acquisition of visual discriminations.

The Anatomic Basis of Visual Agnosia in Man

According to Bodamer (1947), inability to recognize familiar objects and people after lesions of the central nervous system was first recorded by Thuycidides in his description of the typhus epidemic of Athens in 430 B. C. Lissauer (1890) offered the first extensive clinical description of a patient, who, after a stroke in the territory of the left posterior cerebral artery, was unable to name, describe, or demonstrate the use of visually presented objects, though he easily named them when he touched them or heard them. He had a right homonymous hemianopia. Although central visual acuity was about one-third of normal, the patient could draw visually presented objects even when he was unable to name them. To describe the syndrome Lissauer employed the term *Seelenblindheit* (psychic blindness)—the same term Munk had used to describe the vision of his destriate dogs. Freud, in his monograph on aphasia (1891), substituted the term *agnosia* for the then current term *asymbolia* (Spamer 1876) and did not consider the term *psychic blindness* in his discussion. Thus, *psychic blindness* or *visual agnosia* (synonymous in the clinical literature) came to denote the conditions of patients who, when faced with a visual object, were unable to name it, show its use, or sort it into a group of morphologically dissimilar objects with identical functions—that is, showed no "recognition" of the object—but nevertheless showed evidence of preserved vision in the usual tests of central visual acuity and peripheral visual fields. The impairment was specific to the visual modality, and performances were normal when the patient touched the object or heard it make its characteristic sound. The syndrome was well defined and has been employed consistently by clinicians interested in the subject in the past 70 years (for example, Dejerine [1914], von Monakow [1914], Pötzl [1928], Lange [1936], Nielsen [1937], Ajuriaguerra and Hécaen [1960], and Brain [1961]). However, in addition to its referring to the above syndrome, *visual agnosia* has come to have another meaning, defined not operationally but in psychological terms. This notion, originating with Lissauer's (1890) attempt to explain the abnormalities in his patient in psychological terms, is that the visual agnosic has intact "perception" but that his percepts have no "meaning." This theoretical concept of visual agnosia is not a satisfactory explanation of the syndrome, for reasons to be discussed later in the chapter. Here, I emphasize that in this paper the term *visual agnosia*, unless otherwise stated, is used to denote the syndrome defined above and not the theoretical concept.

Although studied since the latter part of the nineteenth century, the anatomic basis of visual agnosia in man is less securely established than is the syndrome of impaired visual discrimination in the monkey. This results, of course, from reliance on postmortem neuropathologic study. The number of cases of well-documented visual agnosia is small. With rare exceptions, cases that have been well studied clinically have not had postmortem examinations, whereas cases examined postmortem have often been studied insufficiently during life.

Despite these difficulties, there has been a remarkable degree of agreement among many authors who have tried intensively to establish the localization of visual agnosia (von Stauffenburg [1914], Pötzl [1928], Lange [1936], Nielsen [1937]). A major review is that of Nielsen (1937). Although Nielsen did not distinguish sufficiently between visual agnosia and (the independent syndrome of) visual disorientation, and although he considered only cases with unilateral cerebral disease, the former difficulty leads to exclusion of at most one or two of his cases and the latter can be supplemented with other reviews considering bilateral lesions as well. The "cortical area seemingly essential for the recognition of objects" that emerged from Nielsen's survey is illustrated in Part B of figure 1. This area comprises the ventral convexity portions of occipital and temporo-occipital cortex.

A second review is that of Pötzl (1928), who included cases with both bilateral and unilateral disease and who carefully distinguished visual agnosia from visual disorientation. According to Pötzl, visual agnosia results most frequently from infarction in the territory of the posterior cerebral arteries bilaterally. The crucial cerebral area is the ventral occipital convexity and the fusiform gyrus at the base of the temporo-occipital lobe. Unilateral, left-sided infarction of this area could also produce the syndrome if the corpus callosum was involved. Pötzl emphasized that the crucial area "lies very basally and often reaches far into the inferior portion of the temporal lobes anteriorly." He noted the frequency with which the white matter in these areas is more severely damaged than the overlying cortex.

Subsequent cases confirmed this localization. The majority (Heidenhain 1927; Hoff et al. 1962; Gloning et al. 1970; Lhermitte et al. 1972; Benson et al. 1974; Cohn et al. 1977) resulted from bilateral infarctions in the territory of the posterior cerebral arteries. The lesions involved the basal occipitotemporal regions, extending forward from a centimeter or two anterior to the occipital pole to at least the level of the splenium of the corpus callosum. The infarctions included variable portions of the cortex of lingual, fusiform, and inferior occipital gyri. There was consistent involvement of the white matter deep to these gyri, most often the white matter subjacent to the collateral sulcus and the contiguous lingual and fusiform gyri. This white matter consisted not only of the predominantly radially oriented fibers immediately subjacent to the cortex, but also of the basal portions of the strata sagitalia adjacent to the floor of the lateral ventricle. The affected white matter thus included

• cortico-cortical connections—both short fibers interconnecting gyri locally and longer fibers connecting inferior occipital cortex with temporal and inferior frontal cortex,

• afferent and efferent fibers interconnecting basal occipitotemporal cortex with subcortical structures (these connections include the inferior geniculocalcarine radiations as well as occipitotemporal connections to pulvinar, striatum, midbrain tectum and tegmentum, and basis pontis), and

• commissural fibers interconnecting the basal temporo-occipital regions of each hemisphere (these fibers traverse the ventral portions of the splenium of the corpus callosum).

Although the majority of cases have shown bilateral, roughly symmetric lesions of the basal temporo-occipital regions, one case showed a unilateral, left-sided lesion in this region (Caplan and Hedly-Whyte 1974), one case showed a right-sided temporo-occipital lesion associated with a left-sided lesion of the angular gyrus (Pevzner et al. 1962), and one case (involving a tumor) showed a right temporo-occipital lesion with only minimal involvement of the left hemisphere (Hécaen et al. 1957). The influence of such asymmetric distributions of lesions on the clinical manifestations of visual agnosia will be discussed later in the chapter.

It is thus clear that in man disorders of visual identification can occur in association with bilateral lesions of the cortex and white matter of the basal occipital and basal posterior temporal regions. The precise extent of relevant cortex is still unknown, because few cases are available and they have been relatively uniform in their pathology. For example, the precise lateral extension of relevant cortex beyond fusiform gyrus to inferior occipital and inferior temporal gyrus, or even to more dorsal cortex of the occipitotemporal convexity, remains unknown.

Despite our incomplete knowledge of the relevant human anatomy, the regions of known importance in man are remarkably similar to those in the monkey. In both, the occipital association cortex contiguous with the representation of the fovea in striate cortex appears to be important. In man, where much of the striate cortex has been dislodged from the lateral convexity of the hemisphere, the foveal portion of striate cortex lies at or near the occipital pole. The foveal "prestriate" region, which would correspond roughly with Nielsen's "essential area" (figure 1), is therefore more posterior than in the monkey. In both man and monkey inferior temporal neocortex is also important. In man, it is primarily the posterobasal portion of inferotemporal cortex that is known to be relevant, and the role of more lateral and more anterior inferotemporal cortex is still not clear. In the monkey, the important inferotemporal cortex extends laterally to the superior temporal sulcus and anteriorly toward the temporal pole.

Thus (except for the question of unilateral lesions, to be considered shortly), there is a striking correspondence between the lesions associated with human visual agnosia and the ablations that result in impaired visual discrimination in the monkey. It would thus appear that in man an interconnected system consisting of foveal striate, foveal prestriate, and inferotemporal cortex is necessary to prevent visual agnosia.

Behavioral Parallels

We have suggested that visual agnosia in man and impaired acquisition and retention of visual discrimination in monkeys (see Dean, this volume) have, as far as the available data will allow, identical anatomical substrates. It is now time to compare the behavioral deficits produced by comparable lesions in the two primates to determine to what extent they too are comparable.

The Problem

At the outset, the two syndromes appear different because one usually tests man and monkey differently. The patient is asked to "recognize" a visual stimulus. By "recognition" is meant a classification into one of a group of categories that correspond to those of the surrounding normal population. This classification may be verbal (the patient names the visual pattern) or nonverbal (the patient demonstrates the conventional use of the stimulus objects or sorts visual stimuli into different groups). It is obvious that every such classification is also a discrimination. For example, in naming the stimulus, the human patient is discriminating the object from others that would be labeled by different words in his vocabulary. (If he were severely aphasic so that his vocabulary consisted of a single word, naming would be neither a classification nor a discrimination.) "Recognition" is said to be impaired when no means of response, verbal or nonverbal, yields a set of classifications (discriminations) that corresponds to the conventional. The categories may be too broad, lumping conventionally differently classified patterns together, or they may be too narrow, such that each stimulus pattern is unique to itself. In addition to the above static changes, the classifications may fluctuate excessively, so that a given stimulus pattern, on separate occasions, is classified differently far in excess of normal tendencies. (Bruner [1957] emphasized that some fluctuations occur in the normal individual where classifications are influenced by needs and expectations as well as by the stimulus material.) If such impaired "recognition" of visual stimulus patterns exists in the presence of "sufficient" vision (tested by conventional measures of central acuity, e.g., the Snellen chart, and peripheral fields, e.g., kinetic perimetry) and normal "recognition" by touch and hearing, visual agnosia is said to exist.

The monkey, on the other hand, is usually faced with an apparatus in which there are several visual patterns. He is required to select one of these patterns consistently over successive trials. The number of such trials required to reach a preestablished criterial level of performance is compared with that of the normal monkey, and if it is excessive the discrimination performance is said to be impaired.

Several important differences between the performances demanded of man and monkey are thus evident:

- The monkey is often asked to acquire a new visual discrimination (that is, to form categories that it may never have had occasion to form before), whereas the human is asked to make a classification into conventional, well-established categories.
- The monkey is required to discriminate between only two (or at most among a few) visual patterns, that is, it must form only a twofold categorization system, whereas the human often must assign the pattern to one of a great number of possible categories (for example, in a naming task, all possible namable objects).
- The classification (discrimination) capacities of the monkey are conventionally tested with the very same visual patterns used to form the categories initially, whereas the human is often faced with a visual stimulus pattern not exactly like any he has used to form the category of which this stimulus pattern is an example (for example, he may never have seen a key of this shape before, but is still required to "recognize" it as a key).
- In learning a categorization, the monkey is usually given only the same two patterns, that is, one example per category, whereas the human has usually had a broad range of experience with many members of each category (he has previously classified as "keys" many patterns of different size and shape).
- The monkey is usually faced with all of the choices (in its visual presence is an example of each of the categories among which the discrimination is to be made), whereas the human is often faced with only one visual pattern and must select the proper response (category) from among many of which no examples are present.
- The discriminating (classifying) response of the monkey is a limb or whole-body movement (such as pointing to the correct discriminandum), whereas that requested from the human may be either a limb movement or a specific pattern of oro-linguo-laryngeal movements.

These differences, however, do not present as insurmountable an obstacle to comparing the behavior of man and monkey as might at first be expected. Several attempts to alter the monkey tests to correspond better to the tasks usually given humans demonstrate that deficits persist under the new test conditions. Thus, the work of Klüver and Bucy (1937, 1939) as well as the latter studies of Mishkin and Pribram (1954) established that, in monkeys with inferotemporal lesions, retention of previously acquired visual discriminations is affected in addition to the acquisition of new ones (the first difference listed above). Pribram and Mishkin (1955) showed that deficits also persist when the monkey is presented with only one stimulus pattern at a time and is required to respond discriminatively to it. This "go/no go" task is more similar to the situation of a human confronted with a single visual pattern and asked to respond with its name or its use (the fifth difference above). Butter et al. (1965) have shown that inferotemporally ablated monkeys are impaired in tests of "stimulus generalization," in which the animal, after acquiring a visual discrimination, is asked to respond to a new pair of stimuli resembling, but not identical to, those of the initial training (see the third difference above).

Conversely, if one alters the tests in human agnosics to correspond better to the customary testing situation in the monkey, the behavior remains abnormal. Thus, the agnosic patient reported on in Levine 1978, when tested for learning of a visual discrimination in a two-alternative forced-choice situation, was unable to point to the correct one of two complex visual patterns that differed very subtly (figure 2) though she succeeded with easier discriminations.

Once it is realized that many of the apparent differences between the behavior of the patient with visual agnosia and the monkey with impaired visual discrimination can be minimized by variations in testing procedures, many striking parallels emerge between the behavior of the two primates in tasks of visual form discrimination as well as in other types of visual and nonvisual tasks. Before discussing these parallels, however, we must consider the subdivision of both visual agnosia in man and impaired visual discrimination in the monkey.

Subdivisions of the Syndromes

To this point, we have treated the syndrome of impaired visual pattern discrimination in the monkey with foveal-prestriate and/or inferotemporal cortex damage as a single entity. The purpose of this treatment was to demonstrate its anatomical homology to the syndrome of visual agnosia in man, which we also have not subdivided. It is clear, however, that in both man and monkey the syndrome can be fractionated.

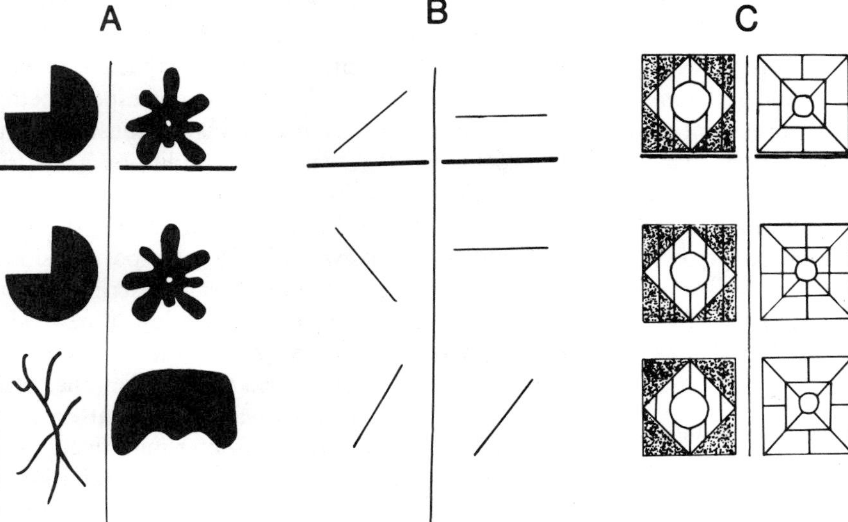

Figure 2. Examples of visual discrimination tasks that were quickly mastered (A, B) or never learned (C) by the visual agnosic reported on in Levine 1978. In each task the patient was presented with a card on which two patterns (below the thick horizontal lines) were displayed. The examiner indicated that one of the two shown above the line was correct. On subsequent trials the same two patterns were shown and the patient was asked to indicate the position of the correct choice verbally. (The relative positions of correct and incorrect choices were varied randomly from trial to trial. The number of trials preceeding 5 consecutive correct responses were recorded). Learning was immediate for 14 tasks similar to the 4 shown in A and B. No learning had occurred, even after 30 trials, for 4 tasks similar to the two shown in C.

In the monkey, Iwai and Mishkin (1968, 1969) and Cowey and Gross (1970) have shown that foveal-prestriate lesions produce a qualitatively different impairment of visual pattern discrimination from inferotemporal lesions. On the one hand, monkeys with foveal-prestriate lesions are more impaired than inferotemporally lesioned animals in acquiring and retaining discriminations between three-dimensional visual objects or two-dimensional visual patterns but are less impaired with color discrimination. Once a discrimination has been acquired, the addition of an extra but irrelevant visual cue distracts (impairs performance of) foveal-prestriate-lesioned but not inferotemporally lesioned animals (Gross et al. 1971). On the other hand, monkeys with inferotemporal lesions are more impaired than those with foveal-prestriate lesions in tasks of "concurrent discrimination." For a procedure of concurrent discrimination only simple pairs of discriminanda are used that would be no trouble, even for the monkey with lesions, if presented alone. However, several such tasks are presented concurrently so that the same task does not appear on successive trials. The greater impairment of inferotemporally lesioned monkeys on tasks of concurrent discrimination has led to the interpretation that inferotemporal lesions produce a deficit in visual "association" or "memory" (Cowey and Gross 1970), whereas the foveal-prestriate deficit is more "perceptual" in nature, amounting to a disturbance in "selective attention" necessary in the orderly construction of a percept.

Wilson et al. (1972) demonstrated that the "memory" defect of the monkey with inferotemporal lesions could not be interpreted in the sense of decay of a trace, because in a matching-to-sample task increasing delay between presentation of the sample and presentation of the choices did not affect the performances of inferotemporal animals any more than it did those of normal or foveal-prestriate monkeys. It is possible that the "memory" deficit may relate to another aspect of the behavior of inferotemporal monkeys demonstrated by Wilson. She showed that these animals have more "intrusion errors" than either foveal-prestriate or normal monkeys in a matching-to-sample problem; they often err by responding in the same manner as on the previous trial. Such proactive interference, or perseveration, in addition to accounting for impaired acquisition of concurrent discrimination, might also explain the beneficial effect of adding punishment for wrong responses to reward for correct responses on the performances of the inferotemporal monkeys (but not the foveal-prestriate animals) in visual discrimination tasks (Manning 1971). The punishment may minimize the tendency to perseverate by approaching the wrong (punished) discriminandum on subsequent trials. A similar explanation may apply to the deterioration in the performances of inferotemporal animals when only intermittent reinforcement is given (Manning et al. 1971).

The perseveration itself, however, may be a result of, or may be associated with, other impairments. Thus, it appears that inferotemporally lesioned animals do not employ a flexible strategy that results in detecting the relevant features in a discrimination problem and in disregarding the irrelevant. That is, the relative values of the component features in determining the response are not those of the normal animal. This distortion of feature values involves not only the various linear and contour features of a shape in a shape-discrimination problem (Butter et al. 1965; Butter 1968) but also a tendency to devalue shape and orientation cues altogether in favor of brightness differences (Iversen and Weiskrantz 1967). Perseveration may at least partially reflect this inflexibility in perceptual strategy, and may represent the stubborn clinging to a distorted set of values of the stimulus features.

In man, cases of visual agnosia have been subdivided into two groups since Lissauer (1890) distinguished "apperceptive" from "as sociative" visual agnosia on a largely theoretical basis. The former group had an abnormality of "apperception," which Lissauer defined as "the seizing by consciousness of sensory impressions." Abnormal "apperception" could be detected, despite adequate central visual acuity and peripheral visual fields, by requiring the patient to make a "judgment" about his perception. Thus, the patient would be unable to draw a visual stimulus pattern or to match it with an identical pattern in an array of stimulus patterns. The "associative" agnosic, on the other hand, had intact (or nearly intact) "apperception" but was impaired in "association," which to Lissauer meant the ability to relate the trace of the visual stimulus pattern in the occipital cortex to past traces left by the object in other sensory areas of the brain (via corticocortical pathways from occipital lobe to other sensory areas). In actual fact, cases of visual object agnosia do vary between two extremes that in the neurological literature are usually classified as either "apperceptive" or "associative." (The further subdivision of associative agnosia into object agnosia and prosopagnosia will be discussed later.) I shall use these terms as descriptive of syndromes, though I do not feel that the psychological or anatomical formulations of Lissauer best describe them.

The cases of "apperceptive" visual agnosia (Goldstein and Gelb 1918; Adler 1944, Benson and Greenberg 1969) have an extremely severe defect in discriminating shapes, but retain nearly normal absolute and differential brightness thresholds and nearly normal visual fields when tested by kinetic perimetry (Benson and Greenberg 1969). The shape-discrimination deficit is so severe that the patient is unable to distinguish, for example, a circle from a cross. A patient examined by the author was an inveterate card player, yet was unable to distinguish a diamond from a club, though visual acuity by testing detection of black dots of different sizes on a white background was at least 20/70 and the upper quadrants of both right and left homonymous visual fields were full. Such patients are completely unable to copy or match visual stimulus patterns. Despite the severe problem with form discrimination, most of these patients have been able to discriminate and to name colors. They are also highly susceptible to distraction by adjacent (Adler 1944) or overlapping (Goldstein and Gelb 1918) visual objects when attempting a visual discrimination performance. Patients with "associative" visual agnosia (see, for example, Lissauer 1890; Heidenhain 1927; Rubens and Benson 1971), on the other hand, are less impaired in shape discrimination. They are, as a rule, able to discriminate and name simple geometric figures such as circles and squares. However, their performances on more difficult discrimination tasks are not normal, and failure can be elicited when the discriminanda are complex patterns that differ from each other subtly (Levine 1978). This point is important, for since the time of Lissauer it has been claimed that accurate performance in matching a visual sample to one of a set of choices by an associative visual agnosic guaranteed that "perception" was intact. However, in fact, these patients match much more slowly than do normals, accomplishing the task by painstakingly comparing components of the discriminanda serially until they detect differences. Thus, they often become hypercritical; that is, their categories become very narrow. For example, Rubens and Benson's patient said that two identical patterns were different because he included slight smudges of printer's ink or irregularities in the texture of the paper in his comparisons. The same procedure is employed in drawing an object. The end product may be good, but drawing is performed slowly, proceeding serially ("slavishly") feature by feature to build up the final product. The inadequacy in discrimination (categorization) is also revealed in tasks of naming and sorting, where underspecification occurs; that is, the patient names an object with a similar overall shape or an identical inner detail (Levine 1978). These patients, as a rule, are less distracted than the apperceptive agnosics by extraneous visual stimuli, but response perseveration—calling an item by the same name that was given to a previous item—is very common.

From the foregoing discussion, it appears that there are parallels in the behavior of the inferotemporally lesioned monkey and the human associative visual agnosic, and in the behavior of the foveal-prestriate-lesioned monkey and the human apperceptive visual agnosic.

Behavioral Parallels Between Human Associative Visual Agnosia and Simian Inferotemporal Visual Discrimination Impairment

The first parallel between the two syndromes is that, in both, the disturbance is reflected in only one sensory sphere: the visual. Monkeys with inferotemporal lesions and impairment in acquiring visual discriminations have shown normal abilities to acquire olfactory discriminations (Brown 1963; Brown et al. 1963), tactile discriminations (Wilson 1957; Pasik et al. 1958), and auditory discriminations (Weiskrantz and Mishkin 1958). In the human visual agnosic this can also be the case (Pötzl 1928; Rubens and Benson 1971), although often there is mild difficulty in naming through other modalities as well (Ettlinger and Wyke 1961; Levine 1978). However, where nonvisual naming difficulties occur, they are much less severe than the visual disturbance.

A second parallel is that disturbances in "elementary" visual functions are not sufficient to account for the inability to make visual form discriminations. "Elementary" visual functions are difficult to define in a manner that will distinguish them precisely from more "complex" functions such as the discrimination of complex forms. Roughly, they comprise discriminations that utilize one or two points of light and can be plotted as a function of the position of these points in the visual fields—such as visual acuity (discrimination of two points from one), absolute and differential brightness thresholds (which determine the "visual fields" of static or kinetic perimetry and amount to discrimination of one point from none), flicker-fusion frequencies, or the closely related tachistoscopic sensation time and adaptation time.

In the inferotemporally lesioned monkey, "elementary" visual function has been assessed in several ways. Visual fields are normal when tested by a method resembling static perimetry in man (Cowey and Weiskrantz 1967). Central visual acuity is also normal when tested by the ability to discriminate alternating black and white vertical stripes (that can be made progressively narrower) from a homogeneous field of the same total luminous flux (Weiskrantz and Cowey 1963). These studies were performed without normal controls, and one cannot assert that the functions were entirely normal; however, they were in all cases better than in animals with lesions of striate cortex, even though the latter perform better on tests of visual form discrimination. Similarly, critical flicker-fusion thresholds in the central visual fields are either slightly (Mishkin and Weiskrantz 1959) or not at all (Symmes 1965) affected by inferotemporal lesions—again different from the case with lesions of striate cortex, where flicker thresholds are worse though form-discrimination performance is better than in inferotemporal animals.

Humans with associative visual agnosia may have normal central visual acuity (see, e.g., Bay 1952 for a report of tests requiring tracing and matching simple forms of progressively smaller size; see also Rubens and Benson, 1971) and normal visual fields (Bay 1952) when tested by kinetic perimetry. Although Bay (1952, 1953) claimed that impaired tachistoscopic sensation time and shortened local adaptation time (probably very similar to elevated flicker-fusion thresholds) are invariably present in human visual agnosics, Ettlinger (1956) and Ettlinger and Wyke (1961) demonstrated that nonagnosic patients may have more severe impairment on such tests than patients with visual agnosia. Unfortunately, in assessing visuosensory efficiency in his patients, Ettlinger did not distinguish impairment in central visual fields from impairment in the peripheral fields. More recently, however, Levine and Calvanio (1980) demonstrated no correlation between impaired identification of pictures of objects and elevated central flicker-fusion frequency in patients with bilateral lesions of the posterior cerebrum. The situation in man thus appears to parallel that in the monkey.

Although disturbances of "elementary" visual functions are not sufficiently severe to entail either associative visual agnosia in man or the inferotemporal discrimination deficit in monkey, it is apparent that stressing these functions will impair performance far more than in normal man or monkey. The effects of reducing visual angle of the discriminanda (stimulus size) in a form-discrimination task is one example. In the inferotemporally lesioned (Pasik et al. 1960) and in the foveal-prestriate-lesioned (Iversen 1973) monkey, reducing the size of the discriminanda adversely affected the ability to discriminate a triangle from a square or a triangle from a plus, though even the smallest stimulus used was well within the range of normal acuity. In the author's human agnosic (Levine 1978) there was a suggestion that larger objects were better described than small objects of similar shape. Moreover, better naming of large than of small letters may occur in agnosic alexia in man (Rubens and Benson 1971; Woods and Poppel 1974). In the human agnosic, other stresses of elementary visual functions also impair form discrimination at levels not affecting normal performance at all. Reduced background illumination, reduced contrast between stimulus and background, or reduced exposure time of the stimulus patterns markedly impaired form discrimination in an agnosic patient (Levine 1978), whereas control subjects were not at all affected in the range of variables used. These studies should be made in the monkey, where lesions can be better controlled.

In addition to modality specificity and to lack of dependence on disturbances of "elementary" visual function, the syndromes of associative visual agnosia in man and of impaired visual discrimination in inferotemporally lesioned monkeys show marked parallels with respect to the nature of the errors made in tasks of visual discrimination:

- Associative visual agnosics characteristically make errors of "underspecification" (Levine 1978). When asked to name a visually presented object, they often give the name of an object that has a roughly similar outline or topological structure to that of the object presented. Or they may name a prominent feature of the presented object, or give the name of another object that shares this feature (and perhaps no others) with the object presented. Thus, Rubens and Benson's (1971) patient called a key a "violin" (topological similarity) and the author's patient called a harmonica a "comb" because she confined her attention to the spaces separated by wooden partitions, which she took to be the teeth of the comb. In the inferotemporal monkey the experiments of Butter et al. (1965) and of Butter (1968) established that the animal also attends excessively to a single feature of the discriminanda in learning visual discriminations. For example, it attends more than the normal monkey to the horizontal base line of a triangle in learning to choose it instead of a circle. Hence, in an equivalence test it will select a semicircle instead of an inverted triangle, whereas a normal monkey will not. This impairment in pattern equivalence thus resembles the behavior in man that has been called underspecification of the discriminandum.

• A very frequent characteristic of humans with associative visual agnosia is perseveration; that is, these subjects name an object shown them with the name of an object that they had previously been shown or thought that they had been shown (Lissauer 1890, Pötzl 1928; Critchley 1964; Levine 1978). The perseveration is specific to tasks of visual discrimination and does not appear in perceptual tasks in other modalities. Thus, the author's patient called most of the objects shown to her in one series of observations a pen. At times the perseveration is so strong that even salient features of the object held before the eyes are disregarded. More often, however, perseveration will occur when the name perseverated (i.e., that of a previous object) denotes an object that is also an underspecification of the object currently presented, and will not occur when the object presented does not at all resemble previous objects morphologically. In the monkey, as previously mentioned, Wilson et al. (1972) showed the presence of more "intrusion" errors (i.e., perseveration) in animals with inferotemporal lesions than in normal monkeys or monkeys with foveal-prestriate lesions.

The syndromes in man and in monkey are further parallel in the beneficial effects of "overtraining" on the performance of visual discriminations. In the monkey, extensive preoperative experience with a form discrimination minimizes the retention deficit after inferotemporal lesions (Orbach and Fantz 1959). In the human agnosic, although the effects of prelesion "overtraining" cannot be readily studied, the relative lack of impairment of visual identification in familiar surroundings has often been mentioned (Pötzl 1928; Critchley 1964). The author's patient (Levine 1978) was able to identify objects better when she saw them utilized in their natural manner (e.g., a toothbrush brushing teeth) than when they were held motionless or were rotated and moved back and forth in front of her eyes.

Several of the above parallels between inferotemporally lesioned monkey and agnosic human can be summarized by the more general parallel that visual discriminations easily acquired by the normal organism are acquired with little difficulty and eventually to the same level of proficiency by the organism with lesions, while tasks difficult for the normal may never be acquired to the normal level of proficiency by the damaged organism or may require extensive and prolonged training. Gross (1972) reviewed this principle for the inferotemporally lesioned monkey. In man this principle is less well established. However, the author's patient (Levine 1978) easily mastered visual discriminations that were obvious to normals, but could not acquire discrimination between subtly different complex forms (figure 2).

Behavioral Parallels Between Human Apperceptive Visual Agnosia and Foveal-Prestriate Visual Discrimination Deficit in the Monkey

Much less can be said about the relationship of these syndromes than about the relationship between associative visual agnosia and the inferotemporal visual discrimination deficit. This ignorance arises from the fact that the significance of the foveal-prestriate region in the monkey has only recently been appreciated and less information about the effects of foveal-prestriate lesions is available than about the effects of inferotemporal (TE) lesions. Even more limiting is the paucity of cases of "apperceptive" visual agnosia in man. Not a single one of the available clinically studied cases has had postmortem examination, in contrast with the situation for associative visual agnosia. Because several of the cases (Adler 1944, 1950; Benson and Greenberg 1969) arose in the context of asphyxiation, where lesions may be widespread, it is unclear to what degree the symptoms reflect foveal-prestriate damage independent of involvement of other areas.

Nevertheless, several parallels between apperceptive visual agnosia in man and foveal-prestriate visual discrimination impairment in monkey are evident when one considers them in relation to associative visual agnosia and inferotemporal visual discrimination deficit, respectively:

• The discrimination deficit is more severe, as mentioned previously. In the monkey, this has been shown for three-dimensional visual objects, for two-dimensional visual patterns, and in pattern-equivalence tests (Gross 1973). Human apperceptive visual agnosics cannot discriminate, name, or draw even simple geometric figures (Benson and Greenberg 1969; Brown 1972), whereas associative visual agnosics can.

• Although form discrimination is more impaired, color discrimination is relatively preserved. Gross et al. (1971) demonstrated this in monkeys with foveal prestriate lesions. Also, the human patients of Adler (1944) and Benson and Greenberg (1969) were able to name colors despite the severe form-discrimination deficit.

• Distraction by irrelevant features of the discriminandum is prominent. Gross et al. (1971) showed that foveal-prestriate-lesioned monkeys performed poorly on a visual form discrimination that they had already mastered when an irrelevant color cue was added to the forms to be discriminated, whereas inferotemporally lesioned animals were less affected. Iversen (1973) showed that irrelevant forms, either surrounding or partially covering the discriminanda, impaired discrimination in foveal-prestriate animals but not in controls. The human apperceptive visual agnosic also is even further impaired in efforts at naming simple visual patterns if a line is drawn over them (Goldstein and Gelb 1918), whereas such need not be the case in associative visual agnosia (Heidenhain 1927). Such distractability may be merely a manifestation of the severity of the form-discrimination deficit in both monkey and man. Thus one might expect similar distractability with inferotemporally lesioned monkeys and human associative visual agnosics if the discriminanda and the overlapping distractions are made more complex.

• The pattern of eye movements during the examination of visual discriminanda is abnormal in foveal-prestriate monkeys (it is also abnormal in inferotemporal animals; see Oscar-Berman et al. 1973), and was abnormal in Benson and Greenberg's (1969) apperceptive visual agnosic. These eye-movement abnormalities may reflect the difficulty of the form discrimination.

The relationship of impaired visual discrimination in foveal-prestriate-lesioned monkeys and of apperceptive visual agnosia in man to disturbances of "elementary" visual function has not yet been clarified. In the foveal-prestriate monkey, Bender (1973) demonstrated normal brightness thresholds under scotopic conditions, but visual-acuity tests (i.e., two-point discrimination), static perimetry, and tests incorporating temporal factors such as flicker fields have not been done, as they have for the inferotemporal animals. In humans, Efron (1968) demonstrated only modest elevation of brightness thresholds, mild decreases in flicker-fusion thresholds, and full perimetric fields in Benson and Greenberg's patient with apperceptive agnosia. Visual acuity was not measured. Clearly more work must be done in both monkey and man in this area.

Thus, it has been established that numerous parallels exist between the syndromes of impaired visual discrimination in monkeys with foveal-prestriate and inferotemporal lesions and the syndromes of visual agnosia (psychic blindness) in man. The analogous behavior and homologous anatomic localization of the syndromes in the two primates makes it likely that similar physiologic processes are impaired in each. In the following section I shall demonstrate that in both man and monkey these syndromes are at least partially dissociable from other syndromes of the temporal lobe and from other disturbances of visual behavior resulting from parietal and parieto-occipital lesions.

Other Syndromes

In this section a number of syndromes that may be found in association with visual agnosia in man or impaired visual discrimination in the monkey will be discussed. The purpose of this discussion is to show that the syndromes are at least partially independent of visual agnosia and impaired visual discrimination. This partial independence suggests that the anatomic substrates of these syndromes are not congruent with those of visual agnosia, though some overlap may occur. The term "visual agnosia," if it is to be applied in its usual sense, should, therefore, not be used in reference to these other syndromes.

The first syndrome that must be distinguished from impaired visual discrimination in the monkey and visual agnosia in man is the portion of the "Klüver-Bucy syndrome" produced by resection of part or all of the territory occupied by the amygdaloid body and adjacent pyriform cortex, neocortex at the tip of the temporal lobe (von Bonin and Bailey's TG), the anterior insula, and the cortex of the orbital surface of the frontal lobe. Monkeys with bilateral lesions of this entire area (Pribram and Bagshaw 1953) demonstrate marked tameness in that they approach or allow themselves to be approached and touched by human observers without displaying fear or aggression. "Hypermetamorphosis" is common, as is ingestion of inedible, unpalatable, and noxious objects such as burning paper, feces, or sharp metal objects. They often approach other monkeys abnormally frequently to groom or to mount, but do not interact normally with their fellows and lose their social status. With more restricted lesions in this area, such as those of amygdala and pyriform cortex alone (Walker et al. 1953; Weiskrantz 1956), the tameness is prominent but hypermetamorphosis either is absent or disappears after a week or two. Instead the animals appear apathetic, sitting in one place with drooping head and arms for prolonged periods and apparently not attending to their environment. Sexual activity is usually decreased, but recovers at a point when tameness and apathy may still be present. The tameness is prominent for visual stimuli (for example, humans or noxious objects), but snarling may be obtained (in some animals) by tail pinch. Conditioned avoidance may be acquired when the reinforcement is electric shock, but not when it is the sight of a man, although acquisition is slower than normal even to electric shock.

It is beyond the scope of this article (and perhaps not possible) to fractionate the components of this "orbitofrontal–anterior temporal" syndrome according to the site of lesion within this system. The major point to be made here is that the results of tests of visual discrimination (Pribram and Bagshaw 1953; Mishkin 1954; Schwartzbaum 1965) have been normal or nearly normal in all such animals. Hearst and Pribram (1964) demonstrated that stimulus generalization with respect to the dimension of background illumination was also normal in animals with bilateral amygdalectomy. To date, there have been no studies of generalization with respect to pattern discrimination analogous to the experiments of Butter et al. (1965) and of Butter (1968) with inferotemporally lesioned monkeys. However, given the information (see below) from human cases with similar lesions, it is predicted that these will be normal as well. If so, it is clear that these animals can discriminate visual patterns normally and can group visual patterns into the usual categories employed by normal monkeys.

In man, similar cases have been reported (see, for example, Terzian and Dalle Ore 1955; Friedman and Allen 1969; Gascon and Gilles 1973); all these cases included lesions of hippocampal formation as well as part or all of the fronto-temporal regions mentioned above). Gascon and Gilles (1973) reported the most detailed study of behavior. After an encephalitic illness, the patient, a young housewife, was left in a state called by the authors "limbic dementia." She wandered continuously about the ward, was found aimlessly searching through other patients' drawers, and often mouthed inedible objects, at one time even feces. Her attention span was very short. She was highly distractable and was unable to sustain goal-directed activity. Although no overt sexual behavior was observed, a psychiatric examiner suggested sexual connotations in her conversation and that she showed "confused courting" of the examiner. In addition to this "limbic dementia" an amnesic syndrome was present. Despite the above permanent changes, after the first few weeks of her illness she was consistently able to name common objects, pictures of common objects, and body parts. She was able to read aloud and to match a printed noun to the appropriate picture. She was also able to name colors well. In short, there was no evidence of the syndrome of visual agnosia. Postmortem examination showed bilateral destruction of amygdala, pyriform cortex, anterior tips of the temporal lobe, and parts of the posterior orbital cortex and the cingulate gyri. The hippocampus and parahippocampal regions were destroyed bilaterally. In addition, the fusiform gyrus on the left and both fusiform and inferior temporal gyri on the right were partially damaged. The latter incomplete damage to the posterior inferotemporal neocortex probably accounted for the transient misnaming of common objects in the first few weeks of illness. This misnaming at that time showed, from the few examples given by the author, the visual underspecification (e.g., thermometer: "needle") characteristic of visual agnosics.

It appears, then, that the orbitofrontal–anterior temporal syndrome of tameness, "hypermetamorphosis" with oral tendencies, and abnormal sexual behavior may occur without impaired visual discrimination in monkey and without the syndrome of visual agnosia in man. The reverse dissociation is also clear. Monkeys with inferotemporal or foveal-prestriate lesions and impaired visual discrimination do not as a rule show the orbitofrontal–anterior temporal syndrome (see, e.g., Mishkin and Pribram 1954; Cowey and Gross 1970).

The independence of the syndromes of striate-prestriate-in-ferotemporal cortex from those of orbitofrontal–anterior temporal cortex in both monkey and man makes it unwise to use the term *visual agnosia* to describe both syndromes. Unfortunately, that term has been applied to many of the symptoms of the orbitofrontal–anterior temporal syndrome, such as hypermetamorphosis, oral tendencies, and indiscriminate sexual behavior. When used in this sense, *visual agnosia* is no longer referring to the syndromes of impaired visual discrimination characteristic of striate-prestriate-inferotemporal lesions; instead it is being used in the theoretical sense of "an intact but meaningless percept." The argument is that, since the organism no longer responds discriminatively to visual objects with respect to the behavioral dimension "to be approached/to be avoided," the objects have lost their "meaning." But, as we have just seen, human patients (and probably monkeys) with the orbitofrontal–anterior temporal syndrome may categorize visual patterns into their conventional groups (for example, by naming, by sorting, or by generalization tests), and in this sense the visual patterns do have "meaning." The loss of "meaning" of visual objects in the orbitofrontal–anterior temporal syndrome is only partial; it is restricted to the behavioral dimension of approach/avoidance. If the term *agnosia* is applied here, one might argue that it should be applied to other syndromes with partial loss of the "meaning" of visual stimuli—for example, to apraxia, where the patient has lost the "meaning" of an object with respect to how to use it; or to aphasia where the patient has lost the "meaning" of an object with respect to how to name it. It would thus seem wise to restrict the term *visual agnosia* to the deficits in visual identification (discrimination) resulting from damage to the foveal striate, foveal prestriate, and inferotemporal portions of the cerebral hemispheres.

Although I would discourage the use of the term *visual agnosia* to describe the orbitofrontal–anterior temporal syndrome, I do not wish to deny that this syndrome may be at least partially modality-specific. Several investigations, as previously discussed, have demonstrated more prominent loss of avoidance for visual stimuli than for stimuli such as electric shock to the skin. Perhaps the modality specificity relates to the strong input from inferotemporal cortex to amygdala, as demonstrated by Whitlock and Nauta (1956). However, one must note that the stimuli used to assess modality specificity in animals with orbitofrontal–anterior temporal lesions may not really be comparable. One should present such animals with complex natural sounds (such as the growl of a leopard) instead of a loud noise, or with complex, natural tactile patterns (such as the crawl of a scorpion) instead of electric shock. If the animals were to respond with avoidance to these but not to complex visual patterns such as the human face, modality specificity would be better established than it is at present. Furthermore, although inputs to basolateral amygdala are particularly heavy from inferotemporal (visual) cortex, Druga (1969–1970) demonstrated in the cat that the heaviest connections seemed to arise from an area corresponding most closely to Woolsey's auditory AII area.

A second temporal-lobe syndrome that is at least partially dissociable from visual agnosia in man is the amnesic syndrome. Patients with amnesia show only mild or no impairment in recall of material that is within the normal immediate span, provided no distracting stimuli are introduced in the interval between presentation and recall. But with the introduction of distracting stimuli, or with lists of items exceeding immediate span, marked deficits in recall occur (Scoville and Milner 1957; Drachman and Arbit 1966). The deficit is not specific to any particular sensory modality of stimulus presentation.

It is beyond the scope of this chapter to deal in detail with the behavioral characteristics of the amnesic syndrome. It is sufficient to point out that such patients, although unable to learn to identify new visual stimuli, do not have difficulty identifying even complex visual patterns with which they have had extensive experience prior to the onset of their lesions. Thus, they display no signs of visual agnosia (Milner and Teuber 1968). Conversely, although patients with associative visual agnosia often perform subnormally on standardized tests of memory (e.g., verbal paired-associate learning subtest of the Wechsler Memory Scale), they do better than patients with the amnesic syndrome. Visual agnosics, to the extent that they can discriminate and classify visual patterns, have little difficulty with subsequent recall, provided that they "see it the same way" (i.e., make the same classification) on representation (Pötzl 1927; Levine 1978).

The neuropathology of the amnesic syndrome is still not entirely clear. Those postmortem examinations that have been conducted have shown that cases associated with temporal-lobe lesions have generally resulted from bilateral infarctions in the territory of the posterior cerebral arteries (Victor et al. 1961; DeJong et al. 1969). Bilateral lesions of Ammon's horn and parahippocampal gyrus have been present, but damage also has extended laterally to the fusiform gyrus and posteriorly to the occipital lobe to a variable degree. Thus, there is considerable overlap with the neuropathology found in associative visual agnosia. Further studies will be required to determine the precise extent to which the amnesic syndrome and the syndrome of associative visual agnosia can be dissociated, both clinically and pathologically.

There remains considerable controversy over the existence of an amnesic syndrome in the monkey with lesions of corresponding structures. Bilateral hippocampectomy in the monkey has not resulted in the expected deficits in discrimination learning (Orbach et al. 1960; Kimble and Pribram 1963). Two explanations of these results have generally been offered: that hippocampal lesions alone are not the basis for amnesia either in monkey or in man (Horel 1978), and that hippocampectomy in the monkey does produce a deficit in memory if appropriate methods of testing (Gaffan 1974) or appropriate interpretation of experimental results (Douglas 1967) are employed. In any event, the behavioral syndrome resulting from hippocampectomy, whatever its relationship to the human amnesic syndrome, appears to be dissociable from impairments in acquisition and retention of visual pattern discriminations. Monkeys with hippocampal lesions are normal in acquiring visual pattern, size, and brightness discriminations (Kimble and Pribram 1963; Douglas and Pribram 1966).

Yet another syndrome that must be distinguished from visual-object agnosia in man and from the syndrome of impaired visual discrimination in the monkey is the syndrome of visual disorientation described initially by Balint (1909), by Holmes (1918), and by Holmes and Horrax (1919). Patients with this syndrome in severe form are unable to localize extrapersonal visual objects by reaching for them with their limbs. Thus, they misreach for objects they wish to grasp, and in drawing or writing they lose the place when the pencil is lifted from the paper. They cannot state which of two objects is nearer to their own bodies or to an external landmark, and cannot traverse a path without colliding with obstacles. Disturbances of eye movement are present. The patients have marked difficulty capturing by fixation objects in the peripheral visual fields, show instability of fixation once it is achieved, and show difficulty in tracking moving objects in a textured visual field. They do not converge or accommodate to approaching visual objects, nor do they blink to an approaching visual threat. Yet visual agnosia is not present. Visual patterns that normally can be recognized without the need for eye movement, including geometric shapes, common objects, and faces, are usually promptly and accurately named (Balint 1909; Holmes 1918; Holmes and Horrax 1919; Hécaen and Ajuriaguerra 1954; Godwin-Austen 1965; Michel et al. 1965). The literature contains six cases of visual disorientation with subsequent postmortem examinations (Balint 1909; Holmes 1981 [2]; Hécaen and Ajuriaguerra 1954 [2]; Michel et al. 1965). The lesions in these cases are more dorsal than those resulting in visual agnosia, and involve the parietal lobes. The cortex of the precuneus, superior parietal lobule, intraparietal fissure, and portions of supramarginal and angular gyri is often affected, and much of the subjacent white matter is usually involved. The area is thus quite distinct from the more ventral temporo-occipital region involved in visual agnosia.

The converse dissociation is also clear—at least with respect to the "associative" type of visual agnosia, in which patients may show no difficulties in orienting their limbs to visual objects, in walking about, in scanning a visual array, or in discriminating lengths of lines (see, e.g., Heidenhain 1927; Rubens and Benson 1971). However, the same may not be true of patients with apperceptive visual agnosia. Although they may navigate adequately in their environment (see Goldstein and Gelb 1918; Adler 1944, 1950; Benson and Greenberg 1969), there are abnormalities of eye movement and disturbances of drawing (Adler 1944; Benson and Greenberg 1969) that resemble features of the syndrome of visual disorientation. Other features of visual disorientation, such as prehension of visual objects and distance discriminations, have not been adequately assessed in these patients. Even if frequently accompanied by features of visual disorientation, the latter may not necessarily be present in apperceptive visual agnosia, for the cases of Adler and of Benson and Greenberg were the result of asphyxiation, in which more widespread lesions were undoubtedly present that those accounting for the visual agnosia. Or the abnormalities in drawing and in eye movement in apperceptive visual agnosia may differ qualitatively from those of visual disorientation. Only further detailed clinical and pathological studies can resolve these questions.

A syndrome resembling visual disorientation can be produced in the monkey by bilateral ablation of Brodmann's areas 5 and 7 on the medial and lateral surfaces of the hemispheres as well as the dorsal portion of the prelunate gyrus (part of areas 18 and 19 of Brodmann). Such animals misreach for visual stimulus objects (Pribram and Barry 1956; Ettlinger and Waegner 1958; Bates and Ettlinger 1960). They have difficulty grading their leaps, so they often collide with obstacles and have trouble finding their own cages among many in the laboratory (Bates and Ettlinger 1960). Pohl (1973), using monkeys with more restricted lesions (sparing area 5 but including area 7 and dorsal 18 and 19), showed impairments in discriminating which of two identical food wells was closer to a given extrapersonal landmark. Inferotemporally lesioned animals show none of these disturbances (Bates and Ettlinger 1960; Pohl 1973). Data are not yet available concerning the effects of foveal-prestriate lesions on these tasks. Conversely, monkeys with superior parietal lesions do not show any impairment in visual shape discrimination when compared with unoperated controls (Bates and Ettlinger 1960; Pohl 1973). Thus, this syndrome is doubly dissociable from the syndrome of impaired acquisition and retention of visual shape discrimination produced by inferotemporal lesions, and is at least singly dissociable from the impaired visual form discrimination produced by foveal-prestriate lesions. Further experiments comparing foveal-prestriate and superior posterior parietal lesions with respect to tasks of visual orientation would be informative (see Ungerleider and Mishkin, this volume).

Finally, visual-object agnosia is also doubly dissociable from the disturbances associated with damage to the angular gyri of either the dominant or the nondominant hemisphere in man. Constructural apraxia, the inability to construct copies of visual patterns, was first described by Kleist (1934). He emphasized the independence of these constructional disturbances from those characteristics of visual disorientation and localized the syndrome to cortex of the angular gyrus. (Deeper lesions involving the strata saggitalia produce visual disorientation.) Later, Paterson and Zangwill (1944) established that, at least with lesions of the nondominant hemisphere, the analysis of spatial relations of elements of a compound visual structure is impaired even when no complex praxic task is required. Thus, the terms *visuo-spatial agnosia* and *apractagnosia for spatial relations* have been used in the English literature to denote this disturbance in the analysis and synthesis of spatial relations. Both early investigations (Lange 1936) and extensive later studies (e.g., Ettlinger et al. 1957) established the lack of visual-object agnosia in patients with severe constructional apraxia. Conversely, a defining feature of associative visual agnosia is the ability of the patient to copy even complex visual patterns accurately, albeit slowly. Thus, associative visual agnosia constructional apraxia are independent syndromes.

The same is probably true with regard to apperceptive visual agnosia. In apperceptive visual agnosia, although copying of visual patterns is extremely poor (Adler 1944; Benson and Greenberg 1969), the nature of the impairment resembles that of severe visual disorientation (constant losing of place resulting in "piecemeal drawings") far more than it does constructional apraxia (no losing of place, rotational errors prominent). The relationship of the drawing disturbances in the syndromes of apperceptive visual agnosia, visual disorientation, and visual spatial agnosia needs further study.

In the dominant hemisphere, lesions of angular gyrus produce, in addition to constructional disturbances, the elements of Gerstmann's syndrome: right-left confusion, finger agnosia, acalculia, and agraphia. This syndrome may occur in severe form without visual agnosia (Gerstmann 1931; Stengel 1944), and, conversely, associative visual agnosia occurs independent of the Gerstmann syndrome (Rubens and Benson 1971). Data on "apperceptive" visual agnosia are not available.

One feature distinguishing the above syndromes of the angular gyrus from visual-object agnosia is the multimodal nature of the former. Constructional apraxia (visuospatial agnosia) probably involves difficulties in spatial analysis not only of visual patterns but of tactile patterns as well (Ettlinger et al. 1957; Levine, unpublished observations). Finger agnosia is also characteristically a supramodal deficit (Lange 1936; Kinsbourne and Warrington 1962). This lack of modality specificity is understandable in view of anatomical studies (Pandya and Kuypers 1969; Jones and Powell 1970) demonstrating that in the rhesus monkey the cortex in the walls of the superior temporal sulcus —presumably a rudimentary homologue of the human angular gyrus—receives converging projections from visual, auditory, and somesthetic association areas.

Thus, in man, the syndromes of visual agnosia produced by foveal-prestriate and inferotemporal lesions are at least partially dissociable from the orbitofronto-anterior temporal syndrome, the amnesic syndrome, visual disorientation, and spatial apractagnosia. Correspondingly, in the monkey, impaired visual discrimination from foveal-prestriate and inferotemporal lesions is dissociable from the fronto-temporal syndrome, the hippocampal syndrome, and parietal-lobe syndromes.

The Question of Dominance

To this point I have demonstrated the striking anatomic and behavioral parallels between the syndromes of impaired visual discrimination in the monkey and the syndromes of apperceptive and associative visual agnosia in man. A possible exception to this parallelism is that unilateral lesions may produce visual agnosia in man, whereas serious impairment in visual discrimination in the monkey requires bilateral lesions.

Ettlinger and Gautrin (1972) studied the effects of unilateral inferotemporal lesions on retention and acquisition of form discrimination in the monkey. Mild impairment in retention of a circle-versus-triangle discrimination and in acquisition of a plus-versus-square discrimination were found. The performances were worse than those of monkeys with unilateral superior temporal lesions and better than those of monkeys with bilateral inferotemporal lesions. No differences were found between animals with unilateral inferotemporal lesions on the right and left sides.

The overwhelming majority of humans with visual agnosia have bilateral lesions. However, in several cases with postmortem examination (Nielsen 1937) and in many more clinically studied cases visual agnosia resulted from unilateral lesions. In those cases where sufficient data were available (Lissauer 1890; Nodet 1899; Poussepp 1923; Caplan and Hedley-Whyte 1974) the agnosia was found to be of the associative type. In one case (Poussepp 1923) the lesion involved the ventral occipital convexity (in addition to a lesion of the angular gyrus). In the other cases, the medial and basal portions of the occipital and occipitotemporal lobes were involved by infarction in the territories of one posterior cerebral artery (see Hahn's [1895] analysis of Lissauer's case).

In those cases of associative visual agnosia resulting from unilateral temporo-occipital lesions, it was at first not clear which hemisphere was more important. Early authors (Heilbronner 1910; Mingazzini 1922; Pötzl 1928) asserted that the left hemisphere was the one usually affected. In Nielsen's (1937) series of twelve cases with unilateral lesions, eight had left-hemisphere damage.

Modern studies in which the visual-stimulus material and the required responses have been varied systematically have elucidated the nature of hemisphere specialization and cooperation in the perception and memory of forms. Agreement between various investigators, however, is not complete. Milner (1958, 1971) and her colleagues (Kimura 1963), comparing patients with unilateral anterior temporal lobectomy, found poorer recall of printed (or spoken) language in a group with left-side lesions and poorer recognition of nonsense shapes (recurrent figures paradigm) in a group with right-side lesions. In tests of matching after tachistoscopic presentation of a sample stimulus, the two groups did not differ when the stimuli were multiple familiar objects, multiple letters, or overlapping pictures of familiar objects. However, the patients with right-side lesions were more impaired when the stimuli were scattered dots or overlapping nonsense forms. On the basis of these experiments, supplemented by studies demonstrating superiority of the normal right visual field in identifying tachistoscopically presented letters and pictures of familiar objects (Mishkin and Forgays 1952; Heron 1957; Wyke and Ettlinger 1961), these authors concluded that the crucial difference appeared to be whether the visual-stimulus pattern had a short verbal description—a name. If so, its "perception" and "memory" would be affected by left-side lesions; if not, by right-side lesions. Sperry and his colleagues (Levy et al. 1972), studying patients with section of the forebrain commissures, came to a somewhat different conclusion. They demonstrated superiority of the left hemisphere (and thus the right visual field) for identification of tachistoscopically presented chimeric stimuli only in tasks where a verbal response such as naming was required. When the required response was only to point to the correct stimulus with either hand, the right hemisphere was superior even when the stimuli were namable objects.

Levine and Calvanio (1980b) studied identification of tachistoscopically presented arrays of visual stimuli in the right and left visual fields of an adult woman with an acquired lesion of the posterior third of the corpus callosum and evidence of little or no extracallosal damage. They found marked right-visual-field superiority for identification of groups of letters, numbers, and colors, whether the required response was naming, drawing what was seen, or matching. There was, however, no difference between the visual fields when the stimuli were simple geometric shapes or letterlike nonsense forms. These results are more consistent with the conclusions of Milner and Kimura than with those of Levy. In further experiments, utilizing partial report, Levine and Calvanio demonstrated that increasing the number of simultaneously presented letters enhanced right-visual-field superiority, even when response requirements remained constant. In this sense, the right-visual-field superiority was one of letter "perception," and not merely one of generating a response to what was perceived. However, this stimulus-specific perceptual superiority of the right visual field was also task-specific. It was present when a group of letters had to be identified (by naming, drawing, or pointing), but was much less marked when the patient had only to indicate how many different letter shapes were present in the array. The presence of such task specificity begins to resemble some of the results of Levy et al. (1972). However, important differences remain, which may be the result of testing procedures (chimeric stimuli splitting the midline vs. whole stimuli lateralized to one visual field), extent of interhemispheric disconnection, and presence of cerebral lesions with onset in childhood.

The marked superiority of the left hemisphere in the perceptual identification of letters, numbers, and colors is also evident from the differing effects of left and right temporo-occipital lesions on reading and identifying colors. Numerous cases of agnosic alexia and color agnosia with unilateral left temporo-occipital damage have been reported (see, for example, Lissauer 1890; Dejerine 1892; Pötzl 1928; Geschwind and Fusillo 1966; Mohr et al. 1971). Though the deficit in alexia and color agnosia has often been described in terms of a naming disability (Geschwind 1965), recent experiments (Kinsbourne and Warrington 1962; Levine and Calvanio 1978) suggest that letter perception itself is affected in these patients. Thus, they match or draw tachistoscopically presented letter arrays no better than they name them. No such deficits are found in patients with right temporo-occipital lesions.

In contrast to the marked advantage of the left hemisphere in the identification of letters, numbers, and colors, there appears to be a definite though considerably smaller advantage of the right hemisphere in the identification of faces. Numerous studies comparing patients with unilateral lesions of either the right or the left hemisphere (De Renzi et al. 1968), the right or the left temporal lobe (Milner 1968), and the right or the left retrorolandic area (Newcombe and Russell 1969; Yin 1970) demonstrated more impairment in tasks of face recognition with right-hemisphere lesions than with left hemisphere lesions. However, the deficits in these cases were not severe. All postmortem examinations of cases with severe prosopagnosia revealed bilateral lesions (see, for example, Heidenhain 1927; Gloning et al. 1970; Rubens and Benson 1971; Lhermitte et al. 1972). Thus, it would appear that the recognition of faces, though performed better by the right hemisphere than by the left, is shared by the two sides.

These studies allow a better understanding of how the various manifestations of associative visual agnosia are related to the corresponding lateralization of the cerebral lesions. As we have seen, the critical zones within the hemispheres are the inferior occipital and posterior infero-temporal lobes. This localization is consistent with the greater ease of demonstrating hemispheric visual perceptual asymmetries with posterior unilateral lesions than with more anterior lesions, such as anterior temporal lobectomy. The same areas are of importance in the monkey; however, in man one must consider the laterality of the lesion as well as its intrahemispheric localization.

Left temporo-occipital lesions, or lesions that simultaneously disconnect the two hemispheres and deprive the left hemisphere of visual input, impair identification of arrays of letters, numbers, and colors (agnosic alexia and color agnosia). Identification of common objects and faces may be less impaired, although with larger lesions (Lissauer 1890; Caplan and Hedly-Whyte 1974) the identification of common objects may be abnormal (visual object agnosia). Right temporo-occipital lesions produce no overt identification deficits as a rule, although careful testing reveals deficits in face identification with little or no impairment in letter or color identification. Bilateral lesions will greatly intensify the difficulties in face identification (prosopagnosia) and object identification, while deficits in identification of letters, numbers, and colors appear to depend on the extent of the left-hemisphere lesions or disconnection. Thus, bilateral lesions, in which the left-side lesion is not massive enough to produce severe letter, number, and color identification deficits, may result in prosopagnosia and moderate object agnosia without severe alexia or color agnosia (Levine 1978).

The psychological principle (if there is one) underlying the asymmetric perceptual performances of the two human hemispheres has been the subject of much speculation, and is far from clear. Sweeping dichotomies, such as "analytic versus synthetic," "categorical versus appositive," and "serial-temporal versus parallel-spatial," abound. Each may be partially true. I prefer as a point of departure the incontrovertible fact that speech production and comprehension are strongly lateralized to the left hemisphere in the overwhelming majority of right-handed people. The anatomic and physiologic bases for this speech dominance are not clear, though they have been the subject of intensive investigation in recent years (for a review see Harnad et al. 1977). In any event, by the time a child begins to read, he has mastered an elaborate system of audio-orolingual communication that is largely under the control of the left hemisphere. Furthermore, he learns to read by using speech to identify (discriminate) certain visual forms (letters and letter groups). The ability to make such discriminations increases steadily throughout childhood (Hoffman 1927); that is, the visual span of apprehension for letters increases. If this form of perceptual learning were under the control of the left hemisphere, the entire process, including input and output, would be intrahemispheric. If the right hemisphere were involved, input to this hemisphere would have to be integrated with speech output from the left hemisphere across the corpus callosum. Myers (1965b), however, has shown that in animals the corpus callosum is a channel of limited capacity. Learning that is entirely intrahemispheric is stronger than learning that requires transfer across the corpus callosum. Thus, it may be the case that the perceptual learning resulting in an increasing span of visual letter identification occurs more strongly in the left hemisphere than in the right as a direct result of the left hemisphere's superiority for speech. A similar explanation may underlie the left hemisphere's superiority in number and color identification.

The basis for the right hemisphere's more modest advantage in identification of faces is less clear. It is true that the preverbal infant is capable of discriminating familiar from unfamiliar faces. So it is no surprise, in view of the remarks above, that there is no left-hemisphere advantage in face identification, since the latter is not learned in intimate relationship with speech. But the reasons for a right-hemisphere advantage, however modest, remain unknown. The advantage is probably not limited to faces. Prosopagnosic patients have difficulty identifying not only faces, but also species of animals, birds, trees, or landscapes (see Brown 1972 for a brief review). Kimura (1963), as previously mentioned, showed that patients with right anterior temporal lobectomy performed more poorly than patients with left temporal lobectomy in matching tachistoscopically presented nonsense figures and dot patterns. It seems that the right hemisphere's advantage is most evident for the discrimination of complex forms that differ from each other not because of distinctive, salient features, but because there are numerous, small differences, along multiple, not obviously separable dimensions (Garner 1974), that cannot be concisely described with words. Is this right-hemisphere advantage merely the result of commitment of the left hemisphere's perceptual apparatus to the processing of language-facilitated visual material, or is its specialization independent of the left? The answer is still unknown.

It appears that the asymmetry of hemispheric function in human visual perception is intimately associated with the asymmetry in the production and comprehension of speech. It is, therefore, not surprising that such asymmetry has not appeared in the monkey. However, as we have seen, the intrahemispheric locations of the lesions producing visual agnosias in man and disorders of visual discrimination in the monkey are highly similar. The variations in human (associative) visual agnosia are better explained on the basis of how the lesions are distributed *between* left and right temporo-occipital regions than by the assumption

(Pötzl 1928) of special regions *within* the left human temporo-occipital lobe for perception of objects, letters, colors, etc.

Conclusions

In man, as in the monkey, a system of corticocortical pathways linking striate cortex, the foveal region of ventrolateral visual association cortex, and the inferobasal temporal neocortex is necessary for intact visual-form classification. Bilateral lesions of this system that allow no connections, ipsilateral or crossed (via corpus callosum), between striate and inferotemporal cortices produce visual agnosia in man and impaired visual-discrimination performance in the monkey. These syndromes are highly comparable with respect to their behavioral features, and it seems entirely appropriate to regard monkeys with bilateral inferotemporal lesions as models of "associative" visual agnosia in man. Bilateral lesions of foveal-prestriate visual-association cortex may also be a model of "apperceptive" visual agnosia in man, but this conclusion must remain tentative until the pathologic anatomy of apperceptive visual agnosia is better established. The major difference between monkey and man concerns the effects of unilateral lesions of the foveal-prestriate inferotemporal system. Because of specialization of the left hemisphere for language in man, disturbances in the visual identification of letters, numbers, colors, and at times common objects can be severely impaired with only a unilateral (left-side) lesion. I postulate that this perceptual specialization is the result of use of previously lateralized speech processes in acquiring more efficient perception of these materials. The right hemisphere is better than the left in visual identification of complex familiar and unfamiliar forms (such as faces), for which facility in discrimination is not dependent on left-lateralized language processes. Unilateral right-sided lesions may modestly impair identification of such forms, while identification of letter and number arrays may remain normal. Because of this asymmetry in man, the comparability of the behavior of man and monkey with lesions in the foveal striate–foveal prestriate–inferotemporal system emerges most clearly when one considers the effects of bilateral lesions in each.

References

Adler, A. 1944. "Disintegration and restoration of optic recognition in visual agnosia." *Arch. Neurol. Psychiatr.* 51: 243–259.

———. 1950. "Course and outcome of visual agnosia." *J. Nerv. Ment. Dis.* 111: 41–51.

Ajuriaguerra, J. de, and H. Hécaen. 1960. *Le cortex cerebrale*. Paris: Masson.

Allman, J. M. 1977. "Evolution of the visual system in the early primates." *Progr. Psychobiol. Physiol. Psychol.* 7: 1–53.

Allman, J. M., and J. H. Kass. 1971. "A representation of the visual field in the caudal third of the middle temporal gyrus of the owl monkey (*Aotus trivirgatus*). *Brain Res.* 31: 85–105.

———. 1974a. "The organization of the second visual area (V2) in the owl monkey: A second order transformation of the visual hemifield." *Brain Res.* 76: 247–265.

———. 1974b. "A crescent-shaped cortical visual area surrounding the middle temporal area (MT) in the owl monkey (*Aotus trivirgatus*)." *Brain Res.* 81: 199–213.

———. 1975. "The dorsomedial cortical visual area: A third tier area in the occipital lobe of the owl monkey (*Aotus trivirgatus*)." *Brain Res.* 100: 473–487.

———. 1976. "Representation of the visual field on the medial wall of occipital-parietal cortex in the owl monkey." *Science* 191: 572–575.

Allman, J. M., J. H. Kass, R. H. Lane, and F. M. Miezin. 1972. "A representation of the visual field in the inferior nucleus of the pulvinar in the owl monkey (*Aotus trivirgatus*)." *Brain Res.* 40: 291–302.

Balint, R. 1909. "Seelenlahmung des 'Schauens,' optische Ataxie, raumliche Storung der Aufmerksamkeit." *Monats. Psych. Neurol.* 25: 57–71.

Bates, J. A. V., and G. Ettlinger. 1960. "Posterior biparietal ablations in the monkey." *Arch. Neurol.* 3: 177–192.

Bay, E. 1952. "Analyse eines Fall von Seelenblindheit." *Deutsche Z. Nervenheilkunde* 168: 1–23.

———. 1953. "Disturbances of visual perception and their examination." *Brain* 76: 515–550.

Bender, D. B. 1973. "Visual sensitivity following infero-temporal and foveal prestriate lesions in the monkey." *J. Comp. Physiol. Psychol.* 84: 613–621.

Benson, D., and J. Greenberg. 1969. "Visual form agnosia." *Arch. Neurol.* 20: 82–89.

Benson, D. F., J. Segarra, and M. L. Albert. 1974. "Visual agnosia-prosopagnosia." *Arch. Neurol.* 30: 307–310.

Blum, J. S., K. L. Chow, and K. H. Pribram. 1950. "A behavioral analysis of the organization of the parieto-temporo-preoccipital cortex." *J. Comp. Neurol.* 93: 53–100.

Bodamer, J. 1947. "Die Prosop-Agnosie (Die Agnosie des Physiognomieerkennens). *Arch. Psych. Z. Neurol.* 179: 6–53.

Brain, W. R. 1961. *Speech disorders: Aphasia, Apraxia, and Agnosia.* London: Butterworths.

Brown, J. W. 1972. *Aphasia, Apraxia, and Agnosia: Clinical and Theoretical Aspects.* Springfield, III.: Thomas.

Brown, S., and E. A. Schafer. 1888. "An investigation into the function of the occipital and temporal lobes of the monkey's brain." *Phil. Trans.* 179: 303–327.

Brown, T. S. 1963. "Olfactory and visual discrimination in the monkey after selective lesions of the temporal lobe." *J. Comp. Physiol. Psychol.* 56: 764–768.

Brown, T. S, H. E. Rosvold, and M. Mishkin. 1963. "Olfactory discrimination after temporal lobe lesions in monkeys." *H. Comp. Physiol. Psychol.* 56: 190–195.

Bruner, J. S. 1957. "On perceptual readiness." *Psychol. Rev.* 64: 123–152.

Butter, C. M. 1968. "The effect of discrimination training on pattern equivalence in monkeys with infero-temporal and lateral striate lesions." *Neuropsychologia* 6: 27–40.

Butter, C. M., M. Mishkin, and H. E. Rosvold. 1965. "Stimulus generalization in monkeys with infero-temporal lesions and lateral occipital lesions." In *Stimulus Generalization*, D. J. Mostofsky, ed. Stanford, Calif.: Stanford University Press.

Campos-Ortega, J. A., W. R. Hayhow, and P. F. de V. Cluver. 1970. "The descending projections from the cortical visual fields of macaca mulatta with particular reference to the question of a cortico-lateral geniculate pathway." *Brain, Behav., Evol.* 3: 368–414.

Caplan, L. R., and T. Hedley-Whyte. 1971. "Cuing and memory dysfunction in alexia without agraphia." *Brain* 97: 251–262.

Chow, K. L. 1950. "Retrograde cell degeneration study of the cortical projection field of the pulvinar in the monkey." *J. Comp. Neurol.* 93: 313–340.

———. 1951. "Effects of partial extirpations of the posterior association cortex on visually mediated behavior." *Comp. Psychol. Mongr.* 20: 187–217.

———. 1952. "Further studies on selective ablation of associative cortex in relation to visually mediated behavior." *J. Comp. Physiol. Psychol.* 45: 109–118.

———. 1954. "Lack of behavioral effects following destruction of some thalamic nuclei in monkey." *Arch. Neurol. Psychiatr.* 71: 762–771.

Cohn, R., M. A. Neumann, and D. H. Wood. 1977. "Prosopagnosia: A clinicopathological study." *Ann. Neurol.* 1: 177–182.

Cowey, A., and C. G. Gross. 1970. "Effects of foveal prestriate and infero-temporal lesions on visual discrimination by rhesus monkeys." *Exp. Brain Res.* 11: 128–144.

Cowey, A., and L. Weiskrantz. 1967. "A comparison of the effects of infero-temporal and striate cortex lesions on the visual behavior of rhesus monkeys." *Q. J. Exp. Psychol.* 19: 246–253.

Critchley, M. 1964. "The problem of visual agnosia." *J. Neurol. Sci.* 1: 274–290.

Dejerine, J. 1892. "Contribution a l'etude anatomopathologique et clinique des differente varietes de cecite verbale." *Mem. Soc. Biol.* 4: 61–90.

———. 1914. *Semiologie des affections du systeme nerveux.* Paris: Masson.

DeJong, R. H., H. H. Itabashi, and J. R. Olsen. 1969. "Memory logs due to hippocampal lesions." *Arch. Neurol.* 20: 339–348.

DeRenzi, E., P. Faglioni, and H. Spinnler. 1968. "The performance of patients with unilateral brain damage on face recognition tasks." *Cortex* 4: 17–34.

Douglas, R. J. 1967. "The hippocampus and behavior." *Psychol. Bull.* 67: 416–442.

Douglas, R. J., and K. H. Pribram. 1966. "Learning and limbic lesions." *Neuropsychologia* 4: 197–220.

Drachman, D. A., and J. Arbit. 1966. "Memory and the hippocampal complex." *Arch. Neurol.* 15: 52–61.

Druga, R. 1969–1970. "Neocortical projections to the amygdala. (An experimental study with the Nauta method)." *J. Hirnforsch.* 11: 467–476.

Efron, R. 1968. "What is perception?" In *Boston Studies in the Philosophy of Science*, R. Cohen and M. Wartofsky, eds. Boston: Reidel.

Ettlinger, G. 1956. "Sensory defects in visual agnosia." *J. Neurol. Neurosurg. Psychiatr.* 19: 297–307.

Ettlinger, G., and D. Gautrin. 1972. "Visual discrimination performance in the monkey: The effect of unilateral removal of temporal cortex." *Cortex* 7: 317–331.

Ettlinger, G., and J. Waegner. 1958. "Somaesthetic alternation, discrimination and orientation after frontal and parietal lesions in monkeys." *Q. J. Exp. Psychol.* 10: 177–186.

Ettlinger, G., and M. Wyke. 1961. "Defects in identifying objects visually in a patient with cerebrovascular disease." *J. Neurol. Neurosurg. Psychiatr.* 24: 254–259.

Ettlinger, G., E. Warrington, and O. L. Zangwill. 1957. "A further study of visual spatial agnosia." *Brain* 80: 335–361.

Evarts, L. V. 1952. "Effect of ablation of prestriate cortex on auditory-visual association in monkey." *J. Neurophysiol.* 15: 191–200.

Freud, S. 1981. *On Aphasia*, E. Stengel, tr. New York: International University Press, 1953.

Friedman, H. M., and N. Allen. 1969. "Chronic effects of complete limbic destruction." *Neurology* 19: 679–690.

Gaffan, D. 1974. "Recognition impaired and association intact in the memory of monkeys after transection of the fornix." *J. Comp. Physiol. Psychol.* 86: 1100–1109.

Garner, W. R. 1974. *The Processing of Information and Structure.* Potomac, Md.: Erlbaum.

Gascon, G., and F. Gilles. 1973. "Limbic dementia." *J. Neurol. Neurosurg. Psychiatr.* 36: 421–430.

Gerstmann, J. 1931. "Zur Symptomatologie der Herderkrankungen in der Übergangsregion der unteren Parietal- und mittleren Okzipitalhirnwindung." *Deutsche Arch. Nervenheilk.* 116: 46–49.

Geschwind, N. 1965. "Disconnexion syndromes in animals and man." *Brain* 88: 237–294.

Geschwind, N., and M. Fusillo. 1966. "Color naming defects in association with alexia." *Arch. Neurol.* 15: 137–146.

Gloning, I., K. Gloning, K. Jellinger, and R. Quatember. 1970. "A case of 'prosopagnosia' with necropsy findings." *Neuropsychologia* 8: 199–204.

Godwin-Austen, R. B. 1965. "A case of visual disorientation." *J. Neurol. Neurosurg. Psychiatr.* 28: 453–458.

Goldstein, K., and A. Gelb. 1918. "Psychologische Analysen hirnpathologischer Falle auf Grund von Untersuchungen Hirverletzten." *Z. Ges. Neurol. Psychiatr.* 41: 1–142.

Gross, C. G. 1972. "Infero-temporal cortex and vision." In *Progress in Physiological Psychology*, E. Stellar and J. M. Sprague, eds. New York: Academic.

———. 1973. "Visual function of infero-temporal cortex." In *Handbook of Sensory Physiology*, vol. 1, part 3B, R. Jung, ed. Berlin: Springer.

Gross, C. G., A. Cowey, and F. J. Manning. 1971. "Further analysis of the visual discrimination deficits following foveal prestriate and infero-temporal lesions in rhesus monkeys." *J. Comp. Physiol. Psychol.* 76: 1–7.

Hahn, E. 1895. "Pathologisch-anatomische Untersuchung des Lissauerschen Falles von Seelenblindheit." *Arb. Psychiatr. Klin. Breslau* 2: 107–119.

Harnad, S., R. W. Doty, L. Goldstein, J. Jaynes, and G. Krauthammer, eds. 1977. *Lateralization in the Nervous System.* New York: Academic.

Hearst, E., and K. H. Pribram. 1964. "Appetitive and aversive generalization gradients in amygdalectomized monkeys." *J. Comp. Physiol. Psychol.* 58: 296–298.

Hécaen, H., and J. de Ajuriaguerra. 1954. "Balint's syndrome (psychic paralysis of visual fixation) and its minor forms." *Brain* 77: 373–400.

Hécaen, H., R. Angelergues, C. Bernhardt, and J. Chiarelli. 1957. "Essai de distinction des modalites clinique de l'agnosie des physiognomies" *Rev. Neurologique* 96: 125–144.

Heidenhain, A. 1927. "Beitrag zur Kenntnis der Seelenblindheit." *Monats. Psychiatr. Neurol.* 66: 61–116.

Heilbronner, K. 1910. "Die aphasischen, apraktischen, und agnostischen Storungen." In *Handbuch der Neurologie*, vol. 1, F. Lewandowsky, ed. Berlin: Springer.

Heron, H. 1957. "Perception as a function of retinal locus and attention." *Amer. J. Psychol.* 70: 38–48.

Hoff, H., I. Gloning, and K. Gloning. 1962. "Die zentralen Storungen der optischen Wahrnehmung." *Wiener Med. Wochens.* 112: 450–459.

Hoffman, J. 1927. "Experimentell-psychologische Untersuchungen uber Leseleistungen von Schulkindem." *Arch. ges. Psychol.* 58: 325–388.

Holmes, G. 1918. "Disturbances of visual orientation." *Br. J. Ophthalmol.* 2: 449–468, 506–516.

———. 1938. "The cerebral integration of the ocular movements." *Br. Med. J.* 2: 107–112.

Holmes, G., and G. Horrax. 1919. "Disturbances of spatial orientation and visual attention with loss of stereoscopic vision." *Arch. Neurol. Psychiatr.* 1: 385–407.

Horel, J. A. 1978. "The neuroanatomy of amnesia: A critique of the hippocampal memory hypothesis." *Brain* 101: 403–445.

Iversen, S. D. 1973. "Visual discrimination deficits associated with posterior inferotemporal lesions in monkey." *Brain Res.* 62: 89–101.

Iversen, S. D., and L. Weiskrantz. 1967. "Temporal lobe lesions and memory in the monkey. "*Nature* 201: 740–742.

Iwai, E., and M. Mishkin. 1968. "Two visual foci in the temporal lobe of monkey." Japan–U.S. Joint Seminar on Neurophysiological Basis of Learning and Behavior, Kyoto, Japan.

———. 1969. "Further evidence on the locus of visual area in the temporal lobe of the monkey." *Exp. Neurol.* 25: 585–594.

Jones, E. G., and T. P. S. Powell. 1970. "An anatomical study of converging sensory pathways within the cerebral cortex of the monkey." *Brain* 93: 793–820.

Kimble, D. P., and K. H. Pribram. 1963. "Hippocampectomy and behavior sequences." *Science* 139: 824–825.

Kimura, D. 1963. "Right temporal lobe damage: Perception of unfamiliar stimuli after damage." *Arch. Neurol.* 8: 264–271.

Kinsbourne, M., and E. K. Warrington. 1962. "A disorder of simultaneous form perception." *Brain* 85: 461–486.

Kleist, K. 1934. *Gehirnpathologie.* Liepzig: Barth.

Klüver, H., and P. C. Bucy. 1937. "'Psychic blindness' and other symptoms following bilateral temporal lobectomy in rhesus monkeys." *Amer. J. Physiol.* 119: 352–353.

———. 1939. "Preliminary analysis of functions of the temporal lobes of monkeys." *Arch. Neurol. Psychiatr.* 42: 979–1000.

Kuypers, H. G. J. M., M. K. Szwarczbart, M. Mishkin, and H. I. Rosvold. 1965. "Occipitotemporal cortico-cortical connections in the rhesus monkey." *Exp. Neurol.* 11: 245–262.

Lange, J. 1936. "Agnosien und Apraxien." In *Handbuch der Neurologie*, O. Bumke and O. Foerster, eds. Berlin: Springer.

Lashley, K. S. 1948. "The mechanism of vision. XVIII. Effects of destroying the visual 'associative areas' of the monkey." *Genet. Psychol. Monogr.* 37: 107–166.

Levine, D. 1978. "Prosopagnosia and visual object agnosia: A behavioral study." *Brain Lang*, 5: 341–365.

Levine, D., and R. Calvanio. 1978. "A study of the visual defect in verbal alexiasimultanagnosia." *Brain* 101: 65–81.

———. 1980a. "Disorders of visual behavior following bilateral posterior cerebral lesions." *Psychol. Res.* 41: 217–234.

———. 1980b. "Visual discrimination after lesions of the posterior corpus callosum." *Neurology* 30: 21–30.

Levy, J., C. Trevarthen, and R. W. Sperry. 1972. "Perception of bilateral chimeric figures following hemispheric deconnection." *Brain* 95: 61–78.

Lhermitte, F., F. Chain, R. Escourolle, B. Ducarne, and B. Pillon. 1972. "Etude anatomoclinique d'un cas de prosopagnosie." *Rev. Neurologique* 126: 329–346.

Lissauer, H. 1890. "Ein Fall von Seelenblindheit nebst Beitrage zur Theorie derselben." *Arch. Psychiatr.* 21: 222–270.

Manning, F. J. 1971. "Punishment for errors and visual discrimination learning by monkeys with infero-temporal cortex lesions." *J. Comp. Physiol. Psychol.* 75: 146–152.

Manning, F. J., C. J. Gross, and A. Cowey. 1971. "Partial re-inforcement; effects on visual learning after foveal prestriate and inferotemporal lesions." *Physiol. Behav.* 6: 61–64.

Mathers, L. H. 1971. "Tectal projection to the posterior thalamus of the squirrel monkey." *Brain Res.* 35: 295–298.

Michel, F., M. Jeannerod, and M. Devic. 1965. "Trouble de l'orientation visuelle dans les trois dimensions de l'espace." *Cortex* 1: 441–466.

Milner, B. 1958. "Psychological defects produced by temporal lobe excision." *Res. Pub. Ass. Res. Nerv. Ment. Dis.* 36: 244–257.

———. 1968. "Visual recognition and recall after right temporal lobe excision in man." *Neuropsychologia* 6: 191–209.

———. 1971. "Interhemispheric differences in the localization of psychological processes in man." *Br. Med. Bull.* 27: 272–277.

Milner, B., and H. Teuber. 1968. "Alteration of perception and memory in man: Reflections on methods." In *Analysis of Behavioral Change*, L. Weiskrantz, ed. New York: Harper and Row.

Mingazzini, G. 1922. *Der Balken.* Berlin: Springer.

Mishkin, M. 1954. "Visual discrimination performance following partial ablations of the temporal lobe. II. Ventral surface versus hippocampus." *J. Comp. Physiol. Psychol.* 47: 187–193.

———. 1966. "Visual mechanisms beyond the striate cortex." In *Frontiers in Physiological Psychology*, R. Russel, ed. New York: Academic.

Mishkin, M., and D. C. Forgays. 1952. "Word recognition as a function of retinal locus." *J. Exp. Psychol.* 43: 43–48.

Mishkin, M., and K. H. Pribram. 1954. "Visual discrimination performance following partial ablations of the temporal lobe. I. Ventral versus lateral." *J. Comp. Physiol. Psychol.* 47: 14–20.

Mishkin, M., and L. Weiskrantz. 1959. "Effects of cortical lesions in monkeys on critical flicker frequency." *J. Comp. Physiol. Psychol.* 52: 660–666.

Mohr, J. P., J. Leicester, L. T. Stoddard, and M. Sidman. 1971. "Right hemianopia with memory and color deficits in circumscribed left posterior cerebral artery infarction." *Neurology* 21: 1101–1113.

Munk, H. 1881. *Über die Funktionen der Crosshirnrinde—Gesammelte Mitteilungen aus den Jahren* 1877–1880. Berlin: Hirschwald.

Myers, R. E. 1965a. "Organization of visual pathways." In *Functions of the Corpus Callosum*, E. G. Ettlinger, ed. Boston: Little, Brown.

———. 1965b. "The neocortical commissures and interhemispheric transmission of information." In *Function of the Corpus Callosum*, E. G. Ettlinger, ed. Boston: Little, Brown.

Newcombe, F., and W. Russell. 1969. "Dissociated visual perceptual and spatial deficits in focal lesions of the right hemisphere." *J. Neurol. Neurosurg. Psychiatr.* 32: 73–81.

Nielsen, J. M. 1937. "Unilateral cerebral dominance as related to mind blindness." *Arch. Neurol. Psychiatr.* 38: 108–135.

Nodet, V. 1899. "Les agnosies; la cecite psychique en particulier." Thesis, Université de Lyon.

Orbach, J., and R. L. Frantz. 1959. "Differential effects of temporal neocortical resection on overtrained and non-overtrained visual habits in monkeys." *J. Comp. Physiol. Psychol.* 51: 126–129.

Orbach, J., B. Milner, and T. Rasmussen. 1960. "Learning and retention in monkeys after amygdala-hippocampus resection." *Arch. Neurol.* 3: 230–251.

Oscar-Berman, M., S. Heywood, and C. G. Gross. 1973. "The effects of posterior cortical lesions on eye orientation during visual discrimination by monkeys." *Neuropsychologia* 12: 175–182.

Pandya, D. N., and H. G. J. M. Kuypers. 1969. "Cortico-cortical connections in the rhesus monkey." *Brain Res.* 13: 13–36.

Pasik, P., T. Pasik, W. S. Battersby, and M. B. Bender. 1958. "Visual and tactual discrimination by macaques with serial temporal and parietal lesions." *J. Comp. Physiol. Psychol.* 51: 427–436.

———. 1960. "Factors influencing visual behavior of monkeys with bilateral temporal lobe lesions." *J. Comp. Neurol.* 115: 89–102.

Paterson, A., and O. L. Zangwill. 1944. "Disorders of visual space perception associated with lesions of the right cerebral hemisphere." *Brain* 67: 331–358.

Pevzner, S., B. Bornstein, and M. Lowenthal. 1962. "Prosopagnosia." *J. Neurol. Neurosurg. Psychiatr.* 25: 336–338.

Pohl, W. 1973. "Dissociation of spatial discrimination deficits following frontal and parietal lesions in monkeys." *J. Comp. Physiol. Psychol.* 82: 227–239.

Pötzl, O. 1928. *Die Aphasielehre vom Standpunkte der klinischen Psychiatrie*, vol. 1. Leipzig: Franz Deuticke.

Poussepp, L. 1923. "Contribution aux recherches sur la localisation de l'aphasie visuelle." *Presse Med.* 31: 564–565.

Pribram, H. B., and J. Barry. 1956. "Further behavioral analysis of parieto-temporopreoccipital cortex." *J. Neurophysiol.* 19: 99–106.

Pribram, K. H. 1960. "The intrinsic systems of the forebrain." In *Handbook of Physiology: Neurophysiology II*, J. Field et al., eds. Washington, D.C.: American Physiological Society.

Pribram, K. H., and M. H. Bagshaw. 1953. "Further analysis of the temporal lobe syndrome utilizing frontotemporal ablations." *J. Comp. Neurol.* 99: 347–375.

Pribram, K. H., and M. Mishkin. 1955. "Simultaneous and successive visual discrimination by monkeys with infero-temporal lesions." *J. Comp. Physiol. Psychol.* 48: 198–202.

Rosvold, H. E., M. Mishkin, and M. K. Szwarzbart. 1958. "Effects of subcortical lesions in monkeys on visual discrimination and single alternation performance." *J. Comp. Physiol. Psychol.* 51: 437–444.

Rubens, A. B., and D. F. Benson. 1971. "Associative visual agnosia." *Arch Neurol.* 24: 305–316.

Schwartzbaum, J. S. 1965. "Discrimination behavior after amygdalectomy in monkeys." *J. Comp. Physiol. Psychol.* 60: 314–319.

Scoville, W. B., and B. Milner. 1957. "Loss of recent memory after bilateral hippocampal lesions." *J. Neurol. Neurosurg. Psychiatr.* 20: 11–21.

Siqueira, E. B., and L. Franks. 1974. "Anatomic connections of the pulvinar." In *The Pulvinar-LP Complex*, I. S. Cooper et al., eds. Springfield, Ill.: Thomas.

Spamer, C. 1876. "Über Aphasie und Asymbolie nebst Versuch einer Theorie der Sprachbildung." *Arch Psychiatr.* 6: 496–542.

Stengel, E. 1944. "Loss of spatial orientation, constructional apraxia, and Gerstmann's syndrome." *J. Ment. Sci.* 90: 753–760.

Symmes, D. 1965. "Flicker discrimination by brain damaged monkeys." *J. Comp. Physiol. Psychol.* 60: 470–473.

Terzian, H., and G. Dalle Ore. 1955. "Syndrome of Klüver and Bucy reproduced in man by bilateral removal of the temporal lobes." *Neurology* 5: 373–380.

Victor, M., J. B. Angevine, E. C. Mancall, and C. M. Fisher. 1961. "Memory loss with lesions of hippocampal formation." *Arch. Neurol.* 5: 244–263.

von Bonin, G., and P. Bailey. 1947. *The Neocortex of Macaca Mulatta.* Urbana: University of Illinois Press.

von Monakow, C. 1914. *Die Lokalisation im Grosshirn und der Abbau der Funktion durch kortikale Herde.* Wiesbaden: J. F. Bergmann.

von Stauffenberg, W. 1914. "Über Seelenblindheit." *Arb. hirnanat. Inst. Zurich* 8: 1–212.

Walker, A. E., A. F. Thompson, and J. D. McQueen. 1953. "Behavior and the temporal rhinencephalon in the monkey." *Johns Hopkins Hosp. Bull.* 93: 65–93.

Weiskrantz, L. 1956. "Behavior changes associated with ablation of the amygdaloid complex in monkeys." *J. Comp. Physiol. Psychol.* 49: 381–391.

Weiskrantz, L., and A. Cowey. 1963. "Striate cortex lesions and visual acuity in the rhesus monkey." *J. Comp. Physiol. Psychol.* 56: 225–231.

Weiskrantz, L., and M. Mishkin. 1958. "Effects of temporal and frontal cortical lesions on auditory discrimination in monkeys." *Brain* 81: 406–414.

Whitlock, D. G., and W. J. H. Nauta. 1956. "Subcortical projections from the temporal neocortex in *Macaca mulatta.*" *J. Comp. Neurol.* 106: 183–212.

Wilson, M. 1957. "Effects of circumscribed cortical lesions upon somesthetic and visual discrimination in the monkey." *J. Comp. Physiol. Psychol.* 50: 630–635.

Wilson, M., H. M. Kaufman, R. E. Zieler, and J. P. Lieb. 1972. "Visual identification and memory in monkeys with circumscribed inferotemporal lesions." *J. Comp. Physiol. Psychol.* 78: 173–183.

Woods, B., and E. Poppel. 1974. "Effect of print size on reading time in a patient with verbal alexia." *Neuropsychologia* 12: 31–41.

Wyke, M., and G. Ettlinger. 1961. "Efficiency of recognition in left and right visual fields." *Arch. Neurol.* 5: 659–665.

Yin, R. K. 1970. "Face recognition by brain-injured patients: A dissociable ability?" *Neuropsychologia* 8: 395–402.

Zeki, S. M. 1969. "Representation of central visual fields in prestriate cortex in monkey." *Brain Res.* 14: 271–291.

———. 1970. "Interhemispheric connections of prestriate cortex in monkey." *Brain Res.* 19: 63–75.

———. 1971a. "Convergent input from the striate cortex (area 17) to the cortex of the superior temporal sulcus in the rhesus monkey." *Brain Res.* 28: 338–340.

———. 1971b. "Cortical projections from two prestriate areas in the monkey." *Brain Res.* 34: 19–35.

9

C. G. Gross, C. E. Rocha-Miranda, and D. B. Bender

Visual properties of neurons in inferotemporal cortex of the macaque

1972. *Journal of Neurophysiology* 35: 96–111

IN THE LAST DECADE, considerable progress has been made in understanding the physiology of one of the most fundamental aspects of human experience: perception of the visual world. It is now clear that the retina and visual pathways do not simply transmit a mosaic of light and dark to some central sensorium. Rather, even at the retinal level, specific features of visual stimuli are detected and their presence communicated to the next level. In cats and monkeys, the geniculostriate visual system consists of a series of converging and diverging connections such that at each successive tier of processing mechanism, single neurons respond to increasingly more specific visual stimuli falling on an increasingly wider area of the retina (19–21).

How far does this analytical-synthetic process continue whereby individual cells have more and more specific trigger features? Are there regions of the brain beyond striate and prestriate[1] cortex where this processing of visual information is carried further? If so, how far and in what way? Are there cells that are concerned with the storage of visual information as well as its analysis?

There are several lines of evidence suggesting that a possible site for further processing of visual information and perhaps even for storage of such information might, in the monkey, be inferotemporal cortex—the cortex on the inferior convexity of the temporal lobe. First, this area receives afferents from prestriate cortex which itself processes visual information received from striate cortex (26). Second, bilateral removal of inferotemporal cortex has specific effects on visually guided behavior. After inferotemporal lesions, visual discrimination learning is severely impaired but discrimination of auditory, tactile, gustatory, and olfactory stimuli remains unaffected (see review by Gross, ref 15). In spite of this visual learning deficit, other more "basic" visual functions appear intact: inferotemporal lesions do not produce visual field scotomata nor do they affect visual acuity, critical flicker frequency, the threshold for detection of a brief visual stimulus, or backward masking functions (see ref 15). Thus, the impairment appears to be one of some "higher" visual functions. Such a syndrome does not follow ablation of other cortical areas. In fact, large partial lesions of striate cortex itself, while producing scotomata and visual threshold changes, have relatively little effect on visual learning (6). Third, visual-evoked responses can be recorded from macroelectrodes in inferotemporal cortex and single neurons in inferotemporal cortex respond to visual but not to auditory stimuli (13, 16, 18, 37).

Although this evidence establishes inferotemporal cortex as a visual area, it indicates little about its specific roles in vision. In this paper we report the existence of visual receptive fields of inferotemporal neurons and describe some of their properties. In a subsequent paper we will discuss the afferent basis of these properties.

METHODS

Animal preparation and maintenance

Seventeen *Macaca mulatta* weighing between 2.5 and 10 kg were used. Two to four days before the start of recording, the base of the microdrive and two bolts for subsequent fixa-

Received for publication June 28, 1971.

[1] In this paper the terms "prestriate cortex," "circumstriate belt" of Kuypers et al. (26), and "areas OA and OB" of von Bonin and Bailey (2) are used synonymously.

tion of the head were implanted under thiopental sodium or pentobarbital sodium anesthesia. The microdrive and the bolts and their methods of implantation were essentially similar to those described by Evarts (10, 11). After excision of the temporal muscle, a ⅝ inch hole was trephined in the temporal bone and the base of the microdrive mounted over the opening. The dura was left intact and the microdrive base was filled with an antibiotic mixture (bacitracin 200 U/ml, polymixin B sulfate 0.1%, neomycin sulfate 0.5%) and capped. In some animals, microdrive bases were implanted bilaterally. The bolts were implanted in the frontal bone and emerged through stab wounds in the skin. After the animal's galea, muscle, and skin incisions were sutured, nitrofurazone ointment was applied topically and benzathine penicillin G given intramuscularly.

On the first recording day, the monkey was anesthetized intravenously with sodium thiamylal for the duration of a tracheotomy and vein cannulation. It was then immobilized with a continuous infusion of gallamine triethiodide in a solution of 5% dextrose in lactated Ringer solution, artificially respired, and anesthetized with a mixture of 30% oxygen and 70% nitrous oxide. (Succinylcholine chloride was used as the immobilizing agent in a few early experiments.) The stroke volume and rate of the respirator were adjusted to maintain the CO_2 content of the expired air at 3–4% as measured with a Beckman CO_2 analyzer. The animal's temperature was maintained between 37 and 39 C with the aid of a thermostatically controlled heating pad and heart rate continually monitored. The early experiments continued for 3 days and the later ones 4–5 days. The method of holding the animal's head by the implanted bolts provided an unobstructed visual field and facilitated adjustment of the position of the eyes.

The pupils were dilated with 0.25% scopolamine hydrochloride and the eyelids retracted. The eyes were fitted with contact lenses chosen with a slit retinoscope to bring the eyes in focus at a plane 57 cm away to the nearest 0.5 diopter. For each eye, the fovea, the center of the blind spot, and two venous junctions near the blind spot were projected onto the tangent screen with a reversible ophthalmoscope. A line passing through the projection of the center of the blind spot and fovea was taken as the horizontal meridian and an orthogonal line passing through the projection of the fovea was taken as the vertical meridian although, in fact, the precise center of the blind spot usually lies very slightly below the horizontal meridian. The combined errors in locating and projecting these landmarks were 0.5–1.0°. With the immobilizing techniques described above, the position of the eyes sometimes drifted 1–2° over several hours and no attempt was made to reduce this drift by additional techniques. Rather, the position of the eyes was replotted immediately before and after each detailed field plotting. Eye shields were arranged to allow monocular stimulation. Each night the contact lenses were removed, the eyes washed with saline and chlortetracycline hydrochloride ophthalmic solution, and then closed for several hours.

Recording techniques

Glass-coated platinum-iridium microelectrodes similar to those described by Wolbarsht et al. (38) were used. Their tips were cone shaped with about 20 μ from the tip exposed and with a diameter of about 4 μ at a point 22.5 μ from the tip. Their capacitance in agar-saline was between 15 and 30 pf according to a Tektronix LC meter. They were advanced with a microdrive similar to that described by Evarts (10, 11). The signals from the electrode were led to a cathode follower mounted on or near the microdrive, and then to a preamplifier, displayed on an oscilloscope, put through an audio amplifier into a speaker, and recorded on magnetic tape. Only signals that clearly came from an isolated single neuron as determined by constant amplitude and waveform were studied. In addition, EEG was recorded from needle electrodes in the scalp over the occipital lobe, amplified, displayed on an oscilloscope, and recorded on magnetic tape.

Visual stimuli

To prevent adventitious stimulation with stray light, the animal was placed in a tent of black cloth. A 70 cm x 70 cm translucent Polacoat tangent screen was mounted in the tent wall perpendicular to the visual axis, 57 cm from the eyes and adjusted so that the projection of the foveae fell near the center of the screen.

Two types of visual stimuli were used, "light" and "dark." The light stimuli were projected onto the rear of the tangent screen by an optical apparatus consisting of tungsten filament light source, lenses, dove prisms, slides, neutral density filters, and often Wratten color filters, all mounted on a movable optical bench. One dove prism was mounted on a galvanometer coil so that stimuli could be moved across the tangent screen either automatically by a waveform generator, or manually by adjusting a potentiometer. The location of the stimulus on the screen was indicated by photocells mounted on the screen and by a voltage output from the galvanometer. Both the state of the photocells and the galvanometer voltage were recorded on magnetic tape along with the bioelectric signals.

Although a great variety of light stimuli were used, most cells were tested with certain relatively "standard stimuli." The standard background luminance of the tangent screen was 1.5 mL. The standard light slit was 1° wide with a luminance of 1.5 log units greater than standard background. Three color filters were occasionally used: red (Wratten filter 29), green (Wratten filter 40), and blue (Wratten filter 47). When these were used, the background luminance was usually reduced to .1 mL and the luminance of the red light was 1.7 log units greater than this background, the luminance of the green light 1.9 units greater and the luminance of the blue light .6 log units greater. All luminance measures were made with a Pritchard spectra photometer. The standard rate of the automatic sweep was between 5 and 7°/sec.

The standard dark stimuli were cardboard cutouts moved manually on the back of the tangent screen with standard background illumination. Their luminance was 2.2 log units below the background.

Receptive-field plotting

The method of plotting receptive fields varied with the response characteristics of the neuron. Thus if the neuron responded equally well to horizontal and vertical slits 1° wide, its field boundaries were determined by moving the slits both horizontally and then vertically across the tangent screen. However, if it responded only to a vertical slit moving orthogonally to its long axis, the lateral boundaries of the field were determined by horzontal movement of the slit, and the upper and lower boundaries by varying the length and vertical position of the slit as it moved horizontally. The stimuli were moved and the receptive fields detected with two methods. In the first, the presentation and movement of the stimulus were controlled by hand and the field borders were detected by listening to the discharges of the isolated unit and marking the boundaries on the screen. In the second, the stimulus was automatically moved across the screen synchronously with the sweep of a Mnemotron Computer of Average Transients (CAT), thus providing a plot of the frequency of firing of the isolated unit as a function of the location of the stimulus. Usually such histograms were generated by 10 sweeps of the stimulus in each direction. For units responsive to standard light stimuli, fields were usually plotted with both methods, which invariably yielded similar receptive fields. With both methods the receptive fields corresponded to the "minimal receptive fields" of Barlow et al. (1). Cells responsive to dark stimuli or nonstandard light stimuli were plotted only with the first method (hand plotting). Plotting with slits of light or edges usually yielded rectangular receptive fields, whereas with other stimuli, the shape of the fields were often not rectangular. However, if the unit responded to both types of stimuli, then the receptive field plotted with each had a similar area and similar location of its geometric center. The histograms presented in this paper were generated by reanalysis of tape recordings of the original raw data with a Digital Equipment Corp. PDP-12 computer with close monitoring of both the waveform of the isolated unit to insure absence of contamination by other signals and of the state of the EEG.

As this study progressed, we learned more and more about the optimal conditions necessary to elicit responses from inferotemporal units and altered our methods of plotting receptive fields accordingly. Among the procedures introduced after several experiments were: *1*) use of dark stimuli; *2*) use of colored stimuli; *3*) use of interstimulus intervals up to a few minutes; *4*) use of irregular and highly complex stimuli; and *5*) most importantly, close monitoring of the EEG and its maintenance in a low-voltage, high-frequency state by presenting somesthetic, acoustic, and olfactory stimuli. Such "arousing" stimuli were presented in the intervals between visual stimulation. Indicative of the importance of these factors was that in the earlier experiments many receptive fields could only be plotted by using the CAT, whereas later, almost all fields could be plotted by moving the stimuli by hand and listening to the loudspeaker.

Histological methods

At the conclusion of each experiment, the monkey was perfused through the aorta with saline followed by 10% formalin. A week later the brain was cut in the coronal stereotaxic plane, cast in dental impression compound, and cut in 25-μ frozen sections which were stained with cresyl violet. The approximate site of entry of each electrode was marked on the cast and its path was reconstructured from the serial sections. The cortex through which the electrode passed was classified according to the cytoarchitectonic criteria of von Bonin and Bailey (2). In addition, the site of entry of each pass was marked on a standard brain drawing (Fig. 1).

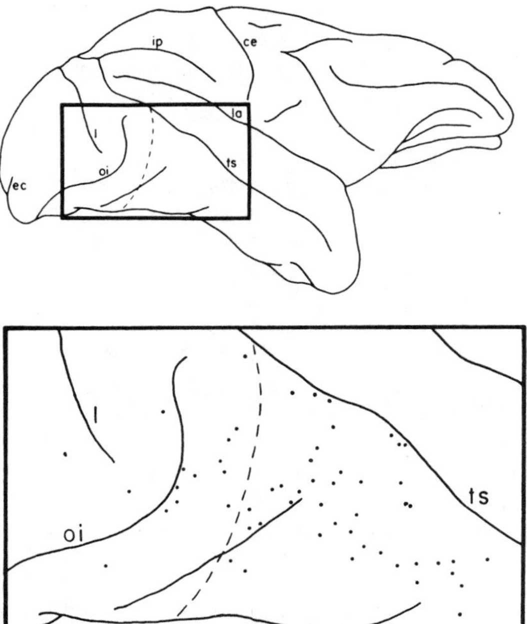

FIG. 1. *Upper:* lateral view of cerebral hemisphere of *Macaca mulatta* showing site of lower drawing. *Lower:* site of entry of electrode passes. Passes made in the left hemisphere are shown in the corresponding sites of the right hemisphere. Passes to the right of the dashed line were in cytoarchitectonic area TE and those to the left were in area OA or in cortex transitional between area OA and area TE (see text). The dashed line represents the typical posterior border of cortex clearly distinguishable as area TE. ce = central sulcus, ec = external calcarine sulcus, ip = intraparietal sulcus, l = lunate sulcus, la = lateral fissure, oi = inferior occipital sulcus, ts = superior temporal sulcus.

RESULTS

Two hundred and sixty-three neurons in the cortex of the inferior convexity of the temporal lobe were studied in sufficient detail to make some statement about their properties. They were divided into two groups, group OA and group TE, on the basis of the cytoarchitectonic criteria of von Bonin and Bailey (2). (They give several distinguishing characteristics of areas OA and TE. We found those pertaining to layers iii and v the most reliable.) Group OA neurons (N = 58) were located in cortex that was either OA cortex or cortex transitional between OA and TE and located within 2 mm of OA cortex. As shown in Fig. 1, these passes were located near the ascending portion of the inferior occipital sulcus, and thus in the most anterior portion of area OA and the circumstriate belt.[1] Group TE neurons (N = 205) were all located in the posterior and middle portions of area TE. The site of entry of the electrode passes on which OA and TE units were recorded is shown in Fig. 1. A coronal section through one pass is shown in Fig. 2. For purposes of exposition, neurons in both groups will be referred to as "inferotemporal neurons," although this term, strictly speaking, should only refer to the TE units.

With the standard background illumination, all neurons encountered were spontaneously active with almost all discharge rates falling in the range 1–30/sec. The activity of 86% of the OA units and 82% of the TE units was altered by visual stimulation.[2] Most of these units responded exclusively by increasing their rate of discharge (72% of TE units, 62% of OA units). For other units only decreased firing to visual stimuli could be demonstrated (20% of TE, 12% of OA units). The remaining ones showed either increased or decreased firing over the spontaneous level depending on the retinal locus, direction of movement, or other stimulus parameters. Significantly more OA units (26%) than TE units (8%) fell in this class (χ^2 test, $P < .005$).

No neurons were found that responded to auditory or somesthetic stimuli. A few passes were made through superior temporal cortex (area TA). Units recorded on these passes responded only to auditory stimuli and not to visual, confirming our earlier observations under different anesthetic conditions (18).

Receptive fields

SIZE. We determined the receptive-field sizes of 116 neurons. The areas of the largest fields were probably often underestimated since fields extending to a border of the tangent screen were taken to end at that border. If receptive fields were plotted for both eyes, the size of the receptive field of

[2] These percentages are probably inflated by the fact that the time required to demonstrate a response was often less than the time required to classify the cell as "unresponsive," and cells were occasionally left or lost before they had been studied sufficiently to be classed as unresponsive and were therefore excluded from our sample.

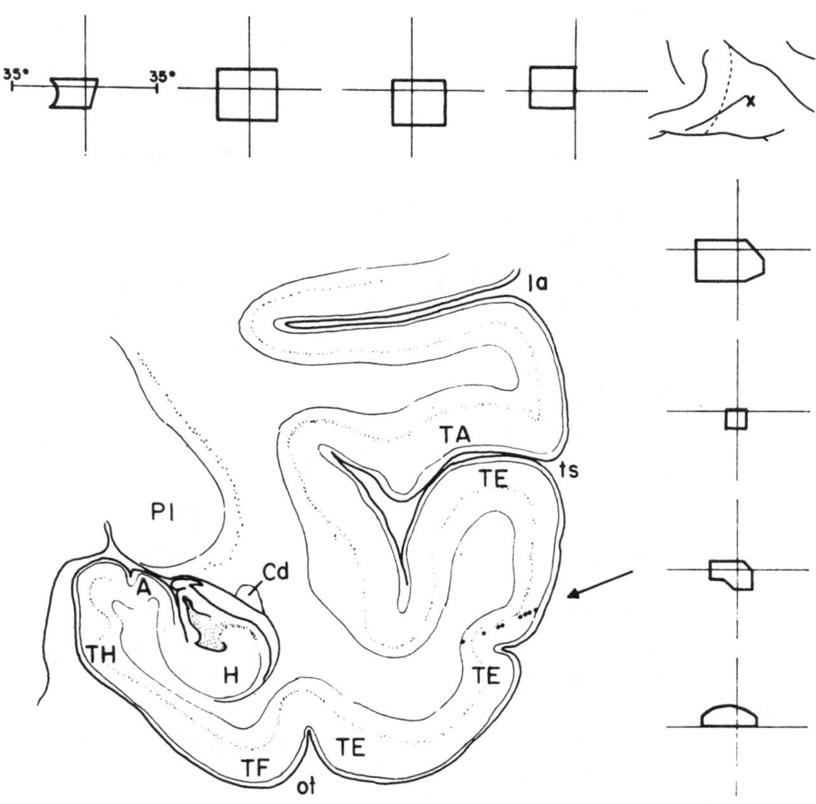

FIG. 2. Coronal section in plane of electrode pass (arrow) in inferotemporal cortex showing approximate location of eight representative cells recorded on the pass and the size and location of their receptive fields. The receptive fields recorded at increasing depth are shown clockwise starting from the top left. In these and all following receptive-field maps, the axes represent the horizontal and vertical meridia of the visual field and the half-field contralateral to the recording electrode is on the left. The scale is in degrees of visual angle. In the inset brain drawing, x marks the site of entry of the electrode pass. la = lateral fissure, ot = occipitotemporal sulcus, ts = superior temporal sulcus, cd = caudate nucleus, H = hippocampus, Pl = pulvinar; TA, TE, TF, TH, and A refer to cytoarchitectonic areas (2).

the dominant eye was used to estimate the size of the neuron's receptive field.

The receptive fields were surprisingly large; those of the TE units were usually larger than those of the OA units. The median area of the receptive fields of TE neurons (N = 86) was 409 deg^2 with first and third quartiles of 145 and 1,410 deg^2, while the median area of the OA fields (N = 30) was 69 deg^2 with the first and third quartiles of 14 and 140 deg^2. This difference in size was significant beyond the .0001 level according to a Mann-Whitney U test. Representative receptive fields are shown in Figs. 2, 4, 5, and 7.

The large size of many of the receptive fields, particularly in group TE, was unlikely to have been the result of some optical artifact, because with the same apparatus and procedures, and often in the same animal, receptive fields of under a square degree were found for units in the circumstriate belt (areas OA, OB) and in striate cortex (area OC). Similarly, scattered light could not easily account for the large size of the fields since there was no difference in the size of the fields when contrast or background illumination was varied over a wide range.

LOCATION. Perhaps the most surprising finding was that, within the accuracy of measurement, the center of gaze or fovea fell within or on the border of the receptive field of every inferotemporal neuron studied.

Unlike those in the geniculostriate system, many receptive fields extended well across the midline into the half-field ipsilateral to the electrode, and some were even confined to the ipsilateral half-field. Lateral borders were determined for 33 OA cells and 95 TE cells. More of the TE cells (56%) than OA cells (30%) had receptive fields which were clearly bilateral (i.e., extended more than 3° into both visual half-fields), although this difference failed to reach significance according to a χ^2 test. Of the essentially unilateral receptive fields (i.e., those extending more than 3° into one half-field and less than 3° into the other half-field) ipsilateral fields were more common in the OA Group (57%) than in the TE Group (20%) according to a χ^2 test ($P < .05$).

The geometric centers of the receptive fields are shown in Fig. 3. Note that for both groups, the centers of the "bilateral" receptive fields were predominantly (79%) located in the contralateral half-field (binomial test, $P < .001$).

About half of the cells responded more strongly when stimulated in one part of their receptive field. This more responsive area always included the fovea and extended, within the receptive field, 3–20° from the fovea. This phenomenon of a stronger response over the fovea is illustrated in Figs. 4 and 5. Among the neurons with bilateral fields, stimulation of the contralateral portion often elicited a stronger response than stimulation of the ipsilateral portion, whereas the converse was very rarely found.

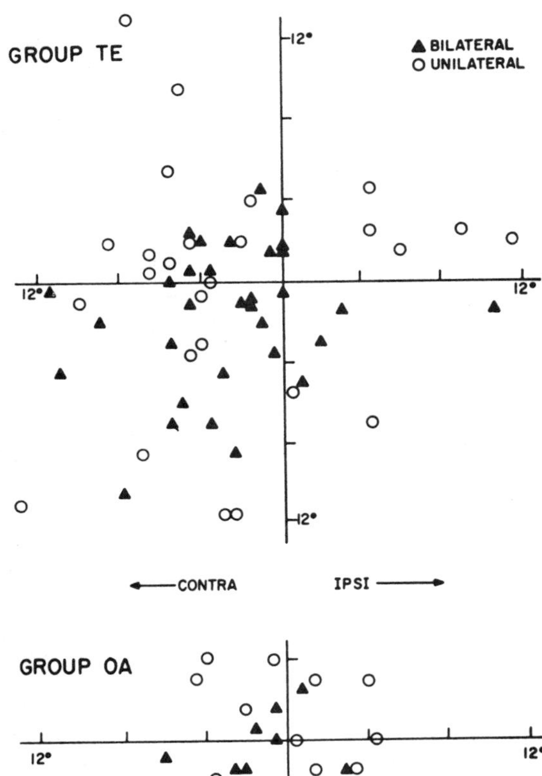

FIG. 3. Geometric centers of receptive fields. Axes represent the horizontal and vertical meridia. The scale is in degrees of visual angle. ipsi is the half-field ipsilateral to the electrode and contra the contralateral half-field. Cells designated as bilateral extended more than 3° into both half-fields and those designated as unilateral extended more than 3° into one half-field and 3° or less into the other half-field. This sample excluded cells whose receptive fields extended to at least one border of the 70° x 70° tangent screen and cells whose receptive fields extended 3° or less into either half-field. (The latter fields, since they included the center of gaze, like all other fields, necessarily had geometric centers within 1.5° from this point.)

Effects of stimulus parameters

MOVEMENT. Almost all the units responded more vigorously to a moving stimulus than to a stationary one. Although rate of movement was not systematically varied for a large number of units, most neurons did seem to respond to the standard rate of 5–7°/sec better than to much higher or lower rates of movement.

LIGHT VERSUS DARK. Of the 226 neurons tested with light stimuli, 71% responded to light stimuli, and of the 186 neurons tested with dark stimuli, 69% responded to dark

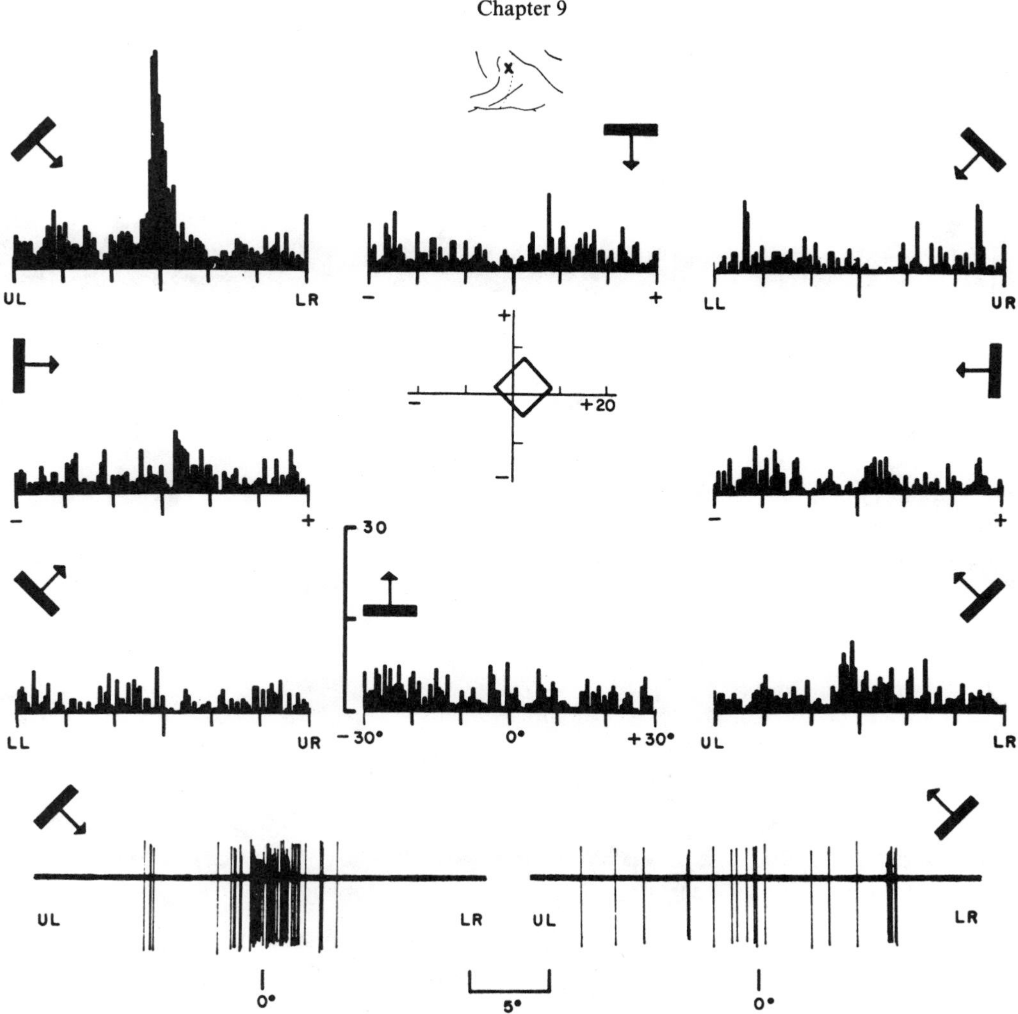

FIG. 4. Receptive field and responses of a group OA neuron which showed unidirectional sensitivity. Histograms indicate frequency of firing of the unit as a function of retinal locus of a 1° x 70° red slit moving at 5°/sec in the direction indicated above each histogram. Each histogram was generated by 10 sweeps of the stimulus. For the eight histograms, the vertical scale indicates number of neuron discharges and the horizontal scale, degrees of visual angle; the middle of each horizontal scale (0°) represents the center of gaze. The receptive field of this unit is shown in the center of the array of histograms. Plus (+) in all parts of the figure inidcates upper or right of the visual field; minus (−) indicates lower or left; UL, upper left; LR, lower right; LL, lower left; UR, upper right. The lower part of the figure shows the discharges of an isolated unit to a single sweep of the stimulus in the indicated direction on an expanded time scale. Histograms and trace in which the arrow is shown on the left were generated from left to right, whereas the converse was true where the arrow is shown on the right. The site of the pass on which this was recorded is shown in the top center of the figure. See also legends to Figs. 1 and 2.

stimuli. Of the 151 neurons studied with both dark and light stimuli, 48% responded to both types of stimulation. These proportions were similar for the OA and TE groups. Whether a neuron responded to dark, light, or both types of stimuli did not appear correlated with its other properties.

SIZE AND SHAPE OF STIMULI. Our set of frequently used stimuli was impoverished relative to the possible set of arbitrary stimuli we could have used or even to a set of stimuli "relevant" to a monkey. Since, in our earlier preparations, circles and rectangles of light were usually much less effective stimuli than light slits, we soon abandoned systematic use of the former stimuli. A few TE neurons, however, did seem to prefer a 3° diameter circle or a 5° x 5° square to the standard 1° slit. 10° x

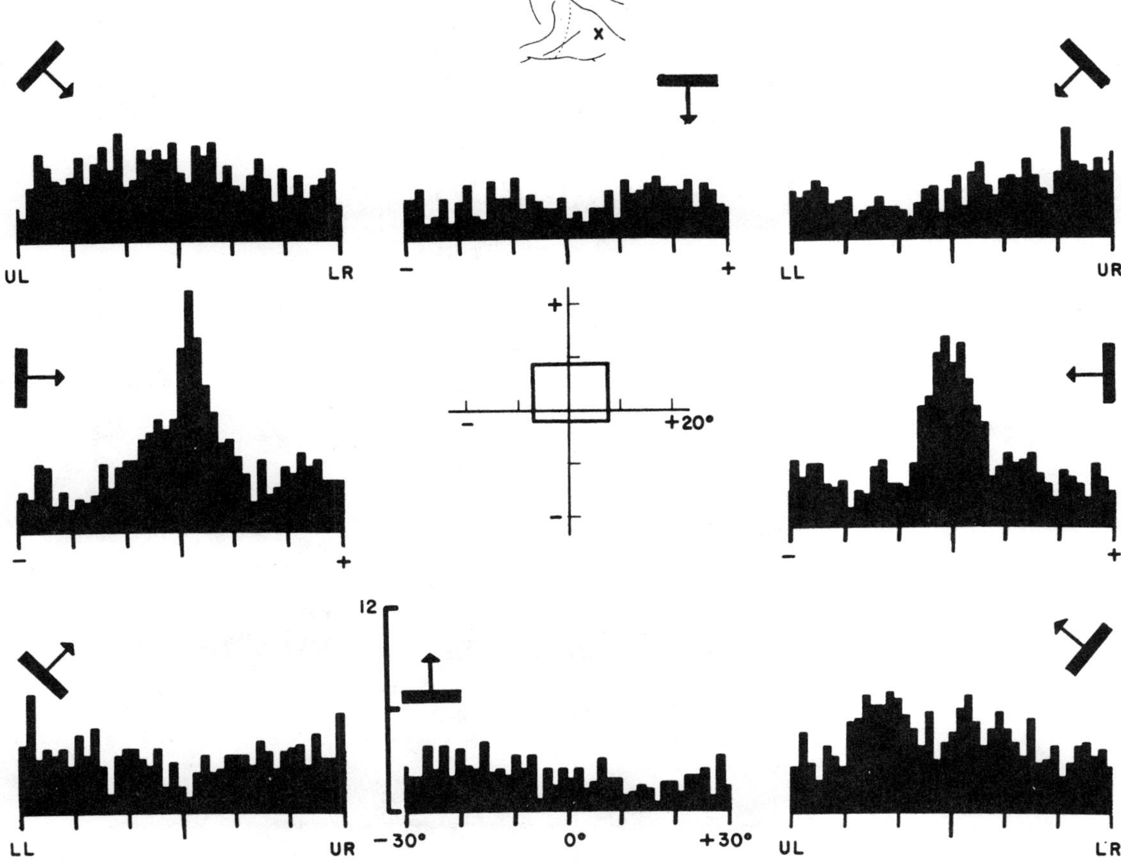

FIG. 5. Receptive field and responses of a group TE neuron which showed bidirectional sensitivity. The stimulus was a white slit 1° x 70° moving at 5°/sec. Each histogram is based on seven sweeps of the stimulus. See also legends to Figs. 1, 2, and 4. Responses of this neuron to single sweeps of the stimulus are shown in Fig. 8.

5° and 5° x 5° checkerboards were good stimuli for several units, but these stimuli were later abandoned because of the difficulty in determining exact field boundaries with them. For most neurons, a light slit 1.0° wide yielded stronger responses than either a much wider or narrower one. Surprisingly, the length of the slit did not appear critical for many neurons in either group. For at least three TE units, complex colored patterns (e.g., photographs of faces, trees) were more effective than the standard stimuli, but the crucial features of these stimuli were never determined. Of the neurons tested to a diffuse light flash, about one-third responded, usually in a very weak fashion.

Our dark stimuli were also less than ideal, both in their poverty and in their lack of correspondence to the standard light stimuli. However, the greater ease of producing dark stimuli (by picking up objects at hand or making paper cutouts) did yield some interesting observations. The most common dark stimuli used were a variety of rectangles or slits with widths of .25–30° and lengths of 1–70°, and the shadow of a human or monkey hand. The use of the latter stimuli was begun one day when, having failed to drive a unit with any light stimulus, we waved a hand at the stimulus screen and elicited a very vigorous response from the previously unresponsive neuron. We then spent the next 12 hr testing various paper cutouts in an attempt to find the trigger feature for this unit. When the entire set of stimuli used were ranked according to the strength of the response that they produced, we could not find a simple physical dimension that correlated with this rank order. However, the rank order of adequate stimuli did correlate with similarity (for us) to the shadow of a monkey hand. The relative adequacy of a few of these stimuli is shown in Fig. 6. Curiously, fingers pointing downward elicited very little response as compared to fingers pointing upward or laterally, the usual orientations in which the animal would see its own hand.

Of the 128 neurons that responded to dark stimuli, about 50 fired best to one of the rectangular stimuli, the smaller ones usually being better. For the remaining neurons, particular complex dark stimuli were the best stimuli we could find.

Several neurons fired much more strongly to three-dimensional objects placed in the plane of the tangent screen than to any stimulus projected onto the screen, including two-dimensional representations of that object. This rather surprising phenomenon was observed with monocular as well as binocular stimulation.

In summary, although our explorations of stimulus size and shape were limited and nonsystematic, certain conclusions can be drawn with some certainty. First, approximately 1° wide light slits were usually more powerful stimuli than light circles, rectangles, wider slits, or diffuse light. Second, there were units whose response depended on the length and width of the light slit. Third, there were units that would respond vigorously to specific and complex dark shapes but not to dark slits or to dark rectangles of similar overall dimensions. (More of the TE units than the OA units responded to unusual stimuli, but this may simply have reflected the greater ease of driving the OA units with the standard stimuli, and the consequent lesser tendency to test them with irregular stimuli.) Fourth, few units responded in identical fashion with one another to a range of stimuli (except for several clusters of two to five units recorded on the same pass at similar depths). Rather, although responses to certain stimuli were common, most units seemed to have their own unique preference spectra. Finally, with the exception of one cell, the optimum stimulus for a cell was optimum throughout the receptive field, even for cells with large bilateral fields.

ORIENTATION AND DIRECTION OF MOVEMENT. Virtually all neurons in both group OA and group TE responded best or only to moving stimuli. Furthermore, if the neuron was sensitive to the orientation of the stimulus, the optimal orientation was almost always orthogonal to the optimal direction of movement. Therefore it was usually not meaningful to distinguish sensitivity to orientation of a stimulus from sensitivity to its direction of movement. Responses to a stimulus moving orthogonally to its long axis in four directions 90° apart were systematically compared for 24 OA units and 64 TE units. If a unit fired differentially to two of these directions of movement it was defined as being "direction sensitive" without implying anything about the underlying mechanism. Some direction-sensitive neurons respond equally well to movements 180° apart (preferred directions) but poorly or not at all to orthogonal directions (null directions). These are termed "bidirection sensitive" units. Other direction-sensitive neurons responded best to one direction of movement and had null directions 90° to the preferred direction. These are termed "unidirection sensitive" neurons.

A far greater proportion of OA units (83%) than of TE units (48%) were direction sensitive (χ^2 test, $P < 0.005$). Of the direction-sensitive neurons most of the ones in group TE (85%) but only half the ones in group OA were bidirection sensitive (difference significant at the 0.01 level, χ^2 test). Responses of a typical unidirection-sensitive OA unit are shown in Fig. 4 and of a typi-

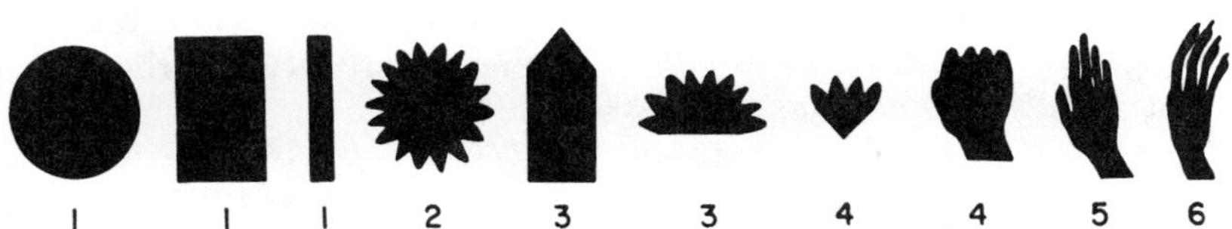

FIG. 6. Examples of shapes used to stimulate a group TE unit apparently having very complex trigger features. The stimuli are arranged from left to right in order of increasing ability to drive the neuron from none (1) or little (2 and 3) to maximum (6).

cal bidirection-sensitive TE unit in Figs. 5 and 8. The directional sensitivity was the same everywhere in the receptive field, with the exception of one cell (ref 16, Fig. 3). For most of the cells tested, directional sensitivity was independent of contrast.

There were a few units that were exceptions to the generalization that the best orientation of a stimulus was orthogonal to its best direction of movement. These included three units that preferred handlike dark stimuli (for which the orientation of the fingers independent of the direction of movement was critical), two that preferred movement of a slit parallel to its long axis, and one that fired best to a moving vertical slit independent of the direction of movement.

We observed only two units for which the preferred direction of movement was different between the two eyes. The receptive-field location and the response properties were similar, as usual, in the two eyes, except that the preferred direction of movement within the receptive field of each eye was mirror symmetric along the vertical meridian (ref 16, Fig. 3).

COLOR. We had not intended to test sensitivity to wavelength. However in an early experiment after the standard dark and light stimuli failed to drive a unit, we tried some colored slides, and elicited strong responses. Subsequent study of this unit revealed that red or orange stimuli were required to drive it. Thereafter, in searching for an adequate stimulus to plot receptive fields we often projected red, green, or blue slits.

Although colored stimuli appeared to be particularly effective in driving many units, we did not plot their spectral sensitivity. However, in 19 of 52 units for which we compared the response to red, green, blue, and white stimuli, the magnitude of the response was not correlated with luminance of the stimuli. Most of these would respond vigorously to a red pattern (luminance 5 mL), but not at all to the same pattern when it was green (luminance 8 mL) or blue (luminance .4 mL). Neither would they respond when the pattern was white even though its luminance was varied over a range of 2.6 log units (.1–40 mL). Only two cells showed such a preference for green light and one did so for blue.

Four of the apparently color-sensitive cells (of 21 tested) were in group OA and 15 (of 31 tested) were in group TE, but no inferences about the incidence of color preferences in the two groups can be made since most of the units studied in any detail were units that were very difficult to drive with white light.

INTERSTIMULUS INTERVAL. Most of the neurons studied showed a decline in response when repeatedly stimulated at less than 5-sec intervals. Response strength could be maintained by increasing this interval. Units requiring more than 15 sec between stimulation for optimum response were more common in the TE group.

The responsiveness of a few of the TE units would decline in the course of a single sweep of an adequate stimulus across the receptive field at the standard (5–7°/sec) rate. Such a unit would fire briskly as a bar sweeping across the tangent screen entered the receptive field, but would show little response by the time it reached the opposite border (see Fig. 7). However, if introduced after several seconds of no stimulation, the bar would elicit an equally strong response any place within the receptive field.

EYE DOMINANCE. For 63 neurons, the relative effectiveness of stimulating the two eyes was determined. For both groups, one-quarter of the units responded more strongly to stimulation of the ipsilateral eye, one-quarter to stimulation of the contralateral eye, and half showed no clear difference between the eyes. The existence and type of eye dominance was not found to be related to the site of the unit or any other response characteristic. If responses could be elicited from both eyes, the receptive field center was approximately the same for both, as were the response properties, with the exception of the two units described above that had opposite directional sensitivity for the two eyes.

Effect of EEG state and barbiturate administration

After several experiments it was observed that, for almost all neurons, variations in the EEG were correlated with variations in

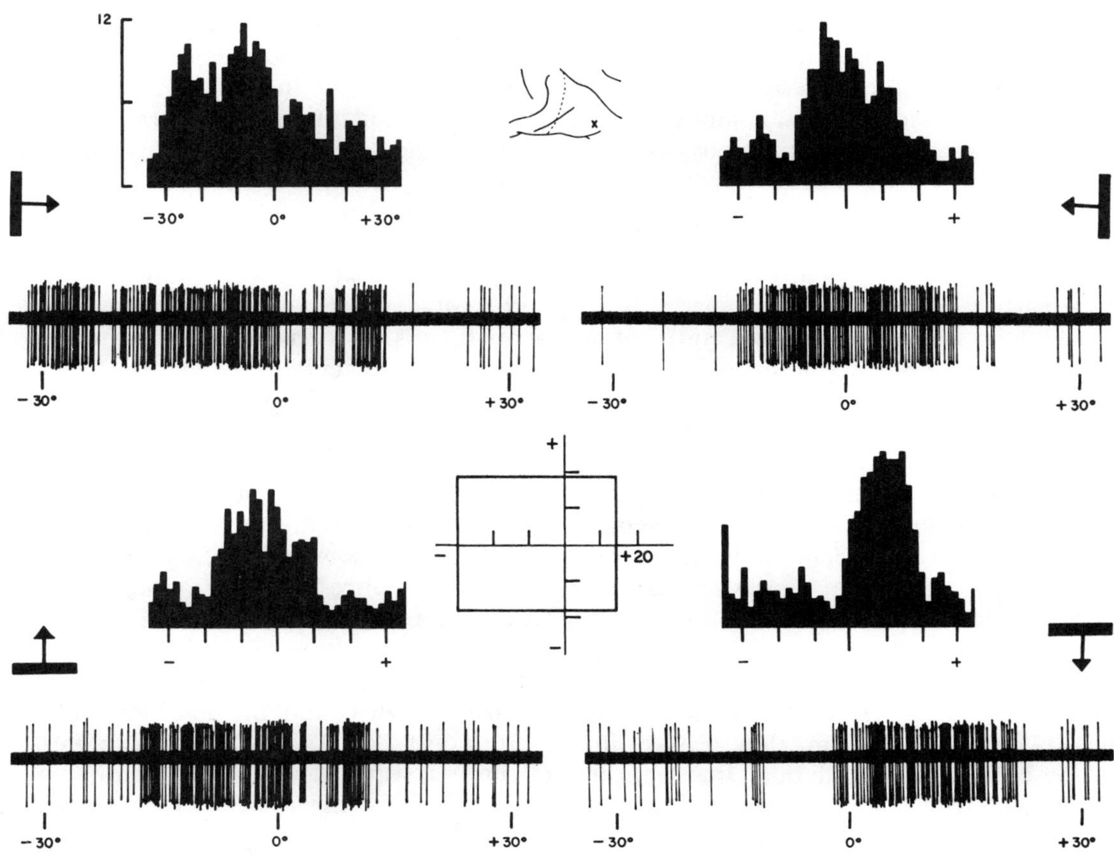

FIG. 7. Receptive field and responses of a group TE neuron which did not respond differentially to the orientation or direction of movement of a 1° x 70° white slit. Each histogram was generated by 10 sweeps of the stimulus moving in the indicated direction at 6.7°/sec. Note that the response is vigorous when the slit enters the receptive field but declines before the slit reaches the opposite border. See also legends to Figs. 1, 2, and 4.

the strength of a neuron's response. Neurons would respond vigorously during periods of low voltage, fast and asynchronous EEG (called hereafter "fast" EEG), but show little or no response during periods of relatively high voltage, slow and synchronous EEG (called hereafter "slow" EEG). This is illustrated in Fig. 8. In some units the pattern of spontaneous activity was different in states of fast or slow EEG, but in

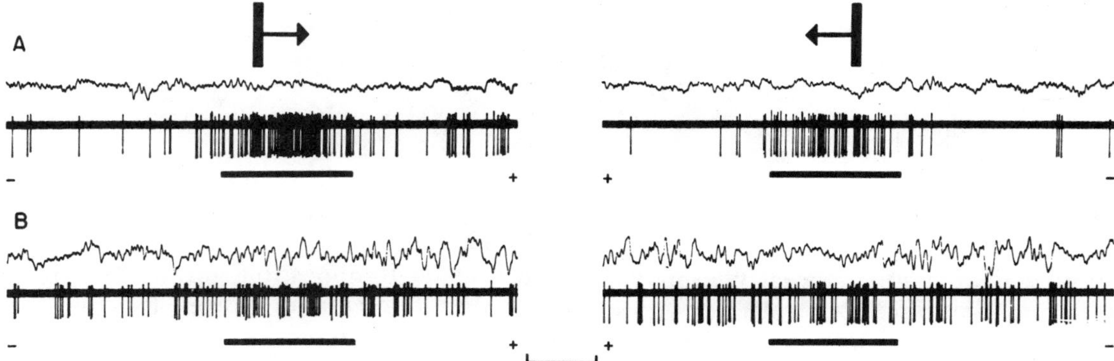

FIG. 8. Responses of a group TE neuron under two EEG conditions, *A,* fast, and *B,* slow (see text), to movement of a 1° x 70° white slit in the indicated direction at 5°/sec. The horizontal bars indicate the receptive-field location. This is the same neuron whose receptive field and histograms are shown in Fig. 5. The marker indicates 3 sec or 15°

others only changes in evoked activity were associated with changes in EEG.

Novel acoustic, somesthetic, and olfactory stimulation would return an animal in a state of slow EEG to its previous state of fast EEG, and simultaneously restore the unit's previous responsiveness. None of these novel stimuli would alter the unit's activity if the EEG was already fast. After these earlier observations were made, EEG was closely monitored during study of a neuron. When the EEG became slow it was returned to its previous fast state by acoustic, somesthetic, or olfactory stimulation before study of the unit continued. Novel somesthetic or auditory stimuli are also often required for full visual responsiveness of area 17 and area 18 neurons in the cat anesthetized with nitrous oxide and oxygen (J. D. Pettigrew, personal communication).

Intravenous injection of sodium thiamylal would totally eliminate first the responsivity of a unit to visual stimuli and then the ability to transform slow EEG into fast by peripheral stimulation. In time, the two phenomena would return in the opposite order.

DISCUSSION

Characteristics of inferotemporal neurons

COMPARISONS WITH OTHER VISUAL NEURONS. The most striking finding of this study was the relatively large receptive fields that invariably included the fovea. Such receptive fields do not appear to be characteristic of neurons in other brain structures. Another unusual finding was the large receptive fields that extended well into both visual hemifields. Cells with similar receptive fields have been found in the pulvinar (14) and anterior middle suprasylvian cortex (AMSS) of the cat (9). Apparently unique were the receptive fields confined to the ipsilateral half-field and extending more than 10° from the vertical meridian.

Two sets of inferotemporal neurons had properties that appeared relatively novel. One would respond only by decreased firing. That is, these cells would fire less when stimulated by particular stimuli (their "adequate" stimuli) but no stimuli could be found that would increase the rate of firing above the spontaneous level. Two similar cells have been previously reported in striate cortex of the cat (30). The other set of cells had opposite directional selectivity in the two eyes. However, both sets were small and similar neurons may turn up elsewhere in the brain. Similarly, although there were a number of inferotemporal neurons with strikingly specific and complex trigger features, the incidence of such cells in inferotemporal cortex and elsewhere is difficult to estimate.

Besides these unusual properties, inferotemporal neurons had many response properties similar to those of neurons in other visual structures. The preference for moving stimuli over stationary ones, preference for bars over spots of light, varying degree of eye dominance, and waning of response with repeated stimulation, typical characteristics of inferotemporal units, have also been reported for neurons in striate cortex, prestriate cortex, and the superior colliculus (e.g., 19–22, 30, 34). Most inferotemporal units resembled superior colliculus and AMSS units in the cat rather than visual cortex units in tolerating considerable variation in stimulus shape and direction of movement without altering their response (e.g., 9, 34). By contrast, other inferotemporal units were similar to visual cortex units and very different from colliculus units in their sensitivity to size, shape, and orientation of a stimulus (e.g., 19–21, 30).

The directional sensitivities of inferotemporal units were very heterogeneous. Many were not direction sensitive at all; while some had null directions 90° to the preferred direction, like units in visual cortex and some AMSS units in the cat; while others had null directions 180° to the preferred direction, like some colliculus and AMSS units in the cat (e.g., 9, 19–21, 30, 34).

The small number and widespread distribution of our passes and the acute angle at which almost all of them entered the brain made it impossible for us to determine if inferotemporal cortex has the columnar organization so characteristic of striate and prestriate cortex. We did observe a clustering of similar properties among neurons successively recorded on the same pass, but this could have reflected a laminar or complex nesting organization almost as well as a columnar one.

COMPARISON OF GROUP TE AND GROUP OA NEURONS. The neurons we studied were in two different cytoarchitectonic areas according to the criteria of von Bonin and Bailey (2). The group OA neurons were in the part of area OA near the ascending portion of the inferior occipital sulcus, thus near the rostral border of circumstriate cortex. The group TE neurons were in the dorsal middle and posterior portions of area TE. Although OA and TE neurons shared many characteristics, the two groups differed in incidence of neurons with certain properties. OA units had smaller receptive fields and were more likely to show differential sensitivity to direction of movement of the stimulus. If direction sensitive, TE units but not OA units were much more likely to be bidirectional. Although both groups included neurons with bilateral, contralateral, and ipsilateral receptive fields, in the TE group, bilateral fields were more common and ipsilateral fields rarer.

Although the exact anterior border of the projection of striate cortex onto the circumstriate belt is unclear, it is likely that at most two passes (the most caudal) fell within it (cf. 7, 39; A. Cowey, unpublished data). Thus except for these two passes, the area we recorded from was connected to striate cortex by a minimum of two synapses. Cowey (unpublished observations) has shown that cells immediately anterior to the inferior occipital sulcus (i.e., in the area of our group OA cells) project diffusely throughout area TE. Therefore the properties of TE units might derive, at least in part, from converging inputs from OA neurons.

Functions of inferotemporal cortex

Bilateral ablation of inferotemporal cortex impairs visual learning while leaving both visuosensory function and learning ability in other modalities intact (see review by Gross, ref 15). Inferotemporal cortex receives direct projections both from the ipsilateral circumstriate belt and, by way of the splenium of the corpus callosum, from the contralateral circumstriate belt (26). In turn, each circumstriate belt receives a projection from both striate cortices (7, 39, 40). Interruption of this corticocortical occipitotemporal pathway impairs visual discrimination learning (5, 24, 28, 29). Therefore we (5, 15, 16, 32) and others (e.g., 4, 28) have hypothesized that this pathway carries visual information to inferotemporal cortex, where it is further processed. Such "processing" is presumed necessary for normal visual discrimination learning.

This hypothesis is directly supported by the present results in that they demonstrate that visual information does arrive at inferotemporal cortex and that this information is both specific and complex. Furthermore, the hypothesis that inferotemporal cortex further processes outputs of the circumstriate belt provides an explanation for two prominent properties of inferotemporal units, viz., the invariable inclusion of the fovea in the receptive fields and the existence of bilateral and ipsilateral receptive fields. The inclusion of the fovea would derive from the fact that inferotemporal cortex receives a heavy projection from the portion of prestriate cortex ("foveal prestriate cortex") onto which the foveal representation in striate cortex projects (7, 39). The ipsilateral and bilateral receptive fields would derive from the connections of the two circumstriate belts through the splenium of the corpus callosum (35) or the connections of the two inferotemporal cortices through the anterior commissure (12) or both connections.

Further support for the importance of the corticocortical input to inferotemporal cortex is the effects of its interruption on the visual properties of inferotemporal neurons. After total removal of one striate cortex, the receptive fields of inferotemporal neurons in both hemispheres are confined to the visual half-field contralateral to the intact striate cortex (unpublished observations). After section of the corpus callosum and anterior commissure, inferotemporal neurons have receptive fields confined to the visual half-field contralateral to the recording electrode (unpublished observations).

The next, and more difficult, question is how inferotemporal cortex processes the visual information it receives from the circumstriate belt. One hypothesis is that inferotemporal cortex is a further stage in the hierarchy of visual mechanisms shown by Hubel and Wiesel (19–21) to extend from the retina through the geniculostriate system to the circumstriate belt. The successive transformations of visual input that Hubel and Wiesel have proposed to occur in this system involve two chief principles. The first is increasing generalization across the retina: cells at higher levels can be driven by their adequate stimulus over wider regions of the retina. The second is increasing specificity of the adequate stimulus: orientation of a slit is not critical for ganglion or lateral geniculate cells but is critical for cortical cells; length of a slit is critical for hypercomplex but not simple or complex cortical cells. Hubel and Wiesel suggest that convergence of outputs from cells at a lower level underlie these transformations.

Virtually all inferotemporal neurons appear to continue the first trend: their receptive fields were much larger than those of complex and hypercomplex neurons with fields in comparable retinal areas. A few inferotemporal neurons appear to continue the second trend: they had more specific trigger features than have been reported for complex or hypercomplex cells. Many cells, however, appeared to be less sensitive to such stimulus parameters as length, width, and orientation than cells in striate and prestriate cortex. This apparent lack of specificity may have been because these cells had complex and specific trigger features that we never found. The existence of other cells in our sample with very complex trigger features supports this possibility. The observation that three-dimensional objects were far more adequate stimuli than two-dimensional patterns for some neurons also suggests that a wider range of stimuli might have revealed a greater stimulus specificity.

It is also possible that "stimulus adequacy" for some inferotemporal neurons may depend on more than the retinal stimulus: it may depend on the orientation of the animal relative to the stimulus or on the meaning of the stimulus for the animal. The former possibility is suggested by the afferent connections of inferotemporal cortex and the latter by both the behavioral effects of inferotemporal lesions and the incredible specificity of the trigger features of a few units.

Besides its input from the geniculostriate system, inferotemporal cortex (and circumstrate cortex) receives a projection from the pulvinar (3, 5) which, in turn, receives a projection from the superior colliculus (29). There is considerable evidence that the superior colliculus is implicated in visual orientation and localization (e.g., 8, 23, 31, 33, 36). Thus, it is conceivable that information about the relation of visual stimuli to the position or movement of the animal's head and eyes may be projected corticopetally from the pulvinar. That is, inferotemporal cortex (and perhaps circumstriate cortex) may integrate pattern analysis functions of the geniculostriate system with orientation functions of the tectofugal system.

The speculation that "adequacy" of a stimulus for inferotemporal neurons might also be a function of the meaning of the stimulus is similar to Konorski's (25) hypothesis of "gnostic units." It was repeatedly suggested by observing units such as the one described above that fired best to the shadow of a monkey hand. Further support for this possibility comes from the analysis of the discrimination deficit that follows inferotemporal lesions: this deficit depends on several nonsensory factors such as the animal's prior experience, the training procedure used, and the type of reinforcement (15 and e.g., 5, 17, 24, 27, 28).

In summary, the present results demonstrate that inferotemporal cortex neurons receive specific and complex visual information. The visual responsiveness of these neurons is dependent on striate cortex and they probably receive visual information over a corticocortical route from striate cortex to the circumstriate belt, and then to inferotemporal cortex. The large receptive fields of inferotemporal neurons and the specific trigger features of some of them suggest that the processing of information in inferotemporal cortex continues the trends seen in the geniculostrate system. However, it is also possible that new types of integration occur in inferotemporal cortex—that the activity of inferotemporal units depends on more than the retinal stimulus. For example, it may also depend on information received from the tectofugal system about the location of the stimulus relative to the animal and on the significance of the stimulus for the animal. We are currently examining these possibilities in behaving monkeys.

SUMMARY

1. The responses to visual stimuli of 263 neurons in inferotemporal cortex were studied in paralyzed monkeys anesthetized with nitrous oxide and oxygen.

2. All had receptive fields that included the fovea and were relatively large. Bilateral, contralateral, and ipsilateral receptive fields were found.

3. Most neurons were sensitive to several of the following parameters of the visual stimulus: contrast, wavelength, size, shape, orientation, and direction of movement. Some had highly specific and unique trigger features.

4. The results were viewed as supporting the hypothesis that inferotemporal cortex further processes visual information received from the geniculostriate system and may be involved in additional visual functions.

ACKNOWLEDGMENTS

We thank L. Frishman, S. Volman, and G. Seiler for their assistance in all phases of the investigation.

This research was begun in the Department of Psychology, Harvard University. It was supported by National Institutes of Health Grants MH-14471 and MH-19420 and National Science Foundation Grants GB 6999 and GB 27612X.

A preliminary account for some of these results has been published (16).

Professor C. E. Rocha-Miranda was a visiting investigator from the Instituto de Biofísica, Universidade Federal do Rio de Janeiro, Brazil.

REFERENCES

1. Barlow, H. B., Blakemore, C., and Pettigrew, J. D. The neural mechanism of binocular depth discrimination. J. *Physiol., London* 193: 327–342, 1967.
2. Bonin, G. von, and Bailey, P. *The Neocortex of Macaca mulatta*. Urbana: Univ. of Illinois Press, 1947.
3. Chow, K. L. A retrograde cell degeneration study of the cortical projection field of the pulvinar in the monkey. J. Comp. Neurol. 93: 313–340, 1950.
4. Chow, K. L. Anatomical and electrographical analysis of temporal neocortex in relation to visual discrimniation learning in monkeys. In: *Brain Mechanisms in Learning,* edited by J. F. Delafresnaye. Oxford: Blackwell, 1961, p. 507–525.
5. Cowey, A. and Gross, C. G. Effects of foveal prestriate and inferotemporal lesions on visual discrimination by rhesus monkeys. *Exptl. Brain Res.* 11: 128–144, 1970.
6. Cowey, A. and Weiskrantz, L. A comparison of the effects of inferotemporal and striate cortex lesions on the visual behavior of rhesus monkeys. *Quart. J. Exptl. Psychol.* 19: 246–253, 1967.
7. Cragg, B. G. and Ainsworth, A. The topography of the afferent projections in the circumstriate visual cortex of the monkey studied by the Nauta method. *Vision Res.* 9: 733–747, 1969.
8. Denny-Brown, D. and Chambers, R. A. Visual orientation in the macaque monkey. *Trans. Am. Neurol. Assoc.* 20: 37–40, 1958.
9. Dow, B. M. and Dubner, R. Single-unit responses to moving visual stimuli in middle suprasylvian gyrus of the cat. *J. Neurophysiol.* 34: 47–55, 1971.
10. Evarts, E. V. Relation of pyramidal tract activity to force exerted during voluntary movement. *J. Neurophysiol.* 31: 14–27, 1968.
11. Evarts, E. V. A technique for recording activity of subcortical neurons in moving animals. *Electroencephalog. Clin. Neurophysiol.* 24: 83–86, 1968.
12. Fox, C. A., Fisher, R. R., and DeSalva, S. J. The distribution of the anterior commissure in the monkey (*Macaca mulatta*). *J. Comp. Neurol.* 89: 245–278, 1948.
13. Gerstein, G. L., Gross, C. G., and Weinstein, M. Inferotemporal evoked potentials during visual discrimination performance by monkeys. *J. Comp. Physiol. Psychol.* 65: 526–528, 1968.
14. Godfraind, J. M., Meulders, M., and Veraart, C. Visual receptive fields of neurons in pulvinar, nucleus lateralis posterior and nucleus suprageniculatus thalami of the cat. *Brain Res.* 15: 552–555, 1969.
15. Gross, C. G. Visual functions of inferotemporal cortex. In: *Handbook of Sensory Physiology*, edited by R. Jung. Berlin: Springer, 1972, vol. 7: part 3.
16. Gross, C. G., Bender, D. B., Rocha-Miranda, C. E. Visual receptive fields of neurons in inferotemporal cortex of the monkey. *Science* 166: 1303–1306, 1969.
17. Gross, C. G., Cowey, A., and Manning, F. J. Further analysis of visual discrimination deficits following foveal prestriate and inferotemporal lesions in rhesus monkeys. *J. Comp. Physiol. Psychol.* 76: 1–7, 1971.
18. Gross, C. G., Schiller, P. H., Wells, C., and

Gerstein, G. L. Single-unit activity in temporal association cortex of the monkey. *J. Neurophysiol.* 30: 833–843, 1967.

19. Hubel, D. H. and Wiesel, T. N. Receptive fields, binocular interaction and functional architecture in the cat's visual cortex. *J. Physiol., London* 160: 106–154, 1962.

20. Hubel, D. H. and Wiesel, T. N. Receptive fields and functional architecture in two nonstriate visual areas (18 and 19) of the cat. *J. Neurophysiol.* 28: 229–289, 1965.

21. Hubel, D. H. and Wiesel, T. N. Receptive fields and functional architecture of monkey striate cortex. *J. Physiol., London* 195: 215–243, 1968.

22. Humphrey, N. K. Responses to visual stimuli of units in the superior colliculus of rats and monkeys. *Exptl. Neurol.* 20: 312–340, 1968.

23. Humphrey, N. K. What the frog's eye tells the monkey's brain. *Brain, Behav., Evol.* 3: 324–327, 1970.

24. Iwai, E. and Mishkin, M. Further evidence on the locus of the visual area in the temporal lobe of the monkey. *Exptl. Neurol.* 25: 585–594, 1969.

25. Konorski, J. *Integrative Activity of the Brain.* Chicago: Univ. of Chicago Press, 1967.

26. Kuypers, H. G. J. M., Szwarcbart, M. K., Mishkin, M., and Rosvold, H. E. Occipitotemporal corticocortical connections in the rhesus monkey. *Exptl. Neurol.* 11: 245–262, 1965.

27. Manning, F. J. Punishment for errors and visual-discrimination learning by monkeys with inferotemporal cortex lesions. *J. Comp. Physiol. Psychol.* 75: 146–152, 1971.

28. Mishkin, M. Visual mechanisms beyond the striate cortex. In: *Frontiers of Physiological Psychology,* edited by R. Russell. New York: Academic, 1966, p. 93–119.

29. Mishkin, M. Cortical visual areas and their interaction. In: *The Brain and Human Behavior,* edited by A. G. Karzsmar and J. C. Eccles. Berlin: Springer, 1972, p. 187–208.

30. Pettigrew, J. D., Nikara, T., and Bishop, P. O. Responses to moving slits by single units in cat striate cortex. *Exptl. Brain Res.* 6: 373–390, 1968.

31. Schneider, G. E. Two visual systems. *Science* 163: 895–902, 1969.

32. Schwartzkroin, P. A., Cowey, A., and Gross, C. G. A test of an "efferent model" of the function of inferotemporal cortex in visual discrimination. *Electroencephalog. Clin. Neurophysiol.* 27: 594–600, 1969.

33. Sprague, J. M. and Meikle, T. H., Jr. The role of the superior colliculus in visually guided behavior. *Exptl. Neurol.* 11: 115–146, 1965.

34. Sterling, P. and Wickelgren, B. G. Visual receptive fields in the superior colliculus of the cat. *J. Neurophysiol.* 32: 1–15, 1969.

35. Sunderland, S. The distribution of commissural fibers in the corpus callosum in the macaque monkey. *J. Neurol. Psychiat.* 3: 9–18, 1940.

36. Trevarthen, C. B. Two mechanisms of vision in primates. *Psychol. Forsch.* 31: 299–337, 1968.

37. Vaughan, H. G., Jr. and Gross, C. G. Cortical responses to light in unanesthetized monkeys and their alteration by visual system lesions. *Exptl. Brain Res.* 8: 19–36, 1969.

38. Wolbarsht, M. L., MacNichol, E. F., and Wagner, H. G. Glass insulated platinum microelectrode. *Science* 132: 1309–1310, 1960.

39. Zeki, S. M. Representation of central visual fields in prestriate cortex of monkey. *Brain Res.* 14: 271–291, 1969.

40. Zeki, S. M. Interhemispheric connections of prestriate cortex in monkey. *Brain Res.* 19: 63–75, 1970.

10

B. C. Motter and V. B. Mountcastle

The functional properties of the light-sensitive neurons of the posterior parietal cortex studied in waking monkeys: Foveal sparing and opponent vector organization

1981. *Journal of Neuroscience* 1: 3–26

Abstract

We describe in this paper the results of a new study of the inferior parietal lobule in 10 waking monkeys combining the methods of behavioral control, visual stimulation, and single neuron analysis. In this study, 1682 neurons were identified; 804 were studied in detail. Neurons insensitive to visual stimuli comprise the fixation, oculomotor, and projection-manipulation classes thought to be involved in initiatives toward action. The largest group of the light-sensitive (LS) neurons were activated from large and frequently bilateral response areas that excluded the foveal region; we term this *foveal sparing*. The remaining cells subtended areas including the fovea, when tested with large stimuli (6° × 6°), but only 8 of 216 cells studied in detail responded to the small fixation target light. We propose that a dynamic central neural process associated with the acts of fixation and visual attention suppresses responses to foveal stimuli.

Parietal LS neurons are sensitive to stimulus movement and direction over a wide range of velocities. The vectors point either inward toward the center or outward toward the perimeter of the visual field, and for neurons with bilateral response areas, the vectors commonly point in opposite directions in the two half-fields; we term this *opponent vector organization*.

The functional properties of area 7 LS neurons are such that they could signal motion in the immediate surround and the apparent motion accompanying head movements and forward locomotion. We surmise that they contribute to a central neural image of immediately surrounding space and to the perceptual constancy of that space obtaining during bodily movement. These properties are suitable for the attraction of gaze and attention to objects and events in the peripheral visual fields. It is this system, together with the classes of parietal neurons concerned with action initiatives, whose destruction is thought to account for the hemi-inattention and neglect of the parietal lobe syndrome in primates.

A number of studies have been made of the homotypical cortex of the inferior parietal lobule in waking monkeys. The animals used in these experiments were in most cases trained to emit stereotyped behavioral acts surmised on other grounds to be controlled or influenced by neural systems of which this cortical region is a part (Goldberg and Robinson, 1977, 1978; Hyvarinen and Poranen, 1974; Hyvarinen and Shelepin, 1979; Leinonen and Nyman, 1979; Leinonen et al., 1979; Lynch et al., 1973a, b, 1977; Mountcastle et al., 1975; Robinson and Goldberg, 1977a, b; Robinson et al., 1978; Sakata et al., 1977, 1978, 1980; Yin and Mountcastle, 1977). The results obtained have been considered in the light of changes in behavior that follow lesions of this region in man and in monkeys. They have led to several different but related concepts of the function of this region of the homotypical cortex.

The first idea is that this region (area 7 in the monkey) functions as an association cortex, in the traditional sense, in which neural abstractions of sensory input signals converge and are "integrated." The resulting neural activity is then regarded as leading to, or itself to be, the neural basis of perceptual experiences. Neurons with convergent properties have been observed in area 7, although cells of this type make up only a small percentage of all the cells identified (Hyvarinen and Poranen, 1974; Leinonen and Nyman, 1979; Leinonen et al., 1979; Lynch et al., 1973a, b, 1977; Mountcastle et al., 1975). Moreover, the studies made so far have shown only the fact of convergence, on which basis alone neurons in many parts of the neuraxis might equally well qualify for an "associative" function. It remains to be shown on quantitative grounds in what way the activities of these cells, evoked by a variety of stimuli, might provide some higher order or abstracted replicate of a complex sensory event, e.g., a pattern of activity uniquely defined by a certain spatial and temporal combination of stimuli in two different sensory domains. Convergence alone does

This work was supported by a grant from the United States Public Health Service (5 RO 1 EY03167) which we gratefully acknowledge. Correspondence and requests for reprints should be addressed to V. B. Mountcastle.

not establish the case. Thus, while it is likely that the parietal homotypical cortex plays an important role in what are called associative functions, the neural mechanisms of those associations are still unclear.

The second general concept is that the inferior parietal lobule is a higher order processing area of the visual system, for it is known to receive convergent inputs from both the geniculostriate and the collicular portions of the visual system. The striate and the prestriate areas are believed to project upon the inferior parietal lobule over a multiple-stage, transcortical system. Area 7 also receives and processes neural signals transmitted via the retino-collicular system and its upward thalamocortical projections, signals thought to provide information about the spatial location of objects, not their contour, orientation, or color. This idea is supported by the fact that neurons activated by visual stimuli were observed in the earliest studies of the inferior parietal lobule (Hyvarinen and Poranen, 1974; Lynch et al., 1973a; Mountcastle et al., 1975) and have since been studied by Goldberg and Robinson (1977, 1978), Robinson and Goldberg (1977a, b), Robinson et al. (1978), and Yin and Mountcastle (1977). The light-sensitive neurons of area 7 make up 25 to 30% of the cells in the region whose functional properties can be identified in experiments of the sort described here.

The third idea is that additional functions of the inferior parietal lobule relate to more complex aspects of behavior and especially to the representation of and operations within immediately surrounding space, i.e., in spatial orientation and perception. For example, the region is thought to be involved in the combined actions of hand and eye within the immediately surrounding behavioral space and, more generally, with maintaining relations between internal bodily and external spatial coordinate systems. There is considerable evidence to suggest that this area, together with the cortical and subcortical structures with which it is linked, plays a role in the direction of attention and in the interested fixation of gaze usually but not always coincident with the direction of attention (Mountcastle, 1976, 1978). These ideas are based upon the behavioral deficits of primates with parietal lesions and the functional properties of several large classes of neurons, other than light-sensitive cells, that have been identified in area 7 (Hyvarinen and Poranen, 1974; Leinonen et al., 1979; Mountcastle et al., 1975; Lynch et al., 1973a, b, 1977; Sakata et al., 1977, 1978, 1980; Yin and Mountcastle, 1977).

The present study is an extension of those made earlier by ourselves and by others of the inferior parietal lobule. It was carried out under experimental conditions that allowed us to define more precisely the functional properties of the light-sensitive neurons of area 7 particularly in regard to the organization of their response areas and their sensitivity to movement and the direction of movement of luminous stimuli. We sought to determine from these properties the suitability of the system for controlling several components of visual behavior: for the attraction of visual attention, particularly for moving objects; for combined visual and manual operations; for spatial orientation and perception. The results obtained are described in the present paper; a short note has appeared (Motter and Mountcastle, 1979).

In the course of these experiments, we discovered a powerful effect of the act of fixation upon the excitability of the parietal light-sensitive neurons and, in addition, we found that their sensitivity to light stimuli is influenced by the angle of gaze, even though the large majority are related to retinotopic response areas (Andersen and Mountcastle, 1980; Motter and Mountcastle, 1980). Therefore, we have examined again the large class of parietal cells found by a number of investigators to be active during the interested fixation of gaze and insensitive to visual stimuli (Hyvarinen and Poranen, 1974; Lynch et al., 1973a, b; Mountcastle et al., 1975; Rolls et al., 1979; Sakata et al., 1977). We have confirmed those properties of the fixation neurons under a number of controlled conditions and compared them with the effects of fixation and the angle of gaze upon the light-sensitive neurons. These results will be described in a later paper.

Methods

The behavioral paradigms used in our previous experiments (Mountcastle et al., 1975; Lynch et al., 1977; Yin and Mountcastle, 1977) were designed with reference to the behavioral deficits produced in man and in monkeys by lesions of the posterior parietal cortex (for review, see Lynch, 1980). We added tests for the present experiments using a variety of visual stimuli that allowed us to study the visual responses of neurons of area 7 during the performance of visuomotor tasks.

Behavioral tasks and test equipment. Macaque monkeys were trained to detect the dimming of a small red target light. Behavioral trials were initiated with computer control, progressed when the monkey closed a response key, and were terminated by release of the key after the monkey detected the dimming of the target light. Constraints upon response times, together with variable foreperiods, eliminated timing as a cue. The monkeys were required to make appropriate eye movements to maintain fixation of the target light if it was displaced and not to break fixation when other visual stimuli appeared. A criterion of 90% correct performance on the visuomotor/detection tasks was reached by successive approximations. One to three weeks before the recording experiments began silver–silver chloride (electro-oculographic, EOG) electrodes were implanted in the orbital rims, and a head restraint device was fixed to the monkey's skull in a sterile operative procedure under anesthesia. Final training with the head fixed and with collection of eye movement records allowed us to set a final performance level. The use of near-threshold dimming detection levels, a wide variety of tasks, and randomly interspersed catch trials ensured continued correct performance of the tasks. For monkeys 84, 86 and 87, eye position was monitored and behavioral trials were terminated automatically through computer control if inappropriate eye movements occurred. In a second operative procedure, 2 to 3 days before recording began, a microelectrode recording chamber was placed over a bony opening centered on the inferior parietal lobule. When study of the first hemisphere was completed, a similar chamber placement was made on the second side, and the experiment continued.

The experimental apparatus for series A of Table I was described earlier (Lynch et al., 1977). It consisted of a tangent screen upon which a laser-generated fixation target could be projected and moved about by galvanometer mirrors. For other tests, the tangent screen could be replaced by a white opaque screen embedded with 17 light-emitting diodes (LEDs) arranged in various spatial patterns. The visual angle subtended by these displays could be varied from 36° to 60°. In addition, a narrow, curved, white opaque board embedded with LEDs could be mounted 31 cm in front of the animal; it would extend 76° into the peripheral visual field. The long axis of the board could be rotated through the visual field in 45° steps.

A second test apparatus was developed for experiments 81 to 83 of series B, listed in Table I. It allowed the presentation of stationary or moving light stimuli of various shapes, sizes, and intensities at positions up to 90° away from the central line of gaze. The monkey viewed binocularly one of three screens arranged like the adjacent sides of a regular hexagon, with the monkey at the center at a viewing distance of 54 cm from each screen center. Each 60° × 60° screen surface consisted of a gray, patternless, back projection material, although only the two side screens were used as projection surfaces. When the monkey faced the center screen, the field of view was free laterally for ±100° and vertically for ±30°. A 0.3° fixation target was generated by a helium-neon laser (λ = 633 nm, 0.5 log unit above background luminance). The laser spot could be directed under program control to any position on any of the three screens by deflection off mirror galvanometers and a rotatable turret located above the animal's head. The monkey could be turned to face either side screen to allow exploration of the visual field near the point of fixation.

For monkeys 84, 86, and 87, the three-screen arrangement was replaced by a single screen measuring 100° × 100°, with the same back projection systems. The animal was placed either 34 or 57 cm from the screen (see Fig. 1).

In each of the experiments of series B, luminous test stimuli were back-projected onto the screen. The test stimulus could be varied in size from a point source to 25° × 25°. It was usually presented at intensities between 0.2 and 0.6 log unit above background, but stimuli up to 2 log units were occasionally used. The projector consisted of a single tungsten source whose light output was collimated, directed through a fast electromagnetic shutter and a photographic slide or slit aperture, reflected off mirror galvanometers and focused on the back of the screen. Program control of the shutter and galvanometers allowed generation of stimulus movements in either direction along any axis at speeds from 0 to 800°/sec. Neutral density filters were used to control stimulus illumination levels; the background illumination of the

TABLE I

The data base for the present experiments

Series A was carried out in the apparatus described by Lynch et al. (1977); series B was carried out using two versions of the apparatus shown in Figure 1 and described in the text.

Series	Exp.	Pen.[a]	Neurons	Quant.	Comp. Runs
A	74-R	14	127	47	163
	74-L	2	25	5	15
	75-R	17	178	65	294
	75-L	8	77	38	183
	76-R	5	63	29	80
	76-L	7	68	18	43
	80-R	11	78	41	125
	80-L	8	92	32	96
		(72)	(708)	(275)	(999)
B	81-R	14	106	59	309
	81-L	13	65	45	254
	82-R	14	78	45	212
	82-L	9	71	35	217
	83-R	8	56	31	119
	83-L	14	111	50	209
	84-R	5	20	15	52
	84-L	9	80	44	196
	86-R	10	73	36	231
	86-L	14	165	73	289
	87-R	10	63	23	150
	87-L	12	86	73	382
	20 Hem.	204	1682	804	3619

[a] The abbreviations used are: Pen., microelectrode penetrations; Hem., hemispheres; Quant., neurons studied in computer-controlled behavioral runs; Comp. runs, total number of such runs.

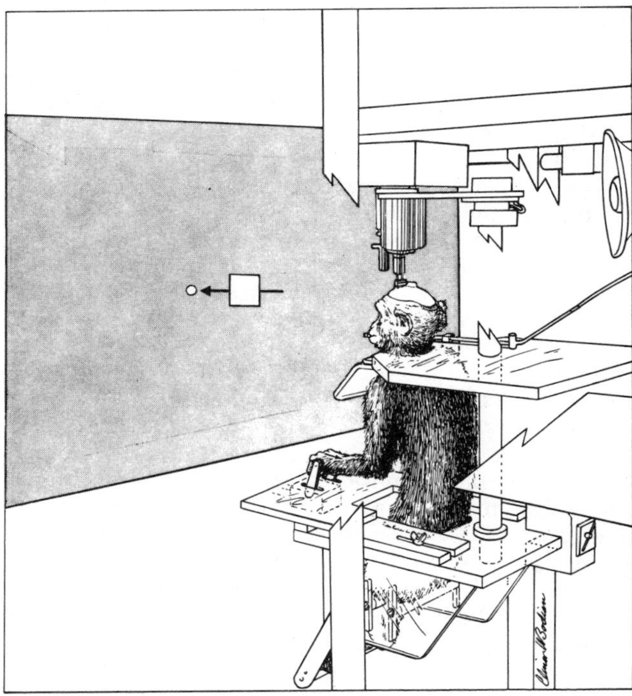

Figure 1. Behavioral task-test stimulus apparatus used for monkeys 84, 86, and 87 of series B of the present experiments (Table I). The head holder allowed positioning in the neutral position shown or at 60° left or right. The head could be freed in the horizontal plane for periods of rest during recording sessions. Microdrive and chamber are not shown. Two back projectors were used. The first positioned the target laser spot at any locus desired and moved in any direction at velocities up to 800°/sec. The second projected light stimuli of variable sizes, intensities, and directions of movement over the same velocity range. A panel of 600 LEDs, on 2-cm centers, could be inserted in front of the screen along guide rails. For monkeys 81 to 84, the monkey faced a screen of three panels, each 60° × 60°; the two lateral panels were angled at 60° to the central one. Projected images could be delivered to either lateral panel as the animal faced either dead ahead or toward one or the other lateral panel. Thus, the entire visual field could be examined over 180° side to side. In this arrangement, the LED panel could be inserted to cover the front panel.

screens was balanced and could be varied from complete darkness to 2 cd/m^2. The entire behavioral apparatus was enclosed in a light-proof chamber.

In addition, a 25 × 27 matrix of LEDs on 2-cm centers could be positioned 34 to 50 cm in front of the monkey in each of the two screen arrangements used. The individual LEDs were under program control and could be turned on, off, or sequenced in any pattern, except that only two LEDs could be on simultaneously. A combination of normal and infrared light video monitor systems allowed observation of the monkey and the projection screens during the experiment.

The sequencing of stimulus and behavioral events and the collection and storage of neural activity and EOG records of eye position were controlled by a PDP 11/20 computer. Interspike interval durations were measured to the nearest 0.1 msec.

Methods of recording. The preparation of the animal for recording sessions and the method of microelectrode recording in waking monkeys were described in a previous paper (Mountcastle et al., 1975). Each daily recording session lasted about 6 hr during which usually one transdural electrode penetration was made. Monkeys initiated between 1000 and 2000 behavioral trials during this period, working to receive their daily water requirement.

Eye position was recorded using Ag-AgCl cup electrodes implanted in the bones of the orbital rims with the leads running subcutaneously to a connector mounted in the acrylic head cap. Electrode pairs were selected for an offset of less than 0.2 mV, measured in 0.9% saline. Slight errors in the attempted orthogonal placement of the electrode pairs across the orbits were electronically corrected to provide true vertical and horizontal eye position records. The eye position records were sampled at rates between 20 and 200/sec depending upon the visuomotor task being studied.

Identification of neurons. The electrical signs of the impulse discharges of single neurons were recorded using glass-coated, platinum-iridium microelectrodes passed through the intact dura. The action potentials thought to be generated by the same single cell were identified by criteria described earlier (Mountcastle et al., 1975). We attempted in the present experiments to study neurons activated by light stimuli, per se, and we frequently terminated penetrations in which neurons with other sets of functional properties were identified. We first used qualitative methods of identification for each neuron brought under study, including manually presented visual stimuli, naturally evoked reaching and manipulation, passive somatic sensory stimulation, etc., and then initiated computer-controlled "diagnostic" runs in which a variety of visual and visuomotor tests were delivered. Further detailed and more quantitative studies of cells determined to be light sensitive were then executed using previously arranged combinations of behavioral and stimulus conditions (control sets); other control sets specifying different conditions could be generated *ad hoc* in a short time.

A computer run consisted of a set of up to 10 different classes, each a particular combination of behavioral and stimulus events; different classes were presented in a randomized order. The stability of the cell's response during long periods of recording was checked by repeating some classes during different sequential runs. Impulse data were stored, sorted on line according to class, and displayed in a raster format on a storage oscilloscope. A printed copy of this display was made by a Tektronix 4631 unit to allow run comparisons. Continuous records of eye position and impulse activity were displayed on other oscilloscopes, digitalized, and stored.

Conventional spike train analysis techniques were used off-line for analysis of the time relations of behavioral, cellular, and eye movement events. Data summaries were generated using incremental plotter and graphics line-printer facilities.

Anatomical studies. Small electrolytic lesions (4 μA for 4 sec, tip positive) were made at the depth of some penetrations. At the conclusion of each experiment, animals were sacrificed with an overdose of sodium pentobarbital. Small guide wires were then inserted into each hemisphere, marking a line for blocking perpendicular to the intraparietal sulcus and normal to the cortical surface. Brains were removed and placed in formalin. The fixed brains were later embedded in celoidin and sectioned serially at 20 μm; every section was mounted and stained with thionine.

Results

General Description

The data base

Observations were made on 20 hemispheres in two series; data summaries are given in Tables I and II. The two series differed only in the test apparatus used, as described above. We averaged 10 successful microelectrode penetrations per hemisphere. A total of 1682 neurons were brought under observation, an average of 8 cells per penetration. A neuron entered this population if its action potential was recorded in isolation from those of others for a time sufficient to allow qualitative tests aimed at identifying its functional properties. Presumptive identifications led to further studies with control sets chosen to confirm or deny them and to elucidate further the properties of the neurons. Under these latter conditions, 804 neurons were studied. We tried to isolate action potentials in the initially negative configuration because of the damage that usually accompanies close approach of the electrode tip to the cell and the inversion of the initial sign of the action potential to positive. Indeed, we commonly observed changes in the dynamic functional properties of parietal neurons to accompany spike inversion. Eight-four percent of the neurons were studied while discharging initially negative action potentials.

Location of recordings. The locations of the microelectrode penetrations made into the inferior parietal lobules of 18 of the 20 hemispheres studied are shown in Figure 2. The penetrations were located in the intermediate and posteromedial parts of area 7 in a region termed by some investigators 7-a; we have not made a general survey of the entire inferior parietal lobule. Many penetrations close to the intraparietal sulcus passed down the cortex of its posterior bank parallel to the cortical layers, but we have not explored the sulcus to its depths. *Solid circles* in Figure 2 indicate penetrations in which any light-sensitive neurons were identified; in the large ma-

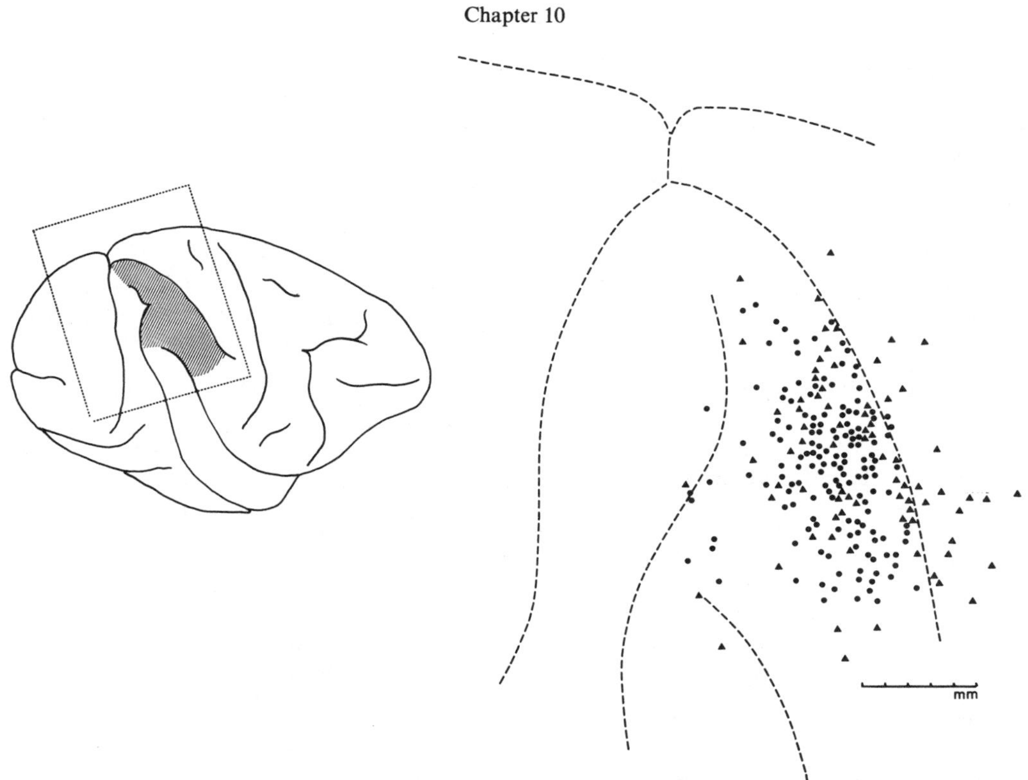

Figure 2. Locations of microelectrode penetrations. The drawing to the *left* shows the lateral surface of the macaque cerebral hemisphere. The *area outlined* is enlarged to the *right*, which is an average drawing of the sulcal patterns of 18 of the 20 hemispheres studied. The location of each penetration is indicated on this drawing. Penetrations marked with *solid circles* are those in which light-sensitive neurons were observed. Neurons of other classes (see Table II) were also encountered in many of these penetrations, often in the *en bloc* distribution compatible with columnar organization. Penetrations marked with *solid triangles* contained no light-sensitive neurons, though in many of them cells of different classes, other than light-sensitive, were frequently encountered in *en bloc* distribution. All penetrations made in front of the intraparietal fissure contained some neurons activated by passive somesthetic stimulation; many also contained cells of the reach-manipulation class, but no light-sensitive cells. No cells activated by passive somesthetic stimulation were identified posterior to the intraparietal sulcus in this portion of area 7-a. The error in positioning a given penetration on such an averaged diagram is 1 to 2 mm. The results indicate that in this portion of the inferior parietal lobule, there is no clear areal segregation of the groups of cells with different properties. The data presented here reveal nothing concerning the detailed functional organization of this region, which is unknown.

jority of them, other classes of neurons were also identified, commonly in blocks with abrupt change from a zone containing cells of one class to a zone with cells of another, in the general mode of columnar organization. *Triangles* indicate penetrations in which no light-sensitive cells were identified; in each of them, the *en bloc* changes from one class to those of another were also common. No neurons activated by passive stimulation of the skin or deep tissues were identified in this region of area 7-a; many such neurons have been described by Hyvarinen and Shelepin (1979) more laterally in area 7-b. We identified no light-sensitive neurons in any of the penetrations made anterior to the intraparietal sulcus.

We made electrolytic lesions in some successful penetrations in early experiments of this series. An analysis of neuronal properties in terms of cytoarchitecture and layer was not our purpose, however, and the results of the studies of the dynamic properties of parietal neurons led us to omit lesions in many penetrations. We observed that even small lesions produce marked changes in the dynamic properties of neurons within a radius of 2 to 3 mm of surrounding cortex and that these changes may last for several days.

The classification of neurons in combined behavioral-electrophysiological experiments

No consistent set of rules has evolved for naming the classes of neurons with different properties that can be identified in the parietal cortex in waking monkeys. This is because the activity of many parietal cells is preferentially related to one or another complex behavioral act; they are not "sensory" or "motor" as cells of the somatic sensory and the motor cortex clearly are. We have therefore labeled parietal neurons by simple empirical correlations between cell activity and behavioral event or, where it is effective, sensory stimulation.

Upon isolation of each action potential, we began a systematic qualitative examination of its properties by evoking reaching movements toward and manipulation of objects; by eliciting oculomotor events such as fixation, tracking, and saccading; by delivering visual stimuli projected upon or moved across the tangent screen as the animal fixated a stationary target; and by passive manipulation of hands and arms. In many cases, identifications made in this way were then confirmed in controlled behavioral task-test stimulus runs. In other cases, equally strong qualitative identifications could be neither confirmed nor proven false in any of the repertoire of behavioral tasks that we could present. In still others, presumptive identifications made in qualitative examinations were shown in controlled runs to be erroneous. Finally, many neurons were observed for which no clear identification was possible using either mode of examination. We conclude that it is not possible to establish with certainty the functional properties of any class of parietal neurons by qualitative ("clinical") examination of a waking monkey.

Definition of Classes of Neurons of the Inferior Parietal Lobule

The classes of parietal neurons that we have identified in the present series of experiments are listed in Table II and are defined as follows.

Unidentified cells (518, 31%). No clear identification could be made for 518 neurons, even though 149 of these were studied in controlled behavioral task-test stimulus runs. Neurons that we could not identify did not differ from those that we could by location in any particular part of area 7-a, by restriction to any particular depth of the cortex, or by a particular pattern of discharge. Like other classes of cortical cells, they were frequently observed sequentially in depth, forming blocks in conformity with the mode of columnar organization. However, unidentifiable cells were also observed in the midst of traverses in which other cells were clearly identified. We do not believe that difficulty in identification was caused by local cell damage, for 81% of the unidentified cells discharged initially negative action potentials, compared with 84% of the identified population. We conclude that there exists a substantial class of cells in area 7-a whose activity is unrelated to the behavioral tasks or test stimulus situations that we could deliver in these experiments; nor were these cells affected by any qualitative test that we could devise.

Fixation (218) and fixation suppression (48) cells. We identified 218 cells of the fixation class previously described by a number of investigators (Hyvarinen and Poranen, 1974; Lynch et al., 1973a, b; Mountcastle et al., 1975; Sakata et al., 1977, 1980). We have confirmed that the activity of these cells is incremented when the animal fixates an object of a rewarding nature, a novel one, or, as Rolls et al. (1979) observed, an object which the animal regards as aversive. The second property that we take as required for identification is insensitivity to light stimuli. All cells with any response to light stimuli of any kind we have classified as light-sensitive cells in one or another of the subclasses shown in Table II. Fixation cells subtend limited gaze fields often located in the contralateral hemifield, confined to its upper or lower quadrants, or, less commonly, to the ipsilateral half of the visual field. The gaze fields of these neurons have been studied recently in a quantitative way by Sakata et al. (1980); we confirmed their observations. A subset of the fixation cells (48 in the present series) is suppressed during fixation; they too are insensitive to light stimuli.

Light-sensitive cells (529, 31%). We identified 462 neurons of area 7-a sensitive to stationary and/or moving light stimuli delivered to the visual fields during active fixations of small target lights. The visual properties of these cells are described in the following sections of this paper. A smaller group of light-sensitive cells (67) showed other properties as well: 47 were active during fixation of targets, not necessarily within their response areas, and 13 were suppressed by fixation of such targets. Seven other neurons were active during hand manipulation in total darkness, were insensitive to passive mechanical stimulation of hand or arm, *and* were related to visual response areas located in the lower quadrants of the visual fields.

Oculomotor cells (163, 10%). We have identified four subclasses of neurons in area 7 that are preferentially active in relation to eye movements. "Saccade neurons" ($n = 60$) are active before and during visually evoked but not spontaneous saccades to targets that do not themselves evoke responses when presented as nontarget visual stimuli, are insensitive to other visual stimuli, and are not active during tracking or fixation. Many light-sensitive cells are also influenced by saccadic movements; e.g.,

TABLE II
The classes of neurons identified in the present series of experiments in area 7-a of the inferior parietal lobule
The classification strategy and the identification parameters used are described in the text. The differences in the proportions of neurons in each class between the total number and the number studied in computer-controlled runs results from our desire to study light-sensitive (LS) neurons in this set of experiments.

		Total		Studied in Computer Runs	
		No.	*%*	*No.*	*%*
Unidentified neurons		518	31	149	19
Fixation (218) and fixation suppression (48)		266	16	139	17
Light-sensitive		529	31	373	46
LS only	462				
Fixation + LS	47				
Fixation suppression + LS	13				
Manipulation + LS	7				
Oculomotor		163	10	114	14
Tracking	23				
Saccade	60				
Re-fixation	25				
Vergence	55				
Projection (126) and manipulation (80)		206	12	29	4
		1682	100	804	100

their responses to visual stimuli may be enhanced or suppressed when those stimuli become targets for saccadic movements (Goldberg and Robinson, 1977; Robinson et al., 1978; Yin and Mountcastle, 1977). There appears to exist a spectrum of cells ranging from those that are activated by light stimuli and unaffected by eye movements, through those with combined properties, to others active with saccades and insensitive to light stimuli. This suggests the possibility that cells with such a gradient change in functional properties may be arranged in a sequential processing chain, but no direct evidence that this is so exists.

"Re-fixation neurons" (25) are active after completion of a visually evoked saccadic movement to a particular zone of the visual field. They are insensitive to light stimuli, are not active during casual fixations in any areas of the visual field, and thus differ from fixation neurons by the requirement for a preceding visually evoked saccadic movement. They differ from saccade neurons only in the relation of the time of discharge to eye movement.

"Tracking neurons" (23) are rare in the region of area 7 which we have studied in these experiments. They are active during slow pursuit movements, are markedly directional in nature, and are frequently suppressed during tracking in the opposite direction (Mountcastle et al., 1975). They are insensitive to light stimuli and are inactive during steadily maintained fixation. Tracking neurons are more common in the posterior part of area 7, particularly in the anterior bank of the superior temporal sulcus. They have been studied in detail by Sakata et al. (1978). Many of these tracking neurons have recently been shown to have vestibular inputs (Kawano et al., 1980).

A newly identified subclass of neurons in area 7 we label "vergence neurons" (55) and tentatively classify them with the oculomotor group. Vergence neurons are active during saccadic or tracking movements evoked by visual targets rapidly displaced or moving slowly in the sagittal plane. Each is preferentially active with movements either toward or away from the face, but not both; they are insensitive to light stimuli. It is likely that a considerable number of neurons of the fixation class, described above, have three-dimensional fixation fields, like those that we tentatively call vergence neurons, for we have not tested them in the third dimension. Neurons with these depth characteristics have been identified in area 7 and studied by Sakata et al. (1977, 1980).

Projection and manipulation cells (206, 12%). Neurons of the first group (126) are active when the animal projects his arm toward a target, those of the second (80) when he manipulates within a small enclosure to obtain the target. We have confirmed our earlier observations that cells of this class are sensitive neither to passive mechanical stimulation of the hands or arms nor to visual stimuli.

On naming and numbers in studies of the homotypical cerebral cortex in waking monkeys

It is clear that the identification and classification of neurons in the parietal lobe is a difficult task and that the classes identified and the proportions of each differ between investigations. This is so because (*a*) qualitative identification of cell types by simple examination cannot be made with certainty in waking monkeys, (*b*) the controlled behavioral task-test stimulus sets that can be delivered in any particular series of experiments are limited by the test apparatus used, and (*c*) the objectives of different investigators differ and will bias the sample of neurons observed. Table III shows that this is true for three successive studies of the inferior parietal lobule from a single laboratory, namely, our own. The three sets of experiments were made using a different test apparatus in each and with different behavioral task-test stimulus control sets. Study I was a general survey of both areas 5 and 7, in which we did not tabulate the "unidentified cells," and concentrated on study of the fixation and projection-manipulation neurons. In study II, we did tabulate unidentified cells, but not the light-sensitive cells, and concentrated on study of the fixation and oculomotor cells. In study III (the present one), we attempted to classify all neurons observed, but have concentrated on detailed studies of the light-sensitive cells. We conclude from this experience, and from the published studies of others, that differences between cell types observed and the proportions in each, in studies from different laboratories, are due to differences in

TABLE III

The classifications of neurons of the inferior parietal lobule as identified in three successive studies

Each investigation had different objectives and was made using different behavioral task and test stimulus apparatus. Study I is from Mountcastle et al. (1975); study II from Lynch et al. (1977); study III is the present investigation.

Class	Study I		Study II		Study III		Total	
	No.	%	*No.*	%	*No.*	%	*No.*	%
Unidentified	NT[a]		369	29	518	31	887	25
Fixation[b]	155	33	521	40	266	16	942	27
Oculomotor[c]	88	19	218	17	163	10	469	14
Light sensitive	73	16	NT		529	31	602	18
Reach and manipulation	128	28	136	11	206	12	470	14
Special	21	4	32	3	—[d]	—	53	2
	465	100	1276	100	1682	100	3423	100

[a] NT, not tabulated.

[b] Includes fixation suppression cells.

[c] Includes tracking, saccade, re-fixation, and vergence cells.

[d] In this study, special cells were classified as subgroups of the light-sensitive class as shown in Table II.

experimental design and objective and provide no ground for polemic controversy (Robinson et al., 1978).

Response of Light-sensitive Neurons to Stationary Stimuli

The response patterns

The light-sensitive cells of area 7-a respond to stationary light flashes in the variety of discharge patterns shown in Figures 3, 4, and 5. A total of 357 cells were tested with stationary stimuli; 17% responded with sustained discharges (Figs. 3*A*, 5, and 6*C*); 52% responded transiently to stimuli delivered anywhere within their response areas, and a few (n = 12) of these discharged a second transient at light-off. The remaining 31% responded too weakly for classification. Sixty-eight cells were suppressed by stimuli at some location, and 12 were suppressed only (Fig. 9*E*) and not activated by stimuli at any locations.

Many LS neurons responded vigorously to small weak lights, e.g., to the 0.3° LEDs used in series A (see Figs. 3*A* and 5). Other neurons responded only to larger stimuli. We examined the requirement for spatial summation in 11 neurons, in the paradigm of series B, using stimuli that were varied from 1 to 200 deg^2. Nine of the 11 reached maximal response with stimuli of 25 to 35 deg^2. We conclude that the 6° × 6° square or the 5° diameter circle used in series B saturated the requirement for spatial summation of most LS neurons.

We tested the responses of 31 LS neurons to stationary light flashes in both light and darkness. The background light condition was between 1 and 2 cd/m^2; 2 min adaptation time was allowed before each test in darkness. The change from light to darkness caused no change in the response of 17 cells, an increase for eight and a decrease for three. For three other cells, we observed a reversal from an "off" to an "on" response.

The latencies of the responses of LS neurons to stationary flashes at the most sensitive loci in their response areas varied from 50 to 290 msec, with a mean of 118 msec (SD = 47 msec, n = 96) and a modal value of 110 msec. The response latency usually increased as the response intensity decreased with shifts in stimulus location within the response area.

Response areas of light-sensitive neurons determined with stationary stimuli: The phenomenon of foveal sparing

The response areas of LS neurons were determined in runs in which single stimuli were delivered during 2- to 5-sec periods of sustained fixation. Stimuli in successive

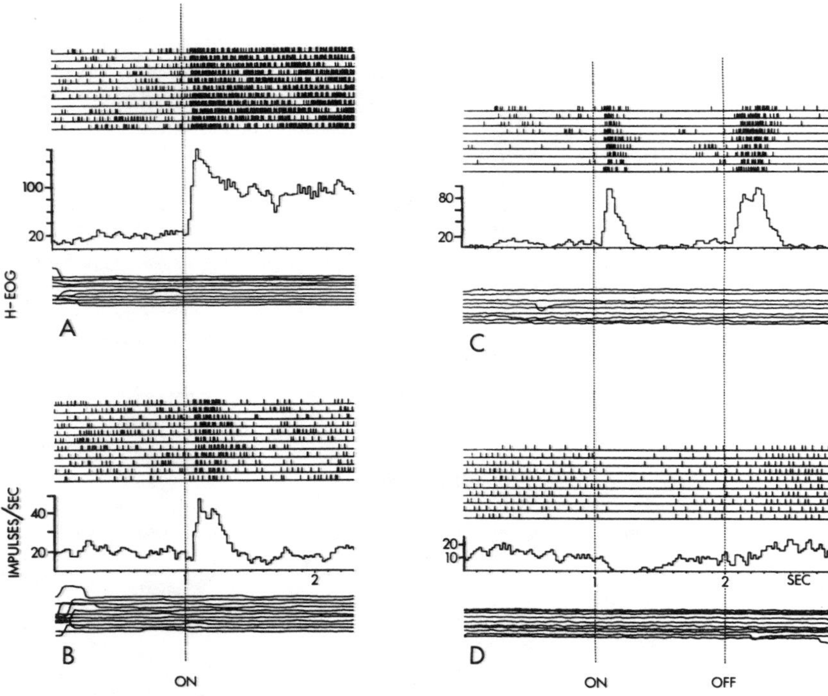

Figure 3. Types of responses of light-sensitive neurons of area 7-a to light stimuli. For each panel, and for many other illustrations that follow, each line of the *upper row* of records represents the time of a single behavioral trial, each upstroke the instant at which the neuron under study discharged an impulse. The histograms *immediately below* average these discharges. The *lower records* are electro-oculograms, one for each of the trials shown above. *Vertical dashed lines* indicate in sequence on and, for some runs, off of the light stimulus. *A*, Discharge pattern of a neuron responding to a LED stimulus, placed within its response area, with a sustained discharge; the stimulus and the discharge continued beyond the length of the record shown here. *B*, Discharge pattern of a neuron responding to a similar LED stimulus with a transient discharge. *C*, The on-off discharge pattern of a neuron elicited by a 6° × 6° square stimulus placed in its response area. *D*, This neuron responded to a similar stimulus with a cessation of discharge. Response type *B* is the most common; types *C* and *D* are relatively rare. Range of stimulus intensive, 0.5 to 1 log unit above background. Time intervals, 100 msec.

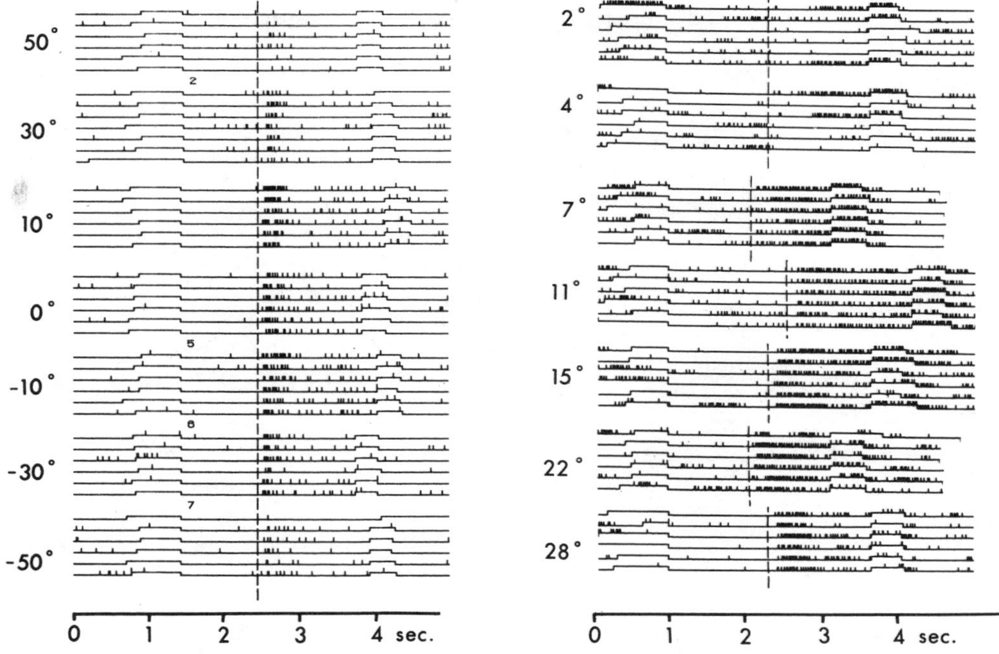

Figure 4. Illustration of the two major classes of response areas of parietal light-sensitive neurons. The impulse replicas to the *left* were obtained in the study of a neuron typical of those with foveal response areas. The maximal response was evoked by stimuli at or close to the central line of vision, and stimuli placed on either side along the horizontal meridian evoked decreasing responses in a nearly symmetrical pattern. Test stimulus 6° × 6° square, about 5 cd/m^2, delivered against a background of about 1 cd/m^2. In each record, the first step displacement indicates target light on, the second the animal's closure of the signal key, the third the dimming of the target light, the fourth the instant of key release by the animal. The *vertical dashed lines* indicate onset of the light stimulus, which remained on for 1 sec. Records to the *right* are those of a neuron related to a response area confined to the contralateral hemifield but which spared the foveal region; the test stimulus was an LED physically identical to the target LED which evoked no response at all. Test stimuli were delivered to the locations indicated, along the contralateral horizontal meridian; no responses were evoked by it when placed at similar locations on the ipsilateral side. All stimuli were delivered as the animal held steady fixation of the target light placed dead ahead.

trials of a run were presented in a pseudorandom sequence at different positions along axes passing through the fixation point. Histograms were constructed for the neural activity evoked by the stimuli at each position.

There are three salient features of these response areas: They are, with few exceptions, very large as compared with those of neurons of either the striate cortex or the superior colliculus; they are frequently bilateral; and many display the characteristic of foveal sparing. The last refers to two observations. Firstly, LS cells rarely (i.e., only eight neurons) respond to the foveally fixated stimulus target even though physically identical stimuli may evoke vigorous responses when delivered close to the fixation point (see Fig. 5). Secondly, perifoveal zones of insensitivity can be demonstrated using other images projected during steady fixation of the target light. Foveal sparing is illustrated further by the discharge replicas of Figure 4 (*right*) and the polar plots of Figure 7, *A*, *B*, and *C*.

We have observed that even a large stimulus (6° × 6°) centered on the fixation point will not evoke a response in about half of the light-sensitive cells. A simple classification of response areas based on this criterion is given in Table IV which shows that even after excluding those neurons that responded to large stimuli centered on the fixation point, but not to the fixation light itself, 127/216 = 59% of the response areas spared the region of the fixation point. Samples of the response areas of cells related to contralateral response areas with foveal sparing are given in Figure 8, and samples of those related to bilateral response areas with foveal sparing are given in Figure 9, *A*, *B*, *C*, and *D*. For some neurons of the latter group, the central zone of inexcitability appeared as a hole in an otherwise continuous response area; in others, it separated two disjointed response areas, one in each half of the visual fields. The examples given in Figure 9 show that the zone of foveal sparing may be large (*A*), may separate two response areas that extend symmetrically to 50° or more into each of the visual half-fields (*B*), may be confined to a narrow zone around the point of fixation (*C*), or may separate zones of unequal sizes (*D*).

The phenomenon of foveal sparing raises the question of whether it results from a dynamic influence of the act of target fixation upon the excitability of the systems linking retina to the parietal lobe, or whether the distribution of response areas can be accounted for on the basis of a connectivity that for this class of LS neurons precisely exempts the point of fixation. We emphasize that the response areas described were determined as the animal fixated a central target, dead ahead, for we have observed two powerful effects that facilitate the re-

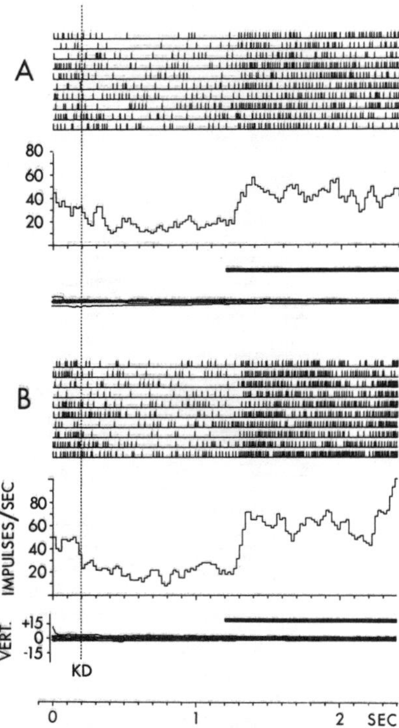

Figure 5. The phenomenon of foveal sparing. Records of a neuron related to a bilateral response area with foveal sparing. The set of records *above* are of responses evoked by an LED light placed 3° above the fixation point along the vertical meridian, those *below* by a similar light 3° below the fixation point. Each trial was initiated by the monkey at *KD* (keydown), the *vertical dashed line*, after which he steadily fixated the target light for 1 sec before the test stimulus was delivered; this target light evoked no response of the neuron. The test stimuli were delivered during the times marked by the *solid bars*; each evoked an intense and sustained cellular discharge. The *lowest* records of each panel are superimposed vertical electro-oculograms, one for each of the trials illustrated above. They show the steadily maintained fixations throughout the trials. Time intervals, 100 msec.

sponses of LS neurons to light stimuli delivered in extrafoveal locations: the act of target fixation and the angle of gaze. We will describe them in detail in later papers.

The second class of response areas of parietal LS neurons we term *foveal-inclusive* (89/216 = 41%), because for them, 6° × 6° stimuli superimposed over the fixation point did evoke responses. A number of these foveal-inclusive neurons are most sensitive to stimuli placed at the fixation point itself, and the response intensity for them declined more or less symmetrically on either side (Fig. 4, *left*). The response areas of these cells are almost reciprocal in their spatial distributions to many of the cells with bilateral fields and foveal sparing. Figure 10 shows that the response areas of foveal-inclusive neurons may vary from small (*B*) to very large and may extend to over the 100° examined along an axis (*D*). For other neurons of this class, the response areas were asymmetrically placed, as shown by the polar plot of Figure 10*E* and the histograms of Figure 6*B*. Response areas confined to the ipsilateral visual field are extremely rare.

We observed for all except eight of the cells which we have classified as foveal-inclusive that even when a 6° × 6° stimulus centered over the fixation point evoked an intense response, fixation of the target light itself evoked nothing (see Fig. 4, *left*). The question then is whether foveal sparing exists also for some of the neurons which we have classified as foveal-inclusive, because of the response to large stimuli, or whether the absence of response to the fixation target light reveals only a requirement for spatial summation. We have not resolved that problem and thus in parsimony, have classified these neurons as having foveal response areas.

The Responses of Light-sensitive Neurons to Moving Stimuli

The LS neurons of area 7-a are particularly sensitive to moving as compared to stationary stimuli in both the intensity of the response and the size and distribution of the response areas. We chose for the majority of our studies to move lights along the axes of the visual fields that cross the fixation point; we define as inward movements toward the fixation point while those in the opposite direction are considered outward. We have studied a smaller number of neurons with stimuli moving along other axes, but we have not used movements along axes centered upon and rotated about the "center" of the response areas, for the latter are large and possess no readily defined centers.

Figure 11 shows two common features of the light-sensitive cells of area 7-a. They are much more sensitive to moving than to stationary light stimuli, and they are, in the majority of cases, differentially sensitive to the direction of stimulus movement. We now wish to document these properties further and to describe the relation to each other of the directional vectors in different sectors of the visual fields.

Sensitivity to the direction of movement

We studied 172 LS neurons in paradigms resembling that of Figure 11; the results are summarized in Table V. Each of these cells was tested with standard light stimuli moving along the horizontal and vertical meridians in both directions. Many cells were also tested along diagonal axes and some along axes that did not intersect the fixation point. Table V shows that 90% of the neurons tested were directionally sensitive in at least one half-sector of either the vertical or the horizontal meridian. The varieties and the degrees of this directionality are illustrated by the sets of histograms of Figure 12. These results, together with those of Figures 13, 14, and 15, are typical of all our observations. We conclude from them that the large majority of LS neurons of area 7-a are sensitive to the direction of stimulus movement and that for most of them, this directionality is very strong. Stimuli moving in a direction opposite to that which excites may elicit suppression of on-going activity for a few cells, but more commonly has no effect. Although some of the histograms of Figure 12 suggest that a response area plotted with moving stimuli may in some cases overlap the fixation point, we believe that for most this is not

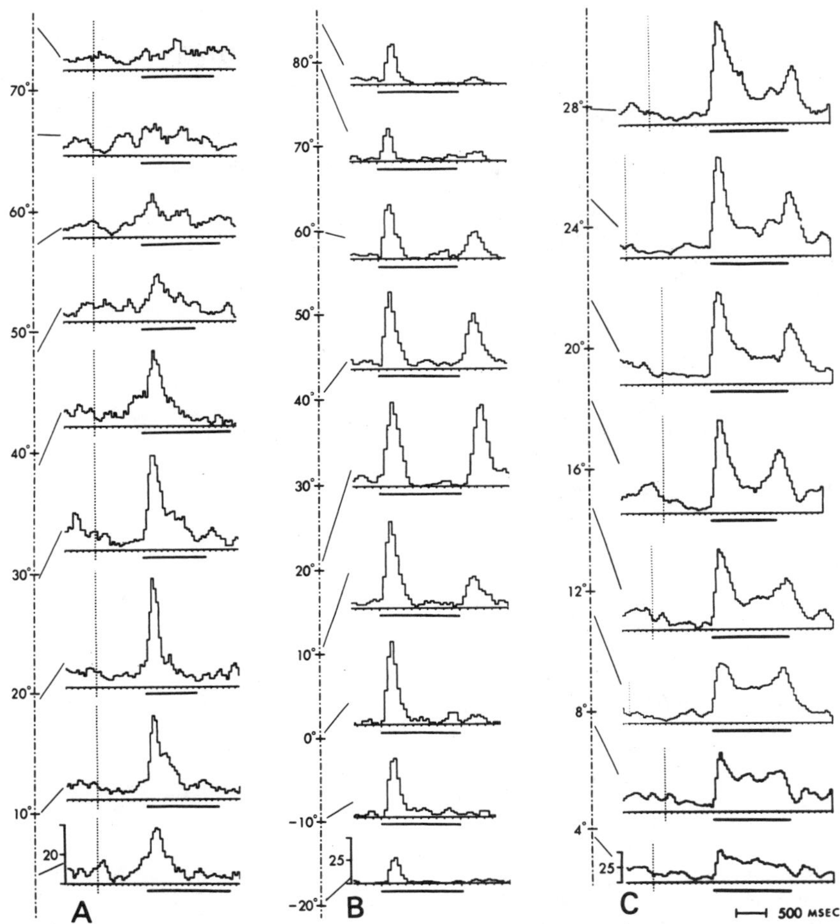

Figure 6. The response areas of three light-sensitive neurons of area 7-a. In each case, the histograms sum the responses of a neuron to 6 to 10 trials of stimuli delivered at each of the locations indicated along the meridian of the visual fields that transected the longest axis of the response area. The *solid bars* indicate the stimulus periods. *A*, Results for a neuron activated from the contralateral visual field with foveal sparing. *Vertical dashed line* indicates switch closure by the animal after which he steadily fixed a target LED dead ahead; this visual stimulus to the foveal region of the retina evoked no response. Then, a physically identical LED came on at one of the locations indicated along the contralateral horizontal meridian. It evoked transient discharges when within an area extending from within 5° of the central line of gaze to at least 60° laterally into the contralateral visual field. *B*, Study of a neuron related to a bilateral, eccentrically distributed response area that included the fovea. Here the trials have begun before the records do; fixation of the target light evoked no response, but the 6° × 6° square light (intensity about 1 log unit above background) evoked an on-off discharge at locations from ipsilateral 20° to at least contralateral 85° along the horizontal meridian. *C*, Study of a neuron that responded with a sustained discharge under circumstances similar to those of *A*. Again, the onset target light evoked no response, and the field extended from as near to the fixation point as 4°, outward along the horizontal meridian, contralaterally; it was tested only to 28°. Study *B* presents an unresolved question: Here the target light evoked no response, but the 6° × 6° square centered on the fixation point did so (see record labeled 0°). We have for reasons of parsimony classified all such neurons as related to foveal response areas, though more detailed studies with small stimuli have revealed for some cells a small zone of foveal sparing, as the absence of response to the fixation light suggests.

true, but that the overlap by the histogram is due to after-discharge. We have observed such an after-discharge of the response when inwardly moving stimuli are stopped and turned off just short of the fixation point. The majority of the movement response areas are laterally placed along the axes examined, and though they may extend close to the center of the visual field, they almost always terminate just short of the fixation point itself.

Sensitivity to the velocity of movement

We have tested the sensitivity of 70 of these parietal LS neurons to stimulus velocity over the range from 10 to 800°/sec. Although a few cells responded over this entire range, the majority had flat velocity sensitivity functions with broad peaks in the range from 30 to 60°/sec. These preliminary studies suggest that while this set of neurons can provide very sensitive signals of stimulus

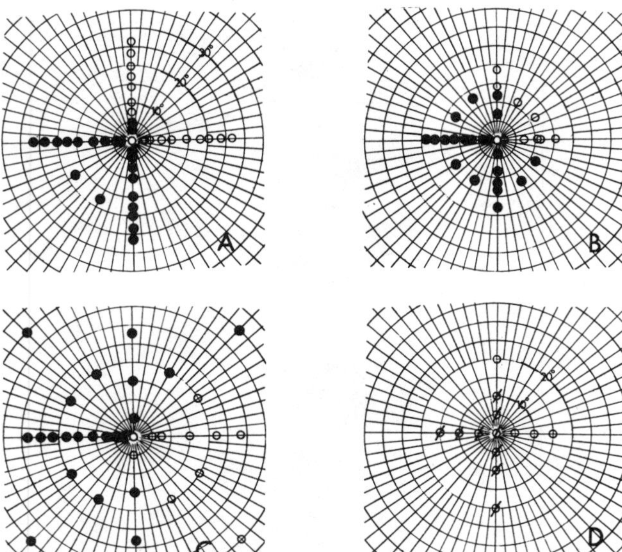

Figure 7. Polar plots of the response areas of light-sensitive neurons of the parietal cortex. Six to 12 trials were delivered at each location, and histograms were constructed summing the evoked activity; stimuli were delivered at the several locations in a pseudorandom sequence. *Solid circles* indicate locations at which stimuli evoked responses; *open circles,* those at which they did not; *open circles with slash,* those at which stimuli evoked suppression. In each case, the animal maintained steady fixation of a LED target light at position 0, 0 throughout each trial. For the neurons of *A, B,* and *C,* the light stimulus was a LED physically identical to the fixation target; for that of *D,* it was a 6° × 6° square. *A, B,* and *C* illustrate large response areas that extend into more than one-half of the visual field, but exempt the central zone of gaze. *D* illustrates the response area of one of the rarely encountered neurons that was suppressed but never excited by the light stimulus.

TABLE IV

Distribution of the response areas of the light-sensitive neurons of area 7-a between those sparing and those including the central zones of gaze

The phenomenon of foveal spring is described in the text.

I. Response areas sparing the fovea		127
A. Unilateral areas	66	
B. Bilateral areas	43	
C. Foveal sparing, laterality undetermined	18	
II. Response areas including the fovea		89
A. Bilateral, symmetrical	32	
B. Bilateral, asymmetrical	31	
C. Bilateral, degree of symmetry undetermined	26	
Total:		216

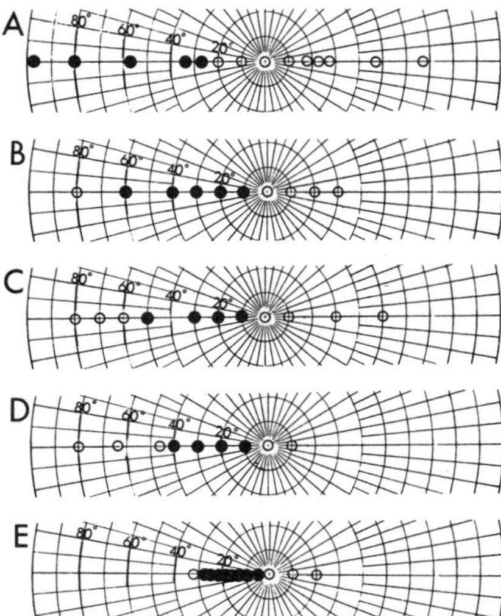

Figure 8. Polar plots of response areas of parietal light-sensitive neurons: unilateral areas with foveal sparing. The distribution of each response area along its major meridian is shown, plotted as in Figure 7. These five neurons were related to contralaterally located response areas of different sizes, with sparing of the foveal and immediately perifoveal regions. *Solid circles,* locations at which stimuli evoked responses; *open circles,* locations at which they did not.

movement over a wide range of velocities, it is not likely to signal accurate information concerning velocity itself.

The opponent organization of vectors in the response areas of light-sensitive neurons

We commonly observed for LS neurons with directionally sensitive response areas in three or four quadrants of the visual field that the vectors in opposite halves of the field pointed in opposite directions. We term this *opponent vector organization.* Of 88 cells that were related to response areas in three or four quadrants, 63 showed opponent organization orientation, and for 75% of these, the directional vectors point toward the fixation point; the remainder point away. Fourteen neurons showed identical vectorial directions in two halves of the visual field, and for 11, the vectorial directions were mixed (Table V, I: A, B, and C). Forty-seven other directionally sensitive neurons were related to response areas in only one quadrant of the visual field, and 18 to two adjacent quadrants. No pattern of vector orientation could be defined for these neurons.

The varieties of vectorial organization that we have observed are illustrated in Figures 13, 14, and 15. Figure 13, *left,* illustrates the directionality typical for a neuron related to a single response sector along the contralateral horizontal meridian. The histograms to the *right* show response properties of a neuron related to two response sectors placed along adjacent half-meridians. The directional sensitivity is strong in each of these two cases, and the vectors point inward toward the fixation point. The histograms of Figure 14 illustrate for two neurons directional sensitivity along each of the four half-meridians of the visual fields; in each, the directional vector points inward, in typical opponent fashion. An instance of four-quadrant, directional sensitivity away from the fixation point is shown by the histograms to the *left* in Figure 15. Finally, a rare instance of a neuron sensitive to moving lights but insensitive to their direction is given to the

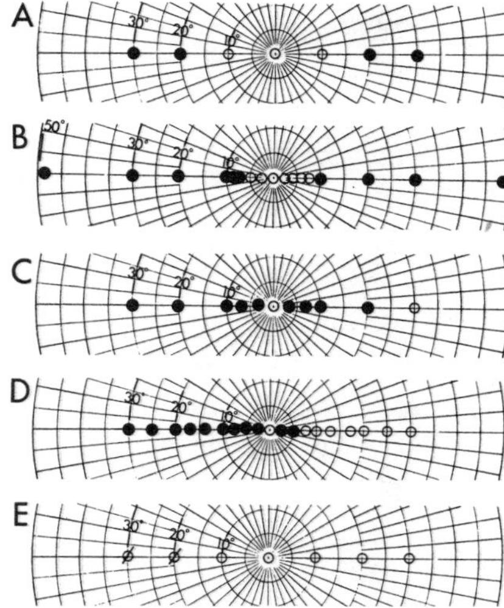

Figure 9. Polar plots of response areas of parietal light-sensitive neurons: bilateral areas with foveal sparing. The distribution of each field is shown along its major meridian, plotted as in Figure 7. The neurons of *A*, *B*, *C*, and *D* were related to bilateral response areas that varied in extent and degree of symmetry; in each, the foveal and immediately perifoveal zones are spared. The neuron of *E* was suppressed from a contralateral response area. Symbols as in Figure 8.

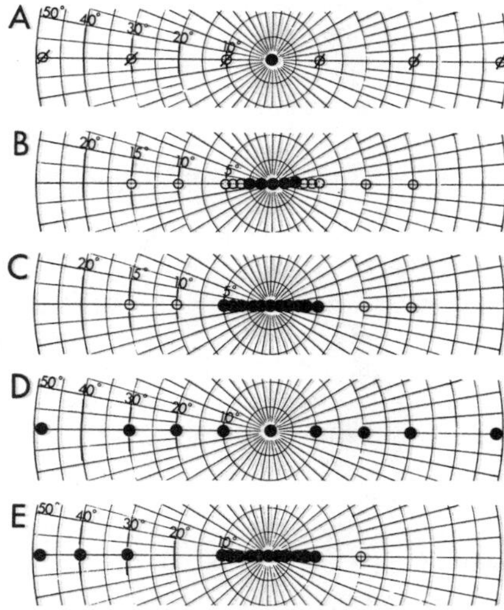

Figure 10. Polar plots of response areas of parietal light-sensitive neurons: bilateral areas including the foveal region. The extent of each area along its major meridian is shown, plotted as for Figure 7. The neurons of *B* and *C* were related to a symmetrical field that extended over at least 100° along the horizontal meridian of the visual field; it also responded to stimuli placed over 100° along the vertical meridian, not shown here. The cell of *E* was related to a typical foveal asymmetrical field. The neuron of *A* was the only one that we ever observed with an excitatory "center" with suppressive flanking zones. Symbols as in Figure 8.

right of Figure 15, which also illustrates that moving lights may evoke a suppression of on-going discharge as they cross the fixation point.

These and other patterns of directional sensitivity and the relation between vectors in different parts of the visual field are illustrated by the cartoons of Figure 16.

Is opponent vector organization radial to the point of fixation?

The data that we have presented indicate that many directionally sensitive LS neurons of area 7 may be activated by stimuli moving through large response areas that frequently include sectors in both the contralateral and ipsilateral visual fields crossed by the opposite halves of the major axes of the visual fields. All our observations suggest that these opposed vectors point either toward the center or outward toward the rims of the visual fields. Observations of neurons tested along four or eight axes (Fig. 16*A*) suggest that for many cells, the directionally opposed vectors are organized in a radial manner around the fixation point. Our findings are not sufficient to establish this point with certainty, and further evidence is needed from experiments in which directional sensitivities are measured along axes that do not intersect the fixation point. Some observations which we made on a few cells are of interest in this regard, for in them, we found vectors pointing toward a meridian; for example, with horizontal vectors aimed toward the vertical meridian at several different vertical levels (Fig. 17). What is certain from our observations is the opponent vector mode of organization, which often occurs in a radial manner around the fixation point, although other forms of organization of the opponent fields exist also.

Comparison of the response areas of light-sensitive neurons determined with stationary and with moving stimuli

We examined 91 light-sensitive neurons to determine the correspondence between their response areas determined with stationary and with moving stiumli. We found a clear mismatch both for size and location for 61 of those cells (67%). This mismatch may be marked, as illustrated in Figure 11 for a neuron directionally sensitive to moving stimuli, and relatively insensitive to stationary ones. An equal lack of correspondence in the reverse direction has been observed for a few cells, and the LS neurons of area 7-a appear to vary over a wide spectrum in regard to the degree of this incongruence.

The relation between excitatory and suppressive response areas

We observed 68 LS cells (13%) whose discharge rates were suppressed by light stimuli. For 12 of these, suppression was the only change evoked by lights placed anywhere in the visual fields, while the remainder were related to a mixture of suppressive and excitatory zones within their total response areas. Moving stimuli in some part of their response areas suppressed the discharge of 54 of the 68 cells, and the majority of these were sensitive to the direction of movement. However, only nine cells were excited by moving stimuli in one direction of movement and suppressed by the reciprocal movement in the same region of the response area. For the remainder, the suppressive and excitatory zones were spatially separate, but no regular relation between the two was established. Figure 10*A* illustrates the only neuron studied that was

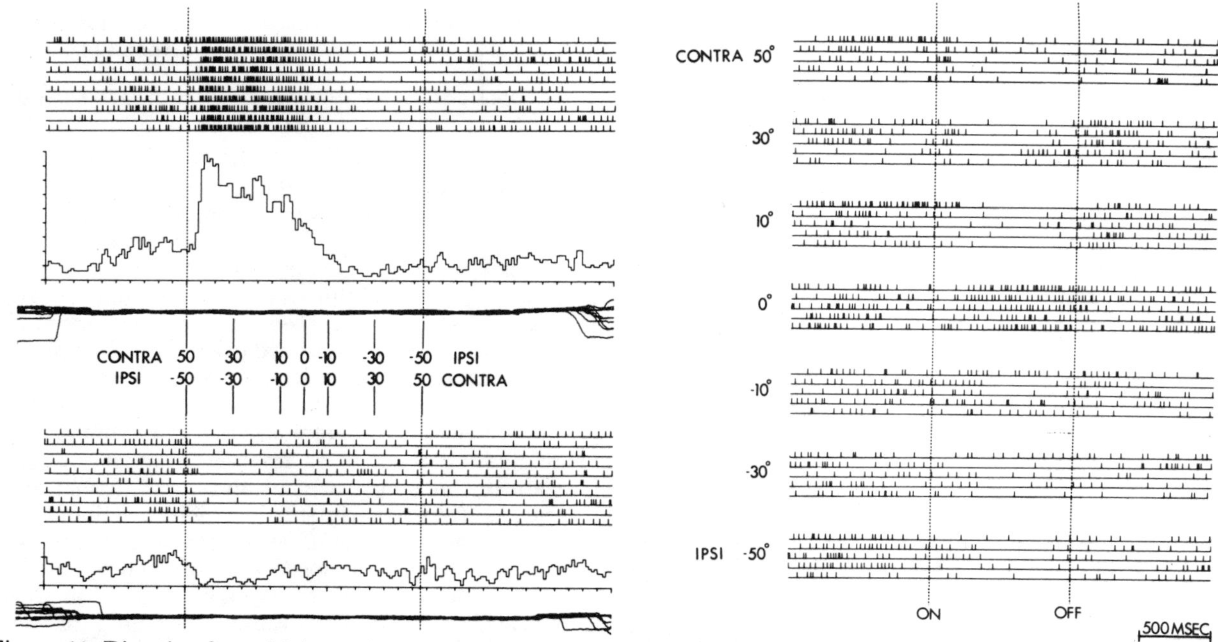

Figure 11. Directional sensitivity and opponent organization. The impulse replicas, histogram, and superimposed electro-oculograms shown at *upper left* illustrate the intense response of this neuron elicited by the stimulus as it moved from a locus 50° contralaterally (*CONTRA*) to one 50° ipsilaterally (*IPSI*) along the horizontal meridian at 60°/sec. The records *below* show the result when the stimulus moved in the reciprocal direction. The neuron was differentially sensitive to the direction of movement in the contralateral field; movements in either direction in the ipsilateral half elicited a mild suppression. The sets of records to the *right* show that physically identical but stationary stimuli elicited little or no change from any of seven locations along the same axis tested with moving stimuli. Stimulus was a 6° × 6° square, about 1 log unit above background.

TABLE V

Distribution of the light-sensitive neurons of area 7-a sensitive to moving stimuli, in regard to the property of directionality

The phenomenon of opponent vector organization is described in the text.

I. Directionally sensitive neurons		153
A. With opponent vector organization	63	
B. Without opponent vector organization	14	
C. With mixed organization	11	
D. Single sector, directional	47	
E. Two adjacent sectors, directional	18	
II. Directionally insensitive neurons		19
	Total:	172

related to an excitatory area with flanking suppressive zones on either side.

Discussion

We first summarize the functional properties of the light-sensitive cells of the inferior parietal lobule (IPL) and the anatomical pathways that link the retina to this cortical region. We then consider to what extent the salient features of parietal LS neurons, foveal sparing and opponent vector organization, can be accounted for by the functional properties of neurons in those parts of the striate and collicular visual systems known to project upon the IPL and whether further processing with elaboration of these features must be assumed to occur within the parietal cortex itself.

Studies of humans and other primates with parietal lobe lesions have revealed a number of complex defects and abnormalities in visual behavior that may occur without changes in visual acuity and with intact visual fields. We discuss what contributions the afferent visual signals to and the processing of them within the IPL, revealed in the functional properties of the light-sensitive cells, may make to these and other complex aspects of visual behavior. These are the direction of attention, especially visual attention; the perception of the spatial relation of objects; and the perception of movement, especially of objects moving in the peripheral fields during fixation, including the apparent movement of the stationary environment during locomotion with eyes fixed on the horizon.

The functional properties of parietal light-sensitive neurons

The LS cells of area 7-a respond to stationary flashing lights with sustained, transient, or on-off discharge patterns. They are related to large response areas in the contralateral half-fields, and two-thirds of these areas extend to include what are usually smaller regions of the ipsilateral visual field (Table IV, IB and II). Fifty-eight percent of all fields, whether uni- or bilateral, do not include the region at and immediately surrounding the fixation point (Table IV, I). This central region of unresponsiveness is frequently quite small, e.g., 3 to 6°, compared to the total area of the bilateral response area

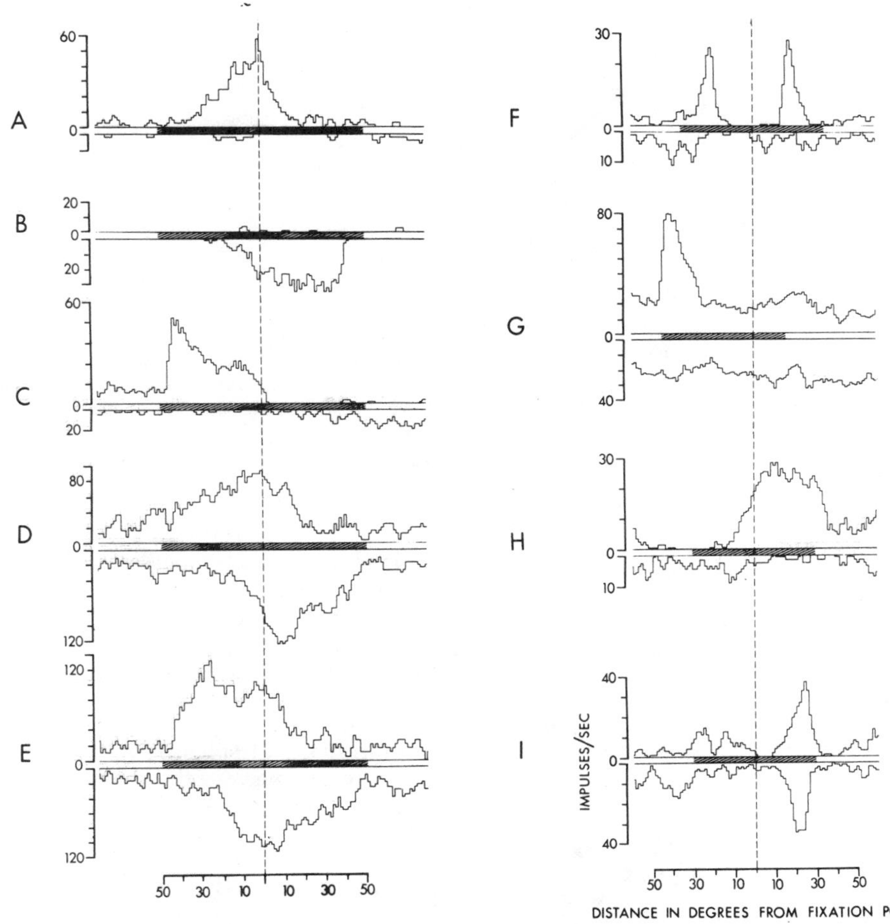

Figure 12. Varieties and degree of directional sensitivity of parietal light-sensitive neurons. The *upper histogram* of each pair sums the discharges of a neuron evoked by a stimulus moving for 100° in one direction along either the vertical or horizontal meridian, whichever was the major axis of the response area. The *lower histogram* of each pair sums the discharges evoked by the stimulus moving in the reciprocal direction, along the same axis. The *lower histogram* is reversed in direction in regard to time, so that the spatial coordinate for the two histograms is identical, as shown by the scales at the *bottom*. The neurons of *A*, *B*, *C*, *G*, and *H* show an absolute directionality, with response areas confined to one-half of the visual field. The small overlap of the fixation point by the histograms of *A*, *B*, *C*, and *H* is thought to be due to after-discharge. *D* and *E* are histogram pairs for the same neuron, *D* for movements along the horizontal meridian, *E* the vertical. The response area for this neuron was very large and included the fixation point; the directional sensitivity was weak, which produced only a skewing of the histograms. *F* shows results for an unusual neuron related to two areas sensitive to the same direction of movement, symmetrically placed in either visual half-field. *I* shows the result for one of the small number of neurons without directional sensitivity. Stimuli were 6° × 6° squares or 5° circles, about 1 log unit above background, moving at either 30 or 60°/sec. *Shaded bars*, segments of the meridians transitted by the stimuli.

disposed around it. The response areas of the remaining 42% of LS cells do include the fovea, at least when neurons that respond to a 6° × 6° light centered on the fixation point are included. All except eight of these neurons did not respond to the fixation light itself, so that the proportion of LS neurons with foveal sparing may actually be much larger than Table IV indicates. The response areas of a significant number of foveal-inclusive neurons are symmetrically arranged around the point of fixation, yield maximal responses to stimuli centered at that point, and vary in size from those 5° in diameter to those that include all of the visual field tested (100° along each meridian). Although many response areas of intermediate size were encountered, the separation into two large classes, one inclusive and one exclusive of the foveal region, seems clear. We observed that a number of neurons tested with stationary stimuli were suppressed by lights in some areas of the visual fields, but no regular relation between excitatory and suppressive zones has been defined. A few neurons were suppressed and never activated by any stationary stimuli. We have not observed orientation sensitivity, but we have not tested with bars longer than 10°.

Parietal LS cells are sensitive to stimuli moving along the axes of the visual fields that intercept the fixation point, and many are differentially sensitive to the directions of movement along those axes. The response areas determined by moving and by stationary stimuli are frequently incongruent, though overlapping, and in the limiting cases, neurons may be insensitive to stationary

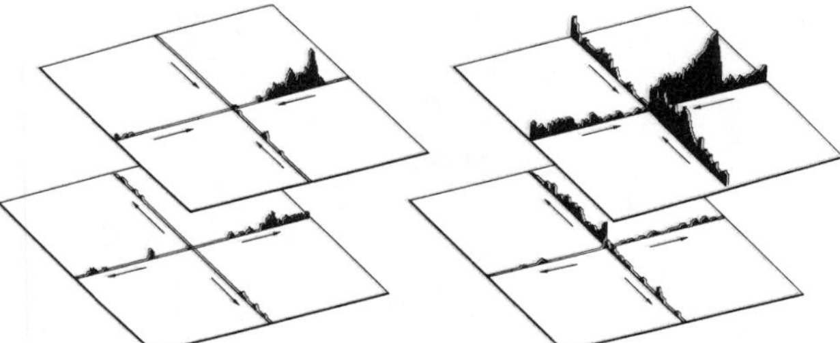

Figure 13. Directional sensitivity of parietal light-sensitive neurons. The histogram displays of this figure and those of Figures 14 and 15 were constructed in the following way. Each histogram, summarizing the discharges of a neuron occurring during movement of the light stimulus along a meridian across the visual field, was cut at the point where the stimuli crossed the fixation point. The halves of the histograms for each of the four directions of motion toward the fixation point were joined and oriented on the *upper plane* of each illustration; the outward motion halves similarly on the *lower plane.* Approximately 100° of visual angle centered at the fixation point is illustrated; stimulus movements covered slightly shorter transits of the visual field. *Left,* histograms of the responses of a neuron related to a response area confined to one quadrant of the contralateral field, with inward directionality. *Right,* histograms of the response of a neuron related to two adjacent quadrants, with inward vector organization. These results, and those of Figures 14 and 15, were obtained with a stimulus of 6° × 6°, about 1 log unit above background, moving at 30°/sec.

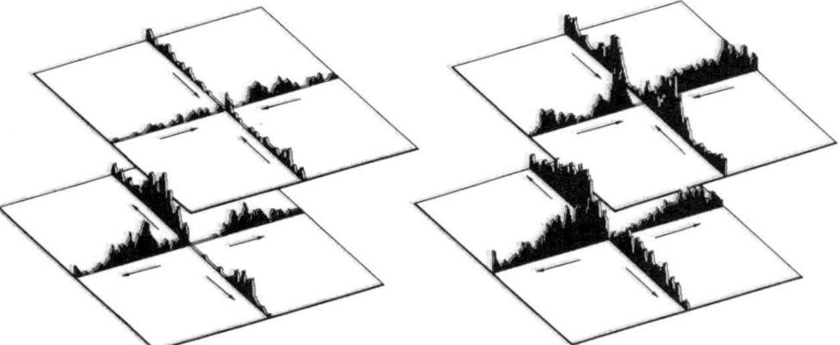

Figure 15. Directional and nondirectional sensitivity of parietal light-sensitive neurons. Directional response planes constructed as described for Figure 13. *Left,* response histograms for a neuron with four-quadrant outwardly directed sensitivity. *Right,* response histograms of a neuron sensitive to stimulus movement in each of the four quadrants, but with very weak directional sensitivity and with foveal suppression.

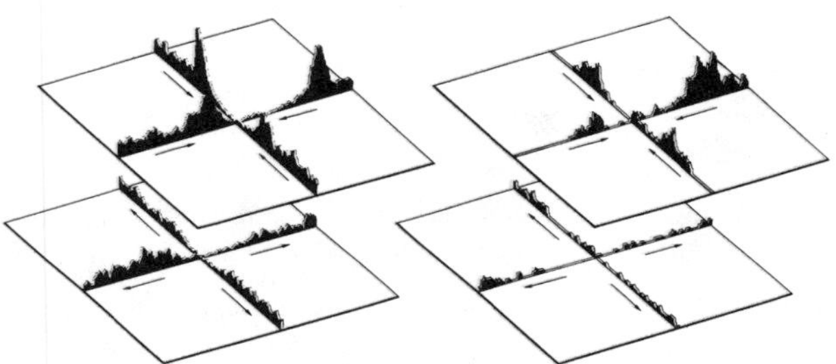

Figure 14. Directional sensitivity of parietal light-sensitive neurons, with opponent vector organization. Directional response planes constructed as described for Figure 13. *Left,* response histograms for a neuron related to response sectors in each of the four quadrants of the visual fields; this result is typical of inwardly directed opponent vector organization. *Right,* a similar result for another neuron, but here the cell is most sensitive to light moving inwardly along the contralateral horizontal meridian, a common pattern.

but respond vigorously to moving stimuli and vice versa. The movement vectors point symmetrically toward the fixation point for 75% of the neurons tested and point outward for the remainder. We term this pattern opponent vector organization. The response areas determined with moving stimuli commonly extend close to but exempt the point of fixation. We discuss below what contributions this system might make to certain forms of visual behavior.

What pathways link the retina and the inferior parietal lobule?

The cortical connections of the IPL dominate its extrinsic projections and receptions, as compared to its direct linkages to the thalamus (Divac et al., 1977; Mesulam et al., 1977; Pandya and Vignolo, 1969; Petras, 1971; Seltzer and Pandya, 1978). The IPL is usually divided into a posteromedial, PG or 7-a, and an anterolateral one, PF or 7-b (von Bonin and Bailey, 1947), but study of serial sections cut perpendicularly to the intraparietal sulcus suggests that it contains a number of fields. Indeed, Seltzer and Pandya (1980) have recently described two new subdivisions, areas POa-i and POa-e. These are long, strip-like zones in the posterior bank of the intraparietal sulcus. Area 7 has been treated as a single unit in many of the anatomical studies in which its extrinsic connections were defined. It is still uncertain whether smaller divisions within this very large cortical area entertain all or only some fraction of the total pattern of connections established for the whole. We consider here only those connections that might account for the properties of the light-sensitive neurons of the IPL.

The retino-striate system. Light-evoked activity may reach the IPL from area 17 either transcortically over a multi-step relay or from the prestriate cortex. Area 17 projects directly upon the cortex of the superior temporal sulcus (STS) (Montero, 1980; Pandya and Kuypers, 1969; Seltzer and Pandya, 1978; Ungerleider and Mishkin, 1979; Weller and Kaas, 1978; Zeki, 1974, 1976) and indirectly to that same STS target through the prestriate zones (Zeki, 1974, 1975). The IPL might then receive relayed light-evoked activity over a projection to it from the cortex lining the banks and floor of the STS. Pandya and Kuypers (1969), using an anterograde degeneration method, and both Mesulam et al. (1977) and Stanton et al. (1977), using tracer methods, have described this projection. Such a transcortical pathway was suggested by Ungerleider and Mishkin (1978) on the basis of their lesion-behavioral studies. They concluded that the spatial aspects of visual behavior measured by the landmark test, thought to depend in part upon the integrity of the IPL, require visual input from both the foveal and perifoveal field regions of area 17 and suggested that the links connecting area 17 and the IPL are transcortical. A zone of cortex within area 19 projects upon area PO-a, in the posterior bank of the intraparietal sulcus (Seltzer and Pandya, 1980) and PO-a is thought to project to other portions of area 7.

In addition to these transcortical pathways, light-evoked neural activity may propagate along pathways linking the prestriate cortex to the IPL via a cortico-

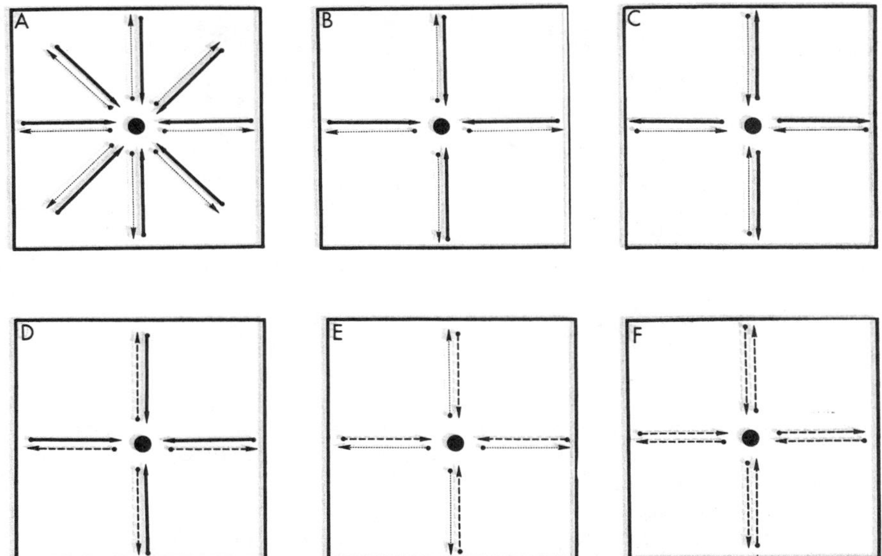

Figure 16. Varieties of the opponent vector organization of parietal light-sensitive neurons. Cartoons illustrating the variety of directional organization. The *arrows* indicate the direction of stimulus movement, but they are unrelated to the intensity of the response or the spatial extent of the response areas. *Solid lines*, excitation; *dashed lines*, suppression; *dotted lines*, no effect. *A*, typical radial opponent vector organization tested along eight axes crossing the fixation point with no reciprocal suppression. *B* and *C*, inwardly and outwardly directed opponent vector organization tested along four axes with no reciprocal suppression; *D*, the same with reciprocal suppression in all directions tested; *E*, suppression for all inwardly moving stimuli in the pattern of opponent vector organization; *F*, suppression by movement in either direction along each of the four axes tested. Types *D*, *E*, and *F* were observed rarely.

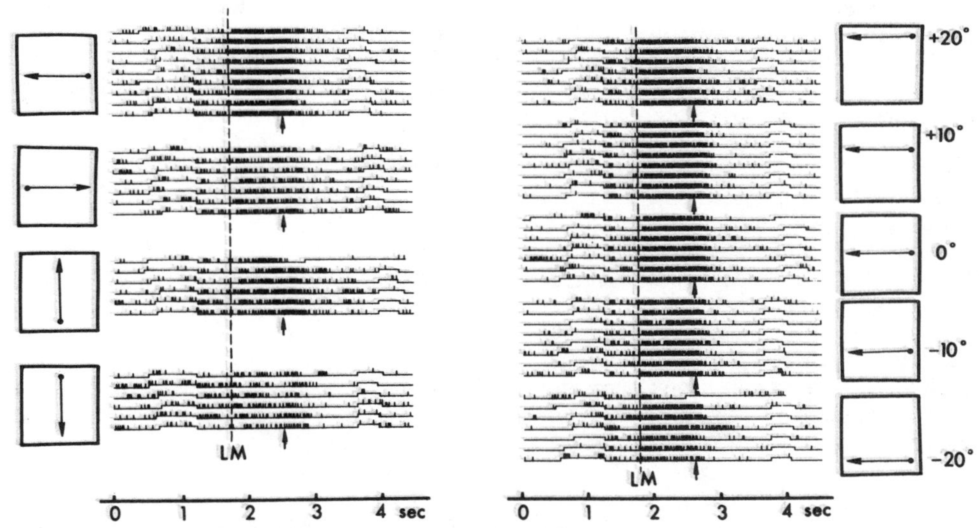

Figure 17. Nonradial opponent vector organization for a parietal light-sensitive neuron. Impulse replicas illustrated were obtained in a study of the opponent vector organization of an unusual type. The records on the *left* were obtained when the light stimulus moved in each direction along the vertical and horizontal meridians as indicated. A discharge was evoked for each movement, most intense for that from right to left (contralateral to ipsilateral) and weakest for movement from above downward. The slight overlap of the fixation point by the discharge (*arrows*) is thought to be due to after-discharge. The records on the *right* were obtained when the stimulus was moved from the contralateral to the ipsilateral side in the horizontal direction, at five different vertical positions. The vector organization appears to be inward toward the vertical meridian. Less intense discharges were evoked by inward movements from the ipsilateral side, as shown by the second set of records on the *left*. Velocity of movement, 60°/sec; stimulus 6° × 6°, about 1 log unit above background; *LM*, onset of light and its movement.

thalamocortical loop. The prestriate cortex projects in a retinotopic manner upon the inferior pulvinar (PI) and the immediately adjacent region of the lateral pulvinar called PL-α (Benevento and Davis, 1977; Rezak and Benevento, 1977) and to the lateral posterior (LP) and lateral dorsal (LD) nuclei as well; these latter projections are only weakly retinotopic. LP and LD are major sources of thalamocortical afferents to the parietal lobe. The IPL also receives fibers from the medial pulvinar nucleus and from the intralaminar group, most densely from the paracentral nucleus (Baleydier and Mauguiere, 1977; Divac et al., 1977; Kasdon and Jacobson, 1978; Trojanowski and Jacobson, 1976; Pearson et al., 1978). Thus, the inferior parietal lobule may receive relayed activity from the retino-striate system over a pathway involving a multi-step transcortical path and, in addition, over the cortico-thalamocortical loops described.

The retino-collicular and pretectal systems. The topographic projection of the retina upon the superficial layers of the superior colliculus and the upward thalamocortical projections from them provide another pathway over which light-evoked activity might reach the IPL. The superficial layers of the superior colliculus receive convergent, retinotopic projections in register from both the retina and the striate cortex. They project upward upon the retinotopically organized PI and PL-α, as well as upon a number of other thalamic nuclei (Benevento and Fallon, 1975; Benevento and Rezak, 1976, 1977; Benevento et al., 1977; Rezak and Benevento, 1975; Partlow et al., 1977). These nuclei, PI and PL-α, project upon the striate and prestriate cortical areas but not upon the parietal lobe. The link from the prestriate cortex to the STS and thence to the IPL might complete such a convergent projection of collicular and striate systems upon the striate cortex. The deeper layers of the superior colliculus and the retinoreceptive sublentiform and olivary nuclei of the pretectal region project upon common thalamic targets: the intralaminar nuclei, PL-β, and LP, nuclei that do project upon the IPL, but which have a weak if any retinotopic organization (Benevento et al., 1977; Magnuson, et al., 1979).

In summary, the inferior parietal lobule receives convergent projections from the retino-striate and retino-collicular systems, and from the pretectal nuclei as well. There are several pathways from the striate cortex to the IPL; each is characterized by a partial loss of retinotopic organization. The properties of the cells of the intermediate and deep layers of the superior colliculus, and of the two pretectal nuclei that project upon the thalamus, suggest that they may provide signals to the cortex concerning eye position and movement—and some neural activity related to the state of attention, poorly defined as that must be for the present. These two projections from two major sources are convergent with reference to the inferior parietal lobule as a whole. The possibility remains that their projections upon the IPL may be partially segregated in regard to the different zones of this large area or even in regard to more local processing units.

How to account for the static properties of the light-sensitive neurons of the parietal lobe

The large response areas of the parietal LS cells suggest a convergence and further intracortical processing of neural activity relayed from the visual system, for they are an order of magnitude or more larger than are those of neurons of the striate cortex or of the superior colliculus, in the monkey (Goldberg and Wurtz, 1972; Hubel and Wiesel, 1968, 1974; Poggio et al., 1975; Schiller et al., 1976a, b; Schiller and Koerner, 1971). There is a progressive increase in field size and loss of retinotopy at each successive step in the transcortical pathways that project upon the IPL. These properties, however, do not serve to differentiate between striate and collicular sources and may equally well be produced by a convergence within a relayed upward projection from the superior colliculus. No characteristic of either system, moreover, can account for the bilateral response areas of many parietal LS neurons. This bilaterality is most likely due to the dense interhemispheric system that links reciprocally the two inferior parietal lobules via the corpus callosum.

The bilaterality of the visual field representation in area 7-a resembles that of light-sensitive cells of the temporal homotypical cortex, which is known to depend upon callosal connections (Rocha-Miranda et al., 1975). There is no evidence for a direct link between the inferior temporal cortex and the IPL. Somewhat comparable bilateral response areas have been observed for a group of visually responsive cells located dorsal to the inferior temporal cortex in the floor and anterior bank of the superior temporal sulcus (Desimone and Gross, 1979). These neurons possess directional attributes resembling in some respects those of the LS cells of area 7-a; they depend upon the striate cortex for that directionality, but not for light sensitivity per se (Desimone et al., 1979). Reciprocal connectivity between this part of the superior temporal sulcus and area 7 is suggested by the findings of projections in one direction by Jones and Powell (1970) and in the other by Mesulam et al. (1977).

The response areas of foveal-inclusive parietal LS neurons may be produced by a preferential projection relayed from the foveal components of the striate system. Indeed, a foveal domination exists for some prestriate areas (Zeki, 1975) and is exaggerated even further in the striate-prestriate projection target in the posterior bank of the superior temporal sulcus (Dubner and Zeki, 1971; Zeki, 1974). Neurons with foveal-inclusive response areas are unlikely to depend upon a dominant projection from the colliculus, where the foveal representation is much less elaborate than it is in the striate system (Cynader and Berman, 1972; Goldberg and Robinson, 1978; Schiller et al., 1974).

The distribution of bilateral response areas with foveal sparing and the sharp exemption of the foveal region from many large response areas that are confined to the contralateral visual field, cannot be explained by any known properties of neurons of either the striate or the collicular systems. It seems unlikely that such a sharp separation into groups of neurons with response areas that include the fovea and those that spare it is produced by a weak retinotopic mapping in the partially shifted overlap mode. One might then expect to observe an entire spectrum of response areas gradually shifted in location across the visual fields. A large majority should then contain the representation of the foveal region because of the large sizes of the response areas. This is just the pattern observed in studies of the visually related cortex of the temporal lobe (Gross et al., 1969). A mapping function might still explain our observations on the assumption that two selective matrix transformations lead from a complete retinotopic map to sets with and without foveal sparing. Indeed, there is a selective projection from that portion of the prestriate cortex (area 19) containing the representation of the contralateral, peripheral visual field, to the posterior bank of the IPS (Seltzer and Pandya, 1980). On the assumption that this region projects in turn to the exposed surface of the inferior parietal lobule, a convergence within this projection could account for the contralateral fields with foveal sparing that we have observed.

Last among the hypotheses which we consider is that foveal sparing is produced by a dynamic process. The lack of response to the fixation target in all but eight of the LS neurons suggests that a dynamic process suppresses a response to the fixation target without affecting the excitability of the system to eccentrically placed targets. We have found in recent experiments that the fixation of a target raises the excitability of parietal LS neurons to eccentric targets (Motter and Mountcastle, 1980). What is less certain is whether this dynamic control process affects the central and peripheral regions of the visual fields in a differential manner—suppressing one while facilitating the other—and thus underlies the phenomenon of foveal sparing.

How to account for the dynamic properties of the light-sensitive neurons of the parietal lobe

The most striking dynamic property of parietal light-sensitive neurons is their sensitivity to stimulus movement and direction. The elaboration of these properties is a major feature of intracerebral processing of neural activity reaching the striate area from the lateral geniculate nucleus (Hubel and Wiesel, 1968; Poggio et al., 1975; Poggio and Talbot, 1980; Schiller et al., 1976a, b). Zeki has shown that these properties are further and selectively elaborated in a striate/prestriate target zone in the posterior bank of the superior temporal sulcus, a region thought to form the last step in one transcortical pathway linking the visual cortex and the inferior parietal lobule (Zeki, 1974, 1976). Directionality is an uncommon property of light-sensitive cells of the superior colliculus of the primate (Cynader and Berman, 1972; Goldberg and Robinson, 1978; Goldberg and Wurtz, 1972; Marrocco and Li, 1977; Schiller and Koerner, 1971; Updyke, 1974). It seems likely, therefore, that the striate system is the major source of light-evoked afferent input to the directionally sensitive neurons of the parietal lobe of the monkey.

Certain of the dynamic properties of the light-sensitive neurons do not appear in any of the candidate afferent inputs to the IPL and must be attributed to intracortical processing. The first is the wide range of velocities to which parietal neurons respond (up to 800°/sec). The second is the opponent organization of the movement vectors for neurons related to bilateral response areas. The first requirement for the construction of opponency in the *horizontal* dimension is the presence in each parietal lobe of neurons related to strictly contralateral response areas, with either inwardly or outwardly directed directional sensitivity. Numbers of cells with these properties were identified in area 7-a (Fig. 13 and Table V). The second requirement is an interhemispheric convergence of neurons with strictly contralateral fields and with identical directional sensitivities, perhaps via the corpus callosum. The target cells of this convergence, in either hemisphere, would then respond as do the parietal cells with bilateral response areas that we have observed, i.e., with sensitivity to movement in one direction in one half of the visual field and to opposite movements in the other. Opponency in the *vertical* direction could result from processing of afferent input within the parietal lobe itself.

In summary, it seems reasonable to attribute certain properties of the light-sensitive neurons of the inferior parietal lobule to a relayed and convergent projection of afferent signals from the striate and the collicular components of the visual system and others to further processing within the parietal cortex itself and, in addition, to the effects of a powerful state control system. These properties are the very large response areas, with and without foveal sparing; the acute sensitivity to stimulus movement over a wide range of velocities and to direction of that movement; and opponent vector organization. It remains to be determined how universal and how balanced such a putative convergence might be upon the several classes of parietal neurons with "visual" properties or, indeed, whether different functional modules of the area that contain one or another of the identified classes of parietal cells might receive projections with different degrees of dominance from striate or collicular sources. A reasonable set of working hypotheses might be these: (*a*) that LS neurons receive visual input largely from the striate system, but perhaps not exclusively so; (*b*) that the several classes of oculomotor neurons receive input mainly via ascending projections originating in the intermediate and perhaps also the deeper layers of the superior colliculus and the pretectal nuclei but not exclusively so; (*c*) that the smaller numbers of neurons that display visual as well as other properties may receive a more balanced input from the two sources, in regard to that part of their input that is visual in nature; and (*d*) that those classes of neurons that appear to be independent of direct or closely linked afferent drive and more closely related to initiatives toward action, the fixation, reach, and manipulation classes of parietal neurons, receive no direct input originating in the visual system.

Relations to behavior

The visual stimuli that we used to determine the response areas and functional properties of parietal LS neurons were not used to initiate, guide, or terminate the behavior of the monkey subjects. On the contrary, the animals were trained to maintain fixation of a target light that did control behavior and to ignore flashing or moving test lights even when the latter crossed the point of fixation at high velocity. A break in fixation and eye movement greater than a pre-set threshold, e.g., 1 to 2°, during the test period was penalized as an error trial in the latter animals of the series. Thus, we do not attempt to make direct "behavioral correlations." We do address the question of which aspects of visual behavior might, by virtue of their own parametric requirements, depend, at least in part, upon a light-driven system with the properties that we have observed, particularly those classes of visual behavior and visually guided motor behavior disturbed by lesions of the parietal homotypical cortex.

We consider these candidate functions of the parietal light-sensitive system in the context of the distinction made by Trevarthen (1968) between focal and ambient vision. *Focal vision* is that which serves with the greatest spatial acuity refined discriminative acts in regard to the shape, size, color, etc., of objects and which has evolved to a high degree of proficiency in primates. Linked to it is a motor apparatus for maintaining the line of gaze upon objects of interest, for saccadic movements to new targets, and for smooth pursuit tracking of moving ones. Focal vision guides praxic operations upon objects in the local environment, particularly manual operations. There is commonly associated with focal vision a co-linear direction of visual attention, though the two can be partially dissociated under laboratory conditions (Posner et al., 1978), and certainly under natural ones, attention is sometimes shared between focal and ambient vision.

Ambient vision relates to what Trevarthen (1968) defined as behavioral space (the "immediate extrapersonal space," Mountcastle, 1976); it is a spatial frame with head as center, symmetrically distributed in the frontal plane, and polarized in the antero-posterior direction disproportionately in the forward direction. The immediate behavioral space is defined by the extent of manual operations, which may of course be extended by tools, but behavioral space obviously extends many meters to include interactions with objects and individuals. Ambient vision is the vision of relations within this space; it extends over the entire visual field but is differentially more effective in the periphery, including the monocular crescents. It operates effectively in daylight illumination and is, compared to focal vision, greatly enhanced in dim surroundings as focal vision fades. Motor operations thought to depend mainly upon ambient vision are head and body orientations, postural adjustments, and locomotory displacements that change the relation between the body and the surrounding spatial configurations of contours, surfaces, events, and objects. This will include manual operations upon objects in the immediate behavioral space, but outside the area of focal vision, that are made during fixation and intense foveal work.

The properties of parietal LS neurons appear suitable to serve several aspects of vision and visual behavior that fall under the rubric of ambient vision. The properties are the large and frequently bilateral response areas of the LS neurons, many of which exclude the foveal region; the striking sensitivity of LS neurons to both stationary and moving stimuli, particularly to the direction of motion; and the opponent organization of the movement vectors. The aspects of visual behavior relate to the central representation of apparent motion of the environment during locomotion and during head movements and to the movement of objects in the periphery of the behavioral space when the eyes are fixed. Both are thought important for the continual updating of a continuing image of the immediately surrounding spatial frame. Finally, we consider the properties of the parietal LS cells in relation to directed visual attention.

Concerning apparent motion, forward locomotion at rates from walking to sprinting (2 to 10 m/sec) will produce angular velocities of apparent motion of objects, passing within 1 to 2 m, that range from very low values when distant 10 m or more to several hundred degrees per second as they pass by and out of the visual fields through their peripheral edges. Parietal LS neurons are sensitive to movement over just that range of velocities, from 10 to 800°/sec. Thus, forward locomotion will activate in an optimal manner the movement-sensitive parietal LS neurons. The flow of the environment by the head will be most heavily represented in the contralateral parietal lobe, but the presence of a significant number of LS neurons with bilateral response areas and opponent vector orientation ensures that the apparent motion of the environment is represented to some degree in both hemispheres. We are uncertain whether this system can provide discriminable signals of the velocity of movement of objects, for the cells that we have studied possessed flat and broad velocity/impulse frequency functions. It may be that the optimal stimuli for these cells are accelerating visual images which we have not used in this study. It is the relative insensitivity to different velocities of the parietal LS cells that leads us to question whether this system plays a significant role in motion perception or in the discrimination between different velocities of motion when these are considered as visual perceptive functions. Whether defects of this discriminative capacity appear in primates after parietal lobe lesions is uncertain and, if present, may be difficult to differentiate from the pervasive visual inattention.

It is obvious that the apparent inward and outward motions of the environment induced by reciprocal movements of the head will activate alternatively the inward and outward sets of directionally sensitive parietal LS neurons. We suggest that these signals of apparent motion of the environment during head movements and during forward locomotion play a role in spatial orientation and perception, considered in the context of ambient vision, and may provide signals used in preserving a perceptual constancy of the environment during movement and in updating a putative neural construct of the surrounding behavioral space and of objects within it. No direct evidence exists for such a neural construct; nevertheless, it is some such neural apparatus that appears to be severely impaired by parietal lobe lesions.

The cardinal signs of the parietal lobe syndrome in primates are contralateral inattention and neglect. The inattention obtains for all major sensory systems and strikingly so for vision. The neglect includes both that to sensory stimuli and a poverty of and errors in motor initiatives into the contralateral behavioral space. That neglect is, however, more a defect in spatial awareness and perception than it is a specific sensory or motor defect. Visual inattention and spatial neglect may occur with intact visual fields and normal visual acuity. We consider them to reflect the loss of the fixation and oculomotor neurons of the parietal lobe and the resulting deficiency in the function of the distributed neural system of which they are parts (Mountcastle, 1976; 1978). These sets of neurons are thought to be involved in the direction of gaze and its accompanying attention to objects of interest. The parietal LS neurons have properties eminently suitable for the afferent elements of such a neural mechanism, particularly because of the large number sensitive to movement of objects inward across the peripheral edges of the visual fields toward the center of gaze. Such a stimulus obviously has a powerful capacity for attracting attention. In addition, the neural activity set in motion by it could have an important survival value. This is so because the attentive primate, sitting or standing and concentrating intently on foveal work, would be vulnerable to threatening events unless he possessed a system for detecting signs of them in the far periphery of the visual fields where focal vision, weak in any case, is thought to be suppressed during foveal work. The afferent system leading to the parietal light-sensitive neurons, by contrast, retains its excitability during interested fixation. Indeed, as we shall show in a future paper, that excitability is increased for many neurons during interested fixation. Such a system seems ideally suited to provide signals evoking a shift of attention and gaze from one object to another.

Studies of mammals other than primates have led a number of investigators to suggest that the two components of the visual system are to a certain degree independent and parallel (see, e.g., Schneider, 1969; Sprague et al., 1979). This duality and independence was suggested by Trevarthen (1968) to have its functional parallel in those aspects of visual function that he called focal and ambient. Such a separation of neural mechanisms seems less likely in the primate than it may in other mammals for two reasons. Firstly, there is a greater corticalization of the collicular system in the primate, with a clear cortical projection from the colliculus and the pretectal nuclei, via the dorsal thalamus. Secondly, especially concerning the parietal lobe as a projection target and thus the aspect of visual function in which it is thought to play a part, there is convergence between striate and collicular projections.

However, convergence between systems cannot automatically be taken to mean convergence between elements or between modular groups of elements. This bears on the body of evidence developed in recent years that supports the idea of parallel processing in the visual system (for review, see Stone et al., 1979). This is envisaged to begin with the three classes of ganglion cells labeled Y, X, and W that project separately upon different neural elements of the lateral geniculate nucleus and the striate cortex and, indeed, transcortically through this area to certain of its efferent pathways. This model of the visual system does not exclude either a certain degree of convergent interaction among Y, X, and W elements nor a certain degree of hierarchical organization, but it does emphasize separate projections and parallel processing. The superior colliculus is thought to receive retinal input mainly from Y and W ganglion cells and only sparsely from X ganglion cells. The functional properties of the Y and W cells, together with other evidence obtained in studies of mammals with collicular lesions, led Stone et al. (1979), like Trevarthen (1968), to suggest a parallel functional dependence of focal and ambient vision upon the striate and collicular components of the visual system, respectively.

It has not yet been possible to examine the functional properties of the parietal LS neurons in sufficient detail in waking monkeys to submit them to the criteria of either the Y-X-W or the simple-complex-hypercomplex classification schemes. The extraordinary movement sensitivity, predominantly transient pattern of response, and large response areas recall some of the properties of Y neurons, but no more certain statement can be made at this time. Thus, we leave open the question to what degree the participation of the parietal lobe in certain aspects of visual function depends upon one or another of the major components of the visual system, or indeed upon both, as the marked convergence between its collicular and striate inputs suggests.

Summary and Conclusions

We describe in this paper the results of a new study of the inferior parietal lobule in waking monkeys, in which the methods of behavioral control and visual stimulation have been combined with that of single neuron analysis. In the course of this research, 204 successful microelectrode penetrations were made into area 7-a (PG) of the inferior parietal lobule. More than 1600 neurons were identified by isolation of the electrical signs of their action potentials, and more than 800 were studied further in a programmatic manner. A new classification strategy was adopted in which every neuron that responded in any way or under any circumstances to visual stimuli was termed a light-sensitive (LS) neuron, regardless of other properties. Of the cells brought under study, 31% (529) were thus classified as LS neurons; of these, a small proportion (67/529) displayed other properties as well; under our earlier classification schemes, they would have been called "complex" cells. Neurons found insensitive to visual or to any other form of passive stimulation fell into classes defined in our previous studies of the parietal lobe: the fixation neurons (17%), the oculomotor neurons (14%), and the projection-manipulation neurons (12%). We emphasize that for each of these latter classes, one of the defining characteristics is the *absence* of response to visual stimuli. Of the neurons that we brought under study, 31% escaped identification even though they were examined intensely, all by "clinical" examination and many in programmed behavioral runs with tests for oculomotor and visual correlations.

The light-sensitive cells of area 7 were studied under low photopic to mesopic conditions, with stimuli usually about 1 log unit above background. They fell into two classes in regard to the spatial distribution of their response areas, when tested with relatively large stimuli (6° × 6°). The largest group (59%) was activated from very large areas that were frequently bilateral and which exhibited the property of *foveal sparing*; i.e., stimuli centered over the point of fixation evoked no responses. The remainder were related to response areas which we term *foveal-inclusive*; for them, 6° × 6° stimuli centered on the fixation point did evoke responses, and for some, the intensity of response was maximal for foveally centered lights and decreased symmetrically on either side. However, only eight of 216 cells that we examined in detail showed any response to the fixation target light itself. This suggests that the large majority of cells that we have classed as foveal-inclusive on the basis of studies with large stimuli may also have small central zones of inexcitability, like neurons with foveal sparing.

The most striking characteristic of parietal LS neurons is their sensitivity to the movement of visual stimuli, particularly to the direction of movement. The velocity sensitivity range varies from 10 to 800°/sec, but parietal neurons provide only a poorly discriminable signal of differences in velocity. The directional vectors of parietal neurons are arranged in a systematic way, pointing either inward toward the center of the visual field or outward toward the perimeter. For neurons that subtend bilateral response areas, the directional vectors in the two half-fields most commonly point in opposite directions and are frequently arranged in a radial manner. We term this arrangement *opponent vector organization.*

The results obtained are discussed in relation to defects in visual and visuomotor behavior that occur in primates with parietal lobe lesions, particularly those of hemi-inattention and neglect. The light-sensitive neurons of area 7 possess properties well suited for signaling motion in the immediate behavioral surround and of the apparent motion that accompanies head movements and forward locomotion. Thus, they are surmised to contribute to a continual updating of a central neural image of the spatial frame of the immediate behavioral surround and to the perceptual constancy of that space that obtains during body movement. The light-sensitive neurons possess properties suitable for the attraction of gaze and attention toward objects and events in peripheral visual fields.

It is this system together with the sets of parietal neurons concerned with initiatives toward action, the fixation, oculomotor, and projection-manipulation neurons, whose destruction is thought to account, at least in part, for the cardinal features of the parietal lobe syndrome.

References

Andersen, R. A., and V. B. Mountcastle (1980) The direction of gaze influences the response of light sensitive neurons of the inferior parietal lobule (area 7) in waking monkeys. Soc. Neurosci. Abstr. *6:* 673.

Baleydier, D., and F. Mauguiere (1977) Pulvinar-latero posterior afferents to cortical area 7 in monkeys demonstrated by horseradish peroxidase tracing technique. Exp. Brain Res. *27:* 501–507.

Benevento, L. A., and B. Davis (1977) Topographical projections of the prestriate cortex to the pulvinar nuclei in the macaque monkey: An autoradiographic study. Exp. Brain Res. *30:* 405–424.

Benevento, L. A., and J. H. Fallon (1975) The ascending projections of the superior colliculus in the rhesus monkey (*Macaca mulatta*). J. Comp. Neurol. *160:* 339–362.

Benevento, L. A., and M. Rezak (1976) The cortical projections of the inferior pulvinar and adjacent lateral pulvinar in the rhesus monkey (*Macaca mulatta*): An autoradiographic study. Brain Res. *108:* 1–24.

Benevento, L. A., and M. Rezak (1977) Further observations on the projections of the layers of the superior colliculus in the rhesus monkey with autoradiographic tracing methods. Soc. Neurosci. Abstr. *3:* 553.

Benevento, L. A., M. Rezak, and R. Santos-Anderson (1977) An autoradiographic study of the projections of the pretectum in the rhesus monkey (*Macaca mulatta*): Evidence for sensorimotor links to the thalamus and oculomotor nuclei. Brain Res. *127:* 197–218.

Cynader, M., and N. Berman (1972) Receptive-field organization of monkey superior colliculus. J. Neurophysiol. *35:* 187–201.

Desimone, R., and C. G. Gross (1979) Visual areas in the temporal cortex of the macaque monkey. Brain Res. *178:* 363–380.

Desimone, R., C. Bruce, and C. G. Gross (1979) Neurons in the superior temporal sulcus of the macaque still respond to visual stimuli after removal of striate cortex. Soc. Neurosci. Abstr. *5:* 781.

Divac, I., J. H. LaVail, P. Rakic, and K. R. Winston (1977) Heterogeneous afferents to the inferior parietal lobule of the rhesus monkey revealed by the retrograde transport method. Brain Res. *123:* 197–207.

Dubner, R., and S. M. Zeki (1971) Response properties and receptive fields of cells in an anatomically defined region of the superior temporal sulcus in the monkey. Brain Res. *35:* 528–532.

Goldberg, M. E., and D. L. Robinson (1977) Visual responses of neurons in monkey inferior parietal lobule: The physiologic substrate of attention and neglect. Neurology (NY) *27:* 350.

Goldberg, M. E., and D. L. Robinson (1978) Visual systems: Superior colliculus. In *Handbook of Behavioral Neurology.* Vol. 1: *Sensory Integration*, R. B. Masterton, ed., pp. 119–164, Plenum Press, New York.

Goldberg, M. E., and R. H. Wurtz (1972) Activity of superior colliculus in behaving monkey. I. Visual receptive fields of single neurons. J. Neurophysiol. *35:* 542–559.

Gross, C. G., D. B. Bender, and C. E. Rocha-Miranda (1969) Visual receptive fields of neurons in inferotemporal cortex of the monkey. Science *166:* 1303–1306.

Hubel, D. H., and T. N. Wiesel (1968) Receptive fields and functional architecture of monkey striate cortex. J. Physiol. (Lond.) *195:* 215–243.

Hubel, D. H., and T. N. Wiesel (1974) Uniformity of monkey striate cortex: A parallel relationship between field size, scatter, and magnification factor. J. Comp Neurol. *158:* 295–306.

Hyvarinen, J., and A. Poranen (1974) Function of the parietal associative area 7 as revealed from cellular discharges in alert monkeys. Brain *97:* 673–692.

Hyvarinen, J., and Y. Shelepin (1979) Distribution of visual and somatic functions in the parietal associative area 7 of the monkey. Brain Res. *169:* 561–564.

Jones, E. G., and T. P. S. Powell (1970) An anatomical study of converging sensory pathways within the cerebral cortex of the monkey. Brain *93:* 793–820.

Kasdon, D. L., and S. Jacobson (1978) The thalamic afferents to the inferior parietal lobule of the rhesus monkey. J. Comp. Neurol. *177:* 685–706.

Kawano, K., M. Sasaki, and M. Yamashita (1980) Vestibular input to visual tracking neurons in the posterior parietal association cortex of the monkey. Neurosci. Lett. *17:* 55–60.

Leinonen, L., and G. Nyman (1979) II. Functional properties of cells in anterolateral part of area 7 associative face area of awake monkeys. Exp. Brain Res. *34:* 321–333.

Leinonen, L., J. Hyvarinen, G. Nyman, and I. Linnankoski (1979) I. Functional properties of neurons in lateral part of associative area 7 in awake monkeys. Exp. Brain Res. *34:* 299–320.

Lynch, J. C. (1980) The functional organization of the posterior parietal association cortex. Behav. Brain Sci., in press.

Lynch, J. C., C. Acuna, H. Sakata, A. Georgopoulos, and V. B. Mountcastle (1973a) The parietal association area and immediate extrapersonal space. Soc. Neurosci. Abstr. *3:* 244.

Lynch, J. C., H. Sakata, A. Georgopoulos, and V. B. Mountcastle (1973b) Parietal association cortex neurons active during hand and eye tracking of objects in immediate extrapersonal space. Physiologist *16:* 384.

Lynch, J. C., V. B. Mountcastle, W. H. Talbot, and T. C. T. Yin (1977) Parietal lobe mechanisms for directed visual attention. J. Neurophysiol. *40:* 362–389.

Magnuson, D. J., M. Rezak, and L. A. Benevento (1979) Some observations on the organization of the retinal projections to the pretectum and superior colliculus in the macaque monkey as demonstrated by the combined use of laser beam lesions of the retina and autoradiography. Soc. Neurosci. Abstr. *5:*

794.

Marrocco, R. T., and R. H. Li (1977) Monkey superior colliculus: Properties of single cells and their afferent inputs. J. Neurophysiol. *40:* 844–860.

Mesulam, M. M., G. W. Van Hoesen, D. N. Pandya, and N. Geschwind (1977) Limbic and sensory connections of the inferior parietal lobule (area PG) in the rhesus monkey: A study with a new method for horseradish peroxidase histochemistry. Brain Res. *136:* 393–414.

Montero, V. M. (1980) Patterns of connections from the striate cortex to cortical visual areas in superior temporal sulcus of macaque and middle temporal gyrus of owl monkey. J. Comp. Neurol. *189:* 45–59.

Motter, B. C., and V. B. Mountcastle (1979) Afferent visual signals for directed visual attention. Soc. Neurosci. Abstr. *5:* 118.

Motter, B. C., and V. B. Mountcastle (1980) Active directed gaze controls the excitability of the light sensitive neurons of the inferior parietal lobule in the waking monkey. Soc. Neurosci. Abstr. *6:* 673.

Mountcastle, V. B. (1976) The world around us: Neural command functions for selective attention. Neurosci. Res. Program Bull. *14:* 1–47.

Mountcastle, V. B. (1978) Brain mechanisms for directed attention. J. R. Soc. Med. *71:* 14–28.

Mountcastle, V. B., J. C. Lynch, A. Georgopoulos, H. Sakata, and C. Acuna (1975) Posterior parietal association cortex of the monkey: Command functions for operations within extrapersonal space. J. Neurophysiol. *38:* 871–908.

Pandya, D. N., and H. G. J. M. Kuypers (1969) Cortico-cortical connections in the rhesus monkey. Brain Res. *13:* 13–36.

Pandya, D. N., and L. A. Vignolo (1969) Interhemispheric projections of the parietal lobe in the rhesus monkey. Brain Res. *15:* 49–65.

Partlow, G. D., M. Colonnier, and J. Szaba (1977) Thalamic projections of the superior colliculus in the rhesus monkey, *Macaca mulatta.* A light and electron microscopic study. J. Comp. Neurol. *171:* 285–318.

Pearson, R. C. A., P. Brodal, and T. P. S. Powell (1978) The projection of the thalamus upon the parietal lobe in the monkey. Brain Res. *144:* 143–148.

Petras, J. M. (1971) Connections of the parietal lobe. J. Psychiatr. Res. *8:* 189–201.

Poggio, G. F., and W. H. Talbot (1980) Mechanisms of static and dynamic stereopsis in foveal cortex of the rhesus monkey. J. Physiol. (Lond.), in press.

Poggio, G. F., F. H. Baker, R. J. W. Mansfield, A. Sillito, and P. Grigg (1975) Spatial and chromatic properties of neurons subserving foveal and parafoveal vision in rhesus monkey. Brain Res. *100:* 25–59.

Posner, M. I., M. J. Nissen, and W. C. Ogden, (1978) Attended and unattended processing modes: The role of set for spatial location. In *Modes of Perceiving and Processing Information,* H. L. Pick and I. J. Saltzman, eds., pp. 137–157, Lawrence Erlbaum Associates, Hillsdale, NJ.

Rezak, M., and L. A. Benevento (1975) Cortical projections of corticorecipient and tectorecipient zones of the pulvinar in the macaque monkey. Soc. Neurosci. Abstr. *1:* 63.

Rezak, M., and L. A. Benevento (1977) A redefinition of pulvinar subdivisions in the macaque monkey: Evidence for three distinct subregions within classically defined lateral pulvinar. Soc. Neurosci. Abstr. *3:* 574.

Robinson, D. L., and M. E. Goldberg (1977a) Functional properties of posterior parietal cortex of the monkey. I. Sensory responses. Soc. Neurosci. Abstr. *3:*574

Robinson, D. L., and M. E. Godberg (1977b) Visual properties of neurons in the parietal cortex of the awake monkey. Invest. Opthalmol. Vis. Sci. *16* (Suppl.): 156.

Robinson, D. L., M. E. Goldberg, and G. B. Stanton (1978) Parietal association cortex in the primate: Sensory mechanisms and behavioral modulations. J. Neurophysiol. *41:* 910–932.

Rocha-Miranda, C. E., D. B. Bender, C. G. Gross, and M. Mishkin (1975) Visual activation of neurons in inferotemporal cortex depends on striate cortex and forebrain commissures. J. Neurophysiol. *38:* 475–491.

Rolls, E. T., D. Perrett, S. J. Thorpe, A. Puerto, A. Roper-Hall, and S. Maddison (1979) Responses of neurons in area 7 of the parietal cortex to objects of different significance. Brain Res. *169:* 194–198.

Sakata, H., H. Sibutani, and K. Kawano (1977) Spatial selectivities of "visual" neurons in the posterior parietal association cortex of the monkey. Proc. IUPS XIII 652.

Sakata, H., H. Shibutani, and K. Kawano (1978) Parietal neurons with dual sensitivity to real and induced movements of visual target. Neurosci. Lett. *9:* 165–169.

Sakata, H., H. Shibutani, and K. Kawano (1980) Spatial properties of visual fixation neurons in posterior parietal association cortex of the monkey. J. Neurophysiol. *43:* 1654–1672.

Schiller, P. H., and F. Koerner (1971) Discharge characteristics of single units in the superior colliculus of the alert rhesus monkey. J. Neurophysiol. *34:* 920–936.

Schiller, P. H., M. Stryker, M. Cynader, and N. Berman (1974) Response characteristics of single cells in the monkey superior colliculus following ablation or cooling of visual cortex. J. Neurophysiol. *37:* 181–194.

Schiller, P. H., B. L. Finlay, and S. P. Volman (1976a) Quantitative studies of single-cell properties in monkey striate cortex. I. Spatiotemporal organization of receptive fields. J. Neurophysiol. *39:* 1288–1319.

Schiller, P. H., B. L. Finlay, and S. F. Volman (1976b) Quantitative studies of single-cell properties in monkey striate cortex. II. Orientation specificity and ocular dominance. J. Neurophysiol. *39:* 1320–1333.

Schneider, G. E. (1969) Two visual systems. Science *163:* 895–902.

Seltzer, B., and D. Pandya (1978) Afferent cortical connections and architectonics of the superior temporal sulcus and surrounding cortex in the rhesus monkey. Brain Res. *149:*1–24.

Seltzer, B., and D. N. Pandya (1980) Converging visual and somatic sensory cortical input to the intraparietal sulcus of the rhesus monkey. Brain Res. *192:* 339–351.

Sprague, J. M., M. A. Berkley, and H. C. Hughes (1979) Visual acuity functions and pattern discrimination in the destriate cat. Acta Neurobiol. Exp. *39:* 643–682.

Stanton, G. V., W. L. R. Cruce, M. E. Goldberg, and D. L. Robinson (1977) Some ipsilateral projections to areas PF and PG of the inferior parietal lobule in monkeys. Neurosci. Lett. *6:* 243–250.

Stone, J., B. Dreher, and A. Leventhal (1979) Hierarchical and parallel mechanisms in the organization of visual cortex. Brain Res. Rev. *1:* 345–394.

Trevarthen, C. B. (1968) Two mechanisms of vision in primates. Psychol. Forsch. *31:* 299–337.

Trojanowski, J. Q., and S. Jacobson (1976) Areal and laminar distribution of some pulvinar cortical efferents in the rhesus monkey. J. Comp. Neurol. *169:* 371–392.

Ungerleider, L. G., and M. Mishkin (1978) Interactions of striate and posterior parietal cortex in spatial vision. Soc. Neurosci. Abstr. *4:* 649.

Ungerleider, L. G., and M. Mishkin (1979) The striate projection zone in the superior temporal sulcus of *Macaca mulatta:* Location and topographic organization. J. Comp. Neurol. *188:* 347-366.

Updyke, B. V. (1974) Characteristics of unit responses in superior colliculus of the *Cebus* monkey. J. Neurophysiol. *37:*

896–909.

von Bonin, G., and P. Bailey (1947) *The Neocortex of Macaca mulatta.* University of Illinois Press, Urbana.

Weller, R. E., and J. H. Kaas (1978) Connections of striate cortex with the posterior bank of the superior temporal sulcus in macaque monkeys. Soc. Neurosci. Abstr. *4:* 650.

Yin, T. C. T., and V. B. Mountcastle (1977) Visual input to the visuomotor mechanisms of the monkey's parietal lobe. Science *197:* 1381–1383.

Zeki, S. M. (1974) Functional organization of a visual area in the posterior bank of the superior temporal sulcus of the rhesus monkey. J. Physiol. (Lond.) *236:* 549–573.

Zeki, S. M. (1975) The functional organization of projections from striate to prestriate visual cortex in the rhesus monkey. Cold Spring Harbor Symp. Quant. Biol. *40:* 591–600.

Zeki, S. M. (1976) The projections to the superior temporal sulcus from areas 17 and 18 in the rhesus monkey. Proc. R. Soc. Lond. (Biol.) *193:* 199–207.

11

J. Allman, F. Miezin, and E. McGuinness

Direction- and velocity-specific responses from beyond the classical receptive field in the middle temporal visual area (MT)

1985. *Perception* 14: 105–126

Abstract. The true receptive field of more than 90% of neurons in the middle temporal visual area (MT) extends well beyond the classical receptive field (crf), as mapped with conventional bar or spot stimuli, and includes a surrounding region that is 50 to 100 times the area of the crf. These extensive surrounds are demonstrated by simultaneously stimulating the crf and the surround with moving stimuli. The surrounds commonly have directional and velocity-selective influences that are antagonistic to the response from the crf. The crfs of MT neurons are organized in a topographic representation of the visual field. Thus MT neurons are embedded in an orderly visuotopic array, but are capable of integrating local stimulus conditions within a global context. The extensive surrounds of MT neurons may be involved in figure-ground discrimination, preattentive vision, perceptual constancies, and depth perception through motion cues.

1 Introduction

We perceive the visual world as an unitary whole, yet one of the guiding principles of more than four decades of neurophysiological research on the visual system has been that neurons respond to stimulation within their classical receptive fields (crfs), which are usually discrete small portions of the total visual field (Hartline 1938). The crfs are organized into a series of topographic representations of the visual field. At least ten areas, each containing a separate map of the visual field, are present in the visual cortex in the owl monkey (see figure 1). It has been widely assumed that perceptual functions that require the integration of inputs over large portions of visual space must be either collective properties of arrays of neurons representing the visual field or else be features of those neurons at the highest processing levels in the visual system, such as those neurons in inferotemporal or posterior parietal cortex that typically possess very large receptive fields and do not appear to be organized in visuotopic maps. These assumptions have been based on results of studies in which receptive fields were mapped with conventional stimuli, spots or bars of light, presented on a featureless background. However, unlike the neurophysiologist's tangent screen, the natural visual scene is rich in features (see figure 2). We thought it would be especially appropriate to study the effects of background motion since the visual field is filled with moving stimuli as the viewer moves through or scans its environment. Neurons in the middle temporal visual area (MT) are specialized for the analysis of moving stimuli, and possess well defined crfs that are organized in a topographic representation of the visual field (Allman and Kaas 1971a; Baker et al 1981; Maunsell and Van Essen 1983a). We have found that the direction and velocity of background textures moving outside the classical receptive field have a profound and selective influence on the responses of MT neurons to stimuli presented within the crf.

2 Methods

2.1 *Subjects*

We recorded from Area MT in three owl monkeys (*Aotus lemurinus griseimembra*: Brumback 1973; Hershkovitz 1983). This is a new taxonomic designation which supersedes the term *Aotus trivirgatus* used in our earlier papers. Our procedures for recording through a chronically implanted chamber were described in detail in Allman et al (1979) and Baker et al (1981). Under aseptic conditions and general anesthesia (ketamine HCl, 25 mg kg^{-1}), a stainless steel chamber was cemented around an opening in the skull exposing the dura over MT. At the beginning of each experimental session the monkey was tranquilized with a single dose of triflupromazine (2 mg kg^{-1}), and small doses of ketamine (2 mg kg^{-1} h^{-1}) were used to maintain sedation. The monkey's head was fixed

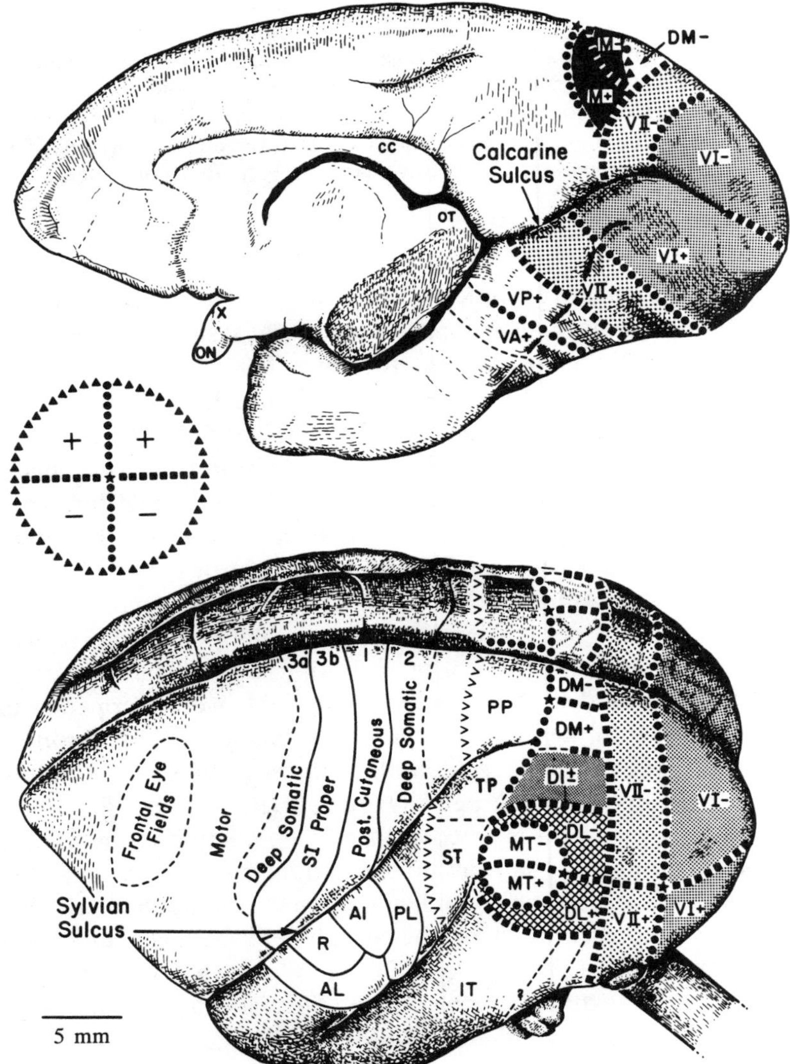

Figure 1. The representations of the sensory domains in the cerebral cortex of the owl monkey. Above is a ventromedial view; below is a dorsolateral view. On the left is a perimeter chart of the visual field. The symbols on this chart are superimposed on the surface of the visual cortex. Pluses indicate upper quadrant representation; minuses, lower quadrants. The row of Vs indicates the approximate border of visually responsive cortex in the parietal and temporal lobes. AI, first auditory area; AL, anterolateral auditory area; CC, corpus callosum; DI dorsointermediate visual area; DL, dorsolateral visual area; DM, dorsomedial visual area; IT, inferotemporal visual cortex; M, medial visual area; MT, middle temporal visual area; ON, optic nerve; OT, optic tectum; PL, posterolateral auditory area; PP, posterior parietal visual cortex; R, rostral auditory area; ST, superior temporal visual area; TP, temporoparietal visual cortex; VA, ventral anterior visual area; V-I first visual area; V-II second visual area; VP, ventral posterior visual area; X, optic chiasm. The cortical visual areas were mapped by Allman and Kaas (1971a, 1971b, 1974a, 1974b, 1975, 1976), and Newsome and Allman (1980); the somatosensory areas by Merzenich et al (1978); and the auditory areas by Imig et al (1977).

with a circular clamp tightened around the steel recording chamber. This clamp was attached to a specially designed chair in which the monkey was restrained in the normal owl monkey sitting posture. The cornea, sclera, and eyelids were topically anesthetized with a long-acting local anesthetic (0.5% dibucaine HCl in contact lens wetting solution), and the pupils were dilated with 1% cyclopentolate HCl solution. After allowing the local anesthetic to take effect, the eyelids were retracted. An eye ring, which was machined to fit the contour of the eye and mounted by an adjustable joint to the apparatus, was cemented to the margin of the cornea with Histoacryl tissue adhesive (n-butyl cyanoacrylate). This method effectively eliminated eye movements during the course of the experimental session. The adhesive was easily removed from the eye without damage at the end of each session. Eye position was monitored by projecting the image of retinal blood vessels in the optic disk onto the screen with an ophthalmoscope (Fernald and Chase 1971). Contact lenses were used to protect the cornea from drying and bring the eye into focus on the television screen which was normally 28.5 cm from the eye.

2.2 *Video stimulator*

We developed a video display system with John Power and Michael Walsh of the California Institute of Technology Biology Electronics Shop. The system was based on an Intel 8085 microprocessor and could be controlled either manually through switches and a joystick or through a Nova 2 computer. The display was presented on a Sony KX-2501 RGB monitor (39 cm × 52 cm). The display consisted of a central region of adjustable length, width, and orientation which contained an array of dots. The direction and speed of movement of the dot array could be varied. The dot arrays were produced by a pseudorandom binary sequence generator (PRBS), the motion parameters were generated by the microprocessor. We positioned the central region so that it corresponded to the crf for each neuron. The dots subtended approximately 0.4 deg at a viewing distance of 28.5 cm and the display consisted of 50% bright and 50% dark dots. The surround region contained the same size and density of dots, which were produced by a second PRBS, and the movement of the surround array was controlled by the micro-

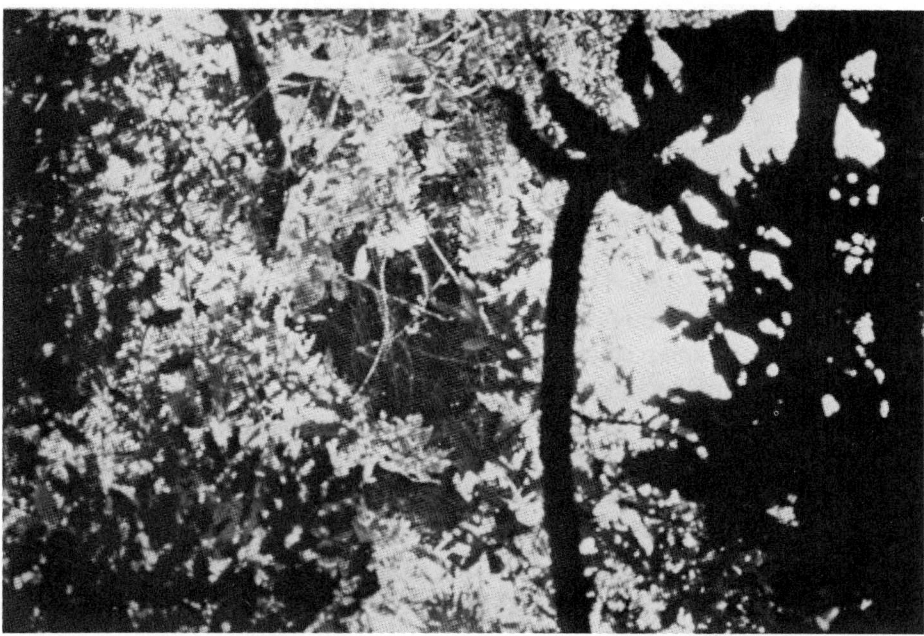

Figure 2. Tropical forest habitat of the owl monkey. A family of owl monkeys resides in the tangle of vines, which is viewed from the ground. This photograph was taken by Dave Sivertsen in the Manu National Park in the Peruvian Amazon.

processor independently from the center array. The rectangular border of the center region remained stationary during both center and background movement, and fresh dots continually appeared at the edges of the center and surround so that the screen was continually filled with dots. In addition, we could present more conventional stimuli such as solid bright or dark bars on dark, bright, or random-dot backgrounds.

2.3 *Single neuron recording and analysis*

We penetrated the dura and recorded the activity of single neurons in MT with sterilized glass-insulated platinum-iridium microelectrodes (Wolbarsht et al 1960) advanced with a stepping motor microdrive mounted on a movable stage attached to the chamber. When a neuron with a stable waveform was isolated with a window discriminator, we plotted its crf with hand-controlled stimuli while listening to the neuron's activity over an audio monitor, and then proceeded with the computer-controlled quantitative characterization of the neuron's response properties described in section 3. Each stimulus condition was presented five times, and in each series the stimuli were presented in pseudo-random order. For a 2 to 3 s foreperiod before each stimulus presentation the computer monitored the neuron's firing to measure the rate of spontaneous activity. The neuron's response was calculated by averaging the spikes that occurred during the foreperiod and subtracting this spontaneous rate from the average firing rate during the stimulus presentation period. To allow for response latency, the period for the response calculation ran from 40 ms after the beginning of the stimulus presentation to the end of the presentation. In addition, when we tested with bar stimuli sweeping at the higher speeds, we found that the response often occurred after the end of the brief stimulus-presentation period. So for calculating the response we allowed a minimum period of 250 ms commencing 40 ms after the beginning of the stimulus presentation. The 40 ms delay and 250 ms minimum period were used by Maunsell and Van Essen (1983a) in their study of MT in macaque monkeys.

When we tested the effect of the direction of background movement, we continuously stimulated the cell with a field of random dots moving in its preferred direction and confined to its crf. We calculated the cell's average firing rate during the five 2 s periods before the presentation of each direction of movement of the random-dot background and compared this firing rate, which contained both driven and spontaneous components, with the average firing rate during background movement. These measurements require that the background firing rate resulting from the stimulation of the crf and spontaneous activity be reasonably constant. We excluded from analysis those cells in which the highest firing rate for a foreperiod was more than double the lowest firing rate of all the foreperiods. Sixty-one of the seventy-five MT cells tested for the influence of direction of background movement were acceptable by this criterion, and the data from these 61 cells are described in section 3.1.

When we tested the effect of velocity of background movement in a cell, we first determined the preferred direction and velocity for the optimally shaped bar stimulus, and then we presented the bar moving in the preferred direction at the preferred velocity while simultaneously presenting background movements in the same direction of varying velocity. Instead of driving the cell continuously with the bar stimulus, we presented the optimal bar stimulus together with various background velocities and compared these responses with those obtained when the background was stationary. The background stationary trials were interleaved in the pseudorandom sequence with the other stimulus presentations. This method enabled us to monitor the spontaneous activity during the foreperiod, and thus assess the effect of the velocity of background movement on spontaneous activity separately from the response resulting from the bar stimulus.

In the course of these experiments we derived a visuotopic map for each monkey from the crfs that enabled us to identify the cortical visual areas from which we were recording by making use of extensive mapping done earlier in owl monkeys (Allman and Kaas 1971a, 1974b). The areal assignment of recording sites was confirmed in two monkeys by identifying recording sites marked with microlesions in MT, which is highly distinctive in histological sections stained for nerve fibers (Allman and Kaas 1971a). These monkeys were deeply anesthetized with a lethal dose of sodium pentobarbital and then perfused with 0.9% saline followed by 3.7% formaldehyde in 0.9% saline. Alternate forty micra frozen sections were stained with cresyl violet for cell bodies and with the Gallyas (1979) method for fibers. The third monkey is in good health and is a successful breeder in our colony.

3 Results

3.1 *Effects of moving stimuli outside the classical receptive field*

For each MT neuron we first mapped its crf with bar and random-dot stimuli and determined its preferred velocity. The term *classical receptive field* (crf) is used instead of *excitatory receptive field* because for many cells the discharge rate is inhibited below the spontaneous rate by conventional stimuli moving against the preferred direction (see the left graph in figure 3 where the response at − 180° was nearly 20% below the level of spontaneous activity). We electronically positioned on the screen a rectangular window of adjustable length, width, and orientation so that it closely corresponded to the crf. We

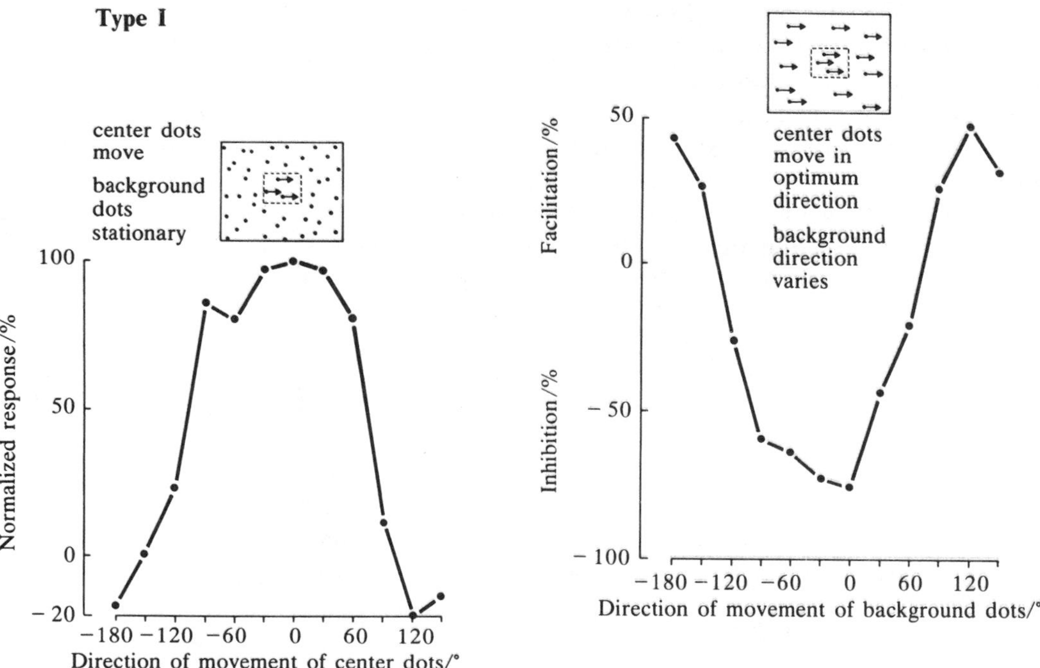

Figure 3. Response properties of a type I neuron (antagonistic direction-selective surround). The left graph depicts the response of the cell, HCMT32B, to twelve directions of movement of an array of random dots coextensive with its crf. The response is normalized so that 0% is equal to the average level of spontaneous activity sampled for 2 s periods before each presentation. Negative percentages in the left graph indicate inhibition relative to the level of spontaneous activity. The response in the optimum direction is 100%. The right graph depicts the response of the cell to different directions of movement in the surround while the crf was simultaneously stimulated with an array moving in the cell's preferred direction. In the right graph the crf was stimulated by the array moving in the optimum direction during the 2 s sample periods preceding background movement; thus a response of 100% in the left graph is equivalent to 0% in the right graph. A value of − 100% in the right graph indicates that the movement in the surround reduced the neuron's firing rate to zero. The stimulus conditions are depicted schematically above each graph. In the experiment the dots were much denser and the background much larger relative to the center than depicted schematically.

examined the neuron's directional preference within its crf by moving random-dot arrays in twelve directions within the window, which was fixed in place and was surrounded by a background of stationary random dots. These data are depicted in the graphs on the left side in figures 3 through 8. To obtain the graphs on the right side of figures 3 through 8, we excited each neuron by presenting random dots moving in its preferred direction within the window and determined the influence of background movement by stimulating the hitherto apparently silent surround with arrays of random dots moving in each of twelve directions. Only the center movement was displayed within the window, and only the background movement was displayed elsewhere on the screen. Both the center and the background dots moved at the same speed, which was approximately the speed for eliciting the optimum response from the crf. Figure 3 illustrates a type I neuron, which possessed a directionally selective crf and an antagonistic directionally selective surround. For type I neurons the preferred direction for the center was the same as the direction of maximum inhibition by movement in the surround.

Figure 4 illustrates a type II neuron, which resembled the type I cell but in addition possessed a strong facilitatory peak when the background moved in one direction 90° to the preferred direction for the center.

Figure 5 illustrates a type III neuron, which also possessed a directionally selective crf but was suppressed by all directions of background movement. In this cell we also tested the effect of having the background move in all directions at once like 'snow' on the television screen. This did not suppress the response to center stimulation and suggests that coherent movement of an array of random dots is required for suppression.

Figures 6 through 8 illustrate all of the data points obtained for the three types. In each graph lines connect the median response obtained for each stimulus condition. The data for the three types are summarized in table 1. The three types cannot be distinguished on the basis of the responses from their crfs. Types I and II have directionally selective surrounds with the maximum suppression obtained for background movements in the preferred direction for the center. Type III was suppressed by all directions of background movement with no directional preference. Type II neurons were strongly

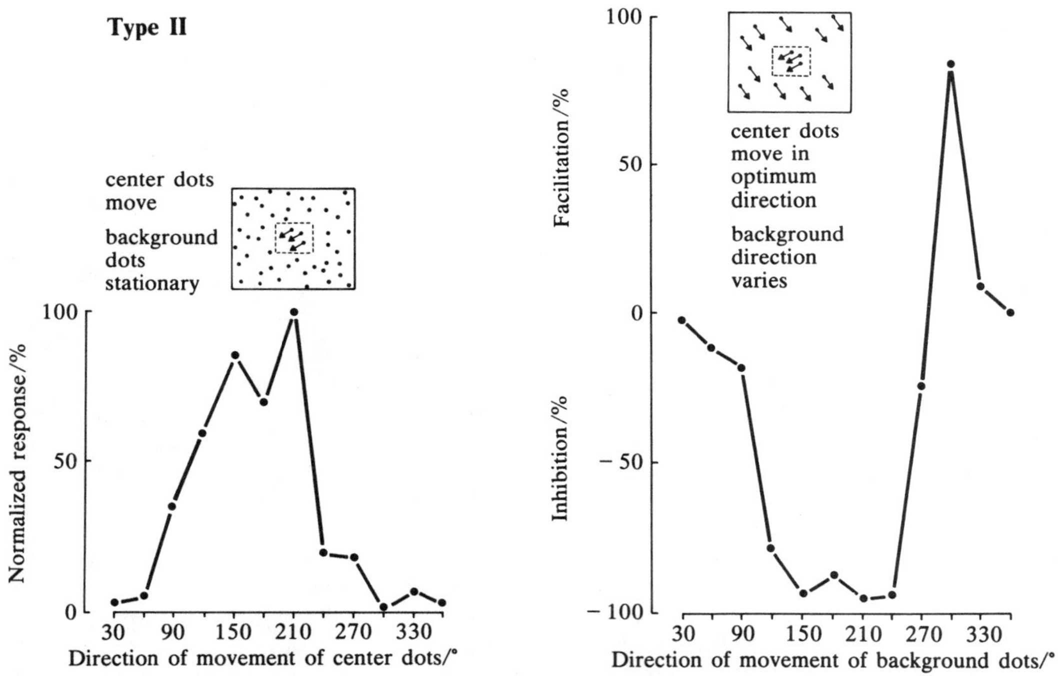

Figure 4. Response properties of a type II neuron, HCMT24E (90° surround facilitator). The schematic diagrams above the graphs depict the optimum stimulus conditions.

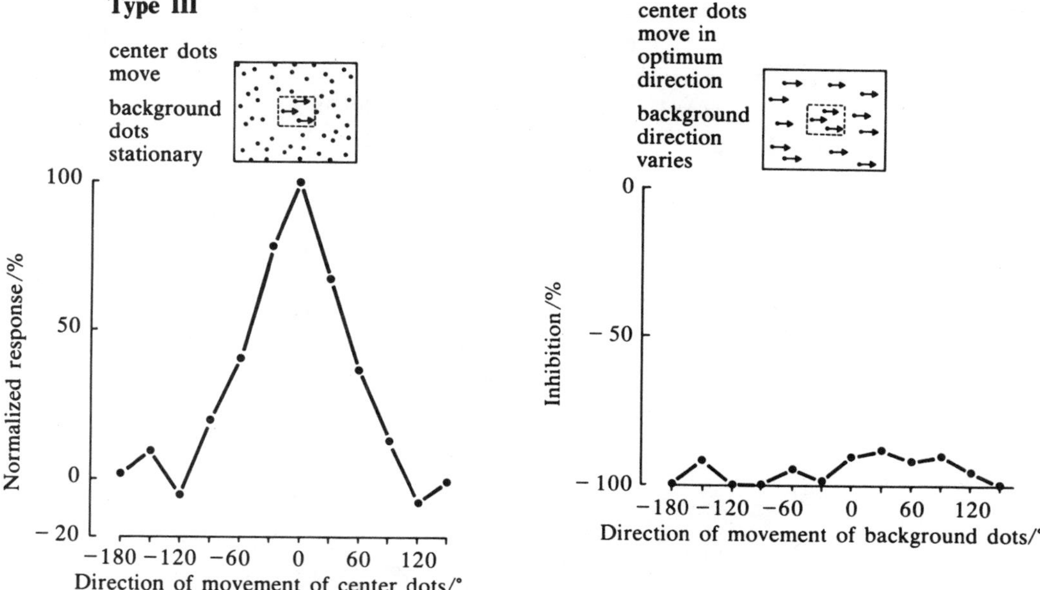

Figure 5. Response properties of a type III neuron, HCMT21K (nondirectional surround inhibitor).

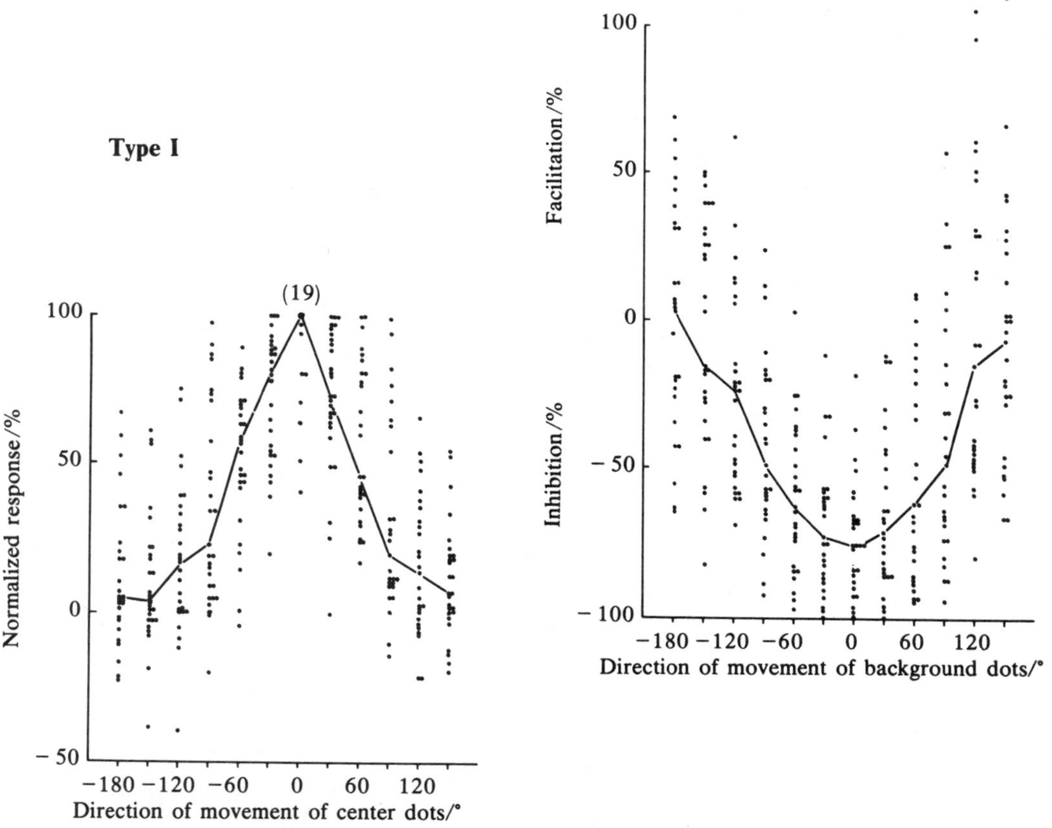

Figure 6. Responses of twenty-seven type I neurons (antagonistic direction-selective surrounds). In the left graph, which depicts responses from the crf with the background stationary, the data have been plotted so that the preferred direction of movement for each cell is set equal to 0° or, in cells with a broad band of preferred directions, the direction in the middle of the band is set equal to 0°. This direction, which also corresponds to the direction of movement driving the center during the presentation of background movements, is also set equal to 0° for each cell in the right graph. A line connects the median responses for each direction in each graph.

facilitated by one direction of shearing background movement that was 90° to the cell's preferred direction. The majority of type I neurons were facilitated by background movement opposite to the preferred direction (180°). In each microelectrode penetration, either type I or type III cells tended to predominate. The five type II cells were found in five separate penetrations mixed with the other types.

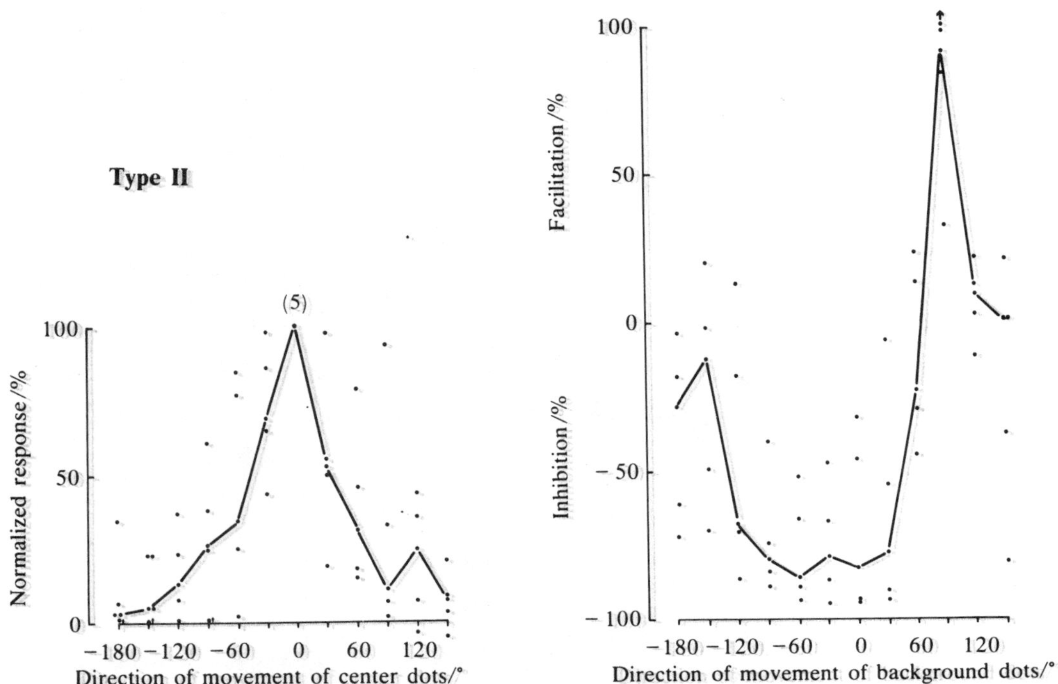

Figure 7. Responses of five type II neurons (90° surround facilitators). The directions have been normalized as in figure 6, but, in addition, the facilitatory peaks have been placed at + 90° although three cells actually had their peaks at − 90°, and the other directions from these three cells have been similarly reversed in both graphs. Small arrows indicate responses falling beyond the limits of the graph.

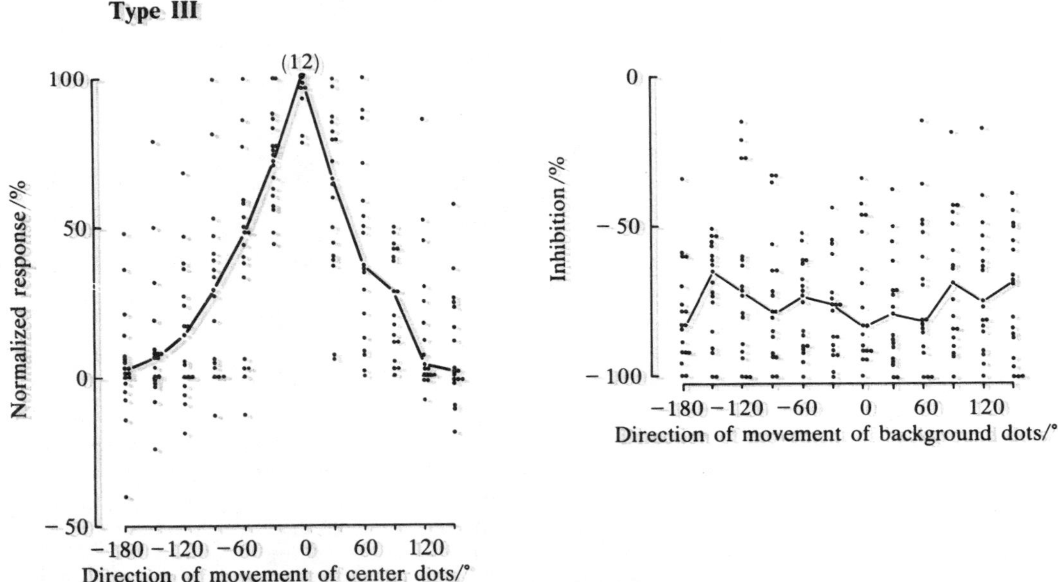

Figure 8. Responses of eighteen type III neurons (nondirectional background inhibitors). The directions have been normalized as in figure 6.

In addition to the three main types, we recorded a cell which responded well to all directions of movement in its crf. When we excited the crf with movement in the preferred 0° direction, the cell behaved like type I with direction-selective background suppression greatest at 0°; when we drove the crf with movement in the 180° direction, the background suppression was greatest at 180°. In another cell the response from the crf was abolished by the presence of a static random-dot surround. In still another cell stimulation of the crf with random dots produced only inhibition. Three cells had irregular mixed patterns of inhibition and facilitation as a result of background stimulation.

Table 1. Types of responses from beyond the crf in MT neurons

Type	Distinguishing features	Number of cells	Percentage of cells
I	directionally selective surround	27	44
II	sharp facilitatory peak for shearing movement in surround in one direction 90° to preferred direction for crt	5	8
III	equal suppression by all directions of movement in the surround	18	30
IV	unresponsive to moving random dots in the surround	5	8
Miscellaneous surround responses		6	10
	Total	61	100

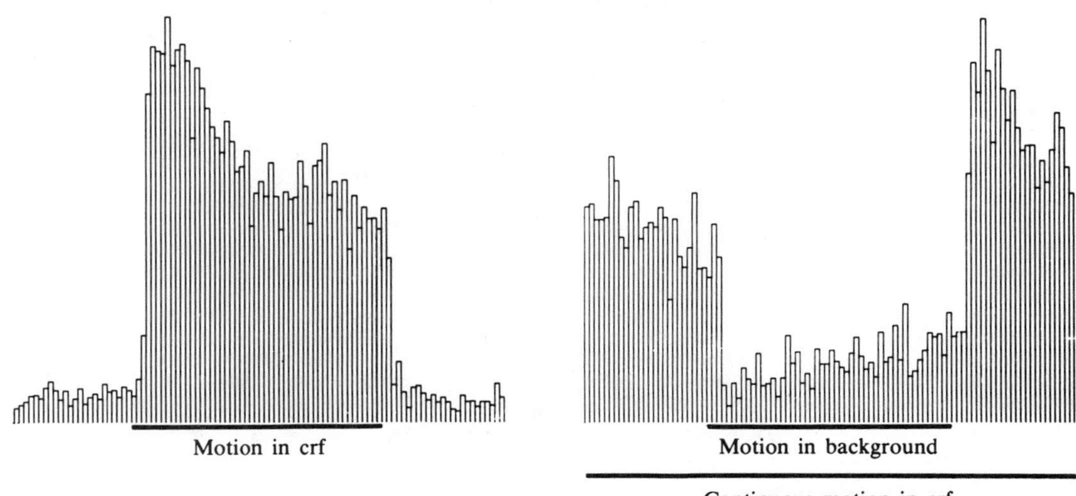

Figure 9. The left histogram illustrates the combined responses of forty-two MT neurons (types I, II, and III) to random dots moving for a 2 s period in the preferred direction within their crfs with the background stationary. In the right histogram the same MT neurons were stimulated continuously with random dots moving in the preferred direction within their crfs and then tested for a 2 s period in which the random dots in the surround also moved in the same direction. Each bin represents 40 ms. The data were based on five stimulus presentations of both conditions to each cell. All of the cells tested with a 2 s period of center and surround stimulation were included in this analysis. The histograms were constructed by normalizing the largest 40 ms bin in the histograms for each cell and then combining the histograms. We were limited in precision for measuring the latency of responses by the cycle time of the video stimulator since the actual beginning of the random dot movement could occur at any time within the 33 ms cycle rather than at the beginning of the cycle as registered by the computer; thus the average latency from the beginning of movement was probably about one half cycle (16.5 ms) shorter than the times illustrated. This delay applies to both the left and right histograms and does not affect the relative delay of the surround response of 40 ms.

Type IV consisted of five cells that showed no effect from surround stimulation; three of these were recorded in their respective penetrations immediately adjacent to type I cells sharing the same crfs and the same directional preferences within their crfs. It is possible that at a higher stage of neural processing the outputs of the type I and type IV cells are compared. Such a comparison would enable the system to determine whether a particular stimulus movement was an isolated occurrence or part of a larger pattern of stimuli moving in one direction (see section 4.4).

3.2 *The latency of the surround response*

The histogram in the top half of figure 9 illustrates the combined responses of forty-two MT neurons (types I, II, and III) to random dots moving in the preferred direction within their crfs with the background stationary. In the lower histogram in figure 9, the same MT neurons were stimulated continuously with random dots moving in the preferred direction within their crfs and then tested for a 2 s period in which the random dots in the surround also moved in the same direction.

The upper histogram in figure 9 indicates that the responses from the crfs began abruptly in the third bin after the onset of movement and ceased just as abruptly in the third bin after the offset of movement. Each bin represents 40 ms. There was a transient response lasting about 600 ms followed by a response subtained through the remainder of the stimulus presentation in the crf. The lower histogram in figure 9 indicates that the inhibitory responses from the surround began abruptly in the fourth bin after the onset of surround movement and ceased just as abruptly in the fourth bin after the offset of surround movement. Thus the response from beyond the crf required somewhat less than 40 ms additional processing time beyond that required for the crf. The lower histogram also indicates that there was a transient rebound in the response from the crf after the offset of background movement.

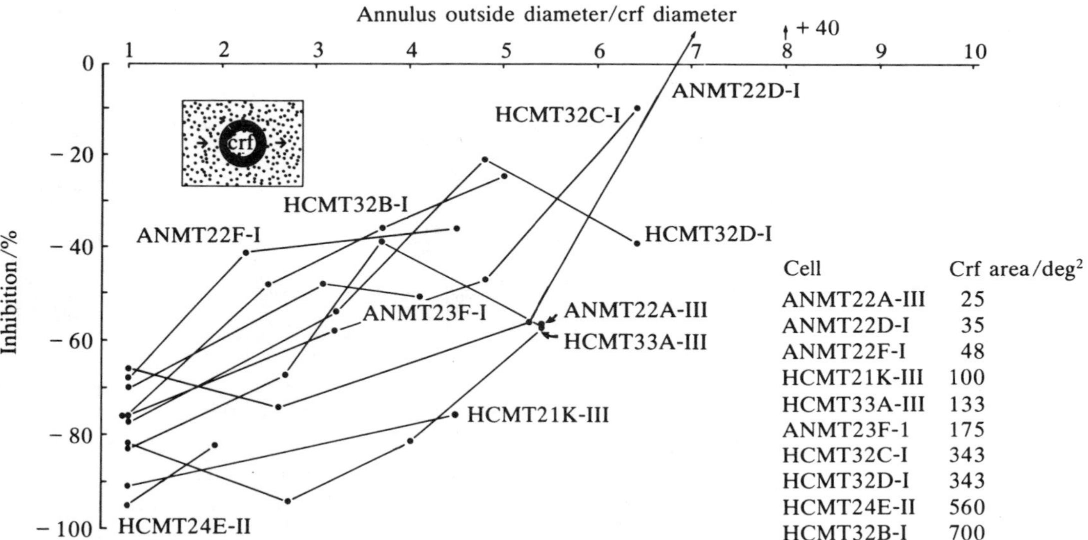

Figure 10. The effects of varying the outside diameter of masking annuli on background inhibition of the response from the crf in ten MT neurons. The stimulus conditions are depicted schematically, but in the experiments the dots were much denser and the surround much larger than are depicted. The dots in the center and background moved in the optimum direction for the crf. The inside diameter of the masking annulus corresponds approximately to the diameter of the crf. The abscissa corresponds to the ratio of the outside diameter of the masking annulus to the diameter of the crf. A value of 1 is equivalent to stimulation without the masking annulus. The cell type is indicated by the roman numeral following the identifying code for each cell. One cell, ANMT22D-I, was facilitated by 40% when a background masking annulus 8 times the diameter of the crf was used. In order to test the larger annuli in some cells we moved the screen to 14.25 cm from the eye.

3.3 *The extent of the surrounds*
We mapped the extent of the surround in eleven cells by systematically masking off parts of the screen with black paper while stimulating both the center and surround with random dots moving in the preferred direction for the center (the direction of maximum inhibition for the surround). In figure 10 the results for ten cells are illustrated in which the crf was surrounded by a masking annulus of variable outside diameter. In only one cell, ANMT22D-I, were we able to create an annulus sufficiently large to eliminate the suppressive effect of movement in the surround, and this was with an annulus 8 times the diameter of the crf. The data suggest that the surrounds are 7 to 10 times the diameter of their crfs. The areas of the crfs of these cells increased with eccentricity and ranged from 25 to 700 deg^2. The smallest surround in this sample would thus be about 1200 deg^2 and some of the others would be enormous (see legend for figure 10). The total hemispherical visual field is approximately 20000 deg^2. Even allowing for considerable tangent error and the possibility that the surrounds were not radially symmetrical about their crfs, it is clear that the surrounds occupied very large portions of the visual field. Finally, in an eleventh cell that is not plotted in figure 10 we found a small but potent suppressive zone less than 4 deg wide flanking the temporal half of a crf 10 deg wide and 5 deg high. This indicates that the surrounds for MT neurons generally, but not always, occupy large portions of the visual field.

3.4 *The influence of background movement on responses to bar stimuli*
In natural conditions stimuli such as bars or edges are often seen against a moving background. We tested bar stimuli moving in twelve different directions on a background of random dots that was stationary or moved in or against the preferred direction for the crf.

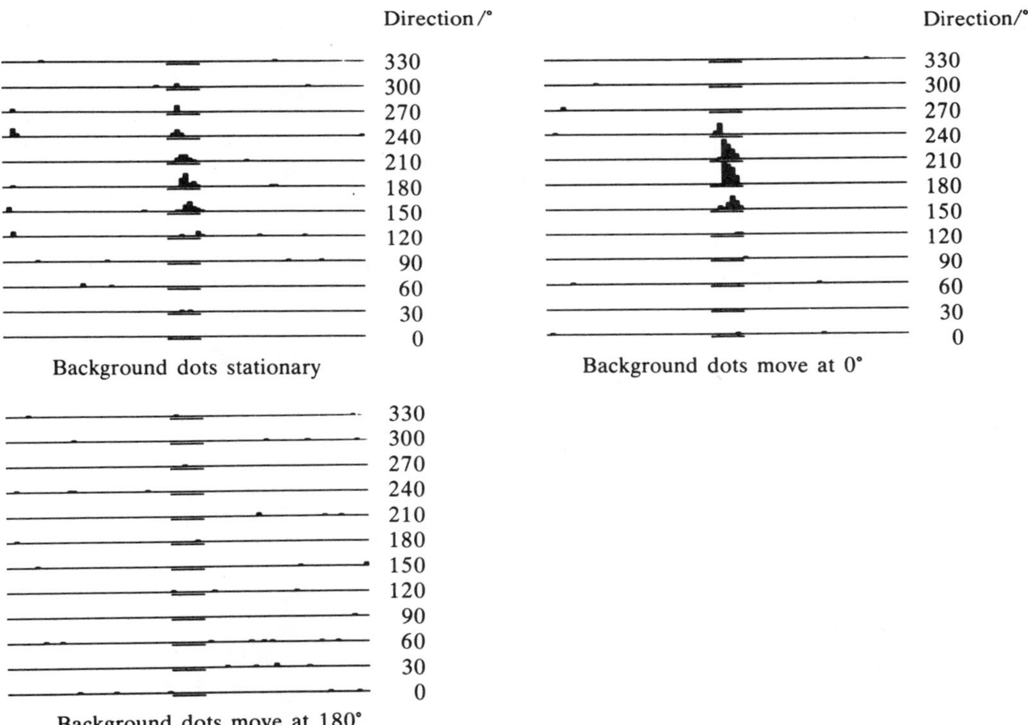

Figure 11. Responses of neuron ANMT17A to a bar moving in different directions superimposed on a background of random dots. The bar was oriented orthogonally to the direction of movement. The results of each of the twelve directions (0° through 330°) are shown in histograms consisting of a fore period, an underscored stimulus presentation period, and an after period. The stimuli were presented in pseudorandom order with each stimulus presented five times. The largest histogram bin contains twenty-six spikes.

This set of stimulus conditions differed from those in sections 3.1 through 3.3 in that both the crf and the surround were stimulated by a continuous sheet of random dots moving in the same direction. In figure 11 the top set of histograms illustrates the response of a MT cell to different directions of bar movement against a stationary random-dot background. The preferred direction of bar movement was 180°. In the middle set of histograms, the background dots were moved against the preferred direction (0°); the response to bar stimuli moving at 180° was enhanced by 110%. The lower set of histograms illustrates that the responses to bar stimuli were abolished by background movement in the preferred direction (180°).

Figure 12 is a two-dimensional plot of the responses of forty-eight MT neurons that were stimulated with a bar moving in the preferred direction superimposed on a random-dot background that was moving either in or opposite to the preferred direction. All but one of the cells were inhibited by the background moving in the preferred direction. 56% were inhibited by the background moving against the preferred direction; the remaining 44% were facilitated. The data in figures 11 and 12 indicate that background movement has a profound influence on the responses of MT neurons to moving bar stimuli. Figure 11 also shows that background movement in the opposite direction can influence the *sharpness of tuning* of the responses to bar stimuli moving in different directions since the responses to the non-optimal directions of 120°, 270°, and 300° that were present when the background was stationary were virtually abolished when the background dots moved at 0°. By applying a tuning index developed in an earlier paper (Baker et al 1981) it was found that this effect was characteristic of MT neurons. Baker et al (1981) found an average tuning index of 0.567 with a standard deviation of 0.246 for one hundred and twenty-nine owl monkey MT neurons. Maunsell and Van Essen (1983a) found an average tuning index of 0.557 with a standard deviation of 0.329 for one hundred and

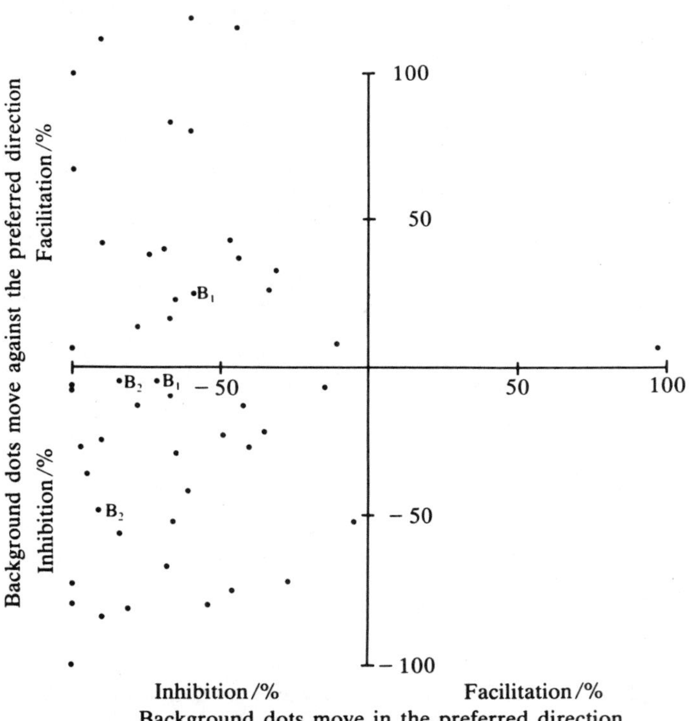

Figure 12. The effect of background movement in and opposite to the preferred direction on the responses of forty-eight MT neurons to a bar moving in the preferred direction. Two cells (B_1 and B_2) were bidirectional and had two preferred directions of motion that were opposite (180°) to one another. Two points were plotted for each of these cells since they were tested with both of their preferred directions of bar movement.

sixty-three macaque monkey MT neurons. Both of these studies were done with conventional bar stimuli moving in different directions against a featureless background. We tested the influence of the background in forty-six MT cells. With a stationary random-dot background, the average tuning index was reduced to 0.44 with a standard deviation of 0.14. With the background moving opposite to the preferred direction for the center (180°), the tuning index was 0.51 with a standard deviation of 0.14. The average tuning index was statistically significantly higher with the background moving opposite to the preferred direction than when the background was stationary ($p < 0.005$), but it was still significantly lower than when the stimuli were presented on a featureless screen ($p < 0.05$). Thus the presence of a stationary random-dot background reduces the sharpness of tuning for direction of bar movement in MT neurons, but this reduction is much less if the background is moving against the preferred direction.

3.5 *Effects of the velocity of background motion*

We also tested the effects of varying the velocity of background motion on the response to a bar moving in the preferred direction. In figure 13 the left graph illustrates the velocity tuning curve for a neuron tested with a bar stimulus of optimum length, width, and contrast moving in the cell's preferred direction against a background of stationary random dots. The cell's preferred velocity was 16 deg s^{-1}. In the right graph in figure 13, we presented the bar at 16 deg s^{-1} and tested the effects of varying the velocity of the random-dot background, which was moving in the same direction. The result was profound inhibition produced by background stimulation at the preferred velocity of 16 deg s^{-1}. Five of the eighteen MT cells tested exhibited this V-shaped pattern with the maximum inhibition resulting when the background dots moved at the preferred velocity for the bar stimulus. However, as is illustrated in figure 14, for the population of eighteen MT neurons, inhibition tended to increase with increasing background velocity. Interestingly, the V-shaped pattern with maximum inhibition at the preferred velocity was found in the majority (20/39) of cells tested in the second visual area (V-II) in the owl monkey (Allman et al 1985b).

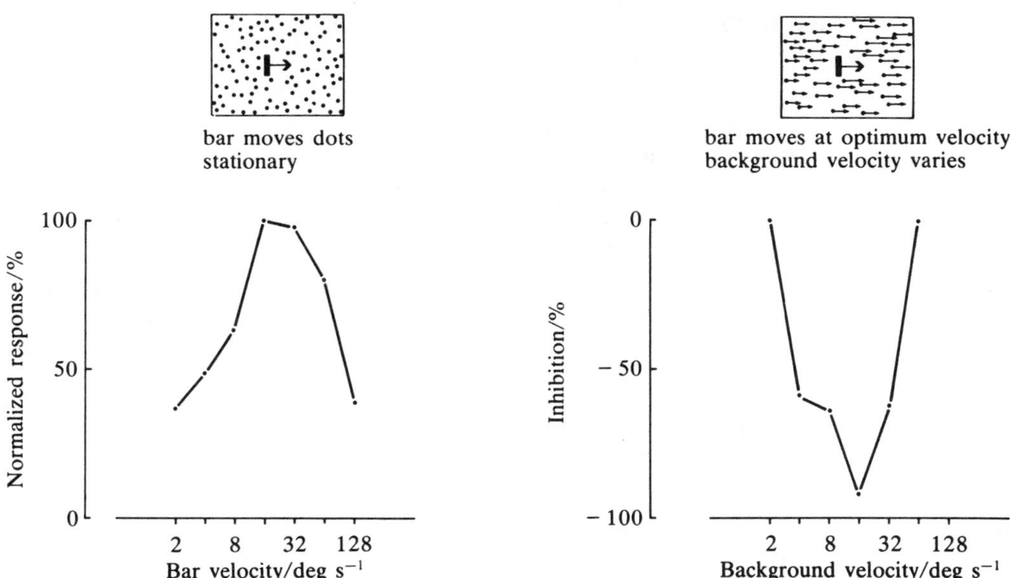

Figure 13. The effect of bar and background velocity on neuron HCMT33C. The left graph is a velocity tuning curve for a bar moving in the optimum direction with the background stationary. The right graph is a velocity tuning curve for background movement in the same direction while simultaneously presenting the bar moving at the optimum velocity (16 deg s^{-1}). The stimulus conditions are depicted schematically above the graphs, but in the experiment the dots were much denser and the surround larger.

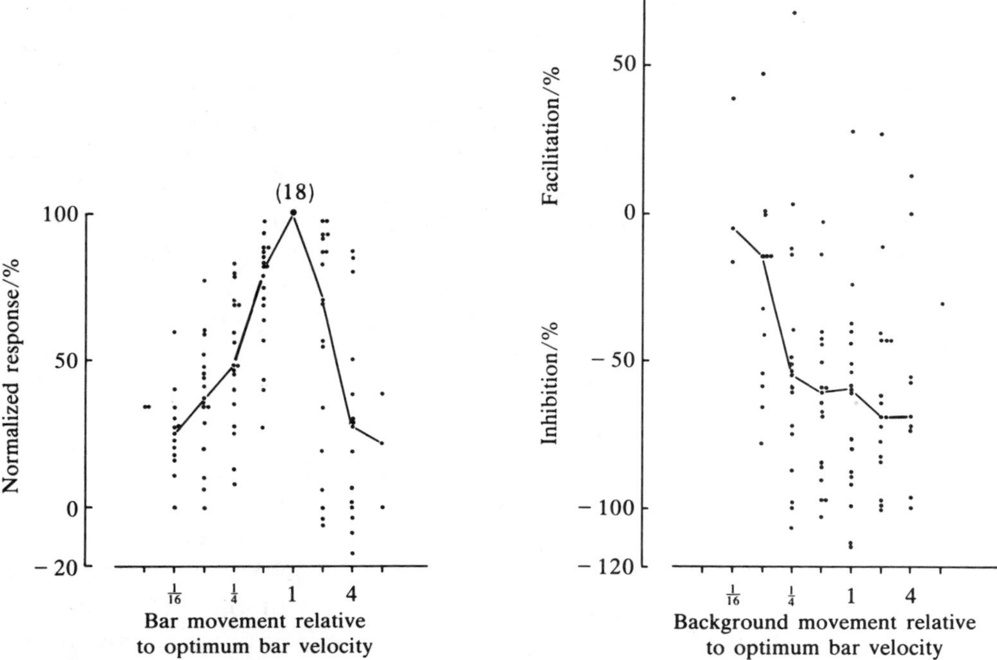

Figure 14. Center and surround velocity responses for eighteen MT neurons. The preferred velocities for these cells ranged from 8 to 32 deg s^{-1} with an average of 25.3 deg s^{-1}. In both graphs a line connects the median response for each velocity. In both the left and right graphs spontaneous activity was sampled during a period prior to the presentation of each stimulus. In the data collection for each cell in the right graph, the bar moving at the preferred velocity against the stationary background was presented interleaved among the other stimulus conditions in which the background moved at different velocities. In the right graph the response to the control condition of the bar moving at the preferred velocity against a stationary background was set equal to zero. Thus it is possible to calculate the response and the spontaneous activity separately, and in the right graph values below − 100% indicate that the response to the bar was entirely suppressed and in addition there was some inhibition below the spontaneous firing rate. In the background velocity experiments, the background dots stimulated both the crf and the surround; however, in these experiments covering the surround usually eliminated or greatly reduced the inhibitory effect of background movement.

4 Discussion

4.1 *Stimulus selectivity beyond the classical receptive field*

The first evidence for directional selectivity for responses to stimuli presented beyond the crf was discovered by Sterling and Wickelgren (1969) in the optic tectum of the cat. This cell was stimulated with a bar moving in the preferred direction within the crf and a second bar just outside the crf. When the bar outside the crf moved in the preferred direction for the center, the cell was more suppressed than when it moved in the opposite direction. In the intermediate and deep layers of the optic tectum of the pigeon Frost et al (1981) stimulated the crf with a moving spot and tested the effect of presenting different directions of movement of random-dot patterns in the surround. They found that the surrounds were directionally selective and were more than 100 deg in diameter. Many of the cells were facilitated by background movement opposite to the direction of spot movement in the center. The responses from the crf *with the background stationary* were very broadly tuned for direction, and Frost and Nakayama (1983) found that the surround effect depended on the direction of movement of the center stimulus such that the direction of greatest suppression by surround movement was the same as that of the movement of the center stimulus.

Neurons in lateral suprasylvian visual cortex in the cat are directionally selective (Hubel and Wiesel 1969; Spear and Baumann 1975), and recently von Grunau and Frost

(1983) have tested surround mechanisms for neurons in this region with the same methods as those used in the pigeon work described above. In nine of eleven cells tested quantitatively they found directionally selective surrounds with the preferred direction for the center being the direction of greatest suppression by the surround and the opposite direction being either less inhibitory or facilitatory. These cells would thus resemble our type I. They concluded that the surrounds were large, although data for only one cell were reported. Portions of lateral suprasylvian visual cortex in the cat have sometimes been considered homologous with MT in primates (see discussion in Baker et al 1981). Very recently Tanaka et al (1984) have recorded from MT in macaque monkeys. The response to a moving bar was suppressed by background movement in the same direction in one half of their MT neurons; one quarter were facilitated by background movement in the opposite direction. In these neurons the effective zone extended well beyond the crf.

We believe that the tuned antagonistic surround effects should be considered distinct from apparently nonspecific facilitatory and inhibitory effects such as those described by McIlwain (1964) and others for cells in the retina and lateral geniculate nucleus. However, these subcortical effects may contribute to the nonspecific effects seen at higher levels. There also is evidence that some of the surround effects observed in the lateral geniculate nucleus may be due to descending inputs from the visual cortex (Marrocco et al 1982). Most of the known response properties described in the studies carried out within the crf of neurons at various levels in the visual system (selectivity for stimulus direction and velocity of movement, orientation, spatial frequency and phase, and color) are matched by antagonistic tuned mechanisms in the surrounding parts of the visual field from which no direct response can be obtained, but which nonetheless exert a strong influence on the responses obtained from stimuli presented within the crf (see Allman et al 1984a for review). One significant parameter—relative depth between the center and surround—has yet to be investigated, but we predict the existence of neurons with antagonistic surround mechanisms tuned for depth. It would be interesting in view of the multiple mechanisms capable of producing depth perceptions (binocular disparity, motion parallax, motion occlusion, perspective, etc) to determine how these different cues for depth might interact in the surround to influence the response from the crf. Opponent processes have a long history in vision research dating back into the nineteenth century with Hering's theory of color vision (see Hering 1879/1942) and to Kuffler's (1953) discovery of antagonistic center-surround organization in retinal ganglion cells, which of course differs from the work under discussion here in that responses can be obtained by stimulation of either the center or the surround and thus both lie within the crf.

Another intriguing issue is the degree to which antagonistic surround mechanisms are 'relativistic' as in the case of the deep optic tectum neurons recorded by Frost and Nakayama (1983) where the directional selectivity of the surround depended on the direction of movement of the stimulus within the crf. We found two cells in MT and three in V-II that were bidirectional with the two preferred directions 180° opposite to one another. These cells possessed directionally tuned antagonistic surrounds that depended on the direction of center movement. This question also arises in the velocity domain, and we are currently investigating whether the velocity of greatest suppression by surround stimulation depends upon the velocity used to stimulate the center. Another 'relativistic' question emerges from the observation that the direction and velocity of the background influences the apparent direction and velocity of the center stimulus. For example, if the center stimulus is moving horizontally and the background is moving vertically upward, the apparent direction of the center stimulus rotates downward by 30° to 40°. We have demonstrated that the movement of the background opposite to the preferred direction significantly sharpens the tuning of the center stimulus relative to the stationary background condition; however, it would be interesting to determine whether direction or velocity preferences for center stimuli ever shift in a manner similar to the perceived changes that occur when background stimuli are altered.

4.2 *Anatomical connections subserving cortical surround mechanisms*

In the first visual area (V-I) in monkeys, horizontal intrinsic fibers in the stria of Gennari extend 3 mm or more from the margins of lesion or injection sites (Fisken et al 1975; Rockland and Lund 1983), which is beyond the 2 mm maximum distance that would be expected for connecting a cell with adjacent cells that would share portions of its crf (Hubel and Wiesel 1974). It is particularly interesting that the horizontal connections are most extensive for V-I in the stria of Gennari since this layer receives an input from the magnocellular laminae of the lateral geniculate nucleus via neurons in layer 4C-alpha (Hubel and Wiesel 1972; Lund et al 1975), contains a high proportion of directionally selective neurons (Dow 1974; Livingstone and Hubel 1984), and projects to MT (Lund et al 1975; Spatz 1977; Tigges et al 1981; Maunsell and Van Essen 1983b). Montero (1980) found by using two separate tracers that the input from V-I to MT terminates in a series of bands within partially overlapping projections from adjacent sites in V-I. These partially overlapping projections may contribute, possibly via interneurons, to the large surrounds in MT. Maunsell and Van Essen (1983b) injected tritiated proline in MT and found intrinsic horizontal connections extending about 3 mm from the margin of the injection site, which because of the relatively small size of MT would cover much of the representation of the visual hemifield, and thus could also contribute to the large surrounds. Although the transcallosal connections of MT are much heavier near the representation of the vertical meridian, they extend throughout most of the area (Newsome and Allman 1980), and thus may contribute to the portion of the surround extending into the opposite half of the visual field as do the transcallosal connections of V4 complex (Moran et al 1983).

The visual system contains many descending pathways (Tigges et al 1981; Maunsell and Van Essen 1983b) which could contribute to surround mechanisms in the recipient structure. The crfs in the higher area typically are larger than those at a comparable eccentricity in the lower area, and thus the crfs in the higher area might match the dimensions of the true receptive field including the surround in the lower area (F Crick, personal communication). Marrocco et al (1982) have demonstrated that interruption of the striate-geniculate pathway by cooling striate cortex eliminates surround responses from regions beyond the crf in many lateral geniculate neurons. Small injection sites in the superior temporal visual area (ST) project to the entire extent of the ipsilateral MT in the owl monkey (Weller and Kaas 1983) and may be another source of the large surrounds present for neurons in MT. Finally another potential source is input from subcortical structures such as the pulvinar.

4.3 *Stimulus selectivity beyond the crf and figure–ground discrimination*

Stimulus-specific responses from beyond the crf seem ideally suited for discriminating figure from ground and preattentive vision (Treisman and Gelade 1980; Julesz 1981). Julesz's elementary units of figure–ground discrimination, the 'textons', are based on differences in motion, color, orientation, etc that are strikingly similar to the tuned antagonistic interactions between the crf and the background in visual cortical and tectal neurons. This preattentive system is capable of guiding focal attention with a latency of about 50 ms (Julesz 1984), which is slightly longer than the time required for the response from the regions beyond the crf to influence the response within the crf in MT neurons (see figure 9).

4.4 *Stimulus selectivity beyond the crf and perceptual constancies*

The function of the visual system is to extract behaviorally significant features embedded in a complex optical array over a very broad range of environmental conditions. Its first task is to discriminate discontinuities in the optic array. Local antagonistic center-surround mechanisms clearly have this role. A second and more difficult task is to make good estimates of the qualities of objects in the visual field, their color and motion for example, on the basis of rather imperfect optical information imaged on the photoreceptor layer of the retina. Thus the wavelength composition of the retinal image will depend on environmental lighting conditions which may vary enormously, yet the behaviorally significant task may involve judging the ripeness of fruit based on its color. Retinal image motion can be produced by movement of the eye, movement of the animal, or movement of the environment, yet the system's task is to determine the motion of objects relative to other objects and the observer. In both cases more than just information restricted to a small locality on the retinal surface is required to make veridical judgements. Land's (1959a, 1959b, 1983) experiments indicate that the system compares the wavelength composition of the light reflected by an object with that of other objects in the surrounding visual field and is able to extract color constancy over a broad range of lighting conditions. The determination of the motion of objects in the environment similarly requires the integration of motion information over a large portion of the visual field, and to determine object motion relative to the observer requires further input concerning eye and head position. These position inputs are usually thought to be derived from motor commands to the eye muscles (Helmholtz 1909/1962), from the vestibular system, and perhaps from proprioceptors in the eye muscles; however another parallel source of position information could be derived from the visual image itself (Gibson 1966; Koenderink 1984) and possibly implemented through comparisons between the crf and its surround.

4.5 *Background motion and depth perception*

Helmholtz (1909/1962) observed:

> "Suppose, for instance, that a person is standing still in a thick woods, where it is impossible for him to distinguish, except vaguely and roughly, in the mass of foliage and branches all around him what belongs to one tree and what to another, or how far apart the separate trees are, etc. But the moment he begins to move forward, everything disentangles itself, and immediately he gets an apperception of the material contents of the woods and their relations to each other in space, just as if he were looking at a good stereoscopic view of it."

Nakayama and Loomis (1974) have suggested a division of labor between *stereopsis* and *kineopsis*:

> "Retinal disparity, based on a relatively small interpupillary distance, probably controls behavior which is directed at the near environment; whereas optical velocity information (kineopsis), based on much greater displacements of a single eye, controls more distantly directed behavior."

Helmholtz (1909/1962) concluded:

> "the apparent angular velocities of objects in the field of view will be inversely proportional to their real distances away; and, consequently, safe conclusions can be drawn as to the real distance of the body from its apparent angular velocity".

Nakayama and Loomis (1974) postulated a simple neural mechanism which could serve as the basis for the analysis of optical flow patterns that occur as a viewer moves through its environment with the images of objects located at different distances from the viewer moving at different velocities across the retina. They hypothesized the existence of a class of neurons possessing a velocity-selective center with an antagonistic velocity-selective surround. Such neurons would be suppressed by an optical flow field of uniform velocity but would detect differential velocities such as would result from sweeping past objects at different distances from the viewer. We have provided the first experimental confirmation of this hypothesis in the discovery of neurons sensitive to the velocity of background movement. It is easy to imagine how an antagonistic velocity-sensitive center–surround mechanism, as first hypothesized by Nakayama and Loomis (1974) and found for some neurons in our study, could subserve the spatial, velocity-discriminating function required for depth perception through motion parallax or optical flow patterns. However, the characteristic symmetrical V-shaped background velocity tuning curves obtained for the majority of V-II and some MT neurons do not discriminate between the condition in which the background movement is faster than the preferred velocity and the condition in which the background movement is slower than the preferred velocity. Thus they could register relative magnitude of the depth difference but not whether the center was nearer or farther than the background. The MT cells in which inhibition simply increases with background velocity might help to resolve this ambiguity.

The velocity–distance relationship postulated by Helmholtz (1909/1962) obtains only when the observer fixates at very distant objects. If the observer fixates on an object at a given depth while he is in motion, objects beyond the fixation plane will move in the same direction as the observer while objects nearer than the fixation plane will move in the opposite direction (Gordon 1965). This cue is utilized in depth perception through motion parallax (Rogers and Graham 1979) and may be analyzed by MT type I neurons, which would be facilitated by stimuli moving in opposite directions nearer and beyond the fixation plane. There exists additional motion-related depth information in the visual scene described so graphically by Helmholtz (1909/1962). As Gibson (1979) has emphasized, the disappearance or emergence of background from behind an occluding surface is a strong cue for depth. The depth percept elicited by kinetic occlusion is very powerful and can override conflicting stereoscopic cues (Royden et al 1984). The antagonistic direction-selective center–surround mechanism may serve the computations for depth perception through kinetic occlusion by helping to identify which surfaces in an array are in motion with respect to other surfaces.

4.6 *Other surround effects*

Recently, von der Heydt et al (1984) have discovered that some neurons in V-II in awake macaque monkeys respond to illusory contours where the real contours evoking the response are located entirely outside the crf. V-I neurons were unresponsive under the same stimulus conditions. This result indicates that under some conditions stimulation of regions beyond the crf is sufficient by itself to evoke an excitatory response. The perception of illusory contours might be considered as a type of constancy function since the visual system is interpolating a continuous contour from an interrupted contour, which under natural conditions would be produced by a partially occluding surface. The tropical forest environment, where primates evolved, abounds with occluding foliage and branches, and the ability to reconstruct surfaces that are partially hidden from view would be very adaptive. Integrative mechanisms extending beyond the crf may underlie a number of possibly related phenomena such as the influence of unambiguous movement in the surround on the perceived direction of ambiguous movement in the center of a display (Ramachandran and Anstis 1983).

Extensive surrounds beyond the crf are not limited to the visual system. Barn owls, which hunt in darkness using sound localization, possess auditory neurons with sharply defined spatial receptive fields which are organized into an orderly representation of auditory space in the midbrain nucleus MLD (Knudsen and Konishi 1978a). These receptive fields are mapped in the owl's auditory space by moving a sound source in an anechoic chamber. Knudsen and Konishi (1978b) probed the regions beyond these receptive fields by stimulating the MLD neurons with a sound source located in the crf and measuring the effect of moving a second sound source through the remainder of the auditory field in a manner analogous to our experiments. By using this technique they demonstrated that the second sound source had an inhibitory effect throughout most of auditory space beyond the crf. Thus neurons in the owl's auditory-space-mapped MLD would be capable of making the same sort of local-global comparisons within a representation of space that exist in MT and other visual structures.

5 Conclusions

The function of the visual system is not merely to create a set of precise neural analogs of the optical image on the photoreceptors, but, beyond this, to reconstruct behaviorally significant features of the visual environment on the basis of imperfect and unconstant optical stimuli. Gibson (1950, 1966, 1979), Land (1959a, 1959b, 1983), and Ramachandran and Anstis (1983) have emphasized the influence of the context of the whole visual field on perception at any one locality within the field. The brain contains many maps of the visual field, as revealed by the topographic organization of crfs, but the true receptive fields for many neurons in these maps may be much larger and even extend throughout much of the visual field. The crfs and their surrounds provide mechanisms for local-global comparisons embedded in visuotopic matrices that may serve as the basis for many functions in vision such as the perceptual constancies, figure-ground discrimination, and depth perception through motion. The surrounds explored thus far usually exert selective antagonistic influences on their crfs, but the existence of more complex surround mechanisms is indicated by the type II neurons in MT, the responses to illusory contours in V-II (von der Heydt et al 1984), and the influence of background color patches on the properties of neurons in the V4 complex (Zeki 1983). The successful exploration of complex surround mechanisms calls for collaboration among psychophysicists, mathematical modelers, and neurophysiologists for which there exist some very promising beginnings (Horn 1974; Nakayama and Loomis 1974; Ballard et al 1983; Land 1983; Reichardt et al 1983). The exploration of surround mechanisms will be vital to our understanding of the role that each cortical visual area plays in perceptual processes.

Acknowledgements. We thank Drs Francis Crick, Bob Desimone, John Maunsell, and Terry Sejnowski for many helpful discussions, Leslie Wolcott for drawing many of the illustrations, and Dave Sivertsen for the photograph of the owl monkey's habitat. This work was supported by grants from the National Institutes of Health (EY-03851), the Pew Memorial Trust and the LSB Leakey Foundation.

References

Allman J M, Campbell C B G, McGuinness E, 1979 "The dorsal third tier area in *Galago senegalensis*" *Brain Research* **179** 355-361

Allman J M, Kaas J, 1971a "A representation of the visual field in the caudal third of the middle temporal gyrus of the owl monkey (*Aotus trivirgatus*)" *Brain Research* **31** 84-105

Allman J M, Kaas J H, 1971b "Representation of the visual field in striate and adjoining cortex of the owl monkey (*Aotus trivirgatus*)" *Brain Research* **35** 89-106

Allman J M, Kaas J H, 1974a "The organization of the second visual area (VII) in the owl monkey: a second order transformation of the visual hemifield" *Brain Research* **76** 247-265

Allman J M, Kaas J H, 1974b "A cresent-shaped cortical visual area surrounding the middle temporal area (MT) in the owl monkey (*Aotus trivirgatus*)" *Brain Research* **81** 199-213

Allman J M, Kaas J H, 1975 "The dorsomedial cortical visual area: a third tier area in the occipital lobe of the owl monkey (*Aotus trivirgatus*)" *Brain Research* **100** 473-487

Allman J M, Kaas J H, 1976 "Representation of the visual field on the medial wall of occipital-parietal cortex in the owl monkey" *Science* **191** 572-575

Allman J, Miezin F, McGuinness E, 1985a "Stimulus specific responses from beyond the classical receptive field: neurophysiological mechanisms for local-global comparisons in visual neurons" *Annual Review of Neuroscience* **8** 407-430

Allman J, Miezin F, McGuinness E, 1985b "Direction and velocity specific responses from beyond the classical receptive field in the first and second cortical visual areas" in preparation

Baker J F, Petersen S E, Newsome W T, Allman J, 1981 "Visual response properties of neurons in four extrastriate visual areas of the owl monkey (*Aotus trivirgatus*): a quantitative comparison of medial, dorsomedial, dorsolateral, and middle temporal areas" *Journal of Neurophysiology* **45** 397-416

Ballard D H, Hinton G E, Sejnowski T J, 1983 "Parallel visual computation" *Nature (London)* **306** 21-26

Brumback R A, 1973 "Two distinctive types of owl monkeys (*Aotus*)" *Journal of Medical Primatology* **2** 284-289

Dow B M, 1974 "Functional classes of cells and their laminar distribution in monkey visual cortex" *Journal of Neurophysiology* **37** 927-946

Fernald R, Chase R, 1971 "An improved method for plotting retinal landmarks and focusing the eyes" *Vision Research* **11** 95-96

Fisken R A, Garey L J, Powell T P S, 1975 "The intrinsic, association and commissural connections of area 17 of the visual cortex" *Philosophical Transactions of the Royal Society of London, Series B* **272** 487-536

Frost B J, Nakayama K, 1983 "Single visual neurons code opposing motion independent of direction" *Science* **220** 744-745

Frost B J, Scilley P L, Wong S C P, 1981 "Moving background patterns reveal double-opponency of directionally specific pigeon tectal neurons" *Experimental Brain Research* **43** 173-185

Gallyas F, 1979 "Silver staining of myelin by means of physical development" *Neurological Research* **1** 203-209

Gibson J J, 1950 *The Perception of the Visual World* (Boston, MA: Houghton Mifflin)

Gibson J J, 1966 *The Senses Considered as Perceptual Systems* (Boston, MA: Houghton Mifflin)

Gibson J J, 1979 *The Ecological Approach to Visual Perception* (Boston, MA: Houghton Mifflin)

Gordon D A, 1965 "Static and dynamic visual fields in human space perception" *Journal of the Optical Society of America* **55** 1296-1303

Grunau M von, Frost B J, 1983 "Double-opponent-process mechanism underlying RF-structure of directionally specific cells of cat lateral suprasylvian visual area" *Experimental Brain Research* **49** 84-92

Hartline H K, 1938 "The response of single optic nerve fibers of the vertebrate eye to illumination of the retina" *American Journal of Physiology* **121** 400-415

Helmholtz H von, 1909/1962 *Physiological Optics* volume 3 (New York: Dover, 1962); English translation by J P C Southall for the Optical Society of America (1924) from the 3rd German edition of *Handbuch der physiologischen Optik* (Hamburg: Voss, 1909)

Hering E, 1879/1942 *Spatial Sense and Movement of the Eye* (Baltimore, MD: American Academy of Optometry, 1942) English translation by C A Radde of "Der Raumsinn und die Bewegung des Anges" in *Handbuch der Physiologie* Ed L Hermann, Band 3, Teil 1 (Leipzig: Vogel, 1879)

Hershkovitz P, 1983 "Two new species of night monkeys, genus *Aotus* (Cebidae, Platyrrhini): a preliminary report on *Aotus* taxonomy" *American Journal of Primatology* **4** 209-243

Heydt R von der, Peterhans E, Baumgartner G, 1984 "Illusory contours and cortical neuron responses" *Science* **224** 1260-1262

Horn B K P, 1974 "Determining lightness from an image" *Computer Graphics and Image Processing* **3** 277-299

Hubel D H, Wiesel T N, 1969 "Visual area of the lateral suprasylvian gyrus (Clare-Bishop area) of the cat" *Journal of Physiology (London)* **202** 251-260

Hubel D H, Wiesel T N, 1972 "Laminar and columnar distribution of geniculocortical fibers in the macaque monkey" *Journal of Comparative Neurology* **146** 421-450

Hubel D H, Wiesel T N, 1974 "Uniformity of monkey striate cortex: A parallel relationship between field size, scatter, and magnification factor" *Journal of Comparative Neurology* **158** 295-306

Imig T J, Ruggero M A, Kitzes L M, Javel E, Brugge J F, 1977 "Organization of auditory cortex in the owl monkey (*Aotus trivirgatus*)" *Journal of Comparative Neurology* **171** 111-128

Julesz B, 1981 "Textons, the elements of texture perception, and their interactions" *Nature (London)* **290** 91-97

Julesz B, 1984 "Toward an axiomatic theory of preattentive vision" in *Dynamic Aspects of Neocortical Function* eds G Edelman, M Cowen (in press)

Knudsen E I, Konishi M, 1978a "Space and frequency are represented separately in auditory midbrain of the owl" *Journal of Neurophysiology* **41** 870-884

Knudsen E I, Konishi M, 1978b "Center-surround organization of auditory receptive fields in the owl" *Science* **202** 778 - 780

Koenderink J J, 1984 "Space, form and optical deformations" in *Brain Mechanisms and Spatial Vision* eds D Ingle, D Lee, M Jeannerod (The Hague: Nijhot)

Kuffler S W, 1953 "Discharge patterns and functional organization of mammalian retina" *Journal of Neurophysiology* **28** 37 - 68

Land E H, 1959a "Color vision and the natural image, Part I." *Proceedings of the National Academy of Sciences USA* **45** 115 - 129

Land E H, 1959b "Color vision and the natural image. Part II." *Proceedings of the National Academy of Sciences USA* **45** 636 - 644

Land E H, 1983 "Recent advances in retinex theory and some implication for cortical computations: Color vision and the natural image" *Proceedings of the National Academy of Sciences USA* **80** 5163 - 5169

Livingstone M S, Hubel D H, 1984 "Anatomy and physiology of a color system in the primate visual cortex" *Journal of Neuroscience* **4** 309 - 356

Lund J S, Lund R D, Hendrickson A E, Bunt A H, Fuchs A F, 1975 "The origin of efferent pathways from the primary visual cortex, area 17, of the macaque monkey as shown by retrograde transport of horseradish peroxidase" *Journal of Comparative Neurology* **164** 287 - 304

Marrocco R T, McClurkin J W, Young R A, 1982 "Modulation of lateral geniculate nucleus cell responsiveness by visual activation of the corticogeniculate pathway" *Journal of Neuroscience* **2** 256 - 263

Maunsell J H R, Van Essen D C, 1983a "Functional properties of neurons in middle temporal visual area of the macaque monkey. I Selectivity for stimulus direction, speed, and orientation" *Journal of Neurophysiology* **49** 1127 - 1147

Maunsell J H R, Van Essen D C, 1983b "The connections of the middle temporal visual area (MT) and their relationship to a cortical hierarchy in the macaque monkey" *Journal of Neuroscience* **3** 2563 - 2586

McIlwain J T, 1964 "Receptive fields of optic tract axons and lateral geniculate cells: peripheral extent and barbiturate sensitivity" *Journal of Neurophysiology* **27** 1154 - 1173

Merzenich M M, Kaas J H, Sur M, Lin C S, 1978 "Double representation of the body surface within cytoarchitectonic areas 3b and 1 in S1 in the owl monkey (*Aotus trivirgatus*)" *Journal of Comparative Neurology* **181** 41 - 74

Montero V M, 1980 "Patterns of connections from the striate cortex to cortical visual areas in superior temporal sulcus of macaque and middle temporal gyrus of owl monkey" *Journal of Comparative Neurology* **189** 45 - 59

Moran J, Desimone R, Schein S J, Mishkin M, 1983 "Suppression from ipsilateral visual field in area V4 of the macaque" *Society for Neuroscience Abstracts* **9** 957

Nakayama K, Loomis J M, 1974 "Optical velocity patterns, velocity-sensitive neurons, and space perception: a hypothesis" *Perception* **3** 63 - 80

Newsome W T, Allman J M, 1980 "Interhemispheric connections of visual cortex in the owl monkey, *Aotus trivirgatus*, and the Bush baby, *Galago senegalensis*" *Journal of Comparative Neurology* **194** 209 - 233

Ramachandran V S, Anstis S M, 1983 "Perceptual organization in moving patterns" *Nature (London)* **304** 529 - 531

Reichardt W, Poggio T, Hausen K, 1983 "Figure - ground discrimination by relative movement in the visual system of the fly. Part II: Towards the neural circuitry 1" *Biological Cybernetics* **46** 1 - 30

Rockland K S, Lund J S, 1983 "Intrinsic laminar lattice connections in primate visual cortex" *Journal of Comparative Neurology* **216** 303 - 318

Rogers B, Graham M, 1979 "Motion parallax as an independent cue for depth perception" *Perception* **8** 125 - 134

Royden C, Baker J, Allman J M, 1984 "Illusions of depth produced by moving random dots" unpublished manuscript

Spatz W B, 1977 "Topographically organized reciprocal connections between area 17 and MT (visual area of superior temporal sulcus) in the marmoset *Callithrix jacchus*" *Experimental Brain Research* **27** 559 - 572

Spear P D, Baumann T P, 1975 "Receptive field characteristics of single neurons in lateral suprasylvian visual area of the cat" *Journal of Neurophysiology* **8** 1403 - 1420

Sterling P, Wickelgren B G, 1969 "Visual receptive fields in the superior colliculus of the cat" *Journal of Neurophysiology* **32** 1 - 15

Tanaka K, Saito H, Fukada Y, Hikosaka K, Yukie M, Iwai E, 1984 "Two groups of neurons responding to local and whole field movements in the macaque MT area" *Neuroscience Abstracts* **10** 474

Tigges J, Tigges M, Anschel S, Cross N A, Letbetter W D, McBride R L, 1981 "Areal and laminar distribution of neurons interconnecting the central visual cortical areas 17, 18, 19, and MT in squirrel monkey (Saimiri)" *Journal of Comparative Neurology* **202** 539–560

Treisman A M, Gelade G, 1980 "A feature-integration theory of attention" *Cognitive Psychology* **12** 97–136

Weller R E, Kaas J H, 1983 "Connections of visual cortex rostral to the middle temporal region in superior temporal cortex" *Neuroscience Abstracts* **9** 958

Wolbarsht M L, MacNichol E F, Wagner H G, 1960 "Glass insulated platinum microelectrode" *Science* **132** 1309–1310

Zeki S, 1983 "Colour coding in the cerebral cortex: the responses of wavelength-selective and colour-coded cells in monkey visual cortex to changes in wavelength composition" *Perception* **9** 767–781

12

R. von der Heydt, E. Peterhans, and G. Baumgartner

Illusory contours and cortical neuron responses

1984. *Science* 224: 1260–1262

Abstract

Figures in which human observers perceive "illusory contours" were found to evoke responses in cells of area 18 in the visual cortex of alert monkeys. The cells responded as if the contours were formed by real lines or edges. Modifications that weakened the perception of contours also reduced the neuronal responses. In contrast, cells in area 17 were apparently unable to "see" these contours.

A basic task in visual perception is to segregate the visual input into objects. Given a flat retinal image of a three-dimensional world, this is not trivial. An object boundary may be defined by a physical discontinuity in the image due to a difference in color or luminance between object and background, although any change in illumination, or a movement of the object or the observer, can change these conditions. Nevertheless, the contours of objects appear to be invariant. Contours may also be seen in the absence of discontinuity in the stimulus (*1*) (for example, Fig. 1, A, B, and D). These illusions (*2*, *3*) show that perceived contours are the result of an image analysis performed in the brain. The nature of this process is not known, and different theories have been proposed (*3*, *4*). We have examined the activity of cells in the visual cortex of monkeys during presentation of conventional stimuli producing contours by luminance gradients and of stimuli producing illusory contours. In area 18 we found responses that paralleled some of the perceptual phenomena. These responses could not be easily predicted from the known receptive-field properties of cells in the visual cortex.

Rhesus monkeys (*Macaca mulatta*) were trained to perform a visual fixation task. To receive a reward they had to pull a lever when a fixation target appeared and to release it upon detecting a 90° turn of the target, which occurred after an unpredictable delay. The target consisted of two parallel short lines whose orientation could be resolved only in foveal vision. It appeared in the center of a display at a viewing distance of 40 cm; the other stimuli were also presented on that display. For recording, the animal's head was fixed by means of a bolt implanted in the skull. Otherwise the animal was free to take a comfortable position in a boxlike primate chair. Single units were recorded with microelectrodes inserted through the intact dura throughout an experimental session.

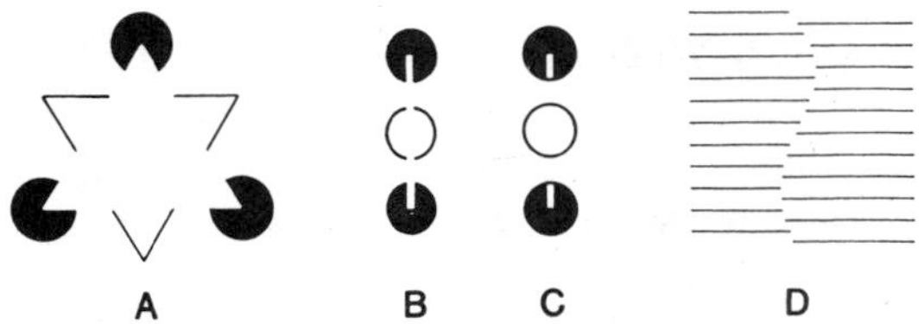

Figure 1. Illusory contours. Such contours are perceived in A, B, and D, at sites where the stimulus is homogeneous. Small alterations in the stimulus can have dramatic effects on the appearance of these contours (C) (*9*).

Figure 2 shows three examples of neurons recorded in area 18. Neuron 1 responded to the lower right edge of a light bar (Fig. 2A). Its responses indicated precisely where, and in which orientation, a light-dark boundary appeared in the visual field: the response field measured 0.9° by 0.4° visual angle and was located 1.8° below the fixation point; only orientations between 46° and 101° produced a response (*5*). We then tested a stimulus in which a strip of 1.3°, covering the cell's response field, was blanked out, thus reducing the bar to a pair of notches (Fig. 2B). If one looks at such a stimulus with the notches moving back and forth together, one has the illusion of a light bar moving in front of two dark bars. The cell responded to this stimulus as it had to the edge of the bar, though less strongly. The response occurred at the same position, and the optimal orientation also remained the same.

In general, illusory contours disappear when only part of the inducing configuration is viewed. When, for example, one of the disk sectors in Fig. 1A is occluded, not only the corner of the triangle disappears, but also the adjacent flanks. The Gestalt psychologists stated that the whole is greater than the sum of its parts. We found a similar effect in the neuronal responses. Neither half of the stimulus of Fig. 2B excited the unit (Fig. 2, C and D; E shows the spontaneous activity), whereas both together did (Fig. 2B). The exact width of the gap between the two halves was not critical for this effect. With 2° instead of 1.3°, the cell still responded, and 4.1, 0.8, and 0.7 spikes per cycle were obtained for the whole figure, the upper and lower halves, respectively. We have tested the influence of the gap width in several other cells; all gave gradually weaker responses when the gap was increased. The largest gap at which a response was still obtained was 4.4° in a cell whose center of response field was

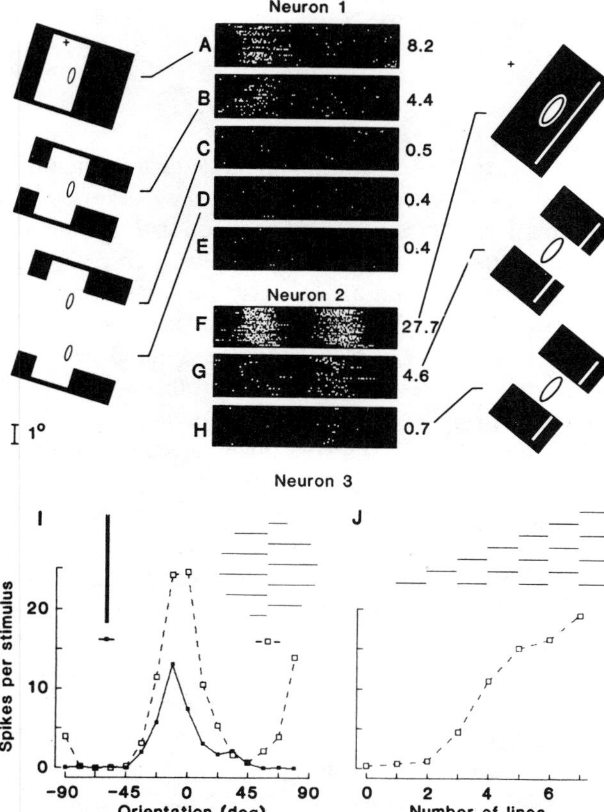

Figure 2. Responses of neurons in area 18 of the monkey visual cortex to edges, bars, and stimuli producing illusory contours. The stimuli (insets) (*10*) were moved back and forth across the receptive fields (neuron 1, 1° at 1 Hz; neurons 2 and 3, 2° at 1 Hz). Each was presented 8 (I), 16 (J), or 24 (A to H) times; blocks of eight repetitions were alternated in pseudorandom order. For neurons 1 and 2, the response fields (the regions in the visual field where the neurons could be activated by a bar or edge) are represented by ellipses, and the fixation point is marked by crosses in A and F; the responses are represented by rows of dots; mean numbers of spikes per stimulus cycle are indicated on the right. Neuron 1, which responded to the lower right edge of the light bar (A), was activated also when only the illusory contour passed over its response field (B). Either half of the stimulus failed to evoke a response (C and D): (E) spontaneous activity. Neuron 2 responded to a narrow bar (F) and, less strongly, to the illusory bar stimulus (G). When the ends of the "bar" were intersected by thin lines, however, the response was nearly abolished (H). In neuron 3, the border between two abutting gratings elicited a strong response. The orientation tuning curves show corresponding peaks for bar and illusory contour (1). When the lines inducing the contour were reduced in number to less than three, the response disappeared (J): compare the lines above the curve (the actual stimuli were centered over the response field). The lines were 1 minute of arc wide and spaced 48 minutes apart.

located 3° from the fixation point. It could be argued that these responses were due to stray light falling into the response field and moving along with the notches and that the light coming from only half the figure might just not reach the cell's threshold. However, we have observed the same nonadditivity in the stimulus-response relationship at a sixfold stimulus intensity. Again, neither half of the stimulus alone produced a response. This result argues against a simple threshold explanation.

Small changes in configuration can have dramatic effects on the appearance of illusory contours. An example is the closing lines in Fig. 1C. A similar effect could be observed in the neuronal responses, as demonstrated by neuron 2. It responded well to a narrow bar (Fig. 2F) and also gave a regular response to the illusory bar stimulus bridging a gap of 2° (Fig. 2G). When the notches were closed by line segments 5 minutes of arc wide, the response was almost abolished (Fig. 2H). Nearly all cells that responded to the illusory bar stimulus showed this reduction; in some cells, lines as narrow as 2 minutes of arc had an effect. Again, the gap width was not critical: as long as the cell responded, closure reduced the response.

The responses so far seem to indicate the ability of the cortex to extrapolate lines to connect parts of the stimulus which might belong to the same object. The abutting gratings of Fig. 1D show an illusory contour which is not an extrapolation of the stimulus since it runs more-or-less perpendicular to the inducing lines. We have tested a contour that was straight and perpendicular to the lines. It could be moved back and forth along the lines, leaving the stimulus margin stationary. Responses were recorded for various orientations. Neuron 3, for example, responded to the illusory-contour stimulus better than to any of the conventional stimuli (Fig. 2I). Furthermore, the peak responses were obtained at virtually the same orientation for contour and bar. The curve of the illusory contour bends upward at both ends, indicating a second peak 90° from the optimum. This can be interpreted as a response to the inducing lines. Other cells showed only the peak related to the contour and thus were not activated by the gratings at all. When the cells also responded to the illusory bar stimulus, the optimal orientations were similar for both types of illusory contour.

To see the contour, a minimum number of lines are required; no contour is visible at the end of just one line, but it is usually perceived with four or more line ends. There was a similar threshold for the neuronal response (Fig. 2J). The density of lines, on the other hand, was not critical. Keeping the overall size of the stimulus constant, the responses were equal for line spacings of 12, 24, and 48 minutes of arc, and slightly less for 72 minutes of arc, but still stronger than the response to the bar.

There was a marked difference between striate and prestriate cortex (*6*). Of 70 cells tested in area 17, none showed responses related to the contour between abutting gratings (*7*), whereas about one-third (21 of 68) of the cells in area 18 did. Also, the results obtained with the other type of illusory contour (Fig. 2. B and G) were negative in area 17 (11 cells) but positive in 13 of 38 cells in area 18. (With this type of stimulus, the demonstration of the effect of closure (Fig. 2, G and H) was taken as a criterion.)

We were not able to relate responsiveness to illusory contour stimuli to the conventional classification of cells. With bars and edges, monotonic length-summation curves were usually obtained, but end-inhibition was also observed.

Responses of cells in area 18 that required appropriately positioned and oriented luminance gradients when conventional stimuli were used could often be evoked also by the corresponding illusory contour stimuli. In this area, one would be able to infer location and orientation of the various types of contours from the responses of single cells. In area 17, this would be possible only for edge or line type contours produced by luminance or color differences. Responses in area 18 showed several other parallels to perception, such as the relation between the responses to a figure and to its parts and the dramatic effect of small elements added to the figure.

Gregory (*4*) formulated an antithesis between physiological and cognitive explanations of illusory contour effects. According to his cognitive approach, the contours are perceived because an illusory object is "postulated" as a perceptual hypothesis to account for the sensory data. The explanation suggested by the present experiment is physiological, but it differs from the one stated in Gregory's antithesis (and criticized by him) that "feature detector cells of the striate cortex are activated by the disk sectors [scilicet of the Kanizsa triangle]... to give the appearance of continuous lines, though only their ends are given by stimulation" (*4*, p. 51). Our results do not support this idea. With stimulus configurations like those of B or G in Fig. 2, cells in area 17 did not respond, some of them not even when the gap was narrowed so that the ends of the bar entered the response field. The responses in area 18 on the other hand cannot be interpreted simply as sub-optimal excitation due to partial stimulation of the response field, since they can be evoked by stimuli well outside that field and are affected by small changes in configuration that are negligible in terms of luminous flux. Also the responses to stimuli with lines perpendicular to the cell's preferred orientation reveal an unexpected new receptive field property. The way widely separated picture elements contribute to a response resembles the function of logical gates. The important elements in our stimuli seem to be corners on opposite sides of the response field (Fig. 2, B and G) and line ends arranged in a row (Fig. 2, I and J). Line ends and corners are in fact emphasized in certain signals of area 17 (*8*), and a number of such signals might converge on neurons of area 18. Corners and line ends play a role in the formation of contours because these picture elements are frequently produced by interposition of objects, that is, when an object partially occludes others. Thus, several such elements aligned in a row are likely to mark an object boundary.

References and Notes

1. F. Schumann, *Z. Psychol.* **23**, 1 (1900).

2. Illusory contours are known also as "Scheinkanten," as "quasi perceptive," "anomalous," "subjective," and "cognitive" contours, or "contours without gradients." See (*3*) for a discussion of the terminology.

3. For a review see G. Kanizsa, *Organization in Vision. Essays on Gestalt Perception* (Praeger, New York, 1979).

4. R. L. Gregory, *Nature (London)* **238**, 51 (1972).

5. The range of orientations was obtained from the orientation tuning curve by determining the points where the regression lines fitted to the flanks of the curve crossed the level of spontaneous activity. The length of response field. *L*, was similarly determined from a response curve obtained by scanning the field with the appropriate edge of a bar, taking as *L* the distance between the bars in the two limiting positions. The correctness of this determination was confirmed by the fact that the stimuli in Fig. 2, C and D, singly did not produce a response: because of the choice of the gap width (1.3°) they were outside the response field ($L = 0.9°$).

6. Most of the cells assigned to area 18 were recorded in the posterior bank of the lunate sulcus. The cortical area was judged also from physiological criteria such as the presence of the typical activity of layer IVc in area 17 [G. F. Poggio, R. W. Doty, Jr., W. H. Talbot, *J. Neurophysiol.* **40**, 1369 (1977)] and the topography of receptive fields; it has been confirmed histologically for part of the data. A few cells recorded near the 17–18 border were not counted.

7. The orientation tuning curves obtained with the illusory contour stimulus in area 17 typically showed a single peak corresponding to the orientation of the grating lines.

8. D. H. Hubel and T. N. Wiesel. *J. Physiol. (London)* **195**, 215 (1968).

9. Part A and D are reproduced from figures 4.2 and 12.12 in (*3*); parts B and C are figures 1, C and D, in A. T. Smith and R. Over [*Percept. Psychophys.* **20**, 305 (1976)].

10. To simplify the figure, stimuli have been reproduced in reversed contrast: the parts shown in black were actually lighter than the background (about 2.5 versus 1 foot lambert). To avoid confusion, the text has been made consistent with the figure.

13

J. A. Movshon, E. H. Adelson, M. S. Gizzi, and W. T. Newsome

The analysis of moving visual patterns

1986. In *Pattern Recognition Mechanisms*, edited by C. Chagas, R. Gattass, and C. Gross. New York: Springer-Verlag

Introduction

There is abundant evidence that the orientation of contours is a feature of considerable importance to the visual system. Both psychophysical and electrophysiological studies suggest that the retinal image is treated relatively early in the visual process by orientationally-tuned spatial filters (see Hubel and Wiesel, 1962; Campbell and Kulikowski, 1966, among many others). Orientational filtering undoubtedly plays a role in the analysis of the structure of a visual *pattern*, but the visual system has other tasks, most obviously that of extracting information about the *motion* of objects. A simple analysis reveals that separating a two-dimensional image into its one-dimensional (that is, oriented) components presents problems for a system concerned with extracting object motion. Here we outline the problem, propose a novel formal solution to it, and consider the applications of this solution to a variety of perceptual and electrophysiological phenomena.

The Ambiguity of Motion of One-Dimensional Patterns

The motion of a single extended contour does not by itself allow one to determine the motion of the surface containing that contour. The problem is illustrated in Fig. 1. The three sections of the figure each show a surface containing an oblique grating in motion behind a circular aperture. In Fig. 1A the surface moves up and to the left; in Fig. 1B it moves up; in Fig. 1C, it moves to the left. Note that in all three cases the appearance of the moving grating, as seen through the window, is identical: the bars appear to move up and to the left, normal to their own orientation, as if produced by the arrangement shown in Fig. 1A. The fact that a single stimulus can have many interpretations derives from the structure of the stimulus rather than from any quirk of the visual system. Any motion parallel to a grating's bars is invisible, and only motion normal to the bars can be detected. Thus, there will always be a family of real motions in two dimensions that can give rise to the same motion of an isolated contour or grating (Wohlgemuth, 1911, Wallach, 1935; Fennema and Thompson, 1979; Marr and Ullman, 1981).

We must distinguish at the outset between what we term *one-dimensional* (1-D) and *two-dimensional* (2-D) patterns. A 1-D pattern is one like an extended grating, edge, or bar: it is uniform along one axis. In general, such a pattern would have to extend infinitely along its axis to be truly 1-D but for the present purposes it is sufficient that the pattern extend beyond the borders of the receptive field of a neuron being studied, or beyond the edge of a viewing aperture. The essential property is that, when a 1-D pattern is moved parallel to its own orientation, its appearance does not change. By convention (and in agreement with its appearance), we will represent the "primary" motion of a 1-D pattern as having the velocity normal to its orientation. 2-D patterns are not invariant with translation along any single axis; they include random dot fields, plaids, and natural scenes. Such patterns change no matter how they are moved, and their motion is not ambiguous in the same way as the motion of a 1-D pattern is.

In this paper we are concerned only with uniform linear motion. For certain other kinds of motion (e.g.

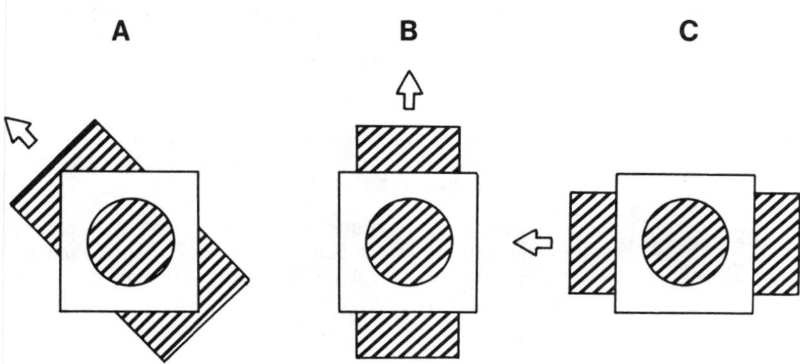

Figure 1. Three different motions that produce the same physical stimulus.

rotation or curvilinear motion, or motion in depth), analogous ambiguities exist and can be described and solved in a manner similar to the one we present here (but see also Hildreth, 1983).

The Disambiguation of Motion If the motion of a 1-D pattern such as an edge is ambiguous, how is it possible to determine the motion of an object at all? It turns out that, although a single moving contour cannot offer a unique solution, two moving contours (which belong to the same object) can, as long as they are not parallel. As Fig. 1 shows, there is a family of motions consistent with a given 1-D stimulus. Naturally, this is also true of the 1-D elements of a 2-D stimulus. Consider the diamonds shown in Fig. 2A. The left-hand diamond moves to the right; the right-hand diamond moves down. Note that in both cases, in the local region indicated on each diamond by the small circle, the border moves downward and to the right. The moving edge in Fig. 2B, which could represent a magnified view of the circled regions of the diamonds' borders in Fig. 2A, can be generated by any of the motions shown by the arrows. Motion parallel to the edge is not visible, so all motions that have the same component of motion normal to the edge are possible candidates for the "true" motion giving rise to the observed motion of the edge. We may map this set of possible motions as a locus in "velocity space", as shown in Fig. 2B. Velocities are plotted as vectors in polar coordinates, starting at the origin. The length of the vector corresponds to the speed of the motion, and the angle corresponds to the direction. As shown in Fig. 2B, the locus of motions consistent with a given 1-D stimulus maps to a line in velocity space. The line is perpendicular to the primary vector representing the motion normal to the 1-D pattern.

It now becomes clear how one may unambiguously assign a velocity to a 2-D pattern, given knowledge only of the motion of its 1-D components. Consider, for example, the diamond moving rightward in Fig. 2C. One edge (viewed in isolation) moves up and to the right; the other moves down and to the right. In velocity space the two edges set up two lines of possible motions. Only a single point in velocity space is consistent with both—namely, the point of their intersection, which corresponds to a pure rightward motion (Fennema and Thompson, 1979; Horn and Schunck, 1981; Adelson and Movshon, 1982).

There are, of course, other ways of combining vectors. For example, one might argue that a simple vector sum would do just as well as the more complex "intersection of constraints" just described. Indeed a vector sum happens to give the correct answer for the diamond of Fig. 2C, but this is only by chance. Consider, for example, the triangle of Fig. 3, which moves straight

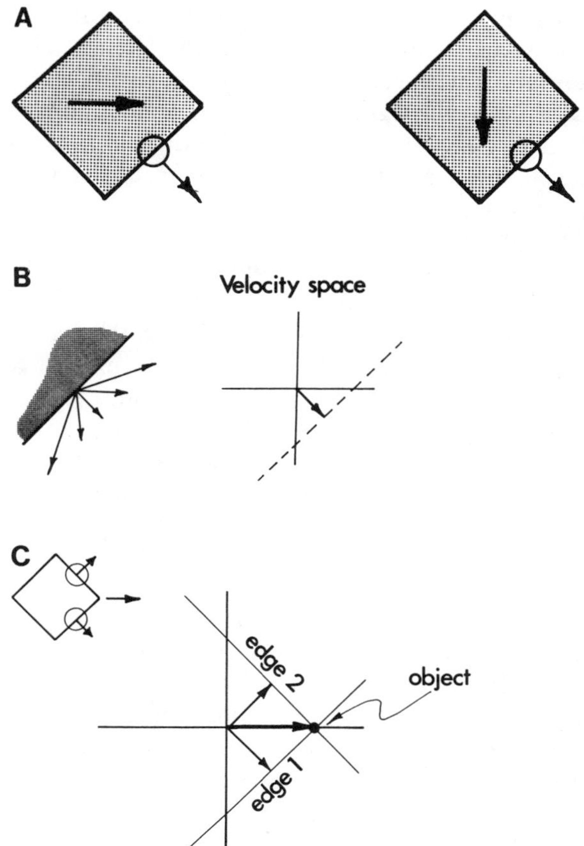

Figure 2. A. Two moving diamonds. The local regions circled on each diamond's border have identical motions. B. A single moving contour, which the representation of its possible motions in a polar "velocity space", in which each vector represents a possible direction and speed. C. The solution to the ambiguity of one-dimensional motion based on an intersection of constraints. Each border's motion establishes a family of possible motions; the single intersection of these two families represents the only possible motion for a single object containing both contours.

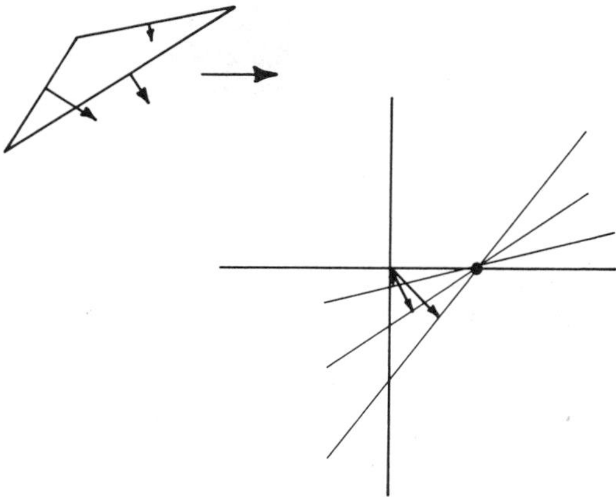

Figure 3. An illustration of the inadequacy of vector summation as a solution to motion ambiguity. All three primary motion of the triangle's borders have a downward component, but the true motion is directly to the right, as given by the intersection of constraints.

to the right. The velocities normal to the edges all have a downward component. Thus, when they are summed, the resultant itself goes down and to the right, instead of straight to the right. On the other hand, applying the intersecting constraints principle leads to the correct solution of a pure rightward motion, as shown in the lower part of Fig. 3.

The solution to motion ambiguity just described is purely formal, and does not imply a particular model of how the visual system actually establishes the motion of objects. In the case of the triangle, there are a number of strategies, such as tracking the motion of the corners, which would not give ambiguous results. But while alternate solutions exist in particular cases, the ambiguity inherent in 1-D motion remains a constant problem when we try to understand how the visual system analyzes motion. 1-D stimuli such as bars and gratings are among the most important stimuli used in studying motion mechanisms. Moreover, the visual system itself seems to analyze the world via orientation selective neurons or channels, which necessarily discard information along one axis in favor of another. In this chapter, we consider some issues this analysis raises in the perception of motion, and describe a series of psychophysical and physiological experiments that address these questions.

Stimuli

We used two kinds of stimuli in our experiments: sine wave gratings and sine wave plaids. The sine wave grating is our 1-D stimulus, and is therefore mathematically ambiguous in its motion. A moving grating can be diagrammed as occupying a line in velocity space, as shown in Fig. 4A. A pair of sine wave gratings, when crossed, produce the "plaid" pattern of Fig. 4B. In this case, there is no ambiguity about the motion of the whole pattern, since the two families of possible velocities (shown by the dotted lines) intersect at a single point. These stimuli have some advantages for experimentation over more conventional patterns like single contours and geometric figures. For one thing, all of our stimuli were identical in spatial extent, and uniformly stimulated the entire retinal region they covered. This sidesteps the issue which arises in considering stimuli like the diamond of Fig. 2, of how the identification of spatially separate moving borders with a common object takes place. Moreover, the plaid patterns were the literal physical sum of the grating patterns, which makes superposition models particularly simple to evaluate.

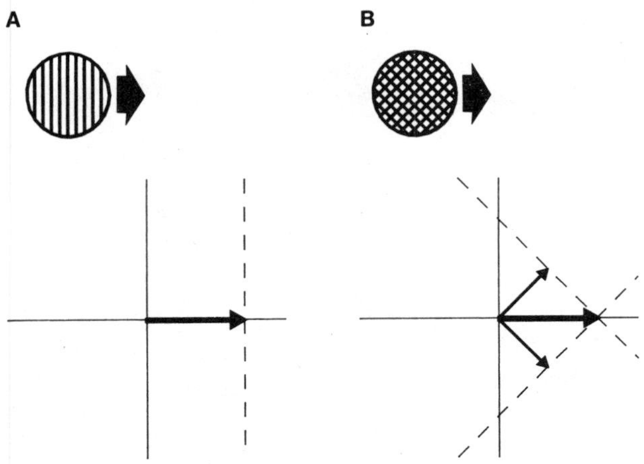

Figure 4. A single grating (A) and a 90 deg plaid (B), and the representation of their motions in velocity space. Both patterns move directly to the right, but have different orientations and 1-D motions. The dashed lines indicate the families of possible motions for each component.

These stimuli were generated by a PDP11 computer on the face of a display oscilloscope, using modifications of methods that are well established (Movshon *et al.*, 1978). Gratings were generated by modulating the luminance of a uniform raster (125 frames/sec, 550 lines/frame) with appropriately timed and shaped signals. The orientation of the raster could be changed between frames, permitting the presentation of superimposed moving gratings on alternate frames. Plaid patterns were generated by this interleaving method at the cost of reducing the effective frame rate of each component of the display. The spatial frequency, drift rate, contrast and spatial extent of the test patterns were determined by the computer.

The same computer was responsible for organizing the series of experimental presentations and collecting the data, using methods detailed elsewhere (Movshon *et al.*, 1978; Arditi *et al.*, 1981). In psychophysical studies, subjects' responses were normally yes-no decisions concerning some aspects of the immediately preceding display; in electrophysiological experiments, the computer collected standard pulses triggered by each action potential and assembled them into conventional averaged response histograms. In both kinds of experiment, all of the stimuli in an experimental series were presented in a randomly shuffled sequence to reduce the effects of response variability.

Psychophysical Studies

When presented with a pair of crossed gratings in motion, the visual system usually chooses the percept of a plaid in coherent motion, rather than the equally consistent percept of two gratings sliding over one another. Informal preliminary observations suggested to us that the likelihood that two gratings would phenomenally cohere was determined by various features of the gratings. We decided to examine the mechanisms that underly this percept of coherent motion. We first established the conditions that produce or prohibit coherence, and then used masking and adaptation techniques to test the hypothesis that the mechanisms responsible for coherence represent a later and different stage of motion processing than the mechanisms responsible for the detection of simple moving patterns.

The Conditions for Coherence

We quickly found that the likelihood that a pair of gratings would cohere depended critically on the similarity between them. The first and most obvious dimension we examined was contrast, and the results of these experiments led to the methodology that we used for subsequent studies (Adelson and Movshon, 1982). Figure 5A shows the results of an experiment on the effect of contrast.

The two gratings were of 1.5 and 2.0 c/deg, and they moved at an angle of 120 deg to one another with a speed of 3 deg/sec. The contrast of the lower-frequency grating was fixed at 0.3, and that of the other was varied from trial to trial. The absolute orientations and directions of the two gratings were varied randomly from trial to trial. We performed two experiments in this situation. In the first (results given by open symbols), we asked the subject to indicate whether the second grating was detectable in the display. For this sequence, 14% of the trials were blank containing only one grating, and the probability that the observer signalled the presence of the second grating in this case was about 0.05 (half-symbol on the ordinate). As the contrast was increased, the probability that the observer detected the grating increased rapidly and monotonically, so that his performance was perfect by a contrast of about 0.008. In the second experimental series (results given by filled symbols), we showed the same family of 120 deg plaids, but now asked the subject to indicate whether the two gratings moved coherently, as a single plaid, or slid incoherently across one another. This judgement is, of course, criterion-dependent, and naive subjects often required several practice sessions before they gave stable data. It was also especially important to maintain stable fixation on the mark at the center of the display, since coherence seems to depend strongly on retinal speed. The data show that as the contrast increased, the likelihood of a coherence judgement also increased. It is clear, however, that there was a considerable range of contrasts (between about 0.01 and 0.07) over which the two gratings were clearly visible, but failed to cohere. As the contrast of the weaker grating was increased (i.e. made closer in contrast to the "standard" grating), the probability of coherence increased. Because of the monotonicity of this kind of data, it is possible to define a "coherence threshold", as the contrast of the weaker grating that produces a 50% probability of coherence. In subsequent experiments, we measured this coherence threshold for various combinations of gratings using a staircase technique.

Figure 5B shows the results of two experiments that tested the dependence of coherence on the relative spatial frequency of the test gratings (Adelson and Movshon, 1982). In these, the spatial frequency of the "standard" grating was set at 1.2 (open arrow and symbols) or 2.2 c/deg (filled arrow and symbols), and the coherence threshold measured for a variety of test spatial frequencies. The two gratings were separated in direction by 120 deg, and their absolute orientation and direction were again varied randomly from trial to trial. The speed of all test gratings was fixed at 3 deg/sec. It is clear that the relative spatial frequency of the gratings importantly influenced coherence: when the test and standard gratings were of similar spatial frequency, the coherence threshold was low, but when they were made more than about a factor of two differ-

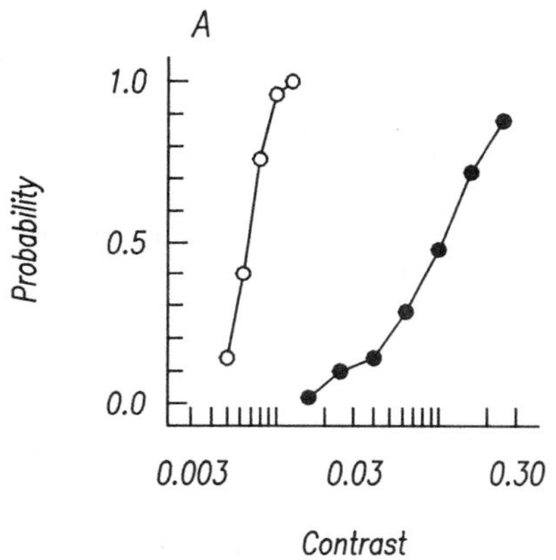

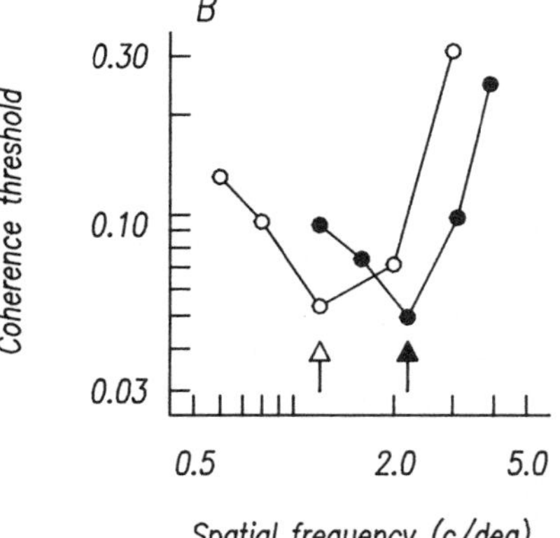

Figure 5. Two experiments on perceptual coherence. A. The effect of contrast on coherence. The two curves show the subject's probability of detecting the second grating (open symbols), and of seeing coherent motion (filled symbols). See text for details. B. The effect of spatial frequency on coherence. The standard grating was of 1.2 (open symbols and arrow) or 2.2 c/deg (filled symbols and arrow), and the data represent the coherence thresholds for a number of gratings of different spatial frequencies. See text for details. From Adelson and Movshon (1982).

ent, threshold rose sharply. The coherence threshold when the two gratings were of the same spatial frequency was about 0.7 log units higher than the detection threshold.

We performed a variety of experiments conceptually similar to these, investigating the effects of the angle between the gratings, their relative speeds, and also the effects of the absolute speeds and spatial frequencies of the gratings. In general, coherence threshold rises as the angle between the gratings is made larger, as their speeds increase, and as the spatial frequency increases, although this latter effect is rather weaker than the others. Under ideal conditions (identical spatial frequencies, low speeds, and a modest angle), the coherence threshold approaches detection threshold so closely as to make the measurements problematic, since coherence is difficult to judge when the observer is not even certain that the second grating is visible.

Models for the Perception of Coherent Pattern Motion The experiments just described gave us a base from which to construct models for various aspects of motion perception. One of the striking features of coherent motion perception is its spatial frequency tuning: two gratings cohere into a moving pattern only if they are of similar spatial frequencies (Fig. 5B). This suggests that the visual system imposes a bandpass spatial filtering on the stimulus before extracting the coherent percept. The filtering could be isotropic—such as the filtering imposed by mechanisms with circularly symmetric receptive fields (e.g. retinal ganglion cells). It could also be oriented—such as the filtering imposed by mechanisms with elongated receptive fields (e.g. cortical simple cells). We consider two models, schematically outlined in Fig. 6.

Model 1: Analyzing Motion without Orientational Filtering The first scheme (Fig. 6A) passes the image through a set of non-oriented bandpass channels. The outputs of these stages are sent to a motion analysis system, which might track salient features such as local peaks, or might perform a cross-correlation between successive views (e.g. Reichardt, 1957; van Santen and Sperling, 1983). This analysis must proceed in parallel in several spatial frequency bands, schematically indicated by the small and large symbols in Fig. 6A. After the determination of motion direction has proceeded within each spatial frequency band, the results are combined (in an unspecified way) to give the final motion percept. The results shown in Fig. 5B would come about in the following way: when two gratings are of similar spatial frequency, they would both pass

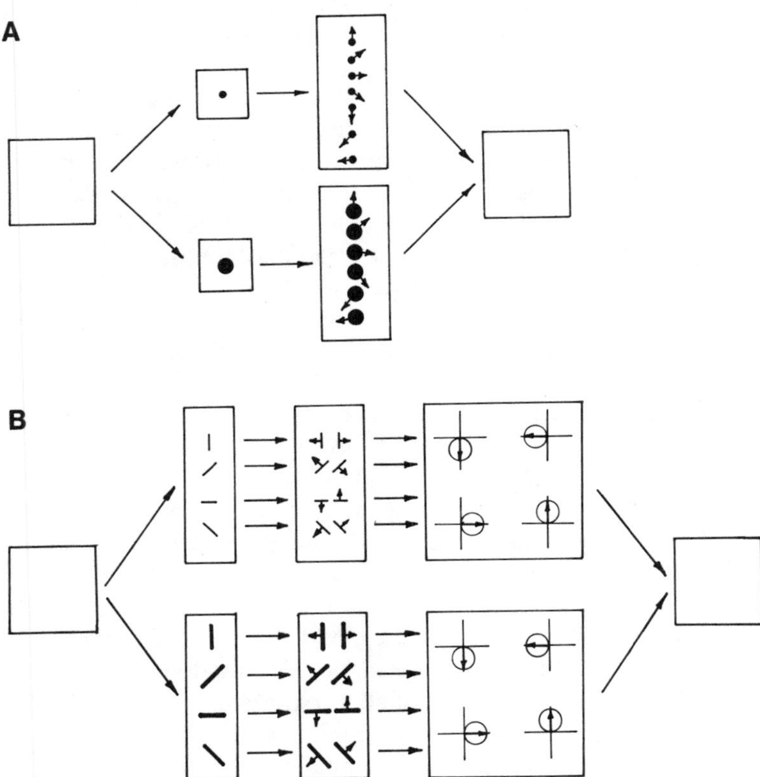

Figure 6. Two models of the mechanisms underlying perceptual coherence. See text for discussion.

the same spatial filter, and so would produce strong local peaks and troughs where their bars crossed. Thus, a feature tracker or a cross-correlator would be able unambiguously to assign a single motion to the whole pattern. If, on the other hand, the two gratings were of different spatial frequencies, they would not pass the same filter, and so would not produce, in the output of any filter, local peaks and troughs that could be tracked. Indeed, within each frequency band, it would be as though there were only a single grating present, and the familiar problem of motion ambiguity would cause this grating to appear to move normal to its own orientation—the motion extraction stages would operate in their default mode, with only 1-D patterns to process. Thus, two separate motions would be seen, rather than a single coherent one. This model, incidentally, bears a close resemblance to one put forward by Marr and Poggio (1979) for stereopsis.

Model 2: Analyzing Motion after Orientational Filtering An alternate scheme (Fig. 6B) would begin by filtering the image with orientation-selective mechanisms (shown as bars), similar to those commonly associated with cortical neurons or psychophysical channels. The outputs of these mechanisms would then pass to motion analyzers, which would not need to track localizable features, because they only provide information about the motion normal to their own orientation (bars with arrows). As we will see below, motion-sensitive cells in striate cortex behave in this way. But here, of course, arises the problem of motion ambiguity —how does one determine the motion of the pattern as a whole, given the velocities of its oriented components? There are several ways in which this problem can be solved, but they are all formally equivalent to the "intersection of constraints" scheme we outlined at the start of this chapter. This might be implemented in neural terms by combining the signals from several appropriately distributed 1-D motion detectors by circuitry similar to a logical "and" or a conjunction detector, requiring the simultaneous activation of several 1-D analyzers before the second-stage 2-D analyzers would respond. The combination rule here corresponds to a cosinusoidal relationship between component velocity and direction; since this relationship maps to a circle in the polar velocity space, we symbolize the second-stage analyzers by these circles. As in model 1, this analysis must take place in parallel in several frequency bands, two of which are symbolized by the small and large symbols in Fig. 6B.

The question of empirical interest is whether the visual system begins with oriented motion channels, and deals with the ambiguity problem later, or begins analyzing motion before orientation in order to avoid the ambiguity problem. Almost all of the psychophysics and physiology available points to the prevalence of oriented filtering at early stages in the visual system, and it would be surprising to find that the task of extracting pattern motion used mechanisms very different from those inferred in other experiments. Yet, on the other hand, it appears that early oriented filtering makes the task needlessly difficult. If the first stage were nonoriented, there should be no problem in finding the local features and using them to infer the pattern's motion.

Affecting Coherence with One-Dimensional Noise To study the role of orientation selectivity in coherent motion perception, we combined sine wave plaid stimuli with one-dimensional dynamic random noise, which appears as a rapidly and randomly moving pattern of parallel stripes of various widths. This noise pattern masks the gratings that compose the moving plaid (e.g. Stromeyer and Julesz, 1972). If coherence depends on the outputs of oriented analyzers, then noise masking should elevate coherence threshold more strongly when the mask is oriented parallel to one of the gratings than when it is oriented differently from either. If, on the other hand, the process involves non-oriented filtering, then the orientation of the noise mask should not matter. Only the noise energy within the frequency band of interest, and not its orientation, should have effects on coherence. Our observations of the effects of one-dimensional noise on the threshold for coherence unambiguously demonstrate an orientation dependence in the masking. If the orientation of the noise pattern is within about 20 deg of the orientation of either component of the plaid, the pattern's coherence is reduced in a manner that seems consistent with the reduction in the apparent contrast of the component masked by the noise. If, on the other hand, the noise orientation is different from that of the components, even if it is normal to the direction of pattern motion, little or no effect on coherence is observed. We conclude from these observations that the mechanisms responsible for the phenomenal coherence of moving plaids belong to a pathway which, at some point, passes through a stage of orientation selective spatial analysis.

The Effects of Adaptation on Coherence

As we have seen, the apparent direction of a pattern's motion can be quite different from the motions of the components that comprise it. We suggested earlier that pattern motion might be extracted in two distinct stages. The first stage is presumably revealed by the many orientationally-selective effects seen in experiments on the detection of moving gratings (e.g. Sekuler *et al.*, 1968; Sharpe and Tolhurst, 1973). The second stage, involving further analysis of complex 2-D motions, reveals itself in our experiments on the coherence of plaids. If these stages are really distinct, it might be possible to affect them differentially in adaptation experiments. That is to say, it should be component motion, rather than pattern motion, that elevates detection threshold, whereas it should be pattern motion, rather than component motion, that affects coherence phenomena. We have presented some preliminary data suggesting that this is the case (Adelson and Movshon, 1981).

It is well established that adapting to a moving grating elevates threshold for the detection of a similar grating moving in the same direction (Sekuler and Ganz, 1963). This adaptation is both direction and orientation selective: an oblique drifting grating has little or no effect on the threshold of a vertical grating (Sharpe and Tolhurst, 1973). Suppose now that we combine two oblique gratings into a plaid, so that the plaid appears to move directly to the right. Suppose further that the oblique gratings have been chosen so that they cause no threshold elevation of a vertical grating (moving rightward), when presented alone. If adaptation is caused by the motion of the components, then threshold for the vertical grating should remain unchanged. If adaptation is caused by the coherent motion of the pattern as a whole, then threshold should be elevated, since the plaid adapting pattern, like the test grating, moves directly rightward. Similarly, the effect on the detection of a rightward moving plaid of adaptation to a vertical, rightward moving grating may be assessed.

Figure 7 shows threshold elevation data for four different test-adapt combinations of this sort. All the stimuli in the experiment moved directly to the right at a constant speed of 1.5 deg/sec. Two kinds of stimuli were employed: single vertical gratings (spatial frequency 3 c/deg), and 120 deg plaids whose component gratings (oriented plus and minus 60 deg from vertical) had a spatial frequency of 3 c/deg. Thus all stimuli were identical in direction and speed of movement, but the orientational components of the plaids and gratings differed by 60 deg. We examined the elevation of contrast threshold for each kind of test stimulus following adaptation by each kind of adapting stimulus; the adapting stimuli were all of high contrast (0.5), and thresholds were measured by the method of adjustment. We tested for threshold elevation both in the adapted and unadapted directions. Inspection of Fig. 7 reveals that the results of these experiments conformed closely to the expectations of a model involving orientation selectivity. The detection threshold for a plaid or grating pattern could be strongly elevated in a directionally-selective manner following adaptation to a similar pattern, but was only slightly changed after adaptation to a different pattern. This result is in line with the ample evidence in the literature concerning the orientation and direction selectivity of the threshold elevation aftereffect (Blakemore and Campbell, 1969; Blakemore and Nachmias, 1971; Sharpe and Tolhurst, 1973), and suggests that the 2-D motion of patterns is not encoded at the level of visual processing where these effects are expressed. There is some reason to suppose that threshold elevation effects of this kind are mediated by neurons in the primary visual cortex (e.g. Maffei *et al.*, 1973; Vautin and Berkley, 1977; Movshon and Lennie, 1979).

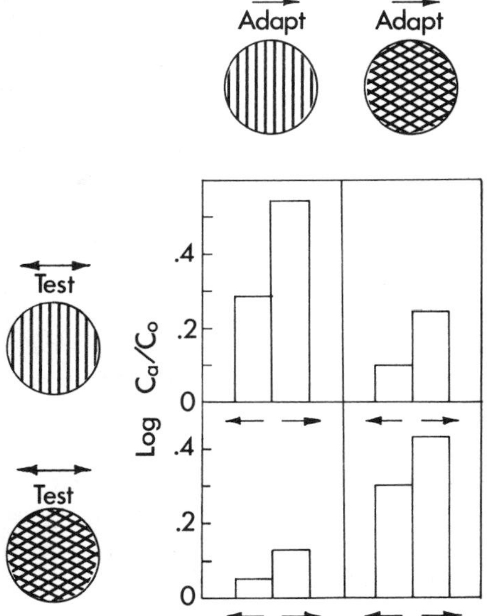

Figure 7. The effects of adaptation to moving gratings and plaids on the detectability of gratings and plaids. Contrast threshold elevation is the ratio of adapted to unadapted contrast threshold, expressed in log units. The two bars of each histogram represent the effects on test stimuli moving in the adapted and unadapted direction, as indicated by the arrows. The data shown are the means of values obtained for three observers; the standard error of the mean was about 0.025 log units.

Adaptation also alters the perception of coherent motion (Wallach, 1976; Adelson and Movshon, 1981). The most interesting case here is one of those used in the threshold elevation experiments described above, in which the adapting stimulus is a rightward moving grating, and the test stimulus a rightward moving plaid. The data in Fig. 7 show that this condition produces no important change in the detectability of the plaid, yet our results show profound effects upon its coherence. We measured this effect by determining coherence thresholds in the manner described earlier above, following adaptation to a high-contrast vertical grating moving to the right. The test plaids had a 120 deg angle, and we varied the spatial frequency of the plaid's component gratings so that either the spatial frequency of the components or the spatial period of the plaid matched the adapting grating. As may be seen from Fig. 8, this paradigm produced very large eleva-

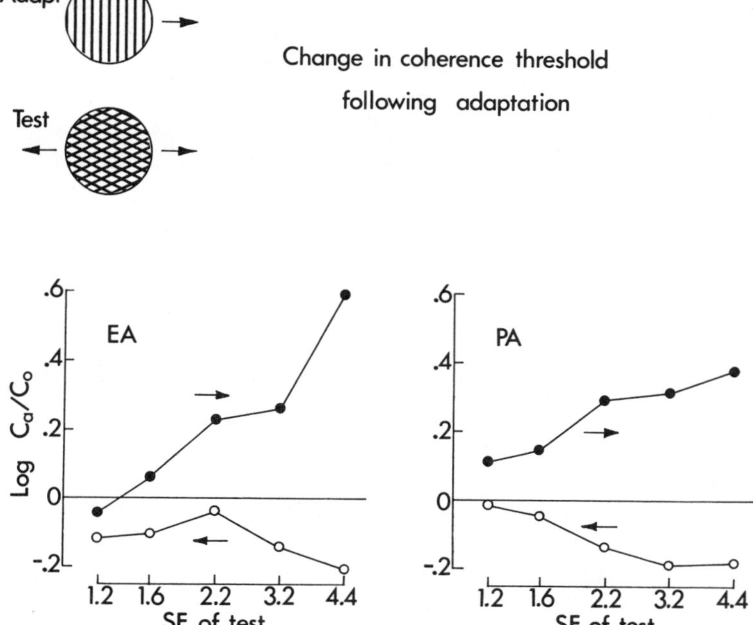

Figure 8. The effect of grating adaptation on the coherence threshold for plaids. The adapting grating was constant, and coherence was tested for plaids of several spatial frequencies moving in the adapted (filled symbols) and unadapted directions (open symbols). Threshold elevation is the ratio of adapted and unadapted coherence thresholds, expressed in log units. The standard error of the mean was about 0.05 log units.

tion of coherence thresholds for patterns that moved in the adapted direction; this effect was most marked for test plaids of relatively high spatial frequency. Conversely, the threshold for coherence of plaids moving in the opposite direction was, if anything, reduced following adaptation.

Evaluation of Psychophysical Models

The results of these two adaptation experiments suggest the existence of two different sites at which the adapting effect of a moving pattern may be expressed. At the first level, presumed to mediate the detection of moving patterns in our conditions, it is the similarity of 1-D motions that determines the effectiveness of adaptation. At the second level, responsible for the coherence of moving plaids, it is the similarity of 2-D motions that is critical. Combined with the evidence from masking experiments, this suggests that our psychophysical model 2, with an initial oriented stage followed by an analysis of 2-D motion, is an appropriate framework within which our data on the perception of moving patterns may be understood. Some issues concerning this model do, however, deserve some further consideration.

The first issue concerns the sequential link between stages 1 and 2 of the model. While our results demonstrate with reasonable clarity that there are two separate systems involved in motion analysis, they do not demonstrate a serial link between the two processes. Some aspects of the results do, however, suggest such a link. For one thing, the effects of one-dimensional noise masks on coherence appear to be related to the effect of the noise on the perceived contrast of the component gratings. That is, the change in coherence seen under masked conditions appears similar to that which would be produced by simply reducing the contrast of the masked grating by a modest amount. If we suppose that the effects of noise on perceived contrast represent a stage 1 effect, this result tends to suggest that the contrast signals from stage 1 feed into stage 2. Similar evidence can be obtained in adaptation experiments, by examining the effect on coherence threshold of adapting to one or another component of the test plaid. Such adaptation reduces the apparent contrast of a single test grating (Blakemore *et al.*, 1973), and causes a small change in coherence threshold that is of roughly the expected magnitude for one due to a change in the effective contrast of one of the plaid components. Thus while we cannot rule out the possibility that we may be studying the effects of two parallel stages, we continue to favor a serial scheme like that of model 2.

Implicit in this serial scheme is that the signals determining the percepts we have studied arise wholly from elements in the model's second stage. The percepts of coherent and incoherent motion are mutually exclusive—when one grating is "captured" by another, it becomes impossible to see the separate motions of the component gratings. In this, the coherence phenomenon resembles such other multistable visual stimuli as the Necker cube and Attneave's triangles (see Kaufman, 1975). It therefore follows that signals related to the "component" stage of processing do not influence the perception of motion when coherence is seen.

Even if the second stage is the only level at which perceptual information is available, our model must explain how it is that signals related to the component motions are ignored when coherence is seen. After all, a single grating is an effective stimulus for both component- and pattern-level analyzers. It seems that we must postulate that the responses of analyzers at the second level to component motion are actively suppressed when coherent motion is seen. Interestingly, we will show electrophysiological data in a later section that reveals precisely this sort of behavior. We may then outline the events that occur in each stage of the model as we alter a parameter (contrast, for example) that influences coherence. When the contrast of one of the two gratings of a plaid is low, signals in the second-stage analyzer sensitive to the pattern direction are weak, while those in an analyzer sensitive to the direction of the components are more prominent. As the weaker component increases in contrast, we suppose that the second-stage analyzers sensitive to the component motions are suppressed, while those sensitive to the pattern motion are activated. Mutual inhibition among these detectors could achieve this result, and assure the mutual exclusivity of the two percepts; this is, of course, only one of several ways in which this might be achieved, so we do not make it a specific feature of our model.

In summary, we believe that our psychophysical studies reveal the existence of two motion-analyzing processes, probably serially linked, having "component-analyzing" and "pattern-analyzing" properties. We now proceed to examine some electrophysiological evidence that suggests the existence of two analogous stages of processing of motion information in the visual cortex.

Electrophysiological Studies

Our electrophysiological studies concerned the motion-analyzing properties of single neurons in the visual cortex of cats and macaque monkeys. It is well-known that neurons both in and outside the primary cortex (V1, area 17) are selective for the direction and speed of motion of visual stimuli (e.g. Hubel and Wiesel, 1962, 1965, 1968; Pettigrew, Nikara and Bishop, 1968; Zeki, 1974; Movshon, 1975; Spear and Baumann, 1975; Hammond, 1978). A distinction emerges from our analysis that had not been carefully studied between what we term "component" and "pattern" direction selectivity. As we have discussed, one may consider the motion of an object in two ways: as the motion of the various 1-D components of the object, or as the motion of the object as a whole. Now, cortical orientation selectivity is typically conceived as part of a process by which cortical neurons break up an image into 1-D constituents. It is natural to ask whether motion signals are similarly parsed, especially since it is from the ambiguities inherent in the motion of isolated 1-D features that our ideas arise. Our results suggest that striate cortical neurons in cats and monkeys are selective only for 1-D motion, and cannot distinguish 2-D motion. We have, however, encountered neurons that appear to be sensitive to 2-D motion in MT, an extrastriate area of the monkey's visual cortex.

Pattern and Component Directional Selectivity

In the course of our experiments on directional processing we have developed definitions and a simple test that allows us to distinguish two types of direction selectivity. We have applied this to the responses of neurons in V1 of both cat and macaque (Movshon, Davis and Adelson, 1980), to neurons in the lateral suprasylvian visual cortex (LS) and superior colliculus of the cat (Gizzi *et al.*, 1981; Gizzi, 1983), and to neurons in MT of the macaque (Gizzi *et al.*, 1983). *Component directional selectivity* corresponds to what previous workers would have termed orientation selectivity with directional selectivity. Neurons showing component direction selectivity respond to the direction of motion of single oriented (1-D) contours presented in isolation, and to the direction of motion of those contours when they form part of a more complex 2-D pattern. *Pattern direction selectivity* corresponds to what previous workers have termed "pure" direction selectivity. Neurons showing pattern direction selectivity, like component neurons, respond to the direction of motion of isolated 1-D contours. When those contours are embedded in a more complex 2-D pattern, however, these neurons respond not to the motion of the contours, but to the motion of the pattern as a whole.

These two kinds of direction selectivity have been of concern for some time in visual electrophysiology, but no satisfactory test has been devised to distinguish them. Previous approaches have relied on two tests designed to establish orientation selectivity; if these tests fail, the neuron is—by default—considered to be "pure" or (in our terms) pattern direction selective (Barlow and Pettigrew, 1971; Zeki, 1974; Spear and Baumann, 1975). First, neurons have been considered orientation selective when they respond to stationary flashed line or grating stimuli in an orientation selective manner. Second, they have been considered orientation selective if their specificity for the direction of motion of a line is more refined than their selectivity for the direction of motion of a spot (Henry *et al.*, 1974). The first of these tests seems to us unimpeachable; its problem lies in the fact that many of the neurons of interest respond poorly to any stationary stimuli. It can also give misleading results if the stimulus is improperly placed in the receptive field. The second test is unreliable for two reasons. Since small spots and random textures contain energy at all orientations, the presence of strong inhibition in the orientation domain (e.g. Blakemore and Tobin, 1972; Nelson and Frost, 1978) can have the effect of making direction selectivity for spots or texture fields as tight as, or tighter than for bars, even in an orientation selective neuron. Moreover, the test specifies no reasonable decision rule—how much difference between the two curves is tolerable before the test fails? And both tests suffer from the problem that they are negative tests when applied to pattern direction selectivity: when a neuron *fails* to show some property it is pattern direction selective, and no positive attribute is associated with this classification.

Our test to distinguish between the two types of direction selectivity relies on the difference in response between moving grating and plaid stimuli. It does not require that the neuron respond to stationary patterns, and it has the further advantage that the stimuli to be compared are identical in spatial extent and physical contrast. It is not applicable to neurons that fail to respond to gratings, but we have found very few neurons in cat or monkey V1, in the cat's lateral suprasylvian visual cortex, or in macaque MT, which will not respond reliably to gratings confined to the central activating region of the receptive field.

Response Predictions Figure 9 illustrates the response of a hypothetical direction selective neuron. In each plot the direction of motion of the stimulus is given by the angle, and the response of the cell to that direction is given by the distance of the point from the origin. The left-hand plot reveals that this "neuron" responded best to gratings moving directly rightward and did not respond to leftward motion. The direction tuning curve for a single grating therefore has a single peak corresponding to the best direction of motion. When one component of a 90 degree plaid (one whose components are oriented at 90 degrees to one another) is within the direction bandwidth of the neuron, the other component will be outside the acceptable range. If the neuron is component direction selective, the predicted direction tuning curve to a plaid then, is the sum of the responses to the two components presented separately. Before the responses are added, however, any spontaneous firing rate (here zero) is subtracted from each. After the two responses are added, the spontaneous rate is added back in. In the right-hand plot, responses are plotted as a function of the direction of motion of a plaid. When the plaid is moving in the optimal direction (as determined with a single grating), the components will be oriented 45 degrees to either side of the optimum (see Fig. 4). Thus the response peaks are also shifted to either side by 45 degrees, and the predicted tuning curve for the plaid is a bi-lobed curve whose peaks straddle the single peak derived from the single grating experiment. This prediction is shown by solid lines in the right-hand plot. The prediction for pattern direction selectivity is even simpler: the neuron's tuning curves for the two stimuli should be similar since their directions of motion are the same. The predicted tuning curve is thus simply the curve derived from the single grating experiment, and is shown by dashed lines in the right-hand plot.

The basis of this test is to dissociate the oriented components of a pattern from the direction in which they move: a single grating always moves at right angles to its orientation, but the plaids move at a different angle to their oriented components (45 deg in

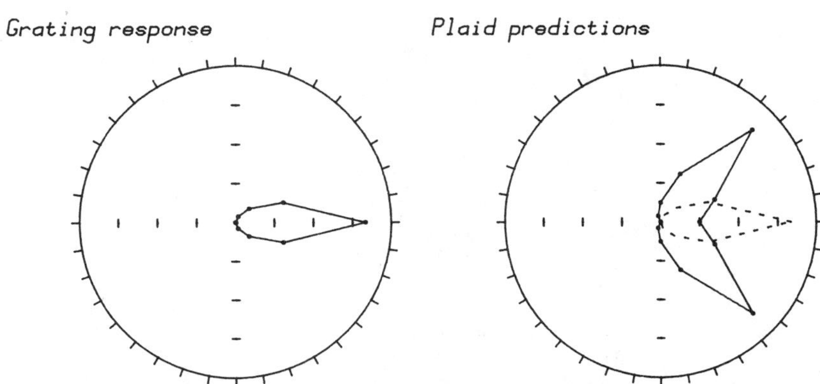

Figure 9. Hypothetical data illustrating component and pattern directional selectivity. See text for details.

the case shown in Fig. 9). The two predictions for the different types of direction selectivity are radically different and one may simply see whether the neuron's response depends on the overall direction of motion, or on the orientation of the moving components. To compare the goodness of fit of the component and pattern predictions, the actual response was correlated with each of the predictions. Since the two predictions are not necessarily uncorrelated themselves, a comparison of the simple correlations might be misleading. In order to make the two predictions independent, we used a partial correlation of the form:

$$R_p = (r_p - r_c r_{pc})/[(1 - r_p)(1 - r_c)]^{1/2}$$

where R_p is the partial correlation for the pattern prediction, r_c is the correlation of the data with the component prediction, r_p is the correlation of the data with the pattern prediction, and r_{pc} is the correlation of the two predictions. A similar partial correlation for the component prediction was calculated by exchanging r_c and r_p. These two correlation values may be used to assign each neuron to a "pattern" or "component" class, or to some intermediate grouping.

At this point the close similarity between linearity of spatial filtering and component direction selectivity should be evident. A neuron that behaves as a linear spatial filter and that possesses orientation selectivity must, in our terms, be component direction selective; our analysis of component direction selectivity here is thus similar to that used by De Valois *et al.* (1979) in their studies of the responses of striate neurons to gratings and checkerboards. Pattern directional selectivity would, however, involve important nonlinearities.

Directional Selectivity in Visual Cortical Neurons

Figure 10 shows typical responses of a component direction selective neuron, in this case a neuron of the "special complex" type (Gilbert, 1977) recorded from area 17 of a cat. The left-hand polar diagram shows the neuron's response to single grating stimuli as a function of direction of motion; the inner circle represents the spontaneous firing level in the absence of a stimulus. The neuron had a marked preference for gratings moving downward and slightly to the right. On the right, the filled symbols show the neuron's response to 90 deg plaids. Two preferred directions are evident, symmetrically displaced by 45 deg from the directional optimal for single gratings. Note that the neuron did not give any response to a plaid that moved downward and to the right, in the direction optimal for single gratings. The dashed lines in the right-hand plot show the component direction selective prediction for the neuron's response, and it is evident that this describes the data very well. In this case, the component correlation value was 0.976 (n = 32), and the pattern correlation value was −0.076. Behavior of this sort was typical of all neurons we studied in area 17 of the cat and in the primary visual cortex of the monkey; this behavior is similar to that observed by De Valois *et al.* (1979) in macaque striate neurons. Cells of the simple type were often sensitive to the relative phase of the two gratings, and variations in phase tended to make one or the other peak enlarge or disappear. No manipulation of phase, however, ever produced pattern direction selective behavior in these neurons.

It is well known that contours of non-optimal orientation may have an inhibitory influence on cortical neurons (Blakemore and Tobin, 1972; Nelson and

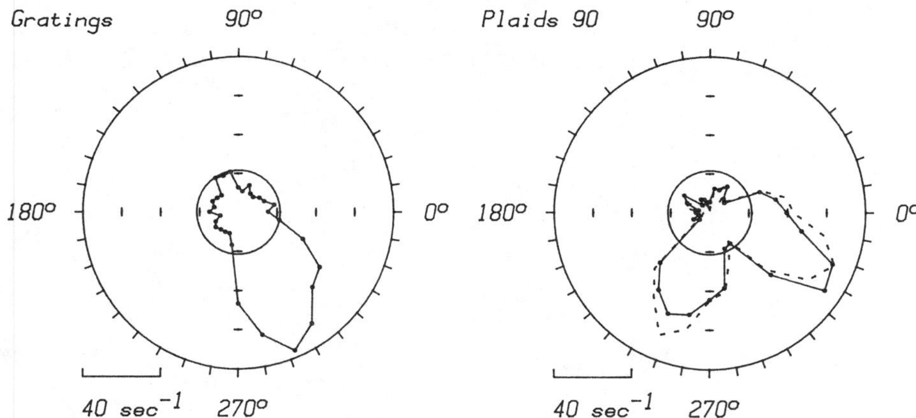

Figure 10. Directional selectivity of a special complex cell recorded in area 17 of a cat. The spatial frequency was 1.2 c/deg, and the drift rate was 4 Hz. On the left is shown the neuron's tuning for the direction of motion of single gratings, and on the right is shown the neuron's response to moving 90 deg plaids. The dashed curve on the right shows the expected response of a component direction selective neuron. The inner circles in each plot show the neuron's maintained discharge level. For this cell the component correlation was 0.976, and the pattern correlation was −0.076 (n = 32).

Frost, 1978). An inhibitory influence of this sort is evident in the single-grating tuning data on the left in Fig. 10, but is visible only because of the relatively high maintained discharge shown by this cell (about 21 impulses/sec). Most cortical neurons have much less spontaneous discharge, and consequently reveal inhibitory influences incompletely; it is therefore not surprising that the magnitude of the responses we observed to plaids tended to be somewhat less than those predicted from simple superposition. The magnitude of the inhibitory effect varied widely, but on average the response to plaids was between 25% and 40% less than predicted. This inhibition was what originally motivated us to use the correlation measure described earlier, since this is insensitive to deviations in response magnitude from the predictions.

We have also studied the behavior of a number of neurons in the lateral suprasylvian cortex of the cat, an area thought to be involved in processing motion information in that species (Spear and Baumann, 1975; Gizzi *et al.*, 1981). Almost all neurons in LS, like those in V1, showed clear component direction selectivity, and none gave a convincingly pattern direction selective response.

In order to examine the distribution of behavior of neurons in different areas, we prepared scatter diagrams in which the values of the pattern and component correlation coefficients were plotted against one another. Figure 11A illustrates the significance of various regions of these plots. The region marked "component" is a zone in which the component correlation coefficient significantly exceeds either zero or the pattern correlation coefficient, whichever is larger. The region marked "pattern" similarly marks neurons that were unambiguously pattern direction selective. The region marked "unclassed" represents cases in which both the pattern and component correlations significantly exceeded zero, but did not differ significantly from one another, or cases in which neither correlation coefficient differed significantly from zero.

Figure 11B shows a scatter plot of data in this space for 69 neurons recorded from cat and monkey V1. It is clear that these cluster around a component correlation value of 1 and a pattern correlation value of zero. While a few neurons lie in the two indeterminate regions of the plot, no clearly pattern direction selective cases exist. Figure 11C shows a similar plot for data from 61 cells recorded in the cat's LS cortex. Here the data are slightly more scattered, but the result is again unambiguous: most neurons lie in the component zone, and only one is (barely) within the pattern zone. It thus appears that neurons in these areas are capable of signalling only the motion of 1-D components, and cannot unambiguously define the motion of whole pat-

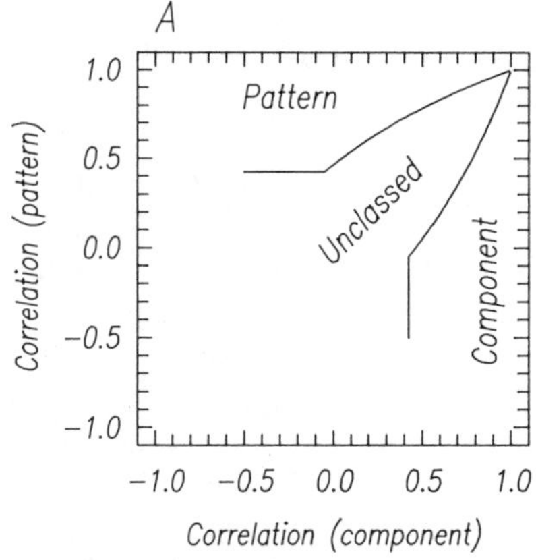

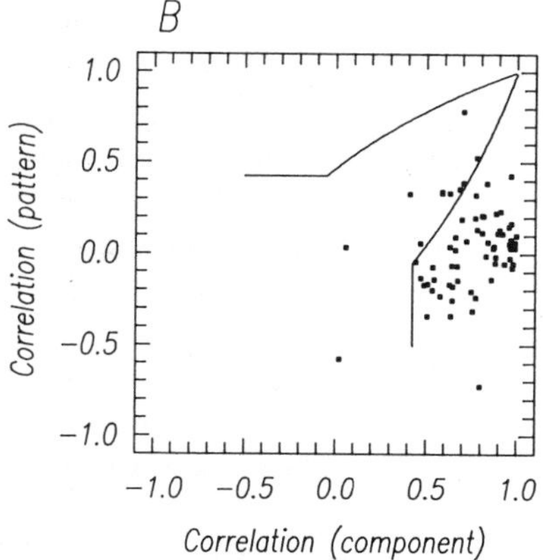

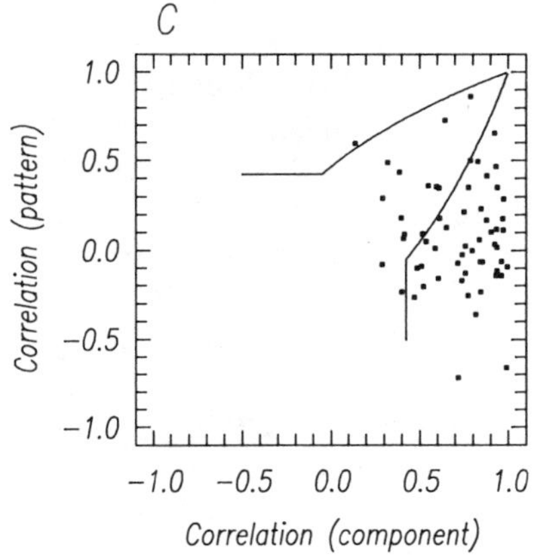

Figure 11. Scatter diagrams of the directional selectivity of neurons in the visual cortex. A. The space within which the data lie (see text for details). B. Diagram of the behavior of 69 cells from area 17 of cats and monkeys. C. Diagram of the behavior of 61 cells from the lateral suprasylvian visual cortex of cats (Gizzi *et al.* 1981).

terns. Our search for pattern direction selective neurons then turned to MT, an extrastriate area in the macaque's cortex thought to be involved in analyzing motion information.

MT is the natural place to study motion sensitivity in primates. In macaque, MT is a heavily myelinated area on the posterior bank of the superior temporal sulcus. It is one of three cortical areas to receive a major projection from striate cortex, the others being V2 and V3 (Zeki, 1978a; Maunsell and Van Essen, 1983). The physiological properties of neurons in macaque MT were first described by Dubner and Zeki (1971; Zeki, 1974), who reported that the area contained a high proportion of directionally selective neurons. This observation is in marked contrast to the very low frequency of directional selectivity in V2 and V3 (Zeki, 1978b). This area was renamed MT by Van Essen (1979) because of its clear homology with the middle temporal area in the owl monkey (Allman and Kaas, 1971; Zeki, 1980; Baker *et al.*, 1981). The areas receive similar projections and contain neurons with similar receptive field properties. Van Essen *et al.* (1981) reported that some cells in macaque MT showed orientation selectivity when tested with stationary stimuli, as has been reported for the majority of cells in owl monkey MT (Baker *et al.*, 1981). Nevertheless, as orientation selectivity distinguishes V1, so direction selectivity distinguishes MT. It is not certain whether this reflects the selectivity of that afferent input or whether direction selectivity is a result of the processing within MT. Only about a quarter of the neurons in macaque V1 are directionally selective (Hubel and Wiesel, 1968; De Valois *et al*, 1982); in V2, the proportion may be even lower (Baizer *et al.*, 1977; Zeki, 1978b). These areas provide the major intracortical input to MT. On the other hand Dow (1974) reported that many neurons in layer IVb of V1 are directionally selective—the projection from striate cortex to MT arises from this layer and layer VI (Lund *et al.*, 1976; Maunsell and Van Essen, 1983). There is also input (which may be directionally selective) to MT from the inferior pulvinar (Trojanowski and Jacobsen, 1976; Benevento and Rezak, 1976).

Figure 12 shows data, in a format similar to that used in Fig. 10, for two neurons recorded from MT. The neuron in Fig. 12A preferred upward movement of single gratings; like its component direction selective counterpart in V1 (Fig. 10), this preference was translated into a dual preference for two directions 45 deg apart when it was tested with 90 deg plaids. As comparison of the data with the dashed lines in the right-hand plot of Fig. 12A reveals, the component direction selective prediction provided a very good description of this behavior. About 40% of the cells we studied in MT were clearly component direction selective. Figure 12B shows data from a neuron in MT whose behavior was rather different. This neuron preferred downward and rightward movement of grating stimuli, and maintained this preference when tested with 135 deg plaids. The actual response to plaids differed very dramatically from the component direction selective prediction. About 25% of the neurons we studied in MT behaved in this way. This apparently simple behavior must involve some remarkable neural circuitry. Consider that the most effective plaid stimulus was composed of two gratings which, in isolation, had directions 67.5 deg different from the optimum; neither direction alone elicited a significant response. Thus the most effective plaid pattern was composed of two gratings which were by themselves ineffective; conversely, when the most effective grating stimulus was combined with another to form a plaid, the response was poor. These features of the tuning characteristics suggest that a combination of suppressive and facilitatory processes must be involved in the generation of pattern direction selectivity. We have some evidence from further experiments that this is the case, and that some neural operation similar to the "intersection of constraints" that we described in the introduction is in fact performed by pattern direction selective neurons in MT.

Figure 13 shows a scatter diagram of the directional behavior of 108 neurons from MT, in the format laid out in Fig. 11A. The data here were derived from experiments using 135 deg plaids. Most neurons in MT are rather more broadly tuned for direction than their counterparts in V1, and in consequence the distinction between the component and pattern predictions cannot often be made very clearly with 90 deg plaids. In contrast to the data from V1 and from cat LS shown in Fig. 11, the distribution of values for MT cells shown here is very broad. About 25% of the cells fall into the pattern category, and 40% into the component category. The significant population of cells that falls in the "unclassed" region deserves comment. Most of these (about 30% of the total) are in the upper right corner of the plot, where both correlation coefficients are different from zero, but do not differ from each other. These cells generally had very broad tuning curves, so that even using 135 deg plaids the variability of the response made statistical distinction between the accuracy of the two predictions difficult. It would thus be a mistake to conclude that these cells were of some "intermediate" type. Rather, the particular standard test conditions and statistics used were insufficiently sensitive to classify them. The remainder of the unclassed cells (about 10% of the total) gave plaid responses that did not correlate well with either prediction. In most of these cases, the response to single gratings was rather weak and variable, resulting in an unsatisfactory pair of predicted tuning curves; in a

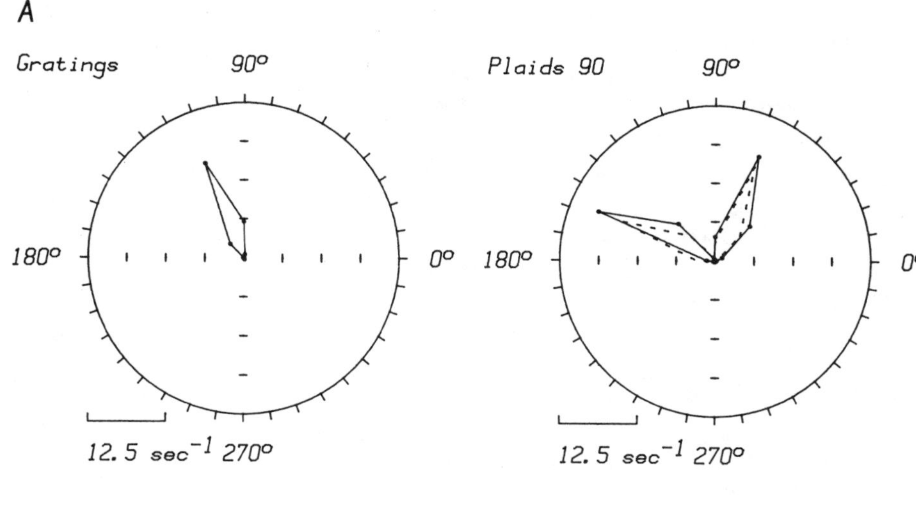

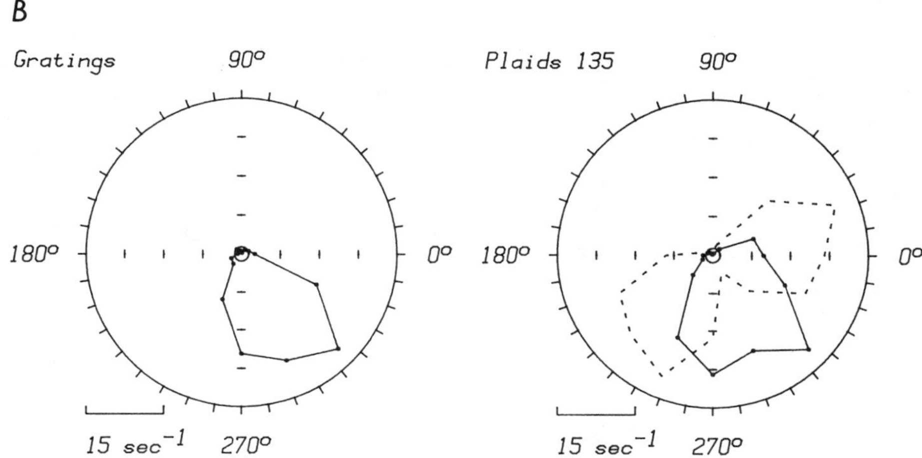

Figure 12. Directional selectivity of two neurons from MT. The format for each figure is the same as in Fig. 10 A. Spatial frequency 3.6 c/deg, drift rate 4 Hz, component correlation 0.991, pattern correlation −0.092 (n = 16). B. Spatial frequency 2.7 c/deg, drift rate 4 Hz, component correlation 0.349, pattern correlation 0.940 (n = 16).

number of these cases, the response to plaids was brisk and reliable.

The continuity of the distribution in Fig. 13 does not immediately suggest the existence of two discrete cell classes in MT. We do, however, have some evidence that the laminar distribution of the component and pattern cells may differ, with the pattern cells primarily encountered in layers II, III and V, and the component cells more often being in layers IV and VI; thus two genuine classes of cell may exist in MT. Regardless of the resolution of this issue, it is clear that information about both types of motion is available in the signals relayed by neurons in MT, including the pattern direction selective type that we have not encountered elsewhere.

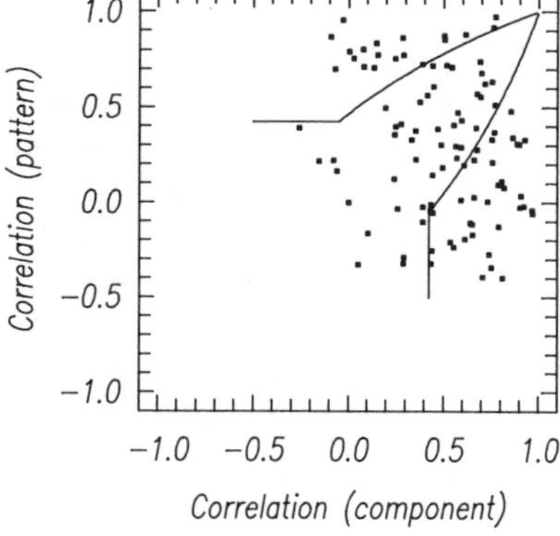

Figure 13. A scatter diagram of the directional selectivity of 108 neurons in MT, tested with 135 deg plaids. The format is the same as in Fig. 11.

Discussion

Our psychophysical studies revealed the existence of two stages in the processing of motion information in the human visual system. The first stage appears to analyze the motion of 1-D patterns, and to be responsible for the detection of simple moving patterns. The second stage seems to be concerned with establishing the motion of complex patterns on the basis of information relayed from the first stage. In our experiments, the action of this stage is most clearly seen in the various coherence phenomena that we have described. These two stages of analysis appear to have natural analogs in our electrophysiological results. The properties of component direction selective neurons in V1 and MT seem to correspond to the first stage, while the pattern direction selective neurons in MT seem to correspond to the second stage.

This parallel between psychophysical and electrophysiological data is gratifying, but it is important to examine in a little more detail the basis for the parallels we draw. Our arguments in both the psychophysical and electrophysiological domain rest on evidence concerning the way in which neural mechanisms represent information. Our knowledge of this representation derives from an examination of tuning characteristics, established with stimuli designed to reveal particular properties of the system we studied. One may ask whether it is legitimate to conclude that the two putative stages genuinely differ simply because their tuning characteristics differ. This issue has been a disputatious one in electrophysiology in recent years, largely as a result of a debate concerning the kinds of signals relayed by striate cortical neurons. On the one hand, traditional descriptions of striate neurons (e.g. Hubel and Wiesel, 1962) have emphasized their sensitivity to contours such as lines and edges, and given rise to the idea that these neurons function as edge-detectors. More recent studies (e.g. Maffei and Fiorentini, 1973; De Valois *et al.*, 1979) have characterized striate neuron responses using sinusoidal gratings, and emphasized their sensitivity to the spatial frequency of these patterns. With the exception of some specific nonlinear models (e.g. Marr, 1982), this debate has centered around matters of interpretation rather than of testable fact. Most available data suggests that striate cortical neurons function as approximately linear spatial filters, and that their responses to aperiodic patterns and to sinusoidal gratings can be simply related to one another (e.g. Movshon *et al*, 1978). Thus the various ways in which striate neurons have been described are probably formally identical, producing an argument about semantics rather than substance.

Our results and claims differ from these in an important respect. Our notion of pattern direction selectivity involves specific nonlinear properties in computing the "intersection of constraints"; the results we have obtained from pattern direction selective neurons in MT are incompatible with a linear model. Now, given the specific nonlinearity present in these neurons, it is natural to argue that they are different in an important way from neurons in the other cortical areas we have studied, whose directional selectivity may be more simply understood. There is also the matter of motion ambiguity with which we began this paper. Our results on striate neurons demonstrate that they provide ambiguous signals about the motion of complex objects. This ambiguity may be resolved by a specific kind of neural computation, and our results from MT show that this computation may be performed there. Thus the signals from pattern direction selective neurons contain an important kind of information not available from the output of any single striate neuron. It is this particular synthesis of information relayed from V1 to MT to which we attribute the greatest significance.

Thus we may plausibly argue from the way in which information is represented in V1 and MT neurons that the two stages of motion processing are present. We cannot, of course, prove that assertion merely with psychophysical or electrophysiological data, for these only allow the development of reasonable hypotheses. Proof of these must await combined psychophysical and electrophysiological study of the consequences of inactivating MT for the perception of moving visual patterns.

Acknowledgements

This work was supported by grants to J. A. Movshon from the National Institutes of Health (EY 2017) and the National Science Foundation (BNS 82-16950). E. H. Adelson was partly supported by a training grant from NIH (EY 7032) to New York University, and M. S. Gizzi was supported by a grant from the New York State Health Research Council. We thank Harriet Friedman for assistance with histology, and Aries Arditi and Robert Schumer for helpful discussions.

References

Adelson E. H. and Movshon J. A., "Two kinds of adaptation to moving patterns." *Invest. Ophthalmol. Vis. Sci.*, supp. *20*, 17 (1981).

———. "Phenomenal coherence of moving visual patterns." *Nature*, *300*, 523–525 (1982).

Arditi A. R., Anderson P. A. and Movshon J. A., "Monocular and binocular detection of moving sinusoidal gratings." *Vision Res.*, *21*, 329–336 (1981).

Allman J. and Kaas J. H., "A representation of the visual field in the caudal third of the middle temporal gyrus of the owl monkey (*Aotus trivergatus*)." *Brain Res.*, *31*, 85–105 (1971).

Raizer J. S., Robinson D. L. and Dow B. M., "Visual responses of area 18 neurons in awake, behaving monkey." *J. Neurophysiol.*, *40*, 1024–1037 (1977).

Baker J., Peterson S., Newsome W. T. and Allman J., "Visual response properties of neurons in four extrastriate areas of the owl monkey (*Aotus trivergatus*): A quantitative comparison of the medial (M), dorsomedial (DM), dorsolateral (DL) and middle temporal (MT) areas." *J. Neurophysiol.*, *45*, 397–416 (1981).

Barlow H. B. and Pettigrew J. D., "Lack of specificity of neurones in the visual cortex of young kittnes." *J. Physiol., Lond.*, *218*, 98–100 (1971).

Benevento L. A. and Rezak M., "The cortical projections of the inferior pulvinar and adjacent lateral pulvinar in the rhesus monkey (*Macaca mulatta*): An autoradiographic study." *Brain Res.*, 108, 1–24 (1976).

Blakemore C. and Campbell F. W., "On the existence of neurones in the human visual system selectively sensitive to the orientation and size of retinal images." *J. Physiol., Lond.*, *203*, 237–260 (1969).

Blakemore C., Muncey J. P. J. and Ridley R. M., "Stimulus specificity in the human visual system." *Vision Res.*, *13*, 1915–1931 (1973).

Blakemore C. and Nachmias J., "The orientation specificity of two visual aftereffects." *J. Physiol., Lond.*, *213*, 157–174 (1971).

Blakemore C. and Tobin E. A., "Lateral inhibition between orientation detectors in the cat's visual cortex." *Expl. Brain Res.*, *15*, 539–540 (1972).

Campbell F. W. and Kulikowski J. J., "The orientational selectivity of the human visual system." *J. Physiol., Lond.*, *187*, 437–445 (1966).

De Valois K. K., De Valois R. L. and Yund E. W., "Responses of striate cortex cells to grating and checkerboard patterns." *J. Physiol., Lond.*, *291*, 483–505 (1979).

De Valois R L., Yund E. W. and Hepler N. K., "The orientation and direction selectivity of cells in macaque visual cortex." *Vision Res.*, *22*, 531–544 (1982).

Dow B. M., "Functional classes of cells and their laminar distribution in monkey visual cortex." *J. Neurophysiol.*, *37*, 927–946 (1974).

Dubner R. and Zeki S. M., "Response properties and receptive fields of cells in an anatomically defined region of the superior temporal sulcus in the monkey." *Brain Res.*, *35*, 528–532 (1971).

Fennema C. L. and Thompson W. B., "Velocity determination in scenes containing several moving objects." *Comp. Graph. Image Proc.*, *9*, 301–315 (1979).

Gattass R. and Gross C. G., "Visual topography of striate projection zone (MT) in posterior superior temporal sulcus of macaque." *J. Neurophysiol.*, *46*, 621–638 (1981).

Gilbert C. D., "Laminar differences in receptive field properties of cells in cat primary visual cortex." *J. Physiol., Lond.*, *268*, 391–421 (1977).

Gizzi M. S., "The Processing of Visual Motion of Cat and Monkey Central Nervous System." Ph. D. dissertation, New York University (1983).

Gizzi M. S., Katz E. and Movshon J. A., "Orientation selectivity in the cat's lateral suprasylvian visual cortex." *Invest. Ophthalmol. Vis. Sci.*, supp. *20*, 149 (1981).

Gizzi M. S., Newsome W. T. an Movshon J. A., "Directional selectivity of neurons in macaque MT." *Invest. Ophthalmol. Vis. Sci.*, supp. *24*, 107 (1983).

Hammond P., "Directional tuning of complex cells in area 17 of the feline visual cortex." *J. Physiol., Lond.*, *285*, 479–491 (1978).

Henry G. H., Bishop P. O., Tupper R. M. and Dreher B., "Orientation, axis and direction as stimulus parameters for striate cells." *Vision Res.*, *14*, 767–777 (1974).

Hildreth E. C., "The Measurement of Visual Motion." Ph. D. dissertation, Massachusetts Institute of Technology (1983).

Horn B. K. P. and Schunck B. G., "Determining optical flow." *Artificial Intelligence*, *17*, 185–203 (1981).

Hubel D. H. and Wiesel T. N., "Receptive fields, binocular interaction and functional architecture in the cat's visual cortex." *J. Physiol., Lond.*, *160*, 106–154 (1962).

———. "Receptive fields and functional architecture in two nonstriate visual areas (18 and 19) of the cat." *J. Neurophysiol.*, *28*, 229–289 (1965).

———. "Receptive fields and functional architecture of monkey striate cortex." *J. Physiol., Lond.*, *194*, 215–243 (1968).

Kaufman L., *Sight and Mind*. New York: Oxford University Press (1975).

Lund J. S., Lund R. D., Hendrickson A. E., Bunt A. M. and Fuchs A. L., "The origin of efferent pathways from the primary visual cortex, area 17, of the macaque monkey as shown by retrograde transport of horseradish-peroxidase" *J. comp. Neurol.*, *164*, 287–304 (1976).

Maffei L. and Fiorentini A., "The visual cortex as a spatial frequency analyzer." *Vision Res.*, *13*, 1255–1268 (1973).

Maffei L., Fiorentini A. and Bisti S., "Neural correlate of perceptual adaptation to gratings." *Science*, *182*, 1036–1038 (1973).

Marr D., *Vision*. New York: Freeman (1982).

Marr D. and Poggio T., "A computational theory of human stereo vision." *Proc. R. Soc. Lond. B.*, *204*, 301–328 (1979).

Marr D. and Ullman S., "Directional selectivity and its use in early visual processing." *Proc. R. Soc. Lond. B.*, *211*, 151–180 (1981).

Maunsell J. H. R. and Van Essen D. C., "Functional properties of neurons in the middle temporal visual area of the macaque monkey. I. Selectivity for stimulus direction, speed, and orientation." *J. Neurophysiol.*, *49*, 1127–1146 (1983a).

———. "The connections of the middle temporal visual area (MT) and their relationship to a cortical hierarchy in the macaque monkey." *J. Neurosci.*, (1983b).

Movshon J. A., "The velocity tuning of single units in cat striate cortex." *J. Physiol., Lond.*, *249*, 445–468 (1975).

Movshon J. A., Davis E. T. and Adelson E. H., "Directional movement selectivity in cortical complex cells." *Soc. Neurosci. Abs.*, *6*, 670 (1980).

Movshon J. A. and Lennie P., "Spatially selective adaptation in striate cortical neurons." *Nature*, *278*, 850–852 (1979).

Movshon J. A., Thompson I. D. and Tolhurst D. J., "Spatial summation in the receptive fields of simple cells in the cat's striate cortex." *J. Physiol., Lond.*, *283*, 53–77 (1978).

Nelson J. I. and Frost B. J., "Orientation selective inhibition from beyond the classic visual receptive field." *Brain Res.*, *139*, 359–365 (1978).

Pettigrew J. D., Nikara T. and Bishop P. O., "Responses to moving slits by single units in cat striate cortex." *Expl. Brain Res.*, *6*, 373–390 (1968).

Reichardt W., "Autokorrelationsauswertung als Funktionsprinzip des Zentralnervensystems." *Z. Naturforsch.*, *12B*, 447–457 (1957).

Sekuler R. W. and Ganz L., "A new aftereffect of seen motion with a stabilized retinal image." *Science*, *139*, 419–420 (1963).

Sekuler R. W., Rubin E. L. and Cushman W. H., "Selectivities of human visual mechanisms for direction of movement and contour orientation." *J. Opt. Soc. Am.*, *68*, 1146–1150 (1968).

Sharpe C. and Tolhurst D. J., "The effects of temporal modulation on the orientation channels of the human visual system." *Perception*, *2*, 23–29 (1973).

Spear P. D. and Baumann T. P., "Receptive field characteristics of single neurons in lateral suprasylvian area of the cat." *J. Neurophysiol.*, *38*, 1403–1420 (1975).

Stromeyer C. F. and Julesz B., "Spatial frequency masking in vision: critical bands and spread of masking." *J. Opt. Soc. Am.*, *62*, 1221–1232 (1972).

Trojanowski J. and Jacobson S., "Areal and laminar distribution of some pulvinar cortical efferents in rhesus monkey." *J. comp. Neurol.*, *169*, 371–396 (1976).

Van Essen D. C., "Visual areas of the mammalian cerebral cortex." *Ann. Rev. Neurosci.*, *2*, 227–263 (1979).

Van Essen D. C., Maunsell J. H. R. and Bixby J. L., "The middle temporal visual area in the macaque: Myelaorchitecture, connections, functional properties and topographic organization." *J. comp. Neurol.*, *199*, 293–326 (1981).

van Santen J. P. H. and Sperling G., "A temporal covariance model of motion perception." *Invest. Ophthalmol. Vis. Sci.*, supp. *24*, 277 (1983).

Vautin R. G. and Berkley M. A., "Responses of single cells in cat visual cortex to prolonged stimulus movement: neural correlates of visual aftereffects." *J. Neurophysiol.*, *40*, 1051–1065 (1977).

Wallach H., "Ueber visuell wahrgenommene Bewegungsrichtung." *Psychol. Forschung*, *20*, 325–380 (1935).

———. *On Perception.* New York: New York Times Books (1976).

Wohlgemuth A., "On the aftereffect of seen movement." *Brit. J. Pyschol., Monogr.*, supp. *1* (1911).

Zeki S. M., "Functional organization of a visual area in the posterior bank of the superior temporal sulcus of the rhesus monkey." *J. Physiol., Lond.*, *236*, 549–573 (1974).

———. "The cortical projections of foveal striate cortex in the rhesus monkey." *J. Physiol., Lond.*, *277*, 227–244 (1978a).

———. "Uniformity and diversity of structure and function in rhesus monkey prestriate visual cortex." *J. Physiol., Lond.*, *277*, 273–290 (1978b).

———. "The response properties of cells in the middle temporal area (area MT) of owl monkey visual cortex." *Proc. R. Soc. Lond. B.*, *207*, 239–248 (1980).

14

D. Marr and H. K. Nishihara

Visual information processing: Artificial intelligence and the sensorium of sight

1978. *Technology Review* 81: 2–23

For human vision to be explained by a computational theory, the first question is plain: What are the problems the brain solves when we see?

Modern neurophysiology has learned much about the operation of the individual nerve cell, but unpleasantly little about the meaning of the circuits they compose in the brain. The reason for this can be attributed, at least in part, to a failure to recognize what it means to understand a complex information-processing system; for a complex system cannot be understood as a simple extrapolation from the properties of its elementary components. One does not formulate, for example, a description of thermodynamical effects using a large set of equations, one for each of the particles involved. One describes such effects at their own level, that of an enormous collection of particles, and tries to show that in principle, the microscopic and macroscopic descriptions are consistent with one another.

The core of the problem is that a system as complex as a nervous system or a developing embryo must be analyzed and understood at several different levels. Indeed, in a system that solves an information processing problem, we may distinguish four important levels of description. (We here are following a formulation published in 1977 by Marr and Tomaso Poggio.) At the lowest, there is basic component and circuit analysis — how do transistors (or neurons), diodes (or synapses) work? The second level is the study of particular mechanisms: adders, multipliers, and memories, these being assemblies made from basic components. The third level is that of the algorithm, the scheme for a computation; and the top level contains the *theory* of the computation. A theory of addition, for example, would encompass the meaning of that operation, quite independent of the representation of the numbers to be added — say Arabic versus Roman. But it would also include the realization that the first of these representations is the more suitable of the two. An algorithm, on the other hand, is a particular method by which to add numbers. It therefore applies to a particular representation, since plainly an algorithm that adds Arabic numerals would be useless for Roman. At still a further level down, one comes upon a mechanism for addition — say a pocket calculator — which simply implements a particular algorithm. As a second example, take the case of Fourier analysis. Here the computational theory of the Fourier transform — the decomposition of an arbitrary mathematical curve into a sum of sine waves of differing frequencies — is well understood, and is ex-

The beginning of vision: a gray-level intensity array which will serve to approximate an input to the retina. The processing of such an image by the brain proceeds so naturally — so unconsciously, in a sense — that we are seldom aware that it begins with only this: a two-dimensional play of light upon the receptors of either eye. Our facility suggests the existence of a well-defined computational method, and makes vision a promising field of investigation in artificial intelligence. The image shown here was originally an array of 128 by 128, with each of its elements — numbers, actually — signifying one of 256 possible brightnesses. But the actual image as seen in this magazine is affected by the process by which it first was displayed on the screen of an imaging system resembling the technology of television, then by the processes that copied and printed it, and finally by limitations in human discrimination of brightness. The largest dots in the image are noise in the imaging system: each serves to suggest the actual size of each picture element, or "pixel." Smaller dots are patterns of stippling used in this figure to denote the shades of gray.

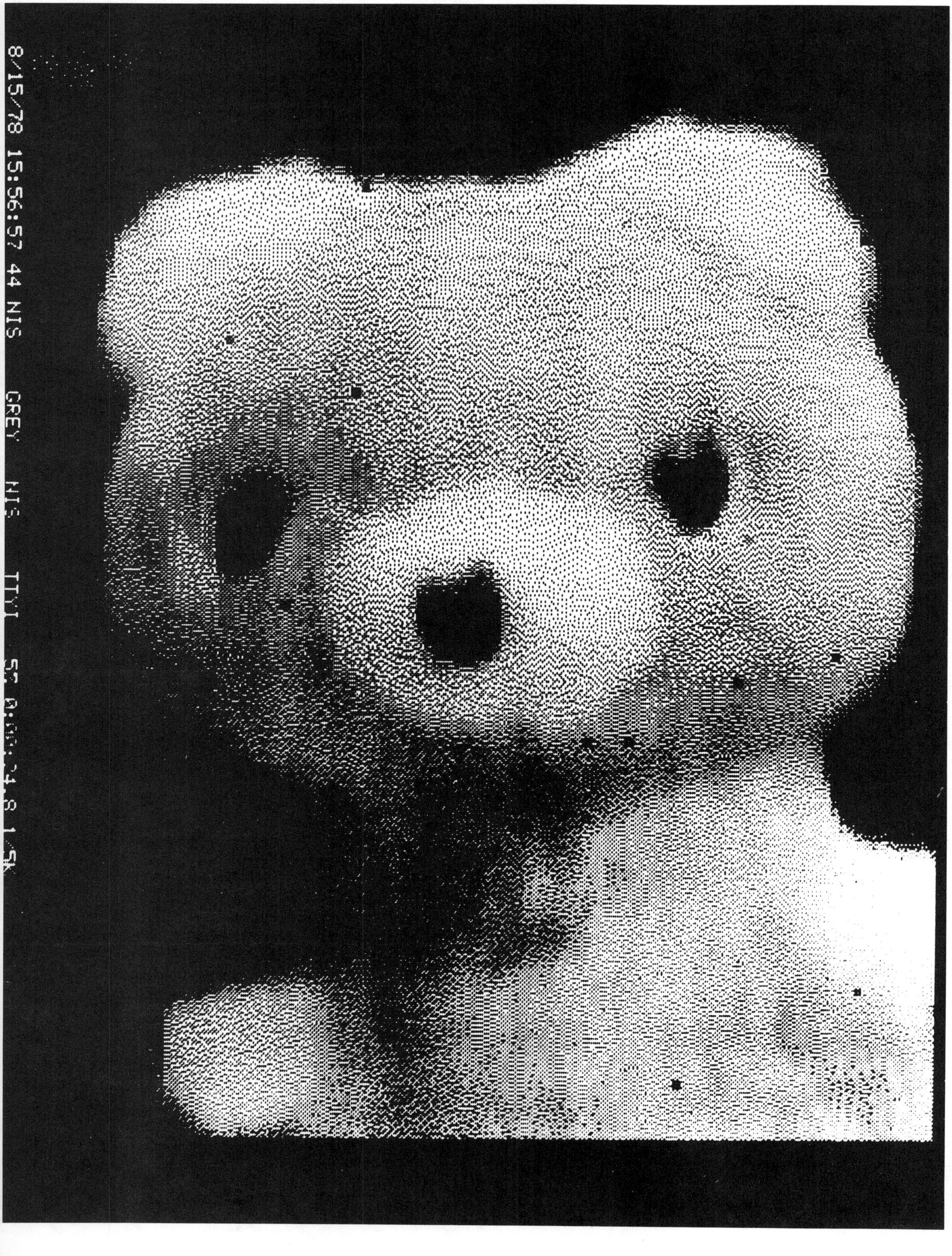
8/15/78 15:56:57 44 NIS GREY NIS

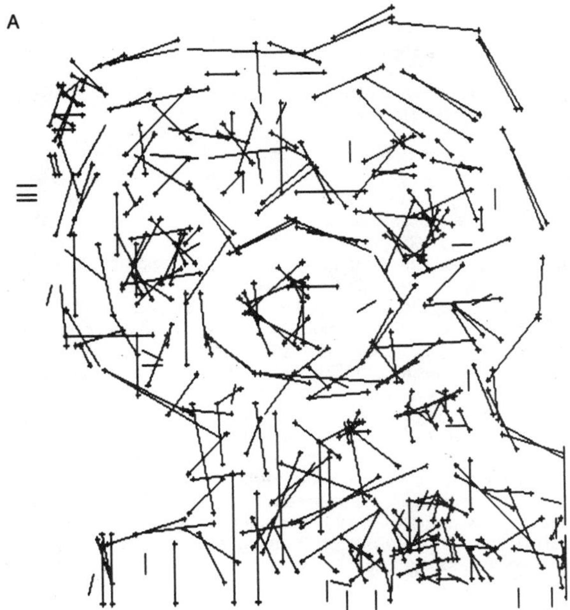

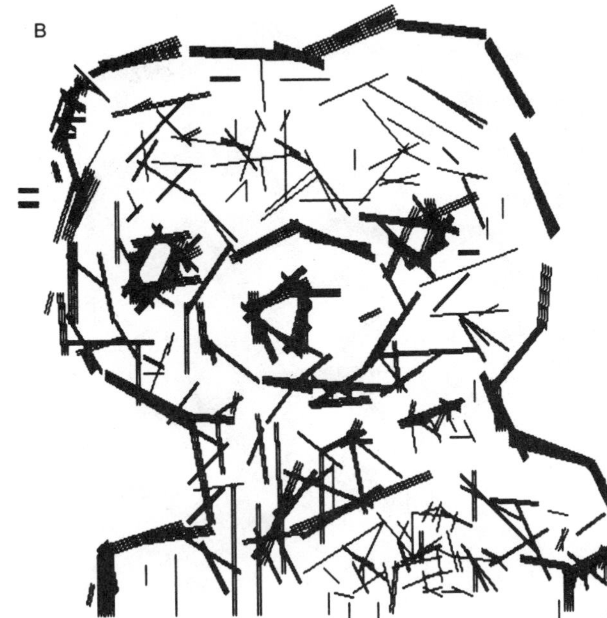

pressed independently of the particular way in which it might be computed. One level down, there are several algorithms for computing a Fourier transform, among them the so-called Fast Fourier Transform (FFT), which comprises a sequence of mathematical operations, and the so-called spatial algorithm, a single, global operation that is based on the mechanisms of laser optics. All such algorithms produce the same result, so the choice of which one to use depends upon the particular mechanisms that are available. If one has fast digital memory, adders, and multipliers, one will use the FFT, and if one has a laser and photographic plates, one will use an "optical" method.

Now each of the four levels of description will have its place in the eventual understanding of perceptual information processing, and of course there are logical and causal relations among them. But the important point is that the four levels of description are only loosely related. Too often in attempts to relate psychophysical problems to physiology there is confusion about the level at which a problem arises — is it related, for instance, mainly to the physical mechanisms of vision (like the after-images such as the one you see after staring at a lightbulb) or mainly to the computational theory of vision (like the ambiguity of the Necker cube as it appears on page 6)? More disturbingly, although the top level is the most neglected, it is also the most important. This is because the nature of the computations that underlie perception depend more upon the computational *problems* that have to be solved than upon the particular hardware in which their solutions are implemented. To phrase the matter another way, an algorithm is likely to be understood more readily by understanding the nature of the problem that it deals with than by examining the mechanism (and the hardware) by which it is embodied. There is, after all, an analog to all of this in physics, where a thermodynamical approach represented, at least historically, the first stage in the study of matter: it succeeded in producing a theory of gross properties such as temperature. A description in terms of mechanisms or elementary components — in this case atoms and molecules — appeared some decades afterwards.

Our main point, therefore, is that the topmost of our four levels, that at which the necessary structure of computation is defined, is a crucial but neglected one. Its study is separate from the study of particular algorithms, mechanisms, or hardware, and the techniques needed to pursue it are new. In the rest of this article, we summarize some examples of vision theories at the uppermost level. We will conclude with some remarks on the development of the field of which these theories are part: the field called artificial intelligence.

Conventional Approaches

The problems of visual perception have attracted the curiosity of scientists for many centuries. Important early contributions were made by Newton, who laid the foundations for modern work on color vision, and Helmholtz, whose treatise on physiological optics maintains its interest even today. Early in this century, Wertheimer noticed the apparent motion not of individual dots but instead of wholes, or "fields," in images presented sequentially, as if in a movie. In much the same way we perceive the migration across the sky of a flock of geese, the flock somehow constituting a single entity, and not individual birds. This observation started the Gestalt school of psychology, which was concerned with describing the qualities of wholes, including solidarity and distinctness, and trying to formulate the laws that governed their creation. The attempt failed for various reasons, and the Gestalt school dissolved into the fog of subjectivism. With the death of the school, many of its early and genuine insights were unfortunately lost to the mainstream of experimental psychology.

The next developments of importance were recent and technical. The advent of electrophysiology in the 1940s

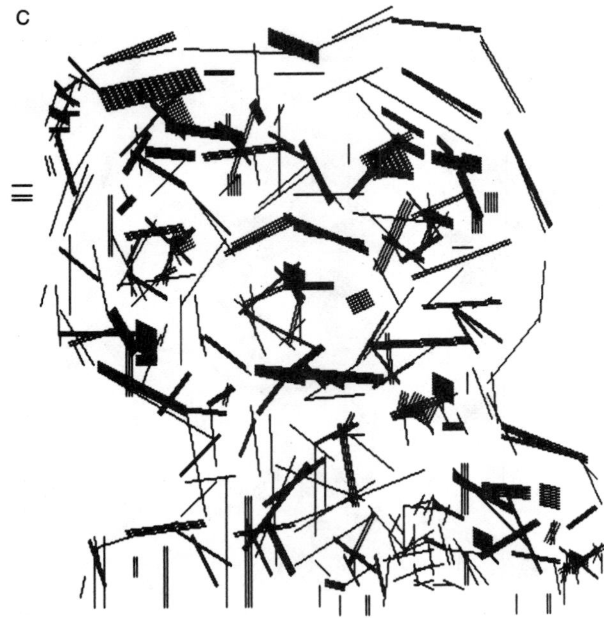

The so-called primal sketch is shown in three of its aspects; each is a representation of intensity changes in a gray-level image such as appears on page 3. Its creation constitutes the earliest stage in the authors' theory of visual information processing. Sketch A shows only "edge-assertions": each line represents the position and orientation at which a change in intensity is found. The cross-bars at the ends of each line show the terminations of the change. This is not to say that each line necessarily denotes a sharp edge in the gray-level array, but rather that each denotes the existence of a gradient in intensity. Sketch *B* adds information about differing contrasts: each line in *A* is transformed into a set of parallel lines in proportion to the logarithm of the intensity change. In other words, a large magnitude of transition from light to dark or dark to light leads to a bolder edge-assertion. Notice, accordingly, that the margin of the bear tends to have more prominent assertions than those to be found within. In the displays shown here, the spacing between parallel lines in a set is simply proportional to their length. For short assertions, therefore, the multiple lines have tended to overlap, so as to create the impression of a single, thick bar. Sketch *C* shows the fuzziness of each of the edge assertions — that is to say, the widths of the variations in intensity, as opposed to their magnitudes. The thicker sets of lines now tend to lie in the interior of the image, which reflects the circumstance that broad gradients in shading tend not to appear at its edges. As held in computer storage, the primal sketch includes the information shown in *A*, *B*, and *C* alike: that is to say, the positions, directions, magnitudes, and spatial extents of intensity gradients in the gray-level array.

and '50s made single cell recording possible, and with Stephen W. Kuffler's study of retinal ganglion cells — the neurons of the eye that give rise to the optic nerve — a new approach to the problem was born. Its most renowned practitioners are David H. Hubel and Torsten N. Wiesel, who since 1959 have conducted an influential series of investigations on single cell responses at various points along the visual pathway in the cat and the monkey.

Hubel and Wiesel used the notion of a cell's "receptive field" to classify cells in the so-called primary and secondary visual areas of the cerebral cortex into simple, complex, and hypercomplex types. Simple cells are orientation-sensitive and roughly linear. That is to say, the simple cell monitors a particular district of visual space, a so-called receptive field, in this case divided into parallel elongated excitatory and inhibitory parts; events in the first of these promote the cell's electrical activity, events in the second tend to inhibit it; the two opposing phenomena act simultaneously on the cell — in a word, they summate; and finally, a simple cell's response to a stimulating pattern is roughly predictable from its receptive field's geometry. Complex cells, on the other hand, apparently respond to edges and bars over a wider range than a simple cell's field. Hypercomplex cells seem to respond best to points where an edge or bar terminates. How the different types of cell are connected and why they behave as they do is controversial.

Students of the psychology of perception were also affected by a technological advance, the advent of the digital computer. Most notably, it allowed Bela Julesz in 1959 to devise random-dot stereograms, which are image pairs constructed of dot patterns that appear random when viewed monocularly, but which fuse when viewed one through each eye to give a percept of shapes and surfaces with a clear three-dimensional structure. An example is shown on page 9. Here the image for the left eye is a matrix of black and white squares generated at random by a computer program. The image for the right is made by copying the left image and then shifting a square-shaped region at its center slightly to the left, providing a new random pattern to fill in the gap that the shift must create. If each of the eyes sees only one matrix, as if they were both in the same physical place, the result is the sensation of a square floating in space. Plainly such percepts are caused solely by the stereo disparity between matching elements in the images presented to each eye.

Very recently, considerable interest has been attracted by a rather different approach. In 1971, Roger N. Shepard and Jacqueline Metzler made line drawings of simple objects that differed from one another either by a three-dimensional rotation, or by a rotation plus a reflection (see the illustration on page 14). They asked how long it took to decide whether two depicted objects differed by a rotation and a reflection, or merely a rotation. They found that the time taken depended on the 3-D angle of rotation necessary to bring the two objects into correspondence. Indeed, it varied linearly with this angle. One is led thereby to the notion that a mental rotation of sorts is actually being performed: that a mental description of the first shape in a pair is being adjusted incrementally in orientation until it matches the second, such adjustment requiring greater time when greater angles are involved.

Interesting and important though these findings are, one must sometimes be allowed the luxury of pausing to reflect upon the overall trends that they represent, in order to take stock of the kind of knowledge that is accessible through these techniques. For we repeat: perhaps the most striking feature of neurophysiology and psychophysics at present is that they *describe* the behavior of cells or of subjects, but do not *explain* it. What are the visual areas of the cerebral cortex actually doing? What are the problems in doing it that need explaining, and at what level of description should such explanations be sought?

A Computational Approach to Vision

In trying to come to grips with these problems, our group at the M.I.T. Artificial Intelligence Laboratory has adopted a point of view that regards visual perception as a problem primarily in information processing. The problem commences with a large, gray-level intensity array, which suffices to approximate an image such as the world might cast upon the retinas of the eyes (an example appears on page 3), and it culminates in a *description* that depends on that array, and on the purpose that the viewer brings to it. Our particular concern in this article will be with a description well suited for the recognition of three-dimensional shapes.

The Primal Sketch. It is a commonplace that a scene and a drawing of the scene appear very similar, despite the completely different gray-level images to which they give rise. This suggests that the artist's symbols correspond in some way to natural symbols that are computed out of the image during the normal course of its interpretation. Our theory therefore asserts that the first operation on an image is to transform it into a primitive but rich description of the way its intensities change over the visual field, as opposed to a description of its particular intensity values in and of themselves. This yields a description of markedly reduced size that still captures the important aspects required for image analysis. We call it a *primal sketch.* Consider, for example, an intensity array of 1,000 by 1,000, or a million points in all. Even if the possible intensity at any one point were merely black or white — two different brightnesses — the number of all possible arrays would still be $2^{1,000,000}$. In a real image, however, there tend to be continuities of intensity — areas where brightness varies uniformly — and this tends to eliminate possibilities in which the black and white oscillate wildly. It also tends to simplify the array. Typically, therefore, a primal sketch need not include a set of values for every point in an image. As stored in a computer, it will instead constitute an array with numbers representing the directions, magnitudes, and spatial extents of intensity changes assigned to certain specific points in an image — points that tend to be places of locally high or low intensity. The positions of these points, particularly their arrangement amongst their immediate neighbors — that is to say, the local geometry of the image — must also be made explicit in the primal sketch, as it would otherwise be lost. (It was implicit, of course, in the 1,000-by-1,000 array, but we are no longer retaining data for each of those million places.) One way to do this is to specify "virtual lines" — directions and distances — between neighboring points in the sketch.

The process of computing the primal sketch involves several important steps, but let it suffice that the first of them is comparable with the measurements that are apparently made by simple cells in the visual cortex. A well-defined interaction then takes place between simple-cell-type measurements made at the same orientation and position in the visual field but with different receptive field sizes, so that any given intensity gradient can be succinctly described by measurements made with receptive fields of commensurate size. This is in direct contrast to theories which assert that every simple cell acts as a "feature detector" whose output is freely available to subsequent processes.

Modules of Early Visual Processing. The primal sketch of an image is typically a large and unwieldy collection of data, even despite its simplification relative to a gray-level array; for this is the unavoidable consequence of the irregularity and complexity of natural images. The next computational problem is thus its decoding. Now the traditional approach to machine vision assumes that the essence of such a decoding is a process called *segmentation,* whose purpose is to divide a primal sketch, or more generally an image, into regions that are meaningful, perhaps as physical objects. Tenenbaum and Barrow, for example, applied knowledge about several different types of scene to the segmentation of images of landscapes, an office, a room, and a compressor. Freuder used a similar approach to identify a hammer in a simple scene. Upon

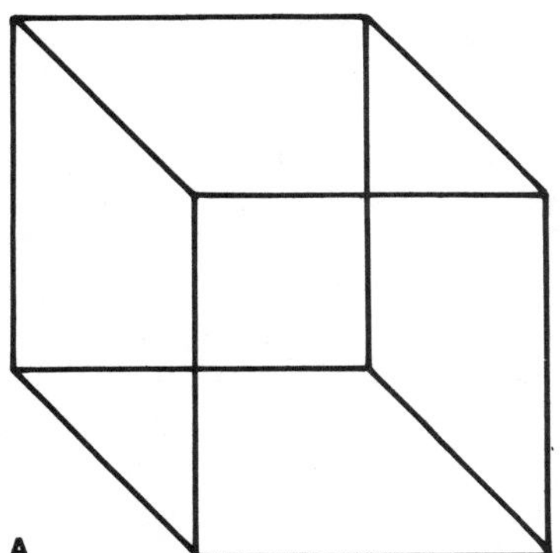

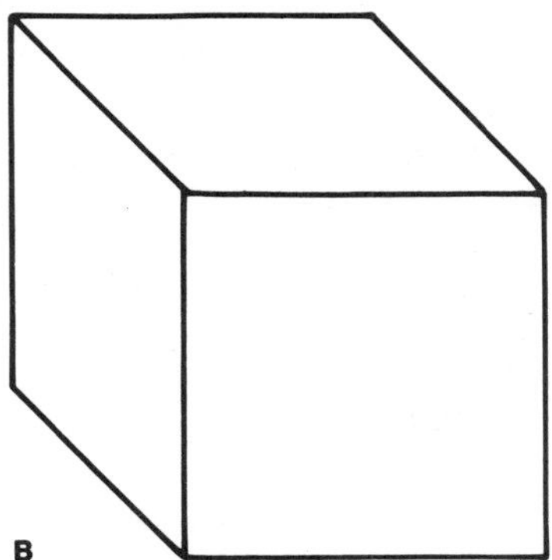

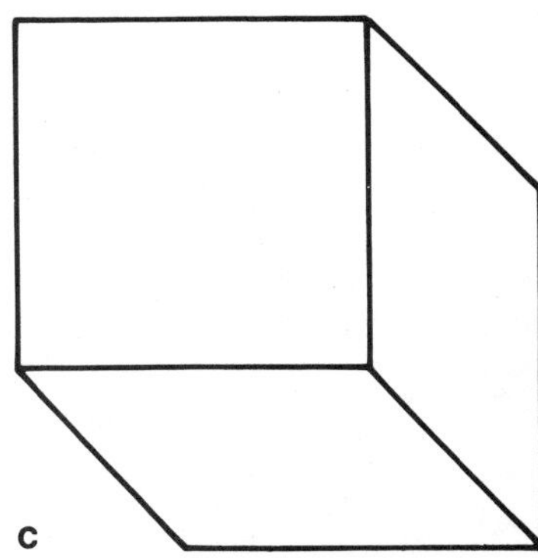

The so-called Necker illusion, named after L. A. Necker, the Swiss naturalist who developed it in 1832. The essence of the matter is that the two-dimensional representation which appears as part (a) of the figure has collapsed the depth out of a cube, and that a certain aspect of human vision is thus to recover this missing third dimension. It develops that the depth of the cube (or rather in its image) can indeed be perceived, but only to the extent that two interpretations are possible: the two shown as (b) and (c). Your perception of (a) characteristically "flips" from one to the other. Understanding why this should be so is a part of devising a computational theory of vision. By contrast, the understanding of the afterimage that you see when you stare at a lightbulb seems simply to be a matter of understanding the characteristics of the visual "hardware" — in this instance, that a sustained stimulus will fatigue the light-receptive cells of the retina.

finding a blob, his computer program would tentatively label it as the head of a hammer, and begin a search for confirmation in the form of an appended shaft. If this approach were correct, it would mean that a central problem for vision is arranging for the right piece of specialized knowledge to be made available at the appropriate time in the segmentation of an image. Freuder's work, for example, was almost entirely devoted to the design of a system that made this possible. But despite considerable efforts over a long period, the theory and practice of segmentation remain rather primitive, and here again we believe that the main reason lies in the failure to formulate precisely the goals of this stage of the processing — a failure, in other words, to work at the topmost level of visual theory. What, for example, is an object? Is a head an object? Is it still an object if it is attached to a body? What about a man on horseback?

We shall argue that the early stages of visual information processing ought instead to squeeze the last possible ounce of information from an image before taking recourse to the descending influence of "high-level" knowledge about objects in the world. Let us turn, then, to a brief examination of the physics of the situation. As we noted earlier, the visual process begins with arrays of intensities projected upon the retinas of the eyes. The principal factors that determine these intensities are (1) the illuminant, (2) the surface reflectance properties of the objects viewed, (3) the shapes of the visible surfaces of these objects, and (4) the vantage point of the viewer. Thus if the analysis of the input intensity arrays is to operate autonomously, at least in its early stages, it can only be expected to extract information about these four factors. In short, early visual processing must be limited to the recovery of localized physical properties of the visible *surfaces* of a viewed object — particularly local surface dispositions (orientation and depth) and surface material properties (color, texture, shininess, and so on). More abstract matters such as a description of overall three-dimensional shape must come after this more basic analysis is complete.

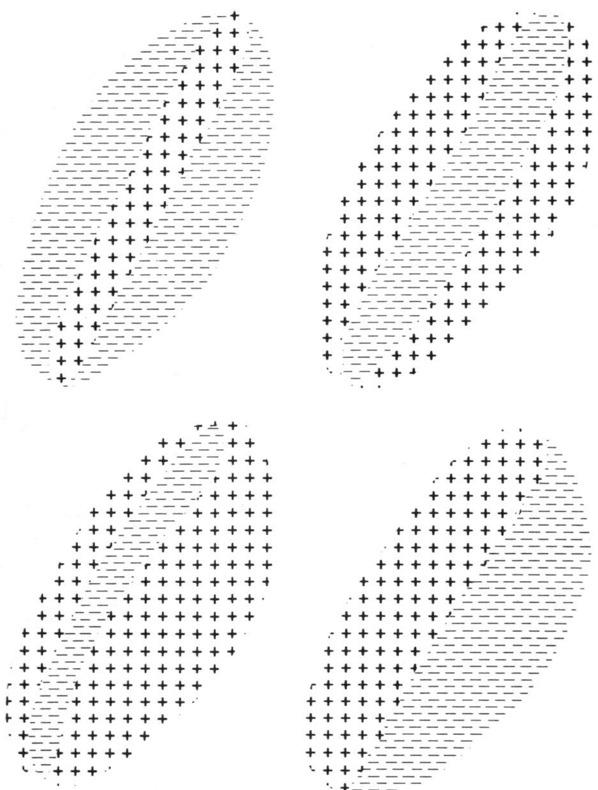

Four examples of "receptive fields" for so-called simple cells of the primary visual cortex. Each field circumscribes the part of the world that is monitored, so to speak, by the cell. But within that locus are bands in which the appearance of light will excite the neuron's ongoing electrical activity (plus signs) and parallel bands that inhibit it (minus signs). The best possible stimulus for the fourth of these examples is a sharp edge in an image with brightness at the left and darkness at the right; for the shining of light on the right-hand side of the receptive field would inhibit, not excite, the associated neuron.

An example of early processing is stereopsis. Imagine that images of a scene are available from two nearby points at the same horizontal level — the analog of the images that play upon the retinas of your left and right eyes. The images are somewhat different, of course, in consequence of the slight difference in vantage. Imagine further that a particular location on a surface in the scene is chosen from one image; that the corresponding location is identified in the other image; and that the relative positions of the two versions of that location are measured. This information will suffice for the calculation of depth — the distance of that location from the viewer. Notice that methods based on gray-level correlation between the pair of images fail to be suitable because a mere gray-level measurement does not reliably define a point on a physical surface. To put the matter plainly, numerous points in a surface might fortuitously be the same shade of gray, and differences in the vantage points of the observer's eyes could change the shade as well. The matching must evidently be based instead on objective markings that lie upon the surface, and so one has to use changes in reflectance. One way of doing this is to obtain a primitive description of the intensity changes that exist in each image (such as a primal sketch), and then to match these descriptions. After all, the line segments, edge segments, blobs, and edge termination points included in such a description correspond quite closely to boundaries and reflectance changes on physical surfaces. The stereo problem — the determination of depth given a stereo pair of images — may thus be reduced to that of matching two primitive descriptions, one from each eye; and to help in this task there are physical constraints that translate into two rules for how the left and right descriptions are combined:

Uniqueness. Each item from each image may be assigned at most one disparity value — that is to say, a unique position relative to its counterpart in the stereo pair. This condition rests on the premise that the items to be matched have a physical existence, and can be in only one place at a time.

Continuity. Disparity varies smoothly almost everywhere. This condition is a consequence of the cohesiveness of matter, and it states that only a relatively small fraction of the area of an image is composed of discontinuities in depth.

In the case of random-dot stereograms, the computational problem is rather well-defined, essentially because of Julesz's demonstration that random-dot stereograms, containing no monocular information, still yield stereopsis. In 1976 Marr and Poggio developed a method for computing local disparities in a pair of random-dot stereograms by an iterative, parallel procedure known technically as a cooperative algorithm. This sort of algorithm has the property that it can be defined completely in terms of simple local interactions because at each of its iterations, each point is affected only by a calculation performed on its immediate neighborhood. Yet all points are so affected during each successive iteration, so the transformations take on a complex global nature. Subsequent comparison of the algorithm's performance with psychophysical data showed that it did not hold up well as a model for human stereopsis. To be sure, it performed better than people do on the standard stereograms like that shown at the right; but it did not explain people's ability to see stereograms in which one of the two images is defocused slightly or enlarged slightly relative to the other. These observations led Marr and Poggio in 1977 to devise another algorithm, this one based on the human use of so-called vergence eye movements, in which the two eyes cross to a greater or lesser extent without changing their average direction of view. This algorithm is consistent with all of the currently known psychophysical data.

A second example of early visual processing concerns the derivation of structure from motion. It has long been known that as an object moves relative to the viewer, the way its appearance changes provides information that we use to determine its shape. The problem decomposes into two parts: matching the elements that occur in consecutive images; and deriving shape information from measurements of their changes in position. Shimon Ullman has shown that these problems can be solved mathematically. His idea is that in general, nothing can be inferred about the shape of an object given only a set of sequential views of it; for some extra assumptions have to be made. Accordingly, he formulates an assumption of rigidity, which states that if a set of moving points has a *unique* interpretation as a rigid body in motion, that interpretation is correct. (The assumption is based on a theorem which he proves, stating that three distinct views of four non-coplanar points on a rigid body are sufficient to determine uniquely their three-dimensional arrangement in space.) From this he derives a method for computing structure from motion. The method gives results that are quantitatively superior to the ability of humans to determine shape from motion, and which fail in qualitatively similar circumstances. Ullman has also devised a set of simple algorithms by which the method may be implemented.

Recovering the Depth of the Three Dimensional World

The following pages provide two pairs of so-called random-dot stereograms as developed at Bell Telephone Laboratories by Bela Julesz. The reader is urged to experiment with them; all that you need, in addition to the images themselves, is a hand mirror that you can hold against either side of your nose. First an explanation: Hold your thumb at various distances from your eyes against a more distant background. Closing first one eye and then the other will then convince you that objects in the world have somewhat different positions in the images that the world casts upon each of your retinas. (The magnitude of the difference is inversely proportional to the distance of the object.) The point of the stereo pair is to show that such disparities are sufficient for your brain to recover the lost third dimension from such two-dimensional images (except for a small percentage of people who lack stereo vision). After all, each of the patterns printed on subsequent pages shows nothing recognizable. Each is a computer-generated assembly of black and white picture-elements ("pixels"). The pair labelled A, however, have a square-shaped region shifted in one of the images several pixels relative to its placement in the other. In short, then, the stereo pair contains *no information whatever about visible surfaces* — except for left-right disparities of the aforementioned sort.

Will this be sufficient for 3-D perception? First of all, cut out the images. Place the pair labelled A on a table-top with a few inches between them. Adhere to "left" and "right" as printed beneath the arrays. Position your head a foot or more above them. Hold the mirror with its back against the left side of your nose, in such a way that your right eye looks directly at the right member of the pair, but your left eye sees the mirror reflection of the left. By suitable maneuvering of the images, your head, and the mirror, get the left and right images to appear to be in the same place — in a word, to coincide. (They would coincide, too, if they were placed in a stereo viewer, but these images have been designed to be used with a mirror, and thus take account of a mirror reflection. They therefore won't work in a stereo viewer.) A few minutes of trying are likely to be required before the image-fusion occurs. Try to relax, and not to strain your eyes. If you achieve stereopsis, there will be no mistaking the effect: it is a striking one. With the mirror reflecting the left image into your left eye, your perception is of a square floating in space above the plane of the background. With the mirror reflecting the right image into the right eye (or alternatively by turning both images upside-down and keeping the mirror as before), the square floats behind. (Many people find this harder to see.) For the effect involving the left-right pair labelled B, consult the illustration and caption on page 12. We wish to express our appreciation to Bela Julesz for the suggestion that a mirror might be used in place of more complicated apparatus to achieve stereopsis.

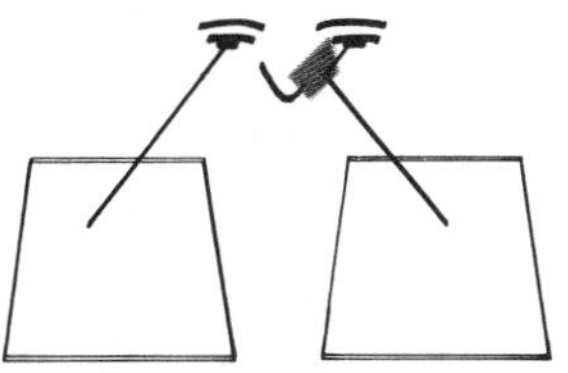

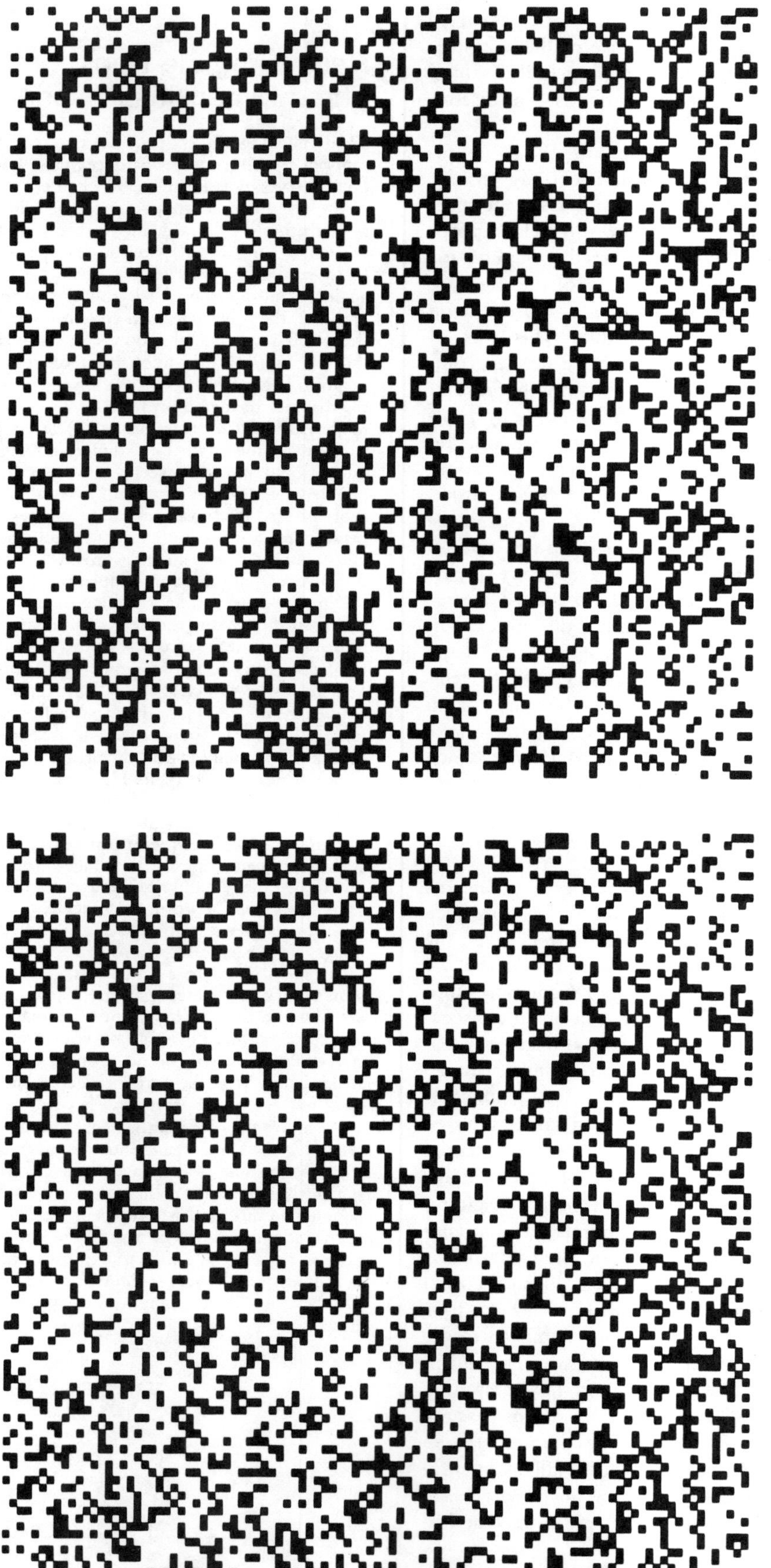

Pair A: Right

Pair A: Left

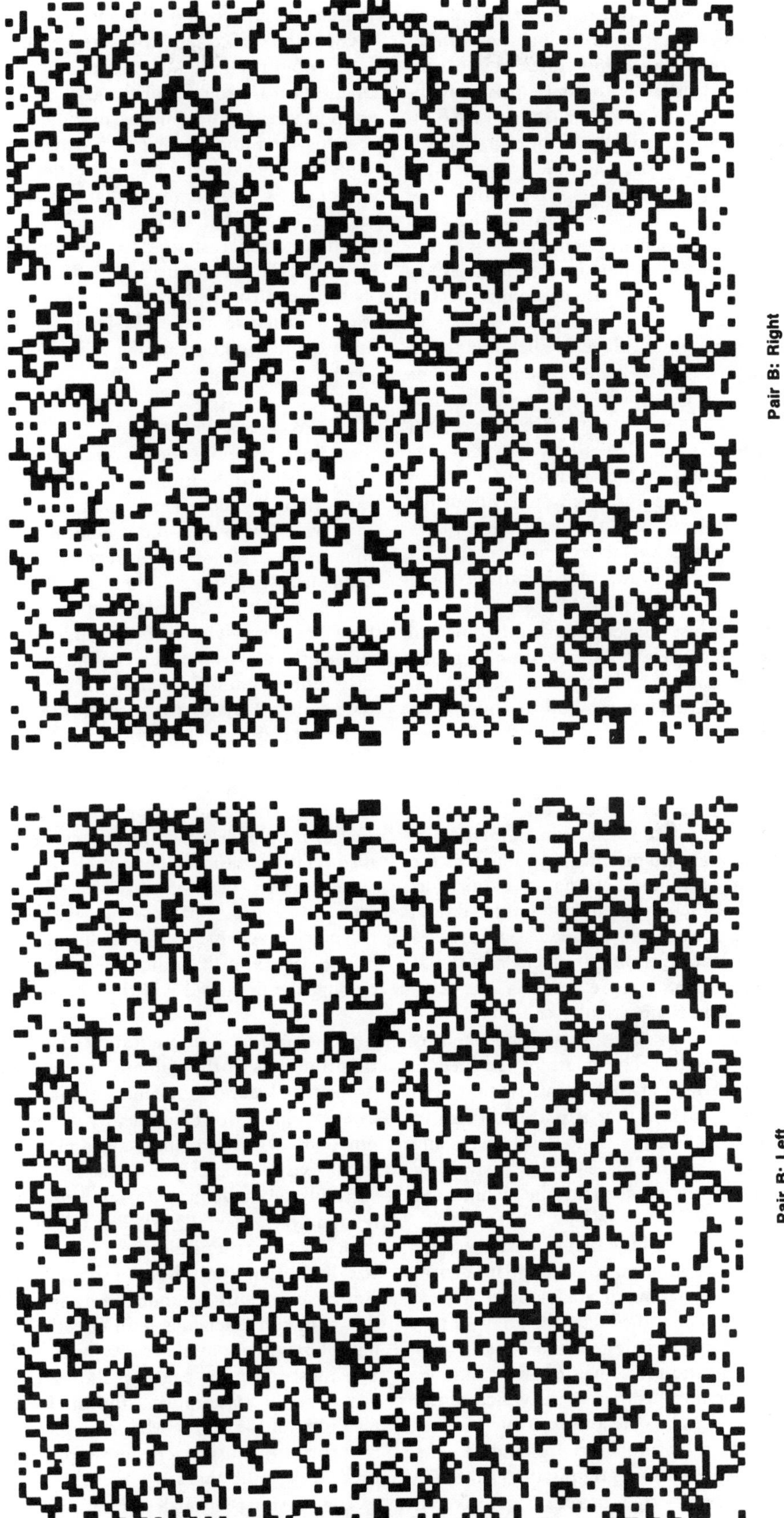
Pair B: Right
Pair B: Left

The 2½-Dimensional Sketch. Both of the techniques of image analysis discussed in the preceding paragraphs provide information about the relative distances to various places in an image. In the case of stereopsis, it is the matching of points in a stereo pair that leads to such information. In the case of structure from motion, it is the matching of points in successive images. More generally, however, we know that vision provides several sources of information about shapes in the visual world. The most direct, perhaps, are the aforementioned stereo and motion, but texture gradients in a single image are nearly as effective. Furthermore, the theatrical techniques of facial make-up reveal the sensitivity of perceived shapes to shading, and color sometimes suggests the manner in which a surface reflects light. It often happens that some parts of a scene are open to inspection by some of these techniques, and other parts to inspection by others. Yet different as the techniques are, they all have two important characteristics in common: they rely on information from the image rather than *a priori* knowledge about the shapes of the viewed objects; and the information they specify concerns the depth or surface orientation at arbitrary points in an image, rather than the depth or orientation associated with particular objects.

In order to make the most efficient use of different and often complementary channels of information deriving from stereopsis, from motion, from texture, from color, from shading, they need to be combined in some way. The computational question that now arises is thus how best to do this, and the natural answer is to seek some representation of the visual scene that makes explicit just the information these processes can deliver. We seek, in other words, a representation of surfaces in an image that makes explicit their shapes and orientations, much as the Arabic representation of a number makes explicit its composition by powers of ten. It might be contrasted with the representation of a surface as a mathematical expression, in which the orientation is only implicit, and not at all apparent. We call such a representation the 2½-dimensional sketch, and in the particular candidate for it shown on page 15, surface orientation is represented by covering an image with needles. The length of each needle defines the dip of the surface at that point, so that zero length corresponds to a surface that is perpendicular to the vector from the viewer to the point, and increasing lengths denote surfaces that tilt increasingly away from the viewer. The orientation of each needle defines the local direction of dip.

Our argument is that the 2½-D sketch is useful because it makes explicit information about the image in a form that is closely matched to what image analysis can deliver. To put it another way, we can formulate the goals of this stage of visual processing as being primarily the construction of this representation, discovering, for example, what are the surface orientations in a scene, which of the contours in the primal sketch correspond to surface discontinuities and should therefore be represented in the 2½-D sketch, and which contours are missing in the primal sketch and need to be inserted into the 2½-D sketch in order to bring it into a state that is consistent with the nature of three-dimensional space. This formulation avoids the difficulties associated with the terms "region" and "object" — the difficulties inherent in the image segmentation approach; for the gray level intensity array, the primal sketch, the various modules of early visual processing, and finally the 2½-dimensional sketch itself deal only with discovering the properties of *surfaces* in an image. One is pleased about that, for we know of ourselves as perceivers that surface orientation can be associated with unfamiliar shapes, so its representation probably precedes the decomposition of the scene into objects. One is thus free to ask precise questions about the computational structure of the 2½-D sketch and of processes to create and maintain it. We are currently much occupied with these matters.

Later Processing Problems

The final components of our visual processing theory concern the application of visually derived surface information for the representation of three-dimensional shapes in a way that is suitable specifically for recognition. By this we mean the ability to recognize a shape as being the same as a shape seen earlier, and this in essence depends on being able to describe shapes consistently each time they are seen, whatever the circumstances of their positions relative to the viewer. The problem with local surface representations such as the 2½-D sketch is that the description depends as much on the viewpoint of the observer as it does on the structure of the shape. In order to factor out a description of a shape that depends on its structure alone, the representation must be based on readily identifiable geometric features of the overall shape, and the dispositions of these features must be specified relative to the shape in itself. In brief, the coordinate system must be "object-centered," not "viewer-centered." One aspect of this deals with the nature of the representation scheme that is to be used, and another with how to obtain it from the 2½-D sketch. We begin by discussing the first, and will then move on to the second.

The 3-D Model Representation. The most basic geometric properties of the volume occupied by a shape are (1) its average location (or center of mass); (2) its overall size, as exemplified, for example, by its mean diameter or volume; and (3) its principal axis of elongation or symmetry, if one exists. A description based on these qualities would certainly be inadequate for an application such as shape recognition; after all, one can tell little about the three-dimensional structure of a shape given only its position, size, and orientation. But if a shape itself has a natural decomposition into components that can be so described, this volumetric scheme is an effective means for describing the relative spatial arrangement of those components. The illustration on page 17 shows a familiar version of this type of description, the stick figure. The recognizability of the animal shapes depicted in the illustration is surprising considering the simplicity of representation used to describe them.

The reason such a description works so well lies, we think, in (1) the volumetric (as opposed to surface-based)

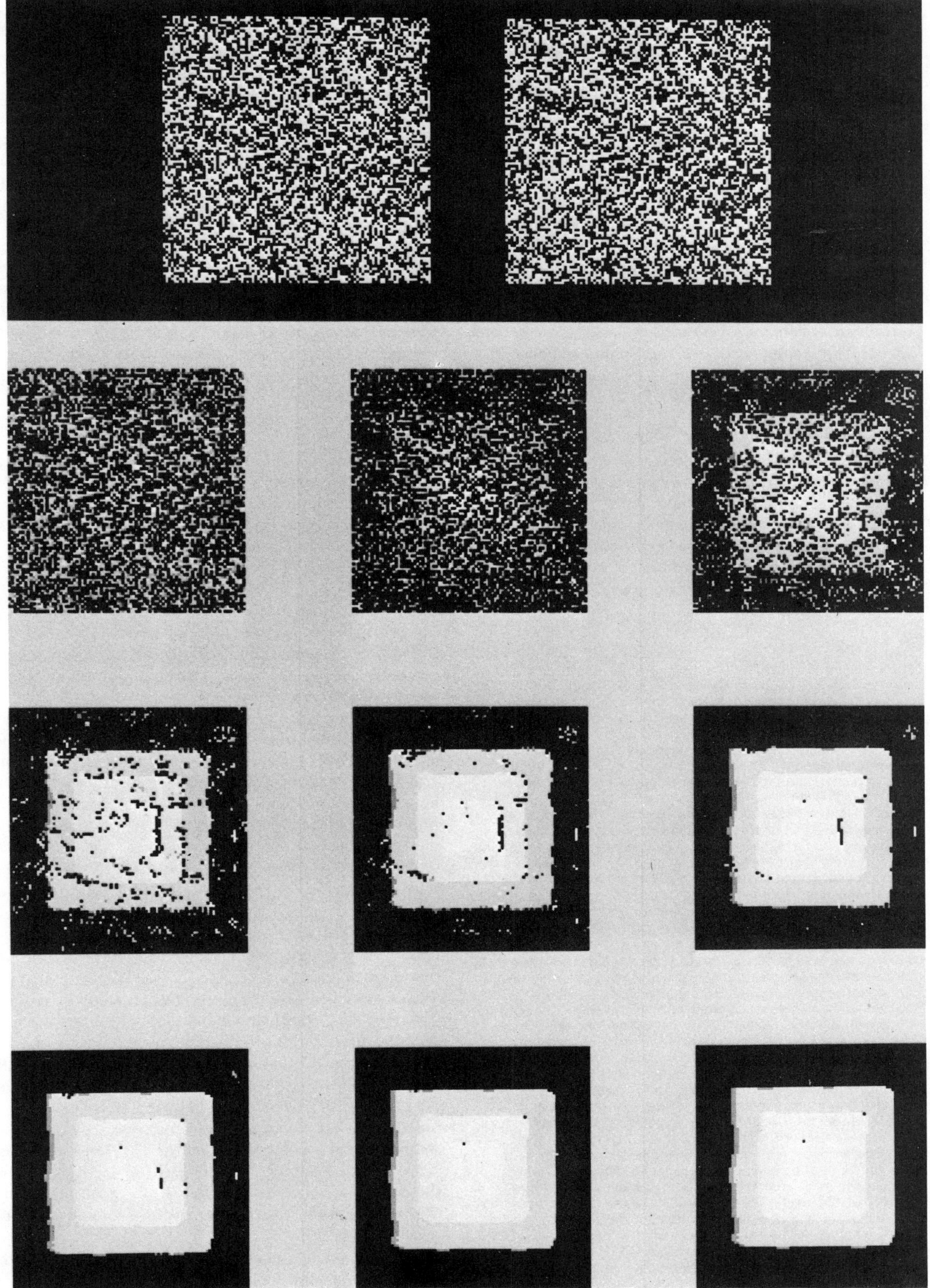

definition of the primitive elements — the sticks — used by the representation; (2) the relatively small number of elements used; and (3) the relation of elements to each other rather than to the viewer. In short, this type of shape representation is volumetric, modular, and can be based on object-centered coordinates. The figure on page 18 illustrates the scheme of representation that was developed from these ideas. Here the description of a shape is composed of a hierarchy of stick-figure specifications we call 3-D models. In the simplest, a single axis element is used to specify the location, size, and orientation of the entire shape; the human body displayed in the illustration will serve as an instance. This element is also used to define a coordinate system that will specify the dispositions of subsidiary axes, each of these specifying in turn a coordinate system for 3-D models of "arm," "hand," and so on. This hierarchical structure makes it possible to treat any component of a shape as a shape in itself. It also provides flexibility in the detail of a description.

Shapes Admitting 3-D Model Descriptions. If the scheme for a given shape is to be uniquely defined and stable over unimportant variations such as viewpoint — if, in a word it is to be canonical — its definition must take advantage of any salient geometrical characteristics that the shape inherently possesses. If a shape has natural axes, then those should be used. The coordinate system for a sausage should take advantage of its major axis, and for a face, of its axis of symmetry.

The decoding of a random-dot stereogram pair, as performed by an algorithm devised by David Marr and Tomaso Poggio in 1976. The nature of the problem is to determine which point in one image is a match to any given point in the other. (Remember that the same surface markings have differing placements in the images cast upon either retina.) After that, a depth can be assigned for any given stereo disparity. The algorithm begins by creating a series of parallel planes to represent possible depths — that is to say, possible distances of various surfaces from the viewer. It then marks this three-dimensional matrix to indicate each location where a local patch of surface could conceivably lie, based on varying construals of the patterns of picture elements in the stereo pair. To phrase it another way, any given pixel in one stereogram is temporarily assumed to match with any of a number of candidate pixels in the other, within a limit of wide angular differences. At this stage, a pair of conditions are applied to each mark in the array thus created: first, that only a single match for any one point in either stereogram will ultimately be accepted; and second, that real 3-D surfaces tend to be continuous in depth. More particularly, at each iteration of the processing that now takes place, the number of marks at a given position but various depths is compared with the number of marks that lie nearby at similar depth. The more of the former, the more likely it is that the mark is incorrectly placed. The more of the latter, the more likely it is that its placement is correct. Thus a weighting of these two factors determines if the mark will be preserved to the next iteration. The illustration shows the original stereo pair, the original matrix computed therefrom, and also the results after one, two, three, four, five, six, eight, and fourteen iterations. Shades of gray are employed to signify marks at greater or lesser depths in the 3-D matrix. The algorithm therefore progressively reveals a nested set of tiers — the pattern, in essence, of a rectangular wedding cake. The reader who succeeds in achieving stereopsis with stereo pair B (printed on page 10 of this article) will see the actual effect that the algorithm here uncovers. It turns out that the algorithm fails under conditions in which human vision is known to succeed — for example, a slight defocusing of the left or right stereogram. In 1977, Marr and Poggio devised a second algorithm, based on different principles, that closely matches human abilities.

Highly symmetrical objects, like a sphere, a square, or a circular disc, will inevitably lead to ambiguities in the choice of coordinate systems. For a shape as regular as a sphere this poses no great problem, because its description in all reasonable systems is the same. One can even allow other factors, like the direction of motion or spin, to influence the choice of coordinate frame. For other shapes, the existence of more than one possible choice probably means that one has to represent the object in several ways, but this is acceptable provided that their number is small. For example, there are four possible axes on which one might wish to base the coordinate system for representing a door, namely the midlines along its length, its width, and its thickness, and also the axis of its hinges. (This last would be especially useful to represent how the door opens.) For a typewriter, there are two reasonable choices, an axis parallel to its width, because that is usually its largest dimension, and the axis about which a typewriter is roughly symmetrical.

In general, if an axis can be distinguished in a shape, it can be used as the basis for a local coordinate system. One approach to the problem of defining object-centered coordinates is therefore to examine the class of shapes having an axis as an integral part of their structure. Consider, accordingly, the class of so-called *generalized cones,* each of these being the surface swept out by moving a cross-section of constant shape but smoothly varying size along an axis, as shown on page 20. Thomas O. Binford has drawn attention to this class of constructions, suggesting that it might provide a convenient way of describing three-dimensional surfaces for the purposes of computer vision. We regard it as an important class not because the shapes themselves are easily describable, but because the presence of an axis allows one to define a canonical local coordinate system. Fortunately, many objects, especially those whose shape was achieved by growth, are described quite naturally in terms of one or more generalized cones. The animal shapes on page 43 provide some examples; the individual sticks are simply the axes of generalized cones that approximate the shapes of parts of these creatures. Many artifacts can also be described in this way — say a car (a small box sitting atop a longer one) or a building (a box with a vertical axis).

It is perhaps worth mentioning the following curious point that has emerged from this way of representing three-dimensional shapes. In 1973 Warrington and Taylor described patients with right parietal lobe lesions (that is to say, damage to a particular part of the cerebral cortex) who had difficulty in recognizing objects seen in "unconventional" views, such as the view of a water pail seen from above in the figure on page 19. The researchers did not attempt to define what makes a view "unconventional." But according to our theory, the most troublesome views of an object will likely be those in which its intrinsic coordinate axes cannot easily be recovered from the image. Our theory therefore predicts that unconventional views in the Warrington and Taylor sense will correspond to those views in which an important axis in the object's 3-D model representation is foreshortened. Such views are by no means uncommon. If a 35mm camera is

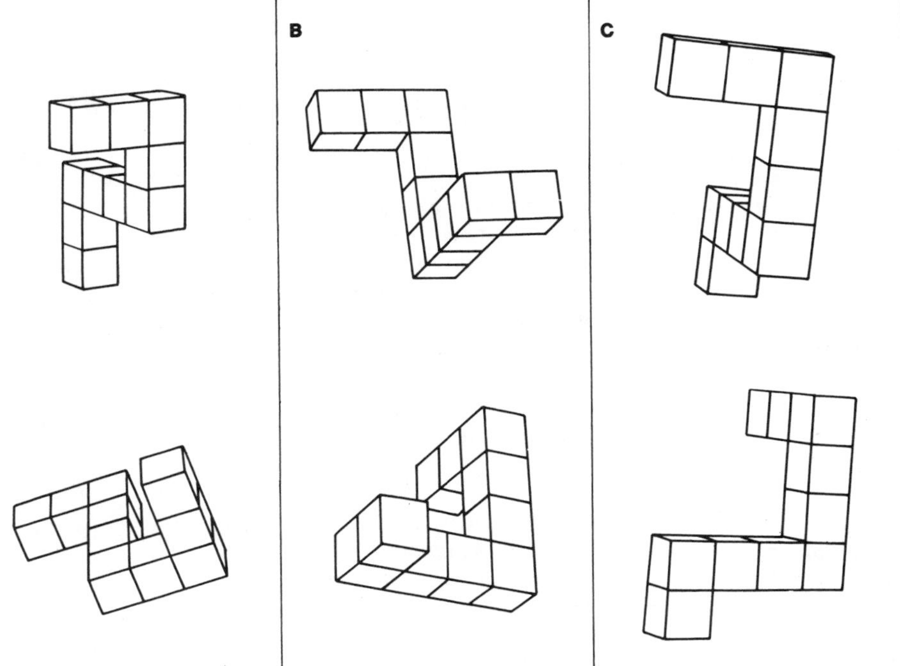

Some drawings similar to those used in Shepard and Metzler's 1971 experiments on mental rotation. The ones shown in (A) are identical, as a clockwise turning of this magazine by 80 degrees will readily prove. Those in (B) are also identical, and again the relative angle between the two is 80 degrees. Here, however, it is a rotation in depth that will make the first coincide with the second. Finally, those in (C) are not at all identical, for no rotation will bring them into congruence. The time taken to decide whether a pair is the same was found to vary linearly with the angle through which one figure must be rotated to be brought into correspondence with the other. This suggested to the investigators that a stepwise mental rotation was in fact being performed by the subjects of their experiments.

directed towards you, you are seeing an unconventional view of it, since the axis of its lens is foreshortened.

It is important to remember, however, that there exist surfaces that cannot conveniently be approximated by generalized cones, for example a cake that has been transected at some arbitrary plane, or the surface formed by a crumpled newspaper. Cases like the cake could be dealt with by introducing a suitable surface primitive for describing the plane of the cut, in much the same way as an axis in the 3-D model representation is a primitive that describes a volumetric element. But the crumpled newspaper poses apparently intractable problems.

Finding the Natural Coordinate System. Even if a shape possesses a canonical coordinate frame, one still is faced with the problem of finding it from an image. Our own interest in this problem grew from the question of how to interpret the *outlines* of objects as seen in a two-dimensional image, and our starting point was the observation that when one looks at the silhouettes in Picasso's "Rites of Spring" (reproduced here on page 22), one perceives them in terms of very particular three-dimensional shapes, some familiar, some less so. This is quite remarkable, because the silhouettes could in theory have been generated by an infinite variety of three-dimensional shapes which, from other viewpoints, would have no discernible similarities to the shapes we perceive. One can perhaps attribute part of the phenomenon to a familiarity with the depicted shapes, but not all of it, because one can use the medium of a silhouette to convey a new shape, and because even with considerable effort it is difficult to imagine the more bizarre three-dimensional surfaces that could have given rise to the same silhouettes. The paradox, then, is that the bounding contours in Picasso's "Rites" apparently tell us more than they should about the shape of the figures. For example, neighboring points on such a contour could in general arise from widely separated points on the original surface, but our perceptual interpretation usually ignores this possibility.

The first observation to be made is that the contours that bound these silhouettes are contours of surface discontinuity, which are precisely the contours with which the 2½-D sketch is concerned. Secondly, because we can interpret the silhouettes as three-dimensional shapes, then implicit in the way we interpret them must lie some *a priori* assumptions that allow us to infer a shape from an outline. If a surface violates these assumptions, our analysis will be wrong, in the sense that the shape we assign to the contours will differ from the shape that actually caused them. An everyday example is the shadowgraph, where the appropriate arrangement of one's hands can, to the surprise and delight of a child, produce the shadow of a duck or a rabbit.

What assumptions is it reasonable to suppose that we make? In order to explain them, we need to define the four constructions that appear in the figure on page 21. These are (1) a three-dimensional surface Σ; (2) its image or silhouette S_V as seen from a viewpoint V; (3) the bounding contour C_V of S_V; and (4) the set of points on the surface Σ that project onto the contour C_V. We shall call this last the *contour generator* of C_V, and we shall denote it by Γ_V.

Observe that the contour C_V, like the contours in the work of Picasso, imparts very little information about the three-dimensional surface that caused it. Indeed, the only obvious feature available in the contour is the distinction between convex and concave places — that is to say, the presence of inflection points. In order that these inflections be "reliable," one needs to make some assumptions about the way the contour was generated, and we choose the following restrictions:

1. *Each point on the contour generator Γ_V projects to a different point on the contour C_V.*
2. *Nearby points on the contour C_V arise from nearby points on the contour generator Γ_V.*
3. *The contour generator Γ_V lies wholly in a single plane.*

The first and second restrictions say that each point on the contour of the image comes from one point on the surface (which is an assumption that facilitates the analysis but is not of fundamental importance), and that where the surface looks continuous in the image, it really is continuous in three dimensions. The third restriction is simply the demand that the difference between convex and concave contour segments reflects properties of the surface, rather than of the imaging process.

It turns out that the following theorem is true, and it is a result that we found very surprising.

Theorem. If the surface is smooth (for our purposes, if it is twice differentiable with continuous second derivitive) and if restrictions 1 through 3 hold for all distant viewing positions in any one plane, as illustrated on page 21, then the viewed surface is a generalized cone. The converse is also true: if the surface is a generalized cone, then conditions 1 through 3 will be found to be true.

This means that if the convexities and concavities of a bounding contour in an image are actual properties of a surface, then that surface is a generalized cone or is composed of several such cones. In brief, the theorem says that a natural link exists between generalized cones and the imaging process itself. The combination of these two must mean, we think, that generalized cones will play an intimate role in the development of vision theory.

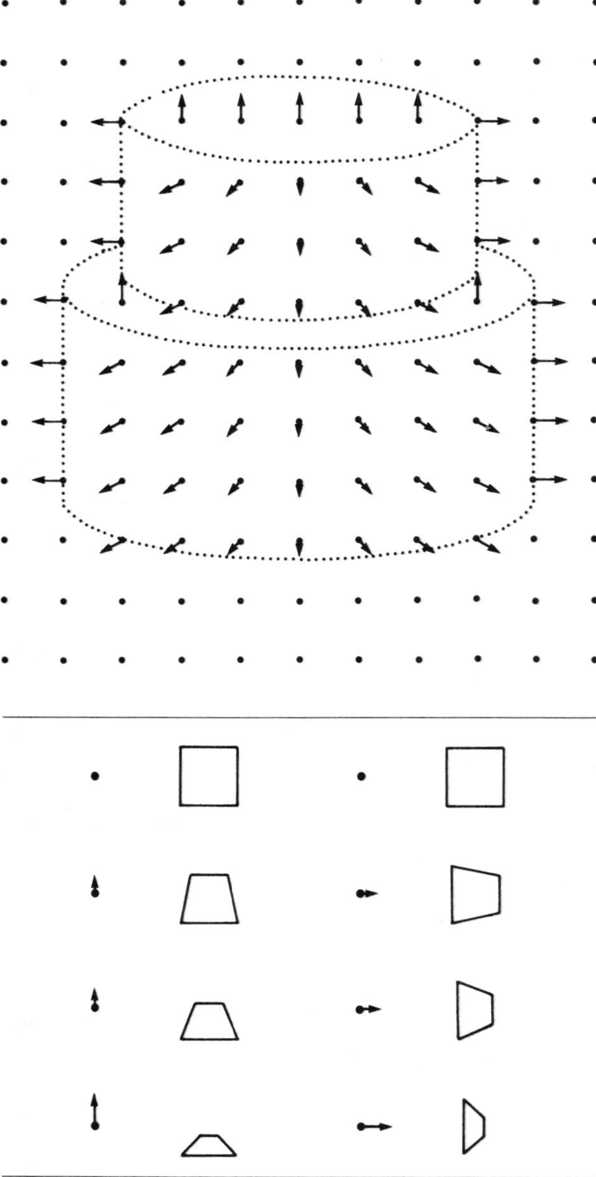

A candidate for the so-called 2½-dimensional sketch, which encompasses local determinations of the depth and orientation of surfaces in an image, as derived from processes that operate upon the primal sketch or some other representation of changes in gray-level intensity. The lengths of the needles represent the degree of tilt at various points in the surface; the orientations of the needles represent the directions of tilt — some examples are shown in the insert. Dotted lines show contours of surface discontinuity. No explicit representation of depth appears in this figure.

The Search for a Theory

We have tried in this survey of visual information processing to make two principal points. The first is methodological: namely that it is important to be very clear about the nature of the understanding we seek. The results we try to achieve should be precise ones, at the level of what we call a computational theory. The critical act in formulating computational theories turns out to be the discovery of valid constraints on the way the world is structured — constraints that provide sufficient information to allow the processing to succeed. Consider stereopsis, which presupposes continuity and uniqueness in the world, or structure from visual motion, which presupposes rigidity, or shape from contour, which presupposes the three restrictions just discussed. The discovery of constraints that are valid and universal leads to results about vision that have the same quality of permanence as results in other branches of science.

The second point is that the critical issues for vision seem to us to revolve around the nature of the representations and the nature of the processes that create, maintain, and eventually interpret them. We have suggested an overall framework for visual information processing that includes three categories of representation upon which the processing is to operate. The first encompasses representations of intensity variations and their local geometry in the input to the visual system. One among these, the primal sketch, is expressly intended to be an efficient description of these variations which captures just that information required by the image analysis to follow. The second category encompasses the representations of visible surfaces — the descriptions, in other words, of the physical properties of the surfaces that

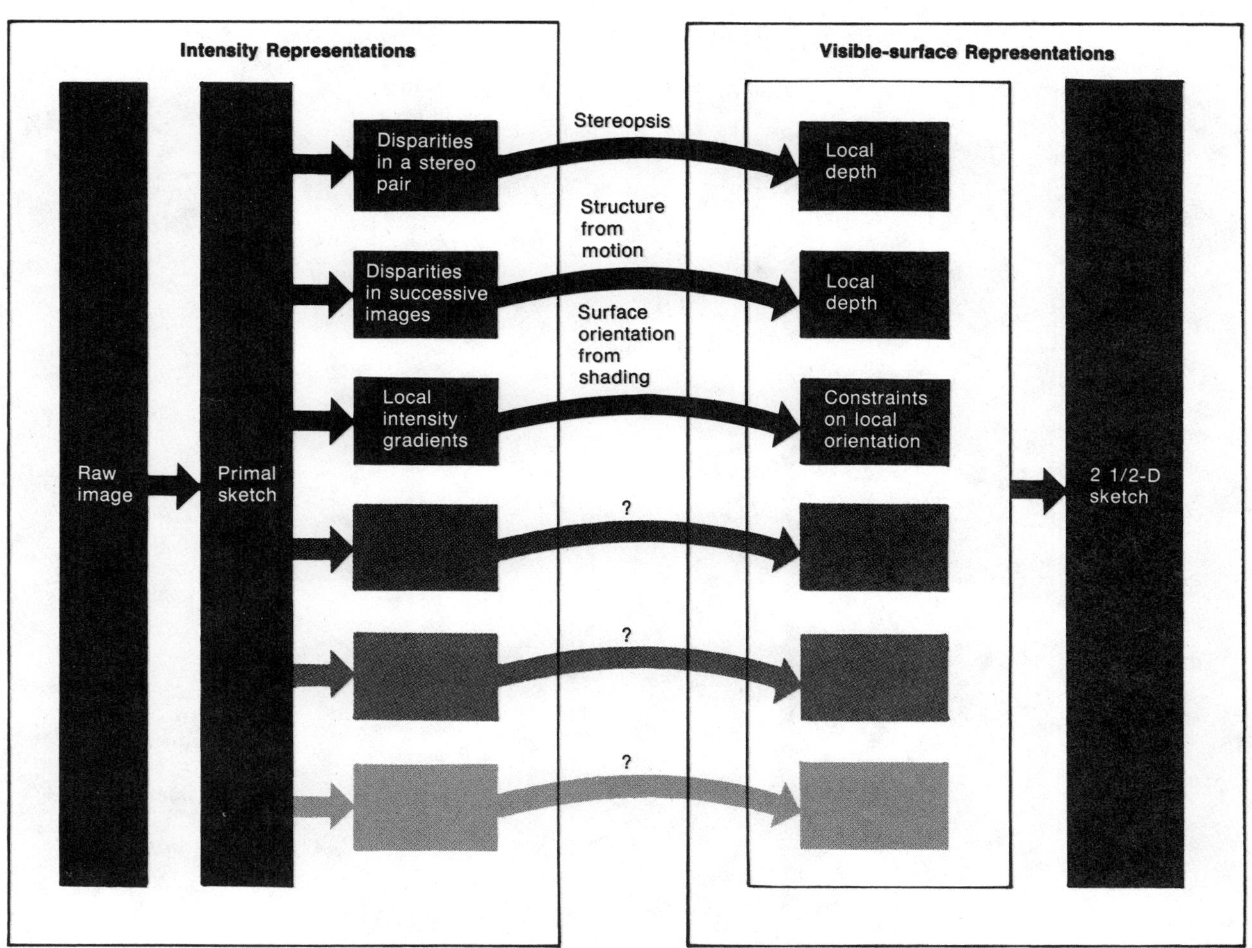

A framework for early and intermediate stages in a theory of visual information processing as proposed by the authors. The computations begin with representations of the intensities in an image — first the image itself, such as the gray-level intensity array shown on page 3, and then the primal sketch, a representation of spatial variations in intensity. Next comes the operation of a set of modules, each employing certain aspects of the information contained in the image to derive information about local orientation, local depth, and the boundaries of surfaces (Further details on the two uppermost modules are supplied in the text.) From this is constructed the so-called 2½-dimensional sketch, as shown on page 15. Note that no "higher-level" information is yet brought to bear: the computations proceed by utilizing only what is available in the image itself.

caused the images in the first place. The nature of these representations — the 2½-dimensional sketch in particular — is determined primarily by what information can be extracted by modules of image analysis such as stereopsis and structure from motion. Like the primal sketch of the previous category, the 2½-dimensional sketch is intended to be a final or output representation: this is where the separate contributions from the various image-analysis modules can be combined into a unified description. The third category encompasses all representations which are subsequently constructed from information contained in the 2½-D sketch. The designs of these tertiary representations are determined largely by the use to which they are to be put, as was the case for the 3-D model representation, to be used for shape recognition. If one had wanted instead, for example, to represent a shape simply for later *reproduction,* say by the milling of a block of metal, then the 2½-D sketch would itself have been sufficient, as the milling process depends explicitly on information about local depth and orientation, such as that sketch can provide.

We conclude with some observations on artificial intelligence in general. First a definition: "Artificial Intelligence" is (or ought to be) the study of information processing problems that characteristically have their roots in some aspect of biological information processing. The goal of the subject is to identify useful information processing problems, and give an abstract account of how to solve them. Such an account is essentially what we have been calling a computational theory — the uppermost of the four levels of understanding described at the outset of this article — and it corresponds to a theorem in mathematics. Once a computational theory has been discovered for solving a problem, the final stage is to develop algorithms that suit it. The choice of an algorithm usually depends upon the hardware available, and there may be many algorithms that implement the same computation. This is not to say that devising suitable algorithms will typically be easy once the computational theory is known, but it is to insist that before one can devise them, one has

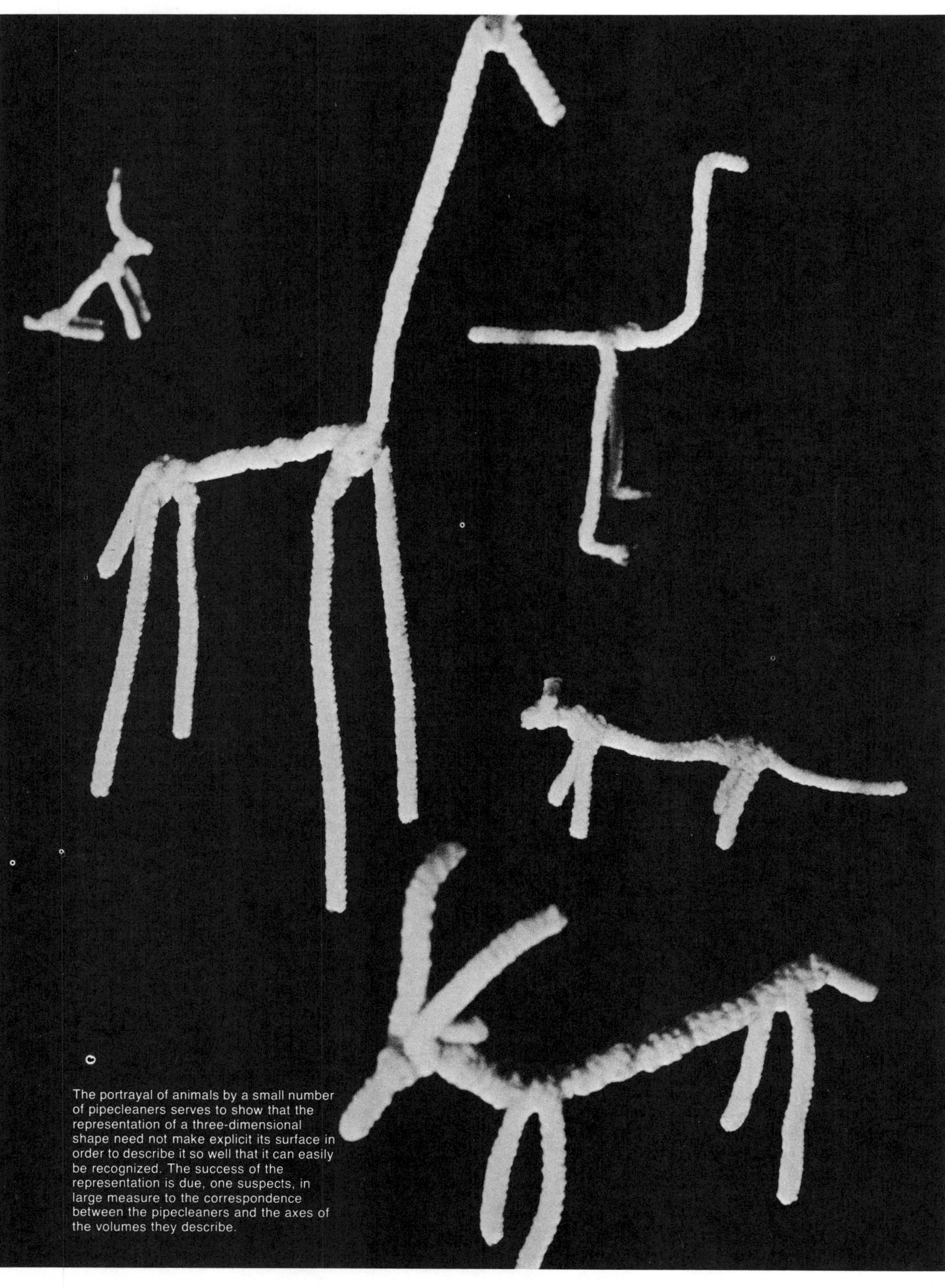

The portrayal of animals by a small number of pipecleaners serves to show that the representation of a three-dimensional shape need not make explicit its surface in order to describe it so well that it can easily be recognized. The success of the representation is due, one suspects, in large measure to the correspondence between the pipecleaners and the axes of the volumes they describe.

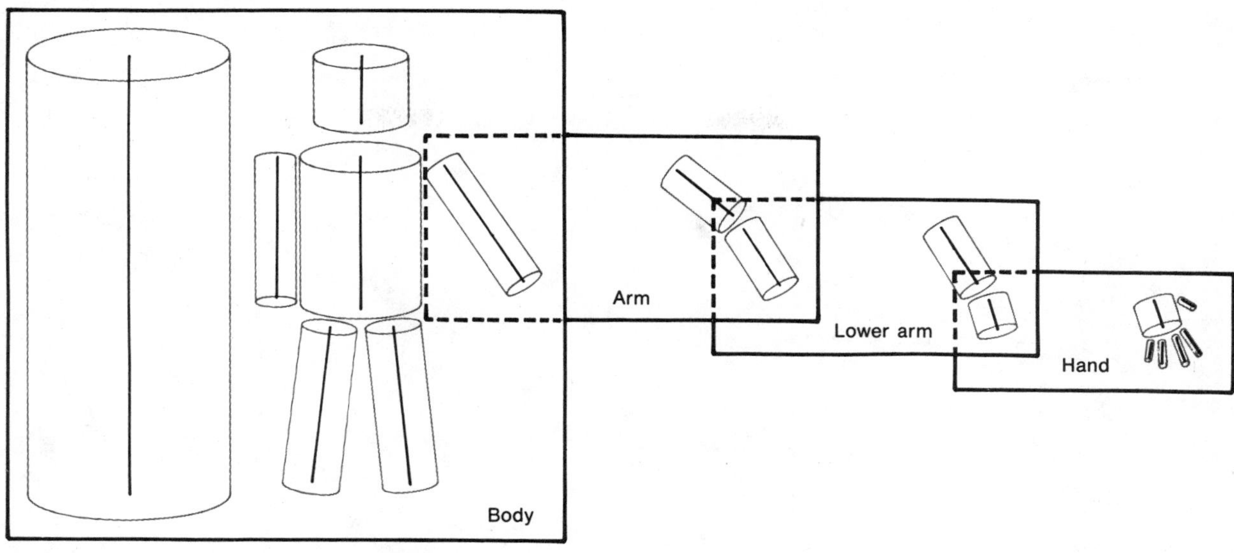

		Origin location			Part orientation		
Shape	Part	ρ	r	θ	i	ϕ	s
Human	head	DE	AB	NN	NN	NN	AB
	arm	DE	CC	EE	SE	EE	BC
	arm	DE	CC	WW	SE	WW	BC
	torso	CC	AB	NN	NN	NN	BC
	leg	CC	CC	EE	SS	NN	CC
	leg	CC	CC	WW	SS	NN	CC
Arm	upper arm	AA	AA	NN	NN	NN	CC
	lower arm	CC	AA	AA	NE	NN	CC
Lower Arm	forearm	AA	AA	NN	NN	NN	DD
	hand	DD	AA	NN	NN	NN	BB
Hand	palm	AA	AA	NN	NN	NN	CC
	thumb	AA	BB	NN	NE	NN	BC
	finger	CC	BB	NN	NN	NN	CC
	finger	CC	AB	NN	NN	NN	CC
	finger	CC	AB	SS	NN	NN	CC
	finger	CC	BB	SS	NN	NN	CC

The arrangement of 3-D models into the representation of a human shape. First the overall form — the "body" — is given an axis. This yields an object-centered coordinate system which can then be used to specify the arrangement of the "arms," "legs," "torso," and "head." The position of each of these is specified by an axis of its own, which in turn serves to define a coordinate system for specifying the arrangement of further subsidiary parts. This gives us a hierarchy of 3-D models: we show it extending downward as far as the fingers. The shapes in the figure are drawn as if they were cylindrical, but that is purely for illustrative convenience: it is the axes alone that stand for the volumetric qualities of the shape, much as the pipecleaners on page 17 serve in themselves to describe the various animals. The illustration also includes a printout of the 3-D model representation as it is stored for use in a computer. The essence of the coding is to express how the various subsidiary axes relate to the shape as whole: where are they, which way are they pointing, and how long are they? For each of the modules, the first three quantities shown in the computer code specify the location of the proximal end of the axis: ρ gives its position along the length of the axis of the overall shape, r gives its distance outward therefrom, and θ gives the angle at which it is found. The last three quantities specify the orientation of the subsidiary axis. Two angles, i and ϕ, serve to give its direction, and a number, s, gives its length. In all cases, angles are specified by a set of compass directions, and lengths by a system of line-segment names; the details need not concern us. Note, however, that there is no *a priori* reason why this scheme ought to be favored; it is simply a possible way to describe a shape in a form that is volumetric, modular, and independent of vantage point.

to know what exactly it is that they are supposed to be doing. When a problem in biological information processing decomposes in this way, we shall refer to it as having a *Type I* theory.

The fly in the ointment is that while many problems of biological information processing may turn out to have a Type I theory, there is no reason why all of them should. Consider in particular a problem that is solved by the simultaneous activity of a considerable number of processes *whose interaction is their own simplest description.* One possible example is the problem of predicting how a protein will fold, since it appears that a large number of influences act concurrently upon a large polypeptide chain as it flaps and flails in a medium. To be sure, only a few of the possible interactions will be important at any one moment, and any attempt to construct a simplified theory must ignore some of the conceivable interactions; but if most interactions are crucial at some stage during the folding, then the simplified theory will prove to be inadequate. As it happens, the most promising studies of protein folding are currently those that take a brute-force approach, setting up a rather detailed model of the amino acids, the geometry associated with their sequence, interactions with the circumambient fluid, random thermal perturbations, *etc.*, and letting the whole set of processes run until a stable configuration is achieved. We shall refer to such a situation as a *Type II* theory.

Now the principal difficulty in artificial intelligence is that one can never be quite sure whether a problem has a Type I solution. If one is found, well and good; but failure to find one does not mean that it does not exist. In particular, if one produces a large and clumsy set of processes that solves a problem, one cannot always be sure that there isn't a simple underlying computational theory whose formulation has somehow been lost in the fog. This danger is most acute in premature assaults on a high-level problem, for which few or none of the concepts that underlie its eventual decomposition into Type I

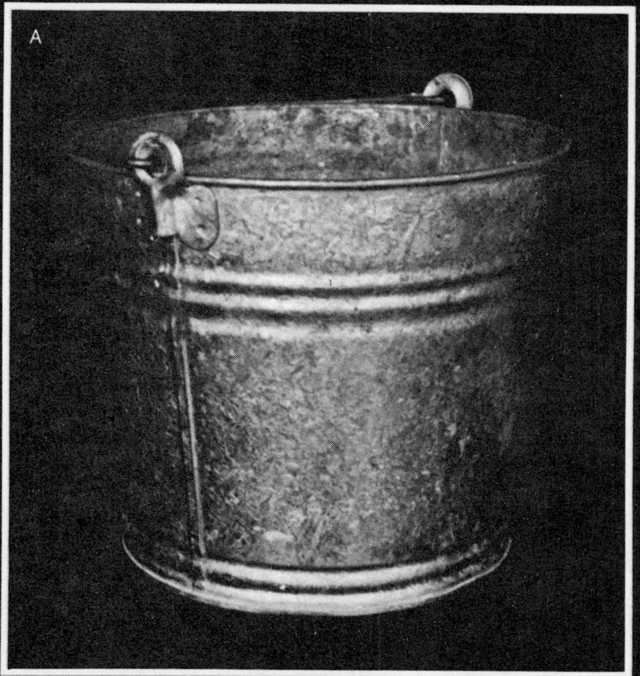

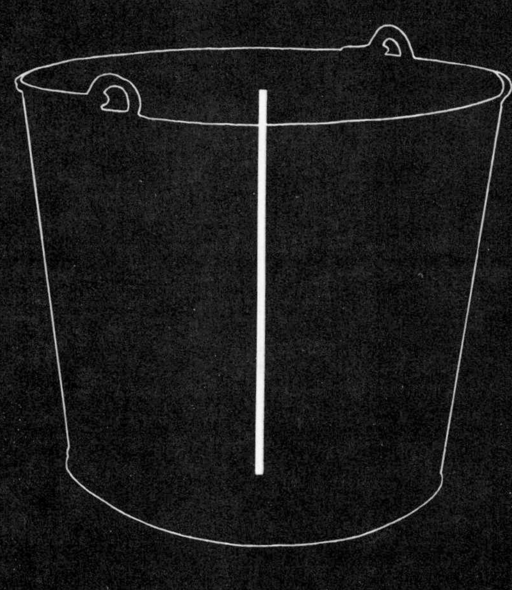

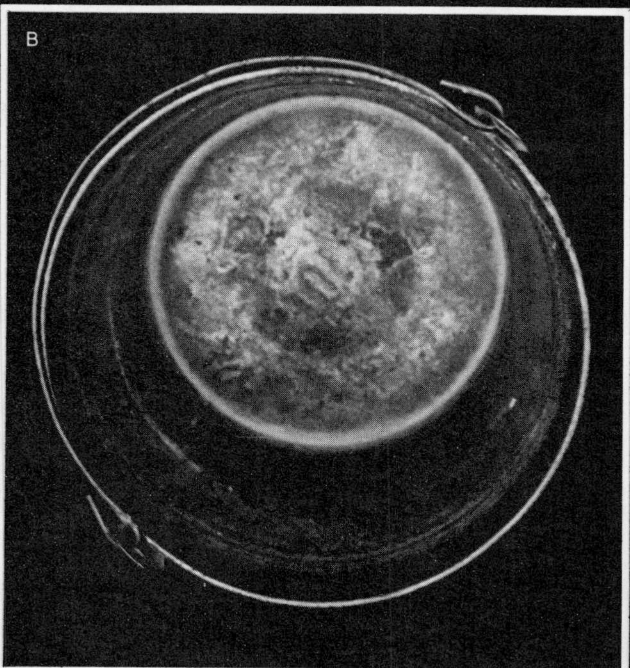

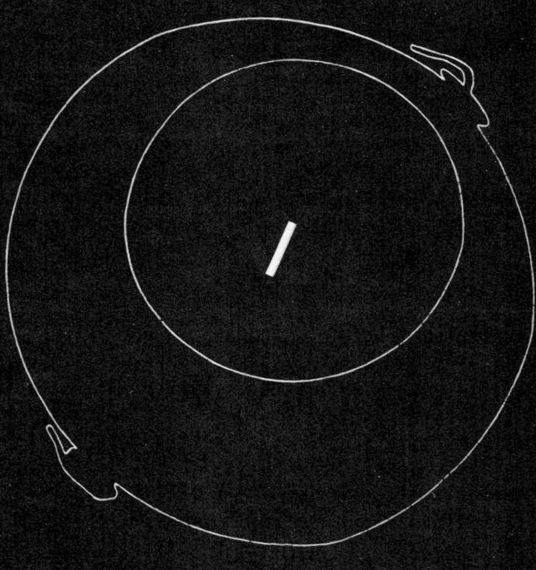

Two views of a water-pail. We display them because Warrington and Taylor reported in 1973 that patients with certain lesions in the right parietal lobe have difficulty in recognizing objects in views such as the one shown in (B). Consider, therefore, that the axis of the water-pail is directly recoverable from an image such as (A), but not from (B), where it is severely foreshortened, as shown by the line drawings that compose the right half of the figure. Consider also that in the 3-D model representation the recognition of a three-dimensional shape relies on the explicit representation of just such an axis. One thus is led by the theory itself to conclude that the recognition of views such as (B) will require considerably more computation than that required for (A).

theories have yet been developed, and one runs the risk of failing to formulate correctly the problems that in fact are involved. In the work of our own group, it first appeared, for example, that image analysis would require a Type II theory. But as more information came to light, we began to see how the analysis might decompose into separate modules for computing certain aspects of visual information — motion, stereoscopy, fluorescence, color — each one of *these* with a theory of Type I. After all, there is no reason why a single theory should encompass the whole. Indeed, one would *a priori* expect the opposite; that as evolution progresses, new modules come into existence that can cope with yet more aspects of the data, and as a result keep the animal alive in ever more widely ranging circumstances. The only important constraint is that the system as a whole should be roughly modular, so that new facilities can be added easily.

Yet even if there turns out to be a Type I theory, or a set of Type I theories, for the extraction of information from sensory data, there would still be no reason why that theory or theories should bear much relation to the theory of more central phenomena. In vision, for example, the theory that says 3-D representations are based on stick-figure coordinate systems and shows how to manipulate them is independent of the theory of the primal sketch, or for that matter of most other stages *en route* from the image to that representation. In short, it is dangerous to suppose that a theory of a peripheral process has any significance for higher level operations.

What, then, shall we say of intelligence? Many people in the field expect that, deep in the heart of our understanding, there will eventually lie at least one and probably several important principles about how to organize and represent knowledge that in some sense captures what is important about the *general* nature of our intellectual abilities. While still somewhat cloudy, the ideas that seem to be emerging are the following:

1. *That the "chunks" of related knowledge for reasoning, language, memory, or perception ought to be larger and have more flexibility in their structure than most recent theories in psychology have allowed.*
2. *That the perception of an object or of an event must include the simultaneous computation of several different descriptions — descriptions that capture diverse aspects of the use, purpose, or circumstances of the object or event.*
3. *That the various descriptions include coarse versions as well as fine ones; for the coarse descriptions are a vital link in establishing correctly the roles played by objects and events.*

An example will help to make these points clear. If one reads

A. *The fly buzzed irritatingly on the window-pane.*
B. *John picked up the newspaper.*

the immediate inference is that John's intentions towards the fly are fundamentally malicious. If he had picked up

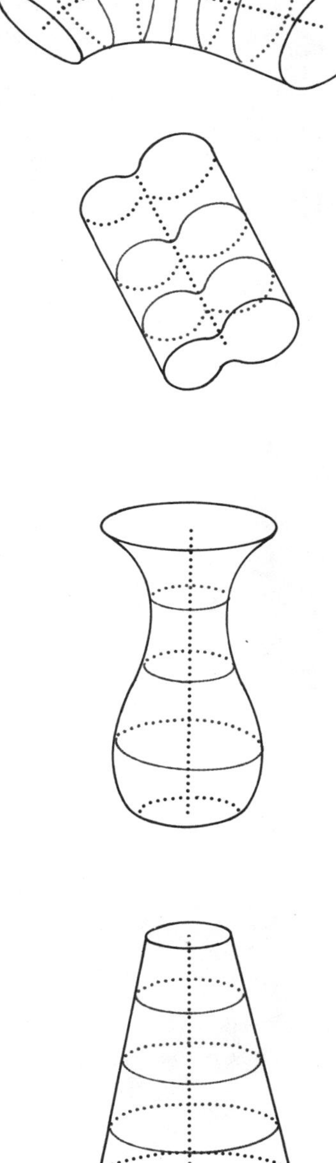

The definition of a generalized cone. In this article, it is the surface created by moving a cross-section along a given straight axis. The cross-section may vary smoothly in size, but its shape remains constant. We here show several examples. In each, the cross-section is shown at several positions along the trajectory that spins out the construction.

the telephone, the inference would be less secure. It is generally agreed that an "insect-damaging" scenario is somehow deployed during the reading of these sentences, being suggested in its coarsest form by the fly buzzing irritatingly. Such a scenario will contain a reference to something that can squash an insect on a window's brittle surface — a description which fits a newspaper but not a hammer. We might therefore conclude that when the newspaper is mentioned (or in the case of vision, seen) not only is it described internally as a newspaper, and some rough 3-D description of its shape and axes set up; it also is described as a light, flexible object with area. Indeed, because sentence (B) might have continued with the words "and sat down to read," the newspaper may also be being described as reading-matter; similarly, as a combustible article, and so forth. It follows that most of the time, a given object or event will give rise to several different coarse internal descriptions. After all, one seldom knows in advance what aspect of an object or event is important. Notice that the description of fly-swatting or reading or fire-lighting does not have to be attached to the newspaper; merely that a description of the newspaper is available that will match its role in each scenario.

The importance of a primitive, coarse catalogue of objects and events lies in the role such coarse descriptions play in the ultimate construction of exquisitely tailored specific scenarios, rather in the way that a general 3-D model description of a shape — one in which only the first level in a hierarchy of stick axes has been specified — can be elaborated as further visual information becomes available to produce eventually a very specific interpretation. What after sentence (A) existed as little more than malicious intent towards the innocent fly becomes, with the additional information about the newspaper, a very specific case of fly-squashing.

Exactly what descriptions should accompany different words or perceived objects is not yet known. In fact, the problems to which we now are led have yet to be precisely formulated, let alone satisfactorily solved. But it seems certain that some problems of this kind do exist and are important; and it seems likely that a fairly respectable theory of them will eventually emerge.

One last observation. It sometimes happens that researchers postulate a particular mechanism or programming style as a central element of the human processor. They then use this mechanism to mimic some small aspect of human performance, for example by writing a language-understanding program, a problem-solving program, or an associative-memory program — each of these applicable only in a highly specialized domain. We believe that such studies are misguided, and the reason is this. If one believes that the aim of information-processing studies is to formulate and understand particular information-processing problems, then it is the structure of those problems that is central, not the mechanisms through which their solutions are implemented. Therefore, the first thing to do is to find operations that we as human beings perform well, fluently, reliably, and hence unconsciously, since it is difficult to see how reliability could be achieved if there were no sound underlying

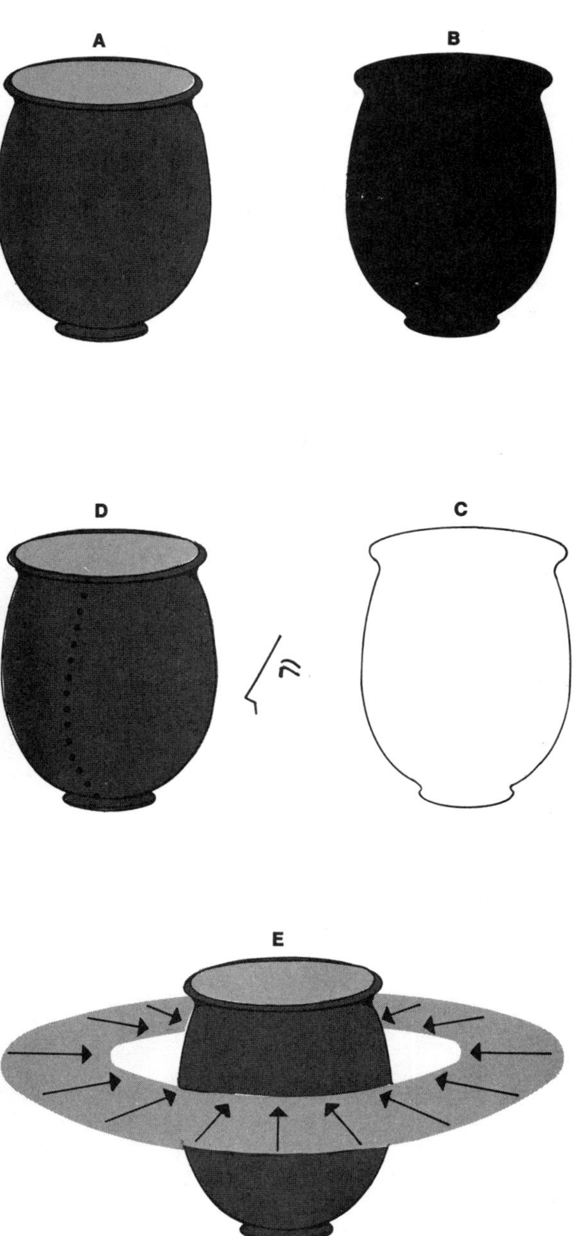

Four structures of importance in studying the *a priori* conditions that we bring to bear on the analysis of a contour. Part (A) shows a three-dimensional surface, Σ. Part (B) shows its silhouette S_V as seen from viewpoint V. Part (C) shows the contour C_V of S_V. Part (D) shows the set of points Γ that project onto the contour. A further part of the illustration shows a condition for a theorem discussed in the text. Here, in particular, the meaning of "all distant viewing directions that lie in a plane" is schematically shown.

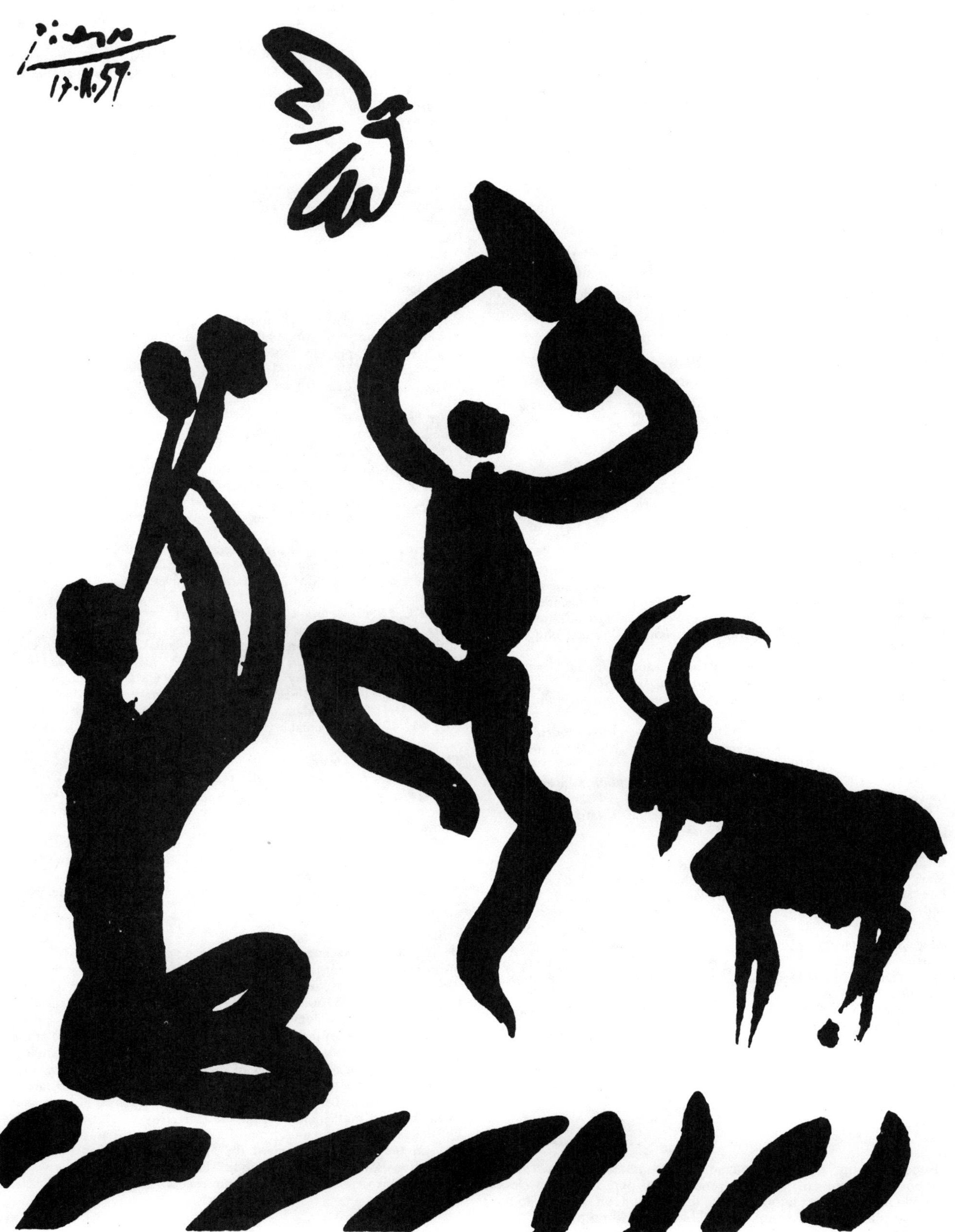
Picasso
17.11.57

computational theory. The next thing is to find out how to do them, and the next after that is to examine our performance in the light of our new understanding. In contrast to all this, current problem-solving research has tended to concentrate on problems that we understand well intellectually, but in fact *perform* poorly, such as mental arithmetic, in which one tries to add, multiply, *etc.* without aids such as pencil and paper; or crypt-arithmetic (for instance, DONALD plus GERALD equals ROBERT, where each letter stands for a digit whose identity is to be found). In other intances the research centers on theorem-proving in geometry or on games such as chess, in which human skills seem to rest on a huge base of knowledge and expertise. We argue that these are exceptionally good grounds for *not* studying how we carry out such tasks — at least not yet. There can be no doubt that when we do mental arithmetic we are doing *something* well, but it is not arithmetic, and we seem far from understanding even one component of what that something is. Let us therefore concentrate on the simpler problems first, for there we have some genuine hope of advancing.

For Further Reading

Levels of Understanding

Marr, D. & Poggio, T. (1977) "From Understanding Computation to Understanding Neural Circuitry." *Neurosciences Res. Prog. Bull. 15,* 470-488. Also available as M.I.T. A.I. Lab. Memo 357.

Conventional Approaches

Newton, I. (1704) *Optics.* London.

Helmholtz, H. L. F. von (1910) *Treatise on Physiological Optics.* Translated by J. P. Southall, 1925. New York: Dover Publications.

Werthheimer, M. (1923) "Principles of Perceptual Organization." In W. H. Ellis, *Source Book of Gestalt Psychology.* London and New York, 1938.

Kuffler, S. W. (1953) "Discharge Patterns and Functional Organization of Mammalian Retina." *J. Neurophysiol. 16,* 37-68.

Kuffler, S. W. & Nicholls, J. G. (1976) *From Neuron to Brain.* Sunderland, Massachusetts: Sinauer Associates.

Hubel, D. H. & Wiesel, T. N. (1962) "Receptive Fields, Binocular Interaction and Functional Architecture in the Cat's Visual Cortex." *J. Physiol., Lond. 160,* 106-154.

Julesz, B. (1971) *Foundations of Cyclopean Perception.* Chicago: The University of Chicago Press.

Shepard, R. N. & Metzler, J. (1971). "Mental Rotation of Three-Dimensional Objects." *Science 171,* 701-703.

A Computational Approach to Vision

Marr, D. (1976) "Early Processing of Visual Information." *Phil. Trans. Roy. Soc. B. 275,* 483-524. Also available as M.I.T. A.I. Lab. Memo 340.

Image Segmentation

Tenenbaum, J. M. & Barrow, H. G. (1976) "Experiments in Interpretation-Guided Segmentation." *Stanford Research Institute Technical Note 123.*

Freuder, E. C. (1975). "A Computer Vision System for Visual Recognition Using Active Knowledge." M.I.T. A.I. Lab. Technical Report 345.

Image-Analysis Modules

Marr, D. & Poggio, T. (1976) "Cooperative Computation of Stereo Disparity." *Science 194,* 283-287. Also available as M.I.T. A.I. Lab. Memo 364.

Marr, D. & Poggio, T. (1977) "A Theory of Human Stereo Vision." To appear in *Proc. Roy. Soc. Lond.* Also available as M.I.T. A.I. Lab. Memo 451.

Marr, D., Poggio, T. & Palm, G. (1977) "Analysis of a Cooperative Stereo Algorithm." *Biol. Cybernetics 28,* 223-239. Also available as M.I.T. A.I. Lab. Memo 446.

Marr, D. (1977) "Representing Visual Information." *AAAS 143rd Annual Meeting, Symposium on Some Mathematical Questions in Biology,* February (in press). Also available as M.I.T. A.I. Lab. Memo 415.

Ullman, S. (1976) "On Visual Detection of Light Sources." *Biol. Cybernetics 21,* 205-212.

Ullman, S. (1977) "The Interpretation of Visual Motion." M.I.T. Ph. D. Thesis, June.

Ullman, S. (1978) "The Interpretation of Structure from Motion." *Proc. Roy. Soc.,* forthcoming.

Ullman, S. (1978) "Two-Dimensionality of the Correspondence Process in Apparent Motion." *Perception 5,* forthcoming.

Ullman, S. (1978) *The Interpretation of Visual Motion.* M.I.T. Press, forthcoming.

Horn, B. K. P. (1975) "Obtaining Shape from Shading Information." In *The Psychology of Computer Vision,* ed. P. H. Winston. McGraw-Hill, New York, pp. 115-155.

Land, E. H. & McCann, J. J. (1971) "Lightness and Retinex Theory." *J. Opt. Soc. Am. 61,* 1-11.

Later Processing Problems

Blum, H. (1973) "Biological Shape and Visual Science (part 1)." *J. Theor. Biol. 38,* 205-287.

Binford, T. O. (1971) "Visual Perception by Computer." Presented to the I.E.E.E. Conference on Systems and Control, Miami, December.

Agin, G. J. (1972) "Representation and Description of Curved Objects." Stanford Artificial Intelligence Project, Memo AIM-173, Stanford University.

Nevatia, R. (1974) "Structured Descriptions of Complex Curved Objects for Recognition and Visual Memory." Stanford Artificial Intelligence Project, Memo AIM-250, Stanford University.

3-D Model Representation

Marr, D. & Nishihara, H. K. (1978) "Representation and Recognition of the Spatial Organization of Three-Dimensional Shapes." *Proc. Roy. Soc. B. 200,* 269-294. Also available as M.I.T. A.I. Lab. Memo 416.

Warrington, E. K. & Taylor, A. M. (1973). "The Contribution of the Right Parietal Lobe to Object Recognition." *Cortex 9,* 152-164.

Marr, D. (1977) "Analysis of Occluding Contour." *Proc. Roy. Soc. B. 197,* 441-475. Also available as M.I.T. A.I. Lab. Memo 372.

The Search for a Theory

Marr, D. (1977) "Artificial Intelligence — A Personal View." *Artificial Intelligence 9,* 37-48.

Levitt, M. & Warshel, A. (1975) "Computer Simulation of Protein Folding." *Nature 253,* 694-698.

Minsky, M. (1975) "A Framework for Representing Knowledge." In *The Psychology of Computer Vision,* ed. P. H. Winston. New York: McGraw-Hill, pp. 211-277.

Newell, A. & Simon, H. A. (1972) *Human Problem Solving.* New Jersey: Prentice Hall.

David Marr is Associate Professor of Psychology at the Massachusetts Institute of Technology. He was educated at Trinity College in the University of Cambridge, receiving his B.A. and M.A. in mathematics and his Ph.D. in neurophysiology, but his education also included training in neuroanatomy, psychology, and biochemistry. After research positions in Britain, he came to the U.S. as an invited visitor at M.I.T. and at the California Institute of Technology. He is author of numerous publications, some of them on theories of neocortex, cerebellar cortex, hippocampus, and the retina. **H. Keith Nishihara** is a Research Associate at the M.I.T. Artificial Intelligence Laboratory. He received his B.A. and M.A., both in mathematics, from the University of Hawaii, and his Ph.D., again in mathematics, from M.I.T., where his thesis, under Marr, was on the "Representation of the Spatial Organization of Three-Dimensional Shapes for Recognition." From 1972 to 1975 he was a National Science Foundation Graduate Fellow.

"Rites of Spring," by Pablo Picasso. We immediately interpret such silhouettes in terms of particular three-dimensional surfaces — this despite the paucity of information in the image itself. In order to do this, we plainly must unconsciously invoke certain a priori assumptions and constraints about the nature of the shapes. Further details are discussed in the text.

15

S. R. Lehky and T. J. Sejnowski

Network model of shape-from-shading: Neural function arises from both receptive and projective fields

1988. *Nature* 333: 452–454

It is not known how the visual system is organized to extract information about shape from the continuous gradations of light and dark found on shaded surfaces of three-dimensional objects[1,2]. To investigate this question[3,4], we used a learning algorithm to construct a neural network model which determines surface curvatures from images of simple geometrical surfaces. The receptive fields developed by units in the network were surprisingly similar to the actual receptive fields of neurons observed in the visual cortex[5,6] which are commonly believed to be 'edge' or 'bar' detectors, but have never previously been associated with shading. Thus, our study illustrates the difficulty of trying to deduce neuronal function solely from determination of their receptive fields. It is also important to consider the connections a neuron makes with other neurons in subsequent stages of processing, which we call its 'projective field'.

The specific task we set for the network was to determine the magnitudes and orientations of the two principal surface curvatures at the centre of each input surface, and to do this independently both of lateral translations of the surface within a small patch of the visual field, and also independently of the direction of illumination. Surface curvature depends upon the direction of travel along a surface. The principle curvatures are the maximum and minimum curvatures for all trajectories through a particular point, which are always perpendicular to each other, and are good descriptors of local shape.

The network had three layers (Fig. 1*a*): an input layer (122 units), an output layer (24 units), and an intermediate hidden layer (27 units). The input layer consist of arrays of units with circular receptive fields (Fig. 1*b*, *c*), similar to neurons found in the retina and the lateral geniculate nucleus. Output units were selective for both the magnitude and orientation of curvature (Fig. 2*d*). Because of its non-monotonic, tuned response, the activity of a single output unit represented the curvature parameters in a degenerate manner; that is, various input images could lead to the same response. To resolve this ambiguity, curvature parameters were encoded by the pattern of activity in a population of output units having different, but overlapping tuning curves, analogous to the way that colour can be encoded by the pattern of activity in three broadly tuned channels. This network was intended to model processing for only a small patch of the visual field, about the size handled by a single cortical column. It would have to be replicated at different locations to cover the entire field, perhaps with all components feeding into a higher level network to integrate the local analyses.

Given this three-layer network architecture, the 'back-propagation' learning algorithm[7] was used to organize the properties of the hidden units to provide a transform between the retinotopic space of the input units and the two-dimensional magnitude and orientation parameter space of the outputs. Images of elliptic paraboloid surfaces were used as inputs (Fig. 2*a*, *b*). Sharp edges were excluded from the images, and so the only cues available for computing curvatures were in the shading. The network was presented with many images, and, for each input, responses were propagated up to the output units. The actual output was then compared with the correct output for that image, and all connection strengths in the network were slightly modified to reduce error in the manner specified by the algorithm. Gradually, the initially random connection strengths became organized. The correlation between the correct and the actual outputs reached a plateau of 0.88 after 40,000 presentations, and the network generalized well for images that were not part of the training set. Increasing the number of hidden units failed to improve the network performance, although it did deteriorate when there were too few hidden units. No biological significance is claimed for the algorithm by which the network developed but, rather, the focus of interest is on the resulting mature network.

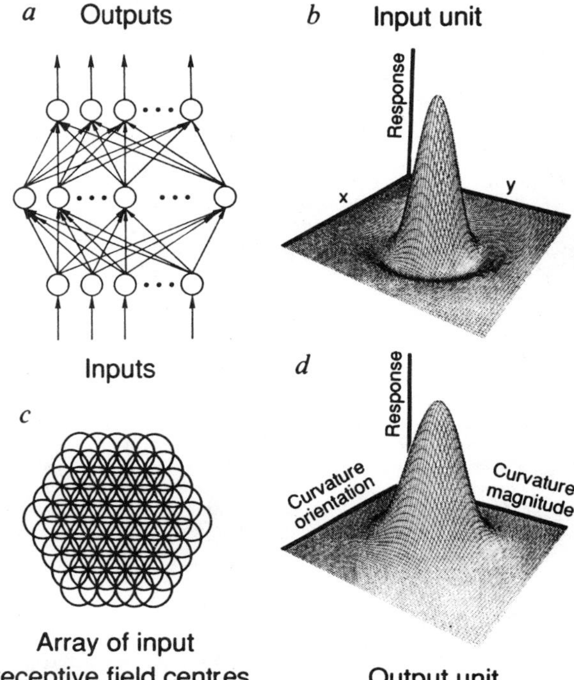

Fig. 1 Organization of neural network that extracts surface curvatures from images of shaded surfaces. *a*, Diagram of three-layer network. Each unit projects to all units in the subsequent layer. The responses of the units in the input layer are determined by the environment. The responses of each unit in the hidden and output layers are determined by summing the activities from all units in preceding layer, weighted by connection strengths which can be positive or negative, and then passed through a sigmoid nonlinearity. Unit activities can assume any value between 0.0–1.0. *b*, Input-unit receptive field, formed by the Laplacian of a two-dimensional guassian. On-centre units have an excitatory centre and an inhibitory surround, while off-centre units have opposite centre/surround polarities. The on- and off-centre terminology does not imply any temporal properties for these units. *c*, Receptive field centres of input units overlapped in a hexagonal array. Images were sampled by both on-centre and off-centre arrays, which were spatially superimposed. *d*, Output-unit response curve, tuned to both curvature magnitude and orientation. The maximum response of each output unit was produced by a different combination of those two curvature parameters. The magnitude axis is on logarithmic scale. Multi-dimensional responses such as this are common in the visual cortex for various parameters, although units selective for surface curvature have not been reported.

An example of the network's response to an image is given in Fig. 2*c* and the network connection strengths underlying this response are shown in Fig. 3. Each of the 27 hourglass-shaped icons represents the connections associated with one hidden unit. The double hexagons in each icon show the connections from all input units to that hidden unit (that is, the receptive field), and the 4×6 array at the top shows the connections between that hidden unit and all output units (that is, the

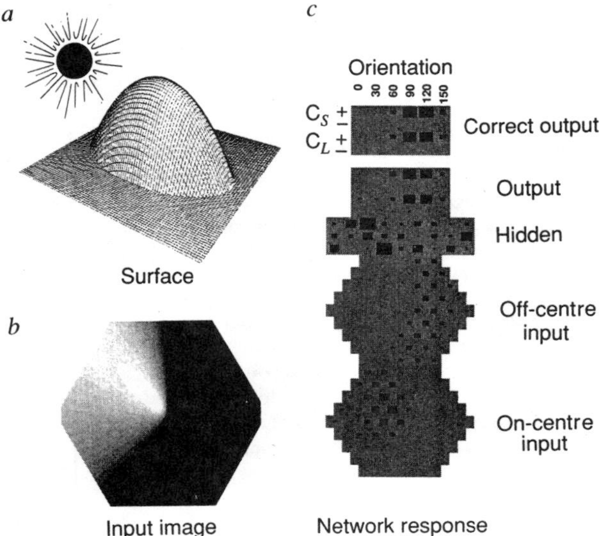

Fig. 2 Typical input image and resulting activity levels within a trained network. *a*, Example of an ellipitcal paraboloid surface. (The flat base did not fall within the input field of the network). *b*, One of 2,000 images used to train the network, synthesized by calulating light reflected from the paraboloid surface. Each image differed in the magnitudes and orientation of the two principal curvatures, in the slant and tilt of illumination, and in the location of the surface centre within the input field. All image parameters were randomly selected from a uniform distribution. The curvature magnitude ranged drom 2 deg^{-1} to 32 deg^{-1} and also −2 deg^{-1} to −32 deg^{-1}, and the curvature orientation from 0° to 180°. The centre of the paraboloid could fall anywhere within the central third of the input field, and the surface normal at the paraboloid centre was always perpendicular to the image plane. Surface reflection was Lambertian, or matte. Illumination came predominantly from one direction but was partially diffused to eliminate sharp shadow edges. The illumination slant fell between 0°–60°. The network was trained to interpret images assuming that illumination came from above (tilt between 0°–180°), and that the signs of both curvatures were the same (that is, the surface was convex or concave). *c*, The network response to an image. The area of a black square indicates a unit's activity. Double hexagons show the responses of 61 on-centre and 61 off-centre input units, calculated by convolving their receptive fields with the image. The responses were rectified, and so they only assumed positive values. These input units cause activity in the 27 hidden units, arranged in a 3×9 array above the hexagons. The hidden units in turn project to the output layer of 24 units, shown in a 4×6 array. This output should be compared with the other 4×6 array at the very top, which shows a correct response to the image. Units within a 4×6 array are arranged as follows. The six columns correspond to different peaks in orientation tuning, at 0°, 30°, 60°, 90°, 120° and 150°. The rows correspond to different curvature magnitudes: the top two rows code for positive (tuning peak: +8 deg^{-1}) and negative (tuning peak: −8 deg^{-1}) magnitudes of the smaller of the two principal curvatures (C_S), while the bottom two rows code the same for the larger principal curvature (C_L) (same tuning peaks). Curvature orientation is unambiguously coded by the pattern of activity in six overlapping orientation-tuning curves. Representation of curvature magnitude, however, remains degenerate because output unit tuning curves in that domain do not overlap. An output can therefore correspond to two curvature magnitudes, which the network cannot distinguish. This remaining ambiguity could be resolved with a larger network containing units that are responsive at different spatial scales.

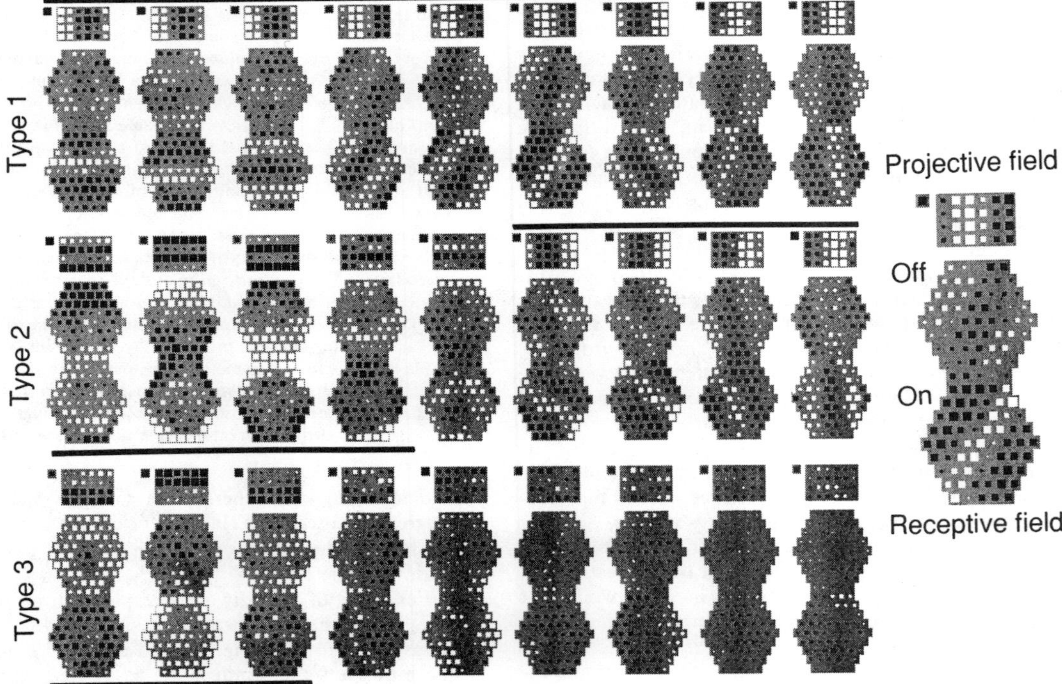

Fig. 3 Connection strength in a typical network. Excitatory weights are white and inhibitory ones are black, and the areas of the squares indicate the connection strengths. Each hidden unit is represented by one hourglass-shaped icon, showing its receptive field (double hexagons) and projective field (4×6 array at the top). The organization of units in the 4×6 array is as described in Fig. 2*c*. The isolated square at the left of each icon indicates the unit's bias (equivalent to a negative threshold). Black horizontal lines group units that have the same type of projective field organization

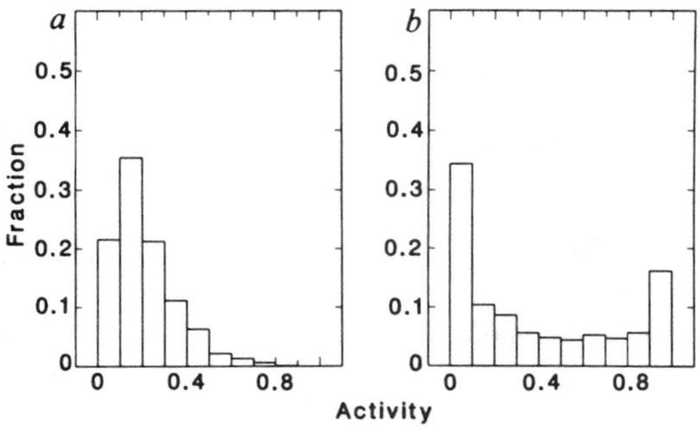

Fig. 4 Distribution of activity levels for two hidden units when the network was presented with the 2,000 images described in Fig. 2*b*. For each image, units gave responses between 0.0 and 1.0, which were grouped into ten bins. *a*, Histogram with a unimodal distribution typical of orientation-selective units (type 1) and of units selective for the relative magnitudes of the principal curvatures (type 3). These units tend to be activated over a range of intermediate levels when presented with many inputs, and appear to act as continuous, tuned filters indicating the values of their respective parameters. *b*, Histogram with typical bimodal distribution for a unit discriminating between positive and negative curvatures (type 2). These units are like feature detectors, tending to be either fully on or off to indicate whether a surface is convex or concave.

projective field). Repeating the learning procedure starting from completely different sets of random weights resulted in essentially the same pattern of connections.

The receptive fields in Fig. 3 are reminiscent of those in the visual cortex[5,6,8]. Excitatory and inhibitory connections are often organized in an orientation-specific and muti-lobed manner, although some are more or less circularly-symmetrical. Upon examining projective fields, however, three types become apparent: type 1 has a vertical pattern of organization to the 4×6 array of weights; type 2 has a horizontal organization with alternate rows being similar; and type 3 has a horizontal organization with adjacent rows being similar. These classes of hidden units appear to provide information to output units about, respectively, the orientation of the principal curvatures (type 1), their signs (convexity/concavity) (type 2), and their relative magnitudes (type 3). The units had different response distributions when presented with many stimuli. Type 1 and type 3 had unimodal distributions (Fig. 4*a*), whereas type 2 units had bimodal distributions (Fig. 4*b*). Based on these distributions, we interpret types 1 and 3 as being filters that indicate values for their respective parameters, and type 2 units as being feature detectors that discrminate between discrete alternatives (convexity and concavity). A few hidden units were difficult to classify, and four failed to develop large weights.

We tried probing the units with simulated bars of light and found that the responses of the hidden units were easily predictable from the pattern of excitatory and inhibitory connections they received from the input units, and that most of these responses appear similar to those of simple cells in the visual cortex[5,8]. In contrast, it required extensive trial and error to find the optimal stimulus for the output units, but this was not surprising as each output unit received convergent inputs from all 27 hidden-unit receptive fields. Some output units had strong 'end-stopped inhibition', similar to that of some complex cells in the cortex[6]. In these units, responses dropped precipitously when the bar length was extended beyond a certain point.

Examination of the receptive fields of individual units does not make apparent what the network is doing, and interpretations other than that of extracting curvatures from shaded images are likely to spring to mind. While this model network obviously does not establish that receptive fields in the cortex which resemble those developed by the network are engaged in shading analysis, it does raise questions about conventional interpretations of the functions of receptive fields, not only in visual pathways, but in other sensory systems as well. Understanding the function of a neuron within a network appears to require not only knowledge of the pattern of input connections forming its receptive field, but also knowledge of the pattern of output connections, which forms its projective field. Indeed, the same neuron may have a number of different functions if it projects to several regions.

This work was supported by an NSF Presidential Young Investigator Award to TJS and a Sloan Foundation grant to TJS and Dr G. F. Poggio.

1. Ramachandran, V. S. *Nature* **331**, 163-166 (1988).
2. Mingolla, E. & Todd, J. T. *Biol. Cyber.* **53**, 137-151 (1986).
3. Ikeuchi, K. & Horn, B. K. P. *Art. Intell.* **17**, 141-184 (1981).
4. Pentland, A. P. *IEEE Transactions on Pattern Analysis and Machine Intelligence* **6**, 170-187 (1984).
5. Hubel, D. H. & Wiesel, T. N. *J. Physiol., Lond.* **160**, 106-154 (1962).
6. Hubel, D. H. & Wiesel, T. N. *J. Neurophysiol.* **28**, 229-289 (1965).
7. Rumelhart, D. E., Hinton, G. E. & Williams, R. J. in *Parallel Distributed Processing: Explorations in the Microstructure of Cognition. Vol.* 1 (eds Rumelhart, D. E. & McClelland, J. L.) 318-362 (MIT Press, Cambridge, 1986).
8. Mullikan, W. H., Jones, J. P. & Palmer, L. A. *J. Neurophysiol.* **52**, 372-387 (1984).

16

D. Zipser and R. A. Andersen

A back-propagation programmed network that simulates response properties of a subset of posterior parietal neurons

1988. *Nature* 331: 679–684

Neurons in area 7a of the posterior parietal cortex of monkeys respond to both the retinal location of a visual stimulus and the position of the eyes and by combining these signals represent the spatial location of external objects. A neural network model, programmed using back-propagation learning, can decode this spatial information from area 7a neurons and accounts for their observed response properties.

THIS article addresses the question of how the brain carries out computations such as coordinate transformations which translate sensory inputs to motor outputs. Visual inputs are collected in the coordinate frame of the retina on which the visual environment is imaged, but motor movements such as reaching are made to locations in external space. Changes in eye position will alter the retinal locations of targets while their spatial locations remain constant. As a result, visual inputs must be transformed from retinal coordinates to coordinates that specify the location of visual objects with respect to the body to perform accurately directed movements.

Lesions to the posterior parietal cortex in monkeys and humans produce profound spatial deficits in both motor behaviour and perception[1-5]. Humans with lesions to this area can still see but they appear to be unable to integrate the position of their bodies with respect to visual inputs. The lesion data further suggest that it is the inferior parietal lobule, which comprises the posterior half of the posterior parietal cortex, which is involved in spatial processes.

Anatomical and physiological experiments in macaque monkeys indicate that the inferior parietal lobule contains at least four separate cortical fields. Area 7a contains visual and eye-position neurons[6-10]; area 7b contains somatosensory and reach-related cells[9,11]; area MST contains visual motion and smooth pursuit eye movement activity (refs 12–14; R. H H. Wurtz and W. T. Newsome, personal communication); and area LIP contains visual and saccade-related activity[15,16]. It has been proposed[10,17,18] that the area most likely to perform spatial transformations is area 7a. Most of the cells in this region were found to receive a convergence of both eye-position and retinal signals. The interaction between eye-position and visual responses was non-linear, and in most cases the visual rsponse could be modelled as a gain that was a function of eye position multiplied by the response profile of the retinal receptive field. Thus the visual receptive field remained retinotopic, but the magnitude of the response was modulated by eye position. This modulation can be shown to produce a tuning for the location of targets in head-centred coordinates that is eye-position-dependent; the cells will fire most for a particular location in craniotopic space, but only when the eyes are at the appropriate positions in the orbits. No cells were found that coded target location over all eye positions (eye-position-independent coding), indicating that this information can only be contained in the pattern of activity of a population of neurons. Here we describe a neural network model that shows how eye-position-independent location can be extracted from a population of area 7a neurons. The model also reproduces the non-linear interactions of eye position and retinal position information seen in actual area 7a neurons, and demonstrates response properties, such as large receptive fields, which are strikingly similar to those observed in single-unit recording studies.

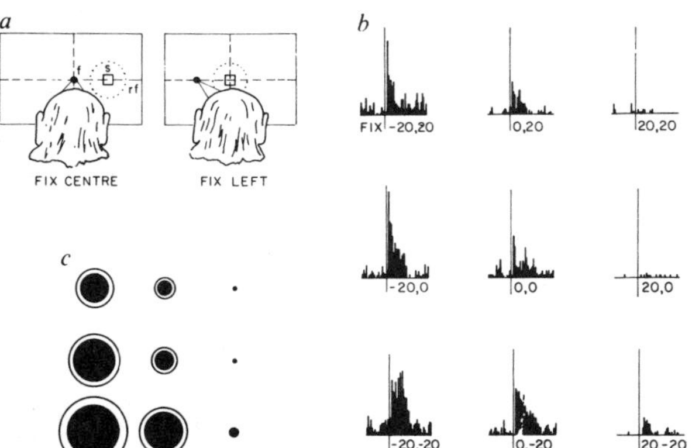

Fig. 1 *a*, Experimental protocol for determining spatial gain fields, with the projection screen viewed from behind the monkey's head. These experiments were carried out several years before the start of the modelling described here[10], but some of the data are being presented for the first time. To determine the effect of eye position, the monkey with head fixed, fixates on a point, *f*, at one of 9 symmetrically placed locations on the projection screen. The stimulus, S, is always presented at the same retinal location, chosen as the maximum-response zone of the retinal-receptive field. The stimulus consists of 1- or 6-degree diameter spots flashed for 500 ms. Each measurement is repeated 8 times. *b*, Peri-stimulus histograms of a typical gain field determination. The nine histograms are located in the same relative positions as the fixations that produced them. The vertical line indicates the time of visual stimulus onset. *c*, A graphic method for illustrating these data in which the diameter of the darkened inner circle, representing the visually evoked gain fields is calculated by subtracting the background activity recorded 500 ms before the stimulus onset from the total activity during the stimulus. The outer circle diameter, representing the total response gain fields, corresponds to the total activity during the stimulus. The annulus diameter corresponds to the background activity that is due to an eye-position signal alone, recorded during the 500 ms before the stimulus presentation.

The neural modelling technique we use differs significantly from most previous approaches, which first found an algorithm to accomplish the computation, and then specified neural models to implement the algorithm. Our approach is based on the use of a neural network training procedure, called 'back propagation', which can programme artificial neural networks to compute arbitrary functions (refs 19–23; S. R. Lehky and T. J. Sejnowski, personal communication). Unlike computer programming, programming by training uses only examples of input and output. This means that it is not necessary to know in advance the algorithm that the network will use; the learning process will discover an appropriate algorithm. Back propagation networks have internal or hidden units that are free to take

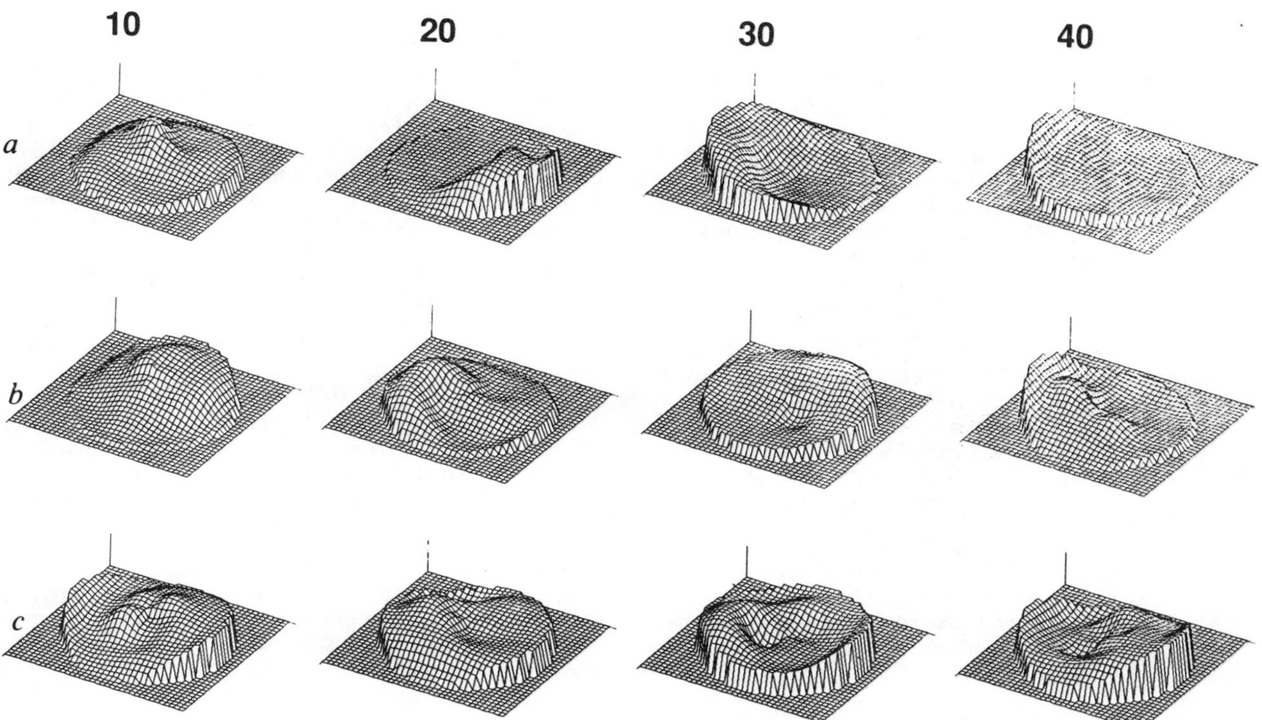

Fig. 2 The receptive fields of spatially tuned neurons from area 7a, arranged in rows with the eccentricity of the field maxima increasing to the right, and in columns with the complexity of the fields increasing downwards. Receptive fields were sampled at 17 radially spaced points, with one sample taken at the centre of the field, and four samples taken on each of four circles of radius 10, 20, 30 and 40 degrees. All the fields in row *a* have single peaks. Those in row *b* have a single large peak but some complexities in the field. The fields in row *c* are the most complex with multiple peaks. The data have been normalized so that the highest peak in each field is the same height.

on the response properties to best accomplish the computational task being learned. It is the properties of these hidden units that we find resemble those of cortical neurons. The back-propagation procedure accomplishes learning by adjusting the strengths of the synapses within the network.

Experimental results from area 7a

The experimental data that must be accounted for by any model of area 7a were collected previously in an extensive series of studies with awake, unanaesthetized monkeys[10]. Here we describe new analyses of these data that facilitate a comparison of area 7a cells with the units generated by training the network model.

Three of the major classes of area 7a neurons are of interest here: the eye-position cells responding to eye-position only (15% of all cells sampled from area 7a), the visual cells responding to visual stimulation only (21%), and the spatially tuned cells responding to both eye position and visual stimulation (57%). Neurons in the first two classes presumably represent the eye position and retinal locaton information available to area 7a as input. The interaction of eye position and visual information found in the third class of cells produces a representation for the head-centred location of visual targets that is eye-position-dependent.

The experimental protocol involved recording neuronal activity extra-cellularly from awake, unanaesthetized monkeys trained in various visuospatial tasks[10] (see Fig. 1). The eye-position sensitivity was tested by having the animal fixate on a small point at different eye positions, with the head fixed in otherwise total darkness. The eye-position cells typically showed a linear increase in activity for a range of horizontal or vertical eye positions, although some cells showed more complex eye-position coding. An ensemble of 30 eye-position unit responses is shown in Fig. 4*c*. The receptive fields of the visual cells were tested by flashing a spot stimulus at different locations in the visual field while the animal fixated on a target at a single eye position. Surfaces were fit to these data points using a gaussian interpolation. These cells typically had large receptive fields equally distributed across the visual field for the population of neurons with a single peak of activity. The shape of the receptive fields approximated a symmetrical gaussian with a $1/e$ width of 15 degrees (see legend to Fig. 4).

The spatially tuned neurons were the largest group and showed a convergence of eye position and retinal position information. The receptive fields are very large (often over 80 degrees in diameter) and have one or more peaks that form a smoothly changing, hilly landscape. A set of 12 retinal receptive

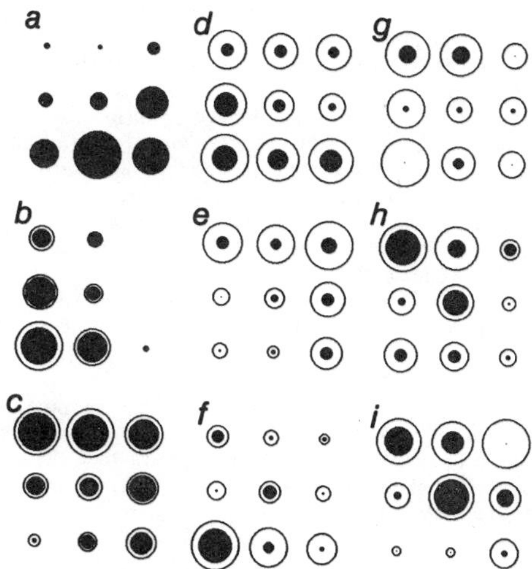

fields from spatially tuned cells, arranged according to peak eccentricity and complexity, is shown in Fig. 2.

As mentioned above, the evoked visual response of spatially tuned neurons varies as a function of eye position. This effect was examined by collecting data under the condition in which the visual stimulus always appears at the peak location in the retinal receptive field, but with the animal fixating at nine different eye positions[10]. These plots are referred to as spatial gain fields. Figure 1 demonstrates the experimental protocol for mapping spatial gain fields.

The majority of the spatial gain fields are roughly planar. This planar behaviour is evident in Fig. 1*c*, where the darkened inner circles are proportional to the magnitude of the visual evoked response, the outer circle diameter to the total activity during the flashed stimulus, and the annulus diameter the background activity due to the eye position alone. The data for the visually evoked response in Fig. 1*c* can be fitted by a plane tilted up for eye positions to the left and also tilted up for downward eye positions. Analysis using linear regressions in the two dimensions of eye position indicated that the gain fields for the visually evoked activity (represented by the dark inner circles) were planar, or had a large planar component, for 55% of the neurons. Interestingly, 80% of the total response gain fields (represented by the outer circles) were planar or largely planar.

A useful way to further characterize the nonlinear combinations of eye and retinal information is to compare the contributions of each to the total response of the cells. This can be done simply by comparing the dark inner circles, which represent the visual contribution to the response, with the white annuli, which represent the eye position contribution to the response. This comparison shows three basic types of gain fields. For 28% the background and evoked activities change in a parallel fashion (Fig. 3*b*, *e*, *f*). In most of the cells (43%), the evoked activity changes with eye position while the background activity, if any, remained constant (Fig. 3*a*, *c*, *d*); three-quarters of these cells had very low or undetectable background activity. The remaining 28% of the neurons showed the interesting property that the background and evoked activities changed in different directions, so that the activity of either alone was grossly non-planar, but the overall activity was planar (Fig. 3*g*, *h*, *i*).

The neural network model

We used a three-layer network (illustrated in Fig. 4) that was trained to map visual targets to head-centred coordinates, given any arbitary pair of eye and retinal positions. The first, or input, layer has two sections, an array of units on which the visual stimulus is represented, and a set of units representing eye position. The second layer consists of the hidden units, which map the input to the output. Each hidden unit receives input from every input unit and projects to every unit in the third output layer. The output of each unit of the hidden and output layers is computed as an S-shaped (logistic) function of the synaptic strength weighted sum of its inputs, plus a bias term.

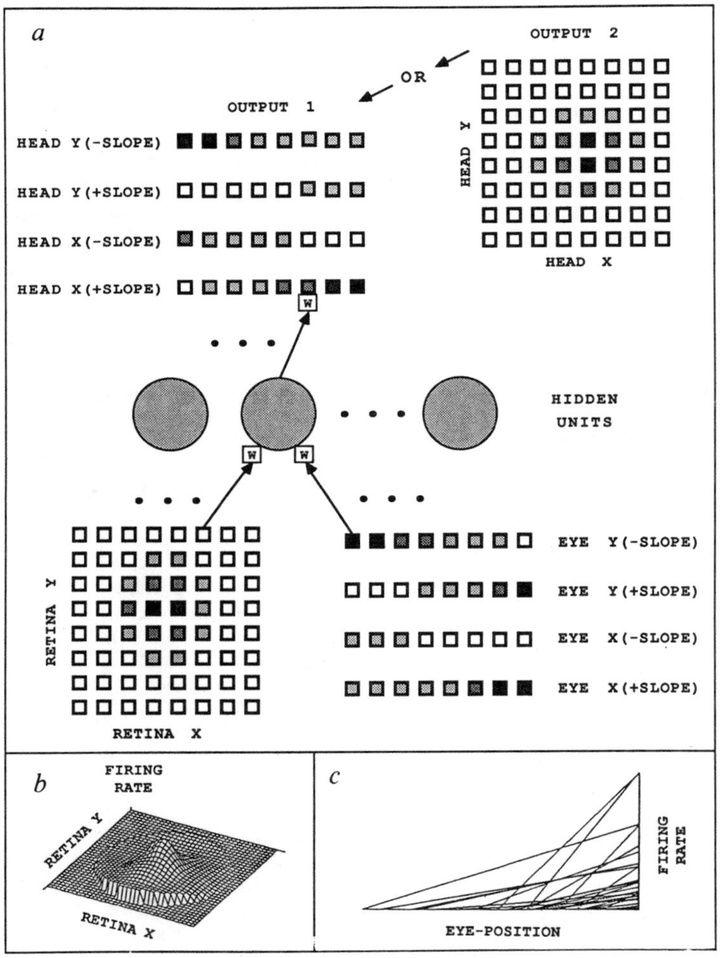

Fig. 4 *a*, Back-propagation network used to model area 7a. The visual input consists of 64 units with gaussian receptive fields with $1/e$ widths of 15 degrees. The centre of each receptive field occupies a position in an 8 by 8 array with 10 degree spacings. The shading represents the level of activity for a single-spot stimulus, with darker shading representing higher rates of activity. The units have been arrayed topographically for illustrative purposes only; this pattern is not an aspect of the model as each hidden unit receives input from every one of the 64 retinal input units. The eye position input consists of 4 sets of 8 units each with two sets coding horizontal position (one for negative slope and one for positive slope) and two sets coding vertical position. Shading represents the level of activity. The intercepts have been ordered for illustrative purposes only and do not represent information available to the hidden layer. Each eye position cell projects to every unit in the hidden layer. Two output representations were used; the gaussian output format is shown on the right and the monotonic format on the left. The gaussian format units have gaussian shaded receptive fields plotted in head-centred coordinates. They have $1/e$ widths of 15 degrees and are centred on an 8 by 8 array in head coordinate space with 10 degree spacings. The monotonic format units have firing rates that are a linear function of position of the stimulus in head-centred coordinates. There are four sets of 8 units with two sets of opposite slope for vertical position and two sets for horizontal position in head-centred coordinates. Again, shading represents the degree of activity and the topographic ordering is for illustrate purposes only. The small boxes containing *W* indicate the location of the synapses whose weights are trained by back propagation. Each hidden unit projects to every cell in the output layer. The output activity of the hidden and output layer units is calculated by the logistic function: $\text{output} = 1/(1+e^{-\text{net}})$, where net = (weighted sum of inputs) + bias. The arrow for the connections represents the direction of activity propagation; error was propagated back in the opposite direction. The back-propagation procedure guarantees that the synaptic weight changes will always move the network towards lower error by implementing a gradient descent in error in the multi-dimensional synaptic weight space. *b*, Area 7a visual neuron receptive field with a single peak near the fovea. Receptive fields were plotted using the same method as in Fig. 3. Visual cells that had no eye-position-related activity or modulation of their responses by eye position were used to model the retinal input to the network. *c*, A composite of 30 area 7a-eye-position units, whose firing rates are plotted as a function of horizontal or vertical eye deviation. The slopes and intercepts are experimental values for eye-position neurons.

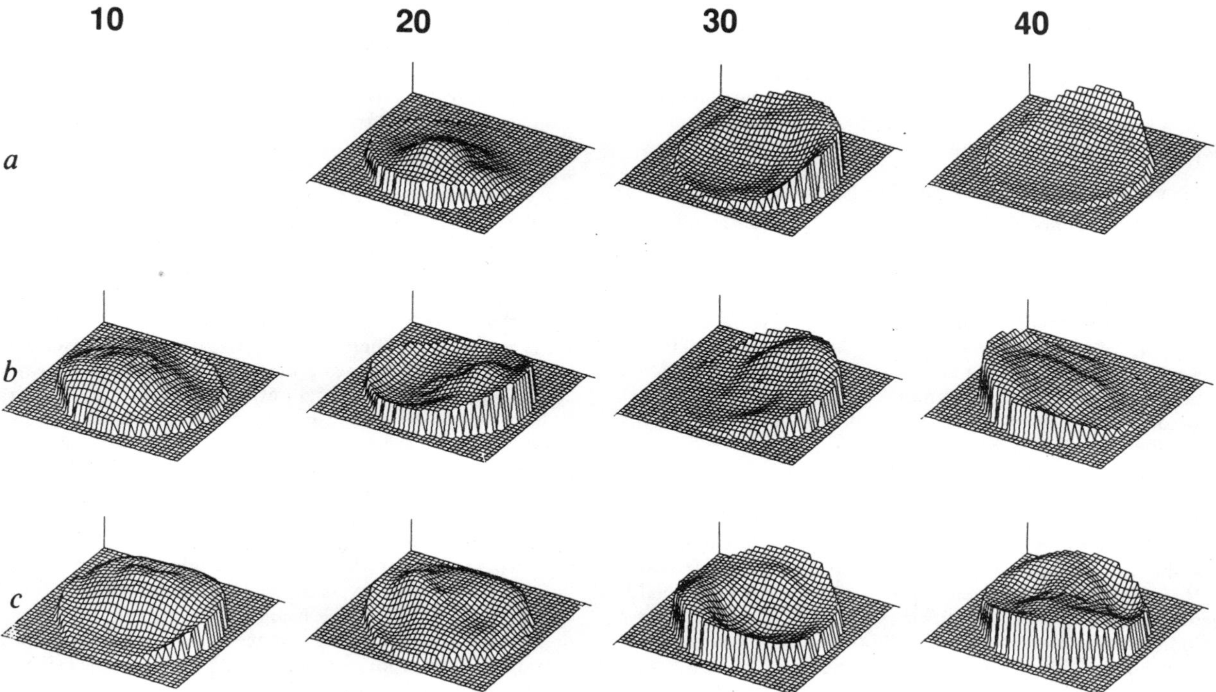

Fig. 5 Hidden unit retinal receptive fields generated by the back propagation model. These plots were generated by holding the eye-position input to the network constant and simulating visual stimulation at the same 17 retinal positions used in the experiments on area 7a. The hidden unit activities were normalized and plotted in the same way as the experimental data shown in Fig. 3. The data shown here are from a series of 4 training sessions using networks with 25 hidden units and the monotonic format output. Similar results were obtained for the gaussian format output. All the fields, except for C-10, C-20 and C-30, are from networks that have received 1,000 learning trials. The remaining three are from untrained networks, resulting only from the random synaptic weights assigned at the start of a training run. Very complex fields are only rarely found in trained networks. No hidden unit with a single peak at 10 degrees appeared in this data set and such units are very rare in trained networks. No spatially tuned neurons with central receptive fields were found in area 7a, and no such fields appeared in the trained model. But central receptive fields are found among the visual neurons in 7a, and this kind of unit was among those used as input to the model network.

The training paradigm uses back propagation learning, which consists of choosing an input and desired output, applying the input to the first layer of the network and propagating the activity it generates through the network to the output units. The actual output is then subtracted from the desired output to generate an error. This error is used to adjust the weights of synapses on the output layer units and hidden layer units in a manner prescribed by the back propagation procedure[19]. Training begins with all weights randomized, resulting in large errors, and the training cycle is repeated until the error is reduced to desired levels.

a b c d e f g h i

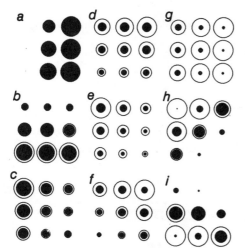

Fig. 6 Hidden unit spatial gain fields generated by the model network. Fields *a*–*f* were generated using the monotonic format output; the rest used the gaussian format output.

The retinal position and eye position inputs to the network are modelled using characteristics of the cells in the posterior parietal cortex that respond to visual stimuli only and eye position only. The visual input consisted of 64 gaussian-shaped receptive fields, with $1/e$ widths of 15 degrees and with each peak separated by 10 degrees in an 8 by 8 array. The eye position input consisted of four sets of 8 units with single sets for positive and negative slopes for horizontal and vertical eye position.

We used two representations of location in head-centred coordinates at the output layer. One (output 2 in Fig. 4*a*) was a gaussian format in which each unit had a gaussian receptive field similar to the representation of the retinal input, but coding location in head-centred rather than retinal coordinates. The other (output 1 in Fig. 4*a*) was a monotonic format, in which the activity of each neuron is a linear function of the location of the stimulus in head-centred coordinates. For the gaussian format, a 64-unit array similar to the retinal input array was used and for the monotonic format, a 32-unit array similar to the eye position input array was used. The gaussian and monotonic formats were chosen because they represent the most common types of coding formats found for brain cells. Also the monotonic format has the interesting feature that it has the same representation as the eye-position code at the input. Thus, if the animal foveates the visual stimulus, the resulting eye-position signal could be used as the teacher to indicate the correct location of the stimulus in head-centred coordinates.

The model network was trained using randomly selected pairs of input eye positions and retinal positions. The teacher signal (desired output) used to train the output units was the true spatial location in head-centred coordinates implied by the inputs, and was represented in either the monotonic or gaussian format. The network trained quickly: after ~1,000 trials, accuracies equivalent to the distance between retinal unit centres were reached. When training was continued, error continued to decrease, but at a lower rate.

Agreement of model with experiment

To evaluate the model, we first compare the experimental and model retinal receptive fields. The model receptive fields were categorized according to their complexity, and the eccentricity of their activity maxima (Fig. 5), as had been done previously for the experimental receptive fields (Fig. 2). Comparison of the top lines in Figs 2 and 5 shows that the trained models generate single-peak receptive fields resembling those observed experimentally at all eccentricities except 10 degrees. The fully trained model also produces moderately complex fields like those found in line 2, but rarely produces receptive fields as complex as those in the bottom line of Fig. 2. This kind of highly complex field is not distinguishable from the untrained model receptive fields shown in the bottom of Fig. 5. The comparison process contains an element of subjectivity, but it demonstrates that the trained model generates retinal receptive fields remarkably similar to the experimentally observed fields. The gain fields generated by the model are shown in Fig. 6. All the total-response gain fields, whether generated by the monotonic or the gaussian output format, were planar in shape. This result compares with 80% of the experimental fields in this planar class. When the model gain fields are examined in more detail, taking into account the non-linearities of the visual response fields, there are significant differences between the eye position and retinal output formats. For example, when trained with the monotonic output format, 67% of the visual response gain fields were planar, but when trained with the gaussian output format only 13% fall in this class. These figures compare with 55% in this class for the experimental data. The irregular visual response gain fields generated by the gaussian output format are more radically irregular than those generated by the monotonic output format. Thus it appears that to account for the details of the visual response gain fields, it may be necessary to use both types of output representation. It should be pointed out, however, that whereas the visual receptive fields and the total gain fields were virtually unaffected by changing parameters of the model, the visual response gain fields were very sensitive to parameters such as threshold value and output representation. The number of hidden units had little effect, giving similar results for simulations ranging from 9 to 36 hidden units.

The striking similarity between model and experimental data certainly supports the conjecture that the cortex and the network generated by back propagation compute in similar ways. As back propagation generates optimal solutions which produce the least error, these results also suggest that the brain chooses optimal solutions with respect to error. The similarity of the model and test results raises the question of what physiological mechanisms could subserve this equivalence. Presently the back-propagation paradigm is structured at a level higher than implementation, and obviously cannot be applied literally to the brain, because information does not travel backwards rapidly through axons. That the back-propagation method appears to discover the same algorithm that is used by the brain in no way implies that back propagation is actually used by the brain. One approach to understanding the physiological significance of these results is to generate models incorporating features found in the brain, such as Hebbian-like learning at synapses and reciprocal back-projection pathways for propagating error, and determine whether these models generate similar results. In this regard it is interesting to note that all cortico-cortical and thalamocortical connections have reciprocal feedback pathways.

An important consideration in interpreting the results is how closely does the model response actually resemble the cortical data? This is a complex issue because there is error in the experimental data, and additional errors introduced by the interpolation process used to produce the full-field views of the receptive fields. Examination of the magnitudes of these errors indicates that they could not account for the various receptive field types, or eye-position gain fields observed experimentally and in the model. The methods of comparison between model and experiment that we have used are to some degree subjective. Perhaps a more objective comparison procedure will eventually be developed, but it is unlikely that, given the complex nature of the data to be compared, any such technique will substantially alter our conclusions concerning the degree of similarity between model and experimental data.

From the physiological perspective these experiments raise the possibility that the posterior parietal cortex learns to associate body position with visual position to localize accurately the position of objects with respect to the body. This idea about the importance of learning is reasonable considering that it would not be practical for spatial representations to be hard-wired because the body dimensions change during development. Furthermore, adaptation experiments show that distortion of space with prisms leads to rapid recalibration, suggesting that these representations are still plastic in adults. As the model, by definition, does not have a topographic organization to localize in space, it shows that the brain does not need a topographic organization to localize in space. The organization of the network is not a product of the spatial position of the cell bodies, but rather is contained in the pattern of the weights of the synaptic connections.

Finally, there is the question of where the output units of the model could exist in the brain. One possible location would be areas that receive projection from area 7a. Although eye position effects on visual responses have been described at several locations in the brain (refs 24–26; S. Funahashi, C. J. Bruce, P. S. Goldman-Rakic; and R. Lal, M. J. Friedlander, personal communication), an eye-position-independent coding has yet to be unequivocally demonstrated. But it is also possible that the final spatial output could only exist in the behaviour of the animal. For example, the muscles innervating the eye or limb are broadly tuned, and the position of the eye or limb is coded in a distributed fashion over the activity of several muscles. Thus the final spatial output may not exist in any single cell in the brain, but rather might be found only in the pointing of the eye or finger accurately to a location in space.

We thank David Rumelhart, Francis Crick and Emilio Bizzi for stimulating discussion during the development of this model and Carol Andersen for editorial assistance. D.Z. was supported by grants from the System Development Foundation, the AFOSR and the Office of Naval Research. R.A.A. was supported by the NIH, the Sloan Foundation and Whitaker Health Sciences Foundation.

1. Critchley, M. *The Parietal Lobes* (Hafner, New York, 1953).
2. Lynch, J. C. *Behav. Brain Sci.* **3,** 484–534 (1980).
3. Andersen, R. A. in *Spatial Cognition: Brain Bases and Development* (eds Stiles-Davis, J., Kritchevsky, M. & Bellugi, U.) (University of Chicago Presss, in the press).
4. Bock, O., Eckmiller, R. & Andersen, R. A. *Brain Res.* (in the press).
5. Andersen, R. A. in *Handbook of Physiology: The Nervous System V* 483–518 (eds Mountcastle, V. B., Plum, F. & Geiger, S. R. (1987).
6. Mountcastle, V. B., Lynch, J. C., Georgopoulos, A., Sakata, H. & Acuna, C. J. *Neurophysiology* **38,** 871–908 (1975).
7. Lynch, J. C., Mountcastle, V. B., Talbot, W. H. & Yin, T. C. T. *J. Neurophysiol.* **40,** 362–389 (1977).
8. Andersen, R. A. & Mountcastle, V. B. *J. Neurosci.* **3,** 532–548 (1983).
9. Andersen, R. A., Siegel, R. M. & Essick, G. K. *Expl Brain Res.* **67,** 316–322 (1987).
10. Andersen, R. A., Essick, G. K. & Siegel, R. M. *Science* **230,** 456–458 (1985).
11. Robinson, C. J. & Burton, H. *J. comp. Neurol.* **192,** 69–92 (1980).
12. Tanaka, K. *et al. J. Neurosci.* **6,** 134–144 (1986).
13. Saito, H. *et al. J. Neurosci.* **6,** 145–157 (1986).
14. Sakata, H., Shibutani, H., Ito, Y. & Tsurugai, K. *Expl Brain Res.* **61,** 658–663 (1986).
15. Gnadt, J. W. & Andersen, R. A. *Expl Brain Res.* (in the press).
16. Andersen, R. A. & Gnadt, J. W. in *Reviews in Occulomotor Research* Vol. 3 (eds Wurtz, R. & Goldberg, M.) (Elsevier, Amsterdam, in the press).
17. Andersen, R. A. in *Neurobiology of Neocortex. Dahlem Koferenzen* (eds Rackic, P. & Singer., W.) (Wiley, Chichester, in the press).
18. Andersen, R. A. & Zipser, D. *Can. J. Physiol. Pharmac.* (in the press).

19. Rumelhart, D. E., Hinton, G. E. & Williams, R. J. in *Parallel Distributed Processing: Explorations in the Microsctructure of Cognition* Vol. 1 (eds Rumelhart, D. E. & McClelland, J. L.) 318–362 (MIT, Cambridge, 1986).
20. Zipser, G. Institute for Cognitive Science, Report 8608 (UCSD, La Jolla, 1986).
21. Zipser, D. & Rabin, D. E. in *Parallel Distributed Processing: Explorations in the Microstructure of Cognition* Vol. 1 (eds Rumelhart, D. E. & McClelland, J. L.) 488–506 (MIT, Cambridge, 1986).
22. Ackley, D. H., Hinton, G. E. & Sejmowski, T. J. *Cognitive Sci.* **9,** 147–169 (1985).
23. Sejnowski, T. J., Kienker, P. K. & Hinton, G. E. *Physica* **22D,** 260–275 (1986).
24. Schlag, J., Schlag-Rey, M., Peck, C. K. & Joseph, J. *Expl Brain Res.* **40,** 170–184 (1980).
25. Peck, C. K., Schlag-Rey, M. & Schlag, J. *J. comp Neurol.* **194,** 97–116 (1980).
26. Aicardi, G., Battaglini, P. P. & Galletti, G. *J. Physiol., Lond.* **390,** 271 (1987).

17

S. M. Kosslyn, C. F. Chabris, C. J. Marsolek, and O. Koenig

Categorical versus coordinate spatial relations: Computational analyses and computer simulations

1992. *Journal of Experimental Psychology: Human Perception and Performance* 18: 562–577.

Results of 4 sets of neural network simulations support the distinction between categorical and coordinate spatial relations representations: (a) Networks that were split so that different hidden units contributed to each type of judgment performed better than unsplit networks; the reverse was observed when they made 2 coordinate judgments. (b) Both computations were more difficult when finer discriminations were required; this result mirrored findings with human Ss. (c) Networks with large, overlapping "receptive fields" performed the coordinate task better than did networks with small, less overlapping receptive fields, but vice versa for the categorical task; this suggests a possible basis for observed cerebral lateralization of the 2 kinds of processing. (d) The previously observed effect of stimulus contrast on this hemispheric asymmetry could reflect contributions of more neuronal input in high-contrast conditions.

Vision, like all other complex mental functions, is accomplished by a method of divide and conquer. Many relatively simple component systems work together to process information (cf. Maunsell & Newsome, 1987; Van Essen, 1985). A major division of labor is achieved by systems in the temporal and parietal lobes, whereby the former encodes object properties (such as shape and color) and the latter encodes spatial properties (such as location and size; see Kosslyn, Flynn, Amsterdam, & Wang, 1990; Maunsell & Newsome, 1987; Ungerleider & Mishkin, 1982). Both of these major systems can be further divided into component subsystems. In this article, we focus on the system that encodes spatial properties and argue that this system is divided into at least two subsystems that compute different kinds of representations of spatial relations.

The research reported here builds on the analyses and findings of Kosslyn (1987) and Kosslyn, Koenig, et al. (1989). We further develop their conception of the two kinds of spatial relations representations by considering implications of the new results reported by Sergent (1991), additional analyses of what is required to build a system that behaves in particular ways (Marr, 1982), and additional facts about the neural substrate. Sergent's findings have led us both to characterize the distinction more rigorously and to link the distinction more tightly to properties of the brain.

Computational considerations suggest that different kinds of representations of spatial relations would be useful for different purposes. Consider two contexts in which people use spatial information. First, people must use spatial information to guide actions, ranging from moving the eyes to reaching and navigating. In fact, many cells in the posterior parietal lobes appear to have some role in movement control, firing either before or after a movement or registering the position of an effector (see Andersen, 1987; Hyvarinen, 1982). For guiding action, metric spatial information must be specified; simply knowing that a table is "next to" a wall does not help one walk right up to it without bumping into the edge.

Second, people often need to encode spatial relations to identify an object or scene. For this purpose, the brain does not need to represent metric information precisely; differences in the precise positions of two objects or parts often are not relevant (and in fact are potentially harmful) for distinguishing them from other objects or parts (cf. Biederman, 1987). Rather, spatial relations are assigned to a category, such as "connected to," "left of," or "above." For some purposes, it may also be useful to assign a spatial relation to a distance category, such as "one inch away," but this sort of category must be distinguished from the kind of analog encoding of metric distance that is necessary to guide action (e.g., see Kosslyn & Koenig, in press; Osherson, Kosslyn, & Hollerbach, 1989).

These considerations lead us to the hypothesis that the brain represents spatial relations in two ways. First, *coordinate* representations specify precise spatial locations in a way that is useful for guiding action. The units of these representations are not equivalence classes; rather, they delineate the finest possible division of space (subject to the resolution limitations of the visual system). These representations do not correspond to particular movements; rather, they specify spatial coordinates in a way that can be used to guide a variety of movements (see Chapter 7 of Kosslyn & Koenig, in press). Second,

---

This work was supported by Grant 88-0012 from U.S. Air Force Office of Scientific Research, Grant BNS 90-09619 from the National Science Foundation, and the National Institute of Neurological Diseases and Stroke Grant 2 P01-17778-09 awarded to Stephen M. Kosslyn. Chad J. Marsolek was supported by a Jacob K. Javits Graduate Fellowship, and Olivier Koenig was supported by Fellowship 81.357.0.86 from the Swiss Science Foundation.

We thank Kris Kirby and Randy O'Reilly for technical assistance; Mark Beeman, Joseph Hellige, and Justine Sergent for helpful comments on an earlier draft; and Robert Rosenthal for valuable statistical advice.

Correspondence concerning this article should be addressed to Stephen M. Kosslyn, Department of Psychology, Harvard University, Cambridge, Massachusetts 02138.

categorical representations assign a range of positions to an equivalence class (such as connected/unconnected, above/below, left/right). For many objects, parts retain the same categorical spatial relations, no matter how the object contorts; thus, the specification of categorical spatial relations is a critical aspect of a robust representation of an object's shape (cf. Marr, 1982). For example, even though its position in space varies widely, a cat's paw remains connected to (a categorical spatial relation) its foreleg regardless of whether the cat is curled up asleep, running, or batting an insect.

We distinguish coordinate representations from those used in recognition partly because the spatial information used to guide action appears to be "encapsulated" (e.g., McLeod, McLaughlin, & Nimmo-Smith, 1985); that is, the information used to guide action is not readily accessible to the systems used to categorize stimuli.

Neuropsychological findings have supported the contention that the two kinds of spatial representations are encoded by separate processing subsystems. Hellige and Michimata (1989), Koenig, Reiss, and Kosslyn (1990), and Kosslyn, Koenig, et al. (1989) all found that subjects judge distances relatively faster when the stimuli are presented initially to the right cerebral hemisphere (i.e., in the left visual field), whereas they evaluate some categorical spatial relations relatively faster when stimuli are presented initially to the left cerebral hemisphere (i.e., in the right visual field) or equally well when stimuli are presented to the left or right hemispheres. Although the left-hemisphere advantage is rarely significant in a single experiment, a trend toward a left-hemisphere advantage for categorical relations was evident in six experiments in which low-contrast stimuli were presented to normal adult subjects (Hellige & Michimata, 1989; Experiments 1, 2, 3, 4 of Kosslyn, Koenig, et al., 1989; Koenig et al., 1990), whereas a trend toward a right-hemisphere advantage was evident only once, in a difference of less than 1 ms (Experiment 4 of Sergent, 1991). According to the binomial distribution (sign test), the probability that this pattern of results is attributable to chance is .06.[1]

More recently, however, Sergent (1991) reported that this dissociation occurs only when stimuli are relatively degraded, and she inferred that this result does not reflect a distinction between two qualitatively different ways of representing spatial relations. Sergent assumed only that when the stimuli are degraded, the right hemisphere can more effectively encode precise spatial location. She offered as one piece of evidence against the distinction the fact that more difficult discriminations (defined by relative distance) affect categorical judgments as well as metric judgments. In addition, Sergent offered arguments that the distinction itself is conceptually flawed.

In this article, we report the results of computer simulations that support three assertions about the distinction between categorical and coordinate spatial relations representation. First, there is a clear conceptual distinction between categorical and coordinate spatial relations representations; second, both sorts of representations are more difficult to compute when fine discriminations must be made, just as was found previously with human subjects; and, third, the effects of stimulus quality can be accounted for easily by reference to a simple computational mechanism. However, Sergent's (1991) findings have led us to reconsider Kosslyn's (1987) original motivation for the distinction between categorical and coordinate spatial representations, which was based on the idea that the left hemisphere is specialized for language and the right is involved in navigation.

Study 1

We have argued that categorical and coordinate spatial relations are qualitatively distinct, and we hypothesized that they are encoded by different processing subsystems. Kosslyn et al. (1990) assumed that these subsystems correspond to separate neural networks, each of which maps an input (in this case, a representation of a pair of locations) to an output (in this case, a representation of a spatial relation). We also hypothesize that separate networks are used to perform qualitatively different types of input/output mappings, such as when different types of spatial relations representations are computed.

Accordingly, it is appropriate to use computer simulations of "neural networks" to investigate whether the two types of computations are in fact qualitatively distinct. These models establish mappings—from sets of input stimuli to correct responses—that appear to share critical features with the corresponding mappings in the brain. For example, Lehky and Sejnowski (1988), O'Reilly, Kosslyn, Marsolek, and Chabris (1990), and Zipser and Andersen (1988) all found that their networks developed an internal organization that mimicked properties of neurons that are thought to be involved in performing the relevant tasks. These networks apparently extracted specific aspects of the input to achieve the mapping, and the brain also extracts those properties when performing the corresponding mapping (for further discussion of this point, see Rueckl & Kosslyn, 1992). It is possible that a simple principle, such as gradient descent or distributed representation, is responsible for such correspondences between the models and the brain, but we need not press this issue further here; for our purposes, all that is important is that these models can be used appropriately to study properties of input/output mappings performed by the brain.

Although we cannot guarantee that the results of studying network simulation models necessarily generalize to the brain, at the very least such results enable us to (a) discover whether

[1] Sergent (1991) reported data from normal subjects for four categorical tasks, three of which involved high stimulus contrast (two tasks from Experiment 1 and one in Experiment 2) and one of which involved low stimulus contrast (Experiment 4). She obtained a 4.5-ms hemispheric difference in one task and differences of less than 1 ms in the other three. Using the Fisher method for combining independent probabilities discussed by Rosenthal (1984, p. 96), we estimated the probability of obtaining differences this small or smaller according to chance. Because some of the F values necessary for this calculation were missing, we estimated them on the basis of the available data; the obtained probability of finding differences this small or smaller was only 0.013, $\chi^2(8) = 19.39$. This finding leads us to suspect that Sergent's findings with high contrast reflect a floor effect for this sort of processing.

certain conclusions or findings can follow from specific assumptions and (b) rule out the possibility that certain conclusions or findings *cannot* follow from specific assumptions.

In the first set of simulations we obtained computational evidence that at least one categorical relation, above/below, is conceptually distinct from the specification of metric location, which is a critical component of coordinate representations.[2] We ran simulations of the bar-and-dot tasks developed by Hellige and Michimata (1989) and also used by Kosslyn, Koenig, et al. (1989, Experiment 3) and Koenig et al. (1990). In these tasks, subjects saw a short horizontal bar and a dot and were asked to determine either whether the dot was above or below the bar (the categorical task) or whether the dot was within a fixed distance from the bar (the coordinate task). In our simulations, the categorical task required the network to judge whether an activated input unit (the dot) was "above" or "below" a landmark (the bar), which consisted of two activated input units flanked by one inactivated input unit to either side. In contrast, the coordinate task required the network to judge whether or not the activated input unit was within four units of the landmark. We considered this a coordinate task because the network had to encode the finest possible distinctions among locations; in contrast, the above/below task required grouping the locations into categories.[3]

We studied these tasks by using the "partition" paradigm developed by Rueckl, Cave, and Kosslyn (1989), in which the efficacies of two types of networks on a pair of tasks are compared; each type performs both tasks simultaneously, using separate sets of output units. In one type of network, all of the hidden units are connected to all of the output units, whereas in the other type, the hidden units are split into two groups. In a "split" network, one group of hidden units is connected exclusively to the output units for one task, whereas the other group is connected exclusively to the output units for the other task. Consequently, the representations developed by the hidden units for one input/output mapping cannot be used for the other, and vice versa. In the "unsplit" networks, in contrast, the hidden units form a single group that is fully connected to all the output units for both tasks.[4]

Following the reasoning of Rueckl et al. (1989), we expected that if two tasks rely on distinct computations, a split network would perform the necessary mapping better than would an unsplit network. The segregation of processing prevents patterns of weights that are useful for accomplishing one input/output mapping from interfering with those that are useful for accomplishing the other mapping. However, this effect may not be evident until the networks have enough hidden units, because a split network has the inherent disadvantage of having fewer connections (and consequently fewer weight space dimensions) than the corresponding unsplit network. With sufficient numbers of hidden units, the advantage of separating distinct representations should overcome the disadvantage of having fewer resources. Accordingly, we systematically varied the number of hidden units.

To establish the input/output mappings, we used the backward error propagation algorithm of Rumelhart, Hinton, and Williams (1986), as modified by Stornetta and Huberman (1987). This algorithm is sometimes characterized as a "learning" procedure, and its behavior is often compared with that of biological systems that learn (e.g., McClelland & Rumelhart, 1986; Rumelhart & McClelland, 1986; Seidenberg & McClelland, 1989). We do not assume that the kind of learning performed by the networks has a direct relation to learning in actual neural networks in the brain. Instead, we use the difficulty of learning in the models solely as a measure of how difficult it is to establish a specific input/output mapping. We treat the amount of error after a fixed number of training trials as a measure of the difficulty of establishing the mapping (cf. Rueckl & Kosslyn, 1992). As noted earlier, we are interested in this type of mapping because it seems to reflect properties of mappings performed by the brain, but we do not regard the *training process* itself as necessarily having any direct correspondence to neural events. If the mappings are distinct, we will have evidence that the conceptual distinction between categorical and coordinate representations is sound, and will be able to rule out the possibility that the two types of representations are logically the same and must be produced by the same computation.

In Part 1 of this study, we compared the ease of establishing categorical and coordinate (metric) mappings in split and unsplit networks with various numbers of hidden units. Each network was trained to establish both types of mappings, and we observed the amount of error after a fixed number of trials. In Part 2, we considered the possibility that any advantage shown by split networks might have nothing to do with the distinct types of representations: Perhaps dividing resources between two tasks is always beneficial, regardless of the nature of the tasks and the degree of similarity between the mappings. To address this question, we compared split and unsplit networks that performed two different variants of the coordinate task, using the same input patterns and network architectures as in Part 1.

Part 1

Method

Materials. We created standard three-level networks that had 28 input units and 4 output units (2 for each task); we parametrically varied the number of hidden units, examining the range from 8 to 17. For each size, we created one unsplit network and split networks

---

[2] We do not mean to imply that a single subsystem necessarily computes all categorical spatial relations. For example, "inside/outside" and "connected/unconnected" may rely on different sorts of mappings than does "above/below." However, we have yet to develop the theory further in this direction.

[3] Although both judgments require a categorization at some level of processing, the above/below judgment requires only approximate localization of the dot, and so the right hemisphere's superior ability to compute precise location is not relevant, whereas the left hemisphere's superior ability to categorize should affect performance. In contrast, although the coordinate task requires categorization to produce the output, the difficult part of the judgment is to evaluate the precise distance. Thus the right hemisphere's abilities should be more important for good performance in this task.

[4] Note that a split network with a hidden units in one partition and b hidden units in the other partition is computationally identical to two separate networks with a and b hidden units.

with 3–6 different ratios of hidden units allocated to the categorical and coordinate tasks. As illustrated in Figure 1, the split networks were identical to the unsplit networks in all respects except for the missing connections across the partition.

As illustrated in Figure 2, the input units were conceptualized as simulating a vertical spatial array. A bar was represented by a four-unit set in which the top and bottom units were always "off" and the middle two units were always "on." This set could appear at any of five positions: at the center of the array, two units up, two units down, four units up, or four units down. A dot was represented by a single activated unit, which could appear at any of eight positions above and eight positions below the bar. Thus there were 5 × (8 + 8), or 80, input patterns in all. Each input pattern was associated with an output pattern, which represented the target values for the four output units, two of which indicated the categorical judgment and two of which indicated the coordinate judgment. For the categorical judgment, one output unit indicated *ABOVE* and the other *BELOW*. For the coordinate judgment, one output unit indicated *IN* and the other *OUT*; the *IN* response was correct if the dot was within four elements of the bar, otherwise the *OUT* response was correct.

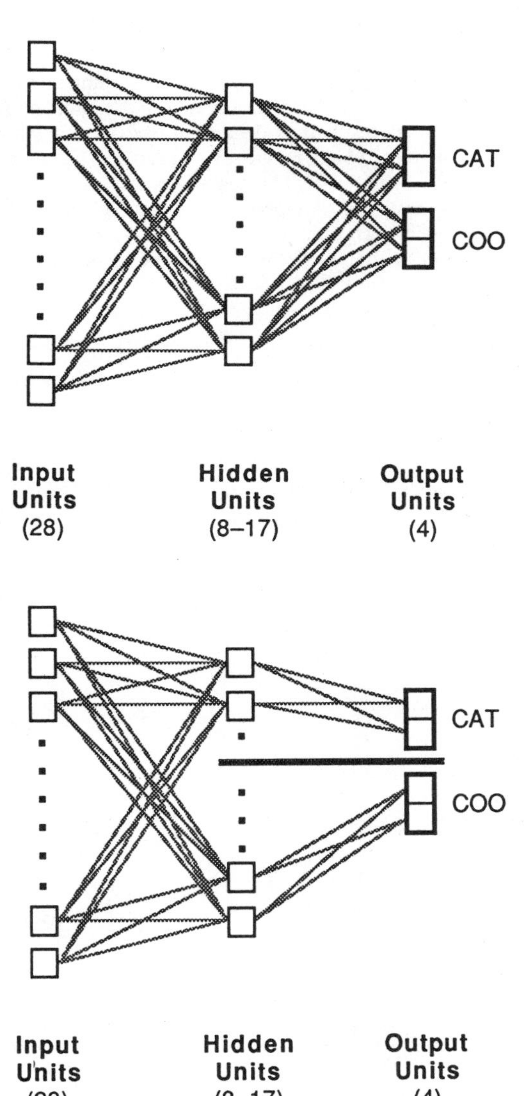

Figure 1. The architecture of the unsplit (top) and split (bottom) networks. (Numbers in parentheses indicate the size of the layers; note that a range of sizes of hidden layers was tested. CAT = categorical; COO = coordinate.)

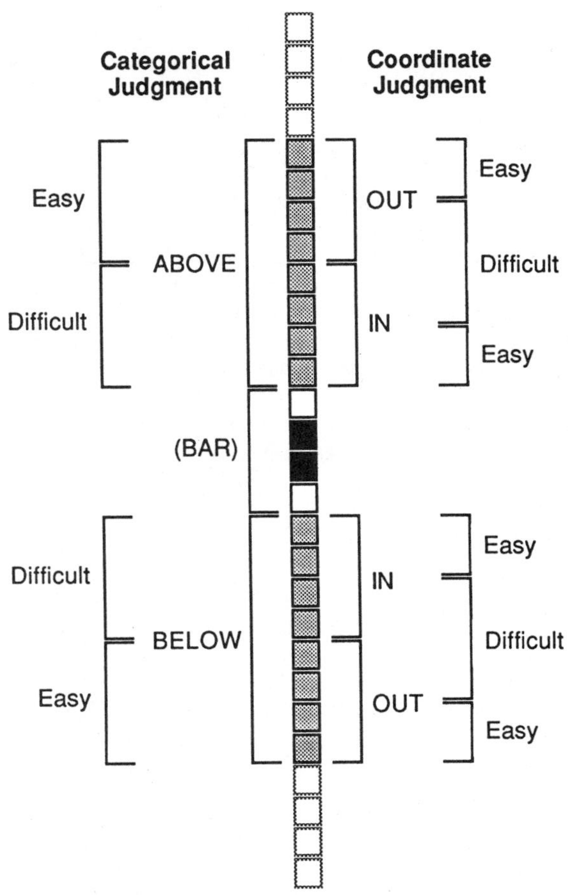

Figure 2. The input to the networks, indicating the bar and possible locations for the dot. (The judgments were based on the relative location of the dot and bar, as noted in the figure. The bar could appear in five distinct locations: at the center and shifted two or four elements up or down from the center.)

Procedure. We tested 18 networks of each type (unsplit and each ratio of split). Testing consisted of training with the backward error propagation algorithm for 50 epochs, at which point we measured the average squared error per output unit per input pattern in the network. An epoch was defined as a complete run through all 80 stimuli in the training set, followed by a single backward error propagation pass. The output signals of the units ranged from −0.5 to +0.5 (in accordance with Stornetta & Huberman's 1987 procedure); for each output unit, a threshold of ±0.4 was used, so that once the output of the unit was within 0.1 of its target, it was considered to have no error at all. Before each new test, the weights on the connections in the network were reset to random values between −0.5 and +0.5. The parameters epsilon ("learning rate") and alpha ("momentum factor") were set to 0.25 and 0.90, respectively.

Results

The results were analyzed in an analysis of variance (ANOVA), with replication (different tests, each using new initial random weights) as the random effect and average squared error per output unit per input pattern as the dependent measure. For each number of hidden units, we compared the unsplit case to the best performer among the split networks; different ratios of categorical to coordinate task hidden units sometimes enabled different-sized networks to perform best. Figure 3 illustrates the results of this analysis and also indicates which ratio was optimal at each network size. As expected, if categorical and coordinate spatial relations computations are qualitatively distinct, the split networks generally produced significantly less error ($M = 0.039$ averaged squared error), than did the unsplit ones ($M = 0.057$), $F(1, 340) = 7.64$, $p < .01$. Furthermore, error decreased linearly with more hidden units, $F(1, 340) = 5.01$, $p < .05$, for the appropriate contrast, but there was no interaction between network type and the number of hidden units ($F < 1$).

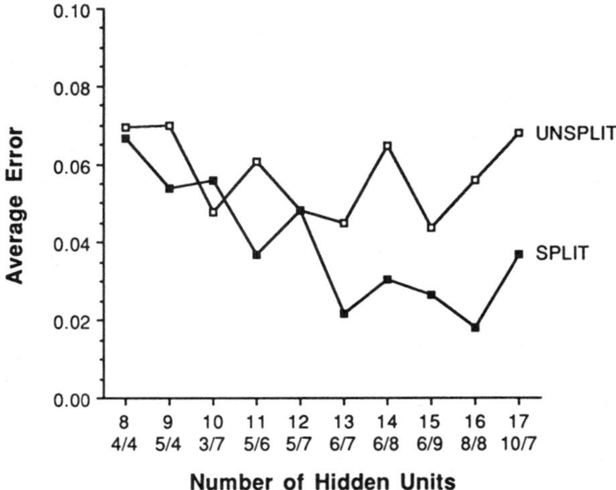

Figure 3. Results from Part 1 of Study 1, illustrating that the split networks established the categorical (CAT) and coordinate (COO) mappings more effectively than the unsplit networks, provided that a sufficient number of hidden units was available. (The ratios under the *x* axis show the numbers of hidden units allocated to the categorical and coordinate tasks, respectively, in the split networks that performed best in each case; in only one case—the 10 hidden unit networks—even the most effective split networks performed worse than the unsplit networks.)

Part 2

Method

Materials. To examine the possibility that split networks generally perform better when two judgments of any type must be made by a single network, we created split and unsplit networks that performed two coordinate judgments. The networks evaluated both whether the dot was within two elements and whether it was within six elements of the bar; thus the only major change from Part 1 was that the output units coded for two distance judgments, rather than the categorical and original distance judgment. The split networks were created by partitioning the hidden units in the same way as in Part 1.

The networks had 10, 12, 14, 16, 18, and 20 hidden units. In order to reduce the number of models that were tested, half of the hidden units in all but one size of the split networks were allocated to each of two tasks; for the 20-hidden-unit size, we also created split networks with ratios of 5:15, 8:12, 12:8, and 15:5 hidden units. On the basis of Rueckl et al.'s (1989) results, we expected that allocating insufficient hidden units to a partition would severely impair the mapping, and thus we chose to manipulate the ratios of the largest split networks to consider this potential problem.

Procedure. Ten networks of each type and size were tested initially; for the 20-hidden-unit size, we tested an additional 6 networks of each type as well as 16 networks of each of the supplementary partition ratios. Testing was conducted as in Part 1, except that the parameter epsilon was set to 0.10 (this modification was necessary because pilot data indicated that the networks would often reach high local minima early in testing with the 0.25 epsilon value).

Results

The data were analyzed as in Part 1. For each network size, we compared the unsplit networks with the even-ratio split networks in an ANOVA with replication as the random effect. Figure 4 illustrates the results of this analysis. In sharp contrast to the results from Part 1, the unsplit networks consistently produced less error ($M = 0.058$) than did the split networks ($M = 0.092$), $F(1, 108) = 63.9$, $p < .001$. Error also decreased linearly with more hidden units, $F(1, 108) = 58.1$, $p < .001$, for the appropriate contrast. However, the interaction between network type and the number of hidden units was not significant, $F(5, 108) = 1.73$, $p > .10$.

One could argue that the poor performance of the split networks was caused by the division of the hidden units into two equal groups. We ruled out this possibility by examining the other ratios tested in the 20-hidden-unit networks. The split networks with 20 hidden units performed worse than the unsplit networks, regardless of the ratio. The mean error was

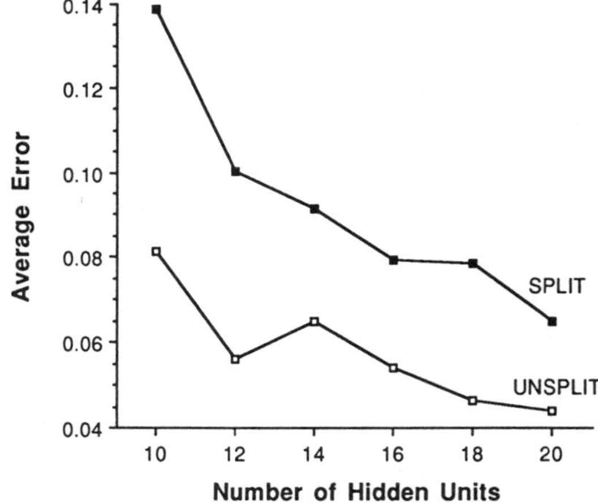

Figure 4. Results of Part 2 of Study 1, illustrating that the unsplit networks established the mappings more effectively when two coordinate judgments were required.

0.042 for unsplit networks, in comparison with mean error of 0.062 for a 12:8 split, 0.068 for a 10:10 split, 0.083 for a 8:12 split, 0.085 for a 15:5 split, and 0.089 for a 5:15 split. Four of the comparisons revealed significant differences according to t tests with the Bonferroni adjustment (adjusted $p < .05$), and the other comparison (between unsplit and 12:8 ratio split networks) approached significance, $t(30) = 2.49$, adjusted $p < .10$.

Discussion

The results of these simulations provide evidence that categorical and coordinate spatial relations are conceptually distinct. In Part 1 we found that networks in which the two types of processing are segregated perform both mappings better than do otherwise equivalent networks in which the representations are intermingled in a single set of units and weights. In Part 2 we found that this result was not merely a consequence of a general advantage for segregating the processing of any two tasks.

For the split networks in Part 1, the optimal ratio of dividing the hidden units was usually close to an even split between the two mappings. This finding may, however, have been an accident of the particular way in which we set up the tasks (e.g., the size of the input array, the amount that the bar moved, and so on), and we do not wish to draw strong inferences from this result; indeed, Kosslyn, Koenig, et al. (1989) manipulated the difficulty of discrimination to make the two kinds of tasks equivalent or either one more difficult than the other. However, it is fortunate that the two mappings were about equally difficult in these networks because it suggests that our results do not somehow reflect an effect of having a difficult task mixed with an easier one.

In addition, the advantage of the unsplit model in Part 2 cannot be ascribed to the "overlap" in outputs between the two tasks; whenever the response for the two-element distance judgment was *IN*, it must also have been *IN* for the six-element judgment and vice versa for the *OUT* judgment. The categorical and coordinate tasks in Part 1 overlapped to the same degree: For half of the input patterns, the output unit targets had the same pattern for both judgments.

These results do not imply that the human brain necessarily has evolved to use separate networks to compute the different types of spatial relations; even though a split network would be better, the brain may not be optimized in this way (we return to this issue in the General Discussion section). Thus these results simply support the contention that the two kinds of representations are not logically intertwined and need not rely on the same computation. Testing a simple prediction of this result would be of interest. If different networks are in fact used for the two tasks, then repetition priming should not transfer well between them. If a subject practices making metric judgments, this practice should prime other judgments in which the same network is used but not judgments in which a different network is used.

Study 2

Sergent (1991) suggested that our theory makes a straightforward prediction: If separate subsystems encode categorical and coordinate spatial relations, categorical judgments should not be influenced by the distance separating the two objects. However, our theory does not imply that distance affects only coordinate judgments; many categorical spatial relations rely on dividing space into discrete bins, and this process may be more difficult when the boundaries of these regions must be delineated more precisely. For example, a dot can be classified as above or below a landmark by observing whether it falls into one of two pockets of space; although any location within each bin is treated as equivalent, it may be more difficult to assign a dot to a category if the bins must be delineated carefully. Furthermore, even after the regions of space are delineated, it may be more difficult to assign a dot to a category if it appears near the boundary. Such center-versus-periphery effects are found in a wide range of categorization tasks (e.g., see Smith & Medin, 1983). Thus we do not assume a pure distinction between "encoding" and "judgment" processes; interactions between the two may influence the speed of response.

In this study, we used networks to discover whether our theory always implies that discriminability has different effects on the two types of computations or whether distance may in fact have similar effects on both computations. We compared the effect of discriminability in individual networks that performed either the categorical or the coordinate mapping (not both simultaneously, as in Study 1). We tested these specialized networks on two complementary subsets of the complete categorical and coordinate tasks: those stimulus patterns that Sergent's (1991) results suggest should be relatively easy and those that her results suggest should be relatively difficult.

In the categorical task, the easy discriminations were those in which the dot was far from the bar, and the difficult discriminations were those in which the dot was near the bar. In the coordinate task, the easy discriminations were those in which the dot was far from the criterion distance (defined in relation to the bar), and difficult judgments were those in which the dot was close to the criterion distance. This simulation enabled us to address directly the prediction that Sergent inferred.

Method

Materials

The networks were identical to those of Study 1, except that we examined only standard unsplit networks with two output units and varied the number of hidden units from 6 to 12. Figure 5 illustrates this network architecture. We chose this range of hidden layer sizes because it was sufficient to enable the mappings to be achieved but still show differences if they are not equally easy; when there are too many hidden units, a "floor effect" may obscure differences in computational difficulty among mappings.

The categorical judgment task was divided into easy and difficult conditions. In the easy condition, the dot was farther than four elements above or below the bar; in the difficult condition, it was within four elements of the bar. Separate networks were trained in the easy and difficult conditions, each receiving a set of 40 input patterns during training. The coordinate judgment task was similarly divided into easy and difficult conditions. In the easy condition, the dot was farther than two elements from the criterion distance (which was four elements from the bar); in the difficult condition, the dot was within two elements of the criterion distance. Again, separate networks were trained to map the easy and difficult conditions; each received 40 input patterns during training.

Procedure

We tested 25 networks of each size in each categorical condition and 25 networks of each size in each coordinate condition. Testing proceeded as in Part 1 of Study 1, except that error was measured after 30 epochs rather than 50 because the amount of error in the easy conditions was too low to compare after 50 epochs.

Results

The data were analyzed as in the previous studies. As is evident in Figure 6, the networks generally performed better when given the easier discriminations ($M = 0.025$ error) than when given the difficult discriminations ($M = 0.078$), $F(1, 532) = 190.9$, $p < .001$, and there was no hint of an interaction between the difficulty of the discrimination and the type of task ($F < 1$). In addition, in this study the categorical mappings were easier than the coordinate mappings (Ms = 0.043 and 0.060 error), $F(1, 532) = 20.9$, $p < .001$, and overall error decreased linearly with more hidden units, $F(1, 532) = 21.1$, $p < .001$, for the appropriate contrast. No other effects or interactions approached significance.

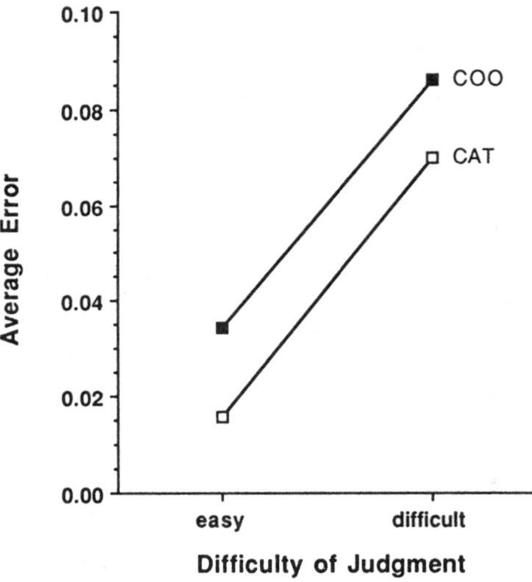

Figure 6. The results of Study 2, showing that both categorical (CAT) and coordinate (COO) judgments are affected by the difficulty of the discrimination (the range of distances).

Discussion

These findings reveal that subtle discriminations can impair both kinds of judgments in networks. This result is important because it is not intuitively clear that a categorical spatial relation should be harder to establish for stimuli that appear in a smaller range of positions. The findings of Study 3 will support our characterization of this sort of categorical spatial relation as delineating regions of space; hence we can interpret the results of Study 2 as suggesting that the more difficult it is to delineate the regions to be related, the more difficult it is to establish the mapping.

In short, the simulation results of Study 2 show that Sergent's (1991) finding that humans display a similar effect does not contradict the distinction between categorical and coordinate representations of spatial relations. It would be of interest to discover whether the effects of the difficulty of discrimination on the categorical and coordinate judgments can dissociate after brain damage; if our interpretation is correct, some brain-damaged patients should show selective deficits for difficult categorical discriminations but not difficult coordinate discriminations, and vice versa for other brain-damaged patients.

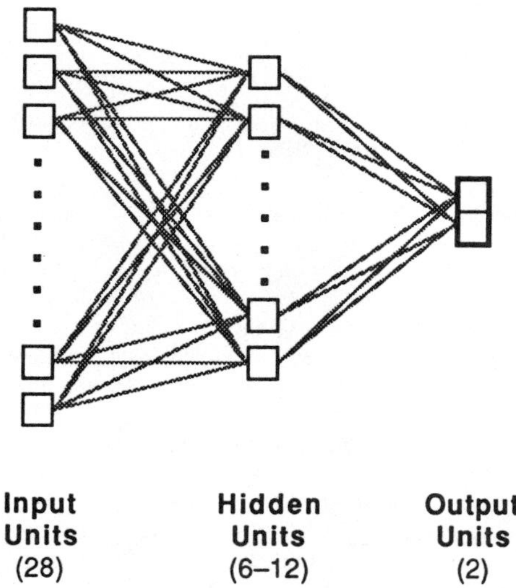

Figure 5. The architecture of the networks used in Study 2. (Only one type of judgment was performed in these models.)

Study 3

The distinction between categorical and coordinate spatial relations representations was formulated on the basis of an analysis of the purposes of spatial representations. We hypothesized that coordinate representations play a special role in action control, whereas categorical representations play a special role in recognition and identification. In this study we considered some implications of these ideas in more detail.

Action control depends on precise representation of spatial location. One way to represent spatial location precisely depends on overlap among rather coarse representations of location (Hinton, McClelland, & Rumelhart, 1986). This sort of *coarse coding* underlies color vision, for example, in which the three types of cones in the retina have overlapping distributions of sensitivity to different wavelengths of light; it is this overlap that enables the three types of cones to encode a wide range of colors. O'Reilly et al. (1990) used network models to show that this mechanism was indeed an effective way of encoding metric spatial location.

It is possible that differences in the use of coarse coding can account for the hemispheric differences in computing the two types of spatial relations. For instance, the right hemisphere may use more input from low-level visual neurons that have relatively large receptive fields (i.e., that receive input from relatively large regions of space), which have a large degree of overlap. These broadly tuned receptive fields would enable effective coarse coding and could be responsible for the right hemisphere's superior ability to encode precise location. In contrast, the left hemisphere may use more input from low-level visual neurons that have relatively small receptive fields, which do not overlap as much. Sets of these receptive fields would define particular areas, which could be used to specify regions that are above or below a reference point, left or right of a reference point, and so on. In the limit, if the receptive fields did not overlap at all and the categories corresponded to discrete regions of space, such mappings would be "linearly separable"—so straightforward that they could be accomplished by direct connections from the input units to the output units, without a hidden layer (see Minsky & Papert, 1969; Rumelhart et al., 1986).

The idea that differences in receptive field properties may be at the root of differences in hemispheric specialization for spatial encoding is intriguing for a number of reasons. First, it is compatible with Sergent's (1982) finding that the left hemisphere encodes smaller, high-spatial-frequency patterns better than the right, and the right hemisphere encodes larger, low-spatial-frequency patterns better than the left (see also Delis, Robertson, & Efron, 1986; Van Kleeck, 1989). Higher spatial frequencies may be encoded more effectively by smaller receptive fields; these fields register smaller variations in space than larger ones. By the same token, lower spatial frequencies may be encoded more effectively by larger receptive fields (cf. De Valois & De Valois, 1988).

Second, neurons with large receptive fields would be useful in preattentive processing, which by definition must monitor large regions of space. Such processing plays a critical role in controlling actions; one often moves one's eyes, head, and body toward a stimulus that suddenly appears, moves, or changes in some other way. Furthermore, one wants to look at or reach toward an object with reasonable accuracy, even if it is seen out of the corner of one's eye. M. Livingstone (personal communication, May 1990) has suggested that the magnocellular ganglia may project preferentially to the right hemisphere (see Livingstone & Hubel, 1988); these neurons have relatively large receptive fields and are thought to be involved in preattentive processing (see also de Schonen & Mathivet, 1989).

Thus it is of interest that overlapping large receptive fields not only enable the system to monitor a large area but also can produce the necessary precision to guide an initial movement, even if a target is seen only out of the corner of one's eye. In keeping with this idea, Fisk and Goodale (1988; see also Goodale, 1988) reported that patients with right hemisphere damage are impaired in the initial phases of reaching toward a visual target.

These findings must be evaluated in the context of Kitterle, Christman, and Hellige's (1990) failure to find any difference in the sensitivities of the two hemispheres to different spatial frequencies in a simple detection task. However, Kitterle et al. did find that high-spatial-frequency gratings were *identified* faster and more accurately when they were presented in the right visual field (and hence were processed initially by the left hemisphere), whereas in some conditions low-spatial-frequency gratings were identified more readily when they were presented in the left visual field (and hence were processed initially by the right hemisphere). Thus, in keeping with Sergent's (1982) ideas, the hemispheric asymmetry cannot be ascribed to low-level processing; rather, it depends on high-level encoding and comparison processes.

In short, we hypothesized that the right hemisphere uses more input than the left from low-level visual neurons that have large receptive fields. These large receptive fields overlap, which enables the right hemisphere to encode coordinate spatial relations better than the left. In contrast, the left hemisphere uses more input from low-level neurons with small receptive fields. These receptive fields have less overlap than do the larger ones, which enables the left hemisphere to specify some categorical relations by delineating discrete sets of locations. For example, if an *X* is "left of" a *Y*, one may be able to represent the relation by defining two regions: one for the left and one for the right.

On this view, if a categorical spatial relation cannot be computed by defining discrete pockets of space, then the left hemisphere will not encode that relation better than the right. This hypothesis is consistent with Sergent's (1991) failure to find left-hemisphere superiority in tasks involving spatially complex stimuli (which had target shapes that could appear in several noncontiguous regions); these stimuli are difficult to delineate into specific regions of space that can be used to categorize stimuli.

These hypotheses rely on subtle distinctions and several steps of reasoning. Thus, they are ideal candidates for computer simulation modeling, which can show whether we have merely engaged in so much hand waving or whether our assumptions can have the consequences that we infer. In this study, we used network models to investigate these hypotheses in two ways. In Part 1, we examined the mappings performed by categorical and coordinate networks by analyzing the "receptive fields" developed by the hidden units of different networks; that is, for each hidden unit, we examined which regions of the input array most strongly influenced its level of activation. The larger the weight on the connection from an input unit to the hidden unit, the more strongly a dot in that location will affect the hidden unit; thus the pattern of weights on the connections to a hidden unit defined its receptive field (Rueckl et al., 1989; see also Lehky & Sejnowski, 1988; O'Reilly et al., 1990; Zipser & Andersen, 1988). Specifically, we tested the possibility that after training proceeds until the network makes no errors, networks that encode coordinate spatial relations will have larger receptive fields than will networks that encode categorical spatial relations. Recall that when a unit's output value was within 0.1 of its target value, it was assigned zero error; otherwise, it was assigned the square of the deviation from the target value. These error scores were then summed over output units and training patterns and divided by the number of each to yield the average error value. In Part 1, we trained the networks until this value was zero.

In Part 2 of this study, adapting the method of O'Reilly et al. (1990), we constructed networks that were "hard wired" to have large or small receptive fields and considered how effectively they performed the two kinds of mappings.

Part 1

Method

Materials. Two network models were constructed in this study: one that performed the categorical mapping and one that performed the coordinate mapping. These networks were identical to those in Study 2, except that they had 10 hidden units each, and they mapped the entire set of stimuli rather than only the easy or the difficult stimuli (as in Study 2).

Procedure. Testing was conducted as in Study 2, except that we continued training on each network until the average error had decreased to zero.

Results

We examined the receptive fields developed by the hidden units of each network. To test the hypothesis that the coordinate network developed relatively large receptive fields, we first normalized the weights on the connections between the input units and the hidden units in the two networks. This was necessary because the two networks developed different patterns of weights and had different maximal and minimal values. We then calculated the radius of a receptive field by determining the average number of contiguous weights from each peak weight value down to the peak value of $1/e$ (cf. Andersen, Asanuma, Essick, & Siegel, 1990; Zipser & Andersen, 1988). For hidden units with multiple-peak receptive fields, we calculated the average crest size. The receptive fields developed by the coordinate network model (average radius 9.7 units) were larger than those developed by the categorical network model (average radius 4.8 units), $t(18) = 2.61$, $p < .05$.

Discussion

As expected, the networks that performed the coordinate task spontaneously developed larger receptive fields than did the networks that performed the categorical task. However, as O'Reilly et al. (1990) found, these receptive fields often tended to have complex shapes (see also Zipser & Andersen, 1988). It is possible that the size differences are somehow related to the various sets of shapes that developed. To examine the effects of size in isolation, we manipulated this variable directly in Part 2 of this Study.

Part 2

Method

Materials. We constructed a new set of network models that were the same as those used in Study 2 except for the following changes. First, as shown in Figure 7, each network had four layers of units. The first layer was conceptualized as a "retinal" array, and the 28 units in this layer received the same input patterns as did the 28 input units in Study 1. The weights on the connections between Layers 1 and 2 were not modified during the training procedure; these weights defined fixed receptive fields of the units in Layer 2. Layers 2, 3, and 4 and the connections among them constituted a three-layer network that was trained with backward error propagation. Thus, only the connections between Layers 2 and 3 and between Layers 3 and 4 were modified during the course of training. There were 14 units in Layer 2, which functioned as the input units for the backward error propagation procedure, and there were 10 hidden units (Layer 3 units). (Layer 2 units can also be referred to as "input units" because these were the input units for the backward error propagation procedure.) As in Study 2, the two output units specified *ABOVE* or *BELOW* for the categorical task and *IN* or *OUT* for the coordinate task.

For half of the networks tested in this study, the Layer 2 units had small fixed receptive fields; for the other half, the Layer 2 units had large fixed receptive fields. For each network, 14 receptive fields were created, one for each Layer 2 unit. All receptive fields were defined by normalized Gaussian distributions that were determined as follows. First, standard Gaussian fields were created according to the formula

$$F_g(y) = \frac{e^{-(y^2/2\sigma^2)}}{2\pi\sigma^2},$$

in which y corresponds to the "vertical" position in Layer 1 and σ is a constant that determines the size of the receptive field. All fields were then normalized to the range of 0–1. We created small receptive fields by setting the value of σ to 0.71, whereas we created large fields by setting the value of σ to 1.42. Figure 8 illustrates the shape and the scope of the two types of receptive fields; as is evident, all receptive field peaks covered two retinal elements. We varied the locations of the receptive field peaks in Layer 1 by modifying the y value in the Gaussian formula; as illustrated in the left panel of Figure 9, the 14 receptive field peaks for each network were tessellated across the retinal array. In all other respects, the networks were constructed like those used in Part 1 of this study.

Procedure. The networks were trained with the stimulus set used in Part 1. Input patterns were presented to the "retinal" units of Layer 1 in the networks, and the receptive fields modulated the input sent to Layer 2. The connection weights between Layer 1 and Layer 2 units (Layer 2 receptive fields) were not modified during training. Thus because the sigmoidal activation function was used to facilitate the modification of connection weights during training, it was not used to modulate the flow of activation from Layer 1 to Layer 2 in this network. Because the sigmoidal activation function was not used, activation values for Layer 2 units were set to the 0–1 range through a linear normalization procedure: Activation was first computed as the sum of the three active connection weights, two from the bar and one from the dot in the retinal array. The maximal possible activation for a Layer 2 unit, given the receptive field size and the constraints of line and dot positioning in the retinal array, was calculated for each network. This value served as the maximal value in the normalization procedure. A minimal possible activation was calculated in an analogous manner, and this value served as the minimum in the normalization procedure.

We tested 10 networks in each of the four conditions, defined by large or small Layer 2 receptive field sizes and the type of judgment. In all other respects, testing was the same as in Part 1.

Results

The results are illustrated in Figure 10. As expected, larger receptive field sizes greatly facilitated the coordinate judgment, whereas smaller sizes were more useful for the categorical judgment, $F(1, 36) = 62.4$, $p < .001$, for the interaction between size of input layer receptive fields and task. Separate tests revealed that the difference for the coordinate judgment

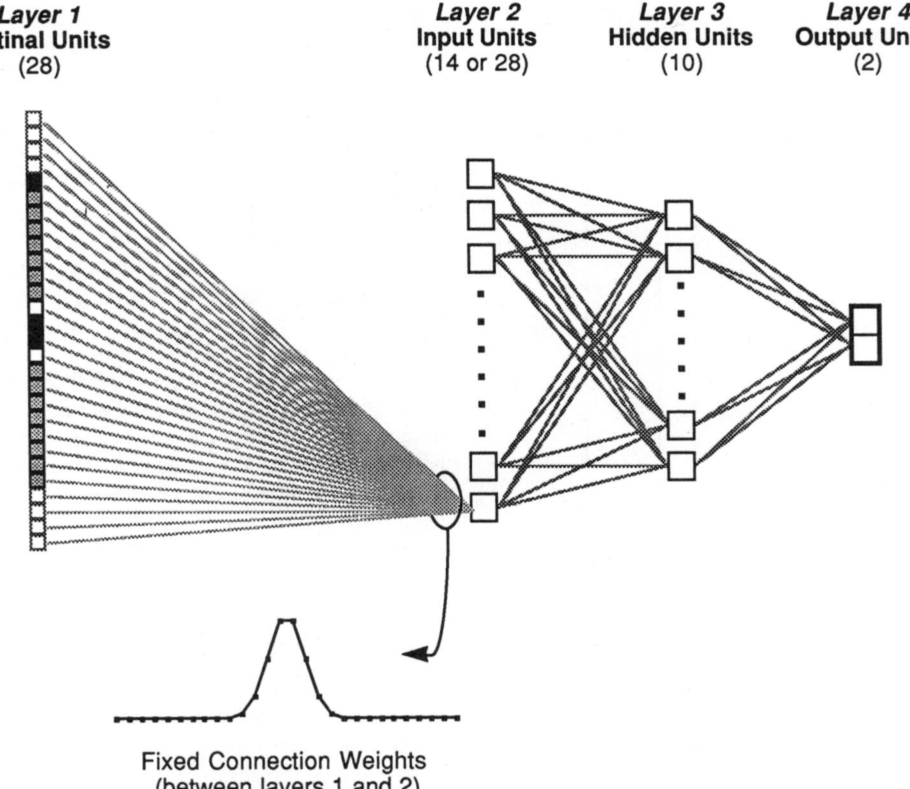

Figure 7. The architecture of the network used in Part 2 of Study 3. (Receptive fields were defined over the input units so that only some elements in the input array fed into units in Layer 2. The connection weights between Layers 1 and 2 were fixed throughout training, whereas the connection weights between Layers 2 and 3 and between Layers 3 and 4 were modified during training according to the standard three-layer back-propagation procedure. Fourteen Layer 2 units were used in Study 3, and 28 were used in Study 4.)

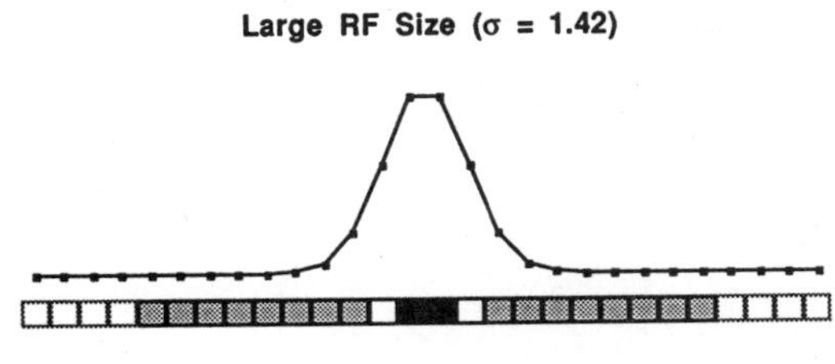

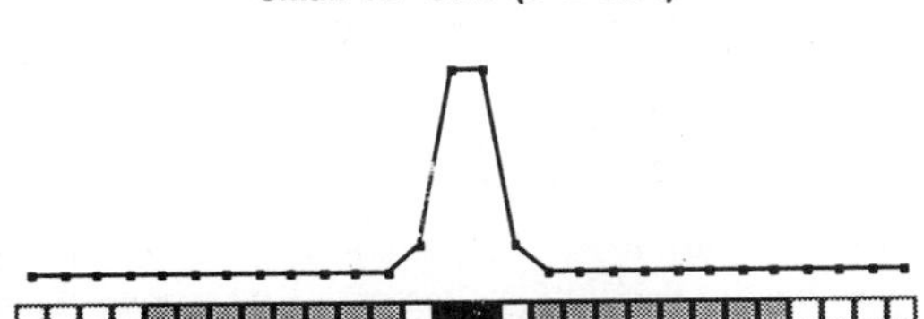

(Ms = 0.057 error for smaller and 0.013 error for larger receptive field networks) was significant, $F(1, 36) = 97.7$, $p < .001$, whereas the corresponding difference for the categorical judgment (Ms = 0.028 and 0.034 error) was not, $F(1, 36) = 2.22$, $p > .10$. Overall, networks with larger receptive fields performed better than those with smaller receptive fields (Ms = 0.024 and 0.042 error), $F(1, 36) = 34.0$, $p < .001$, but under these conditions the two types of judgments did not differ overall (Ms = 0.031 for the categorical task and 0.035 for the coordinate task), $F(1, 36) = 1.60$, $p > .20$.

Discussion

Dovetailing with the results from Part 1 of this study, networks with fixed large receptive fields performed the coordinate task better than did networks with fixed small receptive field sizes, and there was a tendency for the opposite pattern in the categorical task. These findings are like those from the corresponding experiments with human subjects. Indeed, as noted in the introduction, the left hemisphere has only a weak (but consistent) advantage for encoding categorical spatial relations.

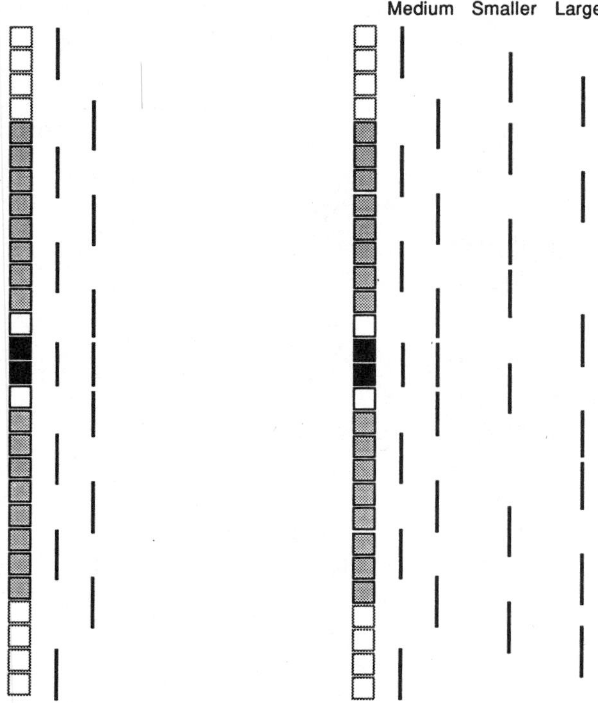

Figure 9. The distribution of receptive field peaks in the networks tested in Part 2 of Study 3 (left) and in Study 4 (right). (For mixed-size networks in Study 4, "medium" peak locations refer to the 14 peak locations for intermediate-sized receptive fields, "smaller" to the 7 peak locations for receptive fields that had relatively smaller sizes, and "larger" to the 7 peak locations for receptive fields that had relatively larger sizes. In the homogeneous networks, peak locations for receptive fields—all of which were the same size—were also distributed across these 28 locations.)

Thus these results provide additional support for the contention that categorical and coordinate spatial relations representations are conceptually distinct. Furthermore, they hint at one possible reason why the hemispheres are specialized for encoding the different types of representations. A prediction of these results is that the left-hemisphere advantage for categorical spatial relations should be present only when the relation can be computed by delineating regions of space. Thus any manipulation that makes this computation more difficult should eliminate this effect.

Study 4

The results of Study 3 may provide an insight into Sergent's (1991) finding that hemispheric differences do not arise when the stimuli have high contrast. In Study 4, we examined networks with narrow or wide ranges of receptive field sizes in the input units. If the hemispheres differ in their sensitivities to input from units with different-sized receptive fields, then any differences in the sizes of the receptive fields of input units may be obliterated if high contrast enables a more varied set of input units to contribute to the computation.

Kosslyn (1987) and Kosslyn, Koenig, et al. (1989) assumed that the hemispheres differ in their *relative* efficacy at encoding the two types of spatial relations; they did not intend to claim that the hemispheres were *exclusively* specialized for the different types of encoding. Indeed, Kosslyn, Sokolov, and Chen (1989) simulated Kosslyn's (1987) "snowball process," in which the relative hemispheric specialization of various subsystems develops gradually over time; at the heart of this model is the idea that the two hemispheres differ in the relative efficacy of individual subsystems. It is unfortunate that we did not state this assumption clearly, as noted by Sergent (1991); this assumption is important because it leads us to expect that the difference in inputs to the two hemispheres is one of degree. Given the previous simulation results, we might expect the left hemisphere to use more input from neurons with relatively small receptive fields and the right hemisphere to use more input from neurons with relatively large receptive fields, but we expect a distribution of inputs from neurons with different receptive field sizes in both hemispheres.

This idea suggests that the "modulation transfer functions" (see Kaufman, 1974) of high-level visual areas may differ in the two hemispheres. We are not considering the modulation transfer functions of low-level areas involved in detection, but rather those of higher areas involved in memory and comparison. Figure 11 illustrates this hypothesis: The modulation transfer functions of the high-level areas are slightly shifted, so that the peak sensitivity for the right hemisphere is at a lower spatial frequency, which could reflect its use of more input from larger receptive fields (and vice versa for the left hemisphere). At low contrast, the performances of the two hemispheres would be well separated, as indicated by the relatively small amount of overlap at the top horizontal dotted line. This difference could arise because the hemispheres differ

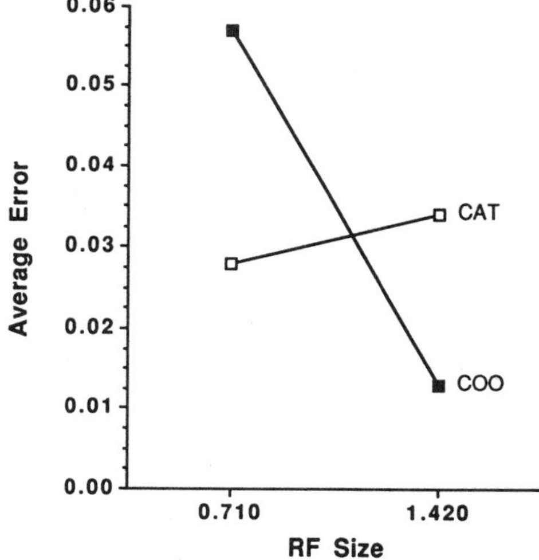

Figure 10. Results of Part 2 of Study 3, showing that the difficulty of establishing the two types of mappings depended on the relative sizes of the receptive fields (RFs). (Receptive field sizes are indicated by σ values for the Gaussian field equation. CAT = categorical; COO = coordinate.)

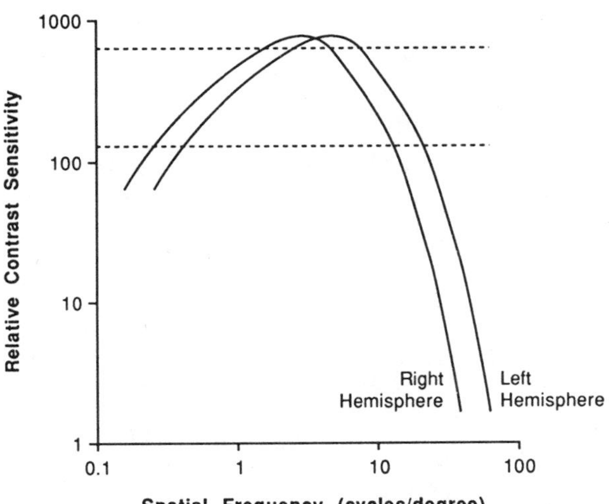

Figure 11. A hypothesized difference between identification modulation transfer functions of high-level visual areas in the left and right hemispheres. (Scales are logarithmic.)

in the degree to which they use inputs from units with different-sized receptive fields. However, at high contrast (when less sensitivity is required, as indicated by the bottom dotted line), both hemispheres use input from units with a wide range of receptive field sizes; hence the two distributions have a large amount of overlap, and the performance of the two hemispheres would not be well separated.

This idea might explain Sergent's (1991) finding that hemispheric differences between categorical and coordinate processing occur only when the stimuli are relatively degraded (i.e., are presented with low contrast). Accordingly, we decided to explore this hypothesis with another set of simulated networks. In these models, we again varied the sizes of the receptive fields of the inputs but now compared networks in which a narrow range of receptive field sizes was used (corresponding to low contrast) with those in which a wider range of receptive field sizes was used (corresponding to high contrast).

In addition, we compared this hypothesis with a simpler one: Perhaps increased contrast does not recruit additional neurons that increase the range of receptive field sizes; rather, it eliminates hemispheric differences simply because more of the same type of low-level neurons are stimulated over threshold. Even if neurons have small receptive fields, enough overlapping outputs would enable coarse coding to be used effectively even in the left hemisphere.

Thus we compared two sets of networks: ones in which greater contrast was assumed to produce outputs from a wide range of sizes of receptive fields ("mixed" receptive-field-size networks) and ones in which greater contrast was assumed simply to produce more input from the lower visual areas ("homogeneous" receptive-field-size networks). If the effect of receptive field size found in Study 3 were eliminated in mixed networks only, the first hypothesis would be supported; if this effect were eliminated in homogeneous networks, the second hypothesis would be supported.

Method

Materials

These networks differed from those used in Study 3 in only two ways: First, Layer 2 was composed of 28 units for all networks, instead of the 14 used before. Second, half of the networks had Layer 2 units with receptive fields of mixed sizes within a single network, whereas the other half had Layer 2 units with receptive fields of one size.

Half of the networks with homogeneous Layer 2 receptive field sizes were created so that all the units in Layer 2 had small receptive fields ($\sigma = 0.71$) and half so that all of these units had large receptive fields ($\sigma = 1.42$). These networks were designated *homogeneous/small* and *homogeneous/large* networks, respectively. Half of the networks with mixed Layer 2 receptive field sizes were created so that 14 of the Layer 2 units had small receptive fields ($\sigma = 0.71$), 7 had even smaller receptive fields ($\sigma = 0.36$), and the other 7 had large receptive fields ($\sigma = 1.42$). These networks were designated *mixed/small* networks. The other half of the networks with mixed Layer 2 receptive field sizes were created so that 14 of the Layer 2 units had large receptive fields ($\sigma = 1.42$), 7 had even larger receptive fields ($\sigma = 2.84$), and 7 had small receptive fields ($\sigma = 0.71$). These networks were designated *mixed/large* networks.

The receptive field peak locations for the 28 Layer 2 units in these networks were tessellated across the retinal array, as illustrated in the right panel of Figure 9. For mixed/small and mixed/large networks, all three receptive field sizes were evenly distributed across the retinal array; Figure 9 also indicates the peak locations for the three receptive field sizes.

Procedure

The procedure was the same as in Study 3, except that eight conditions were tested; we produced these conditions by orthogonally combining categorical and coordinate mappings with homogeneous/small, homogeneous/large, mixed/small, and mixed/large networks. Ten networks were tested in each condition.

Results

The results from this study are shown in Figure 12. To investigate whether mixed or homogeneous networks more accurately paralleled the behavioral findings, we analyzed the results from the two types of networks in separate ANOVAs. The mixed networks performed the mappings differently when they had different-sized receptive fields, as indicated by an interaction between receptive field size and task, $F(1, 36) = 5.37$, $p < .05$. Specifically, mixed networks performed the categorical task better when they had a majority of small receptive fields ($M = 0.0116$ error) than when they had a majority of large fields ($M = 0.0179$ error), $F(1, 36) = 8.98$, $p < .01$, but performed the coordinate tasks equally well with both receptive field sizes (*M*s = 0.0051 and 0.0045 for small and large receptive field networks), $F < 1$. In addition, the mixed networks generally performed the coordinate task better than the categorical one (*M*s = 0.0048 and 0.0148), $F(1, 36) = 45.1$, $p < .001$. These findings thus do not mirror Sergent's (1991) behavioral results, which did not reveal a difference in the categorical task with high contrast.

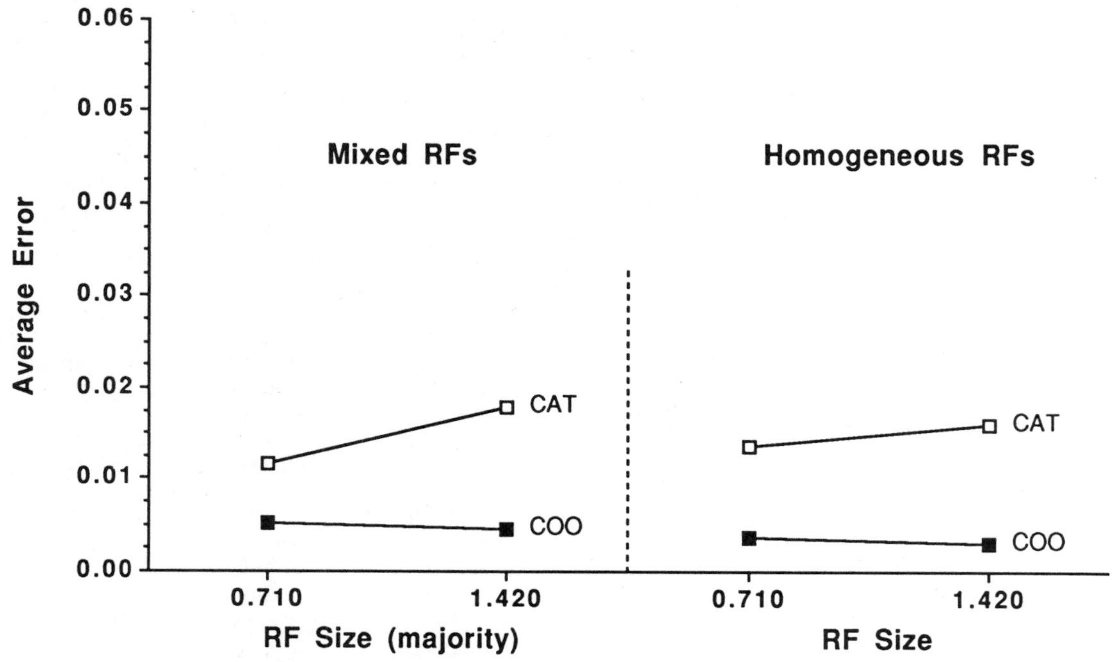

Figure 12. Results of Study 4, showing that adding inputs eliminated the advantage of large receptive fields (RFs) for accomplishing the coordinate mapping. (Moreover, if additional inputs with same-sized receptive fields were added, small receptive fields no longer allowed the network to establish the categorical mapping more easily than did large receptive fields. CAT = categorical; COO = coordinate.)

In contrast, homogeneous networks did produce the same pattern of results found in Sergent's experiments with high contrast. In these networks, there was no interaction between receptive field size and task, $F(1, 36) = 1.14$, $p > .25$. In addition, the categorical task was performed equally well with small and large receptive fields (*M*s = 0.0135 and 0.0159), $F(1, 36) = 1.55$, $p > .20$, as was the coordinate task (*M*s = 0.0036 and 0.0030), $F < 1$. Finally, these networks performed the coordinate task better than the categorical task (*M*s = 0.0033 and 0.0147), $F(1, 36) = 68.5$, $p < .001$.

Discussion

We were best able to model Sergent's (1991) findings if we simply assumed that more contrast leads to more output from low-level neurons. Adding inputs to the network effectively eliminated the advantage of large receptive fields for encoding precise location; the networks apparently used coarse coding effectively, even if the receptive fields were relatively small. This observation makes sense when one considers that coarse coding is an effective strategy only when both sufficient and systematic (but not excessive) overlap exists in the distribution of response profiles. (It has previously been demonstrated that overlap in receptive fields must be staggered in order to encode precise locations; O'Reilly et al., 1990; see also Ballard, 1986.)

Presenting stimuli with higher levels of contrast probably caused more units with overlapping receptive fields to enter the distribution. Therefore, if the added receptive fields represent areas distributed fairly evenly across the input space, a higher and more effective degree of overlap is obtained even among relatively small receptive fields.

General Discussion

Our results provide additional support for the conceptual distinction between categorical and coordinate representations of spatial relations. We not only found that at least in some circumstances different computations encode the two kinds of spatial relations, and hence they are not logically bound together, but also described a simple mechanism that can explain why coordinate representations are computed more effectively in the right cerebral hemisphere and categorical representations are computed more effectively in the left cerebral hemisphere, as well as why these hemispheric differences are not evident when stimuli are presented with high contrast.

Specifically, our networks evaluated whether a dot was above or below a line or whether a dot was within four elements of a line; thus they mimicked the categorical and coordinate tasks developed by Hellige and Michimata (1989). We found that the two judgments were performed more effectively in a neural network model when the hidden units were segregated into two separate subsystems, whereby one provided input to the categorical judgment output units and the other provided input to the coordinate judgment output units. When a single, unsplit network was used to perform both mappings, there apparently was interference between the different types of internal representations needed to accomplish the two mappings. In contrast, the reverse pattern was found when a network made two metric judgments; there, common representations could be used for both mappings, and dividing the networks made it more difficult to establish the mappings.

In addition, we found that both sorts of mappings were more difficult when finer discriminations were required. Sergent (1991) took the corresponding finding with human subjects as evidence against the distinction; our results suggest that her findings do not contradict the contention that the two mappings are qualitatively distinct. Our most general point is that a subset of shared properties does not imply that entities are exactly the same; different species of mammals, for example, share many properties (such as warm blood, hair, and so on), but other characteristics individuate them.

Furthermore, we found that the coordinate mapping was easier if the input was filtered through larger overlapping receptive fields, whereas the categorical mapping was easier if the input was filtered through smaller receptive fields. The idea that the right hemisphere monitors large receptive fields is consistent with its possible role in encoding locations to initiate an action.

Finally, the network models suggested an account of Sergent's (1991) finding that contrast alters the observed pattern of lateralization. When a relatively large number of units contributed input to a network, as may occur with high-contrast stimuli, the sizes of their receptive fields did not affect performance.

These findings suggest that the distinction between categorical and coordinate spatial relations encoding is both conceptually sound and computationally plausible. In some ways, our conceptualization of this distinction is now closer to Sergent's (1991) interpretation of her results than to the original formulation of Kosslyn (1987), and we are grateful to Sergent for leading us to characterize the distinction more rigorously. However, Sergent accounted for the right-hemisphere advantage in the distance task by assuming that it is generally superior at making efficient use of lower quality information and apparently assumed that there is no hemispheric difference in the above/below task because precise location need not be encoded or because high-quality information is not needed to compute this relation. This interpretation fails to account for the fact that people judge categorical relations better when the stimulus is presented initially to the left hemisphere than when it is presented initially to the right hemisphere (as we reviewed in the introduction). Furthermore, patients with Gerstmann's syndrome cannot judge left from right, and these patients typically have damage to the left parietal lobe (e.g., Levine, Mani, & Calvanio, 1988).

Sergent (1991) argued against the idea that each hemisphere computes only one type of representation (either categorical or coordinate). Although we apparently have not been clear about our position previously, we have always agreed with this view; we assume that both hemispheres can compute both types of spatial relations, but not equally effectively. Indeed, one of the reasons why we find neural network simulation models attractive is that they are consistent with five principles that Kosslyn and Koenig (in press) inferred about actual neural computation in the brain, one of which posits that the brain has only "weak modularity." We exploited these five principles in the following way.

First, *division of labor*: It is more efficient for separate networks to perform different types of mappings. Because the same patterns of weights on connections are used to accomplish different input/output mappings, different types of mappings interfere with each other. This principle does not, however, imply that the brain always does things in the most efficient way. Nevertheless, we assume that basic perceptual/motor processing, such as we studied, has become relatively efficient through the course of evolution; hence it is plausible that these sorts of processing often are performed efficiently. Second, *weak modularity*: The subsystems of the brain are not like electronic parts, with completely discrete functions. Rather, there is some overlap in the operation of the different components. For example, neurons in many visual areas are sensitive to more than one stimulus dimension (e.g., Van Essen, 1985). The fact that both categorical and coordinate mappings are sensitive to the distances between objects being judged may suggest that the mappings include a common underlying component (but this does not imply that the mappings are the same any more than the fact that dogs and bears have fur means that they are the same). Third, *constraint satisfaction*: Precise information is computed by satisfying a variety of weak constraints simultaneously. Coarse coding is one mechanism that carries out such computations. Furthermore, we assume that categorical spatial relations are encoded in conjunction with information about the identity of parts during object identification, and it is the combination of the two sorts of information that places strong constraints on what object is being viewed (see Kosslyn et al., 1990). Fourth, *concurrent processing*: We do not expect the system to "decide" which kind of representation to compute; rather, we expect it simply to compute whatever it can on the basis of the input. If so, separate subsystems operating in parallel may often be used to compute independent mappings; our experiments suggest that this would be a feasible arrangement for computing the two kinds of spatial relations representations. Finally, *opportunism*: Mechanisms that originally evolved for one purpose may be recruited later for another (cf. Gould & Lewontin, 1978). We have suggested that hemispheric differences in spatial relations encoding may have arisen because of mechanisms used in preattentive processing. Once the receptive field differences were present for this purpose, they could be exploited by processes that perform other tasks.

It is important to note that we have used network models in an unusual way in these studies; we are interested in them solely in terms of how well they perform specific input/output mappings. We were careful to design the tasks given to the networks to parallel the important features of the tasks given to humans, and we used the models to study the difficulty of establishing the necessary input/output mappings under different conditions. We made minimal assumptions about the psychological reality of the details of the models, and we did not use weights as parameter estimates or the like (see Massaro, 1988, for problems with some more common uses of such models). Rather, we argue that differences in the ease of establishing input/output mappings in these networks are of interest because these mappings capture—at a rather abstract level—certain aspects of corresponding mappings in the brain. The results provide evidence that the two kinds of mappings are distinct within these kinds of networks and enable us to formulate a hypothesis that is sufficient to account for how the hemispheric differences arise.

We have not shown that the same patterns of results would occur with all possible parameter values in the models. For our purposes, however, this is not a very interesting question; it is likely that some parameter settings would allow networks to perform all of the tasks very easily (displaying a floor effect, of the sort seen in Study 4), whereas others (e.g., including only a couple of hidden units) would hamstring them in all of the tasks. The fact that we found selective differences in performance under any conditions is evidence that the mappings are distinct. A critical part of this logic is that we were able to demonstrate not only simple main effects, in which one network configuration was better than another, but also interactions: Depending on the precise task, one network performed better or worse than another. Hence the performance of the network could not be ascribed to a combination of parameter settings that simply made it effective or ineffective in general.

Intuitively, it is easy to question whether the distinction between categorical and coordinate spatial reiations is coherent, let alone plausible. In fact, Kosslyn (1987) and Kosslyn, Koenig, et al. (1989) characterized the distinction slightly differently than we did, partly because they had not yet had to grapple with the problems of implementing simulation models and interpreting the results. It is clear that models such as these are a useful supplement to intuition, providing further bases for formulating and evaluating hypotheses about human information processing.

References

Andersen, R. A. (1987). Inferior parietal lobule function in spatial perception and visuomotor integration. In F. Plum (Vol. Ed.) & V. B. Mountcastle (Sec. Ed.), *Handbook of physiology, Section 1: The nervous system, Volume 5. Higher functions of the brain* (pp. 483–518). Bethesda, MD: American Physiological Society.

Andersen, R. A., Asanuma, C., Essick, G., & Siegel, R. M. (1990). Cortico-cortical connections of anatomically and physiologically defined subdivisions within the inferior parietal lobule. *Journal of Comparative Neurology, 296,* 65–113.

Ballard, D. H. (1986). Cortical connections and parallel processing: Structure and function. *Behavioral and Brain Sciences, 9,* 67–120.

Biederman, I. (1987). Recognition-by-components: A theory of human image understanding. *Psychological Review, 94,* 115–147.

Delis, D. C., Robertson, L. C., & Efron, R. (1986). Hemispheric specialization of memory for visual hierarchical stimuli. *Neuropsychologia, 24,* 205–214.

De Schonen, S., & Mathivet, E. (1989). First come, first served: A scenario about the development of hemispheric specialization in face recognition during infancy. *European Bulletin of Cognitive Psychology, 1,* 3–44.

De Valois, R. L., & De Valois, K. K. (1988). *Spatial vision.* New York: Oxford University Press.

Fisk, J. D., & Goodale, M. A. (1988). The effects of unilateral brain damage on visually guided reaching: Hemispheric differences in the nature of the deficit. *Experimental Brain Research, 72,* 425–435.

Goodale, M. A. (1988). Hemispheric differences in motor control. *Behavioral Brain Research, 30,* 203–214.

Gould, S. J., & Lewontin, R. C. (1978). The spandrels of San Marco and the Panglossian paradigm: A critique of the adaptationist programme. *Proceedings of the Royal Society of London B, 205,* 581–598.

Hellige, J. B., & Michimata, C. (1989). Categorization versus distance: Hemispheric differences for processing spatial information. *Memory & Cognition, 17,* 770–776.

Hinton, G. E., McClelland, J. L., & Rumelhart, D. E. (1986). Distributed representations. In D. E. Rumelhart & J. L. McClelland (Eds.), *Parallel distributed processing: Explorations in the microstructure of cognition. Volume 1: Foundations* (pp. 77–109). Cambridge, MA: MIT Press.

Hyvarinen, J. (1982). Posterior parietal lobe of the primate brain. *Physiological Review, 62,* 1060–1129.

Kaufman, L. (1974). *Sight and mind.* New York: Oxford University Press.

Kitterle, F. L., Christman, S., & Hellige, J. B. (1990). Hemispheric differences are found in the identification, but not the detection, of low versus high spatial frequencies. *Perception & Psychophysics, 48,* 297–306.

Koenig, O., Reiss, L. P., & Kosslyn, S. M. (1990). The development of spatial relations representations: Evidence from studies of cerebral lateralization. *Journal of Experimental Child Psychology, 50,* 119–130.

Kosslyn, S. M. (1987). Seeing and imagining in the cerebral hemispheres: A computational approach. *Psychological Review, 94,* 148–175.

Kosslyn, S. M., Flynn, R. A., Amsterdam, J. B., & Wang, G. (1990). Components of high-level vision: A cognitive neuroscience analysis and accounts of neurological syndromes. *Cognition, 34,* 203–277.

Kosslyn, S. M., & Koenig, O. (in press). *Wet mind: The new cognitive neuroscience.* New York: Free Press.

Kosslyn, S. M., Koenig, O., Barrett, A., Cave, C. B., Tang, J., & Gabrieli, J. D. E. (1989). Evidence for two types of spatial representations: Hemispheric specialization for categorical and coordinate relations. *Journal of Experimental Psychology: Human Perception and Performance, 15,* 723–735.

Kosslyn, S. M., Sokolov, M. A., & Chen, J. C. (1989). The lateralization of BRIAN: A computational theory and model of visual hemispheric specialization. In D. Klahr & K. Kotovsky (Eds.), *Complex information processing: The impact of Herbert H. Simon* (pp. 3–29). Hillsdale, NJ: Erlbaum.

Lehky, S. R., & Sejnowski, T. J. (1988). Network model of shape-from-shading: Neural function arises from both receptive and projective fields. *Nature, 333,* 452–454.

Levine, D. N., Mani, R. B., & Calvanio, R. (1988). Pure agraphia and Gerstmann's syndrome as a visuospatial-language dissociation: An experimental case study. *Brain and Language, 35,* 172–196.

Livingstone, M., & Hubel, D. (1988). Segregation of form, color, movement, and depth: Anatomy, physiology, and perception. *Science, 240,* 740–749.

Marr, D. (1982). *Vision.* New York: W. H. Freeman.

Massaro, D. W. (1988). Some criticisms of connectionist models of human performance. *Journal of Memory and Language, 27,* 213–234.

Maunsell, J. H. R., & Newsome, W. T. (1987). Visual processing in monkey extrastriate cortex. *Annual Review of Neuroscience, 10,* 363–401.

McClelland, J. L., & Rumelhart, D. E. (Eds.) (1986). *Parallel distributed processing: Explorations in the microstructure of cognition.*

Volume 2: Psychological and biological models. Cambridge, MA: MIT Press.

McLeod, P., McLaughlin, C., & Nimmo-Smith, I. (1985). Information encapsulation and automaticity: Evidence from the visual control of finely timed actions. In M. I. Posner & O. S. M. Marin (Eds.), *Attention and performance XI* (pp. 391–406). Hillsdale, NJ: Erlbaum.

Minsky, M. L., & Papert, S. A. (1969). *Perceptrons.* Cambridge, MA: MIT Press.

O'Reilly, R. C., Kosslyn, S. M., Marsolek, C. J., & Chabris, C. F. (1990). Receptive field characteristics that allow parietal lobe neurons to encode spatial properties of visual input: A computational analysis. *Journal of Cognitive Neuroscience, 2,* 141–155.

Osherson, D. N., Kosslyn, S. M., & Hollerbach, J. M. (Eds.) (1989). *An invitation to cognitive science, Volume II: Visual cognition and action.* Cambridge, MA: MIT Press.

Rosenthal, R. (1984). *Meta-analytic procedures for social research.* Beverly Hills, CA: Sage.

Rueckl, J. G., Cave, K. R., & Kosslyn, S. M. (1989). Why are "what" and "where" processed by separate cortical visual systems? A computational investigation. *Journal of Cognitive Neuroscience, 1,* 171–186.

Rueckl, J. G., & Kosslyn, S. M. (1992). What good is connectionist modelling? In A. Healy, S. M. Kosslyn, & R. M. Shiffrin, (Eds.), *Essays in honor of W. K. Estes* (pp. 249–266). Hillsdale, NJ: Erlbaum.

Rumelhart, D. E., Hinton, G., & Williams, R. (1986). Learning internal representations by error propagation. In D. E. Rumelhart & J. L. McClelland (Eds.), *Parallel distributed processing: Explorations in the microstructure of cognition. Volume 1: Foundations* (pp. 318–362). Cambridge, MA: MIT Press.

Rumelhart, D. E., & McClelland, J. L. (Eds.) (1986). *Parallel distributed processing: Explorations in the microstructure of cognition. Volume 1: Foundations.* Cambridge, MA: MIT Press.

Seidenberg, M. S., & McClelland, J. L. (1989). A distributed, developmental model of word recognition and naming. *Psychological Review, 96,* 523–568.

Sergent, J. (1982). The cerebral balance of power: Confrontation or cooperation? *Journal of Experimental Psychology: Human Perception and Performance, 8,* 253–272.

Sergent, J. (1991). Judgments of relative position and distance on representations of spatial relations. *Journal of Experimental Psychology: Human Perception and Performance, 17,* 762–780.

Smith, E. E., & Medin, D. (1983). *Categories and concepts.* Cambridge, MA: Harvard University Press.

Stornetta, W. S., & Huberman, B. A. (1987). *An improved three-layer back propagation algorithm.* Paper presented at the Proceedings of the IEEE First International Conference on Neural Networks, San Diego, CA.

Ungerleider, L. G., & Mishkin, M. (1982). Two cortical visual systems. In D. J. Ingle, M. A. Goodale, & R. J. W. Mansfield (Eds.), *The analysis of visual behavior* (pp. 549–586). Cambridge, MA: MIT Press.

Van Essen, D. (1985). Functional organization of primate visual cortex. In A. Peters & E. G. Jones (Eds.), *Cerebral cortex* (Vol. 3, pp. 259–329). New York: Plenum Press.

Van Kleeck, M. H. (1989). Hemispheric differences in global versus local processing of hierarchical visual stimuli by normal subjects: New data and a meta-analysis of previous studies. *Neuropsychologia, 27,* 1165–1178.

Zipser, D., & Andersen, R. A. (1988). A back-propagation programmed network that simulates response properties of a subset of posterior parietal neurons. *Nature, 331,* 679–684.

II
Auditory and Somatosensory Systems

Introduction to Part II

The recent advances in technology that have helped us to understand the neural mechanisms of vision have also promoted progress in other areas. This part contains reports of recent and important advances in our understanding of audition and somatosensation.

Audition

The paper by Brugge and Reale is a review of important discoveries about the auditory cortex of mammals. Whereas visual inputs have a rather direct route to the cortex via the thalamus, the auditory pathway proceeds through several brainstem and midbrain structures before entering the auditory thalamus. Thus the auditory input to the cortex is much more highly processed than the visual input. One reason for the earlier processing in audition may be the need to extract stimulus time and intensity differences between the ears. These cues are used for auditory localization and require specialized neural mechanisms for their analysis. However, there are also many similarities between the auditory and visual pathways that are reviewed in this article. These include multiple topographic representations of the sensory epithelium in the cortex. In the auditory cortex the cochlea is systematically represented in the primary (area AI) and several secondary auditory cortical areas. Since high frequencies are encoded at the apical end of the cochlea and low frequencies at the basal end, the representation of the cochlea in the cortex results in a systematic map of frequency specificity. This map consists of change in frequency along one dimension and relatively constant frequency along the other dimension, producing "isofrequency" slabs. One important question in auditory physiology is what stimulus attribute is represented along the isofrequency dimension. Recent findings show bands of different interaural interactions running across the isofrequency slabs. One set of bands contains cells that are excited by inputs from both ears and are interdigitated with a second set of bands which are excited by the contralateral ear and inhibited by the ipsilateral ear. These interaural interaction bands may play a role in sound localization and they have also been found in the auditory thalamus. These properties are reminiscent of the eye dominance segregation found in both the visual thalamus and primary visual cortex.

Sounds play an important role in helping us to locate objects, and the neural mechanisms underlying this process are now understood in considerable detail. A key strategy in this research is to study animals that are particularly adept at auditory localization. The papers by Knudsen and Konishi and by Suga and O'Neill are good examples of this approach. Knudsen and Konishi study the barn owl, which uses its exquisite ability to localize sounds to hunt small prey at night. Knudsen and Konishi find that neurons in the midbrain auditory nucleus respond to sounds only when they originate from small regions in space; furthermore, the receptive fields of these neurons vary systematically in their preferred spatial location, providing a map of auditory space within the nucleus. This representation is remarkable because it must be computed from interaural intensity and amplitude difference cues; in contrast, retinotopic representations arise from the approximately point-to-point projections from the retina to the visual cortex.

Suga and O'Neill study bats, whose auditory systems are specialized for echolocation. Bats estimate the distance from a target by comparing the time between a sound they emit and its echo. Suga and O'Neill record from an area in the auditory cortex where the cells are rather unresponsive to either a sound or its echo alone but respond well to a combination of the two sounds with an intervening delay. They find evidence of a map that represents target distance. This research in the bat nicely complements the findings of reseach in the barn owl, showing how the brain can compute representations of space from different auditory cues.

Kaufman and Williamson take a very different tack. They record magnetic fields from the human auditory cortex. Because magnetic waves are not distorted as they pass through the skull or scalp, the source of a magnetic field is more easily isolated than that of an electrical field. Thus magnetic scalp recordings from humans show great promise for localizing functional areas in the human brain. Kaufman and Williamson find that the source of magnetic activity moves systematically along the auditory cortex as the pitch of a tone is changed. They also review experiments in which this technique is used to investigate visual, somatosensory, and motor cortices. sensory, and motor cortices.

Somatosensory System

Recent microelectrode recording experiments in monkeys have also revealed multiple representations of the sensory epithelium in the somatosensory cortex. It has long been known that each part of the body is represented by a separate part of the somatosensory cortex, and these representations are arranged systematically; Woolsey and Fairman (1946) labeled this representation SI. This area spans four anatomically distinct cortical areas, Brodmann's areas 3a, 3b, 1, and 2. The paper by Merzenich, Kaas, Sur, and Lin shows that there are three and perhaps four separate representations of the body surface within area SI. Perhaps not surprisingly, these representations conform to Brodmann's anatomical subdivisions. These findings, taken together with results from the visual and auditory cortex, show that the presence of multiple representations of the sensory epithelium is a general organizing principle for the cerebral cortex. An important challenge for neurophysiologists is to delineate the different processing mechanisms that exist within these different cortial fields.

Reference

Woolsey, C. N., and D. Fairman. 1946. Contralateral, ipsalateral and bilateral representation of cutaneous receptors in somatic area I and II of the cerebral cortex of pig, sheep, and other mammals. *Surgery* 19:684–702.

18

J. F. Brugge and R. A. Reale

Auditory cortex

1985. In *Cerebral Cortex*, edited by A. Peters and E. G. Jones. New York: Plenum Publishing

1. Introduction

Auditory cortex refers, in the classical sense, to the temporal region of cerebral cortex that receives a major ascending afferent input from the medial geniculate body of the thalamus and contains neurons responsive to acoustic stimulation. Anatomical, physiological, and behavioral studies, some dating back to the last century, have shown repeatedly that auditory cortex, so defined, is a complex structure made up of not one field, but several fields that can be distinguished from one another on the bases of cytoarchitecture, connectivity patterns, functional maps, and the coding properties of single neurons. In a more general sense, the definition of auditory cortex may be expanded to include those areas referred to as "polysensory," "nonspecific," or "associational," areas whose major ascending inputs are derived mainly from sources outside of those making up the main auditory lemniscal pathway (Graybiel, 1973, 1974; Irvine and Phillips, 1982; see Pandya and Yeterian, this volume). This so-called "diffuse" or "lemniscal adjunct" system is characterized by poor frequency selectivity, little tonotopic organization, and considerable convergent input from other sensory systems.

Systematic work on the functional organization of auditory cortex began with the classical 1942 study of Woolsey and Walzl in which they mapped on the ectosylvian region of cat cerebral cortex the distribution of slow-wave potentials evoked by focal electrical stimulation of auditory nerve fibers in the osseous spiral lamina of the cochlea. By 1961, Woolsey had developed a scheme of organization of cat auditory cortex that was based largely on evoked potential studies carried out by him and his colleagues over nearly two decades (Woolsey, 1960, 1961). The scheme was consistent with both the cytoarchitectonic analysis of Rose (1949) and the results of studies of retrograde degeneration patterns following regional auditory cortical lesions (Rose and Woolsey, 1949, 1958). Woolsey (1971; Woolsey and Walzl, 1982) later applied this model to other mammalian cortices, especially that of the monkey. His scheme, in which auditory cortex is parcelled into a primary field (AI) and several surrounding fields, has remained essentially intact although in recent years a number of refinements and modifications have been made based on the results of detailed microelectrode mapping studies (Merzenich and Brugge, 1973; Merzenich *et al.*, 1975; Imig *et al.*, 1977; Knight, 1977; Andersen *et al.*, 1980a; Reale and Imig, 1980).

With the boundaries and frequency organizations of several auditory cortical fields firmly established in cat and monkey and with the recent developments of powerful neuroanatomical tracer methods, attention turned again to the patterns of connections these fields have with one another and with the thalamus, midbrain, and basal ganglia. Some of these connectivity patterns are closely related to the functional maps determined electrophysiologically. Single-unit studies of auditory cortex carried out over the past 30 years have revealed some of the coding properties of AI neurons and, most recently, of cells in surrounding fields. In this chapter we review some of the major developments in these areas. We proceed by first outlining the locations and boundaries of auditory cortical fields. We then go on to describe the coding properties of single auditory cortical neurons, paying particular attention to cells in AI. Next we discuss the functional organization of auditory cortex based on the spatial distribution of neurons having particular coding properties. Finally, we take up the relationships between the functional organizations of these fields, as determined electrophysiologically, and the patterns of connections these areas have established with each other and with subcortical structures. The material is necessarily selective and we have omitted, because of space limitations, a discussion of all work not relevant to our understanding of auditory cortex. Some of the gaps can be filled by referring to other reviews (Goldstein, 1968; Goldstein and Abeles, 1975; Brugge, 1975; Imig and Morel, 1983; Aitkin *et al.*, 1984; Masterton and Imig, 1984; Phillips and Brugge, 1985).

2. Parcellation of Auditory Cortex

2.1. Auditory Cortical Fields in the Cat

Woolsey's map of cat auditory cortex is based on evoked potential recordings (Woolsey and Walzl, 1942; Woolsey, 1960, 1961), cytoarchitectonic analysis (Rose, 1949), and studies of the patterns of retrograde degeneration in the medial geniculate body after regional cortical lesions (Rose and Woolsey, 1949, 1958). Four tonotopic (or cochleotopic) fields were recognized by him: the primary auditory field (AI), the second auditory field (AII), the posterior ectosylvian area (EP), and the suprasylvian fringe area (SSF). He also pointed to several other outlying auditory fields, including the temporal field (T), an area in the dog referred to as AIII by Tunturi (1960), the insular field (I), after Goldberg *et al.* (1957), and association cortex, which was studied by Thompson and Sindberg (1960). Auditory evoked potentials have also been recorded under chloralose anesthesia in precentral motor cortex (MI) and in visual area II. The results of fine-grain microelectrode mapping experiments (e.g., Fig. 10A) later added details that required revision of Woolsey's original scheme (Fig. 1).

The location and frequency map of AI has remained largely as Woolsey and Walzl first described it. Neurons with low characteristic frequencies (CFs) are found caudally within the field whereas the representations of higher CFs are found progressively more rostrally. Rostral to AI, on the anterior ectosylvian gyrus, is found another complete and orderly representation of the audible frequency spectrum first mapped by Woolsey (1961) and included by him in the suprasylvian fringe area. Knight (1977) and Reale and Imig (1980) mapped this area in even greater detail and referred to it as the anterior auditory field (A or AAF). The tonotopically organized posterior (P) and ventral posterior (VP) fields discovered by Reale and Imig (1980) lie mainly on the buried banks of the posterior ectosylvian sulcus, a region not explored by Woolsey in his evoked potential work. A portion of Woolsey's area EP probably corresponds to the posterior portions of P and VP. A belt of cortex containing neurons responsive to acoustic stimulation surrounds the core fields of AI, A, P, and VP. These belt areas have not been studied at the single-unit level. One of these areas, AII, which in the cat is contiguous with AI ventrally, has recently been remapped by Schreiner and Cynader (1984). Their observations of broad tuning of single neurons and blurred tonotopy are in accord with those of others and with the anatomical findings that AII, and perhaps other fields in the auditory belt, receives a substantially different thalamic afferent supply than the four tonotopically organized core areas. Neurons in the "association cortex" have been studied systematically and the results of those and related experiments on the thalamus and reticular formation have provided much of the evidence for a diffuse system of afferents arising at the level of the midbrain and projecting forward along pathways separate from those of the lemniscal system (Irvine and Phillips, 1982).

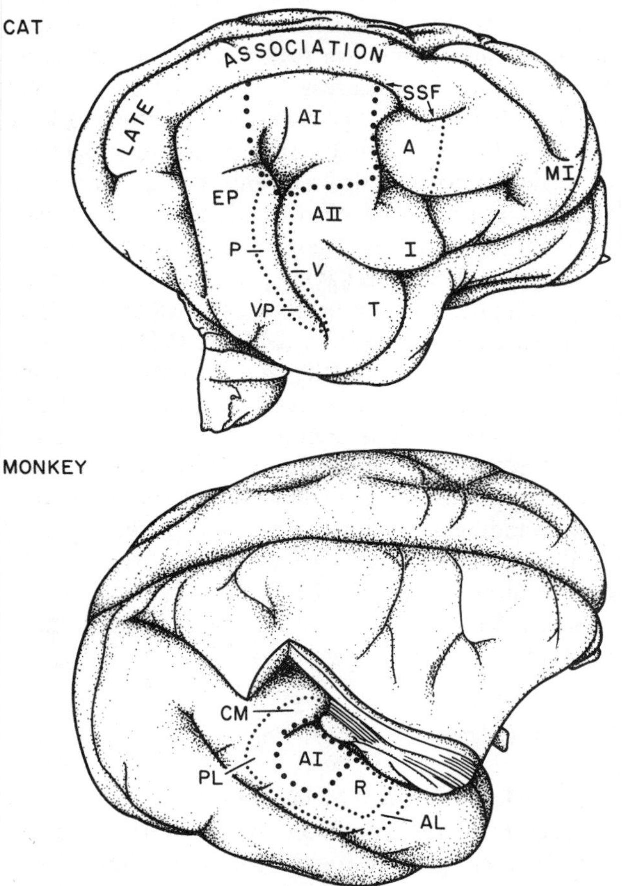

Figure 1. Locations and boundaries of auditory cortical fields in the cat and monkey based on electrophysiological mapping experiments. Shown on the cat brain are the primary (AI), second (AII), anterior (A), posterior (P), ventral posterior (VP), and ventral (V) fields mapped by microtelectrode recording of single neurons or neuronal clusters. The presence of the posterior ectosylvian (EP), temporal (T), insular (I), motor (MI), association, visual cortex (late) fields has been determined by evoked potential mapping. On the monkey brain are outlined the core tonotopically organized areas, the primary (AI) and rostral (R) fields. The auditory belt includes the caudomedial (CM), posterolateral (PL), and anterolateral (AL) fields. All of these fields have been studied by fine-grain microelectrode mapping.

2.2. Auditory Cortical Fields in Primates

The organizational scheme for auditory cortex in the primate has been derived from evoked-potential and single-unit mapping experiments in New World monkeys (Woolsey, 1971; Imig *et al.*, 1977). Old World monkeys (Merzenich and Brugge, 1973; Woolsey and Walzl, 1982), chimpanzees (Woolsey, 1971), and the prosimian primate, *Galago crassicaudatus* (Brugge, 1982). In no single primate species has auditory cortex been mapped in its entirety. The original electrophysiological mapping data, again from the 40-year-old experiments of Woolsey and Walzl, have only recently been published (Woolsey and Walzl, 1982). Microelectrode mapping work has added a great deal to Woolsey and Walzl's results, which were considerably less extensive in the monkey than in the cat. Figure 1 shows a composite map of auditory cortical fields drawn on the superior temporal gyrus of an owl monkey brain. The map is derived from data pooled from microelectrode mapping studies of several primate species.

Like that of the cat, auditory cortex of primates contains multiple fields that are distinguished from one another anatomically and physiologically. Most of the acoustically responsive cortex lies on the superior bank of the superior temporal gyrus, deep within the lateral fissure. Area AI is a tonotopically organized field that is coextensive with an area of koniocortex. It has been referred to in the rhesus monkey as area TC based on cytoarchitectonic analyses (Pandya and Sanides, 1973). AI has been mapped extensively in several primate species and may be considered the homolog of the field by that name in nonprimate species and of that field of temporal cortex in apes and humans identified cytoarchitectonically as koniocortex (von Economo, 1929; Galaburda and Sanides, 1980; Seldon, 1981, and this volume). The fields surrounding AI include the rostral (R), anterolateral (AL), posterolateral (PL), and caudomedial (CM) fields, so named because of their positions relative to AI. In the rhesus monkey, Pandya and Sanides (1973) recognize areas TA and TB adjacent to TC (AI). The correspondence between these areas and the ones mapped electrophysiologically is not entirely clear.

2.3. Auditory Cortical Fields in Other Mammals

About the time that Woolsey and his colleagues were studying the auditory cortex in the cat, Tunturi was mapping the corresponding area in the dog. Using the evoked potential method, he defined four acoustically responsive cortical fields which he named the posterior ectosylvian (PES), middle ectosylvian (MES), anterior ectosylvian (AES), and third auditory fields (Tunturi, 1960). A complete tonotopic map is shown in MES, the apparent primary field in this animal. Evidence for a tonotopic organization exists for AES, a field that occupies the same position with respect to MES as does field A with respect to AI in the cat. PES occupies a region that corresponds to Woolsey's field EP.

An acoustically responsive region of temporal cortex in the gray squirrel has been subdivided on the basis of its electrophysiologic and cytoarchitectonic properties (Kaas *et al.*, 1972; Merzenich *et al.*, 1976). One of these subdivisions contains a complete tonotopic map derived from the responses of sharply tuned neurons; the map is coextensive with a cytoarchitectonic field of koniocortex. Merenich *et al.* (1976) propose that this field be considered the homolog of AI in cat and monkey. Surrounding this field is a belt of responsive cortex the frequency organization of which has yet to be worked out.

In another rodent, the guinea pig, two tonotopically organized auditory cortical fields have been identified (Hellweg *et al.*, 1977). One of them has within it a rostral-to-caudal, low-to-high-frequency gradient similar to that in the presumed primary field of the squirrel. The high-frequency representation of the second of the two areas joins the high-frequency representation of the presumed AI so that together their maps are in a mirror-image relationship.

The auditory region in the rabbit also appears to contain multiple cortical fields which differ in their cellular architecture and tonotopic organization (Woolsey, 1971; Kraus and Disterhoft, 1982; McMullen and Glaser, 1982). Moreover, the relative positions and orientations of the tonotopic maps of the primary and secondary fields differ from those in other mammals studied this way (McMullen and Glaser, 1982). In the presumed AI, neurons with the highest CFs are located in the dorsal part of the field whereas cells having the lowest CFs are found ventrally. The second auditory cortical field in this animal lies dorsal and rostral to the primary field. Its tonotopic sequence is the reverse of that found in AI. The only other species shown so far to possess a dorsal-to-ventral, high-to-low-frequency representation in the primary field is the marsupial possum (Gates and Aitkin, 1982). The available data on this animal are not complete enough to determine whether there are any surrounding auditory cortical fields.

2.4. Homologies

From the available electrophysiological and anatomical data, there seems to be little doubt that areas designated AI in cat and monkey are homologs and that these likely correspond to areas designated AI in dogs, rodents, and rabbits. In the tree shrew (*Tupaia glis*), a field corresponding to the mammalian AI has been defined on the bases of cytoarchitecture and thalamocortical connections (Casseday *et al.*, 1976; Oliver and Hall, 1978).

The parallels between fields surrounding AI are even more problematic and, except perhaps for the dog, can be considered only in the cat and monkey, animals in which extensive mapping data are available. By considering the evolutionary trends in the development of the temporal lobe, the frequency organization of the auditory fields, and the connections these fields make with the thalamus, Woolsey and Walzl (1982) were able to suggest the homologies between the main auditory fields in the cat and monkey. Woolsey considered area A of the cat (the rostral portion of the suprasylvian fringe) the homolog of PL in the monkey. Woolsey also parcelled the area rostral to AI of the monkey into four areas rather than the two (R and AL) suggested by Imig *et al.* (1977). He further suggested that the two of them adjacent to AI are homologs of P and V of the cat. Rostral to these are two others, one of which he labeled the homolog of cat VP. AII does not appear on the recent monkey maps, although Woolsey would put it at the caudal end of the insula, medial to AI.

At this point we postpone further discussion of the organization of auditory cortical fields until later in the chapter. First it is necessary to consider the coding mechanisms of auditory cortical neurons upon which some of this organization is based.

3. Neural Coding Mechanisms within Field AI

For more than three decades, efforts have been made to understand, at the single-neuron level, the cortical mechanisms involved in a listener's ability to detect and discriminate tones of different frequencies or intensities, to locate the sources of sounds in space, and to process more complex acoustic stimuli, such as noises, frequency- or amplitude-modulated tones, clicks, and communication sounds. With few exceptions, the approach has been one of a detailed analysis of the response properties of single cortical neurons recorded extracellularly in anesthetized animals. Most of this work has been carried out in the middle ectosylvian region of the cat cortex, the region designated on Woolsey's map as AI. Unfortunately, the contours of the ectosylvian sulci differ considerably from one cat to the next and, thus, they are poor landmarks for the accurate localization of AI borders (e.g., Merzenich *et al.*, 1975). A similar situation obtains in the monkey, for there are no good gross landmarks on the superior surface of the superior temporal gyrus of this animal's brain to identify unequivocally the boundaries of any of the auditory cortical fields located there (e.g., Merzenich and Brugge, 1973; Imig *et al.*, 1977). Thus, the properties attributed to AI neurons have been derived both from experiments in which the electrode was inserted into the middle ectosylvian area of the cat or supratemporal plane of the monkey assuming the areas penetrated to be AI and from experiments in which the locations of recorded neurons were verified histologically or by electrophysiological mapping of the AI borders.

3.1. Coding for Stimulus Frequency

AI neurons are responsive only within a restricted domain of stimulus frequencies and intensities referred to as the response area of the cell. The frequency selectivity of a neuron may be described by its threshold tuning curve which is derived by determining systematically the sound pressure level required to evoke a threshold response at various stimulus frequencies (Figs. 2 and 8). The frequency at which threshold intensity is lowest, i.e., the tip of the tuning curve, is called the "characteristic" or "best" frequency of that neuron and is related to the place of resonance along the cochlear partition to which the neuron is ultimately connected. For primary auditory nerve fibers, the shape of the tuning curve rather accurately reflects the mechanical tuning properties of the basilar membrane (e.g., Rhode, 1978; Khanna and Leonard, 1982, Sellick *et al.*, 1982). For a neuron within the central auditory pathways, any departure from the primary-like shape of the tuning curve is interpreted to be the result of activation of convergent excitatory and inhibitory inputs to that neuron derived from different afferent sources. The shapes of tuning curves can vary considerably from one AI neuron to the next even for cells of the same CF (Hind *et al.*, 1960; Evans and Whitfield, 1964; Oonishi and Katsuki, 1965, Goldstein *et al.*, 1968; Phillips and Irvine, 1981a; Phillips *et al.*, 1985). Under general anesthesia, the great majority of AI neurons exhibit tuning curves that are narrow and V-shaped, like those of primary auditory nerve fibers (Fig. 2A–C). For other AI cells the tuning curves may be exceptionally broad or contain multiple tips. Some response areas are circumscribed (Fig. 2D–F). Exceptionally broad or multiply tipped tuning curves reflect convergent input from a number of sharply tuned elements whose CFs span a relatively wide spectral range and, hence, are derived from a relatively wide segment of cochlear partition. The fact that some response areas are circumscribed implies that these neurons are selective not only for stimulus frequency but for stimulus intensity as well. Intensity-selective properties of AI neurons are described later in this chapter.

Various proportions of unusually shaped AI tuning curves have been reported from different laboratories. There are at least two possible explanations for the

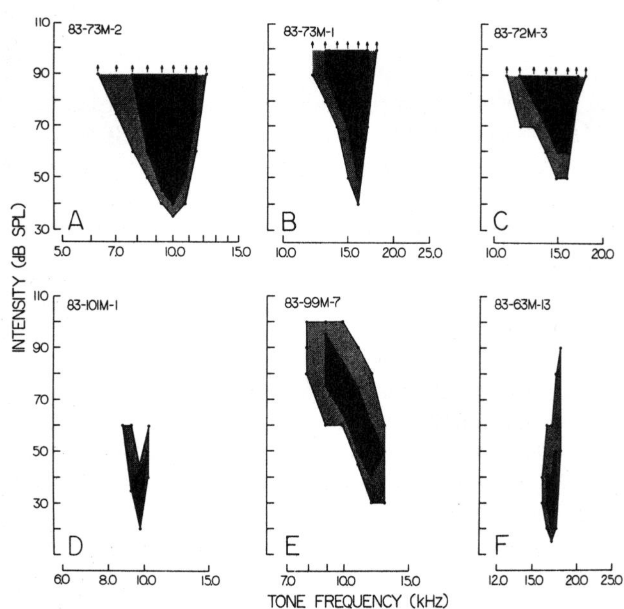

Figure 2. Threshold tuning curves from single AI neurons in the cat. (A–C) V-shaped curves similar to those derived from primary nerve fibers. (D–F) Circumscribed response areas. Stippled area indicates the frequency-intensity domain within which an AI neuron responds to 50% or fewer stimuli. Black area is the region in which fewer than half the stimuli are effective. From Phillips *et al.* (1985).

discrepancies. First, the results attributed to AI neurons may be contaminated with data from adjoining fields where neurons are known to have irregular or broad tuning properties. Second, anesthesia may reduce much of the afferent input to AI cells, other than that arising directly from the thalamus. In this regard, the greatest number of AI cells having nonprimary-like tuning curves are recorded from unanesthetized animals (Evans and Whitfield, 1964; Oonishi and Katsuki, 1965; Goldstein *et al.*, 1968). In the unanesthetized condition, not only are AI neurons more active than under general anesthesia but there is a greater probability of recording from active neurons in cortical layers above and below laminae III and IV which receive the bulk of the thalamic afferent input. The question of proportions aside, it is clear that for a large number of AI neurons, frequency selectivity established at the level of the cochlea is preserved at the level of the cortex (Calford *et al.*, 1983). For other AI neurons, cochlear frequency selectivity is altered by neuronal interactions along the central auditory pathway.

The fact that AI neurons are frequency selective immediately argues for the involvement of this field in a central place mechanism for frequency encoding and, hence, pitch recognition. Although a place principle is clearly supported by many kinds of evidence, it is not possible to explain pitch perception with the simplistic concept that each auditory neuron corresponds to a specific frequency. The shape of even the sharpest tuning curve in cat or monkey AI shows that at moderate suprathreshold sound pressure levels, the neuron associated with that curve would respond over a relatively wide range of frequencies and moreover, that at any one frequency a sizable number of neurons with different CFs would be included in the active neuronal pool. Hence, place theorists must postulate that the central nervous system, for the purpose of pitch identification, ignores all of the activity except the peak or boundary of the array of active neurons.

3.2. Coding for Stimulus Intensity

The sensitivity and dynamic range of hearing are remarkable: a young listener is able to discriminate tones close in frequency, and even understand speech, over an intensity range of more than 100 db on the scale of sound pressure. A primary auditory nerve fiber increases monotonically its discharge rate over a range of no more than about 40 db. How, then, with that dynamic range characterizing individual cochlear nerve fibers, can normal hearing achieve its effective range range of 100–120 db? At the level of the auditory nerve, part of the answer appears to reside in the spread of excitation along the basilar membrane and the recruitment of additional fibers into the active population (see Green, 1976).

The dynamic range for intensity is, as a rule, not extended greatly, if at all, for a single neuron in the central auditory system. Perhaps 75% of the neurons recorded in primary auditory cortex display rate-vs.-intensity functions that are virtually identical to those derived from auditory nerve fibers (Fig. 3A). For them, spike counts increase from threshold over a 10- to 40-db range at which point further increase in stimulus intensity is ineffective in further raising the spike count, i.e., saturation firing is reached. Neurons with V-shaped tuning curves tend to exhibit this property. The responses of other AI neurons to changing intensity may be quite different from this. For these cells, the number of spikes evoked by a tone rises to a maximum as intensity is raised and then, with further increase in sound level, the count falls (Fig. 3B). This property is associated with neurons having the circumscribed response areas previously described. Because cochlear nerve fibers show only monotonic rate-vs.-intensity functions, any nonmonotonic behavior in the rate curve derived from a central auditory cortical neuron may be considered the result of inhibitory processes.

In AI of the anesthetized cat (Brugge *et al.*, 1969; Phillips and Irvine, 1981a) and awake and unanesthetized monkey (Brugge and Merzenich, 1973a, b), the nonmonotonic functions relating spike count to inten-

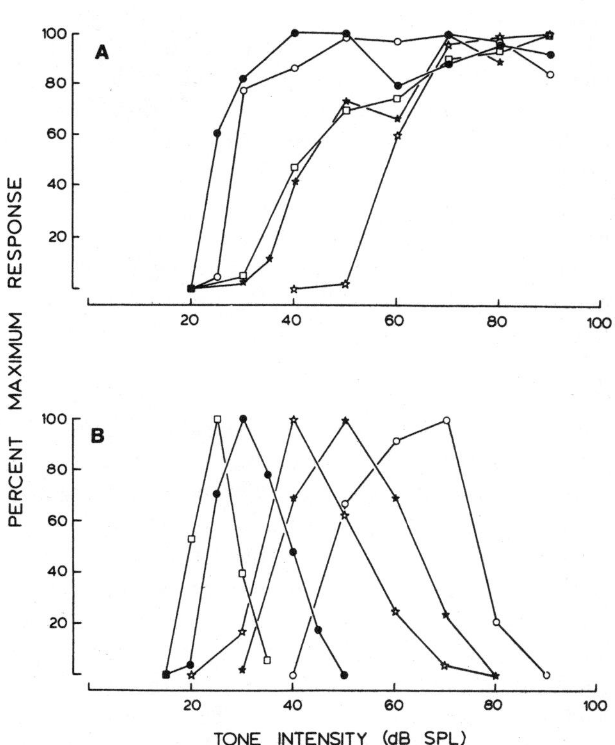

Figure 3. Normalized spike count-vs.-stimulus intensity for repeated tone bursts at CF derived from 10 AI neurons in the cat. Five of the neurons exhibited monotonic (A) and five nonmonotonic (B) behaviors. From Phillips *et al.* (1985).

sity can be sharply peaked and a change of 10 db on either side of the most effective SPL may reduce the count by as much as 90% of its maximum value; other cells have a broad maximum (Fig. 3B). Recent evidence suggests that cells displaying nonmonotonic rate-vs.-intensity functions might represent a class of neurons functionally distinct and spatially separate from those displaying monotonic functions (Phillips *et al.*, 1985). In any given animal, the most effective SPLs differ from one cell to the next. In monkey AI, best SPLs have been recorded between 15 and 94 db whereas in cat the values reported have ranged between 10 and 85 db. The presence of intensity-selective neurons suggests another mechanism, introduced in the central auditory system, whereby the dynamic range of hearing might be accomplished. Namely, regardless of where the stimulus lies within the dynamic range of hearing, there exists a population of cortical neurons that is firing maximally. Other pools of cells will be firing at submaximal rates and still others will be silent or spontaneously active because the sound intensity is too low or too high to evoke from them a vigorous discharge. Changing SPL results in a shift in the active neuronal pool such that many neurons once maximally active become less so and many of those once marginally active or unresponsive are brought to maximal response. Such a finding leads to the hypothesis of a "place" mechanism for intensity coding (Brugge and Merzenich, 1973b). This hypothesis has not yet been tested in either cat or monkey. Evidence for an "amplitopic organization" in the primary auditory cortex of the mustache bat has been obtained, however (see Suga, 1977).

3.3. Coding for Binaural Stimulus

There is abundant evidence that the integrity of AI is necessary for normal azimuthal sound localization behavior (e.g., Jenkins and Merzenich, 1984), although the mechanisms involved are far from being understood. Much of the information concerning the coding of binaural signals and the neural mechanisms of sound localization has been derived from studies of the brain-stem nuclei where activity originating in the two ears first converges and binaural interactions first occur (for recent reviews see Yin and Kuwada, 1984, and Phillips and Brugge, 1985). Brain-stem neurons receiving input from the two ears relay the results of that interaction to higher auditory centers including the cortex. Thus, many neurons within auditory cortical fields are sensitive to the binaural stimulus parameters of interaural time differences (ITDs) and interaural intensity differences (IIDs), two cues used by human listeners for localizing the source of a sound in space.

In order to understand the mechanisms that underlie binaural sensitivity and the possible roles played by cortical cells in sound localization and other binaural phenomena, the discharge properties of neurons in AI have been studied parametrically both under conditions where the stimuli to the two ears are controlled independently and delivered to the two eardrums via speculums sealed into the external ear canals (Hall and Goldstein, 1968; Brugge *et al.*, 1969; Brugge and Merzenich, 1973b; Benson and Teas, 1976; Phillips and Irvine, 1981b, 1983) and under more natural conditions where sounds are generated from speakers located in space around the head (Evans, 1968; Eisenman, 1974; Sovijarvi and Hyvarinen, 1974; Middlebrooks and Pettigrew, 1981). Most studies of binaural interactions carried out under earphone listening conditions have sought to define relationships between neural discharge patterns and variations in the intensities and the times of arrival of the stimuli delivered to the two ears.

3.3.1. Neurons Responding to ITDs In the free field, a difference in the time the stimuli arrive at the tympanic membranes occurs when the sound source is located at a point not equidistant from the two ears. If the stimulus is a pure tone, which it often is in experiments of the kind to be described, then two time disparities are realized: an interaural arrival-time disparity and an ongoing phase disparity. Auditory cortical neurons are sensitive to both temporal cues.

Many AI neurons responding to low-frequency tones, below about 4000 Hz, are exquisitely sensitive to small interaural differences in the interaural phase differences of the tonal stimuli at the two ears (Brugge *et al.*, 1969; Brugge and Merzenich, 1973b; Benson and Teas, 1976). The function relating the number of spikes evoked to the interaural time delay is a periodic one, the period of the function being equal to the period of the stimulating tone (Fig. 4). The periodicity of that function indicates that the neuron is responding to the differences in interaural phase of the stimuli. At favorable interaural delays, the response of a binaural AI neuron may be as strong or stronger than the sum of the two monaural responses. At least-favorable delays, the spike count may fall below that evoked by stimulation of either ear alone, indicating that a suppressive mechanism may be involved in the interaural delay sensitivity of these neurons. Studies of interaural phase sensitivity in the lower auditory brain stem reveal that monaural phase-locked inputs each have an excitatory half-cycle and an inhibitory half-cycle (Goldberg and Brown, 1969; Brugge *et al.*, 1970). When the impulses arriving from the two ears arrive at the cell of convergence at the same time, i.e., when the two excitatory half-cycles are in time register, the output of the binaural neuron is maximal. When the optimal delay is changed, so that the excitatory half-cycle of one input

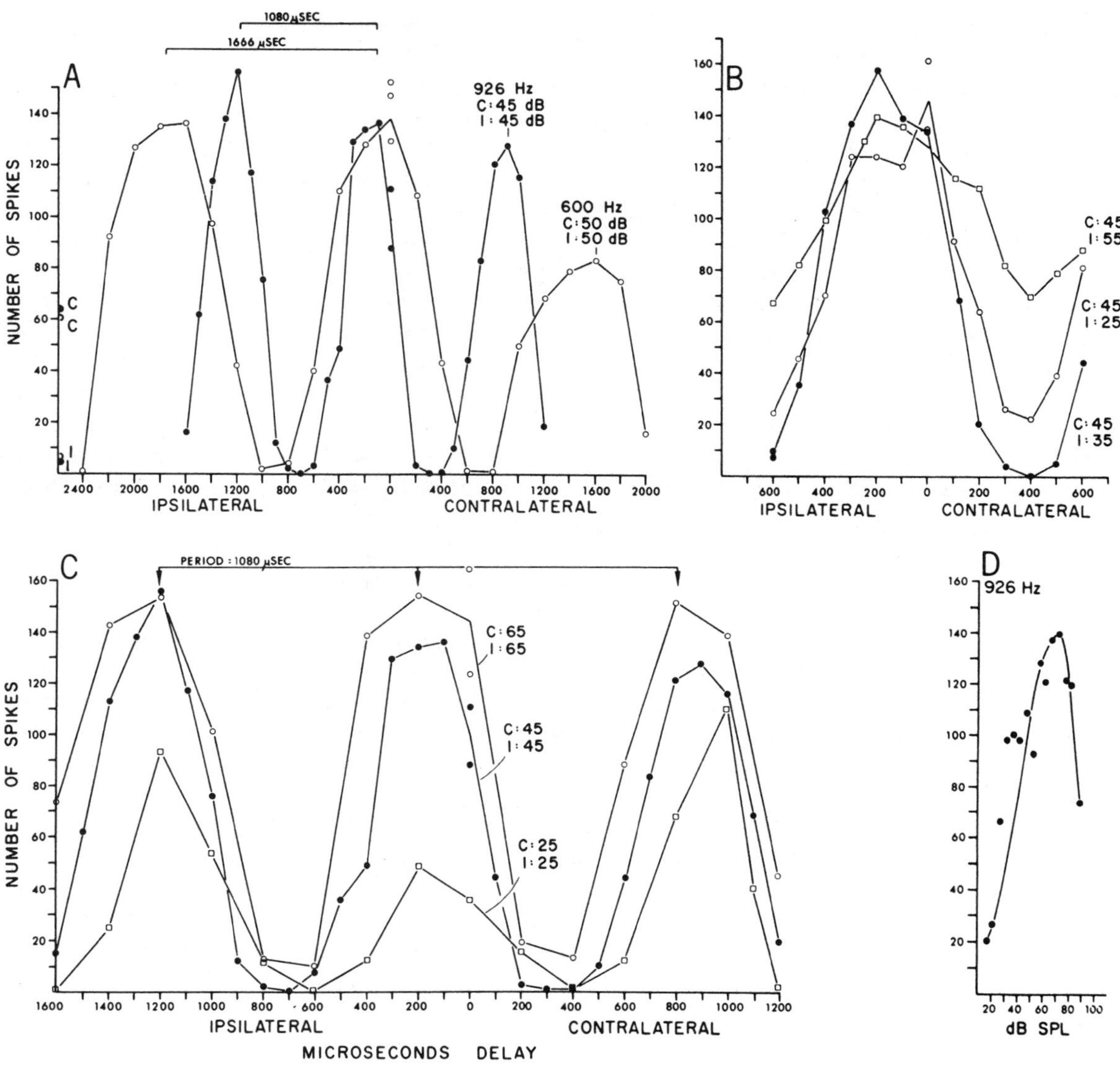

Figure 4. Spike count as a function of interaural time delay of low-frequency tones delivered to the two ears. Data are derived from a single AI neuron in an awake rhesus monkey. (D) Spike count-vs.-intensity function exhibited by this same unit at CF. In (A) the periodic functions obtained at 926 and 600 Hz reach the same maximal values when the tone to the ipsilateral ear lags that to the contralateral ear by around 100 μsec. This preferred time delay is uneffected by changing the interaural (B) or binaural (C) intensity. From Brugge and Merzenich (1973b).

is shifted in a way that makes it coincide in time with the inhibitory half-cycle of the other, the result is cancellation of the monaural response. Thus, the sensitivity to interaural phase delay reflects a temporal interaction of phase-locked excitatory and inhibitory inputs to neurons of the brain stem. The activity that results from this cycle-by-cycle interaction is transmitted faithfully to higher auditory centers including the cortex.

In 1966 Rose *et al.* described a class of binaural neurons in the cat inferior colliculus that detect a specific interaural time delay for all low frequencies to which the neuron is phase sensitive (see also Kuwada and Yin, 1983; Yin and Kuwada, 1983a,b). These cells were said to have a "characteristic delay." This delay would correspond to the interaural phase delay created by a sound lying on the surface of a hyperboloid extending laterally from one ear (the so-called "cone of confusion"). The concept of a "characteristic delay" was attractive and widely accepted despite the fact that until recently there was little experimental evidence to support it. The notion was questioned by some (e.g., Benson and Teas, 1976) largely on the grounds that frequently the characteristic delays recorded were outside of the useful range for animals with small head sizes (e.g., chinchillas and kangaroo rats). The arguments related to this and other issues that take us beyond the scope of this chapter have been discussed recently elsewhere (Phillips and Brugge, 1985). Suffice it to say that many AI neurons in both cat and monkey are phase sensitive and that this interaural phase sensitivity meets the criteria for a characteristic delay as originally put forward by Rose *et al.* (1966). Brugge and Merzenich (1973b) suggested from their studies of AI neurons in the unanesthetized monkey that phase sensitivity may be a column-dependent property of AI. This hypothesis has not been rigorously tested.

The sensitivity of AI neurons to onset-time disparities has received considerably less attention (Brugge *et al.*, 1969; Benson and Teas, 1976; Kitzes *et al.*, 1980). Nonetheless, there is evidence to indicate that this property is not governed by the same phase-locked, cycle-by-cycle mechanisms described previously. Rather, the discharge of such an AI neuron appears determined by the relative times of arrival of the excitatory inputs from one ear and the inhibitory inputs from the other.

Still another group of time-dependent neurons was discovered recently by Kitzes *et al.* (1980). These neurons tend not to be excited by monaural stimulation but respond vigorously when tones are presented to both ears with a zero, or near zero, interaural onset delay (Fig. 5A). This dependence on binaural stimulation prompted Kitzes *et al.* (1980) to refer to these cells as being "primarily binaural" (PB). The PB cells prefer not only an ITD around zero but also a zero, or near zero, IID (Fig. 5B) and hence are good candidates for detecting the location of sound in the vicinity of the median plane.

3.3.2. Neurons Responding to IIDs

IIDs are generated mainly by the acoustic shadow created by the head and pinnae (Moore and Irvine, 1979). They are significant only for high-frequency sound where the wavelengths are smaller than the head diameter or pinna height. The specification of the IID is most accurately and conveniently determined under earphone listening conditions. The IID may be controlled by changing the intensity of a tone delivered to one ear while holding the intensity of the tone to the other ear constant or by differentially changing the intensities of the tones delivered to both ears. For the most part, the connection between sensitivities to IID and absolute intensity has not been thoroughly analyzed at the cortical level despite the fact that both cues are needed to accurately locate the source of sound in space. Thus, it is often not clear from the published data whether and to what extent the apparent IID sensitivity of an auditory cortical neuron is also affected by absolute intensity.

For our present purposes we consider neurons in the high-frequency region of AI as distributed along a continuum based upon the sensitivity of these neurons to changes in the IID of binaurally presented tones. At one end of this distribution are those neurons whose discharge properties are particularly sensitive to changes in the IID. We presume that these neurons participate in the process of detecting the location of a sound in space. At the other end of the spectrum are the IID-insensitive neurons. The position of a neuron along this IID-sensitivity scale is determined to a large

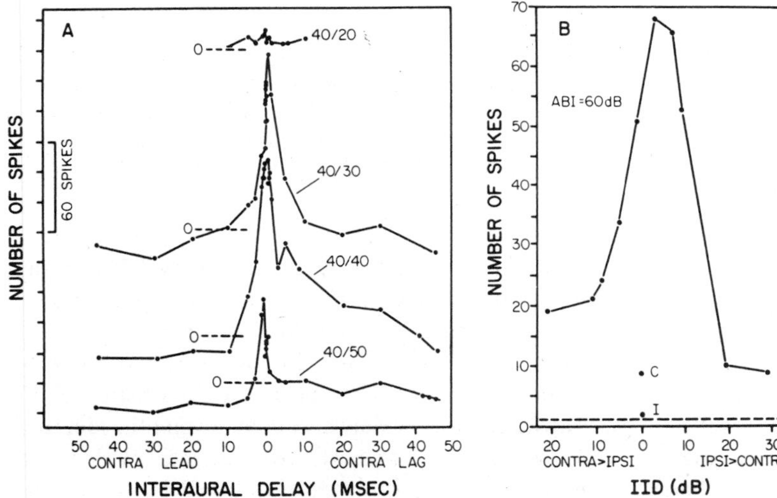

Figure 5. Spike count as a function of interaural time delay (A) or interaural intensity difference (B) for two PB neurons recorded in AI of the cat. (A) Four spike count functions, each at a different IID, are separated along the ordinate for easy comparison. Dashed line on each plot (0) indicates the baseline level of spontaneous activity. Maximal discharge occurs around an interaural delay and interaural intensity difference of zero. Redrawn from Kitzes *et al.* (1980). (B) IID functions obtained while holding the average binaural intensity constant at 60 db SPL. Counts generated by monaural stimulation of the contralateral (C) or ipsilateral (I) ears and the level of spontaneous activity (dashed line) are indicated on the plot. From Phillips and Irvine (1981b).

degree by the extent to which IID sensitivity of the cell is influenced by the absolute intensity of the binaural stimulus.

Neurons that occupy one of the extreme positions near the IID-sensitive end of this continuum are those that are excited by stimulation of one ear (usually the one contralateral to the cortex under study) and inhibited by simultaneous stimulation of the opposite ear the so-called EI neurons after Goldberg and Brown, 1969). Typically, these cells discharge maximally when the IID is adjusted to favor the contralateral ear and may be completely inhibited from discharging when the IID favors the ipsilateral ear. Figures 6A and 7A show the familiar sigmoidal relationship between spike rate and IID exhibited by these kinds of neurons. As shown in Fig. 6A, within the dynamic range of IID sensitivity, the change in discharge rate that accompanies a shift in IID (long arrow) is far greater than the rate change produced by an equivalent decibel shift in absolute intensity (short arrow). Neglecting any front-to-back ambiguity, a neuron with these properties

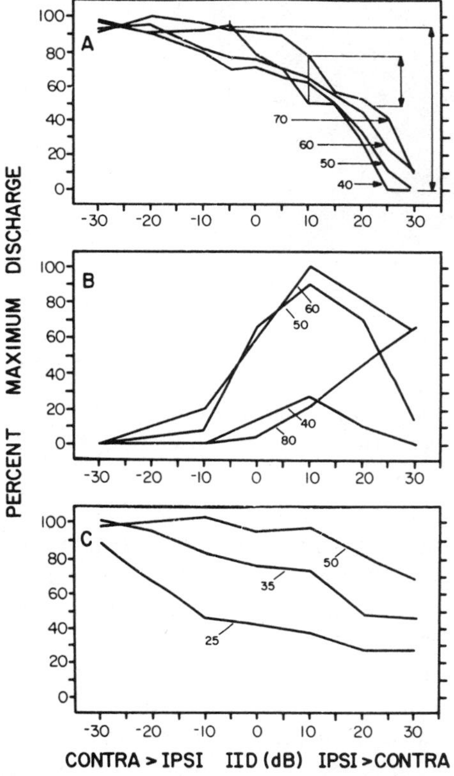

Figure 6. Normalized spike count-vs.-IID functions for three AI neurons in the cat. (A) IID functions derived from an EI cell at the four different average binaural intensities shown on the graph. The sensitivity to change in the IID (long arrow) is far greater than the sensitivity to change in the average level (short arrow) of the CF tone. (B) IID functions derived from a PB cell at four average intensity levels. (c) IID functions derived from a neuron relatively insensitive to IID.

should be able to detect the presence of a sound in the contralateral hemifield and to give information regarding the azimuthal location of that sound, at least in one plane of space (Phillips and Irvine, 1981b). It is also important to note, however, that while such a neuron may provide information about the direction from which a sound emanates, it cannot, because of its relative insensitivity to the overall sound intensity, provide as much information about the distance of the sound source from the head.

A second variant of IID-sensitive AI cell, the PB neuron, exhibits maximal discharge only when the IID and ITD are both around zero (Figs. 5 and 6B). At around zero ITD, there is a gradual reduction in the discharge rate as the IID is increased, until virtually no action potentials are evoked when the IID favors one ear or the other by some 20–30 db (Phillips and Irvine, 1981b). The distribution of IID functions shown in Fig. 6B indicates that the discharge for this PB neuron may also be highly dependent upon change in absolute intensity of the binaural stimulus. The relationship between discharge rate and IID is clearly different when one compares the curves taken at an average binaural intensity of 40 or 80 db with the curves taken with the average binaural intensity at 50 or 60 db. When the average intensity at the two ears is between 50 and 60 db, small changes in IID around the most effective IID result in substantial decreases in spike counts. In contrast, when the average intensity is reduced to 40 db or elevated to 80 db, the sensitivity to IID is greatly diminished or lost. This dual sensitivity to *both* IID and absolute intensity may render to PB neurons the capability of detecting the actual location of a sound source in space if that source is near the midline.

It is not uncommon to find in AI a third variant of IID-sensitive neuron. Cells in this group are excited by monaural stimulation of both ears (so-called EE neurons). When the IID favors one ear over the other, the rate and timing of the binaural response are similar to, if not indistinguishable from, the rate and timing of the response to monaural stimulation of the favored ear. Hence, such neurons not only can detect the hemifield within which the sound source lies but can provide information about the azimuthal location in *both* hemifields.

At this time there are not enough data available to give the complete input–output functions for each variant of AI neuron sensitive to IID. We can, however, suggest that the rules governing binaural interactions involving IID of the kinds previously described may, for many AI neurons responding under dichotic conditions, elicit two simple outcomes. First, if the intensity at one ear far exceeds that at the other, the result-

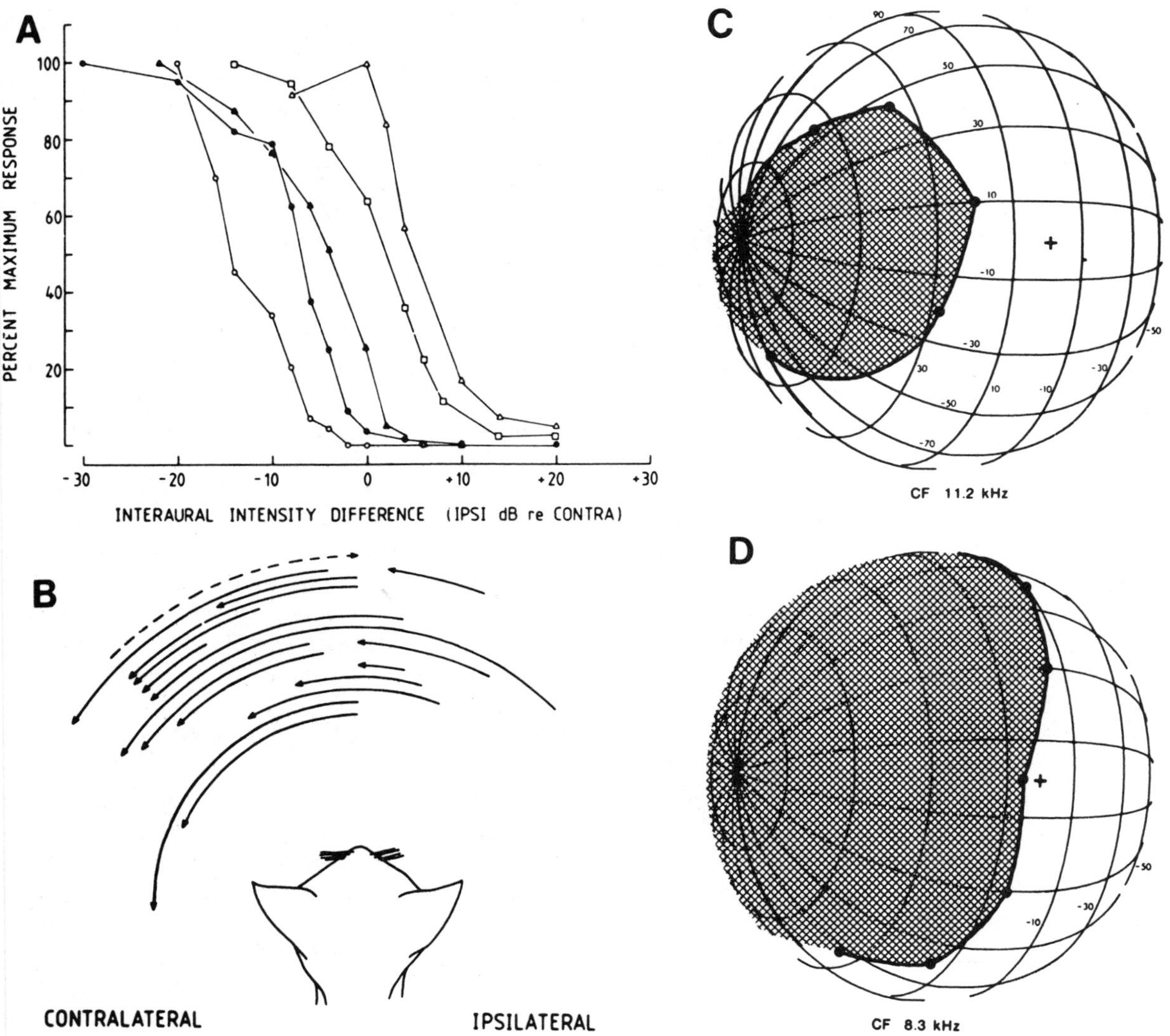

Figure 7. (A) IID functions derived from five AI neurons in cats listening through earphones. (B) Schematic view of a cat's head and sound field viewed from above showing the aximuthal projections of IID functions for 17 cells [including the 5 shown in (A)] isolated in AI. Each arrow represents the azimuthal range corresponding to the IIDs to which an individual unit was most sensitive. (A,B) from Phillips and Irvine (1981b). (C,D) Spatial receptive fields of two AI cells (hemifield units) recorded under free-field listening conditions. (C,D) from Middlebrooks and Pettigrew (1981).

ing discharge pattern is virtually identical to the one evoked by monaural stimulation of the ear receiving the more intense sound. Second, if the intensities of the sounds at the two ears are relatively close to one another, the binaural response is dominated by neither the left ear response nor the right ear response, i.e., the response pattern resembles neither monaural response.

For EI neurons, if the intensity at the excitatory (usually contralateral) ear is much greater than that at the inhibitory (usually ipsilateral) ear, the binaural response pattern is virtually identical to the one evoked by stimulation of the contralateral ear alone. As far as this cell is concerned, the sound is perceived as coming only through the contralateral ear or, extrapolating to the free-field listening condition, from a source in the contralateral hemifield. If, on the other hand, the ipsilateral stimulus is the stronger, then the binaural response may contain no spikes, which is for EI neurons the ipsilateral monaural response.

For EE neurons under conditions of large IIDs, the discharge pattern evoked monaurally by the weaker stimulus does not appear in the joint response. From the neuron's point of view, the relatively weak sound at one ear has been masked by the presence of a more intense sound at the opposite ear and the sound is lateralized to the ear receiving the greater intensity; the sound is perceived as coming through the ear receiving the more intense sound or, extrapolating to the free-field listening condition, from a source in that ear's hemifield. If the IID is reversed, the sound is then lateralized to the opposite ear or localized to the opposite hemifield. PB neurons also obey these rules but, because they produce few or no spikes unless the two ears are stimulated nearly simultaneously and with IIDs near zero, they can only code for stimuli in the vicinity of the midline.

Neurons that are placed near the other extreme of the IID-sensitivity continuum are, because of their relative insensitivity to changes in IID, considered poor candidates for detectors of the locus of a sound in space. Again, stimulation of one ear, usually the contralateral one excites such a neuron whereas monotic stimulation of the opposite ear may or may not evoke spikes. For some of these IID-insensitive neurons, simultaneous stimulation of the two ears results in a rate and temporal pattern of the discharge that are distinct from that recorded from the neuron under monotic conditions regardless of the IID (Brugge *et al.*, 1969; Brugge and Imig, 1978; Phillips and Irvine, 1983). The family of IID curves shown in Fig. 6C illustrates that the discharge of an IID-insensitive neuron changes rather little as a function of IID over a wide range of absolute intensities. Furthermore, the maximal change in discharge rate produced by either small or large changes in IID is virtually identical to the change in discharge rate which can be produced by comparable changes in absolute intensity.

3.3.3. Neurons Reponding under Free-Field Stimulus Conditions The studies mentioned above using dichotic stimulation did not answer directly the questions of whether binaural neurons of any class actually encode the spatial location of sounds and, if they do so, whether these neurons are distributed in a topographic fashion that could be construed to be a neural map of auditory space. These questions have been addressed to some extent in studies of AI neurons carried out under free-field stimulus conditions in both cat (Evans, 1968; Eisenman, 1974; Sovijarvi and Hyvarinen, 1974; Middlebrooks and Pettigrew, 1981) and monkey (Benson *et al.*, 1979). The results of these studies show that, in general, the response strength of a cortical neuron is a graded function of azimuth for sound in the contralateral hemifield and that some neurons show a spatial selectivity to relatively specific locations of the sound source.

In Middlebrooks and Pettigrew's (1981) experiments, an anesthetized cat was held in such a way that its head was in the center of a hemispheric field around which could be moved a loudspeaker. The speaker locations that were effective in eliciting a discharge from an AI neuron were used to determine the locus and extent of a spatial receptive field. About 50% of the neurons isolated in these experiments were selective for the location of sounds. This population could be divided into two subclasses of cells. One contained those cells that responded only to sounds in the contralateral hemifield (hemifield units). The properties of these neurons resemble most closely those of IID-sensitive EI cells recorded under dichotic listening conditions. Figure 7 illustrates the spatial receptive fields of two hemifield neurons and the corresponding rate-vs.-IID curves that such neurons might generate under earphone listening conditions. A second category of location-selective units (axial units) contained cells with small circumscribed receptive fields whose locations were constant for each experiment and which were determined by the orientation of the pinna. The presence of neurons with these properties points to the importance of the pinnae in sound localization mechanisms (Phillips *et al.*, 1982; Calford and Pettigrew, 1984). The remaining half of the AI cells isolated in these experiments were not sensitive to sound location and, thus, were referred to as omnidirectional units. These latter neurons are likely the IID-insensitive cells recorded under dichotic listening conditions. There was no indication of a space map in AI resembling the one discovered by Knudsen and Konishi (1978) in the midbrain of the barn owl. Rather, neurons with similar receptive field properties tend to aggregate into patches similar to those that make up binaural interaction bands in AI mapped under dichotic listening conditions as described later in this chapter.

Sovijarvi and Hyvarinen (1974) discovered in AI of the cat neurons that responded selectively not only to the spatial location of a sound but to the direction of its angular movement. Movement in one direction in the horizontal or vertical direction produced excitation in these neurons whereas motion in the opposite direction evoked inhibition or no change in the spontaneous activity. Although no systematic mapping of these properties was carried out, it is interesting to note that cells whose responses were determined by the location or movement of the sound source were frequently found along the length of an electrode penetration.

3.4. Coding for Complex Sounds

3.4.1. Coding of Species-Specific Vocalizations In certain primates the known repertoires of species-specific vocalizations have provided a wealth of natural acoustic stimuli with which to study the possible roles played by auditory cortical neurons in processing information of communicative significance (Wollberg and Newman, 1972; Newman and Wollberg, 1973; Glass and Wollberg, 1983). In general, however, the stimulus–response relationships derived from primate auditory cortical neurons suggest no simple one-to-one mapping between a neuron's response selectivity and a specific vocalization (Newman, 1978; Newman and Symmes, 1979; Glass and Wollberg, 1983). Neither the specific spectral content nor the communicative significance serves as a feature sufficient to evoke a unique neuronal response. Rather, responses of auditory cortical cells appear to depend in complex ways on specific patterns of acoustic transients embedded in time-varying and spectrally diverse stimuli (Wollberg and Newman, 1972; Newman and Symmes, 1979; Creutzfeldt *et al.*, 1980; Steinschneider *et al.*, 1982, Glass and Wollberg, 1983). Thus, a more suitable model of neural responsiveness may involve mechanisms similar to those proposed for the bat in which neurons are specialized to respond more on the basis of the presence or absence of certain transient components embedded in a species-specific vocalization rather than on the basis of a unique vocalization (Glass and Wollberg, 1983). Such a neural mechanism may also be involved in speech waveform processing since transient components in speech sounds, known to be linguistic parameters of perceptual significance in human communication, are clearly reflected in the temporal responses of primate cortical and geniculate neurons (Steinschneider *et al.*, 1982). Quantitative differences in the selectivities for primate vocalizations and human speech sounds have been documented for neurons believed to be located in different auditory cortical areas (Newman and Wollberg, 1973; Glass and Wollberg, 1983). Such findings would tend to support the idea that different cortical areas detect biologically significant sounds by unique, but not mutually exclusive, processing mechanisms. While there are little data to support this notion (see also Manley and Müller-Preuss, 1978), mechanisms like these are apparently operating at the level of the auditory cortex in the bat.

3.4.2. Repetitive Acoustic Pulses For human listeners, a train of short noise pulses or clicks evokes a pitch sensation at pulse repetition rates that approach several hundred pulses per second. The pitch sensation is not based on spectral cues but, rather, on the temporal waveform, hence its name, periodicity pitch. Monkeys, like humans, can discriminate a train of noise bursts having a rate of 10/sec from one with a rate of 300/sec (Symmes, 1974). This ability is permanently lost in such a trained monkey when the auditory cortex is destroyed bilaterally, suggesting that the cortex is involved in the detection of these temporal cues. De Ribaupierre and Goldstein (1972) discovered in the auditory cortex of the cat several classes of cells responding to click and noise trains. One class contains neurons that could encode the periodicity of clicks or noise bursts that elicit, in human listeners, a strong sensation of periodicity pitch. The single-spike discharge of these cells is precisely time-locked to the click and is perfectly entrained at click rates between 10/sec and 1000/sec. These cells represented 39% of the population of cortical neurons isolated in this experiment. Intracellular recordings of these neurons and neurons in other categories revealed that one mechanism that could limit the rate of locking to repeated acoustic transients is a hyperpolarization that follows a brief depolarization giving rise to the short-latency excitatory onset response. These so-called "locker" neurons resemble functionally certain cells of the cochlear nuclei and, hence, may be part of a neural circuit, originating in the brain stem, that encodes for the periodicity of the acoustic stimulus.

4. Coding Mechanisms in Fields Outside of AI

The publication of fine-grained frequency maps of the organization and boundaries of several auditory cortical fields in the cat (Knight, 1977; Merzenich *et al.*, 1975; Reale and Imig, 1980) was soon followed by several parametric studies in this animal of the coding properties of single neurons in areas outside of AI. These experiments probed the questions of whether and to what extent the different auditory fields divide the labor of encoding the many acoustic features found in the animal's natural environments.

4.1. The Anterior Auditory Field

The anterior auditory field (A) occupies the dorsal part of the anterior ectosylvian gyrus adjacent to (and partially overlapping) the hindquarter representation of the second somatic field. The similarities in the thalamic projections upon this field and AI led to an earlier prediction that the information reaching the two fields would be similar and that the processing of this information by the two fields would be done in parallel (Andersen *et al.*, 1980a). The electrophysiological results of Phillips and Irvine (1982) confirmed these expectations. Like many AI neurons, many cells in field A are sharply tuned to frequency, have dynamic ranges of no more than 30–40 db, and respond to CF tones with latencies as short as 10–12 msec. Their binaural sensitivity to interaural time and intensity differences of tonal stimulation has not been distinguishable from that of AI cells (see also Brugge *et al.*, 1969). Latency data are consistent with the view that the two fields derive parallel inputs directly and mainly from the ventral division of the MGB.

4.2. The Posterior Auditory Field

Field P is located on the caudal bank of the posterior ectosylvian sulcus adjacent to both AI and VP. It receives a widespread distribution of afferent input from its counterpart on the opposite hemisphere, from fields AI, A, and VP on the same side (Imig and Reale, 1980, 1981b), and from at least four subdivisions of the MGB including the ventral and deep dorsal nuclei, the magnocellular division, and those periventral nuclei bordering the ventral division (FitzPatrick *et al.*, 1977; Imig and Reale, 1981a; Morel and Imig, 1984). The physiology of field P cells takes on a character somewhat different from that of neurons in A and AI owing, presumably, to the fact that its thalamic input is weighted in favor of structures other than the ventral division of the MGB. Posterior field neurons have extraordinarily long minimal response latencies, on the order of 50 msec or more (Phillips and Orman, 1984). Such a latency would easily permit input from fields AI and A whose minimal latencies are, on the average, around 12–20 msec (Phillips and Irvine, 1981a). Even longer latencies have been described in field P (Reale and Imig, 1980). More than 85% of the neurons recorded in this area generate spike counts that are nonmonotonic functions of stimulus intensity and for 20% of these the counts fall to nearly zero at high stimulus levels (Phillips and Orman, 1984). This feature is present for all frequencies that excite the neuron and, hence, the response area for this neuron is a circumscribed one (see Fig. 2D–F). Another remarkable property of some of these cells is that the best SPL remains constant across frequency. The mechanisms operating to achieve such intensity selectivity are not known but they must necessarily involve neuronal interactions for the output of the cochlea shows no such selectivity. The high proportion of intensity-selective neurons would suggest that field P may be specialized for encoding intensity shifts by a place mechanism previously suggested for AI neurons. Whether this auditory field, or any other, possesses a map of stimulus intensity, as does one of the cortical fields in the mustache bat (Suga, 1977), is not known.

Field P neurons exhibit binaural interactions of the kind displayed by cells in both A and AI and in many brain-stem auditory nuclei (Orman and Phillips, 1984). Thus, there appear to be striking similarities in the mechanisms of encoding dichotic listening cues between field P cells and cells in other auditory cortical fields. Moreover, the relatively high frequency–intensity selectivity displayed by field P cells has been achieved apparently without cost to the detection of these interaural time and intensity localization cues.

4.3. Second Auditory Field (AII)

Systematic quantitative studies of the discharge properties of single AII neurons have yet to be carried out. Qualitative studies of the responses of neuronal clusters have, however, provided a picture of AII, which is different in several respects from that of AI (Andersen *et al.*, 1980a, Keale and Imig, 1980; Middlebrooks and Zook, 1983; Schreiner and Cynader, 1984). In contrast to AI neurons, AII cells are broadly tuned and have relatively high thresholds to tonal stimulation. These properties may reflect the relatively diffuse afferent input AII cells apparently have from the MGB (Andersen *et al.*, 1980a). Binaural interactions of the kind recorded in AI, A, and P are preserved in AII as well.

4.4. Association Cortex

In unanesthetized cats or in cats under chloralose anesthesia, responses to auditory stimulation are recorded in three regions outside of the ectosylvian auditory area. These fields on the medial suprasylvian gyrus (MSA), anterior lateral gyrus (ALA), and pericruciate gyrus (PCA) receive convergent auditory, visual, and somatic sensory input, hence the name "polysensory" or "nonspecific" cortex. Neurons in these areas are, as a rule, broadly tuned to frequency, respond to tones or noise at each ear with a long-latency (16–54 msec) onset spike which is followed by a 200- to 300-msec suppression of spontaneous activity, and exhibit a binaural interaction described as occlusion (Irvine and Huebner, 1979). The responses to acoustic stimulation of neurons in the medial/intralaminar (M/IL) nuclei of the thalamus are virtually identical to those in association cortical fields, a finding which supports the notion that these areas are reached by a nonspecific projection system that is distinct from the lateral lemniscal pathway reaching ectosylvian fields via the MGB (Irvine, 1980). Input to the intralaminar nuclei comes from the brain-stem reticular formation which contains neurons whose acoustic response properties are similar to those in the M/IL. Another potential source of diffuse input to association cortex is the pulvinar–posterior complex of the thalamus. This work has been reviewed by Irvine and Phillips (1982).

5. Functional Architecture

5.1. Frequency Selectivity and the Cortical Representation of Cochlear Place

Neurons located along a cell column radial to the cortical surface tend to have the same or very similar CFs as illustrated in Fig. 8 (Hind *et al.*, 1960; Abeles and Goldstein, 1970; Merzenich and Brugge, 1973; Merzenich *et al.*, 1975; Phillips and Irvine, 1981a). The frequency organization of a radial cell column has been difficult to determine accurately mainly because of the spatial resolution of the extracellular recording techniques used, the difficulty in obtaining electrode penetrations perfectly aligned with cell columns, and the fact that cells in laminae above and below the thalamocortical target zone are relatively unresponsive under

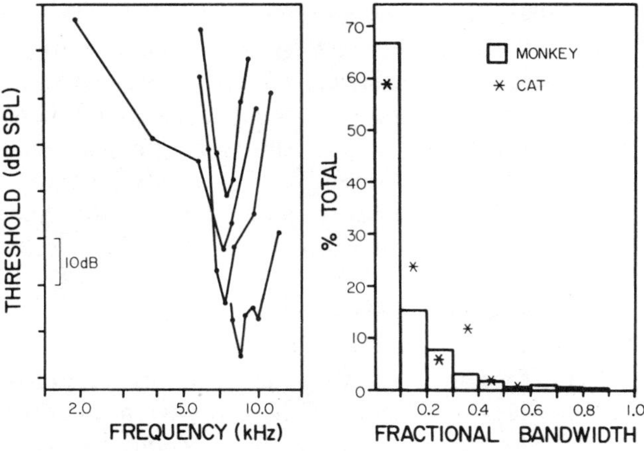

Figure 8. (Left) Threshold tuning curves derived from four AI neurons within a single electrode penetration oriented nearly perpendicular to the cortical surface. The curves are shifted along the ordinate for clarity. From Phillips and Irvine (1981a). (Right) Variation in CF of neurons within a single perpendicular penetration into AI of cat and monkey. Fractional bandwidth = (highest CF − lowest CF)/lowest CF in the penetration. Cat data from Phillips and Irvine (1981a), monkey data from Brugge and Merzenich (1973b).

general anesthesia. Abeles and Goldstein (1970) carefully approached this problem by recording from isolated neurons in AI of unanesthetized cats and correcting the data for the orientation of the electrode path with respect to that of the radial cell columns. They found that almost without exception, narrowly tuned units in the same or close radial cell chains have nearly equal CFs. Although CFs may be more difficult to judge in broadly tuned cells, the response range of frequencies of these neurons overlapped that of neighboring narrowly tuned cells in the same radial penetration. Cell columns representing the same CF are, when projected upon the brain surface, arrayed along what is referred to as an *isofrequency line* (when viewed through the depth of the cortex, the array of elements having the same CF occupies a ribbon of tissue). The presence of isofrequency lines (or ribbons) is the consequence of the projection of points from a one-dimensional linear array (the cochlear partition) to a three-dimensional structure (the cortex). By systematically determining the characteristic frequencies of neurons and neuron clusters in multiple closely spaced microelectrode penetrations, complete CF maps of AI and several surrounding fields have been obtained in a variety of mammalian species as described previously. The isofrequency lines on the cat AI (Fig. 10A) run in a dorsoventral direction; those lines representing high frequencies are found rostrally in the field, those representing lower frequencies are located progressively more caudally. Thus, the isofrequency lines in cat AI, and in surrounding fields, run roughly orthogonal to the high-to-low-frequency gradient of the field, a conclusion reached by Woolsey and Walzl in their evoked potential work more than four decades ago. A similar situation obtains for tonotopically organized fields in other species studies so far.

In 1964 a controversy arose over the question of tonotopic organization in cat AI. At that time Evans and Whitfield (1964) reported that in unanesthetized cats the positions of neurons in what they believed to be area AI were poorly correlated with the neuron's CFs, suggesting that the organization of units in this field was not a tonotopic one. Part of the problem arose from the fact that tonotopy at the level of the cortex has traditionally been linked to a central "place" mechanism for frequency discrimination (see, e.g., Poliak, 1932). As frequency discrimination is not abolished in cats after large auditory cortical lesions, it was not difficult to accept the possibility that tonotopy in this region was blurred or nonexistent. Moreover, it does seem to be the case that general anesthesia reduced substantially the rich and varied afferent input to many cells, thereby rendering them unresponsive to sound or responsive mainly to the more tightly coupled input from the MGB. Third, the CF map of AI is not related in any systematic way to the positions of the sulci of the region. Hence, pooling of CF data from different animals and using sulci as landmarks for the construction of frequency maps can easily blur the organization that might exist there.

5.2. Binaural Sensitivity, Computational Cortical Maps, and the Cortical Representation of Sound in Space

It was discovered several years ago that AI neurons having similar binaural properties tend to form vertical columns through the cortical gray matter and that these columns aggregate into clusters or bands (Imig and Adrian, 1977; Middlebrooks *et al.*, 1980). Detailed microelectrode mapping studies of AI, similar to those that revealed the tonotopic organization of this field, were carried out to determine the distribution of these so-called *binaural interaction bands.*

Some variations may exist in the binaural interactions exhibited by neurons isolated in a single vertical electrode penetration into AI, at least under a limited set of binaural conditions (Phillips and Irvine, 1979). It is also the case that, qualitatively, the binaural response properties of the great majority of neurons and neuron clusters may be assigned to one of two major classes that are easily distinguished from one another simply by visual inspection on the oscilloscope screen of the neural discharge in response to dichotic tonal stimulation. This latter approach was taken by Imig and Adrian (1977) who classified about two-thirds of the neuronal cluster responses as being *summation* responses, i.e., the response to simultaneous binaural stimulation was greater than the response to stimulation of either ear alone. These neurons are generally of the kind referred to as EE (excitatory/excitatory) in the similar study of Middlebrooks *et al.* (1980). *Suppression* responses occurred when the neurons were excited less by binaural stimulation than by stimulation of the more effective monaural stimulus. These are also referred to as EI (excitatory/inhibitory) responses. Other types of responses are recorded but they make up a small proportion of the total recorded.

An electrode penetrating the cortex normal to the pial surface encounters successively units with either suppressive or summative properties (Fig. 9A,C). Systematic mapping of the cortical surface of AI with closely spaced electrode penetrations revealed aggregations of binaural columns, some of which were elongated into bands running nearly orthogonal to the isofrequency contours (Fig. 9B).

Binaural sensitivity, unlike frequency sensitivity, is not a property represented on the basilar membrane. It arises as the result of the interaction of excitatory and inhibitory inputs impinging on target neurons located, presumably, in the lower auditory brain stem. Thus, whereas tonotopy in the auditory cortex is a map of the receptor surface projected topographically upon successive auditory relay nuclei, the binaural map is, in large part, a computational one the elements of which are formed by neuronal interactions.

6. Relationships between the Functional Organizations and Connectivity Patterns of Auditory Cortical Fields

Auditory cortical fields are linked to numerous subcortical areas via axons of thalamocortical, corticothalamic, corticotectal, corticostriatal, and cortico-

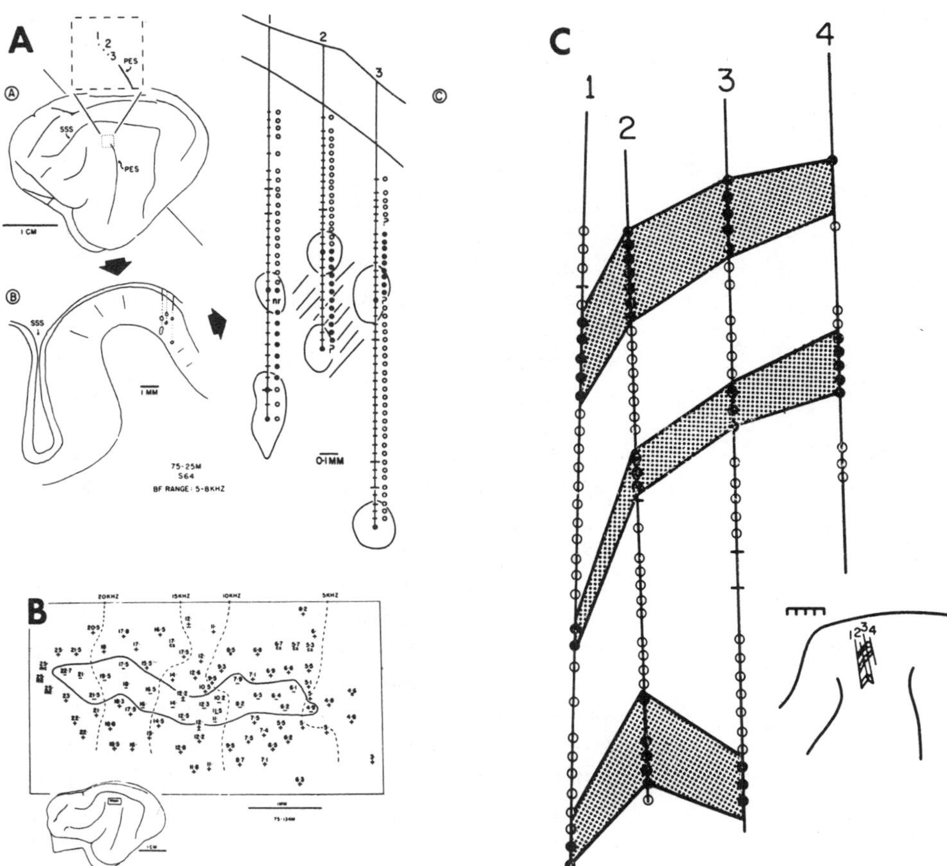

Figure 9. (A) Diagram showing the entry points of three microelectrode penetrations into AI of the cat and the distribution of binaural classes within each penetration. Open circles designate neurons or neuronal clusters classified as generating *summation* (EE) responses; closed circles designate suppression (EI) responses. (B) Surface view of a tonotopic and binaural map. Solid line surrounds a region containing neurons exhibiting only suppression (−) responses. Summation responses (+) are found surrounding this area. Numbers are CFs of neurons or neuron clusters in the penetration at that cortical site. (A, B) redrawn from Imig and Adrian (1977). (C) Distribution of binaural classes of neurons or neuron clusters obtained from four tangentially oriented electrode penetrations through AI of the cat. Open and closed circles represent EE and EI responses, respectively. Shaded areas connect EI zones to form the hypothesized binaural bands running somewhat rostrocaudally across AI. These bands probably correspond to the suppression regions outlined by Imig and Adrian as shown in (B). (C) Redrawn from Middlebrooks *et al.* (1980).

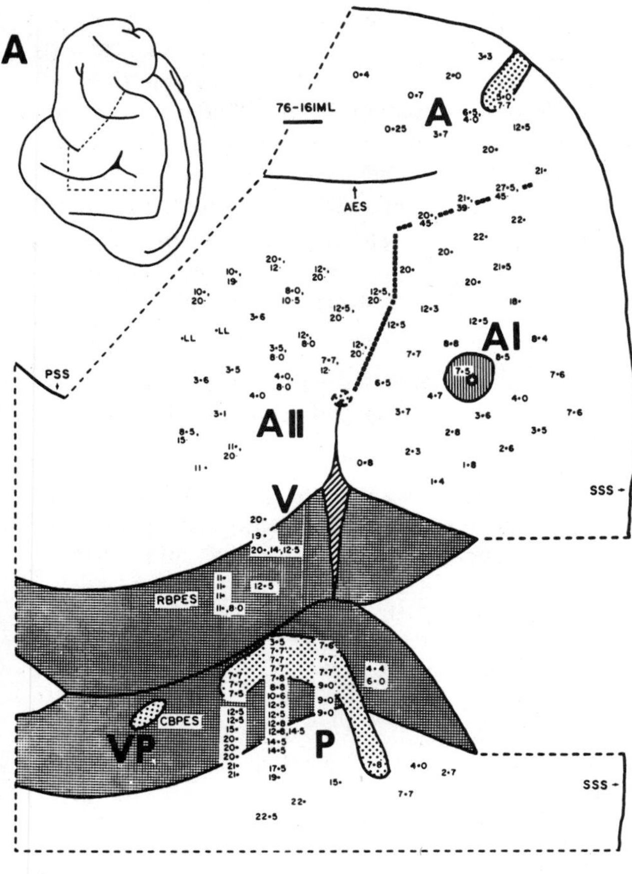

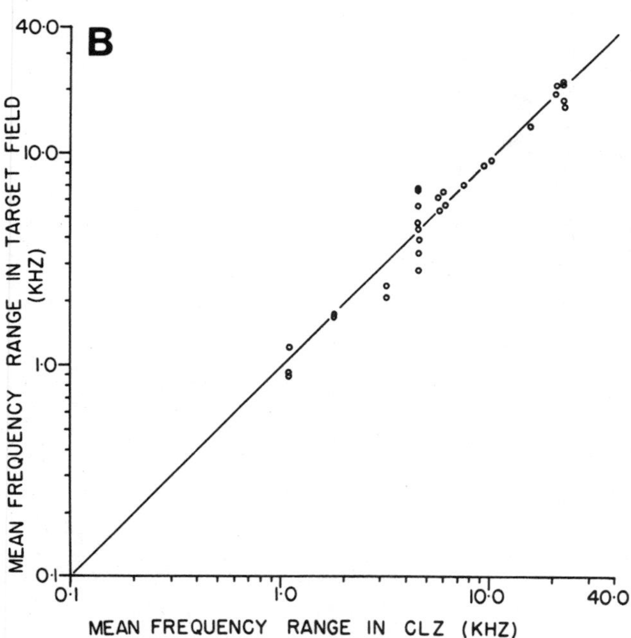

Figure 10. (A) Map of CFs of neurons or neuron clusters in auditory cortex of the cat. Small inset shows lateral view of the cat brain with the rostral end pointed upward and the ventral part to the left. The dashed lines outline the mapped area shown in the exploded view. Numbers are CFs recorded from neurons in penetrations at those points on the brain. Shaded areas represent the depths of the posterior ectosylvian sulcus which has been opened up in this drawing to show portions of the fields normally buried there. Area in AI circled is the site of a small injection of tritiated proline. Stippled areas in A, P, and VP are the sites of terminal labeling that resulted from the injection. (B) Plot of the CF at the site of a tritiated proline injection (CLZ) as a function of the CF at the target site where axonal terminal labeling was detected. From Imig and Reale (1980).

pontine neurons and to each other via a network of corticocortical fibers. A variety of tract-tracing techniques have been employed to study these connections including those of lesion-degeneration and of axonally transported radioactive amino acids or horseradish peroxidase. Figure 11A shows the widespread distribution in the auditory fields around AI of terminal labeling of axons that had transported tritiated proline from the small injection site in AI. The earlier studies of auditory cortical connectivity, in both cat and monkey (Diamond *et al.*, 1968a,b, 1969; Pandya *et al.*, 1969; Heath and Jones, 1971; Kawamura, 1973; Pandya and Sanides, 1973; Sousa-Pinto, 1973; Paula-Barbosa *et al.*, 1975; Winer *et al.*, 1977; Niimi and Matsuoka, 1979), did not use electrophysiological mapping along with tract-tracing to determine the cortical field boundaries or the functional maps within the fields. More recently, several laboratories have combined microelectrode mapping of auditory cortex with anatomical pathway tracing in the same animal. This is a powerful combination of techniques that allows cortical input–output projection patterns to be related directly to the boundaries and functional organizations of cortical fields. Combined microelectrode mapping and tracer studies of auditory cortical connections with the thalamus (Andersen *et al.*, 1980a; Merzenich *et al.*, 1982), midbrain (Andersen *et al.*, 1980b,c), basal ganglia (Reale and Imig, 1983), and neighboring cortical fields (Imig and Brugge, 1978; Imig and Reale, 1980, 1981b) have revealed two outstanding features of these projection systems. First, the cortical auditory system is highly segregated cochleotopically; neurons with similar CFs are strongly connected, often in reciprocal fashion, whereas neurons with dissimilar CFs tend to remain relatively isolated from one another. Second, the projections are both highly divergent and highly convergent.

6.1. Relationships to Tonotopic Organization

6.1.1. Corticocortical Connections Evidence in the cat for a topographically organized system of auditory corticocortical connections was first provided by the

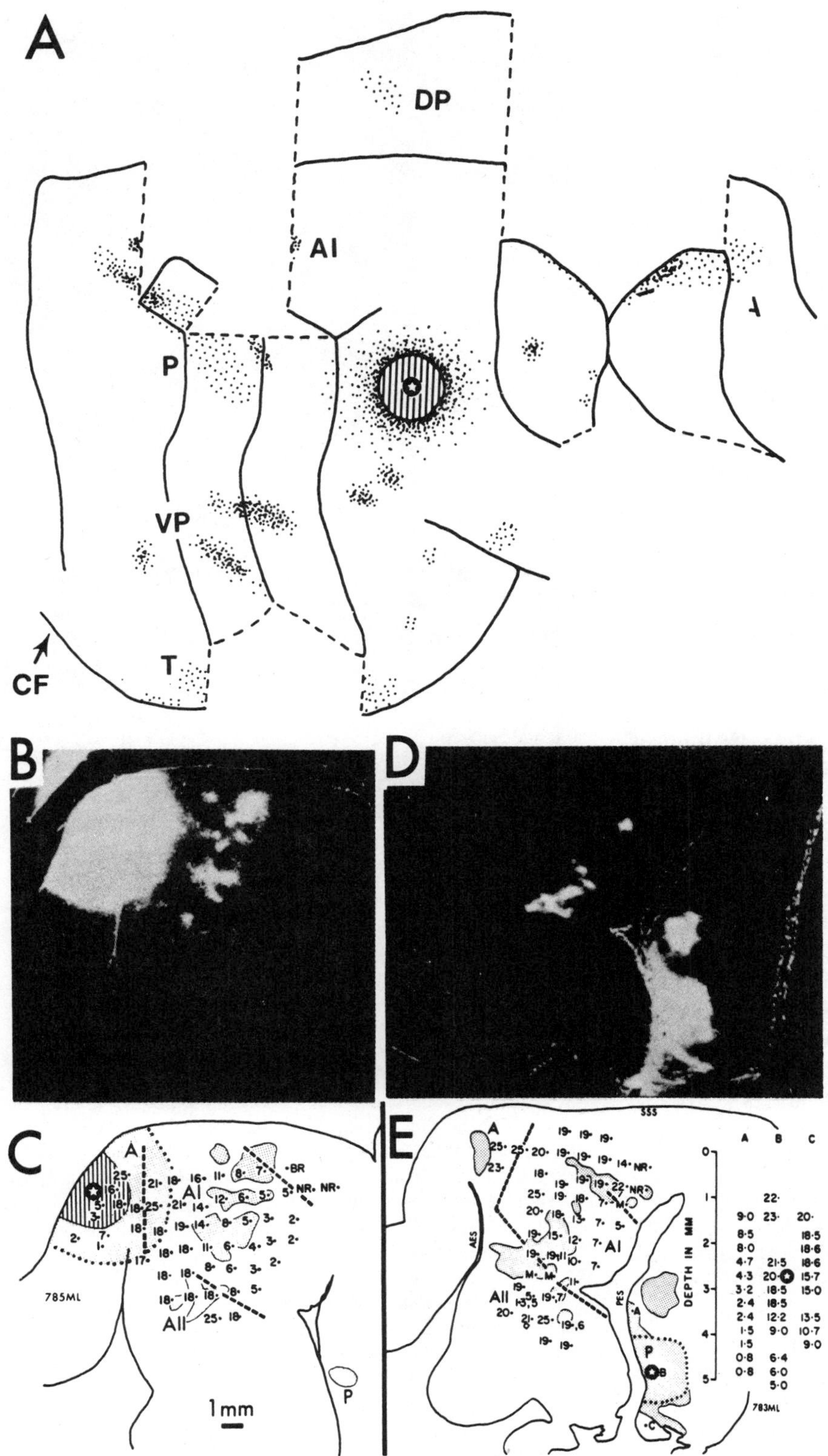

Figure 11. Drawing of the ectosylvian region of the cat, unfolded to show the banks of the sulci within which are found portions of auditory fields. The circle and star mark the center of a small injection of tritiated proline. Stippling indicates the terminal anterograde labeling in the ipsilateral fields to which AI projects. (B, C) Patchy labeling in AI after injection of tritiated proline into A. (D, E) Patchy labeling in AI after injection of tritiated proline into P. In both cases the transported label appears at the same CF region as that of the injection site. Numbers in (C) and (E) are CFs of neurons or neuron clusters.

experiments of Downman *et al.* (1960) in which electrical stimulation of a locus in one auditory field evoked a response in a restricted locus of another. Many of the details of this and other auditory corticocortical pathways were later worked out in studies in which single-unit mapping was combined with autoradiographic and HRP tract-tracing. Examples of results from several of these studies (Imig and Brugge, 1978; Imig and Reale, 1980, 1981b) are shown in Figs. 10–13. In the experiment illustrated in Fig. 10A, large parts of fields AI, A, P, and AII were mapped electrophysiologically and within AI a single small injection of tritiated proline was placed on the 7.5-kHz isofrequency contour. The transported label was later localized to the 7.5-kHz place in A and in P. The results of this experiment illustrate the two features of the auditory corticocortical connections mentioned previously. First, the projection is a topographic one; AI neurons project upon cells in both A and P having the same CF. Second, the projection is a divergent one; a single small injection at a known CF locus in AI produces a terminal labeling pattern that extends along the isofrequency contours in the target fields. Figure 11 illustrates the results of the reverse experiment and another feature of the corticocortical connection patterns. Here small injections of tritiated proline were made into mapped areas of A (Fig. 11B,C) or P (Fig. 11D,E). In both cases, the resultant projection patterns in AI are patchy ones, but within the appropriate CF representation. The uneven distribution of corticocortical connections is most dramatically shown in Fig. 12, which is taken from experiments in which large injections of tritiated proline or HRP were injected into AI of the opposite hemisphere.

The experiments illustrated here are typical of many others in which injections were made in AI, A, P, and VP at many different CF loci. The overall picture is that ipsilaterally fields AI, A, P, and VP appear topographically and reciprocally connected with one another. In addition, each of these fields projects to multiple areas within the peripheral auditory belt. Furthermore, each of the four tonotopically organized areas is reciprocally and topographically connected with the homotopic field on the opposite hemisphere. Figure 10B summarizes the results of many experiments of the kind described. In this figure the abscissa represents the CF at the center of the injection site and the ordinate the centers of the labeled terminal fields that resulted from the injection. The points on the plot cluster around the diagonal line indicating the high correlation between the CFs at the injection and target sites.

The organization of the corticocortical connections in the monkey is far less well understood than that in the cat. Only the projections of AI and the field rostral to it (field R) have been studied in any detail using both

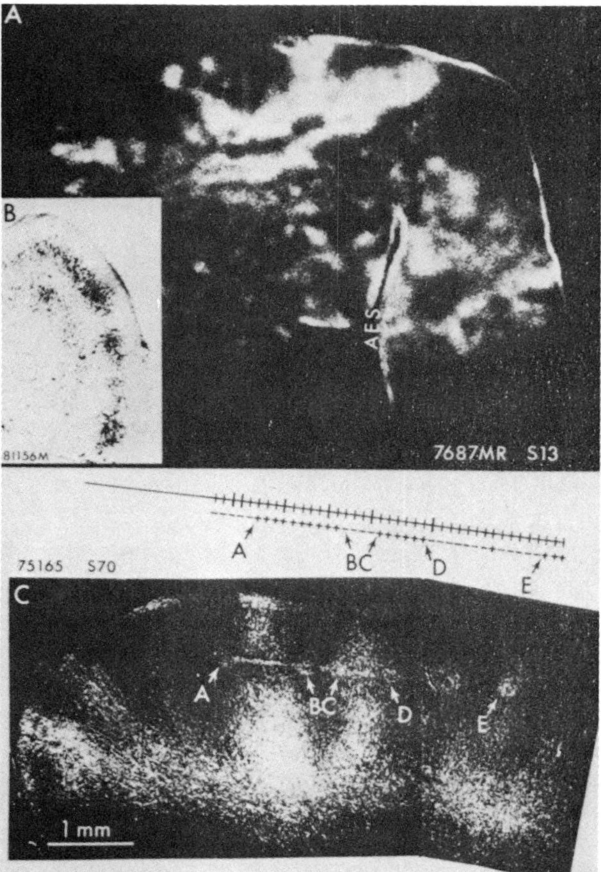

Figure 12. (A) Darkfield photomicrograph of a tangential section through the middle layers of the ectosylvian area of cat brain showing in an autoradiograph the distribution of terminals of the corpus callosum that were labeled as the result of a large injection of tritiated proline into AI of the opposite hemisphere. The suprasylvian sulcus is above, and anterior ectosylvian sulcus (AES) to the lower right. (B) Photomicrograph of a transverse section through AI of the cat showing the pattern of retrograde uptake of HRP following a large HRP injection into AI of the opposite hemisphere. (C) Darkfield photomicrograph through AI of cat showing the labeling of callosal terminals and the relationship of this pattern to the distribution of binaural neurons and neuron clusters recorded in an electrode penetration through that area. In the autoradiographs of both (A) and (C) the white dots are silver grains indicating relatively heavy callosal innervation. Arrows (A–E) point to microlesions produced during the experiment at points where the binaural interactions changed. The reconstructed penetration above shows the clustering of *summation* (EE) responses within areas of relatively heavy callosal innervation and *suppression* (EI) responses in regions of relatively sparse callosal innervation. From Imig and Brugge (1978).

electrophysiological and anatomical tracing methods. According to the results of autoradiographic tracer studies in the owl monkey (FitzPatrick and Imig, 1980, 1982), AI projects ipsilaterally to the five known cortical auditory fields and contralaterally to three fields, including AI. Field R is reciprocally connected to AI and projects to at least three other fields. Contralaterally, field R projects to the same fields as does AI. Like the projections in the cat, those in the monkey auditory cortex are also patchy in nature. In the rhesus monkey, auditory cortex has been shown by Seltzer and Pandya (1978) to be connected in a cascading fashion to the temporal pole and perhaps to a wider segment of the superior temporal gyrus (see Pandya and Yeterian, this volume).

6.1.2. Thalamocortical and Corticothalamic Connections Andersen *et al.* (1980a) mapped the thalamocortical and corticothalamic connections between the MGB and three auditory fields–AI, A, and AII—using both anterograde and retrograde tracing methods. Microelectrode recording guided the cortical placement of the tracers and later was used to correlate the anatomical and CF maps. Restricted loci in AI and A were found to receive coextensive inputs from folded sheets of neurons passing through the ventral division of the MGB, from columns of cells through the deep dorsal nucleus of the dorsal division of the MGB, from the medial division of the MGB, and from cells in the lateral division of the posterior group. Many neurons of the ventral division that project upon field AI also send an axon collateral to field A (Imig and Reale, 1981a; Imig et al., 1981). The main differences between the thalamic connections to fields AI and A are that the input to field AI is stronger from the ventral division whereas that to field A is stronger from the posterior group (Morel and Imig, 1984).

Fields P and VP receive their thalamic input from a different group of thalamic nuclei although the ventral nucleus, deep dorsal nucleus, and medial division of the MGB are also included in this grouping (FitzPatrick *et al.*, 1977; Imig and Reale, 1981a; Imig and Morel, 1983; Morel and Imig, 1984). The projection from the ventral division of the MGB is relatively weak to fields P and VP as compared to AI whereas the projections from nuclei surrounding the ventral division along its dorsal, caudal, and ventral borders are relatively strong. Some neurons in the ventral nucleus, however, have been shown to project via axon collaterals to both fields P and AI and fields P and A (Imig and Reale, 1981a; Imig *et al.*, 1981).

Area AII receives its thalamic input from a different group of MGB sub-divisions including the ventrolateral nucleus and the caudal part of the dorsal nucleus. It also receives from the medial nucleus, as does A and AI. These connectivity patterns are reciprocal in nature.

Imig and Morel (1984) have reconstructed the topography of the entire array of MGB neurons which give rise to the frequency-specific projections destined for fields A, AI, P, and VP. The array is composed of cells located in the ventral and medial divisions of the MGB as well as in the lateral posterior complex. In the ventral nucleus of the ventral division, the precise geometry of an array was found to be dependent on the specific target frequency representation in the cortex and was composed of both planar (sheetlike) and concentric components. This topography is consistent with previous descriptions of the distributions of thalamocortical cells projecting to fields A and AI (Colwell, 1977; Andersen *et al.*, 1980a; Merzenich *et al.*, 1982) and with the tonotopic organization of the ventral nucleus (Imig and Morel, 1985). Taking these data together, Imig and Morel (1984) propose that a single tonotopic representation exists within the ventral nucleus and can be modeled by three-dimensional arrangements of planar and concentric components.

A single cortical locus in either field AI or A having a restricted frequency representation receives input from neurons located in several separate cell aggregates of the ventral division of the MGB (Colwell, 1977; Andersen *et al.*, 1980a; Middlebrooks and Zook, 1983). Together these aggregates of thalamocortical projecting neurons are confined to sheetlike or slablike sectors of the ventral nucleus for a cortical locus representing frequencies near the middle of the acoustic spectrum. This geometry corresponds, in turn, to an MGB isofrequency lamina (Morel, 1980; Imig and Morel, 1985). Similarly, a single cortical locus in either field AI or A projects in a reciprocal fashion to these separate targets in the MGB isofrequency plane (Andersen *et al.*, 1980a). Middlebrooks and Zook (1983) have shown that two different cortical loci located along the same isofrequency strip in field AI receive input from many of the same aggregates of ventral nucleus cells distributed within an MGB isofrequency lamina. These observations are consistent with the findings of Dickson and Gerstein (1974) who recorded simultaneously from neighboring auditory cortical cells and analyzed the spontaneous and sound-evoked spike trains using cross-correlation techniques. Their data suggested that nearly all of the cortical neurons they studied that were located within about 250 μm of one another, and some others that were separated by as much as 1500 μm, received a shared input from some distant source, the most likely one being the MGB. Thus, there appear to be both divergent and convergent connections between similar portions of the thalamic and cortical frequency representations. Later we take up the evidence that points to the relationships between this convergent and divergent pattern of thalamic inputs and the binaural map of AI.

Two functionally separate pathways through the MGB to the cortex have been postulated to account for the physiology and connectivity patterns of the multiple cortical fields described so far in the cat (Reale and Imig, 1980; Andersen *et al.*, 1980a; Imig and Morel, 1983; Schreiner and Cynader, 1984). One pathway preserves cochleotopy through the brain stem, thalamus, and cortex. It would include the central nucleus of the inferior colliculus (ICC) and the pars lateralis and pars ovoidae, deep dorsal nucleus, and medial division of the MGB. Areas AI, A, P, and VP make up the cortical component of this system. A second pathway to the cortex routes the information from neurons that have poor frequency selectivity (e.g., the pericentral nucleus of the inferior colliculus), and, therefore, reside in regions where cochleotopy is blurred. Area AII, and perhaps portions of fields P, VP, and the "temporal" auditory field are the cortical components of this system.

6.1.3. Intrinsic Connections of Field AI Neurons within AI may communicate with one another over local circuits that are intrinsic to AI. The patterns of these connections appear related to the AI cochleotopic organization. Reale *et al.* (1983) deposited iontophoretically small quantities of HRP into AI at a known CF locus within a larger tonotopic map and later traced the courses of neuronal processes that transported the enzyme (Fig. 13). When viewed in a plane tangential to the cortical surface, labeled processes radiated out asymmetrically from the injection site over distances of several millimeters. The heaviest concentrations of labeled fibers were along an axis parallel with the isofrequency line in which the injection was made. In Golgi preparations, neurons in the middle ectosylvian cortex have been shown to have dendritic processes with preferred orientations (Glaser *et al.*, 1979), and while in such preparations no physiological maps were available for comparison, the dorsoventral orientation of the dendritic fields is consistent with the orientation of isofrequency lines in AI. Thus, primary field neurons having the same or similar CFs have the potential of being preferentially interconnected. By the same token, disparate CF representations are unlikely to communicate strongly with one another over this intrinsic fiber system. Recall that along the isofrequency dimensions of AI there are alternating patches of neurons having different binaural properties. Consequently, at any frequency all binaural classes could be activated. It remains to be seen the extent to which the intracortical fiber system of AI interconnects these binaural patches.

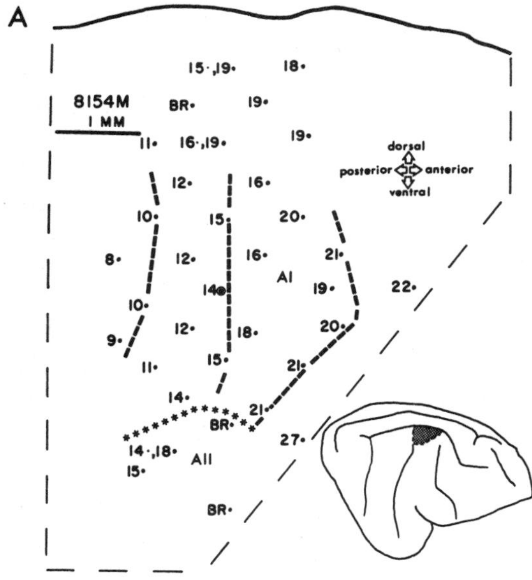

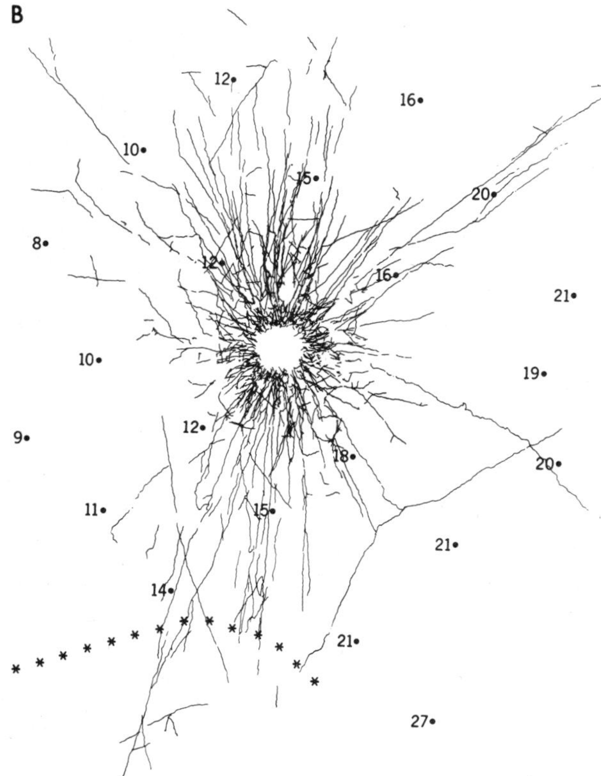

Figure 13. Relationship between the CF map and intrinsic connectivity patterns in field AI of the cat. (A) Reconstructed CF map displayed on the surface of the right hemisphere. Stippling in the inset brain drawing shows the area in which the map was reconstructed. Recording sites are located at decimal points and CFs are in kHz. Thick dashed lines indicate isofrequency contours. Asterisks indicate the border between field AI and AII. BR indicates a response over a broad frequency range. The site of the iontophoretic injection of HRP on the 14-kHz isofrequency contour is shown by the bullseye. (B) Camera lucida tracing of all HRP-labeled processes located within a tangentially cut (90 μm) tissue section showing the orientation of the processes with respect to the orientation of the isofrequency contours. From Reale *et al.* (1983).

6.1.4. Corticotectal Connections The results of the most recent autoradiographic tracer studies of auditory corticotectal connections (FitzPatrick and Imig, 1978; Andersen *et al.*, 1980b,c) are consistent with and extend the earlier observations made with lesion-degeneration techniques (Diamond *et al.*, 1969; Rockel and Jones, 1973). Like the corticocortical and corticothalamic projections, these projections are divergent, convergent, and topographic. In both cat and monkey, corticotectal projections from AI loci terminate as sheets of terminals in the dorsomedial sector of the ipsilateral ICC. The contralateral ICC also receives AI input but to a lesser extent. The sheets of terminals are oriented roughly parallel to the isofrequency contours and to the flattened disk-shaped dendritic fields of neurons in the ventral part of the ICC (see Rockel and Jones, 1973; Merzenich and Reid, 1974; FitzPatrick, 1975). In the cat ICC, AI axons do not appear to project beyond the dorsomedial area of large multipolar neurons, whereas in the owl monkey the corticotectal terminal sheets extend well into the laminated ventral part. The topographic projection patterns are consistent with the cochleotopic organizations of AI and ICC which, considered in light of the tectothalamic and thalamocortical connectivity patterns (Andersen *et al.*, 1980b), means that cochleotopy is maintained throughout the ICC–MGB–AI–ICC loop.

AI of the cat, but apparently not of the monkey, also projects to the pericentral nucleus. The available evidence suggests that the topography and divergence–convergence observed for the AI–ICC pathway obtains here as well. Field A of cat may project sparsely to the dorsomedial area of the ipsilateral ICC. If it does so, then the same CF loci in AI and A may converge upon the same ICC target cells. AII does not send fibers to ICC but does project strongly upon the pericentral nucleus ipsilaterally. Field R of the monkey also projects to the dorsomedial sector of the ipsilateral ICC and to the pericentral and external nuclei.

6.1.5. Corticostriate Connections Using the mapping-tracing methods outlined previously, Reale and Imig (1983) determined in the cat the patterns of projection from the four tonotopically organized fields (AI, A, P, and VP) to the basal ganglia. This subcortical projection system is topographically organized with respect to the relative positions of these four cortical fields. The neurons representing the full high-to-low-frequency axis in fields A and AI were found to project to dorsal striatal targets of the caudate nucleus and the putamen but not to the more ventral lateral amygdaloid nucleus. The field P projections show a low-to-middle-frequency representation in the caudate connections, a complete tonotopic representation in the connections to the putamen, and a middle-to-high-frequency representation in the projection to the lateral amygdaloid nucleus. In the VP projection, the full tonal spectrum is represented ventrally in the putamen and lateral amygdaloid nucleus but no connection is seen dorsally with the caudate nucleus. Moreover, double-tracer experiments in AI and P showed that the projections are also topographically organized with respect to the cortical frequency representation; projections from the high-frequency representations are located more laterally in the striatum than are those from low-frequency areas. Like other auditory cortical projection systems, a restricted locus in each of the auditory fields sends axons to patches of striatal target neurons that are arrayed in a band (Fig. 14).

6.2. Relationships to Binaural Organization: Corticocortical and Corticothalamic Connections Projections from AI of one hemisphere to field AI of the other via the corpus callosum have long been known to exhibit a complex topography (Ebner and Myers, 1965; Diamond *et al.*, 1968a; Pandya *et al.*, 1969; Karol and Pandya, 1971; FitzPatrick and Imig, 1980). Some of this complexity was resolved when Imig and Brugge (1978) combined electrophysiological and anatomical studies in the cat to show that the callosal projection pattern was closely related to the distribution of cells with different binaural properties (Fig. 12). Regions containing neurons that are excited by stimulation of one ear and inhibited by stimulation of the other make relatively sparse interhemispheric connections. From a previous discussion we saw that cells with these properties detect interaural intensity cues for sound localization and are usually sensitive to sound sources located in the opposite auditory hemifield. Cells that are excited by monaural stimulation of each ear, and which are often insensitive to interaural intensity differences, make relatively strong interhemispheric connections.

Fields A and P also project ipsilaterally upon AI in a complex fashion (Fig. 11). Imig and Reale (1981b) demonstrated that, like the callosal connections, the patchy ipsilateral projections are also related to binaural organization. In this case, however, target zones in AI receiving the most dense corticocortical projections are reversed from those of the callosal projection system.

The patchy and divergent–convergent patterns of thalamic inputs are also related to the binaural representation in AI (Middlebrooks and Zook, 1983). A cortical locus containing cells of a binaural class associated with strong interhemispheric connections and weak intrahemispheric connections derives its principal input from a topographically restricted and contiguous region of the ventral division of the MGB. By comparison, AI loci containing cells of the other binau-

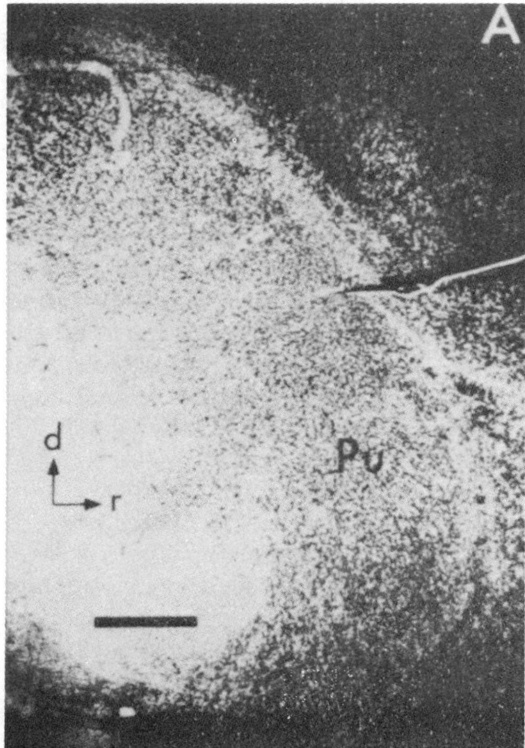

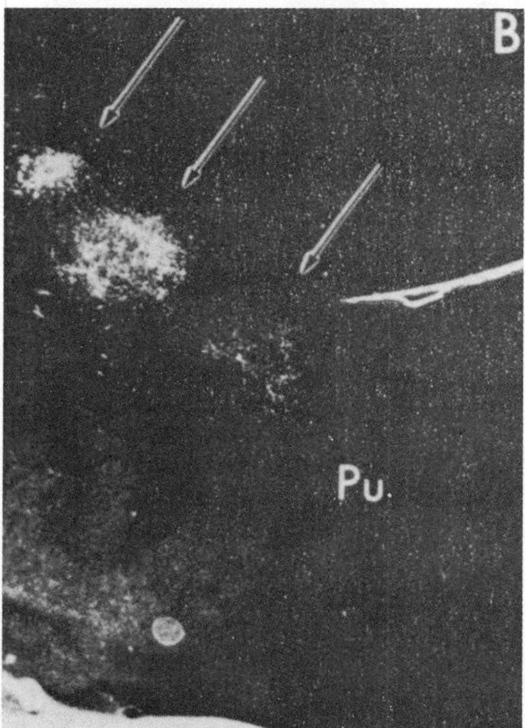

Figure 14. Typical configuration of labeled axonal terminals in the putamen (Pu) of the basal ganglia resulting from an injection of tritiated proline into an auditory cortical field. (A) Brightfield photograph of a Nissl-stained sagittally cut (50 μm) tissue section prepared for autoradiography. (B) Matching darkfield photograph of autoradiograph. Arrows point to divergent targets from a tritiated amino acid injection placed in the anterior (A) cortical field. Bar in (A) = 1 mm.

ral class (i.e., associated with weak interhemispheric and strong intrahemispheric connections) receive a differential input from three separate columns of medial geniculate cells which span the ventral division. Thus, it appears that the two major fiber systems that interconnect directly auditory cortical fields on the same and opposite hemisphere and link these fields with the thalamus are intimately related to representations of both frequency and binaurality.

Acknowledgments We wish to thank Jean Heinz and Carol Dizack for the artwork and Shirley Hunsaker for the photography. Supported by NIH Grants NS-12732 and HD-03352 and NSF Grant BNS-19893.

7. References

Abeles, M., and Goldstein, M. H., Jr., 1970, Functional architecture in cat primary auditory cortex: Columnar organization and organization according to depth, *J. Neurophysiol.* **33**:172–187.

Aitkin, L. M., Irvine, D. R. F., and Webster, W. R., 1984, Central neurai mechanisms of hearing, in: *Handbook of Physiology*, Volume III (I. Darian-Smith, ed.), American Physiological Society, Washington, D.C., pp. 675–737.

Andersen, R. A., Knight, P. L., and Merzenich, M. M., 1980a, The thalamocortical and corticothalamic connections of AI, AII, and the anterior auditory field (AAF) in the cat: Evidence for two largely segregated systems of connections, *J. Comp. Neurol.* **194**:663–701.

Andersen, R. A., Roth, G. L., Aitkin, L. M., and Merzenich. M. M., 1980b, The efferent projections of the central nucleus and the pericentral nucleus of the inferior colliculus in the cat, *J. Comp. Neurol.* **194**:649–662.

Andersen, R. A., Snyder, R. L., and Merzenich, M. M., 1980c, The topographic organization of corticocollicular projections from physiologically defined loci in the AI, AII and anterior auditory cortical fields in the cat, *J. Comp. Neurol.* **191**:479–494.

Benson, D. A., and Teas, D. C., 1976, Single unit study of binaural interaction in the auditory cortex of the chinchilla, *Brain Res.* **103**: 313–338.

Benson, D. A., Heinz, R. D., and Goldstein, M. H., Jr., 1979, Observations on unit activity in monkey auditory cortex and dorsolateral frontal cortex during a sound localization task, *Soc. Neurosci. Abstr.* **5**:16.

Brugge, J. F., 1975, Progress in neuroanatomy and neurophysiology of auditory cortex. in: *The Nervous System: Human Communication and Its Disorders* (D. B. Tower, ed.), Raven Press, New York, pp. 97–111.

Brugge, J. F., 1982, Auditory cortical areas in primates, in: *Cortical Sensory Organization*, Volume 3 (C. N. Woolsey, ed.), Humana Press, Clifton, N.J., pp. 59–70.

Brugge, J. F., and Imig, T. J., 1978, Some relationships of binaural response patterns of single neurons to cortical columns and interhemispheric connections of auditory area AI of cat cerebral cortex, in: *Evoked Electrical Activity in the Auditory Nervous System* (R. F. Naunton and C. Fernandez, eds.), Academic Press, New York, pp. 487–504.

Brugge, J. F., and Merzenich, M. M., 1973a, Patterns of activity of single neurons of the auditory cortex in monkey, in: *Basic Mechanisms in Heanng* (A. R. Moller, ed.), Academic Press, New York, pp. 745–772.

Brugge, J. F., and Merzenich, M. M., 1973b, Responses of neurons in auditory cortex of the macaque monkey to monaural and binaural stimulation, *J. Neurophysiol.* **36**:1138–1158.

Brugge, J. F., Dubrovsky, N. A., Aitkin, L. M., and Anderson, D. J., 1969, Sensitivity of single neurons in auditory cortex of cat to binaural tonal stimulation; effects of varying interaural time and intensity, *J. Neurophysiol.* **32**:1005–1024.

Brugge, J. F., Anderson, D. J., and Aitkin, L. M., 1970, Responses of neurons in the dorsal nucleus of the lateral lemniscus of cat to binaural tonal stimulation, *J. Neurophysiol.* **33**:441–458.

Calford, M. B., and Pettigrew, J. D., 1984, Frequency dependence of directional amplification of the cat's pinna, *Hearing Res.* **14**:13–19.

Calford, M. B., Webster, W. R., and Semple, M. M., 1983, Measurement of frequency selectivity of single neurons in the central auditory pathway, *Hearing Res.* **11**:395–401.

Casseday, J. H., Harting, J. K., and Diamond, I. T., 1976, Auditory pathways to the conex in *Tupaia glis*, *J. Comp. Neurol.* **166**:303–340.

Colwell, S. A., 1977, Corticothalamic projections from physiologically defined loci within auditory cortex in the cat: Reciprocal structure in the medial geniculate body, Ph.D. thesis, University of California, San Francisco.

Creutzfeldt, O., Hellweg, F. C., and Schreiner, C., 1980, The thalamocortical transformation of responses to complex auditory stimuli, *Exp. Brain Res.* **39**:87–104.

De Ribaupierre, F., and Goldstein, M. H., Jr., 1972, Cortical coding of repetitive acoustic pulses, *Brain Res.* **48**:205–225.

Diamond, I. T., Jones, E. G., and Powell, T. P. S., 1968a, Interhemispheric fiber connections of the auditory cortex of the cat, *Brain Res.* **11**:177–193.

Diamond, I. T., Jones, E. G., and Powell, T. P. S., 1968b, The association connections of the auditory cortex of the cat, *Brain Res.* **11**:560–579.

Diamond, I. T., Jones, E. G., and Powell, T. P. S., 1969, The projection of auditory cortex upon the diencephalon and brain stem in the cat, *Brain Res.* **15**:305–340.

Dickson, J. W., and Gerstein, G. L., 1974. Interactions between neurons in auditory cortex of the cat, *J. Neurophysiol.* **37**:1239–1261.

Downman, C. B. B., Woolsey, C. N., and Lende, R. A., 1960, Auditory areas I, II and Ep: Cochlear representatlon, afferent paths and interconnections, *Bull. John Hopkins Hosp.* **106**: 127–142.

Ebner, F. F., and Myers, R. E., 1965, Distribution of corpus callosum and anterior commissure in cat and raccoon, *J. Comp. Neurol.* **124**: 353–366.

Eisenman, L. M., 1974, Neural encoding of sound location: An electrophysiological study of auditory cortex (AI) of the cat using free-field stimuli, *Brain Res.* **75**:203–214.

Evans, E. F., 1968, Cortical representation, in: *Hearing Mechanisms in Vertebrates* (A. V. S. de Reuck and J. Knight, eds.), Little, Brown, Boston, pp. 272–295.

Evans, E. F., and Whitfield, I. C., 1964, Classification of unit responses in the auditory cortex of the unanesthetized and unrestrained cat, *J. Physiol (London)* **171**:470–493.

FitzPatrick, K. A., 1975, Cellular architecture and topographic organization of the inferior colliculus of the squirrel monkey, *J. Comp. Neurol.* **164**:185–208.

FitzPatrick, K. A., and Imig, T. J., 1978, Projections of auditory cortex upon the thalamus and midbrain in the owl monkey, *J. Comp. Neurol.* **177**:537–566.

FitzPatrick, K. A., and Imig, T. J., 1980, Auditory cortico-cortical connections in the owl monkey, *J. Comp. Neurol.* **192**:589–610.

FitzPatrick, K. A., and Imig, T. J., 1982, Organization of auditory connections: The primate auditory cortex, in: *Cortical Sensory Organization*, Volume 3 (C. N. Woolsey, ed.), Humana Press, Clifton, N.J., pp. 71–109.

FitzPatrick, K. A., Imig, T.J., and Reale, R. A., 1977, Thalamic projections to the posterior auditory field in the cat, *Soc. Neurosci. Abstr.* **3**:6.

Galaburda, A., and Sanides, F., 1980. Cytoarchitectonic organization of the human auditory cortex, *J. Comp. Neurol.* **190**:597–610.

Gates, G. R., and Aitkin. L. M., 1982, Auditory cortex in the marsupial possum *Trichosurus vulpecula*, *Hearing Res.* **7**:1–11.

Glaser, E. M., Van der Loos, H., and Gissler, M., 1979, Tangential orientation and spatial order in dendrites of cat auditory cortex: A computer microscope study of Golgi-impregnated material, *Exp. Brain Res.* **36**:411–431.

Glass, I., and Wollberg, Z., 1983. Responses of cells in the auditory cortex of awake squirrel monkeys to normal and reversed species-specific vocalizations, *Hearing Res.* **9**:27–33.

Goldberg, J. M., and Brown, P. B., 1969, Response of binaural neurons of dog superior olivary complex to dichotic tonal stimuli: Some physiological mechanisms of sound localization, *J. Neurophysiol.* **32**:613–636.

Goldberg, J. M., Diamond. I. T., and Neff, W. D., 1957, Auditory discrimination after ablation of temporal and insular cortex in cat, *Fed. Proc.* **16**:47.

Goldstein, M. H., Jr., 1968, Single unit studies of cortical coding of simple acoustic stimuli, in: *Physiological and Biochemical Aspects of Nervous Integration* (F. D. Carlson. ed.), Prentice–Hall, Englewood Cliffs. N.J., pp. 131–151.

Goldstein, M. H., Jr., and Abeles, M., 1975, Single unit activity of the auditory cortex, in: *Handbook of Sensory Physiology*, Volume 5, Part 2 (W. D. Keidel and W. D. Neff), Springer-Verlag, Berlin, pp. 199–218.

Goldstein, M. H., Jr., Hall, J. L., and Butterfield, B. O., 1968, Single-unit activity in the primary auditory cortex of unanesthetized cats, *J Acoust. Soc. Am.* **43**:444–455.

Graybiel, A. M., 1973, The thalamo-cortical projection of the so-called posterior nuclear group: A study with anterograde degeneration methods in the cat, *Brain Res.* **49**:229–244.

Gravbiel, A. M., 1974, Studies on the anatomical organization of posterior association cortex, in: *The Neurosciences: Third Study Program* (F. O. Schmitt and F. G. Worden, eds.), MIT Press, Cambridge, Mass., pp. 205–214.

Green, D. M., 1976, *An Introduction to Hearing*, Erlbaum, Hillsdale, N.J.

Hall, J. L., and Goldstein, M. H., Jr., 1968, Representation of binaural stimuli by single units in primary auditory cortex of unanesthetized cats, *J. Acoust. Soc. Am.* **43**:456–461.

Heath, C. J., and Jones, E. G., 1971, The anatomical organization of the suprasylvian gyrus of the cat, *Ergeb. Anat. Entwicklungsgesch.* **45**:1–64.

Hellweg, F. C., Koch, R., and Vollrath, M., 1977, Representation of the cochlea in the neocortex of guinea pigs, *Exp. Brain Res.* **29**:467–474.

Hind, J. E., Rose, J. E.. Davies; P. W., Woolsey, C. N., Benjamin, R. M., Welker, W. I., and Thompson, R. F., 1960, Unit activity in the auditory cortex, in: *Neural Mechanisms of the Auditory and Vestibular Systems* (G. L. Rasmussen and W. Windle, eds.), Thomas, Springfield, Ill., pp. 201–210.

Imig, T. J., and Adrian, H. O., 1977, Binaural columns in the primary field (AI) of cat auditory cortex, *Brain Res.* **138**:241–257.

Imig, T. J., and Brugge, J. F., 1978, Sources and terminations of callosal axons related to binaural and frequency maps in primary auditory cortex of the cat, *J. Comp. Neurol.* **182**:637–660.

Imig, T. J., and Morel, A., 1983, Organization of the thalamocortical auditory system in the cat, *Annu. Rev. Neurosci.* **6**:95–120.

Imig, T. J., and Morel, A., 1984, Topographic and cytoarchitectonic organization of thalamic neurons related to their targets in low-, middle-, and high-frequency representations in cat auditory cortex, *J. Comp. Neurol.* **227**:511–539.

Imig, T. J., and Morel, A., 1985, Tonotopic organization in ventral nucleus of medial geniculate body in the cat, *J. Neurophysiol.* **53**: 309–340.

Imig, T. J., and Reale, R. A., 1980. Patterns of cortico-cortical connections related to tonotopic maps in cat auditory cortex, *J. Comp. Neurol.* **192**:293–332.

Imig, T. J., and Reale, R. A., 1981a, Medial geniculate projections to auditory cortical fields A, AI, and P in the cat, *Soc. Neurosci. Abstr.* **7**:230.

Imig, T. J., and Reale, R. A., 1981b, Ipsilateral cortico-cortical projections related to binaural columns in cat primary auditory cortex, *J. Comp. Neurol.* **203**:1–14.

Imig, T. J., Ruggero, M. A., Kitzes, L. M., Javel, E., and Brugge, J. F., 1977, Organization of auditory conex in the owl monkey (*Aotus trivirgatus*), *J. Comp. Neurol.* **171**:111–128.

Imig, T. J., Morel, A., and Reale, R. A., 1981. Organization of thalamic neurons projecting to auditory cortical fields in the cat, *International Seminar of Neuroscience*, Algiers, Algeria, pp. 62–63.

Irvine, D. R. F., 1980, Acoustic properties of neurons in posteromedial thalamus of cat, *J. Neurophysiol.* **43**:395–408.

Irvine, D. R. F., and Huebner, H., 1979, Acoustic response characteristics of neurons in non-specific areas of cat cerebral cortex, *J. Neurophysiol.* **42**:107–122.

Irvine, D. R. F., and Phillips, D. P., 1982, Polysensory "association" areas of the cerebral cortex: Organization of acoustic inputs in the cat, in: *Cortical Sensory Organization*, Volume 3 (C. N. Woolsey, ed.), Humana Press, Clifton. N.J., pp. 111–156.

Jenkins, W. M., and Merzenich, M. M., 1984, Role of cat primary auditory cortex for sound–localization behavior, *J. Neurophysiol.* **52**:819–847.

Kaas, J. H., Hall, W. C., and Diamond, I. T., 1972, Visual cortex of the grey squirrel (*Sciureus carolinensis*): Architectonic subdivisions and connections from visual thalamus, *J. Comp. Neurol.* **145**:273–306.

Karol, E. A., and Pandya, D. N., 1971, The distribution of the corpus callosum in the rhesus monkey, *Brain* **94**:471–486.

Kawamura, K., 1973, Corticocortical fiber connections of the cat cerebrum. I. The temporal region, *Brain Res.* **51**:1–21.

Khanna, S. M., and Leonard, D. G. B., 1982, Basilar membrane tuning in the cat cochlea, *Science* **215**:305–306.

Kitzes, L. M., Wrege, K. S., and Cassady, J. M., 1980, Patterns of responses of cortical cells to binaural stimulation, *J. Comp. Neurol.* **192**:455–472.

Knight, P. L., 1977, Representation of the cochlea within the anterior auditory field (AAF) of the cat, *Brain Res.* **130**:447–467.

Knudsen, E. I., and Konishi, M., 1978, A neural map of auditory space in the owl, *Science* **200**:795–797.

Kraus, N., and Disterhoft, J. F., 1982. Response plasticity of single neurons in rabbit auditory association cortex during tone-signalled learning, *Brain Res.* **246**:205–215.

Kuwada, S., and Yin, T. C., 1983, Binaural interaction in low-frequency neurons in inferior colliculus of the cat. I. Effects of long interaural delays, inlensity, and repetition rate on interaural delay function, *J. Neurophysiol* **50**:981–999.

McMullen, N. T., and Glaser, E. M., 1982. Tonotopic organization of rabbit auditory cortex, *Exp. Brain Res.* **75**:208–220.

Manley, J. A., and Müller-Preuss, P., 1978, Response variability in mammalian auditory cortex-objection to feature detection. *Fed. Proc.* **37**:2355–2359.

Masterton, R. B., and Imig, T. J., 1984. Neural mechanisms for sound localization. *Annu. Rev. Physiol.* **46**:275–287.

Merzenich, M. M., and Brugge, J. F., 1973, Representation of the cochlear partition on the superior temporal plane of the macaque monkey, *Brain Res.* **50**:275–296.

Merzenich, M. M., and Reid, M. D., 1974, Representation of the cochlea within the inferior colliculus of the cat, *Brain Res.* **77**:397–415.

Merzenich, M. M., Knight, P. L., and Roth, G. L., 1975. Representation of cochlea within primary auditory cortex in the cat, *J. Neurophysiol.* **38**:231–249.

Merzenich, M. M., Kaas, J. H., and Roth, C. L., 1976, Auditory cortex in the grey squirrel: Tonotopic organization and architectonic fields, *J. Comp. Neurol.* **166**:387–401.

Merzenich, M. M., Colwell, S. A., and Andersen, R. A., 1982, Auditory forebrain organization: Thalamocortical and corticothalamic connections in the cat, in: *Cortical Sensory Organization* (C. N. Woolsey, ed.), Humana Press, Clifton, N.J., pp. 43–57.

Middlebrooks, J. C., and Pettigrew, J. D., 1981, Functional classes of neurons in primary auditory cortex of the cat distinguished by sensitivity to sound location, *J. Neurosci.* **1**:107–120.

Middlebrooks, J. C., and Zook, J. M., 1983, Intrinsic organization of the cat's medial geniculate body identified by projections to binaural response-specific bands in the primary auditory cortex, *J. Neurosci.* **3**:203–224.

Middlebrooks, J. C., Dykes, R. W., and Merzenich, M. M., 1980, Binaural response-specific bands in primary auditory cortex (AI) of the cat: Topographical organization orthogonal to isofrequency contours, *Brain Res.* **181**:31–48.

Moore, D. R., and Irvine, D. R. F., 1979, A developmental study of the sound pressure transformation by the head of the cat, *Acta Oto-Laryngol.* **87**:434–440.

Morel, A., 1980, *Codage des sons dans le corps genouille median du chat: Evaluation de l'organisation tonotopique de ses differents noyaux*, Druckt Verlag. Zurich.

Morel, A., and Imig, T. J., 1984, Neurons in the tonotopic thalamus of the cat are topographically organized with respect to their target fields in auditory cortex, *Soc. Neurosci. Abstr.* **10**:244.

Newman, J. D., 1978, Perception of sounds used in species-specific communication: The auditory cortex and beyond, *J. Med. Primatol.* **7**:98–105.

Newman, J. D., and Symmes, D., 1979, Feature detection by single units in squirrel monkey auditory cortex, *Exp. Brain Res. Suppl.* **2**:140–145.

Newman, J. D., and Wollberg, Z., 1973, Responses of single neurons in the auditory cortex of squirrel monkeys to variants of a single cell type, *Exp. Neurol.* **40**:821–824.

Niimi, K., and Matsuoka, M., 1979, Thalamocortical organization of the auditory system in the cat studied by retrograde axonal transport of horseradish peroxidase, *Adv. Anat. Embryol. Cell Biol.* **57**: 1–56.

Oliver, D. L., and Hall, W. C., 1978, The medial geniculate body of the tree shrew, *Tupaia glis*. **II**. Connections with the neocortex, *J. Comp. Neurol.* **182**:459–493.

Oonishi, S., and Katsuki, Y., 1965, Functional organization and integrative mechanism on the auditory cortex of the cat, *Jpn. J. Physiol.* **15**:342–365.

Orman, S. S., and Phillips, D. P., 1984, Binaural interactions of single neurons in posterior field of cat auditory cortex, *J. Neurophysiol.* **51**:1028–1039.

Pandya, D. N., and Sanides, F., 1973, Architectonic parcellation of the temporal operculum in rhesus monkey and its projection pattern, *Z. Anat. Entwicklungsgesch.* **139**:127–161.

Pandya, D. N., Hallet, M., and Mukherjee, S. K., 1969, Intra- and interhemispheric connections of the neocortical auditory system in the rhesus monkey, *Brain Res.* **14**:49–65.

Paula-Barbosa, M. M., Feyo, P. B., and Sousa-Pinto, A., 1975, The association connexions of the suprasylvian fringe (SF) and other areas of the cat auditory cortex, *Exp. Brain Res.* **23**:535–554.

Phillips, D. P., and Brugge, J. F., 1985, Progress in neurophysiology of sound localization, *Annu. Rev. Psychol.* **36**:245–274.

Phillips, D. P., and Irvine, D. R. F., 1979, Methodological considerations in mapping auditory cortex: Binaural columns in AI of cat, *Brain Res.* **169**:342–346.

Phillips, D. P., and Irvine, D. R. F., 1981a, Responses of single neurons in physiologically defined primary auditory cortex (AI) of the cat: Frequency tuning and responses to intensity, *J. Neurophysiol.* **45**:48–58.

Phillips, D. P., and Irvine, D. R. F., 1981b, Responses of single neurons in physiologically defined area AI of cat cerebral cortex: Sensitivity to interaural intensity, *Hearing Res.* **4**:299–307.

Phillips, D. P., and Irvine, D. R. F., 1982, Properties of single neurons in the anterior auditory field (AAF) of cat cerebral cortex, *Brain Res.* **248**:237–244.

Phillips, D. P., and Irvine, D. R. F., 1983, Some features of the binaural input to single neurons in physiologically defined area AI of cat cerebral cortex, *J. Neurophysiol.* **49**:383–395.

Phillips, D. P., and Orman, S. S., 1984, Responses of single neurons in posterior field of cat auditory cortex, *J. Neurophysiol.* **51**:1028–1039.

Phillips, D. P., Calford, M. B., Pettigrew, J. D., Aitkin, L. M., and Semple, M. N., 1982, Directionality of sound pressure transformation at the cat's pinna, *Hearing Res.* **8**:13–28.

Phillips, D. P., Orman, S. S., Musicant, A. D., Wilson, G. F., and Huang, C.-M., 1985, Primary auditory cortex in the cat: Classes of neurons distinguished by their responses to tones and noise, *Hearing Res.* (in press).

Poliak, S., 1932, Origin, course, termination, and internal organization of the auditory radiation, in: *The Main Afferent Fiber Systems of the Cerebral Cortex in Primates* (H. M. Evans and I. M. Thompson, eds.), University of California Press, Berkeley, pp. 81–104.

Reale, R. A., and Imig, T. J., 1980, Tonotopic organization in auditory cortex of the cat, *J. Comp. Neurol.* **192**:265–291.

Reale, R. A., and Imig, T. J., 1983, Auditory cortical field projections to the basal ganglia of the cat, *Neuroscience* **8**:67–86.

Reale, R. A., Brugge, J. F., and Feng, J. Z., 1983, Geometry and orientation of neuronal processes in cat primary auditory cortex (AI) related to characteristic-frequency maps, *Proc. Natl. Acad. Sci. USA* **80**:5449–5453.

Rhode, W. S., 1978, Some observations on cochlear mechanics, *J. Acoust. Soc. Am.* **64**:158–176.

Rockel, A. J., and Jones, E. G., 1973, The neuronal organization of the inferior colliculus of the adult cat. I. The central nucleus, *J. Comp. Neurol.* **147**:11–60.

Rose, J. E., 1949, The cellular structure of the auditory region of the cat, *J. Comp. Neurol.* **19**:409–439.

Rose, J. E., and Woolsey, C. N., 1949, The relations of thalamic connections, cellular structure and evocable electrical activity in the auditory region of the cat, *J. Comp. Neurol.* **91**:441.

Rose, J. E., and Woolsey, C. N., 1958, Cortical connections and functional organization of thalamic auditory system in the cat, in: *Biological and Biochemical Bases of Behavior* (H. F. Harlow and C. N. Woolsey, eds.), University of Wisconsin Press, Madison, pp. 127–150.

Rose, J. E., Gross, N. B., Geisler, C. D., and Hind, J. E., 1966, Some neural mechanisms in the inferior colliculus of the cat which may be relevant to localization of a sound source, *J. Neurophysiol.* **29**:288–314.

Schreiner, C. E., and Cynader, M. S., 1984, Basic functional organization of second auditory cortical field (AII) of the cat, *J. Neurophysiol.* **51**:1284–1305.

Seldon, H. L., 1981, Structure of human auditory cortex. I. Cytoarchitectonics and dendritic distributions, *Brain Res.* **229**:277–294.

Sellick, P. M., Patuzzi, R., and Johnstone, B. M., 1982, Measurement of basilar membrane motion in the guinea pig using the Mossbauer technique, *J. Acoust. Soc. Am.* **72**:131–141.

Seltzer, B., and Pandya, D. N., 1978, Afferent cortical connections and architectonics of the superior temporal sulcus and surrounding cortex in the rhesus monkey, *Brain Res.* **149**:1–24.

Sousa-Pinto, A., 1973, The structure of the first auditory cortex (AI) of the cat. I. Light microscopic observations on its structure, *Arch. Ital. Biol.* **111**:112–137.

Sovijarvi, A. R. A., and Hyvarinen, J., 1974, Auditory cortical neurons in the cat sensitive to the direction of sound source movement, *Brain Res.* **73**:455–471.

Steinschneider, M., Arezzo, J., and Vaughan, H. G. J., 1982, Speech evoked activity in the auditory radiations and cortex of the awake monkey, *Brain Res.* **252**:353–365.

Suga, N., 1977, Amplitude spectrum representation in the Doppler-shifted-CF processing area of the auditory cortex of the mustache bat, *Science* **196**:64–67.

Symmes, D., 1974, Discrimination of intermittent noise by macaques following lesions of the temporal lobe, *Exp. Neurol.* **16**:201–214.

Thompson, R. F., and Sindberg, R. M., 1960, Auditory response fields in association and motor cortex of cat, *J. Neurophysiol.* **23**:87–105.

Tunturi, A. R., 1960, Anatomy and physiology of the auditory cortex, in: *Neural Mechanisms of the Auditory and Vestibular Systems* (G. L. Rasmussen and W. F. Windle, eds.), Thomas, Springfield, Ill., pp. 181–200.

von Economo, C., 1929, *The Cytoarchitectonics of the Human Cerebral Cortex*, Oxford University Press, London.

Winer, J. A., Diamond, I. T., and Raczkowski, D, 1977, Subdivisions of the auditory cortex of the cat: The retrograde transport of horseradish peroxidase to the medial geniculate body and posterior thalamic nuclei, *J. Comp. Neurol.* **176**:387–418.

Wollberg, Z., and Newman, J. D., 1972, Auditory cortex of squirrel monkey: Response patterns of single cells to species specific vocalizations, *Science* **175**:212–214.

Woolsey, C. N., 1960, Organization of auditory cortical system: A review and a synthesis, in: *Neural Mechanisms of the Auditory and Vestilbular Systems* (G. Rasmussen and W. Windle, eds.), Thomas, Springfield, Ill., pp. 165–180.

Woolsey, C. N., 1961, Organization of cortical auditory system, in: *Sensory Communication* (W. A. Rosenblith, ed.), MIT Press, Cambridge, Mass., pp. 235–257.

Woolsey, C. N., 1971, Tonotopic organization of the auditory cortex, in: *Physiology of the Auditory System* (M. B. Sachs, ed.), National Educational Consultants, Baltimore, pp. 271–282.

Woolsey, C. N., and Walzl, E. M., 1942, Topical projection of nerve fibers from local regions of the cochlea to the cerebral cortex of the cat, *Bull. Johns Hophins Hosp.* **71**:315–344.

Woolsey, C. N., and Walzl, E. M., 1982, Cortical auditory area of *Macaca mulatta* and its relation to the second somatic sensory area (Sm II): Determination by electrical excitation of auditory nerve fibers in the spiral osseous lamina and by click stimulation, in: *Cortical Sensory Organization*, Volume 3 (C. N. Woolsey, ed.), Humana Press, Clifton, N.J., pp. 231–256.

Yin, T. C. T., and Kuwada, S., 1983a, Binaural interaction in low-frequency neurons in inferior colliculus of the cat. II. Effects of changing rate and direction of interaural phase, *J. Neurophysiol.* **50**:1000–1019.

Yin, T. C. T., and Kuwada, S., 1983b, Binaural interaction in low-frequency neurons in inferior colliculus of the cat. III. Effects of changing frequency, *J. Neurophysiol.* **50**:1020–1042.

Yin, T. C. T., and Kuwada, S., 1984, Neuronal mechanisms of binaural interaction, in: *Dynamic Aspects of Neocortical Function* (G. M. Edelman, W. M. Cowan, and W. E. Gall, eds.), Wiley, New York, pp. 263–313.

19

E. I. Knudsen and M. Konishi

A neural map of auditory space in the owl

1978. Science 200: 795–797

Abstract

Auditory units that responded to sound only when it originated from a limited area of space were found in the lateral and anterior portions of the midbrain auditory nucleus of the owl (*Tyto alba*). The areas of space to which these units responded (their receptive fields) were largely independent of the nature and intensity of the sound stimulus. The units were arranged systematically within the midbrain auditory nucleus according to the relative locations of their receptive fields, thus creating a physiological map of auditory space.

One of the primary functions of the auditory system is to locate sound sources in space. How space is represented in the auditory system, however, is not known. One theory originally put forth by von Békésy (*1*) assumes that sound location is encoded by the relative activation of two populations of neurons, one population sensitive to sound on the right and the other to sound on the left. An alternative theory (*2*) proposes that sound location is encoded as "place" in the nervous system, with individual neurons being sensitive only to restricted portions of auditory space. Neurons which respond best to particular interaural time or intensity disparities have been found at several levels in the auditory pathway (*3*). However, the interaural disparities to which these units are "tuned" are too great and the tuning is too crude to account for the auditory angular acuity of animals measured behaviorally. Consequently, some researchers have rejected the proposition that the auditory system encodes space in terms of receptive fields and neural maps, as in the visual and somatosensory systems, and have opted for the population theory of sound localization (*4*). On the other hand, recent neurophysiological studies, in which sound stimuli were presented in real space, have shown that auditory units can have restricted receptive fields (*5*), a finding that tends to support the place theory of sound localization.

We have begun to explore the influence of sound source location on the response properties of central auditory neurons by using a movable speaker to deliver sound stimuli under free-field conditions. With this approach we have found a region in the owl's midbrain auditory area, nucleus mesencephalicus lateralis dorsalis (MLD), that contains units that respond to sound only when it originates from a small area of auditory space (receptive field) (*6*). Furthermore, these units are systematically arranged within the nucleus according to the azimuth and elevation of their receptive fields so that they form a physiological map of auditory space.

Four barn owls (*Tyto alba*) were used in these experiments. Light anesthesia was maintained with intramuscular injections of Ketamine (4 mg per kilogram of body weight). The experiments were conducted in a large anechoic chamber (*7*) specially equipped with a remotely controlled movable speaker (*8*) that could be positioned almost anywhere on a sphere centered at the owl's head (*9*). The owl was oriented so that the intersection of its visual plane and its median plane corresponded to 0° of elevation, 0° azimuth of the speaker (*10*). Sound stimuli included clicks, noise, and tone bursts (*11*). Although the units were tested for sensitivity to visual stimuli (*12*), all auditory tests were conducted with the owl in total darkness.

The auditory units described in this report were recorded from a functionally specialized region of the midbrain that was histologically identified as belonging to the MLD, the avian homolog of the inferior colliculus (*13*). The region forms the lateral and anterior borders of the main, tonotopic portion of the MLD, and extends in a continuous L-shaped strip from the posterolateral to the anteromedial corner of the nucleus (Fig. 1). In all, 182 units were recorded from this region on 47 separate penetrations (*14*).

Units in this region of the MLD shared three salient response properties: (i) they responded only when a sound was located within a well-defined area of space, which was virtually independent of the nature and the intensity of the sound stimulus; (ii) they responded well to clicks, noises, and tone bursts; and (iii) they were tuned to the high-frequency end (5 to 8.7 kHz) of the owl's audible range (*15*).

Auditory receptive fields were plotted in the following manner. After a single unit was isolated, the speaker, while emitting noise bursts, was moved to a location to which the unit responded vigorously. With the speaker at this location the threshold of the unit to noise bursts was determined (*16*). The intensity of the noise bursts was then increased to 10 dB above threshold, and the speaker was moved in azimuth and elevation to positions where the unit just failed to respond. The coordinates of these positions defined the borders of the unit's receptive field (Fig. 2). The same procedure was followed when plotting a field with clicks or tone bursts.

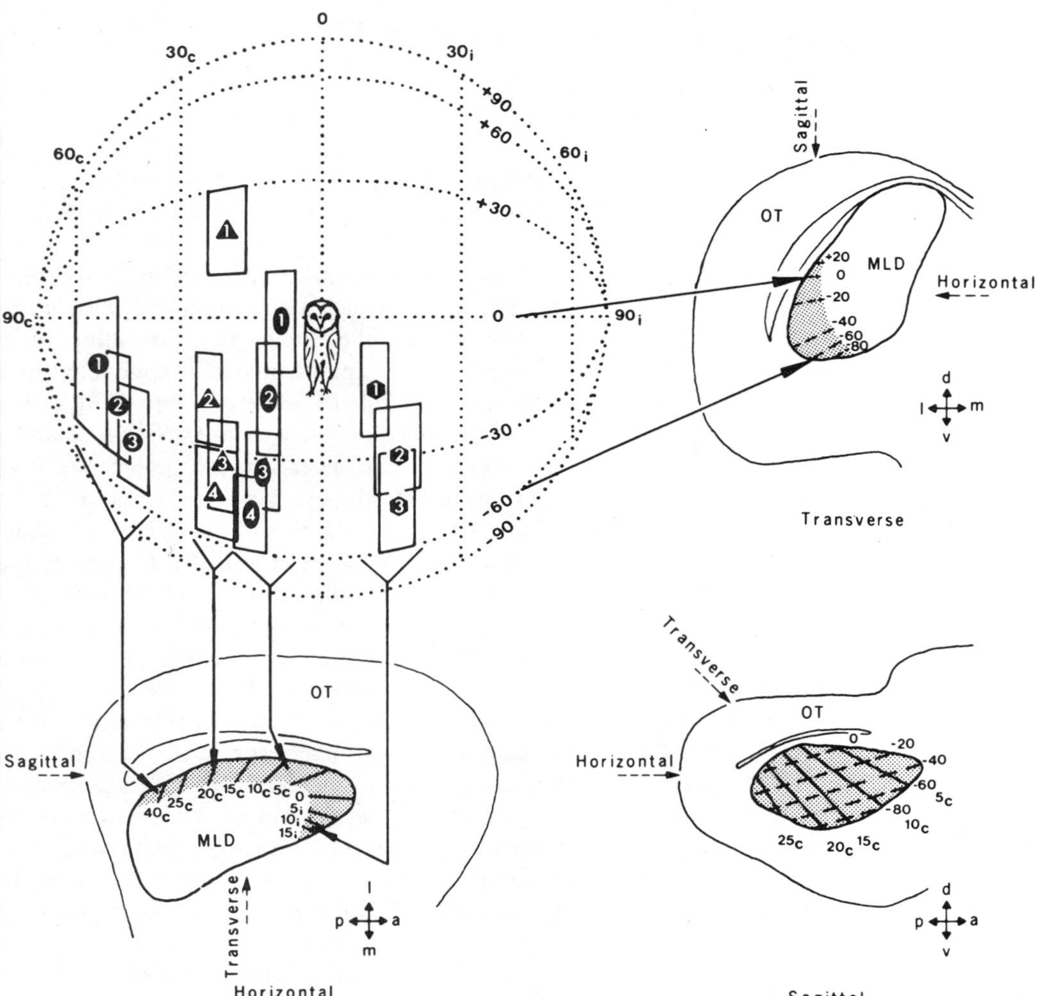

Figure 1. The representation of auditory space in the MLD, as defined by the centers of unit best areas. In the upper left, the coordinates of auditory space are depicted as a dotted globe surrounding the owl. Projected onto the globe are the best areas (solid-lined rectangles) of 14 units that were recorded in four separate penetrations. The large numbers backed by similar symbols represent units from the same penetration; the numbers themselves signify the order in which the units were encountered and are placed at the centers of their best areas. The penetrations were made with the electrode oriented parallel to the transverse plane at the positions indicated in the horizontal section by the soild arrows. Below and to the right of the globe are illustrated three histological sections through the MLD in the horizontal, transverse, and sagittal planes. The stippled portion of the MLD corresponds to the region that contains only neurons with small receptive fields. Isoazimuth contours, based on best-area centers, are shown as solid lines in the horizontal and sagittal sections; isoelevation contours are represented by dashed lines in the transverse and sagittal sections. On each section dashed arrows indicate the planes of the other two sections. Solid, crossed arrows to the lower right of each section define the orientation of the section: *a*, anterior; *d*, dorsal: *l*, lateral; *m*, medial; *p*, posterior; *v*, ventral. The length of the arrows corresponds to 600 μm. The optic tectum (*OT*) is labeled on each section.

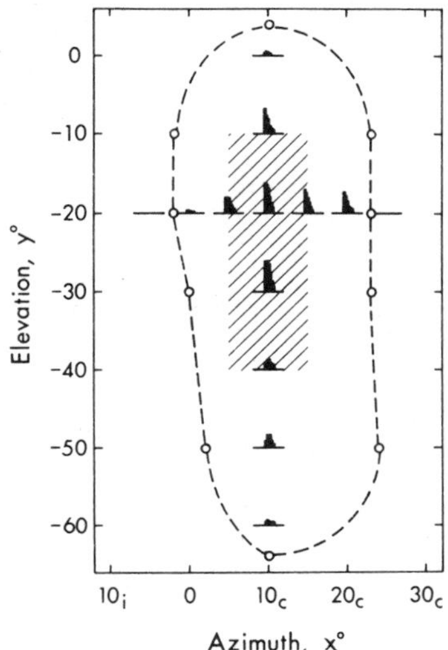

Figure 2. The receptive field and best area of an MLD unit. Dashed lines mark the borders of the unit's receptive field as projected from actual measurement sites (open circles). The receptive field was plotted using noise bursts 10 dB above threshold. The unit's best area (diagonal lines) was derived from the peristimulus time (PST) histograms shown in the figure. Best-area borders were defined by the first test locations that resulted in a submaximum response. Each PST histogram represents a 200-msec sample of the unit's responses to 16 repetitions of a 100-msec noise burst, presented 10 dB above threshold. The position of each histogram corresponds to the location of the speaker during the accumulation of that histogram. Negative degrees indicate locations in the inferior auditory hemifield; subscript *c*, contralateral and subscript *i*, ipsilateral.

The receptive fields of these MLD units were in the shape of vertically oriented ellipsoids (86 units out of 92) or bands (six units), and ranged in size from 7° to 40° (mean, 25°) in azimuth and from 23° to "unrestricted" in elevation. Both ellipsoidal and band-shaped receptive fields cantained a small distinct area within which a sound would induce a maximum response from the unit. This area, which was highly restricted in azimuth and elevation, will be termed the unit's best area. Although a unit's best area could be accurately determined by monitoring spike activity as a test stimulus was moving through its receptive field, more precise measurements of best area were made with the aid of peristimulus time (PST) histograms. The PST histograms were generated through the use of a sound 10 dB above threshold, and were routinely collected at 5° intervals in azimuth and at 10° intervals in elevation, although smaller receptive fields were often sampled at smaller intervals. The extent of a unit's best area was defined by those speaker locations at which the unit first gave a submaximum response (Fig. 2).

Sound intensity had no effect on the location of a unit's best area and had little effect on the size of many receptive fields. When receptive fields plotted with a sound 30 dB above threshold were compared with those plotted with a sound 10 dB above threshold for 63 units, 27 (or 0.4) changed by $\pm 2°$ or less in azimuth and 14 (or 0.2) changed by $\pm 5°$ or less in elevation. Twenty-three (or 0.4) expanded in azimuth by 3° to 11° and 13 (or 0.2) contracted by 3° to 18°.

Changing the test stimulus from noise bursts to clicks or tone bursts did not alter a unit's best area, and usually exerted little influence on its receptive field boundaries. Thus. these MLD units sensed a limited area of space that was largely independent of the intensity or the nature of the sound stimulus.

In plotting the receptive fields of these units, it became apparent that the fields of neighboring units were superimposed and that advancement of the electrode resulted in a systematic shift in receptive field location. During a typical penetration, made dorsoventrally and parallel to the transverse plane (*17*), sequential receptive fields would shift continuously in elevation from high to low while moving little in azimuth.

The impression that the units in this region of the MLD were organized according to the location of their receptive fields was confirmed in a series of three experiments in which both the left and right MLD regions were mapped. In these experiments, a total of 19 penetrations traversed the region, sampling units throughout most of its anteroposterior extent. Lesions placed at the sites of the first- and last-mapped units designated the trajectory of each track. The locations of intervening units were reconstructed from their depths with respect to the two lesion sites, as measured by a hydraulic microdrive.

An ordered representation of auditory space was manifest in both the receptive fields and the best areas of these MLD units. However, variations in receptive field size frequently caused irregularities in the spatial transition of the receptive field borders of sequential units. In contrast, unit best areas shifted smoothly and predictably as the electrode advanced. For this reason, and because the center of a unit's best area could be expressed as a single azimuth-elevation term, best-area centers were correlated with unit location to arrive at the detailed map of auditory space representation (Fig. 1).

Sound azimuths were arrayed in the horizontal plane of the MLD, with most of the region devoted to contralateral auditory space. Best-area centers extended from 60° contralateral ($60°_C$), represented in the posterolateral corner, to 15° ipsilateral ($15°_i$), represented in the anteromedial corner. Azimuths between $20°_C$ and 0° were disproportionately well represented, but azimuths beyond $30°_C$ and $10°_i$ received little representation.

Sound elevation was arranged dorsoventrally in the transverse plane: high best areas were located dorsally;

low best areas were located ventrally. Best-area centers ranged in elevation from $+20°$ to $-90°$ with greatest representation given to the area between $-10°$ and $-60°$.

This map of auditory space is an emergent property of higher-order neurons, distinguishing it from all other sensory maps that are direct projections of the sensory surface. The auditory system must derive its map from the relative patterns of auditory nerve input arriving from the two ears. This requires that (i) there exist unique interaural intensity or time criteria for each area of auditory space, (ii) the auditory input be connected in such a way that each central neuron responds to a slightly different set of criteria corresponding to a slightly different area of space (*18*), and (iii) these neurons be arranged so that the order of their receptive fields conforms to the continuity of auditory space. Because these space-related response properties and functional organization must be specifically generated through neuronal integration by the central nervous system, it seems likely that these neurons in this specialized region of the midbrain are intimately involved in the analysis of spatial aspects of auditory signals.

References and Notes

1. G. von Békésy, *Experiments in Hearing*, E. G. Wever, Transl. and Ed. (McGraw-Hill, New York, 1960). The theory was later expanded by W. A. van Bergeijk [*J. Acoust. Soc. Am.* **34**, 1431 (1962)].

2. L. A. Jeffress. *J. Comp. Physiol. Psychol.* **41**, 35 (1948).

3. For a review of neurophysiological studies on sound localization, see S. D. Erulkar, *Physiol. Rev.* **52**, 237 (1972).

4. J. L. Hall, *J. Acoust. Soc. Am.* **37**, 814 (1965); F. Flammino and B. M. Clopton, *ibid.* **57**, 692 (1975); A. Starr, *Fed. Proc. Fed. Am. Soc. Exp. Biol.* **33**, 1911 (1974).

5. E. I. Knudsen, M. Konishi, J. D. Pettigrew, *Science* **198**, 1278 (1977): B. Gordon, *Sci. Am.* **227**, 72 (December 1972); F. Morrell, *Nature (London)* **238**, 44 (1972); B. G. Wickelgren, *Science* **173**, 69 (1971); E. I. Evans, in *Ciba Foundation Symposium on Hearing Mechanisms in Vertebrates* (Churchill, London, 1968).

6. By analogy to its connotation in contemporary visual research, the term "receptive field" will refer to the area of space within which a sound stimulus can influence the firing of an auditory neuron.

7. The anechoic chamber measured 3 by 3 by 5 m and was free of standing waves due to reflection for the frequency range used; sound attenuation followed the inverse-square law.

8. The speaker (5 cm) was calibrated with a 2.5-cm condenser microphone (Bruel & Kjaer) placed at the position where the owl would be located. The frequency response of the speaker was flat from 4 to 10 kHz. Variation in sound intensity as a function of speaker location was less than ± 2 dB except in a small area directly beneath the owl.

9. The speaker moved in azimuth along a semi-circular track 2 cm wide and 2 m in diameter. The track could be rotated to provide changes in speaker elevation. Azimuth and elevation were controlled independently by two stepping motors located outside the chamber. Thus the speaker could be positioned at any point on a sphere of radius 1 m centered at the owl's head, except for a 20° sector blocked by a supporting post for the owl.

10. The highly pigmented pecten oculi in each eye, which is plainly visible ophthalmoscopically, provided a convenient landmark for aligning the owl's head. The visual plane is the horizontal plane containing the projection from each area centralis through the nodal point of the eye to the horizon. In the barn owl the visual plane is located 8° to 10° below the plane containing the projections of the superior limbs of each pecten into space. The owl's visual plane was adjusted by monitoring the projection angle of the superior limbs of the pectens. Medial plane alignment was achieved by positioning the owl so that its pectens projected symmetrically on either side of the 0° azimuth plane.

11. Noise and tone bursts were 100 msec in duration with 2.5-msec rise and decay times and were repeated at a rate of 0.75 to 1 per second. The noise spectrum was 1 to 10 kHz, and the click spectrum predominately 4 to 8 kHz.

12. Units were tested for sensitivity to visual stimuli by sweeping bars and spots of light across a tangent screen temporarily placed 57 cm in front of the owl. The screen was removed during acoustic stimulation. The MLD units were not responsive to visual stimulation.

13. H. J. Karten, *Brain Res.* **6**, 409 (1967).

14. Units were recorded extracellularly with glassinsulated tungsten electrodes. The electrode penetration angle was 45° to the ear canal-beak hinge axis (that is, in the transverse plane) as measured by a protractor.

15. M. Konishi, *Am. Sci.* **61**, 414 (1973).

16. Unit thresholds ranged from -10 to $+36$ dB sound-pressure level.

17. We have adopted the conventions of H. J. Karten and W. Hodos [*A Stereotaxic Atlas of the Brain of the Pigeon* (Columba livia) (Johns Hopkins Press, Baltimore, 1967)] in defining the planes of section.

18. Attenuation of sound intensity to one ear by earplugging severely altered the receptive fields of these midbrain units.

19. We thank A. J. Hudspeth for critically reviewing the manuscript. This work was supported by an NIH postdoctoral fellowship 1 F32 NS 05529-01 to E.I.K.

20

N. Suga and W. E. O'Neill

Neural axis representing target range in the auditory cortex of the mustache bat

1979. *Science* 206: 351–353

Abstract

In echolocating bats, the primary cue for determining distance to a target is the interval between an emitted orientation sound and its echo. Whereas frequency is represented by place in the bat cochlea, no anatomical location represents target range. Target range is coded by the time interval between grouped discharges of primary auditory neurons in response to both the emitted sound and its echo. In the frequency-modulated–signal processing area of the auditory cortex of the mustache bat (*Pteronotus parnellii rubiginosus*), neurons respond poorly or not at all to synthesized orientation sounds or echoes alone but respond vigorously to echoes following the emitted sound with a specific delay from targets at a specific range. These range-tuned neurons are systematically arranged along the rostrocadual axis of the frequency-modulated–signal processing area according to the delays to which they best respond, and thus represent target range in terms of cortical organization. The frequency-modulated–signal processing area therefore shows odotopic representation.

In the mustache bat (*Pteronotus parnellii rubiginosus*), the auditory cortex has been found to have at least three specialized areas for processing different types of biosonar information: the Doppler-shifted constant-frequency (DSCF), frequency modulated (FM), and CF/CF processing areas (Fig. 1A) (*1–6*). Neurons of the DSCF processing area are arranged along two axes, one representing echo amplitude (target subtended angle), the other representing echo frequency (target velocity information) (*2*). The DSCF processing area consists of two functional subdivisions adapted for target detection or localization (*3*). The FM and CF/CF areas process information carried by different combinations of information-bearing elements in the emitted biosonar signal and its echo (*4–6*). We report that the FM processing area represents target-range information along an anatomical axis without a corresponding anatomical dimension at the periphery.

The mustache bat emits biosonar signals (orientation sounds), each of which contains four harmonics. Each harmonic consists of a CF component and an FM component. Therefore, there are eight components (CF_{1-4}, FM_{1-4}) in each emitted signal (*1, 5, 7*). Echoes that elicit behavioral responses in the mustache bat always overlap with the emitted signal (inset, Fig. 1C). As a result, biosonar information must be extracted from a complex sound with up to 16 components.

Neurons in the FM processing area are maximally excited only when an echo from an orientation sound arrives after a particular delay. The essential elements in such paired stimuli are the first harmonic FM component (FM_1), in the orientation sound and one or more higher harmonic FM components (FM_{2-4}) in the echo. Therefore, these neurons are called FM_1–FM_n facilitation neurons (*4, 5*).

One of the most important aspects of echolocation is ranging. The primary cue for ranging is the delay of the echo from the emitted sound. The FM_1–FM_n facilitation neurons are sensitive to this delay and are therefore range-sensitive. Range-sensitive neurons can be classified into two categories, tracking and range-tuned. The best delays (BD's) (*8*) of tracking neurons shorten and their delay-tuning curves become narrower as the bat changes the signal repetition rate and duration as it approaches a target. These neurons zero in on the target, rejecting echoes from more distant objects (*4, 5*). Range-tuned neurons, on the other hand, are tuned to particular echo delays, regardless of repetition rate and duration of paired stimuli. They respond to the target only when it is within a certain narrow range (*5*). The obvious question is whether range-tuned neurons with different BD's (that is, best ranges) are systematically arranged along an axis in the FM processing area to represent target range information.

Experiments were performed with 12 mustache bats collected in Panama. The activity of single neurons was recorded in unanesthetized bats with a tungsten-wire electrode (5- to 10-μm tip) during the period from 4 days to 4 weeks after surgery to expose the skull. When necessary, local anesthetic (Xylocaine) and tranquilizer (droperidol) were administered. Acoustic stimuli were pure (CF) tones, FM sounds, and combinations of them that mimicked the biosonar signalecho pair in the search, approach, and terminal phases of echolocation in this species (*9*). The stimuli were delivered from a loudspeaker 73 cm in front of the animal in a soundproof, echo-suppressed room. For details of the surgery and the stimulation and recording systems, see (*4*) and (*5*).

In the first stage of our experiment, we inserted an electrode orthogonal to the surface of the FM processing area and recorded single-unit activity at various depths to determine whether there was columnar organization for response parameters, such as best fre-

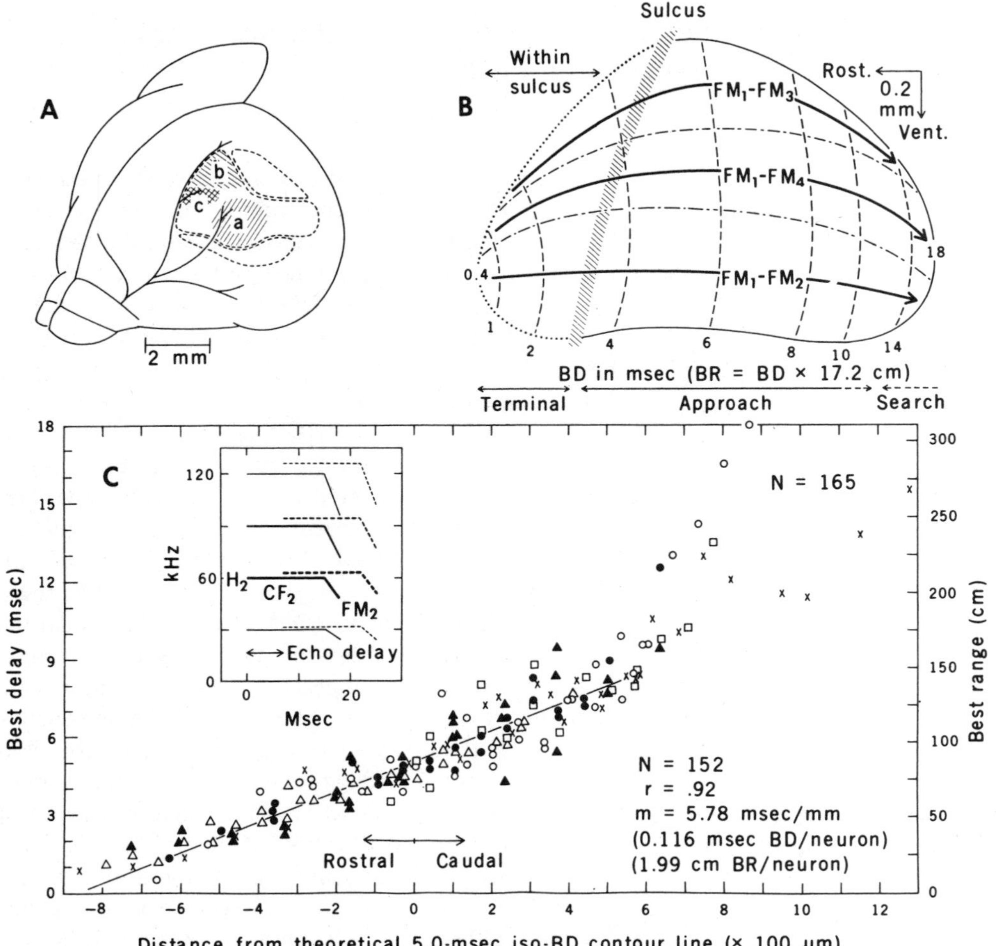

Figure 1. (A) The left cerebral hemisphere of the mustache bat showing (a) Doppler-shifted CF, (b) FM, and (c) CF/CF processing areas. (B) The FM processing area consists of three major clusters of delay-sensitive neurons: FM_1–FM_2, FM_1–FM_3, and FM_1–FM_4 facilitation neurons. Each cluster shows odotopic representation. Iso-BD contours and range axes are schematically shown by dashed lines and solid arrows, respectively. Best delays of 0.4 and 18 msec correspond to best ranges (BR's) of 7 and 310 cm. Range information in the search, approach, and terminal phases of echolocation is represented by activity at different loci in the cerebral hemisphere. (C) The relationship between BD (or BR) and distance along the cortical surface. The data were obtained from six cerebral hemispheres and are indicated by six different symbols. The regression line represents the average change in BD with distance. Since the 5-msec iso-BD contour line always crossed the central part of the FM processing area along the exposed surface of the cortex, the 5-msec BD on the regression line is used as a reference point to express distance (*10*). The inset is a schematized sonagram of an orientation sound and a Doppler-shifted echo in the approach phase of echolocation.

quency, minimum threshold, and frequency bandwidth, with pure tones, FM sounds, and pairs of sounds used to elicit facilitation. We also measured BD, threshold at BD, and width of the delay-tuning curves with pairs of sounds eliciting the strongest facilitation. Neurons at depths between 200 and 1000 μm had nearly identical response characteristics, including BD's. (At depths less than 200 μm, the signal-to-noise ratio was usually small and responses to acoustic stimuli were poor.)

Confirmation of the columnar organization of BD's simplified our study of cortical representation of target range, because we could rely on the uniformity of activity at different depths in the cortex. To gather data from many locations in the cortical plane, we inserted the electrode at a 30° angle into the FM processing area; neuronal responses were studied at 200-μm intervals. We plotted BD's of range-tuned neurons only on a surface map of the cerebral cortex that was drawn prior to the recordings.

The FM processing area consists of three major clusters: FM_1–FM_3, FM_1–FM_4, and FM_1–FM_2 facilitation neurons (*4*), which are usually arranged dorsal to ventral in that order (Fig. 1B). For each electrode penetration through those clusters in the rostrocaudal direction. BD systematically varied. Figure 1B gives a schematic representation of the iso-BD contour lines that comprise a target-range axis. Neurons with extremely short BD's were recorded only at the rostroventral part of the FM processing area. The shortest BD of a range-tuned neuron was 0.4 msec, corresponding to a target range of 6.9 cm. Neurons with very short BD's responded strongly to each paired stimulus even at a rate of 100 repetitions per second (the terminal phase). When BD was shorter than 2.0 msec, the FM component (2.0 msec) of the echo in the terminal phase overlapped that of the orientation sound. The delay-tuning curve for such a short BD is very sharp but nevertheless may cross the 0-msec delay line at 60 to 80 dB SPL. In that case, when the orientation sound is louder than 60 dB SPL, facilitation is evoked by the combination of different harmonics in the sound per se and is further augmented by an echo with a very short delay. Response latencies of range-tuned neurons to the echo FM are short—7 to 10 msec. Thus, the auditory cortex seems to be involved in information processing even in the terminal phase of echolocation.

Neurons with long BD's were recorded at the caudal part of the FM processing area (Fig. 1B). The longest BD obtained was 18 msec, corresponding to a target range of 310 cm. The delay-tuning curves of such neurons are broad, and they responded strongly to each paired stimulus only when delivered at the lower repetition rates characteristic of the search phase. The response was very poor at a rate of 40 repetitions per second and completely disappeared at 100 per second. The role of such neurons in range discrimination may be limited because of their broad delay-tuning curves. The population of neurons with best delay longer than 10 msec is small. The central part of the FM processing area is occupied by neurons with BD's between 4 and 7 msec. Their delay-tuning curves are sharp and their responses are strong and clearly locked to each paired stimulus even at a rate of 100 repetitions per second. Neurons with BD's from 3 to 8 msec are distributed over a disproportionately large area. This suggests that processing of echoes from targets 50 to 140 cm away (the approach phase) is particularly important to the mustache bat.

Best delays were plotted as a function of distance from the 5.0-msec iso-BD contour line (Fig. 1C) (*10*). The correlation coefficient (r) for the BD's between 0 and 10 msec is .92 ($N = 152$). The slope (m) of the regression line is 5.78 msec BD per millimeter of cortical surface. Since the average interneuronal distance in the cortical plane of frozen sections of the brain is about 20 μm, adjacent neurons could express target range in 1.99-cm increments.

There is an interesting correspondence between these results and certain behavioral data. The little brown bat (*Myotis lucifugus*) begins the approach phase for wire obstacles 0.3 cm in diameter at an average distance of 225 cm (*11*), and the horseshoe bat (*Rhinolophus ferrumequinum*) compensates for Doppler-shifted echoes only when delayed less than an average of 17.5 msec (301 cm) (*12*). The finding that bats react when targets are closer than 301 cm corresponds to our finding that the range axis ends at about 310 cm. *Eptescius fuscus*, *Phyllostomus hastatus*, *Pteronotus suapurensis*, and *R. ferrumequinum* are all able to discriminate range differences of 1.2 to 2.5 cm at an absolute distance of 30 to 60 cm (*13*). This also corresponds to our finding if we assume that the rate of change in best range (1.99 cm per neuron) is the theoretical limit of justnoticeable difference in distance.

Delay-tuning curves themselves are sometimes insufficient to express the properties of range-tuned neurons and may even be misleading. Their responses are more appropriately expressed by iso–impulse-count contours plotted on coordinates of echo amplitude against delay. In Fig. 2, for instance, the neuron is

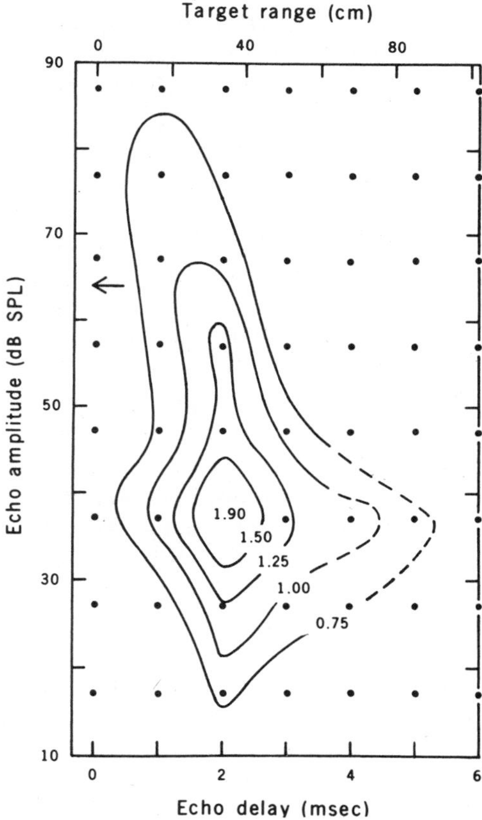

Figure 2. Iso-impulse–count contours representing the response magnitude of range-tune neuron plotted on the coordinates of echo amplitude against delay (or target range). Since the neuron was tuned to targets at a short distance, the orientation sound-echo pair for this plot was delivered at a repetition rate of 100 per second (terminal phase). Dots indicate where an average number of impulses per paired stimulus was obtained by presenting the identical paired stimulus 200 times. The contour lines are drawn on the basis of these data points. The dashed parts of the contour lines indicate where the responses were inflated by background noise associated with animal movement; *SPL*, sound pressure level.

clearly tuned to an echo of 37 dB SPL delayed by 2.1 msec. Range information is apparently processed by a series of such neural filters in both the time and amplitude domains, and as such they may be considered cross-correlators (*14*).

Odotopic representation is the term we use to describe the representation of target range by the location of neurons tuned to different BD's. This representation is the same regardless of wide variations in repetition rate (10 to 100 per second) and signal duration (7 to 34 msec). In the auditory system, the synthesis of a range axis, which has no corresponding anatomical precursor in the periphery, is suggestive of the methods by which sensory information may be extracted and displayed in the brain.

When many conspecific bats echolocate in a confined space, their many orientation sounds and echoes would impair odotopic representation unless some mechanism protected the system from jamming. The fundamental harmonic (H_1, particularly FM_1) of the orientation sound is always critical to the response of range-tuned neurons in spite of the fact that H_1 is always much weaker than the other harmonics and is sometimes barely detectable in laboratory recordings. This means that range-tuned neurons are probably not excited by combinations of orientation sounds and echoes produced by bats flying nearby. To excite range-tuned neurons, H_1 must stimulate the ears prior to an echo in spite of its weakness in the emitted sound. This implies that H_1 produced by the vocal cords stimulates the animal's own ears by bone conduction but is not emitted at a significant amplitude, possibly because of suppression by vocal-tract antiresonance. In nature, range-tuned neurons would be selectively excited only when the animal itself emits orientation sounds and echoes return with particular short delays. Jamming is thereby avoided in most situations.

References and Notes

1. N. Suga, *Fed. Proc. Fed. Am. Soc. Exp. Biol.* **37**, 2342 (1978); ——— and P. H.-S. Jen, *Science* **194**, 542 (1976).

2. N. Suga, *Science* **196**, 64 (1977).

3. T. Manabe, N. Suga, J. Ostwald. *ibid.* **200**, 339 (1978).

4. N. Suga, W. E. O'Neill, T. Manabe, *ibid.*, p. 778.

5. W. E. O'Neill and N. Suga, *ibid.* **203**, 69 (1979).

6. N. Suga. W. E. O'Neill. T. Manabe, *ibid.*, p. 270.

7. A. Novick and J. R. Vaisnys, *Biol. Bull.* (*Woods Hole*) **127**, 478 (1964).

8. The best delay is the echo delay at which the minimum threshold for facilitation is obtained. Best delay corresponds to the best range or a neuron.

9. For mimicking orientation sounds and echoes (inset. Fig. 1C) (*4*, *5*) in the three phases of echolocation, the repetition rate of paired stimuli and the durations of the CF and FM components of the signal were, respectively, 10 per second, 30 msec, and 4 msec (search phase); 40 per second, 15 msec, and 3 msec (approach phase); and 100 per second, 5 msec, and 2 msec (terminal phase). Synthesized echoes were independently varied in frequency, amplitude, and delay from the synthesized orientation sounds. To identify which combination of signal components was essential for excitation of neurons, both the synthesized orientation sounds and echoes were independently simplified by eliminating individual signal components.

10. The sulcus cannot be used as an anatomical reference line since iso-BD contour lines are neither straight nor parallel to it. In each oblique electrode penetration, BD's between 4 and 6 msec were recorded. Therefore, the data for each entire penetration were shifted to be in register with those values. The relative distances between individual data points within each penetration are not affected by this technique.

11. A. D. Grinnell and D. R. Griffin. *Biol. Bull. Woods Hole* **114**, 10 (1958).

12. G. Schuller, *Naturwissenschaften* **61**, 171 (1974).

13. J. A. Simmons, *Ann. N.Y. Acad. Sci.* **188**, 161 (1971); ———, D. J. Howell, N. Suga, *Am. Sci.* **63**, 204 (1975).

14. N. Suga, *Shizen* **79–6**, 70 (1979).

15. We thank J. Jaeger for his assistance in our auditory laboratory and E. G. Jones for kindly providing frozen sections of the brain of the mustache bat. Supported by NSF grant BNS 78-12987 to N.S. and by PHS training grant 1-T32-NS07057-01 to W.E.O.

21

L. Kaufman and S. J. Williamson

Magnetic location of cortical activity

1982. *Annals of the New York Academy of Sciences* 388: 197–213

This paper is a review of recently completed studies of neuromagnetic fields preceding motor activity and following sensory stimulation. Since many of the experiments described here have only recently been submitted for publication, this paper may be considered to be a preview of work to be described in considerably expanded detail elsewhere. Our purpose is to bring together an existing body of facts and ideas supporting the notion that evoked fields complement evoked potentials since they permit a high degree of resolution of the locations of active tissue that are the ultimate sources of evoked potentials. This same degree of resolution, in at least some cases, is not achievable by the study of potentials alone.

The problem of determining the location of a source of potentials on the scalp from an analysis of the distribution of potentials is an instance of the inverse problem. As Helmholtz pointed out long ago,[1] the inverse problem has no unique solution. A large number of possible sources could produce precisely the same distribution of potentials. However, by assuming a particular type of source, e.g., the current dipole, and imagining it to be immersed in a conducting medium within a model representing the head, it is possible to compute the potentials that the hypothetical source would produce on the outer surface of the model. If this solution approximates an observed pattern of potentials on the actual scalp, then it might be assumed that the source of the potentials is located at a place in the brain that corresponds to the place of the current dipole within the model. This general approach has been used with a limited degree of success by Sidman *et al.*,[2] for example, who placed the source of components occurring 20 and 30 msec after somatic stimulation near the central sulcus. This conclusion is consistent with the finding of Goff *et al.*[3] that these components are readily detectable near the posterior bank of the central sulcus when recording from the exposed pial surface.

Most workers studying evoked potentials do not go to the trouble of developing sophisticated models in trying to locate sources. One commonly used criterion is the reversal of polarity of a component. For example, the 30-msec component is electrically positive behind the sulcus and negative anterior to it. If we assume that the source can be represented by a current dipole tangential to the scalp and oriented normal to the central sulcus, then its location coincides with the null point, i.e., the place of polarity reversal.

This procedure seems to be both reasonable and convenient, even though we all recognize that conclusions based on it are ultimately model dependent. Unfortunately, it does not always work. Some evoked potential components as conventionally measured do not display abrupt polarity reversals. Some of them display a gradual change in phase as the active electrode is moved across the scalp. The locations of sources of such components are difficult to determine even when explicit model-building techniques are employed.[4]

One possible reason for such difficulties is that more than one source may be active at a given time. It is widely acknowledged that the evoked potential is mediated by volume currents that flow from a source throughout the intracranial space and into the skin. These currents pass through the pia, the cerebral spinal fluids of the subarachnoid space, through the dura, through and around the skull and, ultimately, into the skin where they produce differences in potential. The boundaries that separate these layers of different conductivities strongly affect the distribution of potentials on the scalp, depending upon the dimensions and depth of the primary source. When two or more sources are simultaneously active, their volume currents are superimposable in the passive conducting media of the head. Moreover, anisotropies in conductivity may well distort the distribution of volume currents in ways that existing models do not attempt to handle. In view of all of this, it is little wonder that source location is so difficult a task.

The situation is not entirely hopeless. For example, Donald[5] was able to recover at the scalp what he called the "Rolandic late wave." This wave is evidently the same as the late somatic response discovered by Goff *et al.*[6] in their pial recordings. The reason for singling out Donald's achievement is that the late somatic response is normally masked at the scalp by the vertex potential. This is an instance of how simultaneously active sources may make it difficult to isolate a relatively unitary source. However, the vertex potential is inherently variable and its variability is independent of the variability of the late somatic response. By selective averaging, when the vertex potential was at its minimum, Donald succeeded in recovering the late somatic response. Moreover, owing to the fact that this response reversed polarity across the central sulcus, he was able to conclude that it originated in the somatosensory cortex.

Unfortunately, it is not clear that all sources of responses are independently variable. Difficulties arise ever when attempting to localize the 20- and 30-msec components from scalp recordings in some subjects.[6] It may not be unreasonable to suggest that other active sources played a role in masking these components in some subjects.

How can magnetic recording be of help? The answer to this question resides in some unique properties of the neuromagnetic response. One of the most important of these is that normal biological tissue is essentially transparent to low-frequency magnetic fields, e.g., less than 1 kHz. Therefore, a field produced by a source inside the head emerges without distortion. Another major feature of the magnetic response is our finding, to be documented below, that the field is relatively unaffected by the volume currents that underly the evoked potential. Rather, the field is due to the relatively high-density intracellular currents flowing in active neural tissue. These two facts taken together, the transparency of tissue to the fields of interest and the intracellular aspect of the current sources, make it possible to resolve spatially separated sources that cannot be resolved by measuring the potentials that arise from these same sources.

We have quite deliberately taken a strong position in this controversial area. For example, Grynszpan and Geselowitz[7] noted that, in principle, when volume currents flow in media separated by boundaries of substantially different conductivity, the boundaries can perturb the volume currents to effectively set up "secondary sources" of fields. Our observations suggest that this theoretical result is not significant in measurements of brain events although it is certainly important in other domains of biomagnetism, e.g., magnetocardiology. In fact, the important theoretical result of Cuffin and Cohen[30] suggesting that volume currents do not contribute to the normal component of the field outside the scalp seems to be applicable to actual measurements.

This introductory section is not the place in which one should fully justify the claims that neuromagnetic fields are unaffected by intervening media and are not generated by the same volume currents that underly the evoked potential. A full justification depends upon a presentation of the data to be reviewed below. For the present, it is sufficient merely to consider the implications of these claims for source resolution. One implication stems from the fact that the strength of the field of a current dipole varies inversely with the square of the distance between the current dipole and the sensor. Now, if the source of the evoked field can be approximated by a current dipole, then the strength of the detected field will be markedly affected by the position of the sensor on the scalp. If it is far from the source, then the field will be dramatically weaker than the field generated by a relatively nearby source. In view of the widespread nature of volume currents and the anisotropies of the conducting medium in which they flow, such a simple distance dependency could not exist for the magnitude of the evoked potential and the distance between its source and the active electrode.

One caveat worth mentioning here is that the field detected outside the scalp must be generated by current that flows tangential to the surface. In spherical models for the head, a current dipole that is not aligned parallel to the radius at the dipole's position has a tangential component and this, in principle, can generate detectable fields. However, a current dipole that is directed radially will not generate a detectable field outside the sphere. The reason is that secondary sources at the boundary of the sphere create a magnetic field outside that exactly cancels the field from the dipole itself (Ampere's law). This theoretical result indicates that field strength outside the head is not only dependent upon the distance between the sensor and the source, but also upon the orientation of the source. The radially oriented current dipole, however, will produce potential differences on the scalp. A dipole that is tilted so that it does not lie along a radius within a sphere can be thought of as being equivalent to two dipoles, one parallel to the radius and the other tangential to the outer surface. The tangential component alone would generate the external field normal to the surface while both the tangential and radial components would affect the pattern of potentials on the surface. As Williamson and Kaufman point out,[8] in a spherical model the external pattern of the normal field remains constant in shape and position as a current dipole is tilted about its center from the tangential orientation, although the field strength will diminish as the dipole is tilted, with a field strength of zero representing the case where the dipole is tilted so that it is radially oriented. This same dipole will produce a potential pattern on the surface that loses symmetry and shifts in position as the dipole is tilted. In the limit, when the dipole is radially oriented, the original dipolar potential field pattern becomes unipolar in appearance. All of this is illustrated in Figure 1 which, though based on a half-space model rather than a spherical model, qualitatively demonstrates the different kinds of behavior to be expected as the current dipole's orientation departs from the tangent to the surface.

Based on such considerations, it seems likely that measured neuromagnetic fields from a single localized source would be distributed in the form of a dipolar pattern, with one member of the symmetrical pair of regions representing the field directed outward from the head and the other field directed inward, as would be produced by an underlying current dipole. The direction of the field, i.e., inward or outward, would depend upon the direction of current flow, in accord with the right-hand rule. Moreover, as illustrated in Figure 1, if the current dipole is strictly tangential to the scalp and if it alone is active, then the resulting

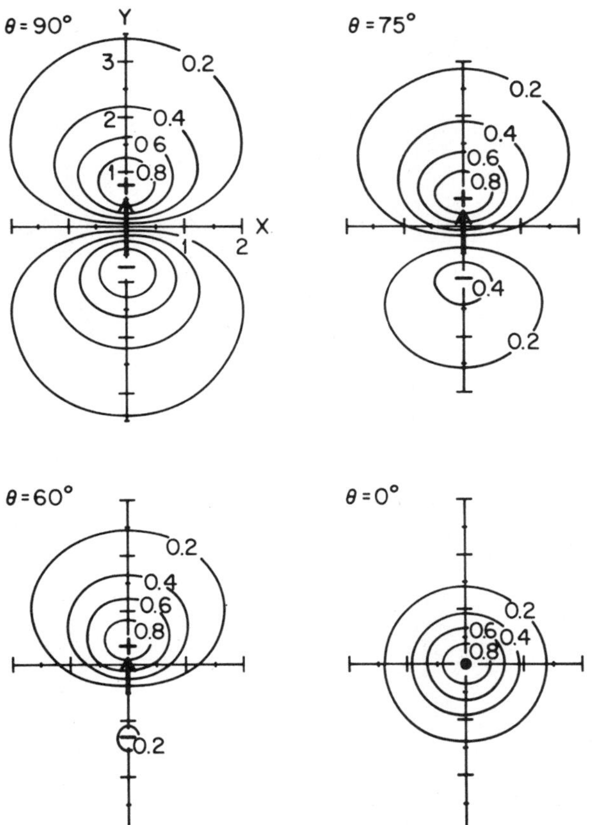

Figure 1. Isopotentials on the flat surface (x–y plane) bounding a half space of uniform conducting material in which a current dipole lies. The dipole is tipped by the angle θ from the surface's normal toward the $+y$ axis. The distances along x and y axes are expressed in units of the depth of the dipole below the surface, and isopotentials are expressed relative to the maximum value of the potential. Isofield contours describing the component of the magnetic field lying nor mal to the surface are identical to the isopotentials for the $\theta = 90°$ case, but the pattern would be rotated by 90° in the x–y plane.

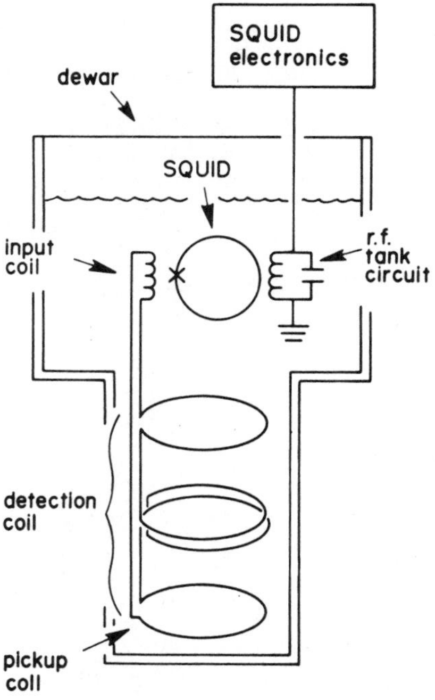

Figure 2. Magnetic field sensor for biomagnetic studied. The net magnetic flux linking the superconducting coil causes a current to flow through the input coil, and that in turn applies a magnetic field to the SQUID. The response of the SQUID is detected by the SQUID electronics, which is magnetically coupled to the SQUID by a circuit resonating at 19 MHz.

potential pattern should also be dipolar in shape but rotated 90 deg relative to the magnetic field pattern. If the current dipole has a radial component as well as a tangential component, then the potential pattern need not have a dipolar appearance while the magnetic field pattern would still be dipolar in character. In any event, all of our field measurements entailed seeking signs of both inward and outward directed fields inasmuch as these should be present if the underlying source can be modelled as a current dipole. We shall now turn to the actual experiments and then conclude with an overview of the accuracy now attainable in source localization by magnetic means.

Methodological Considerations

Before turning to the results of experiments it is of some importance to review the methods used. The first consideration is that the instruments employed must be sufficiently sensitive to low-frequency fields that are typically one billionth the strength of the earth's steady field. This field sensitivity can only be achieved by using a sensor based on the superconducting quantum interference device (SQUID). The SQUID and a superconducting detection coil shown schematically in Figure 2 are kept in a bath of liquid helium within a fiberglass cryogenic Dewar flask. The particular detection coil shown in the figure is known as a second derivative gradiometer since it is wound to be insensitive to uniform fields and to fields with uniform spatial gradient. Consequently, it is relatively immune to fields that arise from distant sources and it is selectively sensitive to fields arising from nearby sources, e.g., those that are close to the bottom-most coil of the gradiometer (the "pick-up coil"). These fields from nearby sources differentially affect the bottom-most coil so that shielding currents are caused to flow in the entire circuit containing the gradiometer to keep the amount of flux trapped within the circuit constant regardless of the external field (the Meisner effect). These shielding currents are magnetically coupled to the SQUID by the input coil shown in the figure. Except for this effect on the SQUID by the input coil, the SQUID itself is isolated from the ambient magnetic field by a superconducting shield placed around it. The

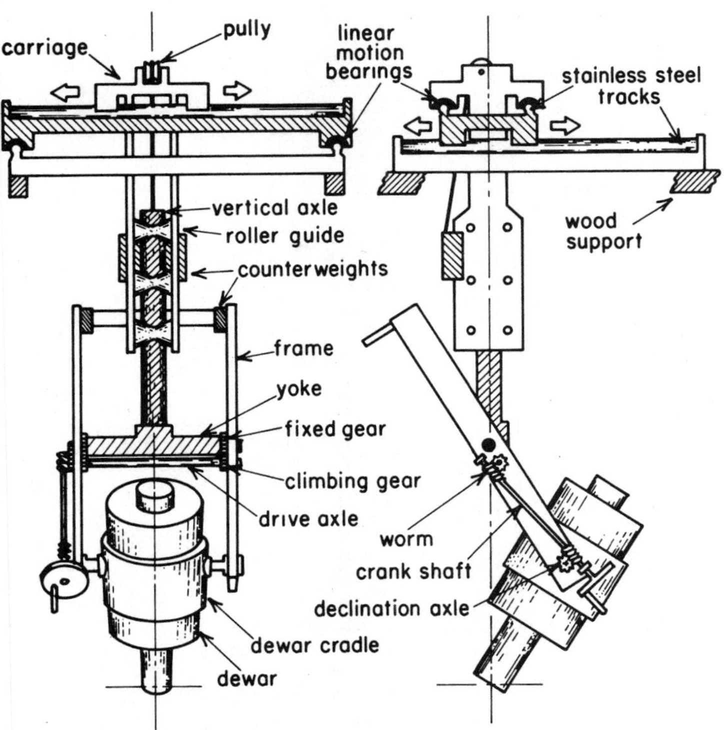

Figure 3. Arrangement for supporting the Dewar flask which contains the SQUID magnetic sensor.

output of the SQUID electronics is a voltage that is proportional to the external field linking the pick-up coil. The details of biomagnetic measurements are described in the review article by Williamson and Kaufman.[9]

As shown in Figure 3, the Dewar flask is mounted in a holder so that it can be displaced in the X, Y, and Z directions and tilted through an angle of 45 deg, with the tip of the Dewar's tail section as the center of rotation. This makes it possible for the experimenter to easily move and tilt the Dewar from one position to the next and keep the bottom-most pick-up coil tangential to the scalp. Therefore, the pick-up coil senses the field that is normal to the scalp. This coil is kept approximately 0.7 cm away from the scalp by the thickness of the bottom wall of the tail section of the Dewar.

In the experiments described here, the Dewar is typically positioned so that the center of the pick-up coil is in the vicinity of the skull where evoked fields are likely to be detected, e.g., over one side of the occipital pole in a vision experiment. The stimulus is then periodically presented for a predetermined period of time, usually 1 or 2 minutes, and the SQUID output is averaged after being applied to a bandpass filter. The particular filter settings and the details of stimulation are described below. The position of the Dewar is then varied in steps of 1 cm from trial to trial until a response is detected that is significantly greater in amplitude than the background noise. Once such a response is found, the trial is repeated to establish the reliability of the measure. The Dewar is then systematically moved in small positional increments until the entire region of the head from which responses of like sign (directed inward or outward) is determined. Such a procedure may take place in sessions that extend over several days. Once the topography of the response is determined, the Dewar is then moved to discover the region from which a response of opposite sign is found. This region is then mapped in the same way as was the other region. When this mapping is completed we generate an isofield graph in which the contours define the loci of fields of equal strength. These maps include the locations on the scalp of the maximum fields directed outward and inward (the "extrema") and repeated measures are made at these points to insure their reliability. This is particularly important since, as we shall see below, the positions of these extrema permit locating the lateral position of the source as well as its depth.

The procedure just described was used in experiments where auditory, somatic, and visual stimuli were employed. A similar procedure was used to locate the source within the motor cortex that became active prior to the voluntary flexion of a finger. The only difference in the latter case was that the reference signal was the electromyogram recorded from the forearm rather than the time of presentation of a stimulus. Moreover, the procedure of Gilden, Vaughan, and Costa[10] was followed in that the response was averaged backward in time from the time of onset of muscle activity as well as forward in time so that events that precede and follow motor action could be recovered.

We will not go into the details here, but will simply indicate that every effort was made to insure that stimulus artifacts did not influence our results. For example, recordings in visual studies were made as a check with the screen of the stimulating display completely masked by a piece of cardboard. In the case of auditory stimulation the earphones were removed from the subjects' ears and responses recorded to insure that we were not picking up an artifact from the transducer in the headset. Similarly, in the case of somatic stimulation, the Dewar was removed from the scalp by a distance of 1 cm to be sure that the pick-up coil was not sensing the electrical stimulus rather than the activity of the brain.

We conclude this section on methodology with a few comments on the procedures used in locating sources from the field patterns. Williamson and Kaufman[8] demonstrated that it is possible to determine the depth of a current dipole within a conducting half-space merely from knowledge of the distance between the extrema of the field pattern measured across the flat surface. This depth is given by dividing the distance between the extrema by $2^{1/2}$. This same method is approximately correct when the current dipole giving rise to the field is near the outer surface of a sphere. In this case, the curvature of the sphere can be ignored and one can assume that the surface is a plane and the dipole is located a short distance beneath it. The results are unaffected if slabs of uniform but different conductivity are interposed between the current dipole and surface to represent the cerebrospinal fluid, skull, and dermis. However, for deeper sources there are strong differences between the sphere model and the half-space model. In the half-space model there is a linear relationship between the distance separating the extrema and the depth of the current dipole. However, in the spherical model the distance separating the extrema increases more rapidly than the depth as the depth increases. This means that small increments of depth can be more easily resolved for deep sources by measuring the distance separating the extrema on the surface. The actual computation of depth in the spherical model merely requires knowledge of the radius of the sphere and a measure of the distance separating the extrema. The appropriate equations can be found in Williamson and Kaufman.[8] In the case of actual applications it is possible to measure the curvature of the head of the human subject to determine its approximate radius and also to measure the distance along the scalp separating the extrema and, by assuming that the head can be approximated by a sphere, compute the depth of the source of the observed field. The depth values given in the following sections were calculated in this way, and, as we shall see, their values are in reasonable correspondence with the depths as given in stereotaxic atlases of the structures most likely to contain the sources of activity affected by the various stimuli employed.

With this background in mind, we shall now turn to consideration of the results of experiments in four different areas of neuromagnetism. These are the auditory evoked field, the somatic evoked field, the visual evoked field, and the field generated by the motor cortex.

The Auditory Evoked Field

The auditory evoked field (AEF) was detected over the temporal region of the scalp by investigators in several laboratories. Reite and Zimmerman[11] were the first to do so using click stimuli. Farrell *et al.*[12] also used clicks as stimuli for evoking a transient response which had a conspicuous 50-msec component. They noted that a similarly conspicuous component had been reported in the literature for the vertex-detected auditory evoked potential.[13] The relative polarity of the magnetic and potential data is consistent with the predictions of a model in which the source of the auditory evoked potential is a current dipole oriented vertically, and therefore the volume currents arising from the current dipole flow downward 50 msec after stimulation, as indicated by the positivity of the component at this time near the vertex. Hari *et al.*[14] observed the AEF for a 1000-Hz tone presented for 800 msec. Elberling *et al.*[15] used a similar stimulus (100 Hz presented for 500 msec) and verified the finding of Hari *et al.*[14] These responses contained clear 100-msec components as well as a sustained component. The fields evoked by these binaural stimuli were of greatest intensity near the two ends of the Sylvian fissure, such as would be produced by two nearly vertically oriented dipoles, with one in each hemisphere. This result was essentially the same as that obtained by Farrell *et al.*[12]

The most interesting aspect of all of these results, however, is that the direction of the field was predictable from a current dipole whose current orientation was opposed to the direction of the current producing corresponding components of the evoked potential. Therefore, the extracellular currents producing the evoked potential could not be the same as the current underlying the AEF. The latter must flow in the opposite direction. Therefore, Hari *et al.* concluded that the source of the AEF is the net intracellular currents evoked by the stimulus while the corresponding components of the evoked potential are due to the extracellular volume current associated with these intracellular currents. This conclusion is consistent with the finding of Farrell *et al.* concerning the 50-msec component of the transient field and potential.

The foregoing results tell us something about the nature of the source of the AEF and that it is located in the vicinity of the Sylvian fissure. Our own concern, however, is with the degree to which it is possible to further refine measures of the location of the source of the AEF. Toward this end, Romani, Williamson, and Kaufman resorted to a very different kind of stimulus.[16] A pure tone of 200, 600, 2000, or 5000 Hz was amplitude modulated by a 32-Hz sinusoid and presented to the subject binaurally by means of an airline headset. The loudness of each tone was adjusted until the subject judged them to be approximately equal. The 32-Hz modulating signal was used as the trigger (reference signal) for signal averaging. Thus, the responses were at 32 Hz and they were all produced by tones that can be described as composed of three frequencies, i.e., the carrier frequency and the sum and difference of the carrier and modulating frequencies. It was assumed that these spectra are sufficiently narrow relative to all of the central carrier frequencies so that they would each affect a relatively uniform population of cells.

During the experiment, the subject lay on his left side and listened attentively to the stimulus. The pick-up coil of the Dewar was positioned with its center over a point in the temporal region of the skull and all four stimuli were presented in repeated trials and in random order. The Dewar was then moved to other locations in small positional increments and the entire series of measurements was repeated at each location. The position of the Dewar and the amplitudes and phases of the responses at 32 Hz obtained in each 30-sec measurement trial were recorded. The results obtained on repeated trials were averaged and all of the data were then plotted in four graphs, one for each of the stimuli. The coordinate system used in plotting the data employed as the horizontal axis the distance along a line connecting the ear canal and the corner of the eye. Distances (in cm) forward of the ear canal are considered positive and those posterior to the ear canal negative. The ordinate of the graph simply represents the distance of the tail section of the Dewar along a meridian connecting the ear canal and the vertex. These two coordinates permit locating the position of the pick-up coil relative to the scalp.

Constant field contours were fit to the data for each tone. These are shown in Figure 4. These are apparently dipolar in character with one region (+) representing the emerging field and the other region (−) the reentering field. These are so designated because responses in the two regions were 180 deg out of phase. The maximum field strengths in the two regions are indeed comparable. The location of the underlying dipole is midway between the maximum emerging and reentering fields. It is obvious that the current dipole deduced from the field pattern evoked by the 200-Hz

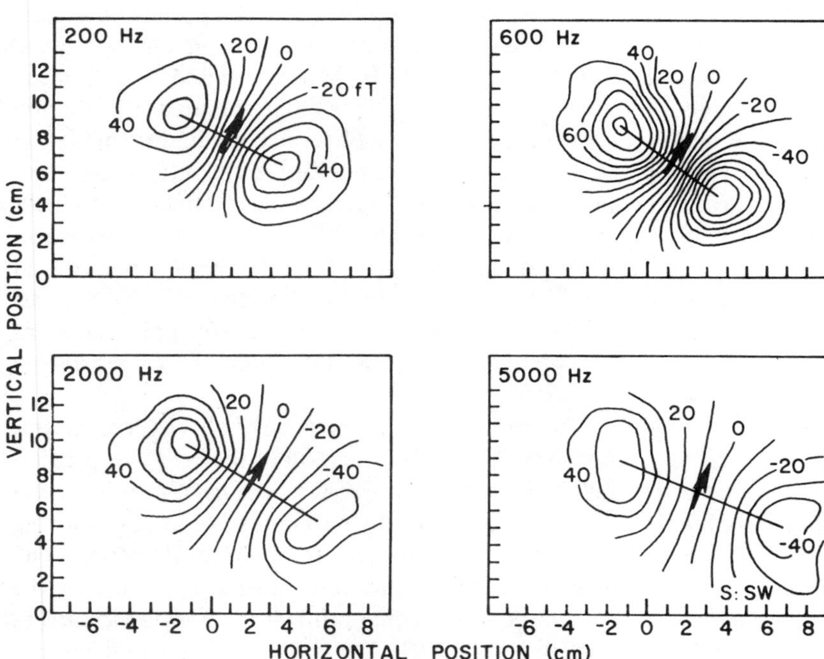

Figure 4. Isofield contours for the component of the auditory evoked field detected normal to the scalp over the right hemisphere. The ear canal serves as the origin, and the corner of the eye lies at a horizontal position of +9 cm. Arrows denote the positions of the equivalent current dipole sources for tones at 200, 600, 2000, and 5000 Hz.

stimulus is nearly directly above the ear canal and that the locations of the other stimuli are increasingly shifted toward the anterior portion of the head with frequency. Morever, the separation between the maxima increases with increasing tonal frequency.

With a correction for the dimensions of the gradiometer, it is possible to compute the depth of a current dipole from the distance separating the maximum emerging and reentering fields for a semi-infinite plane model and also for a spherical model of the head. Using the algorithm for the spherical model, which entails estimating the radius of the head from measurements of its curvature and measurements on the scalp of the distances separating the two maxima of each pattern, the following depths were found: 2.3 cm below the scalp for the 200 Hz; 2.6 cm for the 600 Hz tone; 3.0 cm for the 2000 Hz tone, and 3.3 cm for the 5000 Hz tone. This sequence follows a simple logarithmic progression.

These data for one subject were approximately replicated in another. They show that there is indeed a tonotopic map for the human: cell populations selectively sensitive to different frequencies have a spatial ordering correlated with frequency and, moreover, these populations can be resolved by neuromagnetic means. Thus, the main point of this section is that Romani *et al.*[16] were able to resolve sources within auditory cortex that are separated by distances within the cortex of less than 0.5 cm. Moreover, these regions have different functional properties inasmuch as they are selectively affected by stimuli that differ in their acoustic spectral properties.

It may be worthwhile here to briefly mention one supporting reason for this last assertion, i.e., all of the pure tones were modulated by precisely the same modulating frequency which also served as the trigger. Yet the phase lags of the responses to the modulated stimuli differed by as much as 90 deg from each other. This phase difference could only be due to the difference in the carrier frequencies of the stimuli. Such an effect could only occur if neurons tuned to different spectra of sounds were responding.

Somatic Evoked Fields

Using a SQUID device, Brenner, Lipton, Kaufman, and Williamson[17] detected the steady state response of the somatosensory projection area to stimulation of the little finger of one hand. The response could be detected only over the hemisphere contralateral to the stimulated finger and its topography about the scalp was approximately dipolar in character. The pattern of the somatically evoked field (SEF) was consistent with a current dipole source oriented normal to the central sulcus. A similar pattern was observed when the thumb was stimulated rather than the little finger and the data suggested that the source of this response was at a somewhat lower position along the sulcus. This was confirmed in detail by Okada *et al.*[18] who, in a similar experiment, stimulated the thumb, index finger, little finger or ankle of the subject. Each of these stimuli produced patterns of the SEF whose symmetry allowed the lateral localization of sources. Distinct sources of responses to stimulation of the ankle, thumb, index finger, and little finger were resolved. The positions of these sources are consistent with the known positions along the central sulcus of the representations of the various parts of the body.

Kaufman *et al.*[19] recently detected the transient somatic evoked field in response to stimulation of the median nerve. Responses from the left side of the head of one subject during stimulation of the contralateral or ipsilateral wrists are shown in Figure 5. These responses were measured with a bandwidth of 1–100 Hz and produced by a stimulus presented at about 1.9 Hz. They are typical of responses observed in five subjects. It will be noticed that sharply defined responses are present only when the stimulus was applied to the right (contralateral) wrist. By contrast, the somatic evoked potential (SEP) recorded under similar experimental conditions is quite different in waveform and many of its components are represented with equal strength on both sides of the head.[6] Similarly strong bilateral representation of the evoked field was not encountered in any of our five subjects. It seems likely that the bilaterality of many of the components of the SEP is due to effects of widespread volume currents which do not have the same effect on the SEF. It is perhaps of greater interest to note that there is a strong resemblance between the waveform of the evoked field and that of the electrical response recorded directly from the pial surface of the exposed brain by Goff *et al.*[3] It is also noteworthy that early components occurring 20 and 30 msec after stimulation are visible in the evoked fields of all of our subjects. Although this is not true in scalp recordings, the same components are easily seen in electrical recordings from the pial surface.[6] Such evidence implies that the two responses have a common source, but other sources, perhaps from deeper structures, produce effects that contribute to the evoked potential on the scalp. The effects of these other sources seem to be absent in the SEF. This is one of the major reasons for proposing that the evoked field may be capable of resolving sources that cannot normally be resolved in the evoked potential alone.

A particularly important bit of evidence in this connection is that most components of the somatic response on the pial surface recorded posterior to the central sulcus are opposite in polarity to those of the

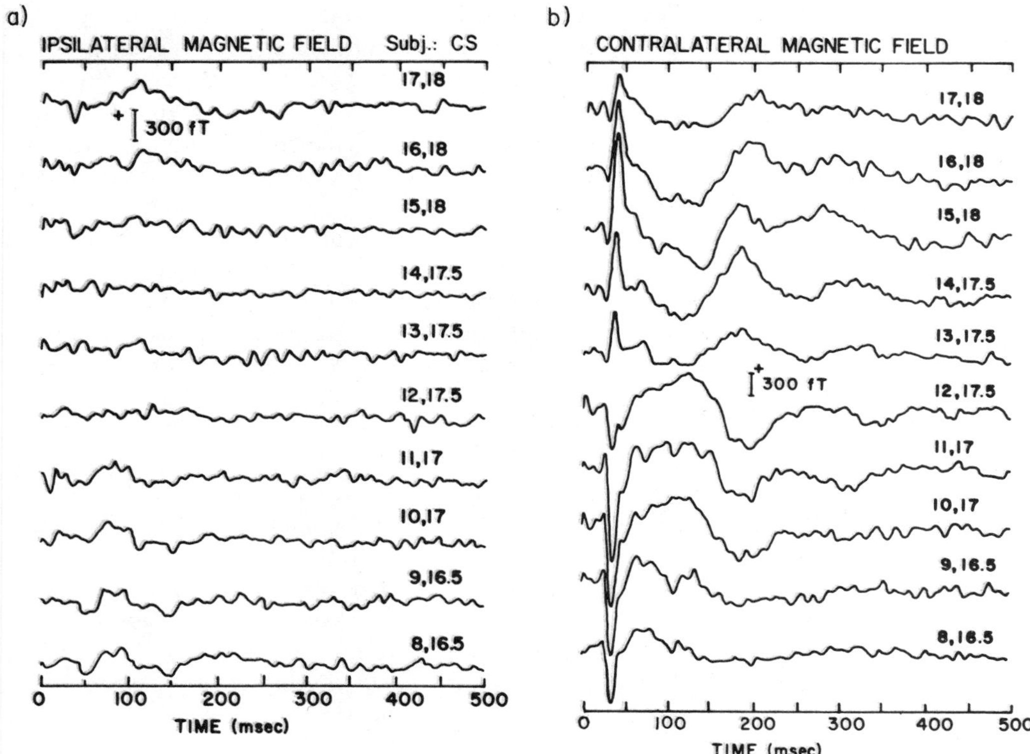

Figure 5. Transient somatically evoked responses over the left hemisphere in response to stimulation of (a) the median nerve of the left wrist and (b) the median nerve of the right wrist. A positive field, indicated by upward deflection, designates a field direction emerging from the head. The pair of numbers indicate the position (in cm) of the recorded response above the ear canal and behind the nasion as measured along the midline.

same components recorded anterior to the sulcuus, including components with latencies as long as ~150 msec. This suggests that the source of these components is at or near the posterior bank of the sulcus. Now, all components of the somatic evoked field abruptly reverse polarity as the pick-up coil is moved rostrally along the projection of the central sulcus onto the scalp. Those components of the somatic evoked potential that did not reverse polarity as the electrode was moved across the central sulcus in the pial recordings of Goff *et al.*[3] were obviously generated by relatively distant sources, and volume currents from these sources contributed to the response. We did not find any components that did not reverse polarity as the probe was moved at right angles to the direction of movement of the active electrode used in the study by Goff *et al.*[3] Consequently, the somatic evoked field seems to be relatively immune to the volume currents that affect the pial response.

We were able to identify three components in the SEF that obviously had counterparts in the pial SEP. These occurred about 20, 30, and 100 msec after stimulation. By way of example, let us consider the 30-msec component. This component in the pial recordings is positive posterior to the sulcus and negative anterior. By the convention that current flows from positive to negative, this may be taken to mean that the volume current related to this component must be flowing anteriorly 30 msec after stimulation. The same is true when this component is detectable in scalp recordings;[4] i.e., the component is conventionally designated as P30 posterior to the projection of the sulcus onto the scalp and N30 anterior. Now, if the evoked field were generated by the same volume current then, by the right-hand rule, the field from the left side of the head should emerge from the head below the source and reenter the head above the source. Figure 5b shows that this is clearly not the case. Upward deflection in the figure indicates an emerging field. The 30-msec component emerges from the head above the source and reenters below. Consequently, the current that gives rise to the evoked field flows in a direction that is *opposite* to the direction of the current that produces this same component in the evoked potential. The same is true of the 20-msec component and the 100-msec component. Now, the only current that could be flowing in opposition to the volume current in the interstitial space is the net intracellular current. It must be concluded, therefore, that the most likely source of the somatic evoked field is the net intracellular current—probably the axial intracellular currents flowing in the apical dendrites of pyramidal cells. More details as to the theoretical reasons for accepting this assertion are provided by Kaufman *et al.*[19]

Our recordings of the transient SEF indicate that the null position—the point at which the external field is tangential to the scalp and, therefore, not sensed by the pick-up coil—defines the lateral position of the source. It is possible to resolve this position with an accuracy of better than 0.5 cm.

The depth of the source of the field evoked by stimulation of the median nerve may be calculated using the same procedure as that used in calculating the depth of the auditory field's source. The distance between the extrema of the 30-msec component of the responses of Figure 5 is about 6 cm. Assuming a head radius of 10 cm, and correcting for the effect of the gradiometer on the response, the depth of the source of this component is approximately 3 cm beneath the scalp. This places the source about half-way into the central sulcus.

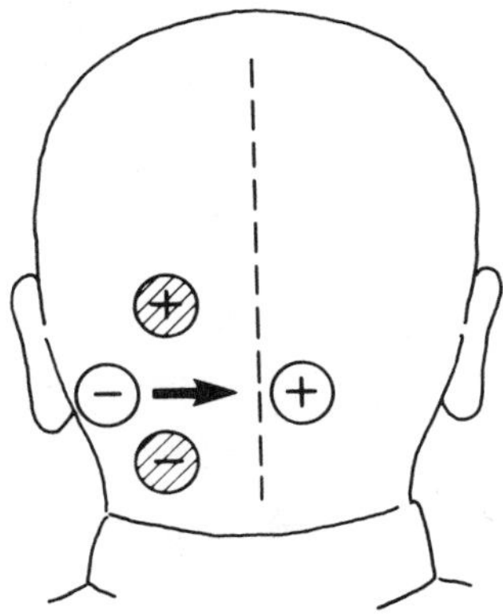

Figure 6. Relative polarities of the visual evoked potential (open circles) and field (hatched circles) for a stimulus pattern in the right visual field. The arrow indicates the direction of the current source responsible for the visually evoked magnetic field.

Visual Evoked Fields

Earlier studies of visual evoked fields indicated that they are relatively sharply localized near the occipital pole.[20,21] Other studies have revealed systematic relations between features of the visual stimulus and the visually evoked field.[22-25] We shall not dwell on such subjects here since our purpose is to discuss neuromagnetic source location.

One of the more interesting of our recent findings is illustrated in Figure 6. Okada *et al.*[24] employed a contrast-reversal grating pattern to stimulate the right visual field. They measured both the steady-state evoked potential and the steady-state evoked field. When the potential reached its maximum positivity to the right of the midline, current associated with it was flowing from right to left in response to stimulation. If this volume current also produced the evoked field, then the field would emerge lower on the scalp and reenter above. However, as shown in the figure, at this time the field was emerging from *above* the source and reentering below. Therefore, as in the case of the auditory and somatic evoked fields, the current that gives rise to the field flows in the direction shown by the arrow, in opposition to the current underlying the evoked potential. This too is consistent with the theory attributing the evoked field to intracellular currents. Moreover, the source in this case is localizable in the left hemisphere, as would be predicted from the hemifield in which the stimulus is placed.

To gain a clearer idea of the possibilities for source localization inherent in magnetic recording, we present some of the data recently collected by Maclin *et al.*[26] In these experiments a grating of 2 cycles/deg was presented either within a hemicircle with a radius of 1.7 deg or within a semiannulus with an inner radius of 4.4 deg and an outer radius of 6.5 deg. With fixation of the left edge of the hemicircle or of the center of the left edge of the semiannulus, the stimuli fell into the right visual field. The hemicircle stimulated the central portion of the hemifield while the semiannulus stimulated a more peripheral region. The contrast-reversal rate of the stimulus was 13 Hz, and this frequency served as the reference signal for measuring the average response at the same frequency. As expected from the basic anatomy of the visual system, the region of the cortex activated by the peripheral stimulus should fall within the longitudinal sulcus while that from the more central stimulus should be at or near the lip of the occipital pole.

The results are shown as isofield contours representing the loci of places that gave equal field amplitudes in response to these stimuli (Figure 7). The equivalent current dipole source that best fits the contours lies between the maximum outward and maximum inward fields. Note that with the central stimulus (Figure 7a) the dipole is about 3 cm to the left of the midline and for the more peripheral stimulus (Figure 7b) it is about 2 cm higher and is closer to the midline. More important is the fact that the distance separating the maxima in the field patterns is greater for the peripheral stimulus than for the central. This separation is not accurately portrayed in Figure 7 since the graphs are plotted into rectangular coordinates with the inion represented as the origin. Actual measurements on the

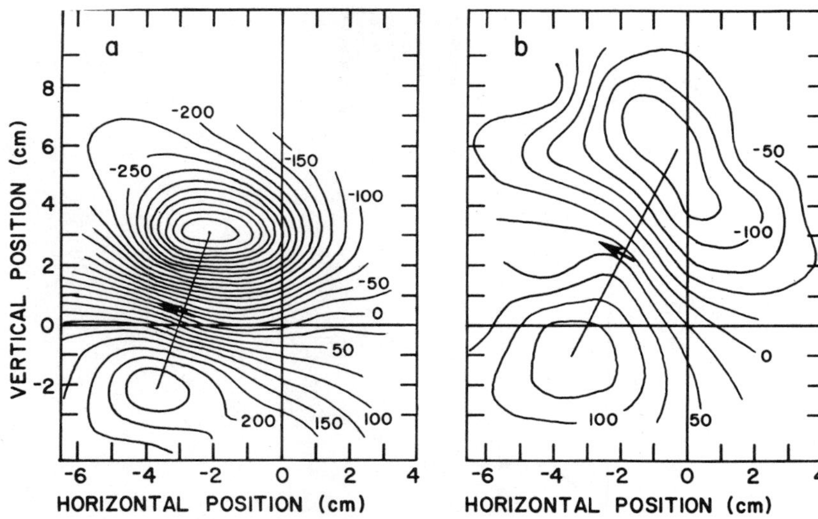

Figure 7. Isofield contours for the visually evoked magnetic field measured normal to the scalp for (a) a central stimulus confined to a hemicircle of 1.7 deg radius in the right visual field and (b) a semiannulus of 4.4 deg inner radius and 6.5 deg outer radious, in the right visual field. Vertical position is measured along the midline with the inion serving as the reference. Horizontal position is measured across the scalp toward the right from the midline, in a plane parallel to the plane defined by the inion and ear canals.

scalp show the separation of the maxima for the central stimulus to be 6.5 cm and for the peripheral stimulus 10.5 cm. These values correspond to depths of 3.3 cm and 5.0 cm, thus confirming that the more peripheral stimulus leads to a field generated by a deeper source than does the more central stimulus. This too illustrates one of the more important features of magnetic studies: a directly measured quantity—the separation between field extrema—is approximately twice as large as the depth of the source. Consequently, small changes in depth can be detected with correspondingly greater sensitivity.

Voluntary Motor Fields

We conclude with a brief account of work by Okada, Williamson, and Kaufman,[27] which is only now being readied for publication. This work is directly related to the study of Gilden, Vaughan, and Costa[10] and Kornhuber and Deecke[28] who succeeded in detecting cortical activity prior to voluntary flexion of the wrist. In our experiment, the subject flexed his forefinger in response to the reversal in contrast of a grating pattern. The EMG recorded during finger flexion served as a reference signal. The pick-up coil of the Dewar was moved along the projection of the central sulcus on the scalp and responses to 100 finger flexions were averaged at each of several positions. The top pair of tracings in Figure 8 show the average time variation of the magnetic field normal to the scalp prior to, during, and after motion of the index finger on the contralateral side. Trace A was obtained 21.5 cm in back of the nasion measured along the midline and 16.0 cm above the line joining the ear canal and the eye. Trace B,

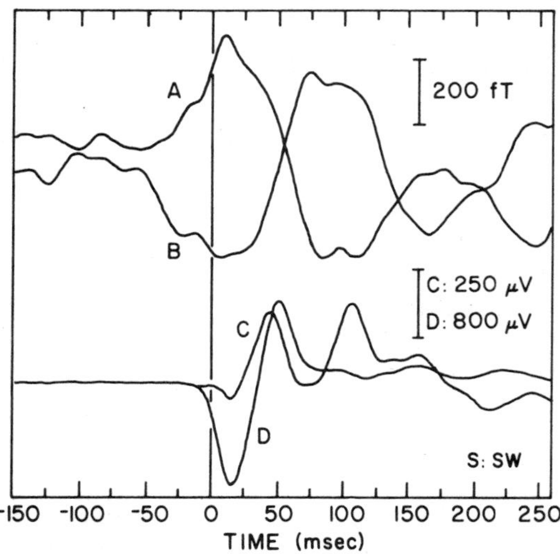

Figure 8. Magnetic field over the right hemisphere preceding and during voluntary flexture of the left index finger, with traces A and B obtained at different positions along the central sulcus showing a reversal in field direction. The lower two traces show the simultaneously recorded electromyograms obtained for the C extensor muscle and D flexure muscle.

which was recorded at a lower position, i.e., 10 cm up and 19.5 cm back, displays the polarity inversion typical of those that occur when recordings are made on different sides of an underlying source. The lowermost traces C and D show the electromyogram obtained simultaneously for the flexor extensor muscles. It is apparent that activity in the motor cortex begins about 40 msec prior to the onset of the myogram. Moreover, when the same finger is moved passively by the subject's other hand (on the ipsilateral side), then the early components of the activity of the motor cortex disappear. This preliminary report suggests the possibility that the source of activity of motor cortex prior to finger flexion can be resolved with an accuracy similar to that obtainable with the somatic evoked response.

Conclusions

The main conclusion to be drawn from this review is that the magnetic technique makes it possible to localize sources of evoked fields with an accuracy of a few millimeters. Thus far, this has been true only of sources of cortical responses since subcortical sources have yet to be detected. However, in view of the fact that cortical sources deep inside the longitudinal fissures have been resolved, it is well within the realm of technical feasibility to study the activity of subcortical sources. In any event, it is apparent that the magnetic technique is a useful complement to conventional potential measures since it provides a noninvasive means for identifying relatively unitary sources that contribute to the complex wave known as the evoked potential.

[**Note added in proof**: Recently, Okada, Kaufman, and Williamson[29] observed magnetic activity that is correlated with the P300 complex detected in the event-related potential at the vertex. The field pattern can be interpreted as arising from an equivalent current dipole source in each hemisphere lying deep within the brain in the hippocampal formation. This finding is evidence that the magnetic technique has the capability of determining the location of subcortical activity, as well as the cortical activity described above.]

Notes

This work was supported by the Office of Naval Research (Contract N00014-76-C-0568) and the National Institutes of Health (Grant 1 RO1 EY02059-03).

References

1. Helmholtz, H. 1853. Uber einige Gesetz der Vertcilung elektrischer Strome in korperlichen Leitern, mit Anwendung auf die thierischelektuschen Versuche. Ann. Phys. Chem (Ser. 3) **89**: 211–233, 353–377.

2. Sidman, R, D., V, Giambalvo, T. Allison & P. Bergey. 1977. A dipole localization method for determination of sources of human cerebral evoked potentials Am. EEG Soc. (Miami).

3. Goff, W. R., P. D. Williamson, J. C. Van Gilder, T. Allison & T. C. Fisher. 1980. Neural origins of long latency evoked potentials recorded from the depth and cortical surface of the brain in man. Prog Clin. Neurophysiol. **7**: 126–145.

4. Goff, W. R., T. Allison & H. E. Vaughan, Jr. 1978. The functional neuroanatomy of event related potentials. *In* Event Related Brain Potentials in Man, E. Callaway, P. Tueting & S. Koslow, Eds. pp. 1–79. Academic Press, New York. N.Y.

5. Donald, M. W. 1976. Topography of evoked potential amplitude fluctuations. *In* The Responsive Brain. W. C. McCallum & J. R. Knott, Eds. pp. 10–14. J. Wright and Sons, Ltd., Bristol, England.

6. Goff, G. D., Y. Matsumiya, T. Allison & W. R. Goff. 1977. The scalp topography of human somatosensory and auditory evoked potentials. Electroenceph. Clin. Neurophysiol. **42**: 57–76.

7. Grynszpan, F. & D. B. Geselowitz. 1973. Model studies of the magnetocardiogram. Biophys. J. **13**: 911–925.

8. Williamson, S. J. & L. Kaufman. 1981. Evoked cortical magnetic fields. *In* Biomagnetism. S. N. Erné, H. D. Hahlbohm & H. Lübbig, Eds. pp. 353–402. Walter de Gruyter, Berlin.

9. Williamson, S. J. & L. Kaufman. 1981. Biomagnetism. J. Magn. Magn. Mat. **22**: 129–202.

10. Gilden, L., H. G. Vaughan, Jr. & L. D. Costa. 1966. Summated human EEG potentials associated with voluntary movement. Electroenceph. Clin. Neurophysiol. **20**: 433–438.

11. Reite, M., & J. E. Zimmerman. 1978. Magnetic phenomena of the central nervous system. Ann. Rev. Biophys. Bioeng. **7**: 167–188.

12. Farrell, D. E., J. H. Tripp, R. Norgren, & T. J. Teyler. 1980. A study of the auditory evoked field of the human brain. Electroenceph. Clin. Neurophysiol. **49**: 31–37.

13. Picton, T. W., S. A. Hillyard, H. I. Krausz, & R. Galambos. 1974. Human auditory evoked potentials. I: Evaluation of components. Electroenceph. Clin. Neurophysiol. **36**: 179–190.

14. Hari, R., K. Aittoniemi, M. L. Järvinen, T. Katila & T. Varpula. 1980. Auditory evoked transient and sustained magnetic fields of the human brain. Exp. Brain Res. **40**: 237–240.

15. Elberling, C., C. Bak, B. Kofoed, J. Lebech & K. Saermark. 1980. Magnetic auditory responses from the human brain. A preliminary report. Scand. Audiol. **9**: 185–190.

16. Romani. G.-L., S. J. Williamson & L. Kaufman. 1982. Tonotopic organization of the human auditory cortex. Science (in press).

17. Brenner, D., J. Lipton, L. Kaufman & S. J. Williamson. 1978. Somatically evoked fields of the human brain. Science **199**: 81–83.

18. Okada. Y.. R. Tanenbaum, L. Kaufman, & S. J. Williamson. 1982. Projection areas of human primary somatosensory cortex determined by neuromagnetic techniques. (In preparation).

19. Kaufman, L., Y. Okada, D. Brenner & S. J. Williamson. 1982. On the relation between somatic evoked potentials and fields. Intl. J. Neurophysiol. (in press).

20. Zimmerman, J. T., N. J. Edrich, J. E. Zimmerman & M. L. Reite. 1978. The human magnetoencephalographic averaged visual evoked field. *In* Proc. San Diego Biomed. Symp. J. I. Martin & E. A. Calvert, Eds. Vol. 17:217–221. Academic Press, New York, N.Y.

21. Brenner, D., S. J. Williamson & L. Kaufman. 1975. Visually evoked magnetic fields of the human brain. Science **190**: 480–482.

22. Teyler, T. J., B. N. Cuffin & D. Cohen. 1975. The visual evoked magnetoencephalogram. Lire Sci. **17**: 683–692.

23. Williamson, S. J., D. Brenner & L. Kaufman. 1978. Biomedical applications of SQUIDs. A.I.P. Conf. Proc. **44**: 106–116.

24. Okada, Y., L. Kaufman, D. Brenner & S. J. Williamson. 1982. Spatial and temporal modulation transfer functions of the human visual system revealed by visually evoked magnetic field. Vision Res. (in press).

25. Brenner, D., Y. Okada, E. Maclin, S. J. Williamson & L. Kaufman. 1981. Evoked magnetic fields reveal different visual areas in human cortex. *In* Biomagnetism. S. N. Erné, H. D. Hahlbohm, and H. Lübbig. Eds. pp. 431–444. Walter de Gruyter, Berlin.

26. Maclin, E., Y. Okada, S. J. Williamson & L. Kaufman. Topography of human visual response revealed by neuromagnetic measurements. (In preparation).

27. Okada, Y., S. J. Williamson & L. Kaufman. 1982. Magnetic field of the human sensorimotor cortex. (Submitted for publication).

28. Kornhuber, H. & L. Deecke. 1965. Hernpotentialanderungen bei Willkeurbewegungen und passiven Bewegungen des Menschen; Bereitschaftspotential und Potentiale. Pflugers Arch. Ges. Physiol. **284**: 1–17.

29. Okada, Y. C.. L. Kaufman, & S. J. Williamson. 1982. Hippocampal formation as a source of endogenous slow potentials. (Submitted for publication).

30. Cuffin, B. N. & D. Cohen. 1977. Magnetic fields of a dipole in special volume conductor shapes. IEEE Trans. Biomed. Eng. BME-**24**: 372–381.

M. M. Merzenich, J. H. Kaas, M. Sur, and C.- S. Lin

Double representation of the body surface within cytoarchitectonic areas 3b and 1 in "SI" in the owl monkey (*Aotus trivirgatus*)

1978. *Journal of Comparative Neurology* 181: 41–73

Abstract

Microelectrode multiunit mapping studies of parietal cortex in owl monkeys indicate that the classical "primary" somatosensory region (or "SI") including the separate architectonic fields 3a, 3b, 1, and 2 contains as many as four separate representations of the body rather than one. An analysis of receptive field locations for extensive arrays of closely placed recording sites in parietal cortex which were later related to cortical architecture led to the following conclusions: (1) There are two large systematic representations of the body surface within "SI." Each is activated by low threshold cutaneous stimuli; one representation is coextensive with Area 3b and the other with Area 1. (2) While each of these representations contains regions of cortex with topological or "somatotopic" transformations of skin surface, the representations have many discontinuities where adjoining skin surfaces are not adjoining in the representations. Thus, the representations can be considered as composites of somatotopically organized regions, but cannot be accurately depicted by simple continuous homunculi. Lines of discontinuity often cut across dermatomes and seldom follow dermatomal boundaries, i.e., neither cutaneous representation constitutes a systematic representation of dermatomal skin fields. (3) While the two cutaneous fields are basically similar in organization and are approximate mirror images of each other, they differ in important details, i.e., lines of discontinuity in the representations and the sites of representations of different specific skin surfaces differ significantly in the two representations. (4) The two cutaneous representations also differ in size and in the relative proportions of cortex devoted to representation of various body parts. Because the proportions in each representation differ, they cannot both be simple reflections of overall peripheral innervation density. (5) All or part of Area 2 contains a systematic representation of deep body structures.

These conclusions are consistent with a view of the anterior parietal region as containing functionally distinct fields at least partially related to different subsets of receptor populations and coding or representing different aspects of somatic sensation. We suggest that the "SI" region of primates be redefined as a *parietal somatosensory strip*, the Area 1 representation as the *posterior cutaneous field*, and, for reasons of probable homology with "SI" of other mammals, the Area 3b representation as SI *proper*.

Over the last four decades, electrophysiological mapping experiments conducted in a number of mammalian species have established the view that the parietal cortex of all mammals contains at least two systematic representations of the body surface, i.e., the first (first discovered) and second somatosensory areas, SI and SII. Many of the early pioneering experiments were on macaque monkeys (Marshall et al., '37; Woolsey et al., '42). These studies demonstrated an orderly progression or representation of body parts in a wide band of post-central parietal cortex that later became known as "SI" (Woolsey and Fairman, '46). From the beginning, it was recognized that this "SI" of macaque monkeys encompassed three of the architectonic fields of Brodmann ('09), Areas 3, 1 and 2. The more caudal parietal Areas 5 and 7, and the precentral motor field, Area 4, were excluded from the representation on the basis of a sharp decline in the amplitude of potentials evoked by somatosensory stimuli whenever the recording electrode was moved onto the surface of these Areas.

Initial reports on the postcentral parietal cortex in macaques emphasized the mediolateral organization. The mediolateral sequence of representation was found to parallel that defined concurrently by electrical stimulation in the anterior parietal cortex in man (Penfield and Boldrey, '37). That is, stimulating the tail evoked surface potentials from recording sites in the extreme medial aspect of the representational region; more laterally, the postaxial leg, then the foot, the preaxial leg, the body, the arm, the hand, and finally the head were successively represented (Woolsey et al., '42). In these studies, the rostrocaudal changes in the body surfaces represented in "SI" were less dramatic; receptive fields tended to remain in the same general body region. Determination of the rostrocaudal order of the representation was aggravated by the fact that the most rostral half of the responsive region including nearly all of Area 3 was buried in the central sulcus, and was accessible for exploration by surface electrodes only after extensive cortical ablations. Possibly for these reasons, the rostrocaudal organization of the responsive zones was not stressed. In later reviews of the organization of somatosensory cortex in mammals, Woolsey ('54, '58, '64) summarized both the mediolateral and rostrocaudal organization of postcentral parietal cortex of macaque monkeys with the now familiar distorted "homunculus" (or "simiunculus") of the contralateral half of the body surface, which was superimposed on a lateral view of the brain to show the major features of "SI" organization. The homunculus portrayed the body on the brain with the distal digits of the hands and feet pointing rostrally along the rostral border of Area 3 (actually, of 3a), the head laterally, and the back of the animal caudally (along the caudal border of Area 2).

A difficulty with the concept of the organization of postcentral parietal cortex as a homunculus overlying three or four major architectonic fields became evident with the publication of the microelectrode studies of the properties of single neurons in parietal cortex, by Powell and Mountcastle ('59a,b) and Mountcastle and Powell ('59). These investigators demonstrated that neurons in each of three architectonic fields (actually, 3b, 1, 2) of "SI" tended to have different modes of response to sensory stimuli. Thus, cells of Area 2 responded almost exclusively to the stimulation of deep rather than cutaneous receptors; neurons in Area 1 responded to both types of stimulation; and cells in Area 3b were predominantly activated by light tactile stimulation of cutaneous receptors. This discovery meant that if the proposed concept of the rostrocaudal organization of postcentral parietal cortex were valid, then different body parts would be subserved by populations of neurons with decidedly different functional properties. However, it was still possible to conclude that distal and proximal body parts have different roles in sensory experience, and to argue that the homunculus made functional sense in that the input from cutaneous receptors would be predominant rostrally in Area 3b, where the highly sensitive finger tips were located in the representation, while neurons activated by the stimulation of joints and deep body tissues would be predominant in Area 2, where the less sensitive proximal parts of the limbs and the back were represented.

The concept of an unequal distribution of receptor inputs to a single cortical representation, "SI," became less attractive as further microelectrode studies of neurons in parietal cortex extended the basic discoveries of Powell and Mountcastle. It gradually became apparent that neurons in Area 2 are principally responsive to the rotation of joints and the stimulation of periosteum for fascia (or other "deep" structures); Area 1 neurons are activated by cutaneous input from quickly adapting receptors; Area 3b derives its input from cutaneous quickly and slowly adapting receptor classes; while Area 3a processes information from muscle afferents and other deep receptors (Mountcastle and Powell, '59; Powell and Mountcastle, '59b; Werner and Whitsel, '68; Phillips et al., '71; Paul et al., '72a; Yumiya et al., '74; Lucier et al., '75; Tanji, '75; Heath et al., '76; Krishnamurti et al., '76). Furthermore, the boundaries between neurons with different response properties were often recognized as being sharp rather than gradual, and were felt to coincide with cytoarchitectonic boundaries. Such stepwise changes in functional zones are obviously less compatible with the concept of a single body representation overlying these fields than was the earlier postulation of gradients of functional change.

A second concept of the organization of the postcentral parietal cortex in primates avoided the apparent inconsistency of the single neuron data with the idea of a single homunculus extending over Areas 3, 1 and 2. Powell and Mountcastle ('59b) first suggested that the afferent fibers relayed from a single dorsal root relate to a narrow rostrocaudal band across all the "SI" architectonic fields. While such a statement is not clearly in conflict with the single homunculus viewpoint, it is not far from the more specific concept that each body part is represented in a band across the three or four architectonic fields, so that each body part is in all fields and can be subserved by all neuronal types. This "rostrocaudal band" concept received support from observations that neurons at the same mediolateral level in the separate architectonic fields were found to have similar receptive field locations (Powell and Mountcastle, '59b; Werner and Whitsel, '71; Pubols and Pubols, '71). However, even strong supporters (Pubols and Pubols, '72) of the "rostrocaudal band" concept recognized evidence for somatotopic organization within "rostrocaudal bands" that was clearly inconsistent with a simple rostrocaudal "isorepresentation" of all body surfaces in the postcentral region (which is, in fact, a topological impossibility).

A third viewpoint on the organization of the "SI" region of primates emerged from an extensive series of microelectrode mapping studies on squirrel and macaque monkeys, first initiated by Werner and Whitsel ('68, '71; Dreyer et al., '74, '75; Whitsel et al., '71). While these authors concentrated on definition of the mediolateral organization of the postcentral parietal cortex (which they described as a dermatomal sequence), they also indicated the general features of their concept of the rostrocaudal organization. As in the original reports of Woolsey et al. ('42), these investigators regarded "SI" as encompassing several architectonic fields, i.e., Areas 3a, 3b, 1 and 2. Larger body units such as the face, arm, hand, trunk, and leg were portrayed as rostrocaudal bands extending across all of these architectonic divisions (fig. 12 of Whitsel et al., '71). In this regard, their viewpoint was similar to the "rostrocaudal band" concept stemming from the experiments of Powell and Mountcastle ('59b). However, in their view, a general somatotopy is preserved within these rostrocaudal bands. The representation of some body surfaces are depicted as extending over several architectonic divisions; others are confined to one or two divisions; still others are duplicated in the representation, so as to occur both rostrally in Areas 3a and 3b and caudally in Areas 1 and 2 (see, for example, fig. 9 in Whitsel et al., '71). For example, the volar surface of the hand is shown as extending over Areas 3a, 3b, 1 and 2 with the distal tips of the digits at the rostral margin of 3a and the proximal part of the hand near the caudal margin of Area 2. By contrast, the representation of the dorsal hand is shown exclusively or mainly in Area 3b. Finally, the abdomen is shown both rostrally in Areas 3a and 3b and caudally in Areas 1 and 2. These two representations of the abdomen are separated by the back, located near the border of Areas 3b and 1. It is clear that even this complicated scheme only partially solves the problem of the incongruency of receptor segregation within distinct architectonic fields and the orderly map of the body surface across these fields.

A quite different possibility for the organization of the postcentral parietal cortex was suggested by the experiments of Paul et al. ('72a,b, '75). In microelectrode mapping experiments of the hand region of Areas 3b and 1 of macaque monkeys, they discovered two separate and topographical representations of the volar hand "in its entirety." Each of the two representations was found to correspond to a separate architectonic subdivision with distinct neural properties. Thus, the rostral representation of the hand was confined to Area 3b and was dominated by input from quickly and slowly adapting cutaneous mechanoreceptors, while the caudal representation was limited to Area 1 and was activated by input from quickly adapting cutaneous mechanoreceptors. Area 2 was not systematically explored, but limited recordings there suggested a third representation of the hand responsive to higher threshold stimulation of "deep" receptors. The results of Paul et al. ('72a) raise the possibility that architectonic subdivisions of the postcentral parietal cortex actually constitute separate representations of the body, each processing input from a distinct subset of receptors. The present mapping experiments were designated to gather evidence for or against this last possibility.

The owl monkey (*Aotus trivirgatus*) was used in these experiments because the central sulcus consists of only a very shallow, short dimple on the cortical surface (e.g., see fig. 15), and because there are no sulci in parietal cortex caudal to the parietal somatosensory cortical region. Thus, the entire surfaces of cytoarchitectonic Areas 4, 3a, 3b, 1, 2, 5 and 7, except those buried in the medial wall or Sylvian fissure, are exposed on the lateral cortical surface. The results demonstrate that there are separate and apparently complete representations of the contralateral body within the separate architectonic fields of the "SI" region.

A preliminary report of some of these results has been published elsewhere (Kaas et al., '76).

Methods

Experiments were conducted with nine adult owl monkeys (*Aotus trivirgatus*). Animals were initially anesthetized with ketamine hydrochloride (50 mg/kg, IM). They were maintained with supplementary injections of ketamine at a surgical level of anesthesia. Body temperature was monitored, and kept at 37° throughout these long (20–50 hours) recording experiments. Parietal cortex was exposed *via* a wide craniotomy. An acrylic dam was constructed around this skull opening to maintain a pool of silicone over the exposed brain surface. A high resolution photograph of the brain surface was then taken. The surface vasculature (observed with a dissecting microscope) was used to site electrode penetrations on this photograph.

Glass-coated platinum-iridium microelectrodes with impedances of 2–3 MΩ were introduced in penetrations perpendicular to the surface of the anterior parietal cortex. The amplified electrode output was fed to an oscilloscope, and to a loudspeaker. Mapping was usually initiated just posterior to a shallow dimple (a poorly developed central sulcus) commonly falling at or near the boundaries of somatosensory cortex and motor cortex. The vertical axis of penetrations was set so that penetrations about midway between the midline and the crest of the Sylvian sulcus were precisely normal to the cortical surface. All penetrations in any given experiment over the relatively flat parietal cortex were parallel with this axis.

In most experiments, an effort was made to map a given sector of the somatosensory cortex in great detail. Up to nearly 500 (usually several hundred) penetrations were made in each hemisphere studied. Electrode penetrations were usually spaced at 200- to 300-μm intervals. The most extensive mapping experiments were within cytoarchitectonic Areas 3b and 1, as later verified in serial sagittal brain sections. More limited recordings were obtained rostrally in motor cortex, and caudally in Areas 2 and 5.

Within Areas 3b and 1, neurons in the middle cortical layers were strongly driven by light tactile stimulation. Receptive fields were defined using fine black glass probes while the relevant body part was carefully stabilized to prevent movement. All receptive fields derived in these maps were minimum fields, defined as the skin region from which a distinct response could be evoked by very light tactile stimulation. There was a consistent attempt to determine whether input arose from cutaneous receptors, or from joint or other deep receptors. Outlines of receptive fields were drawn on enlarged photographs of body surfaces of the owl monkey.

In initial experiments, the receptive field boundaries were determined for different neurons or clusters of neurons at a number of depths across the active depths of cortex within single penetrations. They were found to be remarkably constant throughout vertical penetrations into the cortex, as described by others in other species (e.g., Mountcastle, '57; Powell and Mountcastle, '59b; Werner and Whitsel, '68; Whitsel et al., '71;

Paul et al., '72a; Dreyer et al., '75). In later experiments (in which the most extensive maps were derived), one or two very careful receptive field determinations were made in each penetration. Although receptive fields of isolated neurons were sometimes mapped, any given receptive field in the illustrated maps must be assumed to have been derived for small clusters of neurons (Paul et al., '72a; Allman and Kaas, '74; Merzenich et al., '75). *Without exception,* all neurons studied at any given cortical locus had identical or nearly identical receptive fields.

Following recording experiments, small injections of horseradish peroxidase and/or tritiated proline were introduced at physiological defined locations. At this time, small electrolytic lesions were introduced at physiologically significant landmarks (usually at the borders of representations), and a series of surface locations were marked with carbon black to facilitate transfer of mapping data to photographs of the brain surface in that monkey. The animal was maintained with ketamine anesthesia for 20 to 30 hours after the termination of the recording experiment in order to allow the transport of the anatomical tracers. (Cerebral edema was, surprisingly, not a serious problem in these very long procedures in the owl monkey.) The animal was then perfused intracardially with saline followed by 8% formol-saline. The brain was kept overnight in fixative (at 4°C), passed through several increasing concentrations of sucrose in formalin ending in 30% sucrose, and the cortex cut frozen in the sagittal plane at 25 or 50 μm section thickness. Usually, every fifth brain section was processed for autoradiography and counterstained with cresyl violet. Another set of every fifth section was stained for myelin with hematoxylin. All remaining sections were stained with cresyl violet for cells. Experiments were later reconstructed, so that results of brain cytoarchitecture could be systemically related to mapping and tracer studies. Results of HRP and tritiated amino acid tracer studies are described elsewhere (Lin et al., '78).

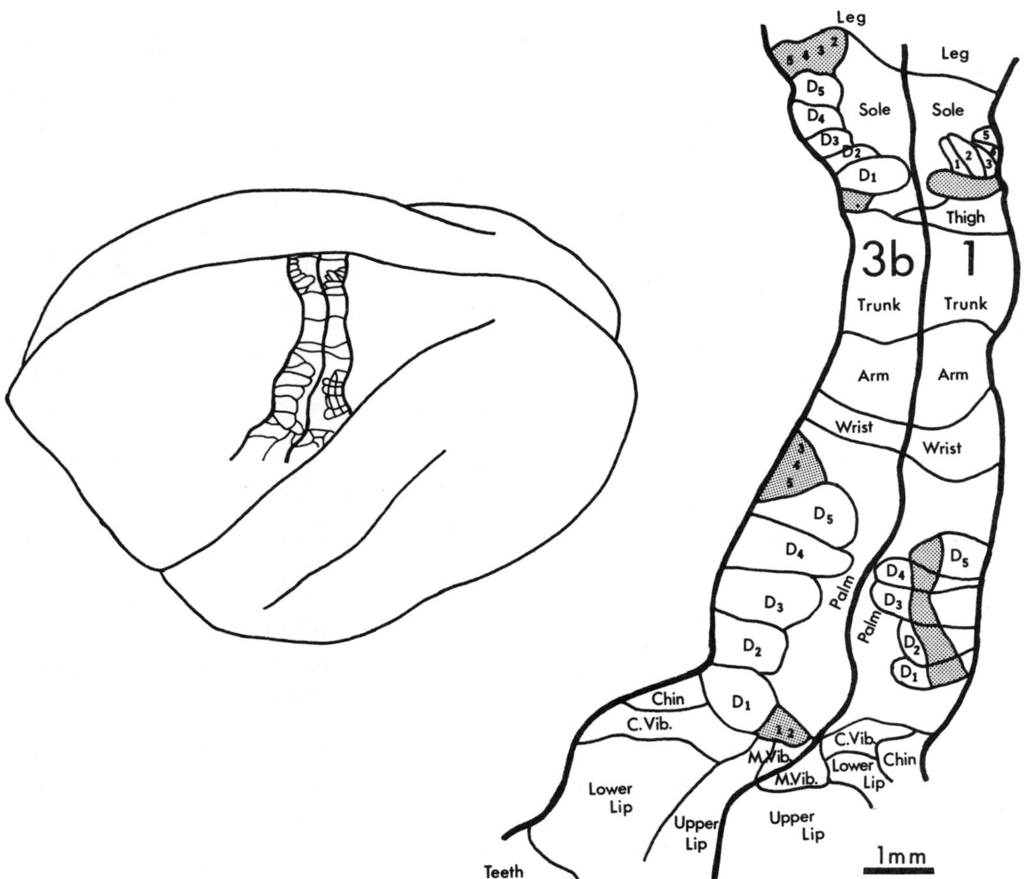

Figure 1. The organization of the two representations of the contralateral body surface within two cytoarchitectonic fields (3b, 1) in the anterior parietal cortex of the owl monkey, *Aotus trivirgatus.* Sectors within each map representing the surfaces of the leg, sole, individual toes, preaxial thigh, trunk, arm, wrist, palm, individual fingers, chin, chin vibrissae, mandibular vibrissae, lower lip and upper lip are demarcated. Cortex representing the dorsal hairy surfaces of the fingers and toes are shaded. This reconstruction is based on receptive fields from 486 electrode penetrations in the "SI" region in a single owl monkey. Similar patterns of organization were found in other monkeys.

Results

There are two highly ordered representations of the contralateral body surface within the "primary somatosensory cortex" ("SI") in the owl monkey. The basic pattern of representation of the body surface within these two large cortical subdivisions is shown schematically in figure 1. The relationship of the two areas is complex when considered in detail, and they are not identical. The two representations have been found to occupy cytoarchitectonic Areas 3b and 1 (as will be described later). In order to appreciate how body surface regions are represented in somatosensory cortex, it is useful to consider in detail the pattern of representation of specific skin surfaces within these two fields.

Representation of the Hand in Cytoarchitectonic Areas 3b and 1

The hand is represented completely within Area 3b and completely within Area 1. The two representations are roughly "mirror images." The tips of the fingers in Area 3b are represented along its anterior border and in Area 1 along its posterior border (fig. 4; figs. 2, 3). The rest of the glabrous skin of the fingers is represented twice in between with a reversal along the palm at the 3-1 border (figs. 2–5).

There is a highly ordered representation of the palmar pads in both representations (figs. 4, 5). The basic pattern of representation, derived from a relatively complete map of the hand obtained in a single experiment, is shown diagrammatically in figure 5. Within each representation, the thenar and hypothenar eminences are displaced from each other and represented in regions lateral and medial (respectively) to the representation of the interdigital pads and fingers. This split representation of the basal palm is more exaggerated in Area 1 than in Area 3. In rows of penetrations extending across the middle of the hand (i.e., the row illustrated in fig. 2), the line of reversal (in fig. 2. between electrode penetrations 4 and 5) runs across the base of the interdigital and insular pads. Thus, the representation of the glabrous surface of the hand is discontinuous. Topological discontinuities were found between

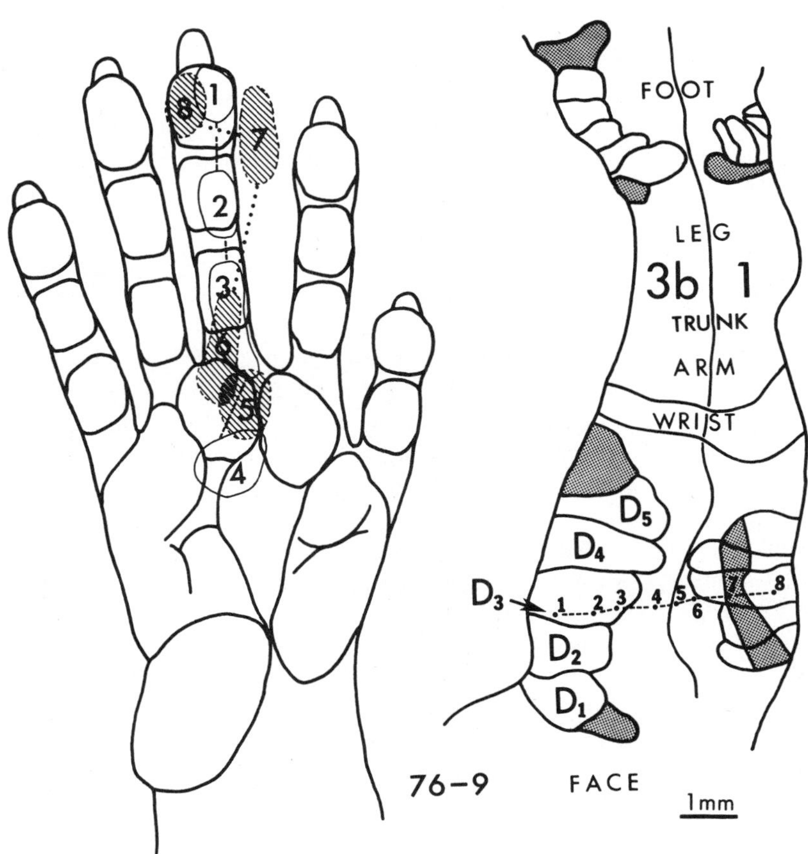

Figure 2. Receptive fields defined within a row of electrode penetrations crossing the regions of Areas 3b and 1 representing the third digit and distal palm. The locations of electrode penetrations are shown on the right on a reconstruction of the mapped portion of Areas 3b and 1. The border between Areas 3b and 1 was defined architectonically. Receptive fields defined within penetrations in Area 3b are outlined with a solid line; those defined within Area 1 are crosshatched. Receptive fields drawn off the digits are on the dorsal hairy surfaces of the fingers at that location. The shaded areas in the reconstruction of the experiment are the regions of representation of the hairy surfaces of the digits.

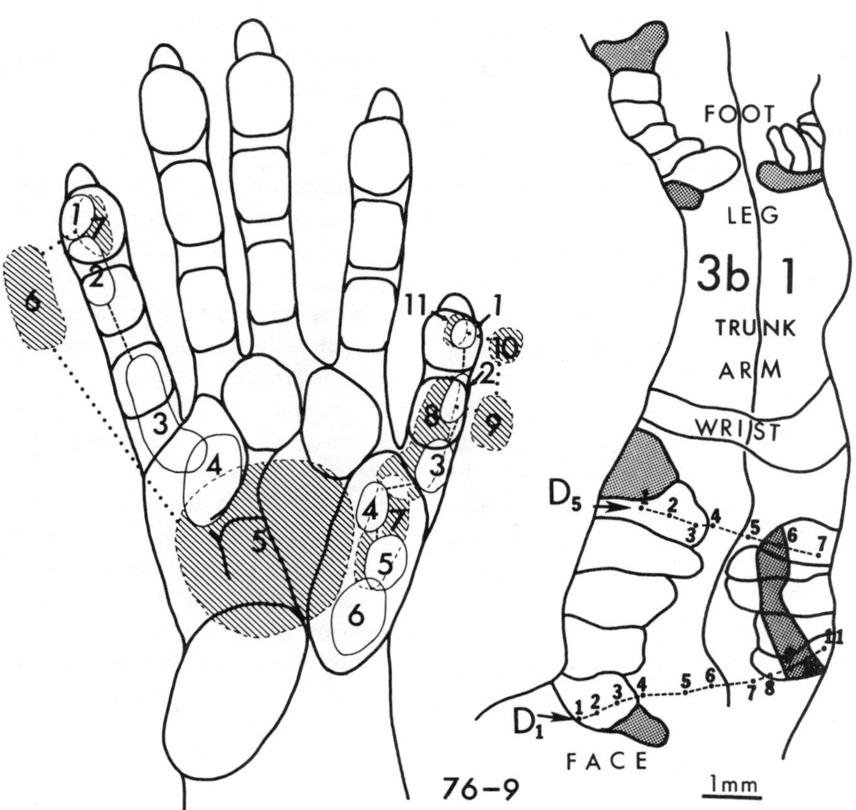

Figure 3. Receptive fields defined for neurons within two rows of penetrations crossing Area 3b and Area 1 in the region representing the thumb and thenar eminence (row D_1 in the reconstruction to the right), and in the region representing the fifth digit and fourth interdigital and insular palmar pads (row D_5).

the adjoining surfaces of the thenar and hypothenar eminences, the radial and ulnar insular parts, part of the border of both thenar and hypothenar eminences with adjacent interdigital pads, and in Area 1, between the most proximal and the more distal aspects of the thenar eminence.

The representation of the glabrous surfaces of the hand in Area 3b is a precisely ordered array. This order is evident in very fine grained mapping, such as that conducted in experiment 76–10, from which receptive fields derived in a continuous row of penetrations across the Area 3b hand representation are shown in figure 4. Penetrations over most of this row were about 200–250 μm apart. In this and similar rows, the centers of successively defined fields shifted in a highly predictable way, usually with significant overlap of minimum receptive fields (like the partially shifted overlap for receptive fields defined in adjacent cortical columns, by Mountcastle, '57, and Powell and Mountcastle, '59b). The representation of the ventral, glabrous surface of the hand in Area 3b was strictly segregated from the representation of the dorsal surfaces of the fingers and hand.

The representation of the glabrous surfaces of the hand in Area 1 was, at first glance, a mirror image of that in Area 3b, but when considered in detail several obvious differences were apparent. The orderliness of the Area 1 representation was not as strict as that of Area 3b. Receptive fields were commonly significantly larger within Area 1 than within Area 3b (see fields illustrated in figs. 2–4). Fields over the palmar pads, for example, frequently extended over an entire pad, or over broad sectors of adjacent pads. Nonetheless, the sequence of representation of the pads was very similar to that of Area 3b, with two exceptions. First, there was a small representation of the basal aspect of the thenar eminence in the extreme medial aspect of the Area 1 hand representation, adjacent to the representation of the wrist, and far from the representation of the rest of the thenar eminence on the extreme lateral side of the hand representation (fig. 5). Second, receptive fields along the base of the palm for neurons in Area 1 commonly included both the glabrous skin and some of the hairy skin of the wrist. Receptive fields for neurons in the Area 3b glabrous representational region never crossed the glabrous-hairy skin boundary.

The most striking difference in the hand representation of the two Areas, however, was in the pattern of representation of the dorsal hairy surface (fig. 5). Within Area 3b, the representation of the dorsal surfaces of

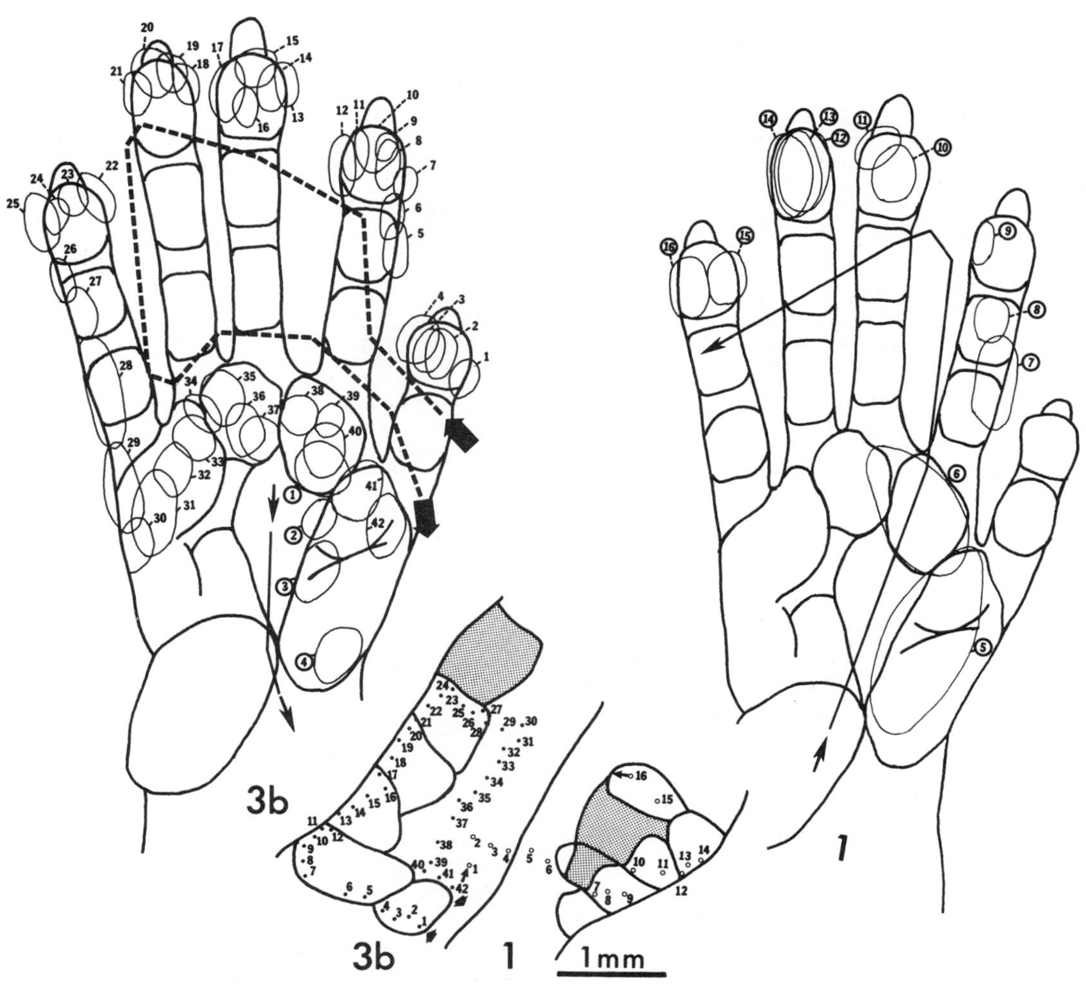

Figure 4. Receptive fields defined for neurons within penetrations along two long rows within the hand representations in Areas 3b and 1. Receptive fields for penetrations in Area 3b are on the left; receptive fields for penetrations in Area 1 are on the right. The locations of penetrations in the two rows (dots and open circles) are shown in the reconstruction of the map derived in this study (bottom).

the fingers was split. The representation of the hairy surfaces of the first and sometimes the second digit were on the far lateral aspect of the hand representation adjacent to the glabrous thumb. The hairy surfaces of the fifth, fourth, third and sometimes the second digits were on the extreme medial aspect of the hand representation adjacent to the glabrous surfaces of the fifth digit. The hairy surfaces were represented as a continuation of glabrous surfaces. Thus, the representation of the outer glabrous margin of the thumb in the lateral region moved onto the dorsal surface and marched across the hairy surfaces of digits 1 and sometimes 2. In the medial region, the representation progressed from the outer glabrous margin of digit 5 and then, in order across the hairy surfaces of digits 5, 4, 3 and sometimes 2. The representation of the back of the hand in Area 3b was continuous with the medial representation of the hairy finger surfaces (digits 5,4,3,2-var.). The representation of the hairy surfaces of the hand within Area 1 was very different. There, the dorsal surfaces of the fingers were represented within a band of cortex between the representation of the distal and middle phalangeal pads (fig. 5), or (in one case see fig. 4) between the representation of the proximal phalangeal pads and the palm. Thus, the dorsal hairy surfaces of the fingers in Area 1 were represented in an island of cortex completely encircled by the representation of the glabrous surfaces of the hand, and thereby creating a discontinuity in their representation by separating fingertips (or fingers) from the rest of the fingers (or palm). The hairy skin of the hand dorsum in Area 1 was represented in a region medial to the representation of the hand and volar wrist, far separated from the representation of the dorsal surfaces of the fingers. The piecemeal representation of the hairy surfaces of the hand in Areas 3b and 1 is again illustrated in detail in the schematic drawing in figure 5.

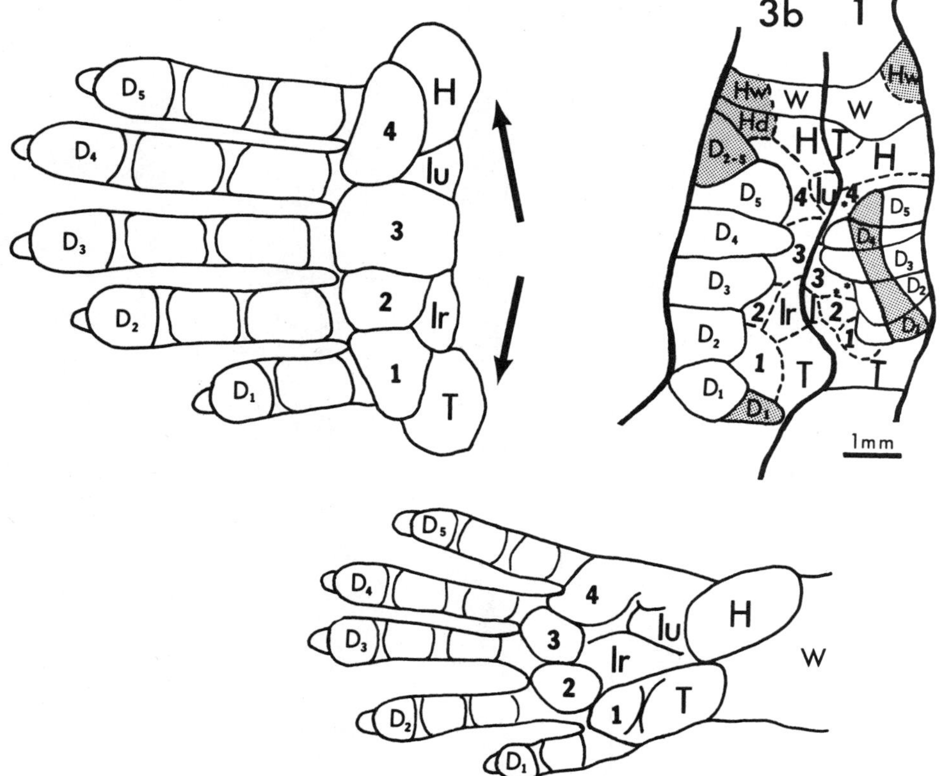

Figure 5. The representations of the glabrous hand in Area 3b and 1. The hand surface (below) is split between the pads of the palm and distorted (upper left) to fit the confines of area 3b in the cortical representation (upper right). The Area 1 representation is roughly a mirror image of the Area 3b representation. The detailed reconstruction of the hand representations shown on the upper right is based on a single extensive experiment. Receptive fields in Area 1 frequently extended over more than one pad, so that the indicated boundaries in the representation are not absolute. Asterisks in Area 1 indicate penetrations with neurons with very large receptive fields suggestive of Pacinian corpuscle input. The representations of the dorsum of the hand are shaded. Receptive fields in Hd (hand dorsum) were restricted to the hand dorsum; receptive fields for Hw (hand and wrist dorsum) included both parts of the wrist and hand dorsum. The digits (D_1–D_5) and interdigital pads (1–4) are numbered in the standard manner. Ir and Iu, radial and ulnar insular pads, T and H, thenar and hypothenar pads.

Representation of the Wrist and Arm in Areas 3b and 1

There are also two separate representations of the wrist and arm in Areas 3b and 1. The pattern of organization is complicated by the fact that the volar wrist surface was represented separately, and by the fact that the order of representation of the arm in Area 1 was often marked by discontinuities which differed in detail from monkey to monkey.

The volar wrist was represented within a narrow strip of cortex immediately adjacent to the representation of the hypothenar eminence, in both Areas 3b and 1. Volar wrist fields were in continuous sequence with fields on the eminence. As noted earlier, in Area 1 fields commonly overlapped the hairy wrist and glabrous hypothenar (or thenar) eminence surfaces, while in Area 3b, fields did not cross the hairy-glabrous skin boundary. The ulnar side of the volar wrist was represented toward the anterior margin of Area 3b, and near the posterior margin of Area 1 (fig. 6). Proceeding toward the 3-1 border in either field, successively defined receptive fields shifted over the wrist toward its radial margin, which was represented along the 3-1 border.

The dorsal wrist was represented within a narrow strip of cortex just medial to the representation of the volar wrist in an ulnar to radial to ulnar sequence identical to that of the volar wrist. Thus, as shown by example in figure 7, the ulnar side of the wrist dorsum was represented near the anterior border of Area 3b and near the posterior border of Area 1. Proceeding toward the 3-1 border in either field, successively defined receptive fields shifted systematically toward the radial margin of the wrist dorsum, which was, again, represented along the 3-1 border. Note that given identical sequences in representation of the dorsal and ventral surfaces of the wrist, much of the representations of the two surfaces are discontinuous. Thus, recording sites 6 in figure 6 and 6 in figure 7 are close to

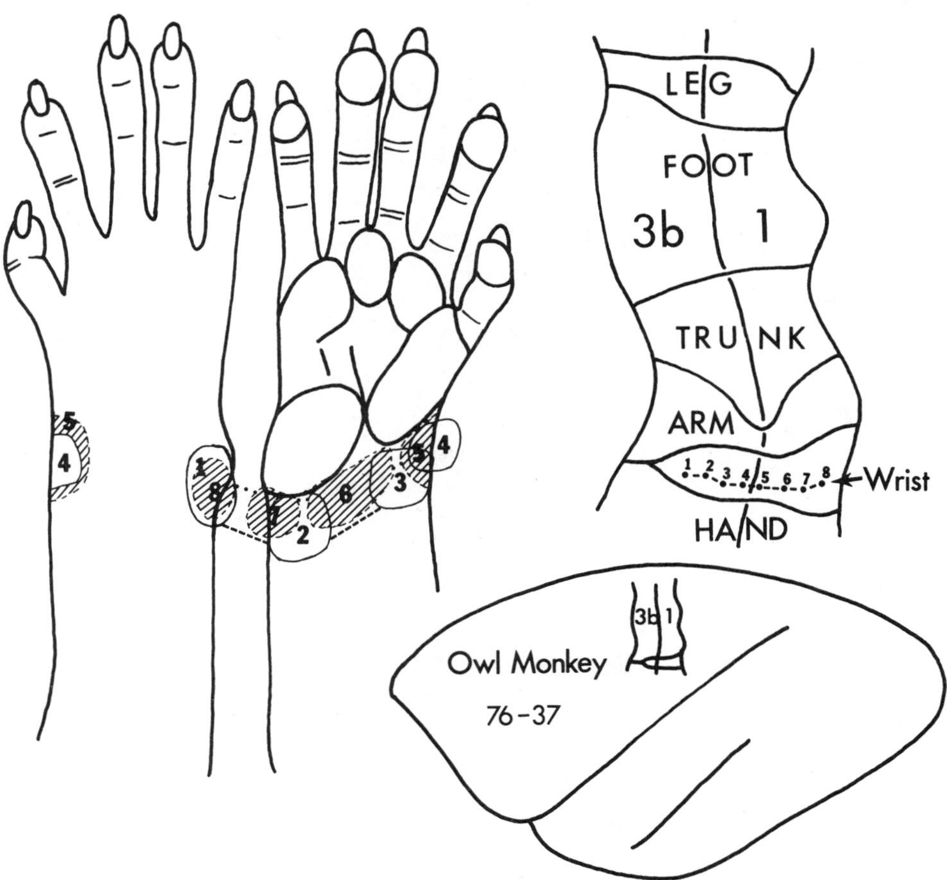

Figure 6. Receptive fields defined within a row of penetrations crossing Area 3b and 1 in the region representing the volar wrist. Details as in figure 2.

each other on the brain but correspond to distant receptive fields located on the middle of the ventral and dorsal surfaces of the wrist, respectively.

The forearm and upper arm were also represented twice within Areas 3b and 1. Receptive fields defined near the anterior border of Area 3b or near the posterior edge of Area 1 were usually found to lie along or near the radial margin of the arm. Proceeding toward the 3-1 border within Area 3b, successively defined receptive fields shifted across the ventral surface of the arm toward the ulnar margin, and moved around the arm over the dorsal surface to return to a location near the radial margin, which was again represented along the 3-1 border. Thus, one can imagine the skin of the arm as being slit down the radial margin and laid out on the cortex of Area 3b with the ventral surface represented more anteriorly and the dorsal surface toward the 3-1 boundary.

The representation of the arm within Area 1 was difficult to reconstruct in detail. For some anterior-posterior recording sequences, successively defined receptive fields for Area 1 marched around the arm a second time in the same direction as was seen in Area 3b (as in the experiment illustrated in fig. 8). In other sequences, reversals or discontinuities in represented skin location were recorded within the Area 1 arm representation. Thus, although it is clear that there is a single and complete representation of arm surfaces in Area 1, as in the more clearly ordered Area 3b, a simple pattern of representation could not be defined that fit all derived mapping data in the several monkeys in which the arm representation was relatively completely mapped. These data indicated that, in fact, there must be significant variation in the way arm surfaces are represented within Area 1 in different individual monkeys.

Representation of the Trunk

The double representation of the trunk was difficult to illustrate completely in most monkeys because we found the representation of the back in Area 1 to be small (as in the case illustrated in fig. 8). Only a small number of receptive fields on the back have been defined in all experiments. On the other hand, the representation of the skin of the chest and abdomen actually appeared to be larger within Area 1 than within Area

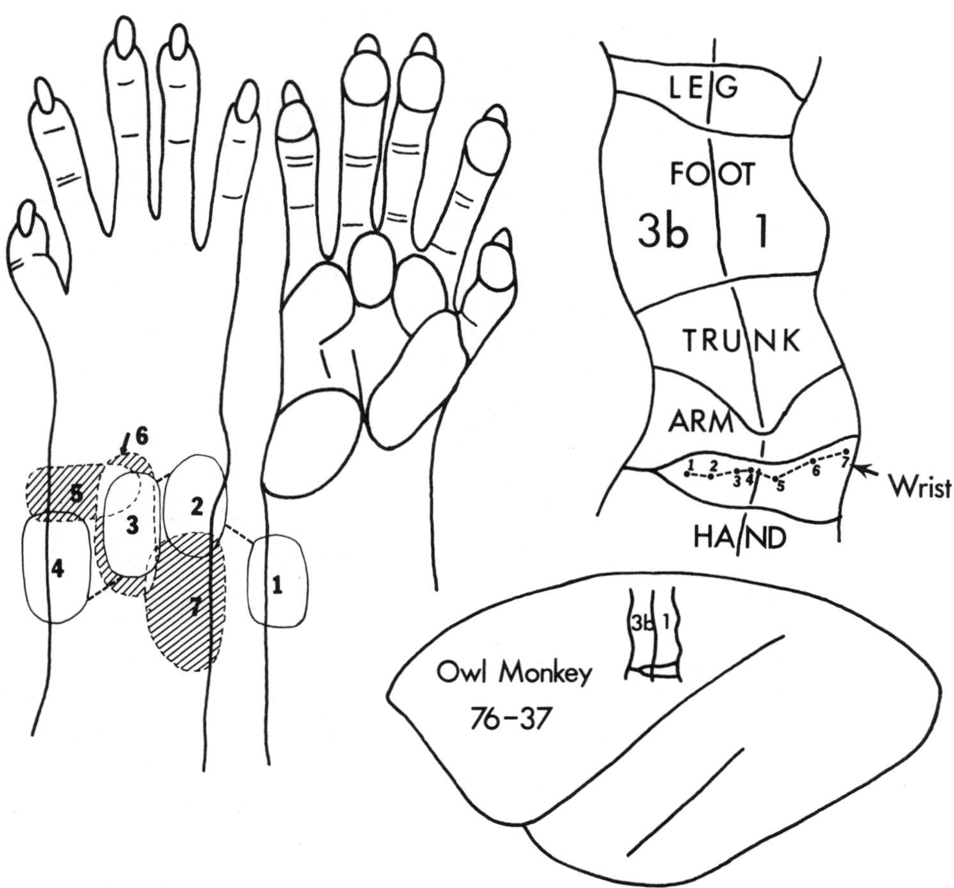

Figure 7. Receptive fields defined within a row of penetrations crossing Areas 3b and 1 in the region of representation of the dorsal surface of the wrist. Details as in figure 2.

3b. However, all mapping data were consistent with a crude mirror-image representation of the trunk, with the top of the back represented along the anterior margin of Area 3b and near the posterior margin of Area 1, and with the skin along the contralateral side of the midline of the chest and abdomen (the line of reversal) represented along the 3-1 boundary (fig. 9). The shoulder and back of head were located in the lateral aspect of the trunk representation, continuous with the arm, and far removed from the topologically adjacent face. In rows of penetrations passing in the lateral to medial direction within the trunk representation of either field, there was a systematic shift of receptive fields down the trunk, from the neck and shoulders and upper chest to the lower back and abdomen.

Representation of the Foot in Areas 3b and 1

Figure 10 is a schematic drawing of the representation of the contralateral foot within Areas 3b and 1. The figure was based upon one of several reconstructions of complete maps of the foot derived in individual monkeys. Again there was a double representation of foot surfaces in the two fields. The representation of the glabrous surfaces of the foot within Area 3b was highly ordered, and was similar in many respects to the Area 3b representation of the hand. The great toe (D1) was in the lateral aspect of the representation. The other digits were represented in order, progressing toward the midline, in a lateral-to-medial sequence. The distal phalanges of the toes were represented along the anterior border of Area 36 (figs. 11, 12). Proceeding toward the 3-1 border, successively defined receptive fields shifted down the digits onto the pads of the sole toward the base of the foot, which was represented along the 3-1 border. The representations of the foot pads in Area 3b were not separated from each other as were those of the palmar pads (fig. 10). The one notable exception was that some of the receptive fields on the thenar eminence were recorded in the medial aspects of foot representations in Areas 3b and 1. Therefore, these recording sites related to the thenar eminence were separated from those related to the representation of the rest of the thenar eminence.

Within Area 1, digits were represented in a largely anterior to posterior sequence, with the great toe near the middle of Area 1 and only the third (variable),

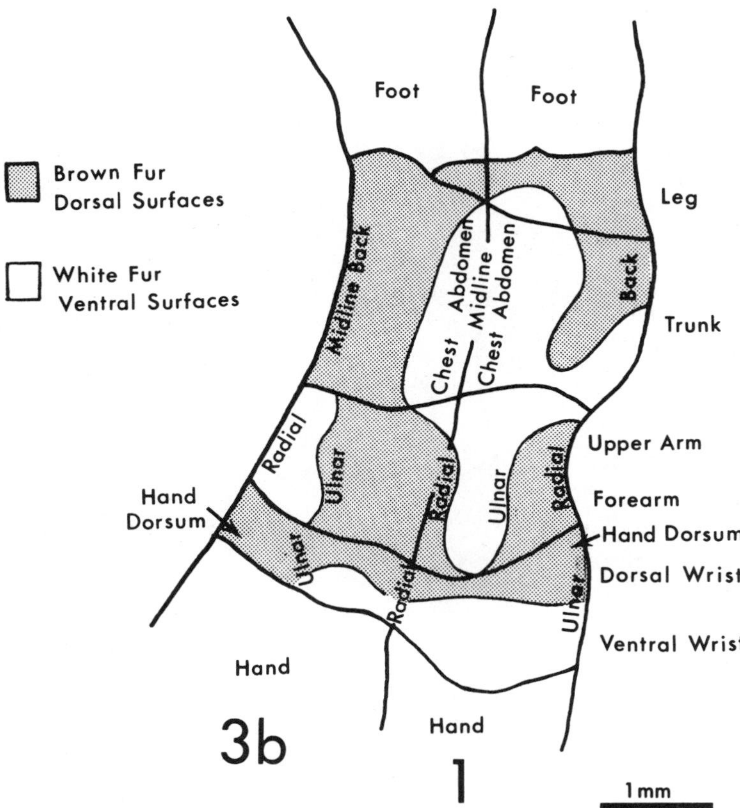

Figure 8. The patterns of representation of the arm and trunk in Areas 3b and 1 in a single monkey (76–9). Representation of the brown fur of the arm dorsum, side and back of the trunk and lateral thigh (shaded region) and of the white fur of the ventral arm, axilla, chest, abdomen and medial thigh (not shaded) are shown. The patterns of representation of the arm and trunk differ in detail among individual monkeys (see text).

fourth and fifth digits in contact with the posterior border of Area 1 (figs. 10–12). Thus, the representation of the foot within Area 1 was not a mirror image of that in Area 3b, although they were topographically very similar. The representation of the sole in Area 1 was like that in Area 3b. As in the hand representations, receptive fields for the pads of the sole were much larger in Area 1 than in Area 3b, and commonly extended over entire pads, or over adjacent pads.

The dorsal surfaces of the toes (as with the fingers) were ordered in a very different way within the two representations. In the Area 3b foot, the representation of the dorsal, hairy surfaces of the toes was split (in a manner similar to the split of the representation of the hairy fingers in Area 3b), with the dorsum of the great toe represented in a region lateral to that of the glabrous surface of the great toe, and with the hairy surface of digits 5, 4, 3 and 2 represented in order in the region medial to the representation of the glabrous surfaces of the fifth digit. As with the hand, the representational sequence moved around the outer surfaces of the first and fifth digits onto the adjacent hairy skin, and then marched over the hairy surfaces of the toe or toes. The representation of the foot dorsum was continuous with that of the fifth, fourth, third and second digits on the medial side of the Area 3 foot representation.

In contrast to the Area 3b representation, the dorsal surfaces of the foot within Area 1 were represented entirely on the *lateral* side of the foot representation, adjacent to the representation of the distal phalanges of digits 1, 2 and 3 (figs. 10–12). Successively defined receptive fields in a lateral-to-medial sequence in this region marched from the proximal foot to the distal foot. Hairy surfaces on the distal phalanges of the toes were represented in the cortex adjacent to the representation of glabrous phalanges.

Representation of the Leg

The region representing the leg on the lateral surface of the cortex was explored, but since much or most of the leg representation was on the medial wall in the owl monkey, derived representational data were fragmentary. Available data were consistent with a re-representation of leg surfaces in Areas 3b and 1. The preaxial surface of the thigh was mapped in entirety within both representations. A few postaxial fields were also defined in Area 1 and 3b in this region.

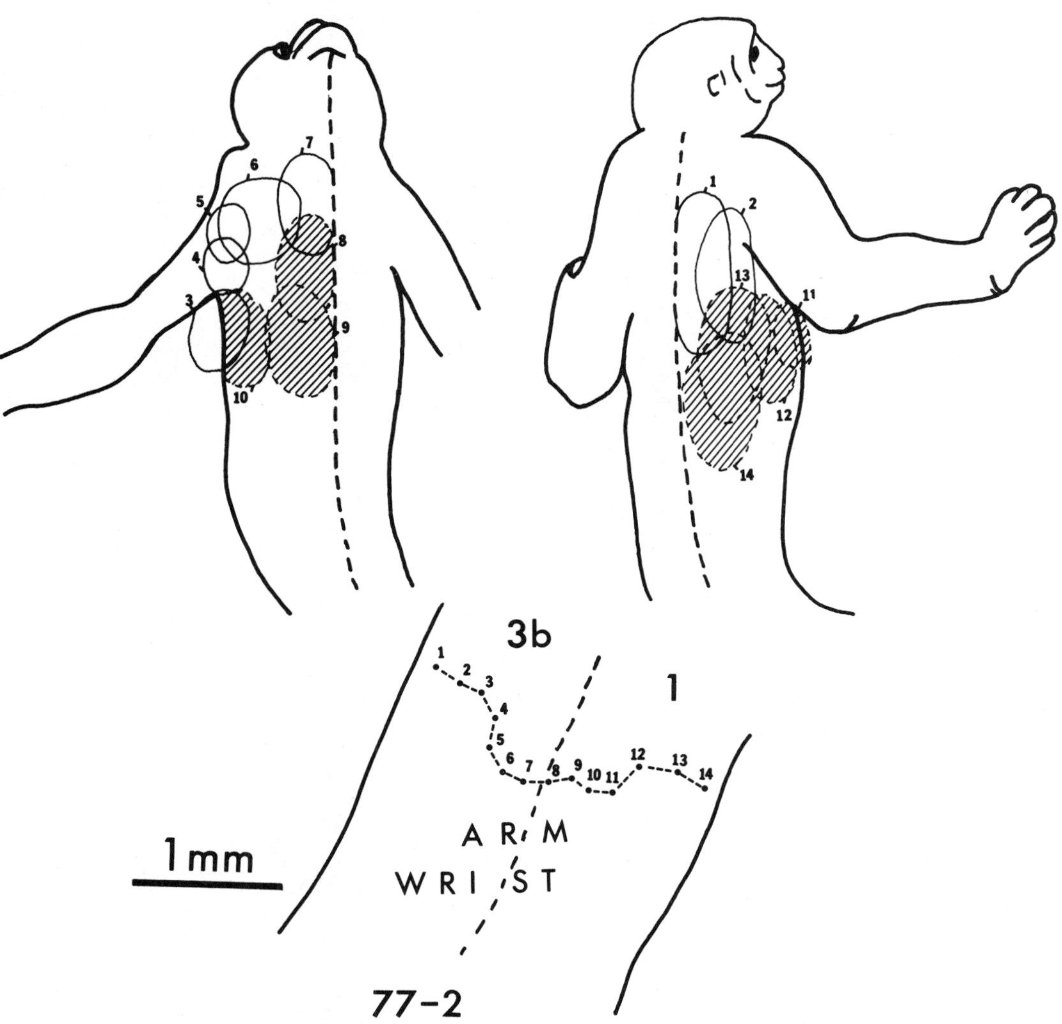

Figure 9. Receptive fields defined within a long row of penetrations crossing Areas 3b and 1 in the region representing the chest and anterior back. Note the reversal in representational sequence across the 3b-1 border. Details as in figure 2.

As in some other species of primates (Discussion), part of the leg was found both medial and lateral to the foot representation in somatosensory cortex of owl monkeys. While most of the leg was represented medial to the foot, significant portions were represented in cortex immediately lateral to the foot in both Areas 3b and 1. Both lateral leg representations were small (table 1), but the leg representation lateral to the foot was consistently larger in Area 1 than in Area 3b (in some experiments, no leg representation could be found lateral to the foot in Area 3b). The lateral representation of the leg in Area 1 was almost totally restricted to the preaxial surface of the thigh, which appeared to be represented there in its entirety. Receptive fields for sequences of recording sites in this region formed continuous sequences with those on the abdomen and lower back, indicating that the representations of the thigh and adjoining abdomen and back, are continuous. In contrast, rows of recording sites never revealed continuous sequences of receptive fields from the thigh to the lower leg. For example, in lateromedial rows of recording sites in the lateral leg representation in Area 1, a discontinuity was consistently found such that skin from the knee was adjacent to the cortical representation of the dorsal foot.

Surprisingly, the complete preaxial thigh in Area 3b was found on the *medial* side of the foot representation, where it has been mapped in detail. Thus, there are double representations of parts of the preaxial thigh in each of Areas 3b and 1, with the two representations lying on different sides of the representation of the foot.

Representation of the Face in Areas 3b and 1

The region of the face representation of the lateral surface of the cortex has been mapped in detail, but the representational area buried within the Sylvian fissure

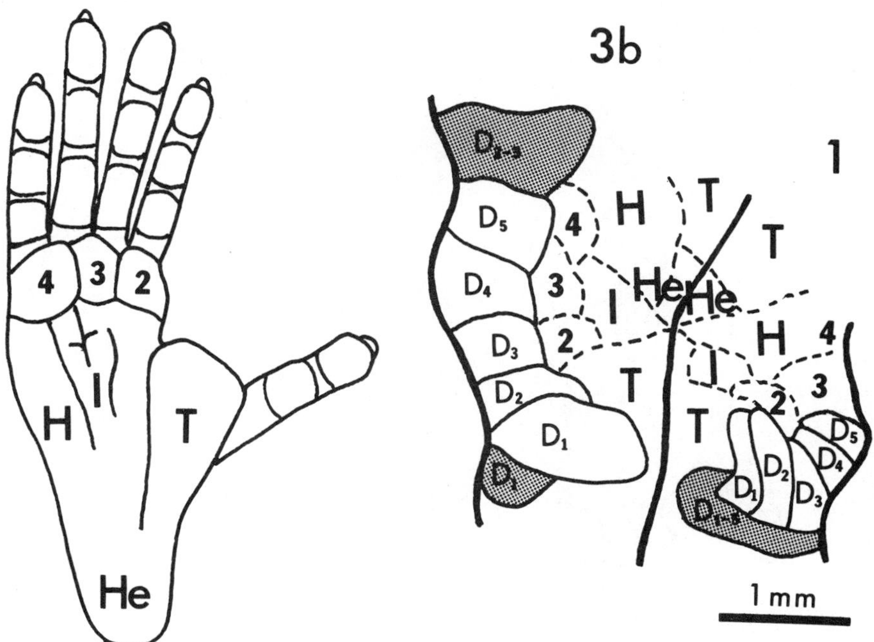

Figure 10. Reconstruction of a detailed map of the representations of the foot, from an experiment in one of several monkeys in which the foot region was completely mapped. The heel and the interdigital, insular, hypothenar and thenar pads are identified on the diagram at the left. Boundaries between the pads of the sole (dashed lines) are not absolute in Area 1 since receptive fields frequently extended over more than one pad.

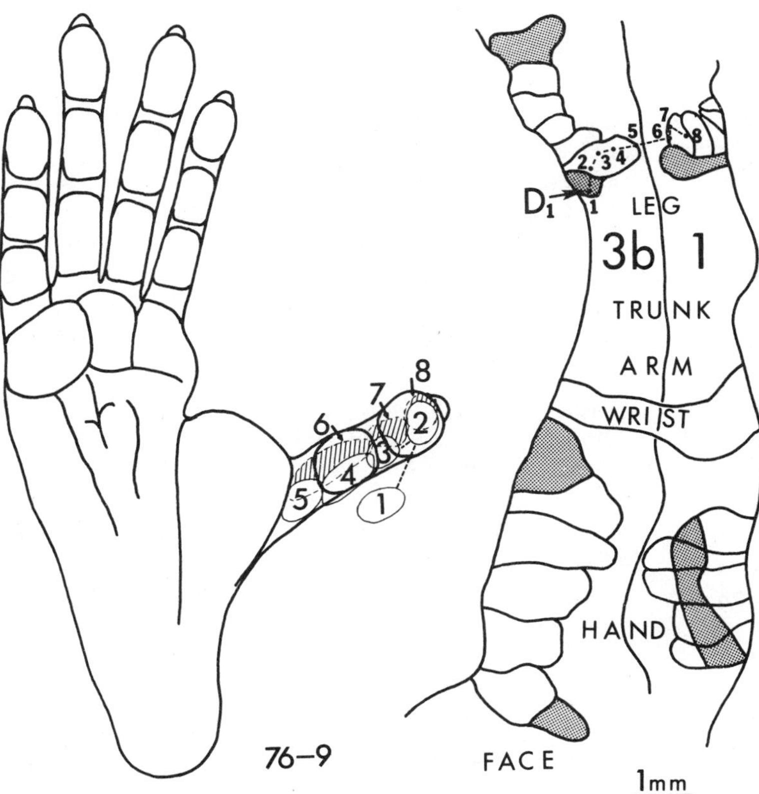

Figure 11. Receptive fields defined within a row of penetrations crossing Areas 3b and 1 in the region representing the great toe. Details as in figure 2.

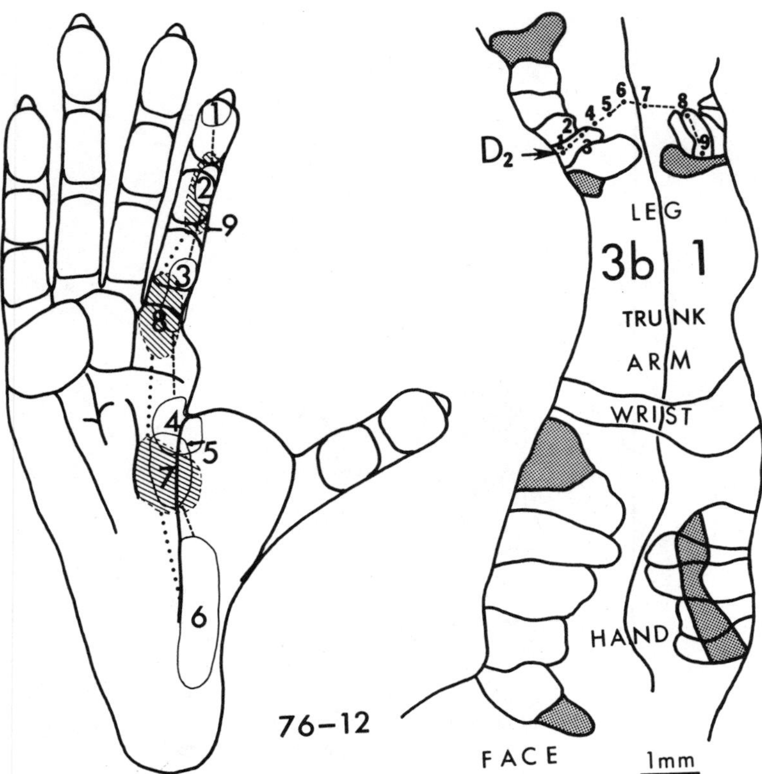

Figure 12. Receptive fields defined within a row of penetrations crossing areas 3b and 1 in the region representing the second pedal digit, second interdigital pad, insular pad and heel. The representational sequence reverses between penetrations 6–7, near the proximal end of the glabrous foot. Details as in figure 2.

has not been systematically explored. The buried portion includes significant parts of the Area 3b and especially the Area 1 face representations. Nonetheless, the general pattern of representation of the face was evident. There is clearly a double representation of the face within the two cytoarchitectonic fields. The midline of the lower face (lower lip, chin vibrissae, chin) was represented at or near the anterior border of Area 3b, and at or near the posterior border of Area 1 (fig. 13). The region of the representation of the contralateral upper lip and mandibular vibrissae at or near the midline was along the 3-1 border. The two representations in Areas 3b and 1 were topographically similar, with areas on the face represented in roughly mirror-image sequence proceeding away from the 3-1 border. An example of this re-representation of the face is illustrated by the receptive fields for a long row of penetrations illustrated in figure 13. Beginning with a receptive field near the midline on the chin in the Area 3b representation (penetration 1, fig. 13), successive receptive fields were located first near the midline on the chin and lower lip, then progressing toward the corner of the mouth on the lower lip, and then toward the midline on the upper lip. A reversal in the sequence of the representation was recorded at the 3-1 border (between penetrations 8 and 9 in fig. 13). Receptive fields for the remaining recording sites crossing Area 1 retraced a sequence similar to that of Area 3b.

It should be noted that the representation of the chin was immediately adjacent to that of the glabrous skin of the first digit in Area 3b, and to the thenar eminence in Area 1 (figs. 5, 13). The representation of the chin vibrissae was adjacent to that of the glabrous thumb in Area 3b, and of the thenar eminence in Area 1. Finally, the representation of the mandibular vibrissae was adjacent to the representation of the dorsum of the finger in Area 3b, and to the thenar eminence in Area 1. No transition from the radial hand to the face *via* intervening skin could be recorded. This step was discontinuous, within the finest possible grain of recording. As noted earlier, contiguous interconnecting skin surfaces (arm, shoulder, side of head) were found to be represented within the cortex in a region medial to the representation of the hand and wrist, and far from that of the face.

A very large representation of the contralateral teeth was mapped within Area 3b. Our maps never extended into the probable location of the Area 1 representation of the teeth, or the tongue. The teeth were represented lateral and rostral to the lower lip in Area 3b. In penetration rows directed rostralward in Area 3b, successive receptive fields shifted from near the midline on

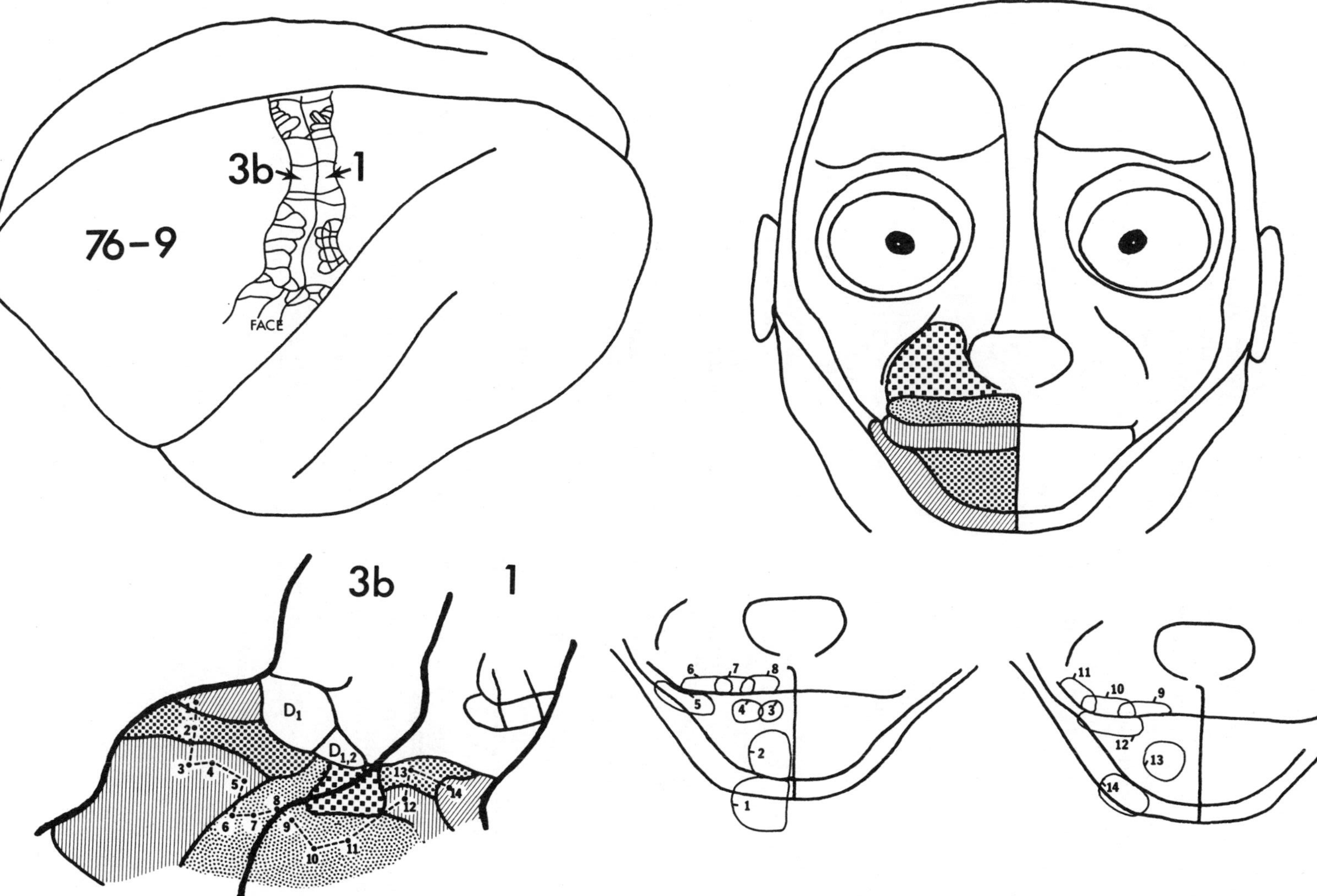

Figure 13. Some features of representations of the face within Areas 3b and 1. As in other primates, there is a disproportionately large representation of the anterior face, especially of the lips and the vibrasse of the chin and upper jaw. These skin surfaces (indicated in the drawing at the upper right) are represented in Areas 3b and 1 as shown in the drawing at the lower left. Receptive fields defined within a long row of penetrations crossing the Area 3b and Area 1 face representations are drawn at the lower right (Area 1 fields, right Area 3b fields, left). Penetrations in this irregular row were chosen to show approximately corresponding lines of receptive fields for both cytoarchitectonic areas.

the lower lip onto the lower incisors and then to the more lateral lower teeth. Still further rostralward, receptive fields crossed to the lateral upper teeth, and then moved medialward toward the upper incisors.

The Proportion Areas of Cortex Devoted to Different Skin Surfaces within Area 3b and Area 1

It is of interest to note that the proportional representation of different body surfaces within the Area 3b representation is similar, but definitely *not* identical to that within the Area 1 representation. These two large body surface representations are *not* scale versions of each other.

To illustrate how the areas of representation of different body surfaces vary in the two fields, areas from maps have been measured planimetrically. Measurements derived from one extensively studied owl monkey (consistent with similar, more fragmentary data derived in other monkeys) are recorded in table 1. Excluding the incompletely mapped face, leg, tail and genital representations, the Area 3b representation was about 35–40% larger than that in Area 1. The representation of the hand was about one and a half times larger in Area 3b than in Area 1. The representation of the foot was nearly twice as large. In contrast, the representation of the trunk and arm were nearly equal in the two Areas, and the representation of the wrist was actually larger in Area 1 than in Area 3b.

It is evident from table 1 that the biggest disparity between Areas 1 and 3b was in the proportional areas of the representations of subdivisions of the hand and foot. The area representing the glabrous surfaces of the hand digits in Area 3b, for example, was over twice as large as that in Area 1; while the areas representing the palm and the dorsal hand were nearly equal in Area 3b and Area 1. As an even more striking example, the area of representation of the glabrous surfaces of the foot digits in the Area 3b representation was over three times as large as in Area 1. In contrast, the representations of the sole and dorsal foot in Areas 3b and 1 were more nearly equal. Thus, it would appear that much of the difference ln the overall sizes of the two representations can be attributed to a proportionately larger representation of the glabrous surfaces of the fingers and toes in Area 3b.

Fields Bordering Areas 3b and 1

Penetrations were introduced into Areas 3a, 4 and 2 in all mapping experiments. The cortical region posterior to Area 1 (including Area 2) was extensively mapped in two experiments.

In penetrations anterior to Area 3b, neurons were not driven by light tactile stimulation. Numerous lesions were introduced along this anterior border of the anterior cutaneous somatosensory representation. Medially, this boundary fell along a distinct Area 3b-3a border; laterally, Area 3a was very narrow or absent, and Area 3b appeared to directly border Area 4. In some penetrations into Area 3a, neurons were driven by deep (never cutaneous) stimuli, while in other penetrations neurons were driven poorly if at all even by stimulation of deep body tissues. If neurons in Area 3a were responsive to deep stimuli, the Area 4 border could be detected by a marked reduction in responsiveness.

In some instance, intracortical stimulation was employed to confirm the position of the caudal border of Area 4. Those experiments were conducted in Area 4 adjacent to the Area 3b representation of the face and hand. Within this region, Area 3a is very narrow or absent. The rostral boundary of Area 3b defined through use of light tactile stimulation corresponded

Table 1. Area of representation of different body surfaces within areas 3b and 1 in Owl Monkey 76-9

Represented body surface	Area 3b representation (mm^2)		Area 1 representation (mm^2)		Area 3b/area 1
Hand	11.5		7.6		1.51
Glabrous digits		5.8		2.3	2.52
Palm		4.6		4.2	1.10
Dorsum		1.1		1.1	1.00
Wrist	0.8		1.5		0.53
Arm	1.9		1.8		1.06
Trunk	2.7		2.3		1.17
Leg (lateral to foot)	0.1		0.7		0.14
Foot	4.9		2.7		1.81
Glabrous digits		1.9		0.6	3.17
Sole		2.2		1.6	1.38
Dorsum		0.8		0.5	1.60
Total[1]	21.8		15.9		1.37

1. Excluding leg lateral to foot, and incompletely mapped face, leg medial to foot, tail and genital representations.

closely (within a few 100 μm) to the caudal border of Area 4 defined by low threshold movements produced by intracortical "microstimulation."

Two classes of responses were encountered in a broad region caudal to Area 1. In a very narrow strip immediately adjacent to Area 1, neurons were commonly driven by light tactile (cutaneous) stimulation over very large receptive fields. These receptive fields commonly extended over the entire body surface region represented in adjacent Area 1. Thus, adjacent to the representation of the abdomen in Area 1, for example, neurons in this narrow zone might have receptive fields that extended over part of the chest, the entire abdomen, and the medial surface of the leg. In a few exceptional cases, such receptive fields appeared to extend across the midline. Input to these neurons appeared to be cutaneous, and not from the Pacinian receptors. These responses were never recorded more than a few 100 μm from the border of Area 1, and frequently neurons in penetrations just posterior to Area 1 could not be driven by cutaneous stimulation. Nonetheless, these data suggest that there might be a very narrow, third cutaneous or mixed modality representation of the body surface in "SI" of the owl monkey.

In a much broader and clearly delimited field behind Area 1 (probably coextensive with Area 2), neurons could be driven by manipulation of joints or other "deep" stimulation, and were *never* excited by cutaneous stimulation. Rows of recording sites revealed that there is an orderly representation of deep body structures within this region, with the sequence of representation paralleling that of skin surfaces represented in the nearby cutaneous sensory strip (fig. 14). Input at many loci within this field appeared to be derived from joint receptors. However, it was not possible to unequivocally define the receptor source of this "deep" input (especially when the effective stimulation required movement of the shoulder girdle, neck, back or hips).

The Relation of Electrophysiological Results to Cortical Architecture

The cytoarchitecture of the somatosensory and motor areas of the cerebral cortex of New World monkeys had been described for marmosets by Brodmann ('09) and Peden and von Bonin ('47), for squirrel monkeys by Rosabal ('67), Sanides ('67) and Jones ('75), and for cebus monkeys by von Bonin ('38). Since characteristics of the somatic fields appear to be very similar in these monkeys and in owl monkeys, the major architectonic features are only briefly reviewed below. These features are apparent in figure 15, which shows photomicrographs of Areas 4, 3a, 3b, 1 and 2 in owl monkeys. Since they have general acceptance, Brodmann's ('09) numbers are used, although Sanides ('68), Peden and von Bonin ('47) and von Bonin ('38) used other nomenclature. The two architectonic fields of most interest for the present study are Areas 3b and 1.

The major features of Area 3b are easy to appreciate in the owl monkey because this subdivision is located in relatively flat cortex (see, for example, fig. 15A). Unlike most primates there is no central fissure to

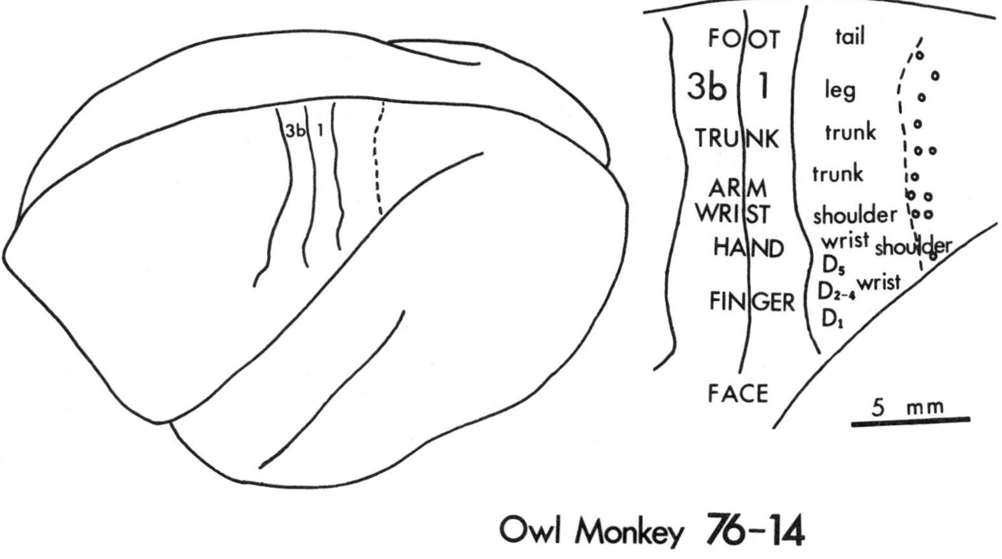

Figure 14. The basic pattern of the representation of deep body structures within the cortical region caudal to Area 1. This schematic drawing summarized results obtained in an extensive mapping experiment conducted in Areas 3b and 1 and the cortex caudal to Area 1. In the caudal representation (including and possibly coextensive with Area 2), neurons responded specifically to stimulation of joint or other "deep" receptors in the indicated body regions (see text). Circles mark penetrations within which neurons were not obviously driven by tactile or deep somatic stimulation.

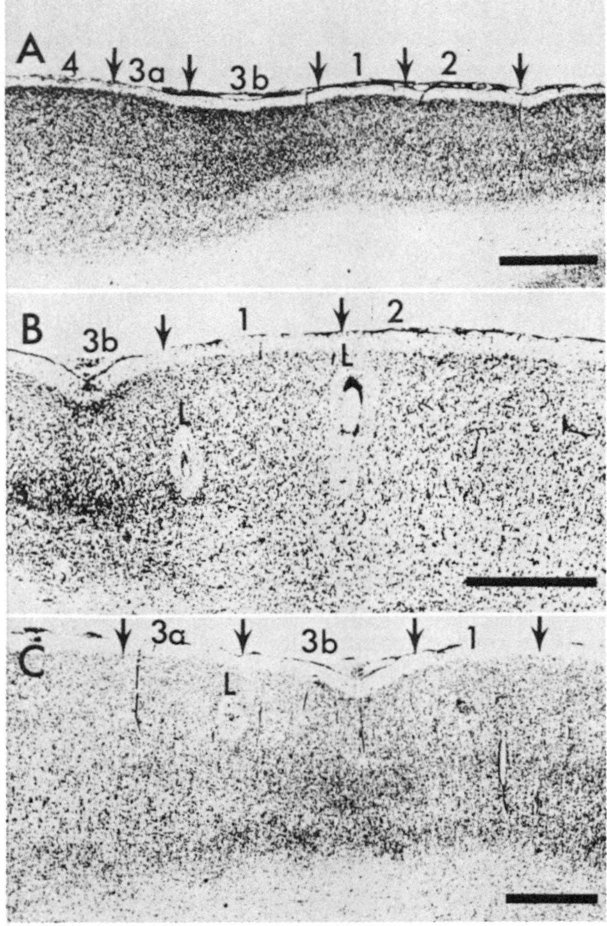

Figure 15. Some features of the cytoarchitecture of the parietal somatosensory strip illustrated in Nissl-stained parasagittal sections. Boundaries of cytoarchitectonic Areas 4, 3a, 3b, 1 and 2 are indicated by arrows. Lesions in B were introduced at locations determined physiologically to mark the approximate boundaries of the posterior body surface representation. In all such instances, these marks fell at or very near the Area 1 boundaries. The lesion in C was one of the many introduced at the site of the first penetration rostral to the anterior body surface representation. All such lesions fell along the 3b-3a (or far laterally, along the 3b-4) boundary. Boundaries of Areas 3b and 1 were defined solely on cytoarchitectonic bases from material like that shown in A-C in all illustrated cases. Note the very shallow, incomplete (absent at the level shown in A) central sulcus. It is rarely deeper than as seen in B and C. Marker bar, 1 mm.

distort the architectonic features. However, owl monkeys generally do have a short, shallow dimple in the expected location of the middle part of the central fissure, and this dimple is shown in figures 15B and C. The dimple is rarely deeper than that shown in figure 15, and it does not significantly alter the laminar pattern of the underlying cortex. When the dimple occurs, it is over Area 3b with usually more of 3b rostral than caudal to the dimple. Therefore the dimple is a good landmark in recording experiments.

Area 3b is a koniocortical or hypergranular field identified by the densely packed granular cells in the outer cell layers. The cell packing in layer IV is most dense, but cells are also tightly packed in layers II and III so that layers II–IV sometimes appear to fuse (fig. 15A). Layer VI is slightly more dense than in adjoining cortex so that the relatively light layer V stands out in contrast to the layers above and below. Area 1 is marked by a less dense but obvious inner granular cell layer, and a less dense layer V. The transition from Area 1 to more caudal parietal cortex, Area 2, is denoted by an increase in layer III and layer V pyramidal cells and more densely packed cells in layer IV. Area 3a has both the larger pyramidal cells in layer V characteristic of motor cortex and a clear inner granular layer characteristic of sensory fields, and therefore has been called a transitional or intermediate field. However, Area 3a has distinct boundaries with Areas 4 and 3b, and does not appear as a gradual transition from motor to sensory fields. Rather, we agree with Sanides ('68) that Area 3a is a separate field with a "character" that does not "allow one to consider it a subdivision of Area 3." The motor field or Area 4 is rostral to the central dimple, and is characterized by large pyramidal cells in layer V, overall low density of neurons, and the lack of a clear granular cell layer. Area 4 is several millimeters wide, and gradually merges laterally with cortex having smaller pyramidal cells. Stimulation experiments suggest that this cortex is also part of the motor representation.

In alternate brain sections stained for myelinated fibers, Area 3b is more densely myelinated than is Area 1, and we found this feature useful in distinguishing between the two fields. The myeloarchitecture of postcentral cortex has been described in detail in the squirrel monkey by Sanides ('68) and Jones ('75) and the overall features are similar in owl monkeys.

In all recording experiments, electrolytic lesions were made along the boundaries of the two body surface representations in order to relate the recording results to cortical architecture. Two examples of brain sections with such marking lesions are shown in figures 15B and C. Cytoarchitectonic field boundaries were completely reconstructed from this histological material. The field boundaries drawn in all illustrations represent such objectively defined lines, drawn solely from histological reconstructions. Coincidence of the distinct cytoarchitectonic and functional boundaries of these fields is remarkable. *In all instances*: (1) Lesions placed at the electrophysiologically defined border between the rostral and the caudal cutaneous representation of body surfaces were later found to be along the border between cytoarchitectonically defined Areas 3b and 1 (fig. 15B); (2) lesions placed along the caudal border of the caudal cutaneous field were between Areas 1 and 2 (fig. 15B); (3) lesions located along the rostral border of the rostral cutaneous field were between Areas 3a and 3b (fig. 15C).

Individual Variations in the Organization of Areas 3b and 1

As has been noted earlier, these mapping studies have revealed that there is unequivocal variation in the detailed pattern of representation in different individual monkeys. Examples include: (1) The arm representation in Area 1 was different in detail in every mapped monkey. In Area 3b, the region of the rostral margin of the arm representation was different in individual owl monkeys. (2) In most owl monkeys, the hairy skin of the dorsal fingers in Area 1 was represented continuously between the representation of the glabrous fingertips and that of the middle and proximal phalanges. In one extensively mapped exceptional case, they were represented in a region between a representation of the entire glabrous surface of the digits and the distal palm. (3) In one monkey, the representation of the back in Area 1 was clearly defined throughout the mediolateral extent of the representation, and the back representation occupied a relatively large proportion of the total Area 1 trunk representation. In all other monkeys, the Area 1 back representation was very small, and receptive fields on the back were defined only a few penetrations in the most posterior aspect of the field. The pattern of representation appeared to differ in fine detail in each owl monkey. Certainly, individual variation in the organization of sensory areas is much greater than has been generally appreciated.

Discussion

The microelectrode mapping results of the present study lead to the conclusions that each of two separate architectonic fields in owl monkeys is occupied by a map of the skin surface, that the two maps differ in organization, and that a third architectonic zone is devoted to non-cutaneous "deep" receptors. The results obviously require modifications and revisions of some of the current concepts of "SI" organization in primates, and new terminology will be needed to reflect these changed concepts. In addition, the results and conclusions raise the important questions: (1) What are the homologues of these separate representations in other mammals, and (2) how did these multiple representations evolve? These issues are considered further below.

1. Current Tenets of Somatosensory Organization

The parietal somatosensory region has been mapped in a number of primate species, including the slow loris, marmoset, squirrel monkey, cebus monkey, spider monkey, macaque monkey, gibbon, chimpanzee, and man. From these studies, a concept of the organization of the primate parietal somatosensory cortex has arisen that includes at least six principal tenets. *First*, there is a single representation of the contralateral body surface ("SI") within the parietal sensory strip. *Second*, this representation overlies more than one clearly delimitable cytoarchitectonic field. *Third*, the two-dimensional organization of "SI" is (a) a somatotopic homunculus; (b) a sequence of rostrocaudal bands each devoted to a single body part; or (c) some combination of these two views. *Fourth*, the representation of the body surface follows a dermatomal sequence. *Fifth*, the proportional representation of different body surface regions is a reflection of peripheral innervation density. *Sixth*, "SI" is the primary functional division of somatosensory cortex. While investigators have derived evidence contrary to almost all of these commonly held tenets, these concepts of somatosensory cortex still dominate. Therefore, it is useful to start by reviewing evidence for and against each of these ideas, and to suggest modifications and revisions that are consistent with present and previous results.

(a) There is a single representation of the body surface in the parietal somatosensory strip in primates

Investigators who have studied the representation of the body surface within the parietal somatosensory strip using microelectrode and surface evoked potential mapping techniques have described a single representation of the body occupying the "SI" region in the New World marmoset (Woolsey, '52, '54), squirrel monkey (Benjamin and Welker, '57; Werner and Whitsel, '68), cebus monkey (Hirsh and Coxe, '58) and spider monkey (Chang et al., '47; Pubols and Pubols, '71, '72); in the Old World rhesus monkey (Marshall et al., '37; Woolsey et al., '42; Mountcastle and Powell, '59; Werner and Whitsel, '68; Whitsel et al., '71; Dreyer et al., '74, '75); in the gibbon (Woolsey et al., '60; Welt, '63); the chimpanzee (Woolsey et al., '43; Woolsey et al., '60; Welt, '63); and in humans (Penfield and Boldrey, '37; Penfield and Rasmussen, '50). However, there have been notable exceptions to the idea of a single "SI" representation. Most importantly, Paul et al. ('72a) presented evidence for two complete and separate cutaneous representations of the glabrous hand surface in "SI" of macaque monkeys (other parts of "SI" were not explored). A second exception is the recent report of a cutaneous body representation completely within only one of the architectonic fields of the "SI" region of the prosimian, slow loris (Krishnamurti et al., '76). While further representations were not identified in these experiments, the finding of a complete representation restricted to only part of "SI" clearly challenges the concept of "SI" as a single representation. Furthermore, cortex adjoining the cutaneous representation was responsive to somatosensory stimulation. A third report which was strongly suggestive of multiple representations was that of Zimmerman ('68). This investigator noted separate rostral and caudal foci of evoked responses to light tactile stimulation of the digit tips in the "SI" region of somatosensory cortex of the squirrel monkey. Zimmerman argued that these foci indicated two "entirely separate and differently organized sensory areas" for three reasons. First, the rostral and caudal foci were discontinuous; second, the two zones differed in response characteristics such as the latency, following frequency and threshold; third, experiments involving spreading depression showed that responses in the two foci were independent. Unfortunately, the experiments of Zimmerman had limited impact, perhaps because he regarded the rostral somatosensory zone as within "somatomotor" cortex rather than as a functional division of "SI" cortex. To us, it appears that both the rostral and caudal foci were within the region commonly considered the "SI" field in squirrel monkeys.

While there are few examples of direct challenges to the concept of "SI" as a single representation, there are many examples of data that are inconsistent with that concept. Starting with the initial pioneering studies on macaque monkeys, Woolsey et al. ('42) described a second representation of the thumb on the caudal bank of the central fissure that was "at some distance" from the representation of the thumb on the dorsal surface of post-central parietal cortex. Likewise, microelectrode single unit and mapping studies (Powell and Mountcastle, '59b; Whitsel et al., '71 Dreyer et al., '75) have consistently noted the activation of nonadjacent cortical locations within "SI" from the stimulation of a single body location. Dreyer et al. got so far as to conclude that, for each body part of "SI," "a single region in the periphery is represented several times in widely separate locations." This viewpoint is not far from a formal rejection of the single "SI" concept.

While there have been a few conclusions and many observations in conflict with the concept of "SI" as a single representation in primates, this concept has persisted. We believe that the present extensive mapping of the "SI" region of the owl monkey presents unequivocal evidence that there are two cutaneous representations in owl monkeys. Furthermore, more limited mapping results indicate a third representation that is devoted to non-cutaneous receptors. Thus, we feel that the concept of a single representation in "SI" must be abandoned for owl monkeys, and in view of these and previous results, must be placed in serious doubt or abandoned for other primates.

(b) The body representation in the parietal somatosensory strip occupies more than one architectonic field

It has been recognized from the first surface evoked potential somatosensory mapping studies (Marshall et al., '37; Woolsey et al., '42) that "SI," as described in macaque monkeys, would include more than one cytoarchitectonic field. These authors concluded that the "SI" representation occupied Brodmann's Areas 3, 1 and 2, but not the adjoining Areas 4 and 5. The viewpoint that "SI" includes Areas 3, 1 and 2 has prevailed for macaques and other primates (Whitsel et al., '71; Whitsel et al., '72; Dreyer et al., '74, '75).

However, it has been puzzling why a single representation should have distinct architectonic subdivisions. Such distinct and different architectonic "subunits" are not found within other cortical sensory representations (although subregions of some structural specialization occur; the monocular and binocular portion of striate cortex can be distinguished, for example). The usual way to account for the architectonic differences within "SI" has been to relate them to varying extents of submodality segregation within the field (Powell and Mountcastle, '59b; Werner and Whitsel, '68; Whitsel et al., '71; Dreyer et al., '75). Such segregation, of course, implies either separate maps or rostrocaudal bands of "isorepresentation" (see below).

Not all investigators have included more than one architectonic field within "SI." In macaque monkeys Paul et al. ('72a,b) argued for a representation of the hand within Area 3b, a second representation of the hand within Area 1, a possible third "deep" representation in Area 2, and other non-cutaneous activation within Area 3a. Krishnamurti et al. ('76) reported a complete body surface representation that was coextensive with somatic koniocortex or Area 3b of the slow loris (Sanides and Krishnamurti, '67). These conclusions agree with the present results, which indicate that there is a large body surface representation that is coextensive with Area 3b and a second somewhat smaller body surface representation that is congruent with Area 1. Area 3a is outside this cutaneous sensory strip. And there is an orderly representation of deep body structures (probably coextensive with Area 2) within the cortical region caudal to Area 1.

(c) The representation of the body surface is a homunculus, or forms rostrocaudal bands of isorepresentation

There have been two different basic viewpoints as to how a single body representation, "SI," lies across the several architectonic fields in primates. Many investigators have summarized the pattern of the representation of the body surface on the parietal cortex by describing or drawing a "homunculus" (or "simiunculus"), a body figure distorted to illustrate the proportional representation of different skin surfaces. The homunculus has been shown or described as having the same overall orientation on the brain of prosimians (Krishnamurti et al., '76, where it was confined to Area 3b), marmosets (Woolsey, '52), squirrel monkeys (Benjamin and Welker, '57), macaques (Woolsey, '58, '64), chimpanzees (Woolsey, '64), and humans (Penfield and Boldrey, '37; Penfield and Rasmussen, '50). The distal limbs and digits are rostral, and back and dorsal midline are caudal, the head is lateral, and the tail medial in these figurative illustrations of representational patterns.

Other investigators have concluded that each different body region is represented (at least for the most part) across "SI" within a rostrocaudal cortical strip extending from margin to margin. The concept of rostrocaudal bands was first introduced in the landmark studies of Powell and Mountcastle ('59b) in describing the functional organization of "SI" in macaque monkeys. The concept has also been advanced in a study of spider monkey somatosensory cortex by Pubols and Pubols ('71, '72), and to some extent for squirrel and macaque monkeys by Werner and Whitsel ('68, '71) and macaque monkeys by Whitsel et al. ('71) and Dreyer et al. ('74, '75).

Both points of view reasonably account for certain sets of observations. For example, progressions of recording sites in "SI" commonly result in simple somatotopic sequences of receptive fields. And recording sites at different positions at the same rostrocaudal level are often activated by the same body part. But most investigators recognized that a strict adherence to either point of view would not account for all the observations. In particular, it has been necessary to admit to some degree of somatotopic organization within "rostrocaudal bands," and major discontinuities and re-representations in "the single somatotopic map" have been noted. We have presented evidence for a third point of view (also see Paul et al., '72a). There are clearly not rostrocaudal strips across the architectonic fields in owl monkeys. Rather, separate architectonic fields have separate representations. Furthermore, the concept of a homunculus does not accurately reflect the organization of either of the two cutaneous representations that we have demonstrated. Rather, the representations are better described as composites of subunits or sectors, each of which is internally somatotopic. Within each sector, progressions of recording sites produce simple progressions of receptive fields. However, adjoining neurons on two sides of a "sector" border might relate to quite distant or discontinuous body parts. Thus, the representations are not simple or topological transformations of the complete contralateral body surface, and therefore are not homunculi. We prefer to consider the representations as *composites of somatotopic regions*.

(d) The representation follows a dermatomal sequence

All three concepts of somatosensory cortex organization could, in principle, be reasonably (but not completely) consistent with a further postulate or organization: that the medial-to-lateral sequence of representation follows the dermatomal order. There has been some disagreement as to the actual order of the medial-to-lateral sequence of body surface representation in primates, but a number of investigators suggested (as did earlier neurologists such as Head, '20, and Benisty, '28) that this sequence follows the dermatomal order (Bard, '38; Woolsey et al., '42; Woolsey et al., '43; Powell and Mountcastle, '59b; Werner and Whitsel, '68, '71). Holding a more extreme form of the concept of dermatomal organization of "SI," Powell and Mountcastle ('59b) and Werner and Whitsel ('68, '71) argued that the representation of the body in "SI" is actually a simple representation of the dermatomes, which are laid out over the rostrocaudal dimension of "SI," and represented in order in its lateral-to-medial dimension.

On the other hand, many investigators have described exceptions to the dermatomal sequence of representation. Woolsey and colleagues ('42) first noted the discontinuity between the representation of the hand and two parts of the head, i.e., the dorsal head is represented in the cortical region medial to the hand, while adjoining head surfaces are represented lateral to the hand. This "splitting of the occiput" has been recorded in nearly all the primate species that have been studied. Other exceptions to dermatomal sequences were reported later in the chimpanzee and gibbon (genitalia adjacent to trunk representation, foot lateral to a complete leg representation) (Woolsey et al., '60); in humans (entire leg lateral to foot) (Penfield and Rasmussen, '50); in cebus monkeys (genitalia represented on both sides of the foot) (Hirsch and Coxe, '58); and in spider monkeys (head lateral to hand) (Pubols and Pubols, 71, '72).

The detailed maps of the two cutaneous fields in the owl monkeys allow us to evaluate the usefulness of considering these representations as "metameric maps", i.e., maps of the dorsal root cutaneous fields. For both representations there are numerous examples, both of regions where the dermatomal sequence is not followed, and where discontinuities between the representations of adjoining skin surfaces are not along "dermatomal boundaries." Among obvious examples are the following: (1) As many others have noted, the representation of the face is immediately adjacent to that of the thumb and thenar eminence in both fields. In the dermatomal sequence, of course, fields on the arm, shoulder and head dorsum should be represented between the hand and face. The skin field represented in the dermatomes innervating the arm and shoulder are actually represented in both cortical fields 3b and 1 in cortex distant from the representation of the hand. This separation of the hand from adjoining skin surfaces has also been described in other species (Woolsey et al., '42; Benjamin and Welker, '57; Woolsey et al., '60; Penfield and Boldrey, '37; Paul et al., '72a; Pubols and Pubols, '72). (2) The representation of the dorsal surfaces of the fingers is separated from that of the rest of their dermatomal fields on the hand and arm. Moreover, the dorsal fingers are represented differently in Areas 3b and 1. Especially in Area 1, lines of discontinuity in the representations of fingers fail to follow even a short part of any dermatomal boundary. A similar segregation of the Area 3b representation of the volar and dorsal hand was also recorded in the slow loris, by Krishnamurti et al. ('76). (3) The representation of the hand and volar wrist is discontinuous with that of the rest of the arm. Given this discontinuity, the dermatomes would be cut off at the wrist, and in the hand-wrist sector there would be fragments of several dermatomes. (4) If dermatomal fields occur in the region of representations of the arm, they are aligned successively in the mediolateral and not the rostrocaudal cortical dimension in both fields. (5) The representation of part of the preaxial leg is found lateral to the foot within Area 1 (the lateral representation in Area 3b is very small or absent). The split of the preaxial and postaxial leg is along dermatomal lines, and this finding in other primates has been one of the major arguments for a systematic representation of dermatomes in cortex (Woolsey et al., '42), i.e., according to the dermatomal sequence, and the preaxial leg should be represented lateral to the foot.[1] However, at least most of the preaxial leg in Area 3 is clearly represented in the cortex *medial* to the foot representation, and out of the dermatomal sequence. (6) The hairy skin of the toes is not represented with the remainder of the dermatomes covering these surfaces, in either Areas 3b or 1. Again, the pattern of representation of the dorsal digits is different for the two fields, and again, in both instances, lines of discontinuity that cut across these skin fields cut through dermatomes. (7) In somewhat different ways in Areas 1 and 3b the representation of the foot is largely discontinuous with that of the leg. However, dermatomes in this region cross the dorsal foot to extend up onto the leg.

Can *any* discontinuities really be described as falling along dermatomal boundaries? It is possible that the lines of discontinuity along the arm and leg representations follow dermatomal boundaries. Our mapping data is not precise enough to define these lines with sufficient accuracy to resolve this question. The lines splitting the hairy skin of the toes (and possibly the fingers) in Area 3b (but not Area 1), and lines of discontinuity which split the palm and which separate off a sector of the thenar eminence could conceivably follow a dermatomal boundary over a short distance. The dermatomal boundaries defining the preaxial thigh may be followed over a part of their length in the Area 1 representation of the thigh. In all of these instances, on the other hand, *the sector of the skin field represented discontinuously would probably never include all of any one dermatome.* We conclude that while both the dermatomal sequence and the body maps reflect in a general way the spatial outlay of the skin surface, the organizations of the body maps are not a consequence of the dermatomal sequence.

(e) The proportion of representation of different body surface regions is a simple reflection of cutaneous peripheral innervation density

As the observation that the parts of body surfaces with the greatest peripheral innervation density occupy proportionately more of "SI" became appreciated, the idea has arisen that there might be a simple relation between numbers of peripheral receptors per unit area and the cortical area representing the peripheral unit. Beginning with the insightful discussion of the somatosensory cortex in the report of Woolsey et al. ('42), most mapping studies have alluded to this basic concept. However, quantitive evidence for the hypothesis that the somatosensory cortical representations are simply a reflection of peripheral innervation density is limited to that presented in the report of Lee and Woolsey ('75). These investigators found a proportional relationship between the numbers of fibers innervating individual vibrissae on the face and the number of neurons in distinct groupings (termed barrels) of cells in layer IV of SI cortex devoted to individual vibrissae. Although the numbers of peripheral fibers and the numbers of layer IV neurons for each whisker varied, there was a constant proportion of 17 central neurons for each peripheral fiber. From these findings, Lee and Woolsey ('75) proposed that the distortion of the body representation is directly related to the quantity of peripheral innervation and is the result of a "peripheral scaling factor."

Attractive as this concept is, it cannot be applied without modification to the parietal somatosensory strip. Since the proportional representations of different skin areas are different in these two fields, the same peripheral scale factor obviously cannot be applied to both. It is also apparent that several features of at least the Area 1 somatosensory representation do not follow overall peripheral innervation patterns. The relatively small representations of the glabrous surfaces of the fingers and toes as compared with the relatively large representations of the palm and sole in Area 1 are examples (table 1). Thus, there is not a simple relationship between peripheral innervation density and cortical expansion. An alternative view is that functional specialization within cortex is a factor in the distortion of the representations, and consequently, the number of cortical neurons related to the peripheral input varies within representations, and from representation to representation. It is also possible that a modified form of the peripheral-central relationship exists, but that it applies for distributions of different specific afferents or submodalities for each cortical representation. Thus, each representation would reflect the differential distribution of a separate set of peripheral receptor or primary fiber types. Nonetheless, any application of the "peripheral scaling" principal to parietal somatosensory cortical fields must await further direct evidence of the kind derived by Lee and Woolsey ('75).

(f) "SI" is the basic functional subdivision of somatosensory cortex

Most anatomical, ablation-behavioral, and electrophysiological studies of "SI" have been predicated on the concept that "SI" is a single large functional unit. As a result, and despite the clear architectonic subdivisions, limited attention has been paid to where recording sites, lesions, or injections have been located within this strip. Perhaps the most compelling argument against considering "SI" of primates as a single functional unit is the evidence that this region of cortex contains separate, complete and detailed representations of receptor surfaces that are coextensive with the separate and distinct architectonic fields. However, three other types of evidence support the hypothesis of functionally separate areas within "SI."

The first type of additional evidence is that the overall response characteristics of neurons differ in each of the "SI" architectonic subdivisions. This difference was noted in the early study of Powell and Mountcastle ('59b), although they regarded "SI" as a functional unit and argued that there was a graded distribution of neurons with different response characteristics across the architectonic fields. Subsequently, a number of investigators have presented evidence that different receptor populations ultimately project to Areas 3a, 3b and 2 (Paul et al., '72a,b; Krishnamurti et al., '76; Tanji, '75; Heath et al., '76). From their studies, it is reasonable to conclude that muscle afferents feed into Area 3a, input from perhaps different types of cutaneous receptors into Areas 3b and 1, and joint and other "deep" receptors into Area 2.

There may be some differences in the overall neuronal response properties of the architectonic fields in different primates. While neurons in Areas 3b and 1 of macaque monkeys apparently differ in adaptation rate to a steady cutaneous stimuli (Paul et al., '72a) we have been unable to demonstrate this segregation of slowly and quickly adapting inputs in the owl monkey. While neuronal responses were not studied in detail for adaptation properties, both fields appeared to have neurons that were basically quickly adapting. (This does not mean, of course, that differences in adaptation rate do not exist or that both populations derive their input solely from quickly adapting receptor classes.) On the other hand, the response properties of neurons in Areas 3b and 1 in owl monkeys were different in receptive field size and numbers of discharges in response to transient stimuli. Furthermore, as in macaque monkeys (Paul et al., '72a), Pacinian-like responses (Mountcastle et al., '69) were limited to Area 1 recording sites and were not found in Area 3b. Also in concurrence with the observations of Paul et al. ('72a), no joint receptor input was recorded in Areas 3b and 1 in anesthetized owl monkeys; joint receptor input was found in Area 2.

A second additional reason for considering "SI" of primates as several functionally distinct fields is that each of the separate representations has a different pattern of anatomical connections. Most significantly, Vogt ('76) found that Areas 3b and 1 are reciprocally interconnected, a finding that might be expected between separate cutaneous representations but would be surprising between parts of a single representation. Similarly, electrophysiological evidence indicates that Area 3a is topographically interconnected with motor cortex (Zarzechi et al., '76). It is also of interest that the commissural connections revealed by lesions restricted to Areas 1 and 2 result in three contralateral bands of degeneration corresponding to Area 3a, the boundary of Areas 3b and 1, and the boundary of Areas 2 and 5 (Shanks et al., '75). Such multiple connections between somatosensory cortex of one hemisphere and somatosensory cortex of the other hemisphere would be puzzling if the region contains only a single representation. The idea of a single representation across the somatosensory architectonic fields also is difficult to relate to other anatomical observations. Thus, the different "SI" architectonic fields project to different loci in the dorsal column nuclei (Weisberg and Rustioni, '76) and spinal cord (Jones, '76; Coulter and Jones, '76). In addition, the results of several types of experiments (Clark and Powell, '53; Jones and Powell, '70; Jones, '75; Lin et al., '78) have suggested that the ventroposterior nucleus projects heavily to Area 3b, and less heavily to Areas 1 and 2. All of these patterns of connections are more readily explained by the present concept of separate representations occupying separate architectonic fields than by the traditional concept of a single body representation and functional field.

A third type of evidence suggesting the subdivision of "SI" of primates into more than one unit of functional significance comes from a recent report of Randolph and Semmes ('74) on the behavioral consequences of ablating parts of Areas 3b, 1, or 2 in macaque monkeys. These investigators trained monkeys on tactile discrimination tasks and found that lesions of the hand region of Area 2 were followed by impairments on tasks involving the discrimination of angles; similar lesions of Area 1 affected discriminations of texture; while lesions of Area 3b led to severe impairments on both types of tasks.

In summary, the electrophysiological mapping data of the present report, studies of the distributions of neurons with different response characteristics, the cortical architecture, the connections of the parietal lobe, and the behavioral effects of ablations of architectonic subdivisions of postcentral cortex all argue against the concept of "SI" as the basic functional subdivision of somatosensory cortex.

2. A Redefinition of the Primate "SI" and Suggested Terminology

Our conclusion that there are two separate representations of the body surface within Areas 3b and 1 of the classically defined "primary somatosensory cortex" or "SI" introduces the problem of redefining the cortical subdivisions of somatosensory cortex in primates. We believe that there are enough similarities between the representation in Area 3b of monkeys and the "SI" representation of most other mammals to argue that Area 3b is the homologue of the non-primate "SI." Therefore, we suggest the term "SI proper" for the 3b subdivision of primate somatosensory cortex, to distinguish it from the traditional primate "SI," which these studies suggest is comprised of as many as four body representations in monkeys, apes and man.

Three types of evidence suggest the homology of "SI proper" of primates with "SI" of other mammals. First, the overall organization of "SI," as generally described for non-primates (see Sur et al., '78, for review), is basically similar to that of "SI proper." For example the representations of the digits of the forepaw and foot are oriented rostrally in both "SI" and "SI proper." The most significant reported difference is that the dorsal trunk is usually portrayed as caudal to the abdomen in "SI" (e.g., see Woolsey, '64), while the reverse order occurs in "SI proper." However, the proportionately small representation of the trunk has been poorly documented in most species, and in "SI" of at least one mammal, the grey squirrel (Nelson and Sur, '77; Sur et al., '78), the representation of the trunk is like that of the owl monkey, with the dorsum rostral and the abdomen caudal in the field.

The cytoarchitecture of "SI proper" and non-primate "SI" is also very similar. Both fields are characterized by a well-developed layer IV with small, tightly packed granule cells. Finally, both "SI" of non-primates (Jones and Powell, '69; Hand and Morrison, '72) and "SI proper" (Jones, '75; Jones and Powell, '70; Clark and Powell, '53) receive a major input from the ventroposterior nucleus, and this input terminates largely in layer IV. For these reasons, we feel that it is probable that Area 3b of primates is homologous with "SI" as described for most non-primates, and that the term "SI proper" both suggests the likely homology, and distinguishes the Area 3b representation from the rest of the postcentral somatosensory strip of monkeys.

With the exception of "SIII" in the cat (Darian-Smith et al., '66), a systematic somatic representation has not been described for cortex caudal to "SI" in nonprimates. Thus, there is little data to suggest that the representation in Area 1 of monkeys is or is not homologous with any field in other mammals. For the present, we prefer the term, "posterior cutaneous field" (PCF) for the Area 1 representation, since it is both non-committal in regard to homologies, and descriptive with regard to location and function.

Finally, we suggest that the "deep" and cutaneous somatosensory fields, 3a, 3b, 1, and 2, of parietal cortex which currently are collectively termed "SI," be renamed the "parietal somatosensory strip" (PSS).

3. Evolution of the Parietal Somatosensory Strip in Primates

The generality of finding a body representation with the same relative location, the same overall orientation and arrangement of the body parts, a characteristic cytoarchitecture, and similar connections from the ventroposterior nucleus in "SI" of a wide range of mammalian species[2] and in "SI proper" of monkeys indicates that this subdivision of neocortex must have arisen early in mammalian or premammalian evolution, and is a basic feature of mammalian neocortex probably common to all mammals. On the other hand, the same argument cannot be made for the posterior cutaneous field. There is a general lack of evidence for a second cutaneous representation (except, perhaps, for cats; see above) that is posterior to "SI" in non-primates. Furthermore, the posterior cutaneous field appears to vary significantly in response characteristics and in organization within the primate order. In the prosimian, slow loris, the somatosensory field on the caudal border of "SI proper" requires rather strong stimuli for activation (Krishnamurti et al., '76), and probably for this reason the organization of the representation remains uncertain. In both New World monkeys (present study) and Old World monkeys (Paul et al., '72a), the PCF responds to low threshold cutaneous stimuli, but the neural responses appear to be more rapidly adapting in Old World monkeys. Finally, the organization of at least part of the PCF appears to be quite different in Old and New World monkeys. The evidence indicates that the hand representation in PCF is oriented with the fingertips caudally in New World monkeys (present study) and rostrally in Old World monkeys (Paul et al., '72a). These variations in PCF characteristics suggest that the field was not well developed in early primates, and perhaps existed as a high-threshold, crudely organized fringe such as it appears to be in present day prosimians.

We know too little about the interspecies comparative features of the Area 3a and Area 2 fields to make reasonable suggestions about their evolution. There is evidence for muscle afferent input to a narrow band of cortex between "SI" and motor cortex in a range of mammals, and the 3a field may be a widespread feature of mammalian brains. The Area 2 "deep" body field is, of course, only known for Old and New World monkeys, and even in these primates, the organization has not been determined in very much detail.

The significance of differences in the organization of the cutaneous fields in the various primates is not known. In reviewing earlier studies, there are difficulties in determining whether the described representational organization applies to Area 3b, to Area 1, or to both fields. Nonetheless, there is no question that quite marked differences in the representational sequence in either or both fields occur. For example, as reviewed earlier, the entire leg is represented lateral to the foot in apes and humans; the leg is represented almost completely on the medial side of the foot in owl monkeys; and the leg is split with the postaxial leg medial and the preaxial leg lateral to the foot in Old World monkeys. Perhaps, other differences among parietal somatosensory strip representations in different primates will be described as the organization of the PSS fields in more primates are mapped in detail. However, it is hardly surprising that species differences exist when the representations differ in organization to some extent from owl monkey to owl monkey. Thus,

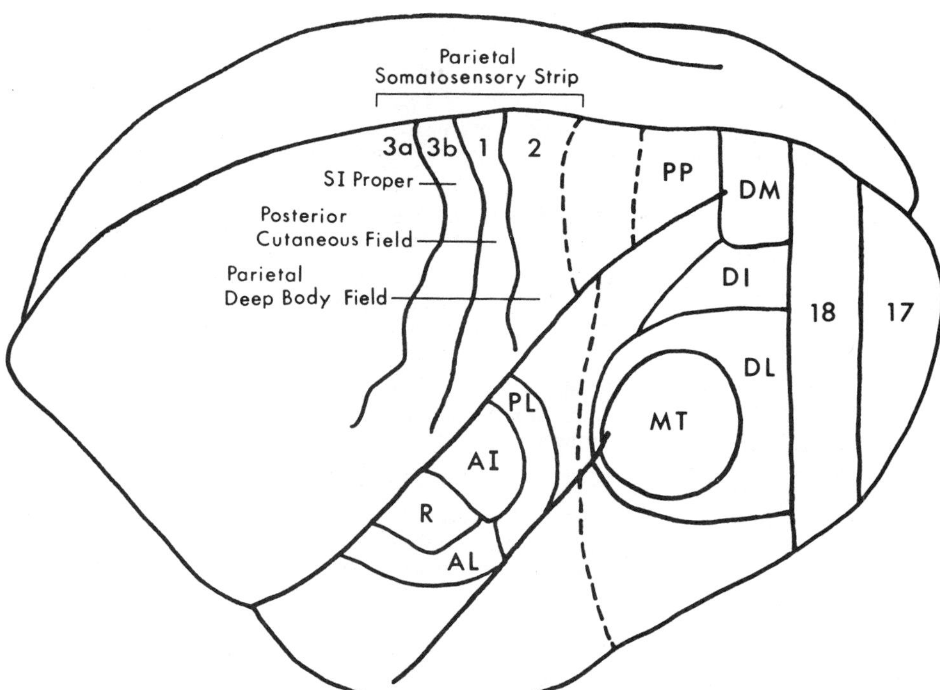

Figure 16. Visual, auditory and somatosensory areas in the owl monkey. The schematic maps of the auditory representations are redrawn from the studies of Imig et al. ('77): the summary of visual mapping studies is redrawn from Allman and Kaas ('76). The posterior broken line marks the approximate boundaries of visually responsive cortex. The anterior broken line marks the posterior border of cortex activated by somatic stimuli in the present experiments. Refer to figure 1 for a detailed reconstruction of Area 3b and Area 1 body surface representations.

field organization in primates appears to be less constant and more subject to intraspecies and interspecies variation than formerly thought.

5. A Note on Multiple Representation of Sensory Epithelia in the Neocortex

With the completion of the present studies, most of the neocortex caudal to the central sulcus has been mapped in the owl monkey. Nearly all of the parietal, occipital, and temporal cortex has been found to be occupied by retinotopically, cochleotopically, or somatotopically organized fields (fig. 16) (Allman and Kaas, '76; Imig et al., '77). For each of the six visual, the three somatic, and the four auditory areas that have been mapped in the owl monkey, there is evidence that the representations occupy delimitable cytoarchitectonic fields. Given the present redefinition of the organization of somatosensory cortex, no representations of the sensory epithelia in the neocortex overlie more than one generally recognized cytoarchitectonic field. There can be little question that the functional subdivisions of neocortex can be distinguished by structural characteristics. And it is of great theoretical significance to concepts of the genesis of perception in the forebrain that *all or nearly all of these fields* in the parietal, occipital and much of the temporal cortex *embody systematic spatial representations of individual sensory epithelia.*

Acknowledgments

The authors gratefully acknowledge the technical assistance of Laura Symonds, Randy Nelson and Leona Wayrynen. In some of these studied animals, Evelynn McGinnis carefully defined the caudal Area 4 border by use of microstimulation. This work was supported by NIH Grant NS-10414 and NSF Grant BNS 76-81824.

Notes

1. The preaxial leg has been described as being represented on the lateral side of the foot representation in squirrel monkeys (Benjemin and Welker. '57; Werner and Whitsel, '68), spider monkeys (Pubols and Pubols, '72) and rhesus monkeys (Woolsey et al., '42; Werner and Whitsel, '68): Investigations of somatosensory cortex organization in apes and man (Penfield and Boldrey. '37; Penfield and Rasmussen. '50; Woolsey et al., '60) report that the entire leg is represented lateral to the foot.

2. Among the more complete maps of non-primate mammals are those derived in the opossum (Lende, '63; Pubols et al., '76), the marsupial wallaby (Lende, '63), the pig and sheep (Woolsey and Fairman, '46, Johnson et al., '74), rabbit (Woolsey, '64), rat (Woolsey, '64; C. Welker, '71), grey squirrel (Sur et al., '78), dog (Pinto Hamuy et al., '56) guinea pig and capybara (Campos and Welker, '76), llama (Welker et al., '76), hyrax (Welker and Carlson, '76), beaver (Carlson and Welker, '76), and raccoon (Welker et al., '64).

Literature Cited

Allman, J. M., and J. H. Kaas 1976 Representation of the visual field on the medial wall of occipital-parietal cortex in the owl monkey. Science, *191*: 572–575.

Bard, P. 1938 Studies on the cortical representation of somatic sensibility. Bulletin N. Y. Acad. Med., *14*: 585–607.

Benisty, M. 1928 Les lesions de la zone Rolandique (Zone motrice et zone sentive) por blessures de querre. Paris (cited by M. Hines, Physiol. Rev., *9*: 462–574.)

Benjamin, R. M.. and W. I. Welker 1957 Somatic receiving areas of cerebral cortex of squirrel monkey (*Saimiri sciureus*). J. Neurophysiol., *20*: 286–299.

Bonin, G. von 1938 The cerebral cortex of the cebus monkey. J. Comp. Neur., *69*: 181–227.

Brodmann, K. 1909 Vergleischende Lokalisationslehre der Grosshirnride. Barth, Leipzig, 324 pp.

Campos, G. P., and W. I. Welker 1976 Comparisons between brains of a large and small Hystricomorph rodent: capybara, *Hydrochoerus* and guinea pig, *Cavia*; neocortical projection regions and measurements of brain subdivisions. Brain Behav. and Evol., *13*: 243–266.

Carlson, M., and W. I. Welker 1976 Some morphological, physiological and behavior specializations in North American beavers. (*Castor canadensis*). Brain Behav. and Evol., *13*: 302–326.

Chang, H.-T., C. N. Woolsey, L. W. Jarcho and E. Henneman 1947 Representation of cutaneous tactile sensibility in the cerebral cortex of the spider monkey. Fed. Proc., *6*: 89.

Clark, W. E. LeGros, and T. P. S. Powell 1953 On the thalamo-cortical connexions of the general sensory cortex of *Macaca.* Proc. Royal Soc. B, *141*: 467–487.

Coulter, J. D., and E. G. Jones 1976 Subcortical projections from cytoarchitectonic fields of the somatic sensory cortex in monkey. Neuroscience Abst., *2*: 1306.

Darian-Smith, I., J. Isbister, H. Mok and T. Yokota 1966 Somatic sensory cortical projection areas excited by tactile stimulation of the cat: A triple representation. J. Physiol. (London), *182*: 671–687.

Dreyer, D. A., P. R. Loe, C. B. Metz and B. L. Whitsel 1975 Representation of head and face in postcentral gyrus of the Macaque. J. Neurophysiol., *38*: 714–733.

Dreyer, D. A., R. J. Schneider, C. B. Metz and B. L. Whitsel 1974 Differential contributions of spinal pathways to body representation in postcentral gyrus of *Macaca mulatta.* J. Neurophysiol., *37*: 119–145.

Hand, P. J., and A. R. Morrison 1972 Thalamo-cortical relationships in the somatic sensory system as revealed by silver impregnation techniques. Brain Behav. and Evol., *5*: 273–302.

Head, H. 1920 Studies in Neurology. Vol. 1. Oxford, London.

Heath, G. J., J. Hore and C. G. Phillip 1976 Inputs from low threshold muscle and cutaneous afferents of hand and forearm to Areas 3a and 3b of baboon's cerebral cortex. J. Physiol. (London), *257*: 199–227.

Hirsch, J. F., and W. S. Coxe 1958 Representation of cutaneous tactile sensibility in cerebral cortex of *Cebus.* J. Neurophysiol., *21*: 481–498.

Imig, T. J., M. A. Ruggero, L. M. Kitzes. E. Javel. and J. F. Brugge 1977 Organization of auditory cortex in the owl monkey (*Aotus trivigatus*). J. Comp. Neur., *171*: 111–128.

Johnson, J. I., E. W. Rubel and G. I. Hatton 1974 Mechanosensory projections to cerebral cortex of sheep. J. Comp. Neur., *158*: 81–108.

Jones, E. G. 1975 Lamination and differential distribution of thalamic afferents within the sensory-motor cortex of the squirrel monkey. J. Comp. Neur., *160*: 167–204.

——— 1976 Cells of origin of afferent projections from the monkey first somatic sensory area. Neuroscience Abst., *2*: 913.

Jones, E. G.. and T. P. S. Powell 1969 The cortical projection of the ventroposterior nucleus of the thalamus in the cat. Brain Res., *13*: 298–318.

——— 1970 Connections of the somatic sensory cortex of the rhesus monkey. III. Thalamic connections. Brain, *93*: 37–56.

Kaas, J. H., M. M. Merzenich, C.-S. Lin, and M. Sur 1976 A double representation of the body in "primary somatosensory cortex" ("SI") of primates. Neuroscience Abst., *2*: 914.

Knight, P. K. 1977 Representation of the cochlea within the anterior auditory field (AAF) of the cat. Brain. Res., *130*: 447–467.

Krishnamurti, A., F. Sanides and W. I. Welker 1976 Microelectrode mapping of modality-specific somatic sensory cerebral neocortex in slow loris. Brain Behav. and Evol., *13*: 367–383.

Lee, K. J., and T. A. Woolsey 1975 A proportional relationship between peripheral innervation density and cortical neuron number in the somatosensory system of the mouse. Brain Res., *99*: 349–353.

Lende, R. A. 1963 Cerebral cortex: A sensorimotor amalgam in the Marsupialia. Science, *141*: 730–732.

Lin, C.-S., M. M. Merzenich, M. Sur and J. H. Kaas (1978, in preparation) Connections of Areas 3b and 1 of the parietal somatosensory strip with the ventroposterior nucleus in the owl monkey (*Aotus trivirgatus*).

Lucier, G. E., D. C. Ruegg and M. Wiesendanger 1975 Responses of neurons in motor cortex and in Area 3a to controlled stretches of forelimb muscles in *Cebus* monkeys. J. Physiol. (London), *251*: 833–853.

Marshall, W. H., C. N. Woolsey and P. Bard 1937 Cortical representation of tactile sensibility as indicated by cortical potentials. Science, *85*: 388–390.

Merzenich, M. M., P. L. Knight and G. L. Roth 1975 Representation of cochlea within primary auditory cortex in the cat. J. Neurophysiol., *38*: 231–249.

Mountcastle, V. B. 1957 Modality and topographic properties of single neurons of cat's somatic sensory cortex. J. Neurophysiol., *20*: 408–434.

Mountcastle, V. B., and T. P. S. Powell 1959 Central nervous mechanisms subserving position sense and kinesthesis. Bulletin Johns Hopkins Hospital, *105*: 173–200.

Mountcastle, V. B., W. H. Talbot, H. Sakata and J. Hyvärinen 1969 Cortical neuronal mechanisms in fluttervibration studies in unanesthetized monkeys. Neuronal periodicity and frequency discrimination. J. Neurophysiol., *32*: 452–484.

Nelson, R. J., and M. Sur 1977 Organization of primary somatosensory cortex (SMI) in the grey squirrel. Anat. Rec., *187*: 666.

Paul, R. L., M. M. Merzenich and H. Goodman 1972a Representation of slowly and rapidly adapting cutaneous mechanoreceptors of the hand in Brodmann's areas 3 and 1 of *Macaca mulatta*. Brain Res., *36*: 229–249.

Paul, R. L., H. Goodman and M. M. Merzenich 1972b Alterations in mechanoreceptor input to Brodmann's areas 1 and 3 of the postcentral hand area of *Macaca mulatta* after nerve section and regeneration. Brain Res., *39*: 1–19.

Paul, R. L., M. M. Merzenich and H. Goodman 1975 Mechanoreceptor representation and topography of Brodmann's areas 3 and 1 of *Macaca mulatta*. In: The Somatosensory System. H. H. Kornhuber and G. Thieme eds. Stuttgart, pp. 262–269.

Peden, J. H., and G. von Benin 1947 The neocortex of *Hapale*. J. Comp. Neur., *86*: 37–63

Penfield, W., and E. Boldrey 1937 Somatic motor and sensory representation in the cerebral cortex of man as studied by electrical stimulation. Brain, *60*: 389–443.

Penfield, W., and T. Rasmussen 1950 The Cerebral Cortex of Man. Macmillan, New York.

Phillips, C. G.. T. P. S. Powell and M. Wiesendanger 1971 Projection from low-threshold muscle afferents of hand and forearm to Area 3a of baboon's cortex. J. Physiol. (London), *217*: 419–446.

Pinto Hamuy, T., R. B. Bromiley and C. N. Woolsey 1956 Somatic afferent areas I and II of the dog's cerebral cortex. J. Neurophysiol., *19*: 485–499.

Powell, T. P. S., and V. B. Mountcastle 1959a The cytoarchitecture of the postcentral gyrus of the monkey *Macaca mulatta*. Bulletin Johns Hopkins Hospital, *105*: 108–131.

——— 1959b Some aspects of the functional organization of the cortex of the postcentral gyrus of the monkey. A correlation of findings obtained in a single unit analysis with cytoarchitecture. Bulletin Johns Hopkins Hospital, *105*: 133–162.

Pubols, B. H., and L. M. Pubols 1971 Somatotopic organization of spider monkey somatic sensory cerebral cortex. J Comp. Neur., *141*: 63–76.

——— 1972 Neural organization of somatic sensory representation in the spider monkey. Brain Behav. and Evol., *5*: 342–366.

Pubols, B. H., L. M. Pubols, D. J. DiPette and J. C. Sheely 1976 Opossum somatic sensory cortex: A microelectrode mapping study. J. Comp. Neur., *165*: 229–246.

Randolph, M., and J. Semmes 1974 Behavioral consequence of selective subtotal ablation in the postcentral gyrus of *Macaca mulatta*. Brain Res., *70*: 55–70.

Rosabal, F. 1967 Cytoarchitecture of the frontal lobe of the squirrel monkey. J. Comp. Neur., *130*: 87–108.

Sanides, F. 1968 The architecture of the cortical taste nerve areas in squirrel monkey (*Saimiri sciureus*) and their relationships to insular, sensorimotor and prefrontal regions. Brain Res., *8*: 97–124.

Sanides, F., and A. Krishnamurti 1967 Cytoarchitectonic subdivisions of sensorimotor and prefrontal regions and of bordering insular and limbic field in slow loris (*Nycticebus coucang coucang*). J. Hirnforsch., *9*: 225–252.

Shanks, M. F., A. J. Rockel and T. P. S. Powell 1975 The commissural fiber connections of the primary somatic sensory cortex. Brain Res., *98*: 166–171.

Sur, M., R. J. Nelson and J. H. Kaas 1978 The representation of the body surface in somatosensory Area I of the grey squirrel. J. Comp. Neur., *179*: 425–450.

Tanji, J. 1975 Activity of neurons in cortical area 3a during maintenance of steady postures by the monkey. Brain Res., *88*: 549–553.

Tigges, J., W. B. Spatz and M. Tigges 1973 Reciprocal point-to-point connections between parastriate and striate cortex in the squirrel monkey (*Saimiri*). J. Comp. Neur., *148*: 481–490.

Vogt, B. A. 1976 The origin, course and termination of intrinsic connections between Areas 3 and 1-2 in the monkey. Anat. Rec., *184*: 554.

Wisenberg, J. A., and A. Rustioni 1976 Cortical cells projecting to the dorsal column nuclei of cats. Anatomical study with the horseradish peroxidase technique. J. Comp. Neur., *165*: 425–437.

Welker, C. 1971 Microelectrode delineation of fine grain somatotopic organization of SmI cerebral neocortex in albino rat. Brain Res., *26*: 259–275.

Welker, W. I., H. O. Adrian, W. Lifschitz, R. Kaulen, E. Caviedes and W. Gutman 1976 Somatic sensory cortex of llama (*Lama glama*). Brain Behav. and Evol., *13*: 284–293.

Welker, W. I., and M. Carlson 1976 Somatic sensory cortex of hyrax (*Procavia*). Brain Behav. and Evol., *13*: 294–301.

Welker, W. I., J. I. Johnson and B. H. Pubols 1964 Some morphological and physiological characteristics of somatic sensory system in raccoons. Am. Zool., *4*: 75–94.

Welt, C. 1963 Topographical organization of the somatic sensory and motor areas of the cerebral cortex of the gibbon (*Hylobates*) and chimpanzee (*Pan*). Ph.D. Thesis, University of Chicago.

Werner, G., and B. L. Whitsel 1968 Topology of the body representation in somatosensory area I of primates. J. Neurophysiol., *31*: 856–869.

——— 1971 The functional organization of the somatosensory cortex. In: Handbook of Sensory Physiology, A. Iggo, ed. Springer, New York, pp. 621–700.

Whitsel, B. L., D. A. Dreyer and J. R. Roppolo 1971 Determinants of body representation in postcentral gyrus of Macaques. J. Neurophysiol., *34*: 1018–1034.

Whitsel, B. L., L. M. Petrucelli, H. Ha and D. A. Dreyer 1972 The resorting of spinal afferents as antecedent to the body representation in the postcentral gyrus. Brain Behav. and Evol., *5*: 303–341.

Woolsey, C. N. 1952 Patterns of localization in sensory and motor areas of the cerebral cortex. In: The Biology of Mental Health and Disease. Milbank Memorial Fund, Hoeber, New York, pp. 193–206.

——— 1954 Localization patterns in a lissencephalic primate (*Hapale jacchus*). Amer. J. Physiol., *178*: 686.

——— 1958 Organization of somatic sensory and motor areas of the cerebral cortex. In: Biological and Biochemical Bases of Behavior. H. F. Harlow and C. N. Woolsey, eds. University of Wisconsin, Madison, pp. 63–81.

——— 1964 Cortical localization as defined by evoked potential and electrical stimulation studies. In: Cerebral Localization and Organization. G. Schalter Brand and C. N. Woolsey, eds. University of Wisconsin, Madison, pp. 17–26.

Woolsey, C. N., and D. Fairman 1946 Contralateral, ipsilateral, and bilateral representation of cutaneous receptors in somatic areas I and II of the cerebral cortex of pig, sheep, and other mammals. Surgery, *19*: 684–702.

Woolsey, C. N., W. H. Marshall and P. Bard 1942 Representation of cutaneous tactile sensibility in the cerebral cortex of the monkey as indicated by evoked potentials. Bulletin Johns Hopkins Hospital, *70*: 399–441.

——— 1943 Note on organization of tactile sensory area of cerebral cortex of chimpanzee. J. Neurophysiol., *6*: 287–291.

Woolsey, C. N., R. Tasker, C. Welt, R. Ladpli, G. Campos, H. D. Potter, R. Emmers and H. Schwassmann 1960 Organization of pre- and postcentral leg areas in chimpanzee and gibbon. Trans. Amer. Neurol. Assoc., *85*: 144–146.

Yumiya, H., K. Kubota and H. Asanuma 1974 Activities of neurons in area 3a of the cerebral cortex during voluntary movements in the monkey. Brain Res., *78*: 169–177.

Zarzechi, P., Y. Shimada and H. Asanuma 1976 The projection of group I afferents to the motor cortex in Area 3a. Neuroscience Abst., *2*: 958.

Zimmerman, I. D. 1968 A triple representation of the body surface in the sensorimotor cortex of the squirrel monkey. Exp. Neurol., *20*: 415–431.

III
Attention

Introduction to Part III

One is aware of only a limited subset of information at any moment in time. This filtering of information is referred to as *attention*; attention is the selective aspect of information processing. Attention ensures that the limited capacity of the system is not overwhelmed. Visual attention can be easily studied at both a psychological and neurophysiological level because it can be relatively easily controlled in behavioral tasks. Typically attention is directed to one of a group of stimuli, and some functional indicator of attention is measured. This measure could be a reaction time in a behavioral task or the activity of a neuron in a recording experiment. Such investigations have told us much about the properties of attention and the locations in the brain in which it operates.

The article by Posner and colleagues is a good example of a behavioral study of attention using a reaction time task. They examined whether visual-spatial attention is a separate "module" in the brain by having subjects perform a visual-spatial orienting task either alone or in combination with a language attention task. They reasoned that if a general attentional mechanism has common links to visual-spatial and language attention mechanisms, then the language task should interfere with shifts in attention. Their data show such a linkage.

Mesulam outlines an anatomical circuit for attention that is derived from the study of attentional deficits following cortical lesions in humans. This circuit involves three cortical areas and the reticular formation. He proposes that the posterior parietal cortex is concerned largely with sensory aspects of attention, the frontal cortex is involved in motor components of attention, the limbic (cingulate) cortex is affected by motivation and directs the attentional focus accordingly, and the reticular system provides a general arousing influence to all of the cortex. Mesulam also reviews the clinical literature that indicates that the attentional system in right-handed humans is lateralized, with the right cerebral hemisphere playing a dominant role. What set Mesulam's ideas apart from many others is that he saw attentional mechanisms as embodied in a distributed circuit. All three cortical areas of his circuit are strongly interconnected by cortico-cortical projections, which is consistent with this hypothesis.

In their articles Richmond and Sato and Moran and Desimone examine the effects of attention on neural activity in awake, behaving monkeys. Richmond and Sato record activity of inferotemporal cortical neurons while monkeys perform different tasks. They find enhanced activity for a dimming detection task and even more activity for a pattern discrimination task. They hypothesize that the further increment in activity in the discrimination task arises because it requires a greater amount of attention. Moran and Desimone examine attentional modulation in areas V4 and IT, which are important in object recognition. They train monkeys to ignore stimuli at one location in the receptive field of a neuron being studied and to focus on stimuli at another location. If the stimulus at the focus of attention is one preferred by the cell being examined, then a large response is recorded. If attention is shifted away from the preferred stimulus and onto a nonpreferred stimulus in the receptive field, however, then the cell responds much less, even though the preferred stimulus is still within the receptive field. These experiments indicate that unwanted visual information is filtered from the receptive field of neurons by visual attention.

Wurtz and colleagues examine the role of visual attention in areas of the brain that are involved in programming saccadic eye movements. In most of these areas they find that the sensory response to a visual stimulus is enhanced if that stimulus is a target for an impending eye movement; however, only in the posterior parietal cortex are responses enhanced when attention is shifted but the monkey does not make an overt eye movement.

Crick proposes a bold first step toward a theory of the neural mechanisms underlying attention. He proposes that the focus, or "searchlight," of attention is regulated by the reticular nucleus of the thalamus. Treisman, Julesz, and others have shown that the attentional searchlight is important when sets of features (such as colors and shapes) must be conjoined, as is necessary to recognize a red ball, for example. Because different conjoined features are often likely to be processed in different cortical areas, Crick proposes that one role of the attentional searchlight is to produce correlated activity in diverse cortical areas that code different features of the same object. His hypothesis can also be considered a solution to the "binding" problem, a term that originated from computer vision and relates to how different attributes can be assigned to a single object. In an addendum to this paper, Crick points out that recent evidence does not support the idea that the attentional searchlight is being regulated by the reticular nucleus; however, his idea that correlated activity solves the binding problem has received considerable attention lately. For example, the results reported by Gray et al., reprinted in Part I, suggest that binding may be mediated by high-frequency oscillations in cortical activity.

All of the papers in this part, then, provide insight into how some information is selected for additional processing whereas other information is not so privileged.

23

M. I. Posner, A. W. Inhoff, F. J. Friedrich, and A. Cohen

Isolating attentional systems: A cognitive-anatomical analysis

1987. *Psychobiology* 15: 107–121

Recently our knowledge of the mechanisms of visual-spatial attention has improved because of studies employing single cell recording with alert monkeys and others using performance analysis of neurological patients. These studies suggest that a complex neural network that includes parts of the posterior parietal lobe and midbrain is involved in covert shifts of visual attention. Is this system an isolated visual attentional module or is it part of a more general attentional system? Our studies employ the dual-task technique to determine whether covert visual orienting can take place while a person's attention is engaged in a language processing task. We find clear evidence of interference between the two tasks, which suggests some common operations. However, the results also indicate that whatever is common to the two tasks does not have the same anatomical location as that of visual-spatial attention.

A fundamental problem in the study of attention is to understand how the unity of conscious experience is related to the many levels of selectivity involved in processing external events. The amount of information of which we are aware at any moment seems remarkably limited, yet it is often efficiently selected from a vast array of input. We are generally unaware of the details of the selection, but without it our subjective experience could not remain unified.

In recent years a more detailed anatomical and physiological analysis of attention has developed within the domain of selection of visual-spatial information (Mountcastle, 1978; Posner, 1980; Wurtz, Goldberg, & Robinson, 1980). This work involves studies of alert monkeys and of normal and brain injured patients orienting to visual events. Since no overt changes (e.g., eye movements) need occur for there to be evidence of selection at the attended location, it is possible that mechanisms revealed by these studies may serve as a model for understanding attention in general.

At the level of computations, one can view a shift of visual attention as involving three more elementary operations isolated from chronometric studies. The first operation is disengaging from the current focus of attention. It is a well established principle that the difficulty of processing influences the amount of time necessary to switch or disengage from that task (LaBerge, 1973). This principle is responsible for much of the use of secondary tasks to measure attention demands (see Kerr, 1973, for a review).

The second operation involves a movement of attention from its current focus to a new location. There is some reason to believe that this movement is analog in the sense of passing through intermediate locations (Shulman, Remington, & McLean, 1979; Tsal, 1983; Ullman, 1984), but this is by no means settled (Hughes & Zimba, 1985; Remington & Pierce, 1984). The move operation could be similar to the operation involved in mental rotation and image scanning (Kosslyn, 1980; Pinker, 1980; Shepard, 1978).

Finally, the subject must engage the new target. The engage operation is likely to differ according to the task required. Some processing (e.g., the registration of features or the looking up of highly familiar responses) may take place without engaging attention (Marcel, 1983; Treisman & Gelade, 1980). However, it appears that attention must be at the target for an arbitrary speeded response of maximum efficiency to occur. Thus faster responses and higher *d*'s are reported for events that occur at locations to which attention has been cued (Bashinski & Bachrach, 1980; Downing & Pinker, 1985; Posner, 1980).

Each of these operations appears to be affected by a different form of brain injury. Damage to the parietal lobe can produce a severe deficit in the ability to disengage attention from a visual location, without any loss in efficiency of the move or engage operations (Posner, Walker, Friedrich, & Rafal, 1984). Our results show only small

This research was supported in part by NIMH Grant R01-3853-02 and in part by the Office of Naval Research under Contract Nos. N 0014-83-K-0601 and N 0014-86-K-0289. Requests for reprints should be sent to Michael I. Posner, Department of Neurology, Box 8111, Washington University School of Medicine, 660 S. Euclid, St. Louis, MO 63110.

differences in reaction time (RT) to targets in either visual field once attention has been brought to that location by a cue (valid trials). Moreover, the improvement in RT to a target following a valid cue is about the same for targets in the contralateral and ipsilateral fields. If this improvement is due to a shift of attention to the cued side, it follows that the ability to move attention must not differ between the two fields. However, if attention is first cued to fixation (or to the visual field ipsilateral to the lesion), there is a massive increase in RT (of several hundred msec) for targets that occur on the side opposite the lesion. Thus, once attention is engaged at fixation (or at another place), the patient seems to have great trouble in disengaging it to deal with targets contralateral to the focus of attention (Posner, Cohen, & Rafal, 1982; Posner, Walker, Friedrich, & Rafal, 1984). We call this result the *extinction-like reaction time pattern* because it resembles what neurologists have called extinction of a contralateral event when it is presented simultaneously with an event on the side of the lesion.

This pattern contrasts with what we have found when there is damage to the midbrain. In progressive supranuclear palsy, patients lose the ability to make voluntary eye movements (saccades). This usually occurs first for vertical eye movements and later for horizontal movements (Posner, Choate, Rafal, & Vaughan, 1985; Posner et al., 1982). We have found that these patients are slower in shifting attention in the vertical direction than in the horizontal (Posner et al., 1985; Posner et al., 1982). For these patients, unlike for normals or other control populations, the advantage of the cued side over the uncued side emerges later when the cue requires a vertical shift of attention than when it requires a horizontal shift. The pattern is quite different for parietal patients, who show a specific deficit to contralateral targets only when they follow invalid cues. The deficit for midbrain patients occurs even for a target at a cued location, as though such patients have difficulty in moving attention either to a cue or to the target. This pattern is consistent with a deficit in the move operation because all shifts of attention in the vertical direction are affected. It is as though the patient simply has increased difficulty in shifting attention in the vertical direction.

These findings fit well with the single-cell recording data from monkeys. These data demonstrate that the parietal lobe contains cells that show enhanced responses to stimuli in their receptive fields when the animal is trained to attend to that location while maintaining fixation at another place (Wurtz et al., 1980).

Cells in the superior colliculus appear to be more closely related to attention when actual eye movements are involved (Wurtz et al., 1980). The human data also suggest the close relation of midbrain damage to eye movements. As described above, damage that affects the ability to move the eyes overtly toward a stimulus also retards the rate of the covert move operation toward that stimulus. In addition, lesions of the midbrain may increase the likelihood of attention's returning to a visual location that has recently been examined either by fixation or covertly (Posner et al., 1985). A bias against such return movements would have obvious importance in favoring novel information during visual scanning.

Thus we can now define one form of visual-spatial attention in terms of relatively precise cognitive operations and also say something about the anatomical locus of these operations. In this paper we ask whether visual-spatial attention shares cognitive operations with other attention senses. Specifically, does attending to a language task interfere with the operations involved in orienting visual-spatial attention, or are these operations independent of the language task? If visual-spatial attention and language share operations, we can use the results from our patients to attempt to establish whether these shared operations involve the parietal lobe.

EXPERIMENT 1

Our strategy was to assess the performance of patients with known deficits due to parietal lesions and that of groups of normal controls. The primary task was the visual-spatial attention orienting task studied previously. Each trial began with a visual cue that drew the person's attention to a location in space. To assess the effectiveness of the cue, we required the person to respond as rapidly as possible to targets that occurred at the cued location 80% of the time (valid trials) and at an uncued location 20% of the time (invalid trials). A single key was pressed irrespective of target location. The advantage of the cued over the uncued location in RT has been confirmed many times (Hughes & Zimba, 1985; Jonides, 1981; Lansman, Farr, & Hunt, 1984; Posner, 1980) and has often been attributed to the covert shift of attention to the cued location.

To study the issue of whether visual-spatial attention is a separate module, we had the subjects perform a visual-spatial orienting task either by itself or combined with one of two secondary tasks. The secondary tasks involved language and were chosen in an effort to ensure the use of separate input and output paths and quite different cognitive operations from those used in visual-spatial orienting. We then examined the ability of the patients and the normals to time-share the primary and secondary tasks. If visual-spatial attention is a separate module, we would expect a general increase in RT due to interference with output or reliance on some very general common resource. However, the advantage of a shift of attention to the cued location would be expected to remain, since, if visual-spatial attention is a separate module, it could operate to shift attention even when the subject was engaged in performing the secondary task. If the secondary task shares some attentional mechanisms with visual-spatial attention, we would expect to find interference with the covert shift of attention (e.g., invalid − valid RTs) as well as an overall increase in RT. There is already some evidence that dual tasks influence the ability to shift attention toward a cue. In one study researchers found that cuing the modality of a probe (visual vs. auditory) produced significantly faster RTs for the cued modality (Lansman et al., 1984), but these cuing effects were reduced or eliminated when performed during a dual task. In another study, when counting backward, the subjects were affected less by spatial cues during a dual task than during a spatial orienting task alone (Posner, Cohen, Choate, Hockey, & Maylor, 1984). It seems likely, then, that dual-task conditions may serve to reduce the effectiveness of the cues.

If attending to the language task reduces the validity effect (invalid − valid RTs), we can conclude that the spatial orienting and language tasks share a common attentional system. The system must be common because the act of processing language interferes with the validity effect; it must be attentional because, according to theory, the validity effect involves a shift of attention.

Our use of parietal patients also makes it possible to say something about the anatomy of the interference. When parietal patients attend to a cue in the good field, or at fixation, they show a specific interference in responding to targets on the side of space contralateral to the lesion. Many of these patients show no difference between ipsilateral and contralateral targets in uncued trials or in trials in which the cue is at the target location. We have interpreted this result as showing that the problem parietal patients have with contralateral targets is due to a specific deficit in their ability to disengage attention from the cue (Posner, Walker, Friedrich, & Rafal, 1984). If attending to the language task involves the same system as does attention to a spatial location, we would expect to observe a similar specific disadvantage for a contralateral target when the patient is engaged in processing the language task. The idea is quite straightforward. When a parietal patient attends to a visual cue, we find a specific disadvantage in detecting contralateral targets, as compared with ipsilateral targets. This appears to be a specific sign of parietal damage. If attending to language uses the same system, parietal patients should show a specific disadvantage in responding to contralateral targets.

If we find that doing the language task reduces the validity effect, we can argue that the patients are attending to language. We can then ask whether attending to language produces a specific disadvantage for contralateral targets. If this occurs, then attending to the language task would be thought to use the same parietal attentional system that we have found to be involved in visual-spatial attention. If attending to language produces no specific disadvantage for contralateral targets, we can conclude that the attention system common to language and spatial orienting is quite different from that used by spatial orienting alone. The common system would not be the parietal system we have identified with visual-spatial attention.

We thus have two indices of the separability of the primary and secondary tasks. The first has to do with whether the secondary task reduces the advantage of valid over invalid RTs when the primary task is performed alone. This index allows us to determine whether the two tasks involve the same or different cognitive operations. The second index tells us whether the secondary task produces a greater specific deficit for invalid targets contralateral to the lesion. This tells us whether attending to the secondary task involves the same anatomical system as does attending to a visual location.

Method

Subjects/patients. Nine parietal patients were studied, using two different secondary tasks. The first, which involved counting backward from a three-digit number, was used with only 5 patients. The second, which involved monitoring a series of auditory words and counting the number of phonemes, was used with all 9 patients. The 9 patients used in this study all had unilateral lesions of the parietal lobe confirmed by computerized tomography (CT) scan: 4 patients had lesions on the left side, and 5 had lesions on the right side. All of the lesions resulted from stroke. Two of the patients with right-hemisphere lesions were 5 or more years poststroke. All of the right-hemisphere patients had aspects of neglect and extinction at the time of the stroke. However, only one of them had clear problems at the time of testing. This patient, J.C., had a field cut that affected visual processing for stimuli more than 5° from fixation. Within the field cut he showed evidence of neglect. The left-hemisphere patients did not appear to have clear neglect problems. However, 3 of them had some form of aphasia as a result of the lesion. Three of 9 patients had damage that extended beyond the parietal lobe into the frontal area; 2 of the 9 patients had temporal damage in addition to the frontal damage. Further data on the lesions of 3 of the patients (J.C., W.K., and E.A.) are presented in Table 1 of Posner, Walker, Friedrich, and Rafal (1984). In that study of 13 patients, we found that the deficit in the disengage operation correlated with the extent of parietal lobe removed, and the best correlation was with the extent of superior parietal lobe removed. Such factors as lesion size and posterior or frontal extent of the lesion did not correlate with the disengage deficit. Because several of these patients were used in the earlier study and because we had only 9 patients for this study, we did not attempt to reexamine these correlations.

Control subjects. Sixteen subjects without documented neurological disorders served as controls for the parietal patients. Eight of the control subjects were in the 19 to 35 age group and were recruited from the staff of Good Samaritan Hospital and Medical Center or Portland State University; the other 8 control subjects were from 60 to 75 years old.

Tasks. In the single-task condition, subjects were required only to detect the visual target and to depress a single key with the index finger as quickly as possible. The basic experimental paradigm was similar to that used in Posner, Walker, Friedrich, and Rafal (1984). Subjects faced a cathode-ray tube (CRT) 80 cm from the eyes. They were instructed to maintain fixation on a central box. Two peripheral boxes were present approximately 8° to the left and right of fixation.

Two types of single-task blocks were used. In cued blocks, one of the two peripheral boxes was brightened for 300 msec by doubling the number of illuminated points that formed the box. After an interval of 100, 500, or 1,000 msec, the onset of the cue was followed by a bright asterisk that filled the box. The target asterisk was presented on the cued side 80% of the time (valid trials) and 20% of the time on the uncued side (invalid trials). In uncued blocks, the cue was omitted and only the target occurred, 1,100, 1,600, or 2,000 msec after the previous response.

In the dual-task condition, one of two secondary tasks was added to the primary task. One secondary task involved phoneme detection. The subjects were required to monitor for the phoneme *p* in a list of words. Specifically, the subjects were played a tape with 30 lists of 20 words each. These lists were spoken by a native speaker at a word presentation rate of approximately one word per 2 sec. Only nouns were used. In each list one to seven words began with the phoneme *p*. Immediately after the last word of a list was pronounced, the command "stop" was given to indicate that the visual-detection task was to be interrupted and that the last item of a list of words had been presented. After the stop command, the patient was asked how many nouns on the presented list of words had begun with the letter *p*. The question was followed by a silent interval of approximately 3 sec within which the subject was required to report the number of words that started with the phoneme *p*. After this, a "ready" command was given to indicate that the visual-detection task was to be continued and that a new list of words was to be presented.

The backward-counting task was similar. Each block of trials was initiated by a three-digit number from which the patient counted backward by ones. In the dual-task blocks, orienting trials were conducted during the counting process. After 15 to 20 trials, the subjects rested before a new number was given.

Performance on the phoneme-monitoring task alone was measured for 5 of the patients.

Procedure. Each subject was tested under all of the conditions in a single session. At the start of the session, each was introduced to the phoneme or backward-counting task. Each then received either three blocks of no-cue trials followed by three blocks of cued trials or the reverse (the order was counterbalanced across subjects). Each block consisted of 100 trials if no cues were involved, or 300 trials for cued blocks. Within each set of three blocks an ABA design was used, so that visual orienting alone came both before and after the dual-task block.

The backward-counting task was run on 5 patients prior to the phoneme-monitoring task. This was done in a single session, and only cued trial blocks were used.

Results

The main results of the experiment are described in terms of RTs for the spatial-attention task when performed alone and in conjunction with the monitoring task. The median RTs for each condition were calculated for each subject. All RTs less than 100 msec or greater than 3,000 msec were excluded (these represented less than 1% of the trials). Overall results were quite similar for the trials in which there was a 100-msec delay following the cue and for the trials in which the delay was longer. Since ⅔ of the trials were run at the 100-msec interval and these trials were free of any eye movements, they seemed most appropriate for discussion. Although the analyses of variance (ANOVAs) reported include all delay intervals, we discuss the longer intervals only in those cases where interval interacted with other effects.

The overall data from the primary task that had phoneme monitoring as the secondary task were cast into two ANOVAs. One involved the patient groups and had side of lesion as the between-subjects condition and attention (focused vs. divided), cue (valid, invalid, no cue), visual field (ipsilateral vs. contralateral to lesion), and interval (short vs. delayed) as the within-subject variables. The second analysis involved only the control subjects and had age as the between-subjects variable (8 old and 8 young), with the same set of within-subject variables except that visual field was left versus right. The data from the 5 subjects who counted backward were also summarized, but were not analyzed statistically.

Figure 1 shows both valid and invalid trials from cued trial blocks for each of the four subject groups. The results confirm the findings of numerous experiments (Hughes & Zimba, 1985; Jonides, 1981; Posner, 1980) that showed advantages for the cued side over the uncued side in all conditions. The younger normal subjects in this experiment showed the smallest advantage of the cued side over the uncued side [$F(1,7) = 5.7$, $p < .05$]. This was clearest at the short interval (36 msec) [$F(1,7) = 12.1$, $p < .01$], but there was no significant interaction with interval. The older normal subjects also showed a significant advantage for the cued side [$F(1,7) = 9.4$, $p < .01$], which was largest (98 msec) at the 500-msec interval, but once again there was no significant interaction with interval. The patients also showed a highly significant effect of validity [$F(1,8) = 15.2$, $p < .01$].

In each group, cued trials showed an advantage over noncued trials. There was no overall interaction with delay interval. In previous studies, where more intervals were used, the advantage of the cued side over the uncued side, attributed to the orienting of attention toward the cue, grew during the first 150 msec following the cue. Possibly because so few intervals were used in the current study, we found no growth of the validity effect (advantage of cued over noncued side) with interval. The presence of a constant validity effect over intervals indicates that the effect could not be due to purely sensory influences caused by the cue, because the effect was present long after the cue went off. Since the validity effects were fully present at a 100-msec interval, there seems to be little likelihood that overt eye shifts were mediating this effect. Moreover, in previous work it was demonstrated explicitly that the eyes remained fixed under conditions similar to those used in this experiment (Posner, 1980).

The data also confirm previous findings with parietal patients (Posner, Walker, Friedrich, & Rafal, 1984). Both left- and right-sided patients showed a markedly greater advantage of valid over invalid trials when the target was contralateral to the lesion than when it was ipsilateral [cue × side interaction; $F(2,14) = 9.3$, $p < .01$]. This has been previously reported (Posner, Walker, Friedrich, & Rafal, 1984) and called the *extinction-like reaction time pattern*, since it is similar to the clinical phenomenon in which patients miss contralateral signals when they occur simultaneously with ipsilateral signals (extinction). Left- and right-sided patients both show normal validity effects on the ipsilateral side (about 50 msec) but markedly larger effects on the contralateral side (200 msec).

In the dual-task performance, 5 of the patients were run on the phoneme-monitoring task alone as well as with the visual task. The mean percentage of 20 trial blocks in which their report of the number of phonemes detected was correct was 68% when performed alone and 36% when combined with the visual task. The 4 patients for whom no separate blocks of phoneme monitoring alone were collected had a mean detection rate of 70% in the dual-task blocks.

Figure 2 shows valid and invalid RTs for both divided and focused conditions for the two secondary tasks. The

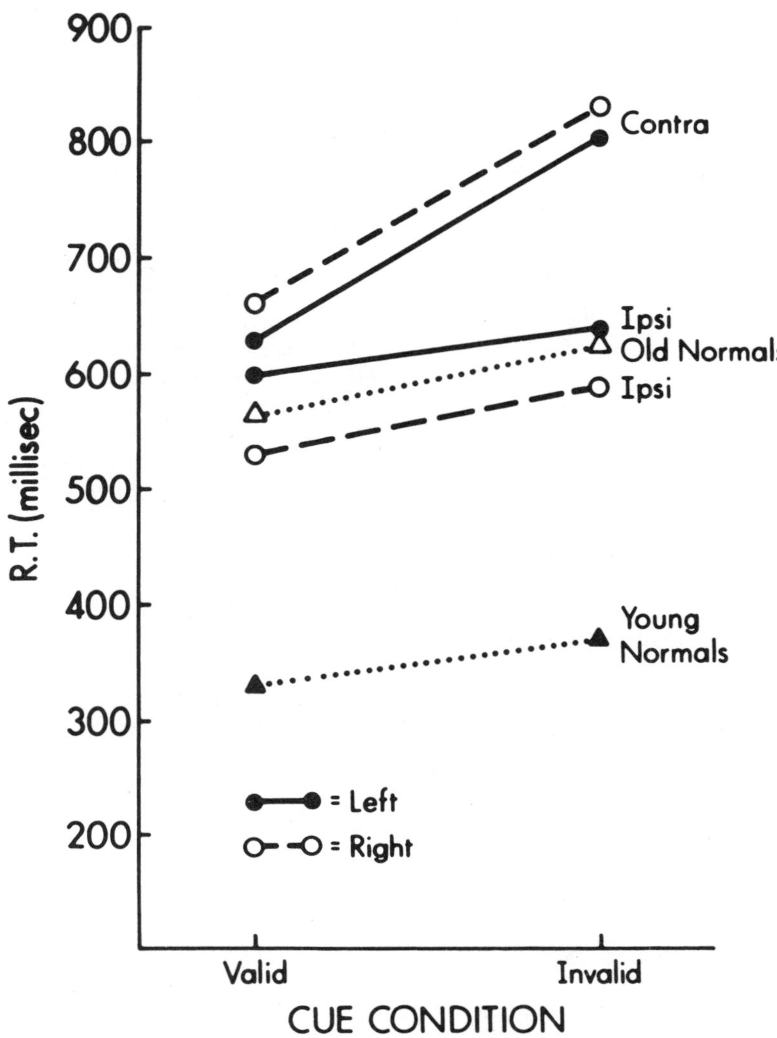

Figure 1. Mean RTs as a function of cue condition (valid vs. invalid) in the single task blocks of Experiment 1. Data are for young and old normal groups and for patients with right and with left parietal lesions. For the patient groups, the data are separated for targets on the side of the lesion (ipsilateral) and on the opposite side (contralateral).

top two lines are for the phoneme-monitoring task. It is clear that dividing attention had a powerful main effect on the spatial task RTs [$F(1,7) = 10.5$, $p < .01$]. Moreover, dividing attention clearly eliminated the validity effect. Valid and invalid RTs were essentially identical under divided-attention (phoneme) conditions. An identical effect was found for the counting task (lower two lines). Under divided-attention conditions, there was no difference between valid and invalid RTs. Only 5 patients were run on the counting task, so no statistical analysis was done.

Figure 2 gives data for the 100-msec delay condition for 9 patients studied in the phoneme-monitoring task. Phoneme monitoring was, however, the only place in which interval interacted significantly. There was a strong attention × cue × interval interaction (shown in Figure 3). Although dividing attention abolished the validity effect at 100 msec (see Figure 2), the effect was clearly present by 500 msec (see Figure 3). Thus divided attention delayed the ability of the patient to shift attention to the cue.

Normal subjects showed similar effects when attention was divided under some circumstances. Figure 4 shows the results for old and young normals in the phoneme-monitoring task (left panel) and for young normals in a previously reported study of counting backward by threes (Posner, Cohen, Choate, Hockey, & Maylor, 1984). In all cases, attention affected primary task performance. However, for phoneme monitoring, divided attention clearly had no effect on the size of the difference between valid and invalid trials. When we examine the backward-counting task (Figure 4, right panel) reported by Posner, Cohen, Choate, Hockey, and Maylor (1984), we find that

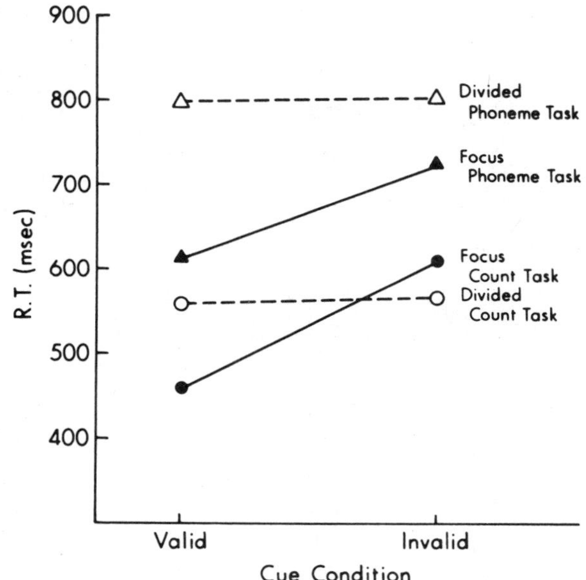

Figure 2. Mean RTs for valid and invalid trials for a spatial-attention task when performed alone (focus) and when done with two types of secondary tasks: monitoring for phonemes and counting backward.

divided attention had a much greater effect on raw RTs and its interaction with validity was of the same type as found in patients. Maylor (1985) examined the dual task of backward counting and visual orienting. She found that early in practice, counting backward eliminated the facilitation due to the cue; later in practice, however, the cue was effective. In another experiment in the same study, she showed that preparation of a saccadic eye movement eliminated the facilitation effect, although pursuit movements did not. These results seem to support the view that when the secondary task involves sufficient difficulty, there is interference with orienting toward the cue.

The results illustrated in Figures 2 and 4 show that under appropriate conditions, divided attention can delay the ability of the cue to draw attention sufficiently, so that neither normals nor patients show a validity effect at 100 msec. This suggests that the spatial orienting system must share some operations with the two secondary tasks, causing a delay in orienting when they are sufficiently difficult.

One might argue that patients use the cue normally under divided-attention conditions, but that no effect is found because the language task delays the keypress. This view would regard the cue effects as being lost because the delayed RT allows the subject to shift attention from cue to target without this attention shift's showing in RT. This view, however, cannot explain the presence of a validity effect in the longer delay trials shown in Figure 3. In this delayed condition RTs were longer due to the secondary task, but now a validity effect is clearly present. If the secondary task reduced the validity effect by delaying output in the 100-msec trials, one would expect a similar effect at longer intervals, since the overall delay in RT due to the dual task is still present. Instead, it appears that the longer intervals provided a differential advantage on valid trials, as one would predict if the secondary task retarded the ability to use the cue.

Why should patients not orient to the cue at the short intervals in the dual-task blocks? Clearly this must be due to the fact that they are engaged in processing the language task. If orienting to the secondary task uses the same parietal system as does visual-spatial orienting, the patients should have specific problems with invalid contralateral targets. Prediction of an extinction-like RT pattern at 100 msec follows both from the view that the patient has oriented to the cue but cannot respond because of the secondary task, and from the view that visual orienting has not taken place because the language task is engaging attention and uses the same parietal mechanism that is used for visual-spatial attention.

Table 1 shows the RTs for focused- and divided-attention conditions at 100 msec for valid and invalid targets in the ipsilateral and contralateral visual fields. Divided attention elevated RTs in all conditions except that of the contralateral invalid cue. According to our earlier theory, RTs in the contralateral invalid cue condition are inflated because damage to the parietal lobe interferes with disengaging from the visual cue when

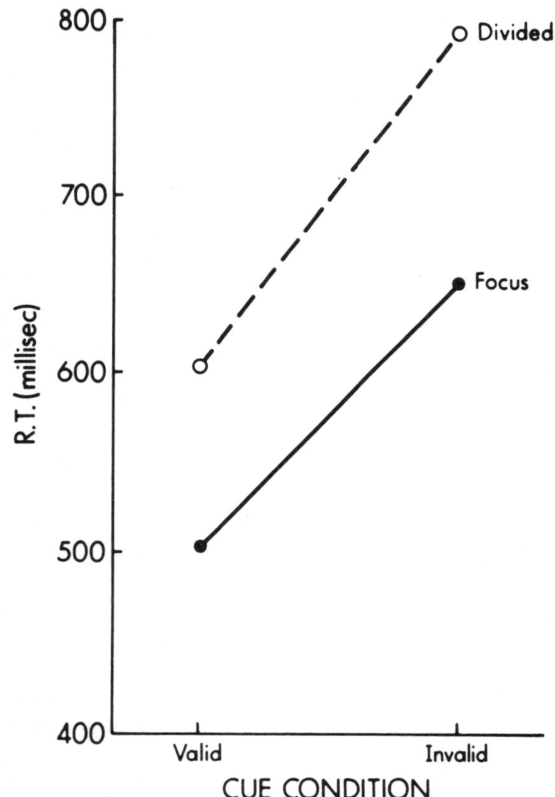

Figure 3. Mean RTs for patient groups with long delay trials (500 or 1,000 msec between cue and target) for both focused and divided blocks as a function of cue validity.

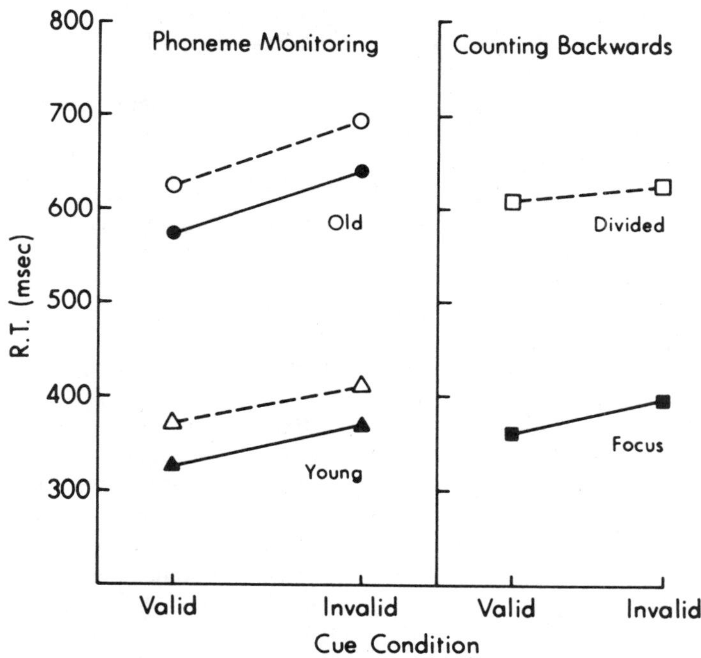

Figure 4. Mean RTs for young and old normals for spatial attention alone (solid lines) and dual task (dashed lines). Left panel involves phoneme monitoring as the secondary task. Right panel refers to data from Posner, Cohen, Choate, Hockey, and Maylor (1984) for counting backward by 3 as the secondary task.

contralateral targets are presented. If the language task prevents engaging the cue, it should also reduce the specific disadvantage for contralateral targets, provided that specific deficit does not also occur when the subject is engaged in a language task.

Divided attention eliminated the extinction-like RT pattern (contra visual field—ipsi visual field) for invalidly cued trials. This result is confirmed by a significant triple-order interaction between validity, attention, and visual field [$F(2,14) = 3.5$, $p < .01$]. The interaction for the 100-msec delay interval is shown in Figure 5. The figure shows that under focused-attention conditions, RTs were greatly lengthened for contralateral invalid trials (extinction-like RT pattern), but there is no evidence of this under divided-attention conditions.

Discussion

When the patient is engaged in a visual task, there is a specific deficit in the ability to disengage to handle a contralateral target. This result, which shows up clearly under the focused condition in Figure 5, confirms our previous work. This extinction-like RT pattern is a distinctive sign of parietal lesions. However, when the patient's attention is drawn to the language task (the divided-attention condition), the increase in RT to contralateral invalid trials goes away. Thus we conclude that engaging in the language task does not involve the parietal system that we have described for visual-spatial attention.

Table 2 shows the results obtained in the no-cue condition. First, the no-cue blocks generally gave faster RTs than did the valid trials for both normals and left-sided patients. Why should this be if, as we have argued, the advantage of valid over invalid trials is due to the presence of attention? Surely valid trials should be better than those without cues, particularly because cued trials allow for increased alerting as well as for the advantages of selective attention to the cued location.

At first we were very puzzled by these results; however, we have come to view them in light of the "emergent properties" argument (Duncan, 1980a). In a simple RT task, subjects often adopt a criterion of responding to any energy change. This works so long as there are no events to which they must inhibit a response. However, in the cued paradigm the subjects must withhold a response to the cue. Thus subjects could raise their response criteria for blocks in which there are cues over those in which

Table 1
Reaction Time as a Function of Validity and Visual Field

	Focused				Divided			
	Valid		Invalid		Valid		Invalid	
	Contra	Ipsi	Contra	Ipsi	Contra	Ipsi	Contra	Ipsi
	642	570	778	622	748	680	778	715
Contra-Ipsi	72		156		68		63	

Note—All data from 100-msec cue-to-target interval.

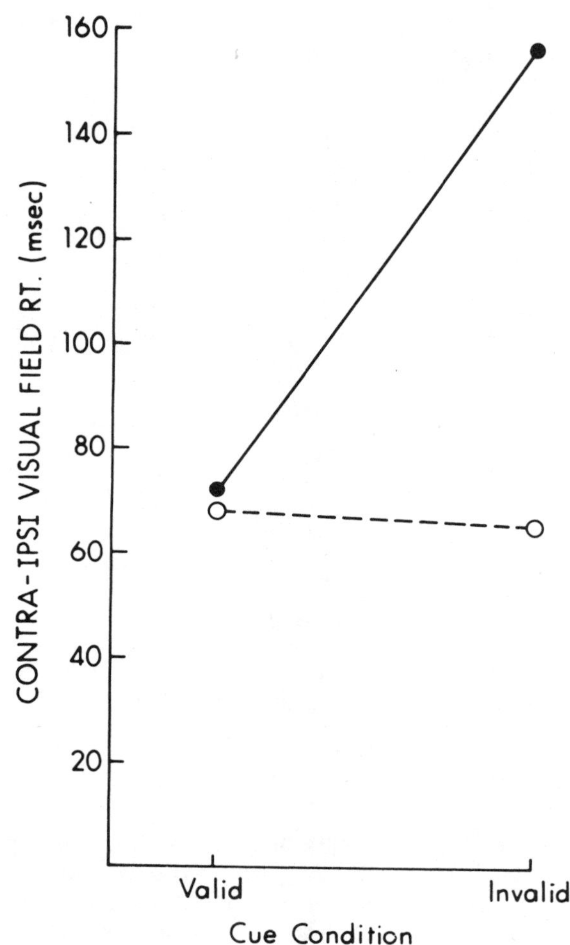

Figure 5. Magnitude of extinction-like reaction time pattern (contralateral minus ipsilateral reaction times) for single (focused; solid line) and dual (divided; dashed line) task blocks of Experiment 1. All data are at 100-msec cue-to-target interval.

no cues are given. We should be able to vary the relationship between valid-cue and no-cue trials, depending on whether they occur in mixed blocks, where a single criterion might be adopted, or in pure blocks, in which different criteria would be allowed.

The second dramatic result of the present experiment was the poor performance of right-sided patients in the no-cue condition. The performance of right-sided patients was clearly worse than that of normals and left-sided patients in the no-cue condition, although they performed virtually identically to the other groups on valid trials. Moreover, even in comparison with their own performance on valid trials, right-sided patients performed poorly in the no-cue condition. Heilman and Van Den Abell (1979) proposed that the right hemisphere is specialized for arousal. They argued that the hypoarousal resulting from damage to the right hemisphere causes patients with right parietal lesions to have more difficulty in spatial tasks than do left parietal patients. A recent theoretical revoew (Tucker & Williamson, 1984) has also supported the idea that the right hemisphere is more important than the left for arousal.

Our results suggest that left- and right-sided patients have equal problems with disengaging attention to deal with targets, but they raise the possibility that patients with right-sided lesions also have a special problem with maintaining alertness.[1] This idea is based on the supposition that, since no-cue trials do not provide a warning, the subjects must act to maintain a high level of alertness if they are to sustain fast RTs. If they fail to do so, their performance will suffer in the no-cue condition. If patients with right-sided lesions have difficulty in maintaining their alertness without a warning, their performance would be at a special disadvantage in this condition.

Experiment 2 concerned the degree of separation between the alerting or arousal produced by the cue and the cue's ability to direct attention to the cued location. In many cognitive theories these are seen as separate aspects of attention. The data shown in Table 2 suggest that the omission of a cue selectively increases RTs for patients with right-sided lesions. These patients do not differ from left-sided patients in the ability of the cue to direct attention (invalid—valid RTs). Thus if we are correct in conjecturing that the performance in the no-cue condition is due to normal subjects' adopting a low criterion in pure no-cue blocks, we could then attribute the performance of right-hemisphere lesioned patients to a specific deficit in alertness that appears quite separate from the deficit found in the ability of the cue to direct attention.

EXPERIMENT 2

To test our conjecture about the nature of the data provided by the no-cue condition, we designed an additional set of experiments with young normal subjects. In Experiment 2a we tested the idea that the relative speed of responding for blocks of cued trials and for blocks of no-cue trials depended on the subject's level of alertness. We compared blocks of trials in which the time between trials was 500 msec (nearly optimal for alertness) with trials with intervals of 5,000 msec (a suboptimal interval for maintaining alertness). Sanders (1977) showed that long foreperiods produce suboptimal alerting, which has much greater effects for visual than for auditory signals.

In Experiment 2b we tested the idea that the advantage of no-cue over valid trials depended on subjects' adopting a low criterion during no-cue blocks. We did this by comparing blocks in which no-cue and cued trials were randomized so that no special criterion could be chosen

Table 2
Mean Reaction Time (in Milliseconds) for No-Cue Blocks Under Focused Task Conditions

Parietal Patients				Normals	
Right		Left		Old	Young
Contra	Ipsi	Contra	Ipsi	Both	Both
820	525	470	430	405	240

for the no-cue trials with pure blocks in which only no-cue or only cued trials were given.

Method

In Experiment 2a, 12 young normal subjects were run for 2 h. Four pure blocks were used. For two of the blocks the time between trials was 500 msec; for the other two, it was 5,000 msec. Within each delay condition, one block consisted of no-cue trials in which only a target was presented, and the other block consisted of cued trials (80% valid and 20% invalid) in which the target followed the cue equally often after 100 and 900 msec. Each block had 100 trials.

In Experiment 2b, 10 young normal subjects were run in a single 1-h session. The experiment was similar to Experiment 2a except that each subject ran in two mixed blocks of 160 trials. Within each mixed block, there were 96 cued trials (50% valid) and 64 uncued trials. One mixed block was run with a 500-msec intertrial interval (ITI) (high alertness) and one with a 5,000-msec ITI (low alertness).

Results

The results of Experiment 2a are shown in Figure 6. The pattern of results in the high-alertness condition was quite similar to that found with normal subjects and left-sided patients in Experiment 1. RTs were fastest in the no-cue condition, intermediate in the valid-cue condition, and slowest in the invalid-cue condition. The low-alertness condition showed a pattern much more like that of the right-sided patients in Experiment 1. The valid trials were slightly faster than the no-cue condition, with the invalid-cue trials the slowest.

A statistical analysis of the overall data showed significant effects of ITI [$F(1,11) = 6.2, p < .05$], of validity [$F(2,22) = 11.1, p < .01$], of cue-to-target interval [$F(1,11) = 67.1, p < .01$], of the interaction of validity with cue-to-target interval [$F(1,11) = 17.8, p < .01$], and of the triple-order interaction of ITI and validity with cue-to-target interval [$F(2,22) = 3.4, p < .01$].

The interaction between ITI (alertness) and validity shown in Figure 6 was present at both cue-to-target intervals, but was stronger with the 900-msec interval. This is mainly because the no-cue trials showed a smaller improvement with interval than did the cued trials, since there was no cue to mark the start of the trial. Figure 6 makes it appear that alertness effects were present for both no-cue and invalid trials. In fact, although 11 of the 12 subjects had longer RTs in the low-alertness, no-cue condition than in the high-alertness, no-cue condition, only

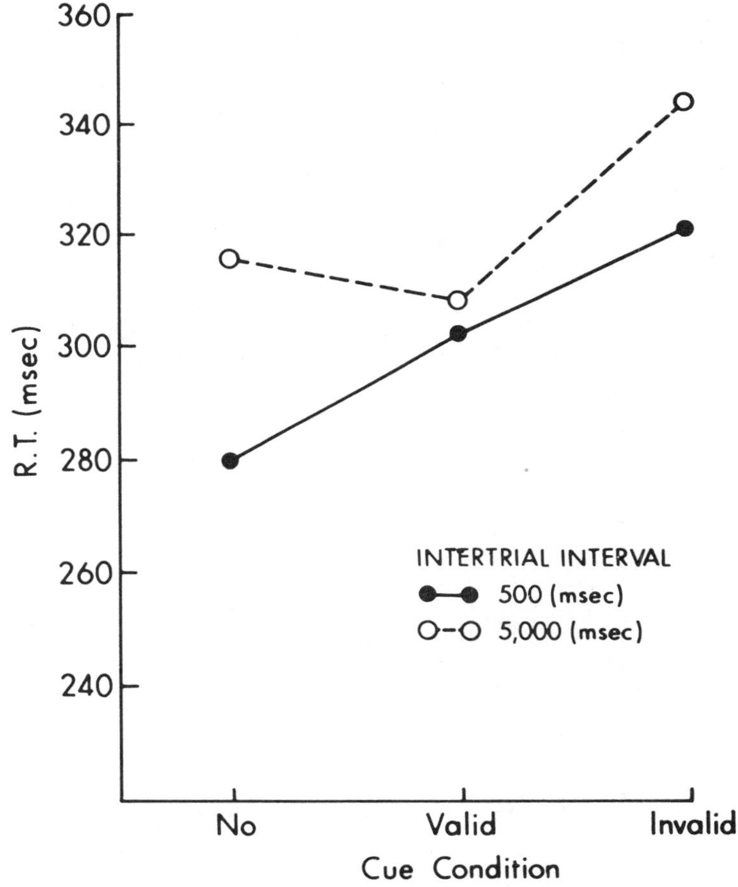

Figure 6. RTs as a function of cue conditions for pure blocks of cued or uncued trials conducted with long (5,000-msec) or optimal (500-msec) intertrial intervals (Experiment 2a).

7 of the 12 showed an alertness advantage for invalid trials. Thus, subjects appeared to compensate for the suboptimal warning interval quite well in a pure block of cued trials, but not in a pure block of uncued trials.

The results of Experiment 2b are shown in Figure 7. In this experiment, ITI, cue-to-target interval, and cue condition all had significant effects. There was also a cue × interval interaction due to the large improvement in RTs when a cue was present ($p < .01$). In both alertness conditions, the valid trials had an advantage over the invalid and no-cue trials. This advantage occurred despite the 50% validity used in the experiment. The no-cue trials had somewhat longer RTs than did the invalid trials, particularly in the low-alertness condition. In comparing the two experiments, it is clear that mixing the block produced a specific disadvantage for the no-cue trials.

Discussion

These results illustrate the complexity of events that occur even under the relatively simple conditions of Experiment 1. Apparently, the RT to a cued event depends in part on the warning properties the cue provides, in part on the location information provided by the cue, and in part on the inhibition produced by raising the criterion set by subjects in order to resist responding to the cue. By comparing valid with invalid trials in mixed blocks, one can hold the alertness and criterion effects relatively constant to compare the directional effect of the cue.

Experiments 2a and 2b generally confirm our conjecture that the advantage of uncued trials for normal subjects in Experiment 1 results from the subjects' adopting a lower criterion for these blocks. Apparently this is done based on the property of the block and not, or at least not as much, on a trial-by-trial basis. This conclusion follows from our finding that, in mixed blocks, performance was much worse on no-cue trials than on valid trials. The results also suggest that right-sided patients have difficulty in maintaining a high enough level of alertness to perform well when a warning signal is absent. Put another way, patients with right-side lesions fail to lower their criterion for no-cue blocks. Since alertness effects usually result in changes in criterion, these two statements may be equivalent. Our results with normal subjects suggest that a failure to maintain alertness would account for the

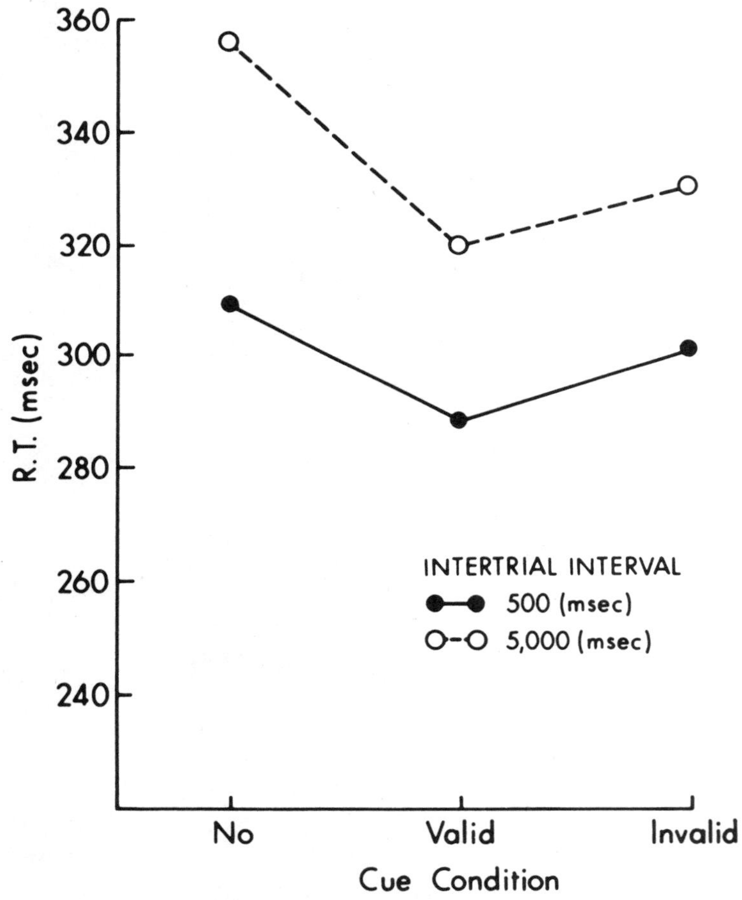

Figure 7. RTs as a function of cue conditions for blocks of mixed cue and no-cue trials with long (5,000-msec) and optimal (500-msec) intertrial intervals (Experiment 2b).

poor performance of right-sided subjects in the no-cue trials, since their performance resembles that of normals at a lowered level of alerting induced by a suboptimal ITI.

It is also possible to ask whether normals show any differences in alerting when cues are presented directly to the right hemisphere. Heilman and Van Den Abell (1979) suggested that cues delivered to the right hemisphere from the left visual field would result in faster RTs than those found when cues go directly to the left hemisphere. Figure 8 shows RTs from Experiment 2b as a function of which hemisphere first received the target or cue. The lower two curves are for high-alertness conditions; the upper two are for low-alertness conditions. When no cue was provided, the subjects had only the time from the last keypress as the mark of the start of a trial. For cued trials we plotted only valid trials where both cue and target went directly to the same hemisphere. The ANOVA for this breakdown shows that the only significant effects were those of alertness and warning interval. There was a small but nonsignificant trend for performance on the left-hemisphere targets to be better than that on right-hemisphere targets under the high-alertness conditions. This trend is in the opposite direction from what would be predicted from a right-hemisphere advantage for alerting. There is no hint that the alerting functions differ for the two hemispheres. Thus, although our patient evidence suggests that right-hemisphere damage reduces the ability to maintain alertness, we are not able to confirm that this effect can be found in normals by varying the location of the warning cue.

CONCLUSIONS

Parietal Deficit

The present experiments confirm previous findings concerning the visual-spatial attention system (Baynes, Holtzman, & Volpe, 1986; Morrow & Ratcliff, 1987; Posner, Walker, Friedrich, & Rafal, 1984). When the attention of patients with parietal lesions is summoned to a visual cue, they have a powerful deficit in handling contralateral targets. When attention is at the cued location or when the target is ipsilateral to the lesion, patients show only a small deficit, if any, over the performance of age-related controls. This supports our finding that parietal lesions are specific to the ability to disengage from a stimulus once attention has been committed.

The present study suggests that the right and left parietal lobes are symmetric for the disengage operations, because the advantage of valid over invalid trials is similar for the two groups. Morrow and Ratcliff (1987) used our task and found similar results for right-parietal patients, but little evidence for an overall deficit for left-parietal

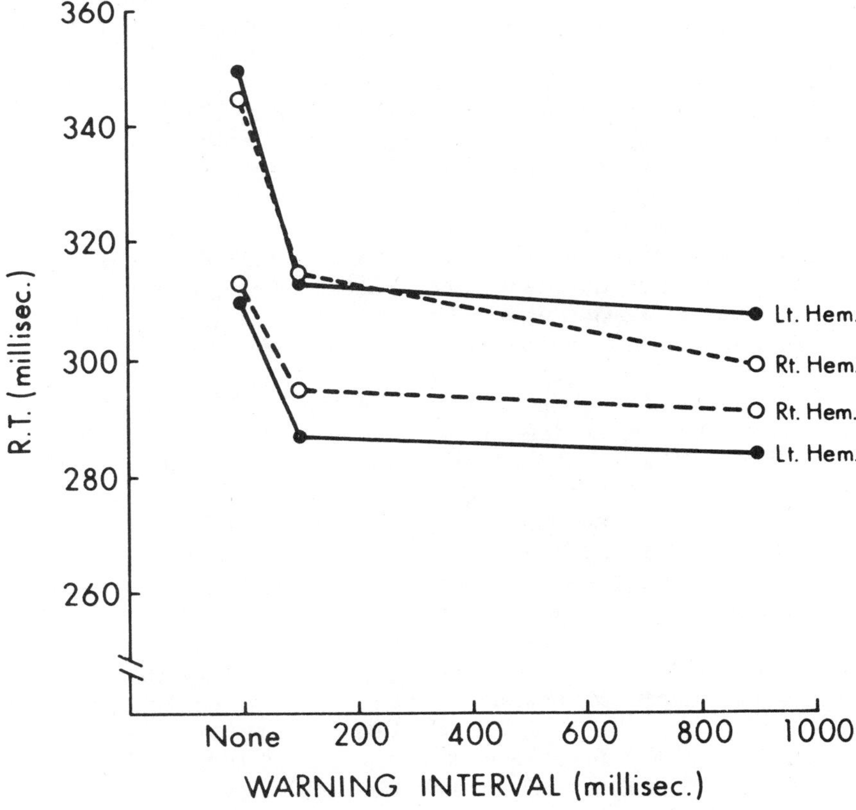

Figure 8. Warning signal function for trials in which the cue or target is presented to the left visual field (right hemisphere) and those for which they are presented to the right visual field (left hemisphere). Data are from no-cue and valid trials of Experiment 2b.

patients. Indeed, in our previous work we also found a weaker effect in left- than in right-parietal patients.[2] It is well known in clinical neurology that right-parietal patients often show more evidence of neglect than do left-parietal patients (DeRenzi, 1982). However, our data from the no-block trials indicate that the difference between the two groups may lie not in the directionally specific effect of the cut but in its arousal effect (see Alerting, below). Morrow and Ratcliff also found a right-frontal patient who had a disengage deficit. Rafal (1987) presented two frontal patients who showed an orienting deficit, but of a kind different from that found in parietal patients. These results suggest that frontal areas may also play an important role in orienting under some circumstances. It is known that elements of neglect can result from frontal lesions (DeRenzi, 1982). We suggest below that frontal areas may be important in the more general functions of attention common to both spatial orienting and language control.

Is Spatial Attention an Independent Module?

Visual-spatial attention is one form of selectivity by which information reaches neural systems responsible for conscious report. The parietal damage must involve only a pathway toward conscious report. This is established by the relatively intact performance of parietal patients on valid trials even to targets whose location is contralateral to the lesion. Thus some systems can compensate for the relative inefficiency of the damaged parietal lobe, which argues that higher level attentional systems must be intact.

How does this visual-attention pathway relate to pathways involved in dealing with other aspects of attention? Experiment 1 shows that processing language stimuli (phoneme monitoring or counting backward) delays orienting to the spatial cue. Since the act of orienting requires no overt movement that might interact with the secondary task, it seems reasonable to suppose that attending to nonspatial stimuli interferes directly with the system that shifts visual attention. We know from other work on interference effects (Posner, 1978) that tasks such as counting backward or phoneme monitoring also interfere with most other types of cognitive operations. Moreover, this interference is quite time locked. It is not that the secondary task completely inhibits the attention shift; it simply delays it so that what is usually quite strong at 100 msec is no longer present at that time. In addition, performance on the secondary task suffers from competition from the primary attention-shifting task. These properties suggest that there is a common command system needed both to issue commands that produce spatial orienting and for some aspects of monitoring (e.g., incrementing the count when a target occurs) (Duncan, 1980b).

If one accepts the interference effects found in our patients during the visual-spatial orienting task as evidence for a common attention system, what can we say about this system? Our main finding is that the anatomy of the common system must be different from that of the visual-spatial pathway, because engaging the subject in a language task produces no specific deficit for targets contralateral to the lesion. Since it appears that damage to the parietal lobe manifests itself in a specific deficit in disengaging to deal with contralateral targets, it follows that engaging attention to the language task must not involve the parietal mechanism involved in visual-spatial attention.

In short, our evidence favors two distinct neural systems: a specific visual-spatial system that involves the parietal lobe, and a more general system common to both visual-spatial and language attention. It seems likely that the more general system operates as a command system to allow orienting of visual-spatial or other forms of attention. Since we know that failure of the visual-spatial system means that the patient will be unaware of the target, this second system could be responsible for the specific operations underlying our ability to report the stimulus subjectively.

From previous work in cognitive psychology (Marcel, 1983), it appears that under some conditions a visual stimulus is processed quite deeply, including the production of semantic activation without the subject's being aware of the stimulus. In anatomical terms, this suggests that a good deal of processing by posterior areas of the brain can occur without the subject's being conscious of the event.

It is possible only to speculate on the anatomical basis of the systems common to visual-spatial attention and attention to language. The parietal lobe is closely connected anatomically to areas of the frontal lobe, both on the lateral surface (the dorsolateral prefrontal cortex; Schwartz & Goldman-Rakic, 1982) and on the medial surface (e.g., the supplementary motor area). In recent studies using positron emission tomography to study regional cerebral blood flow, the supplementary motor area has been found to be active in tasks that involve attention to language (Petersen, Fox, Posner, Mintun, & Raichle, 1987) and in tasks that involve overt eye movements during visual processing and imagery (Fox, Fox, & Raichle, 1985; Roland, 1985).

Alerting

How do the results concerning alerting fit into the operation of selective systems? First, our experiments show that alerting effects are quite independent of the direction of attention. This view arose first from experiments performed many years ago in which primes and warning signals were shown to have additive effects on improvement in RTs (Posner & Boies, 1971). At that time it was pointed out that the source of alerting effects was likely to be subcortical arousal systems, since EEG evidence of alerting was found in both hemispheres of split-brain monkeys even when the signal went only to one hemisphere (Gazzaniga & Hillyard, 1973). These subcortical systems seem to influence stimulus processing by acting on a higher level attention system rather than on input pathways (Posner, 1975). This argument was based on evidence favoring a criterion shift because increased error rates usually accompany faster RTs following warning signals.

The present data extend this view by showing that patients with right-side lesions have special difficulty in maintaining a high level of alertness during a brief delay between trials. This difficulty does not affect their ability to use warning signals or their ability to shift attention in the cued direction.

According to our earlier argument (Posner, 1978), deficits in alerting affect higher level attention systems, rather than the activation of pathways by which information is accumulated. In terms of our present argument, they would affect the frontal attention-command system rather than, or more strongly than, the posterior visual-spatial attention system. In consequence, deficits in alerting would retard the commands needed to activate the posterior system. Such poorly maintained alerting in the absence of specific cues might explain why right-parietal patients show a deficit in performance in natural and clinical situations. In accord with this possibility, recent evidence suggests that the right hemisphere may be more closely involved in the arousal of cortex by norepinephrine and serotonin than is the left hemisphere (Tucker & Williamson, 1984).

Hierarchical Distributed Network

Figure 9 illustrates the view of covert orienting under dual-task conditions that appears to be consistent with our data. The top of the figure shows the task events. Each rectangle in the lower part of the figure contains the mental operations involved in the performance of the task. The last four operations have been discussed in some detail in our previous work on visual orienting (Posner, Walker, Friedrich, & Rafal, 1984). When a cue arrives, the subject's attention is disengaged from its current location. We have shown that damage to the posterior parietal lobe selectively interferes with this operation, which suggests that the parietal lobe is a necessary structure for performing it. Attention is then moved to the location of the cue. We have shown that the speed of moving attention to a cued location is slowed by damage to the midbrain (Posner et al., 1985). We assume, then, that attention must engage the location of the target to generate the arbitrary detection response required by the task (Posner, 1980). When attention is drawn to a location by a cue and is subsequently withdrawn, there is a long-lasting inhibitory effect at the cued location, which we have called *inhibition of return* (Maylor, 1985; Posner & Cohen, 1984).

This paper concerns the three mental operations indicated at the top of Figure 9, namely, alert, interrupt, and localize. The first, we assume, is a general effect of the cue. It is well known that any event that can be used as a warning signal produces a negative shift in the EEG (Donchin, 1984). This negative shift, called the *contingent negative variation* (CNV), is the brain sign most closely associated with a general alerting function. It is thought to involve the reticular activation system and to operate first on prefrontal sites and then move backward over the scalp, the exact details depending on the task to be performed. The frontal distribution to the CNV makes this sign attractive as the basis for interrupting the ongoing language processing in which our subjects are engaged in the dual-task conditions. On the basis of the close anatomical connections of prefrontal cortex to both parietal and language areas and to the cortical origin of the CNV, we speculate that prefrontal cortex is the common site of interference between the language and spatial attention tasks. Because the subjects engaged in the language task showed retarded orienting toward the cue, we believe that an interruption of the ongoing language task must be a necessary condition to produce the four operations listed at the bottom of the figure. In this sense, the system involved in the interrupt operation is in command of the posterior systems involved in the final four operations.

The localize operation is necessary for the coordinates of the cue to direct the covert shift of attention. A model for this operation was described by Koch and Ullman (1985), who assumed that it involves areas of primary visual cortex that must also be directly activated by the

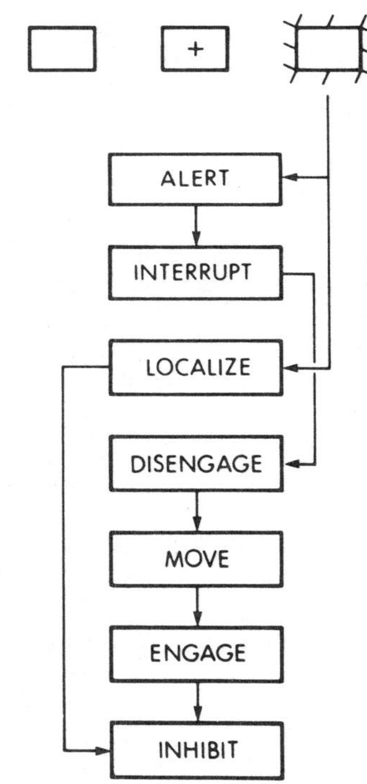

Figure 9. An overview of the hierarchy of attention involved in the covert orienting task described in this paper. The presentation of the cue produces a change in alertness thought to operate via reticular activating system on frontal sites. Alerting can be used to interrupt the current attended activity, which, in our dual-task conditions, is attending to phoneme monitoring. The cue also provides information about its location. Once ongoing language processing is interrupted, the posterior parietal lobe acts to disengage attention from its current focus and move it to the location of the cue. The cue is also known to set up an inhibition of return that leads to slower performance to events at the cued location once attention has been withdrawn (Posner, Choate, Rafal, & Vaughan, 1985).

cue. Koch and Ullman also described how the process of localizing the cue might lead naturally to the inhibition of return.

Mesulam (1981) attempted to distinguish among several views of the way in which brain systems function to control spatial attention. He called these general views *center theories*, *network theories*, and *holistic theories*. The center theory regards spatial attention as the single system. The network theory views components of the function as assigned to quite distinct neural systems. The holistic theory regards attention as a general property of the brain. The data reviewed by Mesulam favor a network theory. Our data also support a network approach. The anatomical separation between the visual-spatial attention system and the higher level common system argues against a single center, and the degree of anatomical specificity found for visual-spatial attention argues against any holistic view. However, our findings suggest two additions to the network view.

First, we try to specify the components of covert orienting of spatial attention (see Figure 9). In this sense, our viewpoint is cognitive as well as anatomical. This is quite similar to what has been done by Kosslyn (1980) for visual imaging. Indeed, some of the operations in covert visual attention may be the same as those used in scanning visual images. It is also in the spirit of recent work in imagery to attempt to relate the mental operations posited by the model to the neural systems that support them (Farah, 1984). In this sense our approach is also anatomical.

Our results favor a second modification of Mesulam's network theory. This modification might be called a *hierarchical network*. We find that some neural systems related to attention seem to coordinate or to control the action of other systems. Thus within the visual-spatial system, the parietal mechanism must act to disengage attention prior to its being moved to the target. The midbrain centers shown to affect the move operation would have to be controlled by the operation of the cortical centers responsible for the disengage operation. Similarly, it appears that the posterior areas responsible for spatial orienting as a whole are controlled by a higher level frontal system.

We believe that the hierarchical network viewpoint is very much in accord with the general spirit of findings in both neurophysiology and cognitive psychology. Neurophysiology often views the operation of higher centers as acting to tonically inhibit lower systems and, through feed-forward mechanisms, to produce phasic potentiation of activity (Mountcastle, 1978). In cognitive psychology, central-attention theories offer a necessary means of coordination among a number of semi-independent codes that are activated by input (Keele & Neil, 1978; Posner, 1978; Treisman & Gelade, 1980).

There are selection mechanisms within each sensory system (Hillyard & Kutas, 1983; Näätänen, 1982) that serve to gate some information and to potentiate other information sources. At the level of the cortex, information from different sensory systems (e.g., vision and audition) must be integrated when it relates to the same cognitive system (e.g., spatial attention, object identification, language). Indeed, Posner and Henik (1983) compared the effectiveness of stimuli in producing mutual interference and facilitation when both were within the same modality (e.g., vision) but in different cognitive systems (e.g., spatial vs. language), and when they were within the same cognitive system (e.g., language) but in different modalities (e.g., vision vs. audition). Our results show that, at least under the conditions of our test, stimuli within the same cognitive system produce more mutual interaction than those that share only input modality. This point argues for a level of selection that integrates separate sensory systems.

It seems reasonable to suppose that stimuli in different cognitive systems (e.g., language and spatial location) must be coordinated at some level. The results of the present study show that the principle of distributed but hierarchical networks can be applied to this problem. Although the disengage operation can be specific to a mechanism within a cognitive system (e.g., visual-spatial attention), it also appears that more general systems are required to permit selection when more than one cognitive system is involved. We find that when a subject is engaged in a language operation, there is a clear reduction in efficiency of spatial orienting. The hierarchical network idea allows us to see why damage to a particular location in the central nervous system produces a deficit in operations specific to one cognitive system (e.g., spatial orienting or language), whereas damage to other locations may produce more widespread attentional deficits that are not specific to any cognitive system.

REFERENCES

Bashinski, H. S., & Bachrach, V. R. (1980). Enhancement of perceptual sensitivity as the result of selectively attending to spatial locations. *Perception & Psychophysics*, **28**, 241-248.

Baynes, K., Holtzman, J. D., & Volpe, B. T. (1986). Components of visual attention: Alterations in response pattern to visual stimuli following parietal lobe infarction. *Brain*, **109**, 99-114.

DeRenzi, E. (1982). *Disorders of space exploration and cognition*. New York: Wiley.

Donchin, E. (1984). Report of Panel III: Preparatory Processes. In E. Donchin (Ed.), *Cognitive psychophysiology* (pp. 179-219). Hillsdale, NJ: Erlbaum.

Downing, C. J., & Pinker, S. (1985). The spatial structure of visual attention. In M. I. Posner & O. S. M. Marin (Eds.), *Attention and performance XI* (pp. 171-188). Hillsdale, NJ: Erlbaum.

Duncan, J. (1980a). The demonstration of capacity limitation. *Cognitive Psychology*, **12**, 75-96.

Duncan, J. (1980b). The locus of interference in the perception of simultaneous stimuli. *Psychological Review*, **87**, 272-300.

Farah, M. J. (1984). The neurological basis of mental imagery: A componential analysis. *Cognition*, **18**, 245-272.

Fox, P. T., Fox, J. M., & Raichle, M. E. (1985). The role of cerebral cortex in the generation of voluntary saccades: A positron-emission tomographic study. *Journal of Neurophysiology*, **54**, 348-369.

Gazzaniga, M., & Hillyard, S. A. (1973). Attention mechanisms following brain bisection. In S. Kornblum (Ed.), *Attention and performance IV* (pp. 221-237). New York: Academic Press.

HEILMAN, K. M., & VAN DEN ABELL, T. (1979). Right hemisphere dominance for mediating cerebral activation. *Neuropsychologia*, **17**, 315-321.

HILLYARD, H. C., & KUTAS, M. (1983). Electrophysiology of cognitive processes. *Annual Review of Psychology*, **34**, 33-61.

HUGHES, H. C., & ZIMBA, L. D. (1985). Spatial maps of directed visual attention. *Journal of Experimental Psychology: Human Perception & Performance*, **11**, 409-430.

JONIDES, J. P. (1981). Voluntary versus automatic control over the mind's eye. In J. Long & A. Baddeley (Eds.), *Attention and performance IX* (pp. 187-204). Hillsdale, NJ: Erlbaum.

KEELE, S. W., & NEIL, W. T. (1978). Mechanisms of attention. In E. C. Carterette (Ed.), *Handbook of perception* (Vol. 9, pp. 3-47). New York: Academic Press.

KERR, B. (1973). Processing demands during mental operations. *Memory & Cognition*, **1**, 401-412.

KOCH, C., & ULLMAN, S. (1985). Selective visual attention: Towards the underlying neural circuitry. *Human Neurobiology*, **4**, 219-227.

KOSSLYN, S. W. (1980). *Image and mind*. Cambridge, MA: Harvard University Press.

LABERGE, D. L. (1973). Identification of two components of the time to switch attention. In S. Kornblum (Ed.), *Attention and performance IV* (pp. 71-85). New York: Academic Press.

LANSMAN, M., FARR, S., & HUNT, E. (1984). Expectancy and dual task of interference. *Journal of Experimental Psychology: Human Perception & Performance*, **10**, 195-204.

MARCEL, A. J. (1983). Conscious and unconscious perception: Experiments on visual masking and word recognition. *Cognitive Psychology*, **15**, 197-237.

MAYLOR, E. A. (1985). Facilitatory and inhibitory components of orienting in visual space. In M. I. Posner & O. S. M. Marin (Eds.), *Attention and performance XI* (pp. 189-289). Hillsdale, NJ: Erlbaum.

MESULAM, M. M. (1981). A cortical network for directed attention and unilateral neglect. *Annals of Neurology*, **10**, 309-325.

MORROW, L. A., & RATCLIFF, G. G. (1987). Attentional mechanisms of clinical neglect. *Journal of Clinical & Experimental Neuropsychology*, **9**, 74-75.

MOUNTCASTLE, V. B. (1978). Brain mechanisms for directed attention. *Journal of the Royal Society of Medicine*, **71**, 14-27.

NÄÄTÄNEN, R. (1982). Processing negativity: An event related potential reflection of selective attention. *Psychological Bulletin*, **92**, 605-640.

PETERSEN, S. E., FOX, P. T., POSNER, M. I., MINTUN, M. A., & RAICHLE, M. E. (1987). Focal brain activity during visual language tasks are measured with averaged PET images of evoked CBF change. *Society for Neuroscience Abstracts*, **12**, 1261.

PINKER, S. (1980). Mental imagery and the third dimension. *Journal of Experimental Psychology: General*, **109**, 354-371.

POSNER, M. I. (1975). Psychobiology of attention. In M. Gazzaniga & C. Blakemore (Eds.), *Handbook of psychobiology* (pp. 441-480). New York: Academic Press.

POSNER, M. I. (1978). *Chronometric explorations of mind*. Hillsdale, NJ: Erlbaum.

POSNER, M. I. (1980). Orienting of attention. *Quarterly Journal of Experimental Psychology*, **32**, 3-25.

POSNER, M. I., & BOIES, S. J. (1971). Components of attention. *Psychological Review*, **78**, 391-408.

POSNER, M. I., CHOATE, L., RAFAL, R. D., & VAUGHAN, J. (1985). Inhibition of return: Neural mechanisms and function. *Cognitive Neuropsychology*, **2**, 211-228.

POSNER, M. I., & COHEN, Y. (1984). Components of visual orienting. In H. Bouma & D. G. Bowhuis (Eds.), *Attention and performance X* (pp. 531-556). Hillsdale, NJ: Erlbaum.

POSNER, M. I., COHEN, Y., CHOATE, L., HOCKEY, R., & MAYLOR, E. (1984). Sustained concentration: Passive filtering or active orienting. In S. Kornblum & J. Requin (Eds.), *Preparatory states and processes* (pp.49-65). Hillsdale, NJ: Erlbaum.

POSNER, M. I., COHEN, Y., & RAFAL, R. D. (1982). Neural systems control of spatial orienting. *Proceedings of the Royal Society of London B*, **298**, 187-198.

POSNER, M. I., & HENIK, A. (1983). Isolating representational systems. In J. Beck, B. Hope, & A. Rosenfeld (Eds.), *Human and machine vision* (pp. 395-412). New York: Academic Press.

POSNER, M. I., WALKER, J. A., FRIEDRICH, F. J., & RAFAL, R. D. (1984). Effects of parietal lobe injury on covert orienting of visual attention. *Journal of Neuroscience*, **4**, 1863-1874.

RAFAL, R. D. (1987). Frontal lobe lesions slow the movement of visual attention. *Neurology*, **37**(Suppl. 1), 128.

REMINGTON, R., & PIERCE, L. (1984). Moving attention and evidence for time-invariant shifts of visual selective attention. *Perception & Psychophysics*, **35**, 393-399.

ROLAND, P. E. (1985). Cortical organization of voluntary behavior in man. *Human Neurobiology*, **4**, 155-167.

SANDERS, A. (1977). Structural and functional aspects of the reaction process. In S. Dornic (Ed.), *Attention and performance VI* (pp. 3-25). Hillsdale, NJ: Erlbaum.

SCHWARTZ, M. L., & GOLDMAN-RAKIC, P. S. (1982). Single cortical neurons have axon colaterals to ipsilateral and contralateral cortex in fetal and adult primates. *Nature*, **299**, 154-156.

SHAW, M. L. (1984). Division of attention among spatial locations. In H. Bouma & D. G. Bouwhuis (Eds.), *Attention and performance X* (pp. 109-124). Hillsdale, NJ: Erlbaum.

SHEPARD, R. N. (1978). The mental image. *American Psychologist*, **33**, 125-137.

SHULMAN, G. L., REMINGTON, R., & MCLEAN, J. P. (1979). Moving attention through visual space. *Journal of Experimental Psychology: Human Perception & Performance*, **5**, 522-526.

TREISMAN, A. M., & GELADE, P. A. (1980). A feature integration theory of attention. *Cognitive Psychology*, **12**, 97-136.

TSAL, Y. (1983). Movements of attention across the visual field. *Journal of Experimental Psychology: Human Perception & Performance*, **9**, 523-530.

TUCKER, P. M., & WILLIAMSON, P. A. (1984). Asymmetric neural control in human self-regulation. *Psychological Review*, **91**, 185-215.

ULLMAN, S. (1984). Visual routines. *Cognition*, **18**, 97-159.

WURTZ, R. H., GOLDBERG, M. E., & ROBINSON, D. L. (1980). Behavioral modulation of visual responses in monkey. *Progress in Psychobiology & Physiological Psychology*, **9**, 42-83.

NOTES

1. Criterion bias has been widely discussed in signal detection theories of attention (Shaw, 1984). In our view, attention might work through a criterion shift or through a change in d'. Indeed, in a multilevel system a bias at one level may be a sensitivity change at some other level. Alertness seems to involve a criterion shift in that it does not affect the rate of information gained from a cue, but only the response of some other system. It is the goal of this study to find out something about the nature of that other system. If patients with lesions of the right hemisphere have a problem in adopting a lowered criterion in no-cue blocks, that would be one sort of constraint on the system involved in establishing the criterion. Elsewhere (Posner & Cohen, 1984) we have discussed other constraints on the kind of criteria that may relate to attention shifts.

2. One has to be cautious about comparisons between small groups of left- and right-lesioned patients. The similarity of the RTs for valid and invalid trials in Figure 1 is quite striking. Moreover, in a previously reported study (Posner, Walker, Friedrich, & Rafal, 1984) we found no significant differences between left- and right-lesioned patients even when we tried to equate lesion size. However, we cannot dismiss the possibility that differences in lesions mask a difference between left- and right-lesioned patients. However, the massive difference between groups in the no-cue conditions suggests that whatever is being measured in that condition is a far more important difference than that found for the attention shift as measured by the difference between valid and invalid trials.

24

M.-M. Mesulam

A cortical network for directed attention and unilateral neglect

1981. *Annals of Neurology* 10: 309–325

Unilateral neglect reflects a disturbance in the spatial distribution of directed attention. A review of unilateral neglect syndromes in monkeys and humans suggests that four cerebral regions provide an integrated network for the modulation of directed attention within extrapersonal space. Each component region has a unique functional role that reflects its profile of anatomical connectivity, and each gives rise to a different clinical type of unilateral neglect when damaged. A posterior parietal component provides an internal sensory map and perhaps also a mechanism for modifying the extent of synaptic space devoted to specific portions of the external world; a limbic component in the cingulate gyrus regulates the spatial distribution of motivational valence; a frontal component coordinates the motor programs for exploration, scanning, reaching, and fixating; and a reticular component provides the underlying level of arousal and vigilance. This hypothetical network requires at least three complementary and interacting representations of extrapersonal space: a sensory representation in posterior parietal cortex, a schema for distributing exploratory movements in frontal cortex, and a motivational map in the cingulate cortex. Lesions in only one component of this network yield partial unilateral neglect syndromes, while those that encompass all the components result in profound deficits that transcend the mass effect of the larger lesion. This network approach to the localization of complex functions offers an alternative to more extreme approaches, some of which stress an exclusive concentration of function within individual centers in the brain and others which advocate a more uniform (equipotential or holistic) distribution.

In human beings, unilateral neglect syndromes are more frequent and severe after lesions in the right hemisphere. Also, right hemisphere mechanisms appear more effective in the execution of attentional tasks. Furthermore, the attentional functions of the right hemisphere span both hemispaces, while the left hemisphere seems to contain the neural apparatus mostly for contralateral attention. This evidence indicates that the right hemisphere of dextrals has a functional specialization for the distribution of directed attention within extrapersonal space.

Mesulam M-M: A cortical network for directed attention and unilateral neglect.
Ann Neurol 10:309–325, 1981

One manifestation of unilateral injury to the human parietal lobe is neglect for events that occur within the contralateral half of extrapersonal space. In severe cases, patients may behave almost as if that half of the universe had abruptly ceased to exist. Thus, one patient may shave, groom, and dress only one side of the body; another may fail to eat food placed on one side of the tray; while still another may omit to read half of each sentence written on a page. In cases of lesser severity, the neglect may not be as obvious during spontaneous behavior but can be elicited in the form of unilateral extinction during bilateral simultaneous stimulation. Since primary sensory or motor deficits are not necessary for the emergence of this syndrome, at least one plausible interpretation has been to assume that the unilateral neglect reflects an underlying attentional deficit for segments of extrapersonal space [14, 21].

The investigation of neglect syndromes in human beings has remained subject to the customary uncertainties inherent in clinicopathological correlations. However, recent physiological and anatomical experiments on the posterior parietal areas of the macaque monkey have provided a wealth of new information, much of which appears directly relevant to an understanding of the mechanisms of neglect and perhaps also of directed attention. This article reviews this evidence from the vantage point of a specific cerebral network that functions to coordinate the different stages of directed attention in macaque monkeys and in humans. An additional purpose is to inquire whether this network could influence

From the Bullard and Denny-Brown Laboratories and the Behavioral Neurology Section, Harvard Neurology Department and Charles A. Dana Research Institute, Beth Israel Hospital, Boston, MA.

Received Dec 31, 1980, and in revised form Mar 10 and Apr 7, 1981. Accepted for publication Apr 7, 1981.

Address reprint requests to Dr Mesulam, Director, Behavioral Neurology, Beth Israel Hospital, 330 Brookline Ave, Boston, MA 02215.

the classification of unilateral neglect syndromes in a fashion that can reconcile the apparently divergent views which have sought to explain the process of unilateral neglect as well as the organization of selective attention.

Experiments in Macaque Monkeys

Physiological Basis of Unilateral Neglect

Contralateral attention hemianopia and sensory extinction can be elicited following unilateral but extensive posterior parietal ablations in macaque monkeys [23, 52]. A physiological substrate for this phenomenon emerged in the course of single-cell recordings in the inferior parietal lobule of awake and behaving monkeys. In these experiments, neurons with response contingencies relevant to attentional processes were encountered predominantly in the dorsal portion of the inferior parietal lobule, a region that corresponds to area PG of von Bonin and Bailey [13]. Neurons in this area increase their activity when the animal reaches toward a desirable object such as food, while equivalent but passive limb displacements do not elicit a similar response [61, 97]. Other neurons react most vigorously when the eyes fixate or track a motivationally relevant object; the high rate of response continues until the animal is rewarded by a drop of sweet liquid but then declines abruptly, even in the absence of any gaze shift [82]. Still other neurons increase their rate of discharge prior to the onset of visually evoked saccades toward meaningful events within certain portions of the visual field but not in conjunction with identical spontaneous saccades [82]. In additional experiments, monkeys were taught to maintain central fixation while spots of light appeared in the peripheral fields. Under some conditions, detection of subsequent dimming of the peripheral spot was rewarded, while under other conditions identically placed stimuli had no such behavioral relevance. Even in the absence of any associated eye movements, the response of PG neurons to the onset of such peripherally placed spots of light was found to be more vigorous when reward was made contingent on accurate detection of subsequent dimming [18]. These experiments suggest that area PG in the monkey contains neurons that respond not only to the presence of a stimulus but also to its current motivational value and to the likelihood of its becoming the immediate target of visual or manual grasp.* It is therefore reasonable to expect that unilateral ablations that include area PG will result in a state of neglect for the contralateral hemispace since the animal will have lost a neural apparatus for registering the impact of motivationally relevant events and for making them the target of subsequent behavior.

Anatomical Basis of Unilateral Neglect

Recent experiments based on axonal transport of tracer substances show that neural connections of area PG, and especially those of its dorsolateral part, provide a pattern of connectivity that is consistent with the physiological properties noted in the preceding section [31, 66, 90, 123]. Although area PG is composed of three subdivisions (intrasulcal, medial, and dorsolateral), the following comments focus on *dorsolateral PG* since this subdivision contains many of the attention-related neurons just described and since it is the most accessible to behavioral and anatomical experiments.

The large number of neural projections which have been shown to reach dorsolateral PG gives the impression of such indiscriminate heterogeneity that the functional contribution of an individual connection may appear irrelevant or impenetrable. However, each of these connections can be placed into one of only four distinct categories such as "sensory association," "limbic," "reticular," and "motor" [90]. This classification highlights the neural convergence of limbic with sensory information, a convergence that may underlie the physiologically demonstrated ability of neurons in this area to recognize motivational clues in sensory events. The group of reticular inputs may provide a means for modulating the regional level of arousal, while the motor output may guide the exploratory and orienting behavior necessary for scanning the environment.

The sensory association afferents reach dorsolateral PG only after undergoing extensive processing in other parts of the cortex (Fig 1). This cortical elaboration of sensory information occurs in orderly succession within specific subtypes of association cortex. Thus, the initial cortical relay for the three major sensory modalities occurs within discrete koniocortical fields in the supratemporal plane (auditory), occipital lobe (visual), and postcentral gyrus (somatosensory). These primary sensory areas send massive connections, either directly or through an intervening relay, to surrounding association areas: auditory cortex to the superior temporal gyrus, visual cortex to peristriate and inferotemporal cortex, and

*Whereas Mountcastle [96] and Lynch [81] conclude that these neurons have a command function for hand and eye movements within extrapersonal space, Robinson et al [106] emphasize their sensory properties, arguing that the change in firing rate that precedes an eye movement reflects enhancement of a sensory response rather than a command signal to perform a saccade. However, both groups agree that neurons in area PG associate complex visual and somatosensory information with the internal drive state, and that an increase in the activity of these units may reflect the psychological state of attention that the stimulus elicits on the basis of its motivational importance.

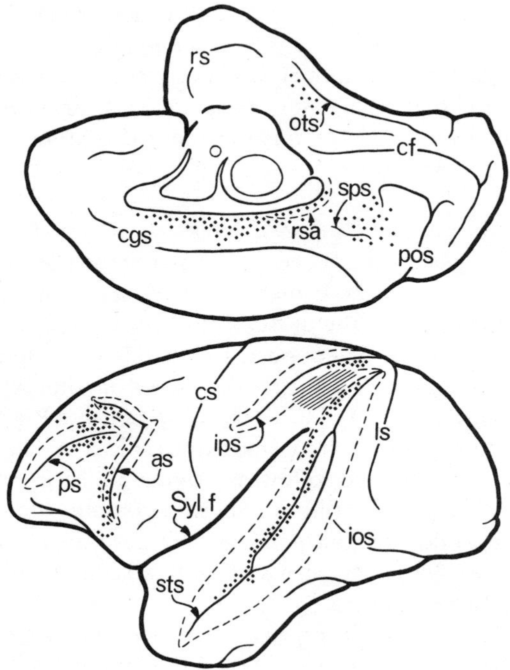

Fig 1. The selective distribution of neurons that send connections into dorsolateral PG in the rhesus monkey. The inferior parietal lobule is bound by the intraparietal sulcus (ips), *sylvian fissure* (Syl. f), *and superior temporal sulcus* (sts). *Dorsolateral PG occupies the dorsal half of the inferior parietal lobule. The cortex along the dorsal half of the caudal bank in the intraparietal sulcus represents the intrasulcal part of PG, while the region bound by the subparietal sulcus* (sps) *and the parietooccipital sulcus* (pos) *contains the medial part of PG. The hatched area in this animal (area virtually confined to dorsolateral PG) was injected with the enzyme horseradish peroxidase. This tracer is transported retrograde to the perikarya of neurons that send axons into the injected area. The distribution of these neurons is indicated by diamonds on the medial and lateral surfaces of the brain. The area between the dashed and solid lines represents the cortex lining sulcal banks.* (as = *arcuate sulcus;* cf = *calcarine fissure;* cgs = *cingulate sulcus;* cs = *central sulcus;* ios = *inferior occipital sulcus;* ls = *lunate sulcus;* ots = *occipitotemporal sulcus;* ps = *principal sulcus;* rs = *rhinal sulcus;* rsa = *retrosplenial area.) (From Mesulam et al* [90], *Brain Res 136:393–414, 1977.)*

somatosensory cortex to the superior parietal lobule [64, 99]. Each of these association regions (and perhaps others) constitutes a *unimodal* association area since its neural input, the behavioral deficits that follow its removal, and the response contingencies of its component neurons are predominantly confined to the one relevant modality. The next stage in processing sensory information occurs when connections from more than one type of unimodal cortex converge (or reside in close proximity) within cortical areas that can be designated as *polymodal.* Periarcuate cortex and the banks of the superior temporal sulcus constitute two of the better-known polymodal areas in the brain of the rhesus monkey [20, 116]. Individual neurons in this type of cortex respond to input in more than one modality, while behavioral consequences of lesions reflect difficulties in detecting multimodal aspects of stimuli [8, 10, 125].

Neuroanatomical experiments led to the somewhat unexpected conclusion that dorsolateral PG receives exceedingly few projections either from primary sensory cortex or from traditional unimodal associated areas. Instead, this part of PG receives the great majority of its cortical sensory association input from polymodal areas [90]. Thus, just as there is at least one obligatory unimodal relay between primary sensory cortex and polymodal areas, there is generally at least one obligatory relay (mostly in polymodal areas) between unimodal cortex and dorsolateral PG [90]. It appears, therefore, that sensory information cannot have access to dorsolateral PG until it is extensively processed in unimodal and then in polymodal cortex. This ensures that dorsolateral PG is in a position to contain an exceedingly elaborate sensory representation of extrapersonal space, a condition that appears desirable for the function of an area involved in distribution of attention.*

Unit recordings indicate the presence of widespread visual responses in dorsolateral PG [97, 106, 135]. The pattern of cortical and subcortical connections is consistent with this pattern of responses. For example, three major sources of projections into dorsolateral PG, area TF in the parahippocampal gyrus, the caudal bank of the intraparietal sulcus, and the medial pulvinar nucleus, have massive connections with unimodal visual association areas and undoubtedly act as relays for visual information [90, 115, 117, 124]. Nevertheless, each of these connections still follows the general principle that there is at least one synapse interposed between traditional unimodal areas and dorsolateral PG. On the other hand, the lateroposterior and intralaminar thalamic nuclei, which have lesser connections with dorsolateral PG, do receive substantial inputs from the superficial (visual) layers of the superior colliculus [7] and may act as more direct relays for visual information. Indeed, a low degree of stimulus specificity and large receptive fields are response properties shared by units in dorsolateral PG and by those in the superficial layers of the superior colliculus but not by components of the geniculocalcarine system [47, 135]. It is interesting to note,

*In a previous publication the term *supramodal* was suggested as a generic name for this type of cortex [90]. Our preliminary observations in the frontal lobes indicate that this profile of sensory connections may be unique to dorsolateral PG. For example, several areas we studied in prefrontal cortex had a substantial unimodal input [2]. With the possible exception of paralimbic areas, dorsolateral PG may thus contain the most extensively processed sensory input.

however, that the medial pulvinar nucleus, which is the major source of thalamic input into dorsolateral PG, receives very few, if any, direct projections from the superficial layers of the superior colliculus [7]. Instead, the medial pulvinar nucleus is probably involved mostly in relaying highly integrated polysensory information (albeit with a bias for the visual modality) into dorsolateral PG. The predominant type of thalamic input therefore parallels the predominant type of cortical input reaching dorsolateral PG from sensory association areas.

The elaborate nature of this sensory input assumes special relevance when it is considered that the limbic projections from the cingulate gyrus are directed predominantly to the dorsolateral part of area PG rather than to its intrasulcal subdivision, which receives the less extensively processed unimodal inputs [90, 100]. In addition to cingulate input, dorsolateral PG also receives additional limbic connections, probably cholinergic, from the substantia innominata and also from the lateral hypothalamic area in the basal forebrain [89]. These limbic connections and their convergence with extensively processed sensory afferents may play a fundamental role in assigning motivational valence to complex events that occur within extrapersonal space. While the basal forebrain may be concerned with a limited set of basic reinforcements such as food or drink [107], the cingulate cortex may subserve the more complex aspects of reinforcement and their modification by learning. Indeed, it was observed that the discharge rate of neurons in area PG did not simply reflect the aversive or desirable properties of food-related stimuli [108]. Thus, it seems that the coding of motivational relevance at the level of dorsolateral PG reflects greater complexity and specificity. Moreover, while the basal forebrain projects widely to many neocortical areas [30, 68, 91], the cingulate cortex has a far more selective efferent field [100]. On the basis of this selectivity, it is reasonable to expect that the cinguloparietal connection is all the more important in shaping the functional specialization of dorsolateral PG.

A third contingent of inputs into dorsolateral PG originates in intralaminar thalamic nuclei, in the nucleus locus coeruleus, and in the brainstem raphe nuclei [90]. I have chosen to combine these projections into a category of reticular inputs. At least in the cat, stimulation of intralaminar thalamic nuclei can elicit cortical recruiting or desynchronization [130], while the nuclei of the locus coeruleus and midline raphe mediate the different phases of sleep [65]. These reticular projections may thus modulate regional cortical activity according to the prevailing level of arousal. Since the effectiveness of attention and the level of arousal are clearly interrelated [58], this group of inputs may be of considerable functional relevance.*

The *efferent* projections of area PG are reciprocally directed to most of the afferent sources already listed here [64, 99]. Of special interest for directed attention are the projections to the frontal eye fields (area 8) and to the superior colliculus [2, 64, 72, 99, 102]. Neurophysiological and behavioral experiments indicate that these areas are crucial for the modulation of head and eye movements. For example, stimulation of each of the two regions elicits contraversive head and eye movements [38, 104, 105]. Unit recordings indicate that the deep layers of the superior colliculus contain neurons active in initiating eye movements [111, 112, 132]. The presence of similar neurons in the frontal eye fields has been questioned [12, 94]. However, there are units in the caudal portion of the frontal eye fields that do show a burst of activity just before a saccade directed to a stimulus in the appropriate part of the visual field. The burst does not occur if the animal merely attends to the stimulus but fails to make a saccade toward it [45]. Furthermore, the receptive fields of these neurons predict the direction of movement that follows their microstimulation [46]. Combined lesions of frontal eye fields and of the superior colliculus result in profound impairment of saccadic eye movements even though destruction of either site alone causes only subtle deficits [95, 113, 133]. Thus, the frontal eye fields and superior colliculus appear to have parallel but complementary and pivotal roles in modulating ocular movements.† The frontal eye fields and surrounding areas may also be involved in limb movements since complex manual tasks are also impaired following lesions that include this area [27, 49, 93, 122]. Thus, the output of dorsolateral PG to the frontal eye fields and to the superior colliculus may coordinate the motor sequences necessary for foveating, scanning, exploring, fixating, and manipulating motivationally relevant events within extrapersonal space.

While none of the projection classes just described is confined to dorsolateral PG, the individual characteristics of each of the four categories and their convergence in this region constitute a unique profile of connectivity that is consistent with functional specialization in the process of directed attention (Fig 2).

*Dorsolateral PG also receives inputs from the claustrum [90]. The claustrum presently defies classification into any single functional category and may have sensory association, limbic, and reticular influences on dorsolateral PG.

†The motor output from the frontal eye fields appears to be mostly nonpyramidal. Thus, there are efferents to the striatum, subthalamic nucleus, and superior colliculus but relatively few to premotor or motor cortex [70, 71, 99].

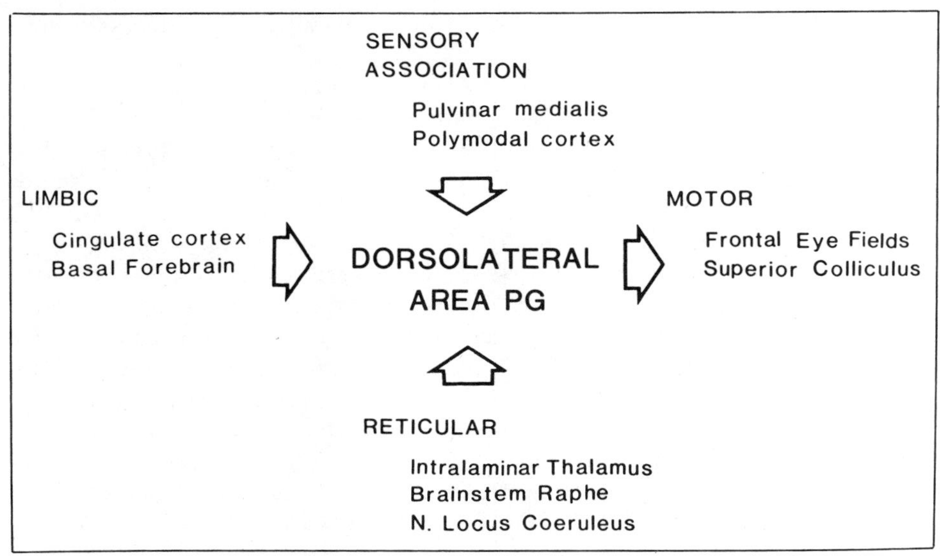

Fig 2. The organization of input and output that is relevant to directed attention.

Unilateral Neglect Syndromes

The two cortical areas that provide pivotal connections for dorsolateral PG, cingulate cortex and the frontal eye fields, are reciprocally connected with each other as well as with dorsolateral PG [2, 64, 90, 99, 100]. Furthermore, reticular input from a similar set of thalamic and brainstem structures reaches not only PG but also cingulate cortex and the frontal eye fields [2, 126]. This intimate coupling among the four regions that are relevant to directed attention raises the possibility that lesions not only in PG but also in cingulate cortex, in the frontal eye fields, and even in reticular structures may disrupt the process of directed attention. Lesions in each individual site of this interconnected network could then be expected to yield a specific clinical picture that reflects the anatomical specialization of the relevant area (Fig 3).

PARIETAL NEGLECT. With respect to directed attention, its sensory connectivity suggests that dorsolateral PG and surrounding areas may provide a stage of *afferent integration* whereby the extrapersonal space becomes transformed into a sensory representational template. The rules for this transformation are not clear. It is reasonable to assume that all three major sensory modalities as well as both sides of space are represented within the dorsolateral PG of each hemisphere. However, there appears to be a bias for the visual modality and for the contralateral hemispace, especially for its peripheral aspects [135]. Furthermore, it is tempting to speculate that the encoding in dorsolateral PG transcends a composite reproduction of actual sensory events and that it contains additional mechanisms for providing an interaction between space and relevance. It is conceivable that area PG contains a fluid template where the transformation of external events into synaptic activity reflects not only the physical properties of the stimulus field but also the distribution of relevance within segments of extrapersonal space. Thus, for a monkey restrained to its chair, a desirable object located beyond an arm's distance is likely to be of far less relevance than an identical object similarly positioned in the visual field but which is also reachable. Indeed, neurons in the dorsolateral PG of awake but restrained animals showed a marked attenuation of response when a motivationally relevant object was moved beyond reach [97]. It appears, then, that under these conditions events inside a sphere with a radius approximately equal to an outstretched arm have a preferential impact value. It is conceivable that relatively more synaptic space is devoted to this segment of the world than would have been the case in the absence of restraints.

Unilateral damage in dorsolateral PG may permanently bias this internal representation in favor of the hemispace ipsilateral to the lesion. In contrast to lesions in primary or unimodal sensory cortex, PG lesions may allow sensory stimuli in any modality and from all parts of extrapersonal space to be analyzed with customary acuity as long as meaningful events occur on one side of space at a time. However, when both hemispaces contain potentially meaningful events of equivalent value, as in the paradigm of bilateral simultaneous stimulation, the contralateral event fades into relative neglect since its synaptic representation within the context of the entire extrapersonal space is markedly attenuated in comparison to the competing events in the ipsilateral hemispace.

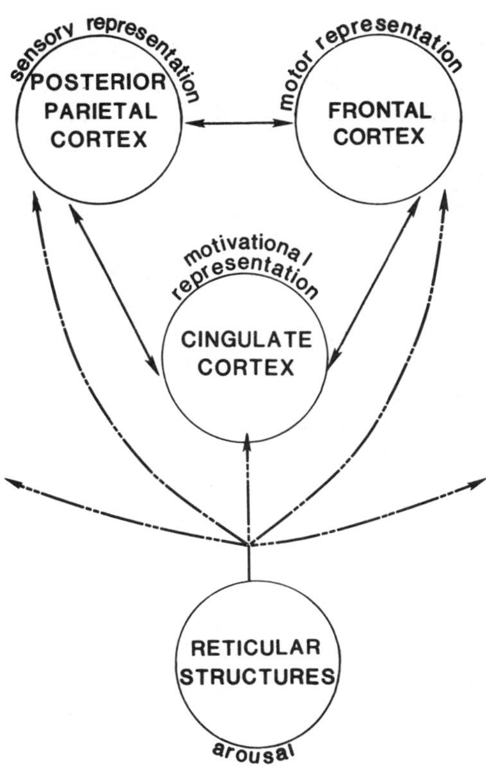

Fig 3. The components of a neural network involved in modulating directed attention.

This hypothesis is consistent with two sets of experimental observations. First, Heilman et al [52] found that rhesus monkeys with unilateral posterior parietal lesions (including area PG) show neglect (extinction) of a contralateral stimulus, predominantly under conditions of bilateral simultaneous stimulation. However, identical stimuli elicited adequate responses when presented unilaterally. Since the authors stressed the absence of primary motor or sensory impairment, the unilateral neglect in these experiments may well have reflected a disturbance in the distribution of attention subsequent to distortion in the inner representation of extrapersonal space. In another set of experiments, by Lamotte and Acuña [73], manual reaching toward a visual target was impaired following unilateral posterior parietal lesions that included PG. The misreaching consisted of deviation toward the side of the lesion with either limb, even when the target was in the ipsilateral hemispace. It is conceivable that the internal representation of space had become skewed in favor of the ipsilateral side and that the motor program for reaching merely reflected this bias, in a fashion somewhat analogous to the behavior of humans subjected to prismatic distortion of visual space.*

FRONTAL NEGLECT. The frontal eye fields (area 8) and surrounding regions may provide a stage of *efferent integration* for the initiation or inhibition of motor mechanisms involved in exploratory or attentive behavior. Unilateral neglect following damage to the frontal eye fields has been known for almost a century [9, 67, 76, 131]. Depending on details of the individual experiment, the neglect encompasses auditory, visual, and tactile stimuli and manifests itself as failure of orienting and reaching toward the contralateral space. Since the animals show no evidence of hemiparesis or conventional sensory loss [67], this phenomenon may be attributed to a distortion in the distribution of attention behavior within extrapersonal space. In contrast to the posterior parietal syndrome, in which bilateral simultaneous stimulation is most effective in eliciting inattention, even unilateral stimulation can be neglected following frontal lesions so that spontaneous behavior displays ongoing contralateral neglect [9, 67].

The predominance of motor over sensory factors in frontal neglect was specifically demonstrated by Watson et al [129]. Macaque monkeys were trained to respond to unilateral tactile stimulation with the contralateral limb. Following unilateral lesions centered around the frontal eye fields, the spontaneous behavior of these animals displayed contralateral neglect even in the absence of hemiparesis. During subsequent retesting in the experimental paradigm, errors were more common when the response was generated by the limb contralateral to the ablation (sensory stimulus being directed to the intact hemisphere). A more accurate performance was obtained when the response was generated by the ipsilateral limb (sensory stimulus directed to the ablated side). These experiments indicate that the unilateral neglect which emerges after frontal lesions reflects a disturbance of motor output rather than of sensory input. Just as PG lesions result in neglect not because of a field cut but because of bias in the internal representation of the sensory space, frontal eye field lesions seem to cause neglect not because of hemiparesis but because of a disinclination to perform motor operations aimed at the contralateral hemispace. Thus, even limbs ipsilateral to the lesion are ineffective in orienting toward meaningful objects in the neglected hemispace [9, 67].

The frontal eye fields and surrounding cortical areas may contain an inner representation of motor programs for the distribution of exploratory sequences within extrapersonal space. In contrast to parietal neglect, which is most active when attention

*Humans rapidly adapt to prismatic distortion, perhaps with the assistance of the neural mechanisms in parts of the brain homologous to dorsolateral PG in the monkey. One would predict that such adaptation is far more difficult in patients with unilateral posterior parietal lesions.

needs to be simultaneously distributed across both hemispaces, frontal neglect may reach maximal expression when the task requires systematic and sequential scanning of the environment.

CINGULATE NEGLECT. The cingulate cortex may provide a locus for *limbic integration* within the network depicted in Figure 3. This area may play a pivotal role in assigning motivational relevance to sensory events according to past experience as well as to present needs. Consequently, events with special motivational meaning can acquire greater impact value, and perhaps a more extensive representation in PG, so that they will be more likely to activate and engage the frontal mechanism for orienting, reaching, and fixating. Thus, a hungry animal may spend a disproportionately long time exploring the area around the door through which the trainer is expected to enter during feeding time. It is conceivable that information concerning the state of hunger and traces related to previous feedings become integrated in the cingulate area. This may cause increased activity in PG neurons representing that portion of space as well as in the corresponding neurons of the frontal eye fields. The net result may be to direct attention preferentially to that part of extrapersonal space. The anatomical basis for this functional property may well be found in the extensive connections of the cingulate region not only with such limbic structures as the hippocampal formation, presubiculum, and amygdala but also with polymodal sensory association areas [100, 109, 126]. Thus, cingulate cortex may participate in directed attention by regulating the spatial distribution of expectation and by assigning impact value to motivationally relevant events. The cingulate area may therefore constitute a third type of parallel and complementary representation of extrapersonal space in a manner that is primarily sensitive to motivational impact.

Unilateral cingulate stimulation in the cat does elicit searching head and eye movements directed at the contralateral space as well as concomitant cessation of all other ongoing activity [63]. Furthermore, Watson et al [127] demonstrated the emergence of contralateral neglect in rhesus monkeys subjected to unilateral lesions in the region of the cingulate. However, the behavioral characterization of this type of neglect requires further delineation.*

*In the rat, unilateral damage to ascending dopaminergic connections elicits contralateral neglect [39, 79, 84]. One target of these projections is the nucleus accumbens. That nucleus provides a major source of neural input to the substantial innominata, which is in turn one of the two sources of limbic input into dorsolateral PG [89]. Furthermore, there seem to be direct corticopetal dopaminergic connections to cingulate cortex, at least in the rat [35]. Thus, the unilateral neglect secondary to interruption of dopaminergic pathways may reflect involvement of the limbic component in the network shown in Figure 3.

RETICULAR NEGLECT. The importance of the reticular formation to arousal and of arousal to attention is a concept that needs no introduction [58]. In the most trivial instance, bilateral lesions within the reticular formation lead to irreversible depression of consciousness that is inconsistent with the operations of selective attention. More selective lesions may also disrupt the distribution of attention. In the rat, for instance, interruption of the ascending noradrenergic bundle from the nucleus locus coeruleus interferes with attentional processes [85, 86]. In the monkey, unilateral lesions in intralaminar nuclei or in the mesencephalic reticular formation result in unilateral neglect [128, 129]. It is conceivable that these lesions interfere with general activation of the relevant cortical regions in the frontal eye fields, dorsolateral PG, and cingulate gyrus by reticular inputs (see Fig 3).

Action and Perception

While the role of dorsolateral PG in directed attention appears to be mostly sensory and that of the frontal eye fields mostly motor, the distinction is by no means absolute. Thus, area PG appears to have some motor properties, and the frontal eye fields have functional aspects that may be characterized as sensory [10, 36, 40, 73, 75, 76, 81, 82, 94, 96, 97, 134]. Therefore, unilateral neglect syndromes are unlikely to be exclusively sensory or motor; rather, they are a mixture of both. This duality becomes more intelligible in light of a recent essay by Droogleever-Fortuyn [32], who challenges the traditional view that sensory input is the primary building block of experience. Instead, he proposes that sense organs are comparable to "feelers of tentacles" used to scan the world in order to update an inner representational map. Thus, perceiving is as much a motor phenomenon as it is sensory, and this is nowhere more understandable than in the process of selective attention.

While these parietal, frontal, cingulate, and reticular components undoubtedly hold pivotal roles in the distribution of directed attention, I do not wish to imply that they account for *all* operations relevant to sensory attention. Indeed, Hubel et al [60] have demonstrated that some neurons even in the primary auditory cortex of cats increase their response to sound when the animal appears to direct attention to its source. In striate cortex and even in the lateral geniculate nucleus, the response to visual stimuli can be enhanced by experimental manipulations which increase the general level of neural activation [4, 44]. Furthermore, in the rhesus monkey, lesions of primary somatosensory cortex may lead to sensory extinction, while unimodal visual areas in inferotemporal cortex appear necessary for inhibiting the impact of irrelevant visual stimuli and for identifying those that are meaningful [34, 50, 120]. However, the role of these areas in attention is probably more limited, being confined to single sensory modalities. It is reasonable to assume that the attention-related responses in these areas predominantly reflect the overall distribution of attention as determined by the network shown in Figure 3. I do not wish to suggest that the regions depicted in Figure 3 are exclusively concerned with functions related to the distribution of attention. For example, the frontal eye fields also appear to play a major role in multimodal sensory integration [125], while dorsolateral PG is essential for complex visuomotor activity [103]. This characteristic functional heterogeneity in areas that are components of an integrated cerebral network will receive further comment.

Human Syndromes

Injuries that result from head trauma, neoplasm, or stroke rarely respect architectonic or topographic landmarks that guide experiments in animals. Moreover, homologies between cortical areas of human beings and other primates are not always clear, and the pattern of intercortical connections that characterizes the human brain is incompletely understood.* It is therefore difficult to compare the details of cerebral organization in different primate species with that of the human. Nevertheless, several independent lines of evidence support the conclusion that the four subtypes of unilateral neglect described in the macaque monkey can also be identified in human patients, suggesting that a cerebral network with a similar organization may be responsible for the coordination of directed attention within extrapersonal space. Since most human unilateral neglect cases reported in the literature consist of patients who have right hemisphere lesions and neglect the left hemispace, the subsequent discussion addresses left-sided neglect exclusively. The assumption that this difference in frequency implies right hemisphere specialization for directed attention will then be analyzed in the light of pertinent evidence.

Parietal Neglect

Severe unilateral neglect in humans is almost automatically attributed to parietal lobe involvement. Indeed, the earlier case reports of this syndrome described patients with lesions in the posterior parts of the right hemisphere [14, 87, 101]. While the parietal lobe was often incriminated as the principal site of damage, localization was hampered because each of the patients in these reports had suffered either multilobar infarcts, head injury, or intracerebral neoplasm. Subsequently, Hécaen et al [51] described the emergence of unilateral neglect in patients subjected to cortical excision of the right inferior parietal lobule (mostly area PG and PF) for control of epilepsy. This localization acquired greater certitude with the help of case reports describing unilateral neglect after infarctions in the area of the intraparietal sulcus and inferior parietal lobule in individuals without a history of prior neurological impairment [22, 23, 54].

Contrary to widespread opinion, the unilateral neglect following an infarction limited to the posterior parietal area is not always severe, and mere observation of spontaneous behavior may fail to reveal consistent deficits. Indeed, bilateral simultaneous stimulation may become necessary for eliciting neglect in the form of extinction while responses to unilateral stimulation may show no abnormality. In more severe cases, however, the tendency to extinction may be so powerful that the mere presence of ambient visual input on the side ipsilateral to the lesion elicits neglect for the contralateral hemispace so that even unilateral stimulation appears to be ignored during bedside examination. In such cases, I have found that presenting brief flashes of light in a darkened room will reveal extinction to be the underlying mechanism of the neglect. Since neither limitation of head and eye movements nor primary sensory loss is a necessary condition, the neglect can be attributed to an attention deficit within the hemispace contralateral to the lesion. Although several authors have already demonstrated that primary sensory loss is not the cause for the neglect [19, 42, 54], one case deserves comment for emphasis. A 74-year-old right-handed man was admitted with a gradually progressive neurological deficit caused by a glioma that included the posterior parietal cortex in the right hemisphere. He showed left-sided extinction to tactile, visual, and olfactory stimuli. Since primary olfactory pathways are not crossed, the olfactory extinction should have occurred on the right rather than on the left if primary sensory loss, however subtle, had been responsible for the neglect.

Although the relevant neural connectivity in humans is less well known than that in the monkey brain, it is likely that parts of the posterior parietal cortex of the human brain have connections similar to those of dorsolateral PG in the rhesus monkey (see Figs 1–3). It is reasonable to assume that this

*According to Brodmann [16, 17], the human inferior parietal lobule consists of areas 39 and 40. Brodmann did not find equivalent achitectonic regions in the monkey. Instead, he designated the inferior parietal lobule in the monkey as area 7. Since area 7 in human beings is situated along the rostral bank of the intraparietal sulcus, this would be the area in the human homologous to the monkey's inferior parietal lobule. According to this scheme, then, the monkey brain contains no architectonic analogue to the human inferior parietal lobule. However, von Economo's [33] work in human beings and that of von Bonin and Bailey [13] in monkeys indicate that the inferior parietal lobules in the two species are far more analogous in that they both consist of areas PG and PF.

region contains an elaborate sensory template of the external world, perhaps obtained through a process similar to the one for which Denny-Brown et al [24] coined the term *morphosynthesis.* Through mechanisms similar to the ones postulated to exist in the monkey, unilateral damage in this region may induce distortion in this representation so that events in the contralateral hemispace lose their relative impact on awareness, thus leading to the phenomenon of extinction.

The role of inner representation in the genesis of parietal neglect has been championed by, among others, Bisiach et al [11]. In their experiments, patients with right hemisphere damage (all of whom had independent evidence of left-sided neglect and most of whom had lesions involving the posterior parietal cortex) were presented with pairs of geometric shapes and asked to judge if the two stimuli in each pair were identical or different. The subjects viewed the stimuli not in their entirety but through a centrally placed slit under which the objects were passed at a constant rate, one at a time. Thus, the subject had to reconstruct the entire object in mind and store it in memory for subsequent comparison with the next object in the pair. The results indicated that the patients were less accurate in detecting differences on the left side of the objects, whether the objects moved leftward or rightward under the slit. Since sensory input during the experiment was centrally situated, the outcome cannot be attributed to neglect of actual events in the extrapersonal space; rather, it was the result of neglect of the inner representation per se, even though the constituent sensory information had originated in the nonneglected parts of the external world [11].

A rather unusual case from our files provides additional support for this position. A right-handed chronic alcohol abuser was admitted with an embolic infarction that included the posterior parts of the right hemisphere. He had severe neglect of the left hemispace. Several days after admission he developed delirium tremens and entered into heated arguments with hallucinated individuals in his room. The hallucinations appeared only on his right, never on his left. It is as if the internal representation of the left hemisphere was so rarefied that it could not even harbor ghosts.

Frontal Neglect

A region in the human frontal lobe has been designated as the frontal eye fields because its stimulation elicits contralateral deviation of the eyes while its destruction leads to transient paralysis of gaze toward the side opposite to the lesion [41]. Unilateral neglect in humans does arise as a consequence of tumors or infarcts in frontal cortex [55, 119]. It is conceivable that the neglect in these patients reflects involvement of the frontal eye fields and immediately surrounding areas. Analysis of frontal neglect in the monkey suggests that these patients should experience greatest difficulty in tasks that depend on exploring, searching, or manipulating objects in the contralateral hemispace. In fact, deficits of active visual scanning have been described with lesions of the frontal lobe [80]. Patients with frontal neglect would therefore be expected to show unilateral neglect in copying figures, route finding, letter cancellation, and even reading, since these tasks require systematic and sequential scanning of the external space. Frontal neglect would also be more likely to result in spontaneous inattention, whereas parietal neglect would be more likely to cause extinction. It is unlikely, however, that either of these two subtypes will be seen in isolation, not only because lesions are rarely that specific but also because effective scanning is likely to require a reliable internal representation, whereas the accuracy of the internal representation probably depends on adequate scanning.

Experiments by DeRenzi et al [25] and by Heilman and Valenstein [56] have demonstrated that one major component of unilateral neglect consists of hypokinesia for exploration and manipulation within the contralateral hemispace. I would suggest that this motor aspect of unilateral neglect reflects involvement of the frontal component in the network that subserves attention (see Fig 3). Just as the sensory aspect of parietal neglect is not the outcome of a multimodal field cut, I believe the motor aspect of frontal neglect does not reflect hemiparesis of limb, head, and eye movements, but rather an underlying disinclination to move within and toward the neglected hemispace, whatever the specific muscle groups required for such activity may be.* Indeed, there is reason to believe that some aspects of motor output in the intact person are also organized according to the hemispace within which the movement occurs. Anzola et al [1] required subjects to make a decision concerning which hand to use in a choice reaction-time experiment depending on the position of a visual stimulus. The experiment was performed with and without hand crossing, and the results showed that the faster hand in the crossed condition was not the one anatomically ipsilateral to the stimulus but the one situated in the same hemispace with the stimulus. Thus, under special condi-

*Bard [3] in 1904 had already suggested that the contraversive head and eye deviation seen in many patients with unilateral lesions reflects not so much motor weakness as diminution in the impact of events emanating from the contralateral hemispace. While Bard did not mention localization, the findings in many of his case studies suggested frontal lesions.

tions requiring concentrated attention to a task, the neural organization of motor output may reflect the part of the extrapersonal space where the movement will be discharged and not exclusively the muscle groups that will be activated.

A relevant case is that of a right-handed man admitted with a stroke in the right hemisphere. He showed left-sided neglect, especially during tasks of visual scanning and figure copying. While no documentation of the lesion site was available, a mild left hemiparesis in the absence of primary sensory loss suggested a frontal localization. During testing he was blindfolded and asked to detect and retrieve, by manual exploration, an object placed on either side of him on the surface of his bed. When the object was placed on his left side, manual exploration with either hand was haphazard and erratic so that failures and delays of retrieval were common. However, performance was virtually intact, even with the mildly hemiparetic left hand, when the object was on his right.

Whereas the salient manifestations of parietal neglect may well be sensory and those of frontal neglect motor, the dichotomy is unlikely to be absolute. Thus, patients with parietal neglect may also show reluctance to project the contralateral limb into the neglected hemispace, while those with frontal neglect may show such diminished reaction to contralateral visual stimuli that the presence of a hemianopia may be suspected in the acute phase. The universality of such sensory-motor duality in attentional mechanisms has been addressed in the preceding discussion.

Cingulate Neglect

Evidence for cingulate neglect in human beings is indirect and speculative. However, one of the patients with unilateral neglect reported by Heilman and Valenstein [55] had a medially situated frontal infarction that could have involved predominantly the cingulate cortex. On the basis of the corresponding connectivity in the monkey, neglect arising from cingulate lesions in humans may reflect a loss in the perception of biological importance associated with events in the contralateral hemispace. If so, the distribution of expectancy for *potential* events and also the attribution of motivational relevance to *actual* stimuli would be impaired on the side contralateral to the lesion. Consequently, the contralateral hemispace would attract less scanning and fixation. The net outcome of these factors may culminate in unilateral neglect. While no specific localization was suggested, the contribution of motivational variables was first stressed by Denny-Brown et al [24], who described one aspect of unilateral neglect as a "diminution in biological stimulus value in the left exteroceptive field." It seems reasonable to attribute this aspect of unilateral neglect to disruption of the limbic component in the network depicted in Figure 3.

Reticular Neglect

It is generally accepted that the overall process of attention refers to at least two different operations [88]. One of these is *tonic* in character and regulates the threshold that a stimulus must exceed before gaining access to consciousness; the second is *phasic* and selects, from among the many stimuli which exceed this threshold, those which will occupy the center of awareness. The parietal, frontal, and cingulate mechanisms already discussed reveal one way in which selective (phasic) attention is coordinated within extrapersonal space. On the other hand, the tonic process of attention is intimately related to the level of vigilance and depends on the integrity of the reticular formation. Thus, focal mesencephalic infarcts that interfere with the reticular formation and its ascending connections result in severe disturbances of vigilance and arousal [15, 114]. In the monkey, the reticular input to the cortical areas implicated in the regulation of selective attention originates in the intralaminar thalamic nuclei, the nucleus locus coeruleus, and the midline raphe nuclei (see Figs 2, 3). Similar connections may exist in the human brain, and it is conceivable that unilateral lesions in these structures may elicit neglect for the contralateral hemispace.

Compound Neglect Syndromes

In naturally occuring lesions that come to clinical attention, damage is rarely confined to one of the four components in Figure 3 so that the patient may simultaneously manifest many aspects of unilateral neglect. The same patient may show marked extinction, a distorted inner representation of external space, failure to scan the contralateral hemispace, devaluation of its biological significance, and even diminution of overall arousal and vigilance. In some cases it appears as if the contralateral side of space has ceased to exist in the patient's consciousness not only with respect to actual sensory stimuli but also as far as potential events are concerned. The deficit is not one of seeing, hearing, feeling, or moving but one of looking, listening, touching, and exploring. The neglect encompasses extrapersonal space, body surface, and even intrapsychic representations. These severe manifestations of unilateral neglect could not be expected to arise from lesions confined to posterior parietal cortex and indicate the involvement of additional components in the network that subserves directed attention.

Agreement with Other Theories of Unilateral Neglect

The preceding account suggests that four distinct contributions to the overall organization of directed attention may be identified in human beings as well as in the monkey. It is likely that lesions which do not directly involve one of these four regions but which interrupt their interconnections may disrupt the effective coordination of directed attention through a mechanism of disconnection. Thus, despite their apparent disagreements concerning the cause of unilateral neglect, the theories of amorphosynthesis [24], extinction [6], disconnection [43], representational distortion [11], hypoarousal [53], and hemispatial hypokinesia [56] each appears valid depending on the anatomical locus of the principal lesion, while none is, by itself, sufficient to explain the entire phenomenon.

Network Approach to Cerebral Localization

Directed attention to extrapersonal space appears to be a compound function based on concerted interaction among at least three major cortical areas. Additional functional specializations characterize each of these areas [22, 51]. For example, anosognosia, dressing apraxia, and construction apraxia are additional major deficits that emerge after right parietal damage. The coordination of one complex function such as directed sensory attention by the interaction of several distinct regions, none of which is exclusively devoted to that function, suggests an approach to functional localization in terms of integrated networks. This network approach offers an alternative to more established views on localization.

To describe it in oversimplified terms, the centrist approach to localization [37] implies that certain complex functions may be integrated by specific cortical areas which are exclusively devoted to that function (Fig 4*A*). While a similar or identical function may also be represented in additional (supplementary) areas, the principle of functional homogeneity applies to these regions as well. Clinical manifestations of lesions are attributed to the destruction of such centers and of their interconnections. There is the expectation that a propitious case will be discovered in which the clinical deficit is confined to the relevant complex function so that the site of the lesion can help delineate the "center" for that function. By contrast, the concept of cerebral equipotentiality [74] minimizes the role of centers and assumes an organization of brain whereby each complex function is, at least potentially, represented widely in cortex even though slight local variations in the concentration of specific functions may be present (Fig 4*D*).

The network approach suggested in this paper (Fig

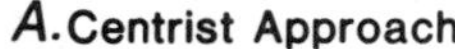

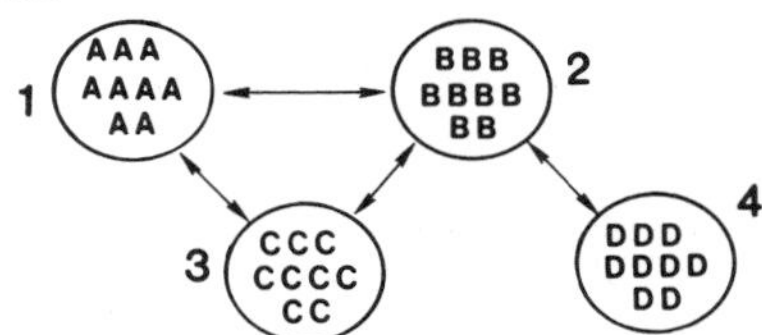

B. Network Approach I

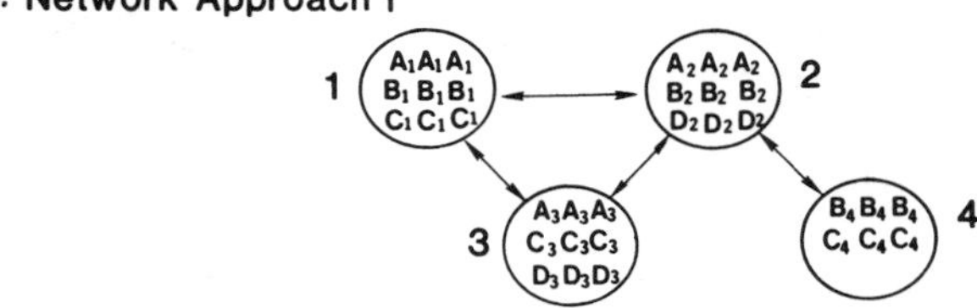

C. Network Approach II

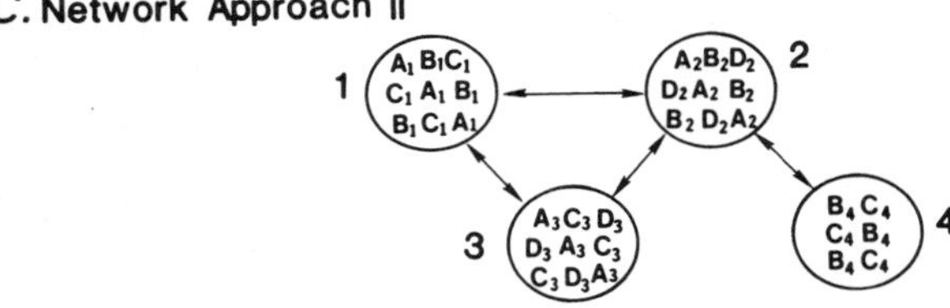

D. Holistic Approach

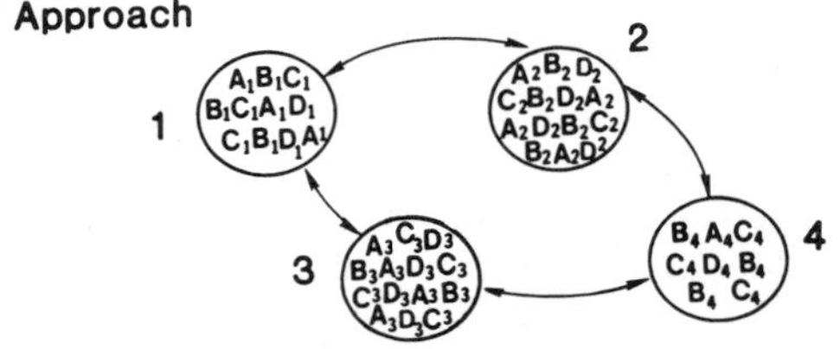

Fig 4. Four approaches to the cortical localization of complex function. B represents a version of the network approach based on the organization of function along discrete cortical columns [48, 96].

4*B, C*) constitutes an intermediate position between these two views. Thus, a complex function such as A in Figure 4*B* is considered in terms of several component processes, A_1, A_2, and A_3, each of which has a distinct localization in sites 1, 2, and 3, respectively. The component sites are intimately interconnected and constitute an integrated network subserving that particular complex function. Each of the sites has a unique set of additional functional specializations, some of which are components of intersecting but distinct networks. For example, function B is confined to sites 1, 2, and 4, a network that partially overlaps with that for function A (Fig 4*B*).

For the sake of illustration, it could be assumed that function A in Figure 4*B* is directed attention. A_1, A_2, and A_3 would correspond to the component functions of scanning, sensory representation, and motivational mapping. Sites 1, 2, 3, and 4 represent the frontal eye fields (site 1), area PG (site 2), the cingulate gyrus (site 3), and the cortex of the superior temporal sulcus (site 4).* Let functions A, B, and D in site 2 (area PG) correspond to directed attention, dressing apraxia, and anosognosia. According to the network approach, the deficits at the highest level of perceptual integration that occur in unilateral neglect, dressing apraxia and anosognosia, become attributed to involvement of area PG (site 2). In the case of directed attention, the relevant neural transformation in area PG is the formation of a template for extrapersonal space, as already discussed; in the case of dressing apraxia and anosognosia, the relevance of area PG may be based on the neural encoding of a body scheme in the same area. The additional affective component of anosognosia (function D) may then reflect the relationship of site 2 (area PG) with site 3 (cingulate gyrus), while the components of dressing apraxia (function B), which indicate difficulties with visual-somesthetic integration, may reflect the interactions of site 2 (area PG) with site 4 (superior temporal gyrus).

This network approach suggests several general principles applicable to the clinicopathological correlation of complex functions: (1) components of a single complex function are represented within distinct but interconnected sites which collectively constitute an integrated network for that function; (2) individual cortical areas contain the neural substrate for components of several complex functions and may therefore belong to several partially overlapping networks; (3) lesions confined to a single cortical region are likely to result in multiple deficits; (4) severe and lasting impairments of an individual complex function usually require the simultaneous involvement of several components in the relevant network; and (5) the same complex function may be impaired as a consequence of a lesion in one of several cortical areas, each of which is a component of an integrated network for that function.

It is likely that different approaches to localization may have validity depending on the function under consideration. Thus, visual acuity within segments of the visual fields is organized in striate cortex according to the centrist point of view. In contrast, generalized attributes such as intelligence, creativity, or personality may well follow the equipotentiality model of organization. On the other hand, functions such as directed attention, language, and memory may be organized according to the network approach.

Corticalization of Attention Functions

In the cat, unilateral ablations of the superior colliculus elicit marked contralateral neglect [121], whereas equivalent lesions in the monkey merely yield subtle delays of contralateral saccades but no evidence of neglect [133]. In the cat, prefrontal ablations do not elicit the contralateral neglect seen in monkeys or humans. Furthermore, the unilateral neglect that follows frontal or parietal lesions is mild and brief in the monkey when compared to that which follows upon analogous lesions in humans. Markowitsch et al [83] have been unable to find substantial connections between posterior parietal lobe and prefrontal cortex in the cat, a projection which is well developed in the rhesus monkey and, undoubtedly, in humans. The corticalization of directed attention may therefore depend upon the development of the relevant cortical connections.

Hemispheric Asymmetry in the Organization of Directed Attention

Most of the cases of unilateral neglect reported in the literature deal with lesions in the right hemisphere. Indeed, it can be shown that left-sided neglect after right hemisphere lesions is more common, more severe, and more lasting than right-sided neglect following lesions in the left hemisphere [19, 25, 42, 98].

Other evidence also implies that the intact right hemisphere is more active and efficient than the left in attentional tasks. Evoked responses to visual and somatosensory stimuli are generally of greater amplitude in the right hemisphere [110]. Furthermore, Dimond [28, 29] tested each hemisphere in a group of split-brain patients and showed that right hemisphere performance was superior in tasks of vigilance. In normal subjects, simple reaction times to ipsilateral visual stimuli are faster with the left hand [1].

Additional experiments show that the attentional function of the right hemisphere is not confined to the contralateral hemispace but may involve the entire extrapersonal space. Active touch exploration with fingers of either hand, for example, elicits specific evoked electrogenesis preferentially in the right hemisphere of intact humans [26]. Similarly, left parietal electroencephalographic leads showed desynchronization mostly after right-sided stimuli, while those over the right parietal area recorded equivalent desynchronization whether stimulation was contralateral or ipsilateral [57]. In another setting, in which patients with unilateral lesions were asked to perform a simple reaction-time task with the hand ipsilateral to the lesion, those with nondominant hemisphere lesions (overwhelmingly right) showed significantly more delays than those with lesions in the dominant (left) hemisphere [59]. Finally, in some cases of prefrontal or posterior parietal infarction in the right hemisphere, the attentional deficit was bilateral and led to the emergence of a confusional state [92].

*The cortex that lines the banks of the superior temporal sulcus, at least in the monkey, is a polymodal area known to have reciprocal connections with area PG [64, 90, 99, 116].

These observations suggest that the right hemisphere of dextrals has a predominant and specialized function in the distribution of attention. This conclusion has often been challenged on the basis of work by Battersby et al [5], who reported a failure to substantiate statistically significant group differences even though 12 out of their 41 patients with right hemisphere lesions showed neglect as opposed to 3 out of 24 testable cases with left hemisphere lesions. The authors argued that even these results reflected a bias in favor of larger lesions in the right hemisphere since equally large lesions in the left hemisphere result in severe aphasias that make patients untestable. They concluded that unilateral neglect may be equally common after lesions in either hemisphere and that primary sensory loss may be an important factor in the genesis of neglect.

Both of these points have been addressed in the course of experiments by Chain et al [19], who measured the distribution of attention by quantitating the amount of time spent looking at each sector of a projected picture. Aphasic patients were not excluded since no verbal responses were required. The results showed that the frequency of contralateral neglect was not significantly different with lesions of the right hemisphere compared to left hemisphere lesions. However, strong qualitative differences emerged. Many patients with a unilateral lesion in the right hemisphere spent virtually all of the 15-second viewing period looking at the far right side of the picture and avoided its left extreme aspect. In contrast, the neglect of patients with left hemisphere lesions was mostly confined to spending a longer time in the left paramedian region, merely exaggerating a tendency shown by subjects without hemispheric lesions. Some patients with lesions in the left hemisphere showed visual neglect of the right side mostly during the first 5 seconds of viewing, whereas those with right hemisphere lesions continued to neglect the left side throughout the entire 15 seconds. Finally, it was shown that the degree of hemianopia was not correlated with the magnitude of neglect. Thus, while there is no doubt that unilateral neglect occurs after damage to the left hemisphere [5, 21, 77], its extent and severity are far less than the neglect resulting from lesions in the right hemisphere.

These observations support a specialized role for the right hemisphere in directed attention, and a simple model may be proposed to explain this functional asymmetry. The model is based on three assumptions: (1) the intact right hemisphere may contain the neural apparatus for attending to both sides of space although the preponderant tendency is for attending to the contralateral (left) hemispace; (2) the left hemisphere is almost exclusively concerned with attending to the contralateral right hemispace; and (3) more synaptic space is devoted to attentional functions in the right hemisphere than in the left, so that most attentional tasks involving either hemispace will generate greater activity of the right hemisphere. According to this model, unilateral lesions of the left hemisphere are unlikely to yield neglect since the intact right hemisphere may take over the task of attending to the right side. By contrast, in the absence of similar compensatory mechanisms in the left hemisphere, right hemisphere lesions will result in marked unilateral neglect. Furthermore, in some patients in whom even ipsilateral attention is predominantly modulated by the right hemisphere, universal neglect (a confusional state) will emerge after a lesion confined to the right hemisphere. This model is consistent with the right hemisphere superiority in vigilance tasks in split-brain patients [28, 29] as well as with the slight tendency of normal persons to pay more attention to the left side [1, 19].

In a review article, Kimura [69] pointed out that the magnitude of left hemispheric superiority for language and related tasks is far greater than the magnitude of right hemisphere superiority in nonlinguistic tasks. This observation is consistent with the supposition that, at some point in primate evolution, each hemisphere shared higher cortical functions more symmetrically. However, with the emergence of language skills, synaptic space in the left hemisphere formerly devoted to other functions was redirected for linguistic abilities. Conceivably, nonlinguistic functions acquired a relative hemispheric specialization in the right hemisphere because the synaptic space for analogous functions in the contralateral hemisphere became devoted to language functions, a view consistent with a proposal by LeDoux et al [78]. Thus, there are great interhemispheric asymmetries in favor of the left hemisphere for language-related functions since these emerged as a left-sided synaptic specialization without having depended on the participation of contralateral neural elements. On the other hand, the differences are not as absolute for nonlinguistic tasks since residues of synaptic space devoted to these functions may still remain in the left hemisphere.

Relevance to Other Aspects of Attention

"Everyone knows what attention is," wrote William James in 1890. "It is the taking possession by the mind, in clear and vivid form, of one out of what seem several simultaneously possible objects or trains of thought. Focalization, concentration, of consciousness are of its essence. It implies withdrawal from some things in order to deal effectively with others, and it is a condition which has a real opposite in the confused, dazed, scatterbrained state . . ." [62].

The effective execution of attention requires a

flexible interplay among intense concentration, inhibition of distractibility, and the ability to shift the center of awareness from one focus to another according to inner needs, past experience, and external reality. The object of attention is not always a sensory event in extrapersonal space but also can include trains of thought or even sequences of skilled movements. In this paper my comments are limited to the factors that influence the spatial distribution of sensory attention within extrapersonal space. Even this portion of attentional functions appears to require the integrated action of a complex network. How much more intricate must be the neural network that also encompasses the additional aspects of attention. One can only agree with Sherrington [118] that "the climax of mental integration would seem to be attention," and with Ferrier [38] that "in proportion to the development of the faculty of attention are the intellectual and reflective powers manifested."

Supported in part by Grant NS-14625 from the National Institute of Neurological and Communicative Disorders and Stroke.

I am grateful to Drs Norman Geschwind and Sandra Weintraub for helpful comments and to Drs M. E. Goldberg and J. C. Lynch for making available preprints of unpublished work. Ms Regina Regan provided unfailing secretarial assistance.

References

1. Anzola GP, Bertoloni G, Buchtel HA, Rizzolatti G: Spatial compatibility and anatomical factors in simple and choice reaction times. Neuropsychologia 15:295–302, 1977
2. Barbas H, Mesulam M-M: Organization of afferent input to subdivisions of area 8 in rhesus monkeys. J Comp Neurol 200:407–431, 1981
3. Bard L: De l'origine sensorielle de la déviation conjuguée des yeux avec rotation de la tête chez les hémiplégiques. Sem Med 24:9–13, 1904
4. Bartlett JR, Doty RW, Choudhury BP: Modulation of unit activity in striate cortex of squirrel monkeys by stimulation of reticular formation (abstract). Fed Proc 29:453, 1970
5. Battersby WS, Bender MB, Pollack M, Kahn RL: Unilateral "spatial agnosia" ("inattention") in patients with cerebral lesions. Brain 79:68–93, 1956
6. Bender MD: Extinction and precipitation of cutaneous sensation. Arch Neurol Psychiatry 54:1–9, 1945
7. Benevento LA, Fallon JH: The ascending projections of the superior colliculus in the rhesus monkey *(Macaca mulatta)*. J Comp Neurol 160:339–362, 1975
8. Benevento LA, Fallon J, Davis BJ, Rezak M: Auditory-visual interaction in single cells in the cortex of the superior temporal sulcus and the orbital frontal cortex of the macaque monkey. Exp Neurol 57:849–872, 1977
9. Bianchi L: The functions of the frontal lobes. Brain 18:497–522, 1895
10. Bignall KE, Imbert M: Polysensory and cortico-cortical projections to frontal lobe of squirrel and rhesus monkeys. Electroencephalogr Clin Neurophysiol 26:206–215, 1969
11. Bisiach E, Luzzati C, Perani D: Unilateral neglect, representational schema and consciousness. Brain 102:609–618, 1979
12. Bizzi E: Discharge of frontal eye field neurons during saccadic and following eye movements in unanesthetized monkeys. Exp Brain Res 6:69–80, 1968
13. von Bonin G, Bailey P: The Neocortex of *Macaca mulatta.* Urbana, IL, University of Illinois Press, 1947
14. Brain WR: Visual disorientation with special reference to lesions of the right cerebral hemisphere. Brain 64:244–272, 1941
15. Brain WR: The physiological basis of consciousness. Brain 81:427–455, 1958
16. Brodmann K: Beitrage zur histologischen Lokalisation der Grosshirnrinde. III: Die Rindenfelder der niederen Affen. J Psychol Neurol (Leipzig) 4:177–226, 1905
17. Brodmann K: Vergleichende Lokalisationlehre der Grosshirnrinde in ihren Prinzipient dargestellt auf Grund des Zellenbaues. Leipzig, Barth, 1909
18. Bushnell MC, Goldberg ME, Robinson DL: Behavioral enhancement of visual responses in monkey cerebral cortex: 1. Modulation in posteriör parietal cortex related to selective visual attention. J Neurophysiol (in press)
19. Chain F, LeBlanc M, Chédru F, Lhermitte F: Négligence visuelle dans les lesions postérieures de l'hémisphere gauche. Rev Neurol (Paris) 135:105–126, 1979
20. Chavis DA, Pandya DN: Further observations on corticofrontal connections in the rhesus monkey. Brain Res 117:369–386, 1976
21. Critchley M: The phenomenon of tactile inattention with special reference to parietal lesions. Brain 72:538–561, 1949
22. Critchley M: The Parietal Lobes. London, Edward Arnold, 1953
23. Denny-Brown D, Chambers RA: The parietal lobe and behavior. Proc Assoc Res Nerv Ment Dis 36:35–117, 1958
24. Denny-Brown D, Meyer JS, Horenstein S: The significance of perceptual rivalry resulting from parietal lobe lesion. Brain 75:434–471, 1952
25. DeRenzi E, Faglioni P, Scotti G: Hemispheric contribution to exploration of space through the visual and tactile modality. Cortex 6:191–203, 1970
26. Desmedt JE: Active touch exploration of extrapersonal space elicits specific electrogenesis in the right cerebral hemisphere of intact right handed man. Proc Natl Acad Sci USA 74:4037–4040, 1977
27. Deuel RK: Loss of motor habits after cortical lesions. Neuropsychologia 15:205–215, 1977
28. Dimond SJ: Depletion of attentional capacity after total commissurotomy in man. Brain 99:347–356, 1976
29. Dimond SJ: Tactual and auditory vigilance in split-brain man. J Neurol Neurosurg Psychiatry 42:70–74, 1979
30. Divac I: Magnocellular nuclei of the basal forebrain project to neocortex, brain stem and olfactory bulb. Review of some functional correlates. Brain Res 93:385–398, 1975
31. Divac I, LaVail JH, Rakic P, Winston KR: Heterogeneous afferents to the inferior parietal lobule of the rhesus monkey revealed by the retrograde transport method. Brain Res 123:197–207, 1977
32. Droogleever-Fortuyn J: On the neurology of perception. Clin Neurol Neurosurg 81:97–107, 1979
33. von Economo C: The Cytoarchitectonics of the Human Cerebral Cortex. London, Oxford University Press, 1929
34. Eidelberg E, Schwartz AS: Experimental analysis of the extinction phenomenon in monkeys. Brain 94:91–108, 1971
35. Emson PC, Koob GF: The origin and distribution of dopamine-containing afferents to the rat frontal cortex. Brain Res 142:249–267, 1978
36. Ettlinger G, Kalsbeck JE: Changes in tactile discrimination

and in visual reaching after successive and simultaneous bilateral posterior parietal ablations in the monkey. J Neurol Neurosurg Psychiatry 25:256–268, 1962

37. Exner S: Untersuchungen über Localisation der Functionen in der Grosshirnrinde des Menschen. Vienna, Braümuller, 1881
38. Ferrier D: Functions of the Brain. New York, Putnam, 1880
39. Fink JS, Smith GP: Mesolimbic and mesocortical dopaminergic neurons are necessary for normal exploratory behavior in rats. Neurosci Lett 17:61–65, 1980
40. Fleming JFR, Crosby EC: The parietal lobe as an additional motor area. J Comp Neurol 103:485–512, 1955
41. Foerster D: The cerebral cortex in man. Lancet 2:309–312, 1931
42. Gainotti G, Messerli P, Tissot R: Qualitative analysis of unilateral spatial neglect in relation to laterality of cerebral lesions. J Neurol Neurosurg Psychiatry 35:545–550, 1972
43. Geschwind N: Disconnection syndromes in animals and man. Brain 88:237–294, 585–644, 1965
44. Godfraind JM, Meulders M: Effets de la stimulation sensorielle somatique sur les champs visuels des neurones de la région genouillée chez le chat anesthésié au chloralose. Exp Brain Res 9:183–200, 1969
45. Goldberg ME, Bushnell MC: Behavorial enhancement of visual responses in monkey cerebral cortex: II. Modulation in frontal eye fields specifically related to saccades. J Neurophysiol (in press)
46. Goldberg ME, Bushnell MC: The role of the frontal eye fields in visually guided saccades. In Fuchs AF, Becker W (eds): Progress in Oculomotor Research. Amsterdam, Elsevier/North Holland, 1981
47. Goldberg ME, Wurtz RH: Activity of superior colliculus in behaving monkey. I. Visual receptive fields of single neurons. J Neurophysiol 35:542–559, 1972
48. Goldman PS, Nauta WJH: Columnar distribution of cortico-cortical fibers in the frontal association, limbic, and motor cortex of the developing rhesus monkey. Brain Res 122:393–413, 1977
49. Goldman PS, Rosvold HE: Localization of function within the dorsolateral prefrontal cortex of the rhesus monkey. Exp Neurol 27:291–304, 1970
50. Gross CG, Rocha-Miranda CE, Bender DB: Visual properties of neurons in inferotemporal cortex of the macaque. J Neurophysiol 35:96–111, 1972
51. Hécaen H, Penfield W, Bertrand C, Malmo R: The syndromes of apractognosia due to lesions of the minor cerebral hemisphere. Arch Neurol Psychiatry 75:400–434, 1956
52. Heilman KM, Pandya DN, Geschwind N: Trimodal inattention following parietal lobe ablations. Trans Am Neurol Assoc 95:250–261, 1970
53. Heilman KM, Schwartz HD, Watson RT: Hypoarousal in patients with the neglect syndrome and emotional indifference. Neurology 28:229–232, 1978
54. Heilman KM, Valenstein E: Auditory neglect in man. Arch Neurol 26:32–35, 1972
55. Heilman KM, Valenstein E: Frontal lobe neglect in man. Neurology (Minneap) 22:660–664, 1972
56. Heilman KM, Valenstein E: Mechanisms underlying hemispatial neglect. Ann Neurol 5:166–170, 1979
57. Heilman KM, Van Den Abell T: Right hemisphere dominance for attention: the mechanism underlying hemispheric asymmetries of inattention (neglect). Neurology 30:327–330, 1980
58. Hernandez-Péon R: Neurophysiologic aspects of attention. In Vinken PJ, Bruyn GW (eds): Handbook of Clinical Neurology. New York, Elsevier, 1969, vol 3, pp 155–186
59. Howes D, Boller F: Simple reaction time: evidence for focal impairment from lesions of the right hemisphere. Brain 98:317–332, 1975
60. Hubel DH, Henson CO, Rupert A, Galambos R: "Attention" units in the auditory cortex. Science 129:1279–1280, 1959
61. Hyvärinen J, Poranen A: Function of the parietal associative area 7 as revealed from cellular discharges in alert monkeys. Brain 97:673–692, 1974
62. James W: The Principles of Psychology. New York, Holt, 1890
63. Jansen J, Andersen P, Kaada BP: Subcortical mechanisms in the "searching" or "attention" response elicited by prefrontal cortical stimulation in unanesthetized cats. Yale J Biol Med 28:331–341, 1955
64. Jones EG, Powell TPS: An anatomical study of converging sensory pathways within the cerebral cortex of the monkey. Brain 93:793–820, 1970
65. Jouvet M: Neurophysiology of the states of sleep. In Quarton CG, Melnechuk T, Schmitt FO (eds): The Neurosciences A Study Program. New York, Rockefeller University Press, 1967, pp 529–544
66. Kasdon DL, Jacobson S: The thalamic afferents to the inferior parietal lobule of the rhesus monkey. J Comp Neurol 177:685–706, 1978
67. Kennard MA: Alterations in response to visual stimuli following lesions of frontal lobe in monkeys. Arch Neurol Psychiatry 41:1153–1165, 1939
68. Kievit J, Kuypers HGJM: Basal forebrain and hypothalamic connections to frontal and parietal cortex in the rhesus monkey. Science 187:660–662, 1975
69. Kimura D: The asymmetry of the human brain. Sci Am 228:70–78, 1973
70. Künzle H: Bilateral projections from precentral motor cortex to the putamen and other parts of the basal ganglia: an autoradiographic study in *Macaca fascicularis*. Brain Res 88:195–209, 1975
71. Künzle H, Akert K, Wurtz RH: Projection of area 8 (frontal eye field) to superior colliculus in the monkey. An autoradiographic study. Brain Res 117:482–487, 1976
72. Kuypers HGJM, Lawrence DG: Cortical projections to the red nucleus and the brain stem in the rhesus monkey. Brain Res 4:151–188, 1967
73. Lamotte RH, Acuña C: Defects in accuracy of reaching after removal of posterior parietal cortex in monkeys. Brain Res 139:309–326, 1978
74. Lashley KS: Brain Mechanisms and Intelligence. Chicago, University of Chicago Press, 1929
75. Latto R: The effects of bilateral frontal eye-field, posterior parietal or superior collicular lesions on brightness thresholds in the rhesus monkey. Neuropsychologia 15:507–516, 1977
76. Latto R, Cowey A: Visual field defects after frontal eye-field lesions in monkeys. Brain Res 30:1–24, 1971
77. Leceister J, Sidman M, Stoddard LT, Mohr JP: Some determinants of visual neglect. J Neurol Neurosurg Psychiatry 32:580–587, 1969
78. Ledoux T, Wilson DH, Gazzaniga MS: Manipulo-spatial aspects of cerebral lateralization: clues to the origin of lateralization. Neuropsychologia 15:743–750, 1977
79. Ljungberg T, Ungerstedt U: Sensory inattention produced by 6-hydroxydopamine–induced degeneration of ascending dopamine neurons in the brain. Exp Neurol 53:585–600, 1976
80. Luria AR, Karpov BA, Yarbuss AL: Disturbances of active visual perception with lesions of the frontal lobes. Cortex 11:202–212, 1966

81. Lynch JC: The functional organization of posterior parietal association cortex. Behav Brain Sci 3:485–499, 1980
82. Lynch JC, Mountcastle VB, Talbot WH, Yin TCT: Parietal lobe mechanisms for directed visual attention. J Neurophysiol 40:362–389, 1977
83. Markowitsch HJ, Pritzel M, Petrovic-Minic B: Prefrontal cortex of the cat: paucity of afferent projections from the parietal cortex. Exp Brain Res 39:105–112, 1980
84. Marshall JF: Somatosensory inattention after dopamine-depleting intracerebral 6-DHDA injections: spontaneous recovery and pharmacological control. Brain Res 177:311–324, 1979
85. Mason ST, Fibiger HC: Noradrenaline and selective attention. Life Sci 25:1949–1956, 1979
86. Mason ST, Iversen SD: Reward, attention and the dorsal noradrenergic bundle. Brain Res 150:135–148, 1978
87. McFie J, Piercy MF, Zangwill OL: Visual-spatial agnosia associated with lesions of the right cerebral hemisphere. Brain 73:167–190, 1950
88. Meldman MJ: Diseases of Attention and Perception. London, Pergamon, 1970
89. Mesulam M-M, Geschwind N: On the possible role of the neocortex and its limbic connections in the process of attention and schizophrenia: clinical cases of inattention in man and experimental anatomy in monkey. J Psychiatr Res 14:249–259, 1978
90. Mesulam M-M, Van Hoesen GW, Pandya DN, Geschwind N: Limbic and sensory connections of the inferior parietal lobule (area PG) in the rhesus monkey: a study with a new method for horseradish peroxidase histochemistry. Brain Res 136:393–414, 1977
91. Mesulam M-M, Van Hoesen GW, Rosene DL: Substantia innominata, septal area and nuclei of the diagonal band in the rhesus monkey: organization of efferents and their acetylcholinesterase histochemistry. Neurosci Abstr 3:202, 1977
92. Mesulam M-M, Waxman SG, Geschwind N, Sabin TD: Acute confusional states with right middle cerebral artery infarctions. J Neurol Neurosurg Psychiatry 39:84–89, 1976
93. Milner AD, Foreman NP, Goodale MA: Go-left go-right discrimination performance and distractibility following lesions of prefrontal cortex or superior colliculus in stumptail macaques. Neuropsychologia 16:381–390, 1978
94. Mohler CW, Goldberg ME, Wurtz RH: Visual receptive fields and frontal eye field neurons. Brain Res 61:385–389, 1973
95. Mohler CW, Wurtz RH: Role of striate cortex and superior colliculus in visual guidance of saccadic eye movements in monkeys. J Neurophysiol 40:74–94, 1977
96. Mountcastle VB: Brain mechanisms for directed attention. J R Soc Med 71:14–28, 1978
97. Mountcastle VB, Lynch JC, Georgopoulos A, Sakata H, Acuña C: Posterior parietal association cortex of the monkey: command functions for operations within extrapersonal space. J Neurophysiol 38:875–908, 1975
98. Oxbury JM, Campbell DC, Oxbury SM: Unilateral spatial neglect and impairments of spatial analysis and visual perception. Brain 97:part III:551, 564, 1974
99. Pandya DN, Kuypers HGJM: Cortico-cortical connections in the rhesus monkey. Brain Res 13:13–36, 1969
100. Pandya DN, Van Hoesen GW, Mesulam M-M: Efferent connections of the cingulate gyrus in the rhesus monkey. Exp Brain Res 42:319–330, 1981
101. Patterson A, Zangwill OL: Disorders of visual space perception associated with lesions of the right cerebral hemisphere. Brain 67:331–358, 1944
102. Petras JM: Connections of the parietal lobe. J Psychiatr Res 8:189–201, 1971
103. Petrides M, Iversen SD: Restricted posterior parietal lesions in the rhesus monkey and performance on visuospatial tasks. Brain Res 161:63–77, 1979
104. Robinson DA: Eye movements evoked by collicular stimulation in the alert monkey. Vision Res 12:1795–1808, 1972
105. Robinson DA, Fuchs AF: Eye movements evoked by stimulation of frontal eye fields. J Neurophysiol 32:637–648, 1969
106. Robinson DL, Goldberg ME, Stanton GB: Parietal association cortex in the primate: sensory mechanisms and behavioral modulations. J Neurophysiol 41:910–932, 1978
107. Rolls ET, Perrett D, Thorpe SJ, Puerto A, Roper-Hall A, Maddison S: Responses of neurons in area 7 of the parietal cortex to objects of different significance. Brain Res 169:194–198, 1979
108. Rolls ET, Sanghere MK, Roper-Hall A: The latency of activation of neurons in the lateral hypothalamus and substantia innominata during feeding in the monkey. Brain Res 164:121–135, 1979
109. Rosene DL, Van Hoesen GW: Hippocampal efferents reach widespread areas of cerebral cortex in monkey. Science 198:315–317, 1977
110. Schenkenberg PH, Dustman RE, Beck EC: Changes in evoked responses related to age hemisphere and sex. Electroencephalogr Clin Neurophysiol 30:163, 1971
111. Schiller PH: The role of the monkey superior colliculus in eye movement and vision. Invest Ophthalmol 2:451–460, 1972
112. Schiller PH, Stryker M: Single-unit recording and stimulation in superior colliculus of the alert rhesus monkey. J Neurophysiol 35:915–924, 1972
113. Schiller PH, True SD, Conway JL: Effects of frontal eye field and superior colliculus ablations on eye movements. Science 206:590–592, 1979
114. Segarra JM: Cerebral vascular disease and behavior. Arch Neurol 22:408–418, 1970
115. Seltzer B, Pandya DN: Some cortical projections to the parahippocampal area in the rhesus monkey. Exp Neurol 50:146–160, 1976
116. Seltzer B, Pandya DN: Afferent cortical connections and architectonics of the superior temporal sulcus and surrounding cortex in the rhesus monkey. Brain Res 149:1–24, 1978
117. Seltzer B, Pandya DN: Converging visual and somatic sensory input to the intraparietal sulcus of the rhesus monkey. Brain Res 192:339–351, 1980
118. Sherrington CS: Man on His Nature. Cambridge, England, Cambridge University Press, 1940
119. Silberpfennig J: Contribution to the problem of eye movements. Confin Neurol 4:1–13, 1941
120. Soper HV, Diamond IT, Wilson M: Visual attention and inferotemporal cortex in rhesus monkeys. Neuropsychologia 13:409–419, 1975
121. Sprague JM, Meikle TH Jr: The role of the superior colliculus in visually guided behavior. Exp Neurol 11:115–146, 1965
122. Stamm JS: Functional dissociation between the inferior and arcuate segments of dorsolateral prefrontal cortex in the monkey. Neuropsychologia 11:181–190, 1973
123. Stanton GB, Cruce WLR, Goldberg ME, Robinson DL: Some ipsilateral projections to areas PF and PG of the inferior parietal lobule in monkeys. Neurosci Lett 6:243–250, 1977

124. Trojanowski JW, Jacobson S: Areal and laminar distribution of some pulvinar cortical efferents in rhesus monkey. J Comp Neurol 169:371–392, 1976

125. Van Hoesen GW, Vogt BA, Pandya DN, McKenna TM: Compound stimulus differentiation behavior in the rhesus monkey following periarcuate ablations. Brain Res 186: 365–378, 1980

126. Vogt BA, Rosene DL, Pandya DN: Thalamic and cortical afferents differentiate anterior from posterior cingulate cortex in the monkey. Science 204:205–207, 1979

127. Watson RT, Heilman KM, Cauthen JC, King FA: Neglect after cingulectomy. Neurology (Minneap) 23:1003–1007, 1973

128. Watson RT, Heilman KM, Miller BD, King FA: Neglect after mesencephalic reticular formation lesions. Neurology (Minneap) 24:294–298, 1974

129. Watson RT, Miller BD, Heilman KM: Nonsensory neglect. Ann Neurol 3:505–508, 1978

130. Weinberger NM, Velasco M, Lindsley DB: Effects of lesions upon thalamically induced electrocortical desynchronization and recruiting. Electroencephalogr Clin Neurophysiol 18: 369–377, 1965

131. Welch K, Stuteville P: Experimental production of unilateral neglect in monkeys. Brain 81:341–347, 1958

132. Wurtz RH, Goldberg ME: Activity of superior colliculus in behaving monkey. III. Cells discharging before eye movements. J Neurophysiol 35:575–585, 1972

133. Wurtz RH, Goldberg ME: Activity of superior colliculus in behaving monkey. IV. Effects of lesions on eye movements. J Neurophysiol 35:587–596, 1972

134. Wurtz RH, Mohler CW: Enhancement of visual responses in monkey striate cortex and frontal eye fields. J Neurophysiol 39:766–772, 1976

135. Yin TCT, Mountcastle VB: Visual input to the visuomotor mechanisms of the monkey's parietal lobe. Science 197:1381–1383, 1977

25

B. J. Richmond and T. Sato

Enhancement of inferior temporal neurons during visual discrimination

1987. *Journal of Neurophysiology* 58: 1292–1306

SUMMARY AND CONCLUSIONS

1. Previous results have shown that spatially directed attention enhances the stimulus-elicited responses of neurons in some areas of the brain. In the inferior temporal (IT) cortex, however, directing attention toward a stimulus mildly inhibits the responses of the neurons. Inferior temporal cortex is involved in pattern discrimination, but not spatial localization. If enhancement signifies that a neuron is participating in the function for which that part of cortex is responsible, then pattern discrimination, not spatial attention, should enhance responses of IT neurons. The influence of pattern discrimination behavior on the responses of IT neurons was therefore compared with previously reported suppressive influences of both spatial attention and the fixation point.

2. Single IT neurons were recorded from two monkeys while they performed each of five tasks. One task required the monkey to make a pattern discrimination between a bar and a square of light. In the other four tasks the same bar of light appeared, but the focus of spatial attention could differ, and the fixation point could be present or absent. Either attention to (without discrimination of) the bar stimulus or the presence of the fixation point attenuated responses slightly. These two suppressive influences produced a greater attenuation when both were present.

3. The visual conditions and motor requirements when the bar stimulus appeared in the discrimination task were identical to those of the trials in the stimulus attention task. However, one-half of the responsive neurons showed significantly stronger responses to the bar stimulus when it appeared in the discrimination task than when it appeared in the stimulus attention task. For most of these neurons, discrimination just overcame the combined effect of the two suppressive influences. For six other neurons, the response strength was significantly greater during the discrimination task than during any other task.

4. The monkeys achieved an overall correct performance rate of 90% in both the discrimination and stimulus attention tasks. To achieve this performance in the discrimination task they adopted a strategy in which they performed one trial type, bar stimulus attention trials, perfectly (100%) and the other trial type, pattern trials, relatively poorly (84% correct). The improved performance in response to the bar stimulus when it appeared in the discrimination task compared with when it appeared in the stimulus attention task suggests that the monkeys increased their level of attention during the discrimination task. Thus the enhancement of the neuronal responses seen in the discrimination task could have been due to either of two influences: the requirement to discriminate patterns or an increased level of attention.

INTRODUCTION

When attention is directed toward a stimulus located within a single neuron's receptive field, neurons in several parts of the brain show responses that are stronger than when attention is directed elsewhere (4, 8, 9, 25). However, in a recent study, when neurons in inferior temporal (IT) cortex were tested in similar experiments, the responses were mildly suppressed when attention was directed to the stimulus (23). This difference in results might have arisen from the difference in the functions of the brain regions studied. IT cortex appears to be specialized for pattern discrimination (13), whereas the other brain regions referred to, parietal cortex, frontal eye fields, and superior colliculus, appear to be specialized for spatial localization of stimuli (4, 8, 9, 16, 25). Thus, if behaviorally induced strengthening of stimulus-elicited responses signifies that a neuron is participating in the function for which that part of cortex is responsible, then pattern discrimination, not spatial attention, should enhance the responses of IT neurons.

In this study, the influence of pattern discrimination behavior on the responses of IT neurons was compared with the influences of spatial attention and the fixation point, both of which caused response suppression in a previous study (23). These two suppressive effects were seen when tasks were used in which two stimuli, a fixation point and a bar of light, appeared. First, neurons responded more weakly to the onset of the bar of light when its dimming rather than the dimming of the fixation point was used as the behavioral cue. Second, the response to the bar stimulus was weaker when the fixation point remained on during stimulus presentation than when the fixation point was turned off for the period of stimulus presentation. These two suppressive influences produced a greater attenuation when both were present. Both suppressive effects were confirmed here. In addition, ~50% of the neurons responsive to visual stimulation showed strengthened responses during pattern discrimination. A brief report of these results appeared previously (22).

METHODS

Procedures in awake monkeys

Awake trained rhesus monkeys were seated in primate chairs 57 cm away from a tangent screen. The tangent screen was made of thin translucent tracing paper taped to a sheet of rigid clear plastic. Slide projectors equipped with high-speed shutters (Uniblitz, Rochester, NY) projected stimuli onto the back of the translucent screen.

While single units were recorded monkeys performed five behavioral tasks, four of which have been described previously (23). For every task, trials began when the monkey touched a plate of metal attached to the primate chair. This caused a fixation point (0.15°) to appear on the tangent screen. The monkey was required to fixate for 500 ms before a visual stimulus, usually a bar of light (Fig. 1*A*) located 3-10° eccentrically, was flashed onto the tangent screen for at least 400 ms.

Throughout these experiments eye position was monitored using the magnetic search-coil technique (14, 24). Eye position was accepted as being correct when it was within 0.75° of the fixation point. Only single-unit responses taken from trials in which the monkey performed correctly were analyzed. The behavioral program and data acquisition were carried out by a laboratory computer with a flexible real-time software system (12).

Modifications of two variables distinguished the five tasks. First, the fixation point could be either on (fixation attention and stimulus attention tasks) or off (blink-fixation attention and blink-stimulus attention tasks) during stimulus presentation. Second, the significance of the bar of light changed, in that it could be ignored (fixation attention and blink-fixation attention tasks), its dimming had to be detected (stimulus attention and blink-stimulus attention tasks), or it had to be discriminated from an outline square of light (Fig. 1*B*). Release of the touch plate at any time during a trial led to the disappearance of the stimuli. At the end of each trial there was a 1-s interval before the next trial could be initiated.

Complete descriptions of the five tasks used during single-unit recording (Fig. 2 and Table 1) follow in the order they were taught to the monkeys.

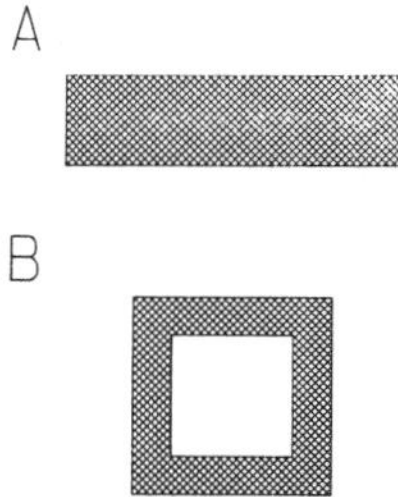

FIG. 1. Schematic illustration of the bar of light and outline square stimuli. The stimuli were matched in brightness and area of illumination. The distance between the stimuli and the fixation point was constant for a set of trials and was 3–10°. These stimuli appeared at the same location. The bar of light appeared in all 5 tasks, whereas the outline square appeared only in the discrimination task. In trials where the bar of light appeared either it or the fixation point dimmed late in the trial, depending on the task, as a behavioral cue. In the discrimination task, appearance of the outline square was a signal for the monkey to release the touch panel within 500 ms.

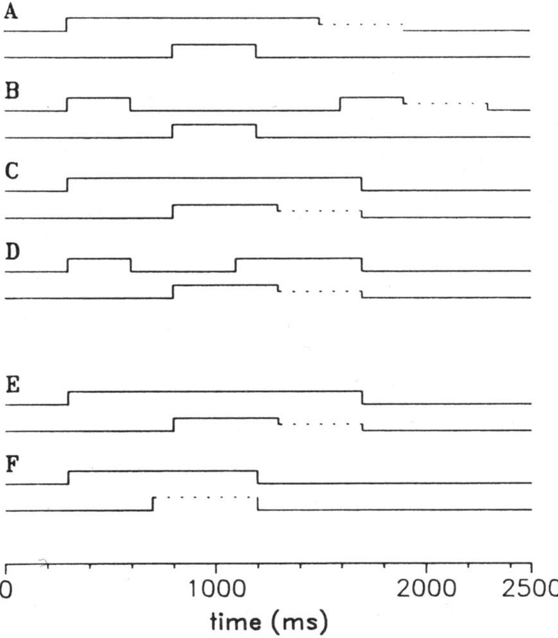

FIG. 2. Schematic outline of tasks. Time goes from left to right. All trials are initiated when the monkey touches a sensitized metal bar. The lines rise to indicate the time of fixation point or stimulus appearance, fall to base line to indicate the time of disappearance, and fall halfway to indicate the time of dimming. The *upper line* of each pair represents the fixation point, and the *lower line* represents the stimulus. The lines are *dashed* to indicate the periods during which bar release caused a reward to be given. *A*: fixation attention task. The monkey responded to the dimming by releasing the bar. During the time the fixation point was on, a stimulus came on and went off. *B*: blink-fixation attention task. The fixation point was turned off or blinked off for 1 s. The stimulus was presented for 400 ms during this blink period. *C*: stimulus attention task. The stimulus dimmed instead of the fixation point, thereby requiring the monkey to attend to the stimulus. *D*: blink-stimulus attention task. The fixation point reappeared 200 ms after the appearance of the bar of light so that the monkeys would not make a saccadic eye movement to the bar of light. The bar of light dimmed. *E*: discrimination task. There were two types of trial. The first trial type was selected from one of the four trial types above, usually a stimulus attention trial. The second, a pattern trial, occurred when an outline square appeared, at which time the monkey had to respond immediately (within 500 ms). All tasks were run in blocks of trials. Intervals that affected the time at which the monkey could successfully obtain a reward were varied unpredictably so the monkey could only succeed by interpreting the stimulus changes correctly (see text).

1) THE FIXATION ATTENTION TASK (FIXATION POINT ON DURING STIMULUS PRESENTATION, FIXATION POINT RELEVANT). While the monkey fixated, the bar of light appeared for 400 ms and then disappeared. Three hundred to 800 ms after the bar of light disappeared, the fixation point dimmed for 400 ms and then also disappeared. If the monkey released the touch-sensitive plate during the dim period, it was rewarded with a drop of juice or water. These trials lasted 1,200–1,700 ms.

2) THE BLINK-FIXATION ATTENTION TASK (FIXATION POINT OFF DURING STIMULUS PRESENTATION, FIXATION POINT RELEVANT). After the initial 500 ms of fixation, the fixation point was blinked off for ~1 s. Beginning 150–300 ms after the fixation point disappeared the bar of light appeared for 400 ms and then disappeared. Three hundred milliseconds later the fixation point reappeared, remained bright for 300–800 ms, dimmed for 400 ms, and then disappeared. If the monkey released the touch-sensitive plate while the fixation point was dim, a reward was delivered. Blink trials, the longest trial type used, lasted 1,450–2,200 ms.

3) THE STIMULUS ATTENTION TASK (FIXATION POINT ON DURING STIMULUS PRESENTATION, STIMULUS RELEVANT). During this task the monkey's attention was directed to the bar of light instead of the fixation point by requiring the monkey to respond to dimming of the bar of light. While the monkey fixated, the bar of light appeared and remained bright for 400 ms. Then, 0–500 ms later, the bar of light dimmed for 400 ms before it disappeared (along with the fixation point). If the monkey released the touch-sensitive plate during the 400-ms dim period a reward was delivered. Stimulus attention trials lasted 900–1,400 ms.

TABLE 1. *Factors that differentiate tasks*

Task	Presence of Fixation Point During Stimulus Presentation	Stimulus Significance
Fixation attn	+	fp dims
Blink-fix attn	–	fp dims
Stim attn	+	bar stim dims
Blink-stim attn	–*	bar stim dims
Discrimination	+†	discriminate bar and bar dims

Two factors vary across the 5 tasks: *1*) whether or not the fixation point remains on during presentation of the bar of light stimulus, and *2*) the significance of the bar of light. The fixation point or bar stimulus could dim as a behavioral cue at the end of the trial, and the bar stimulus could be part of a visual discrimination. +, on; –, off; fp, fixation point; stim, stimulus. * Fixation point appears 200 ms after stimulus appears; † During stimulus attention trials.

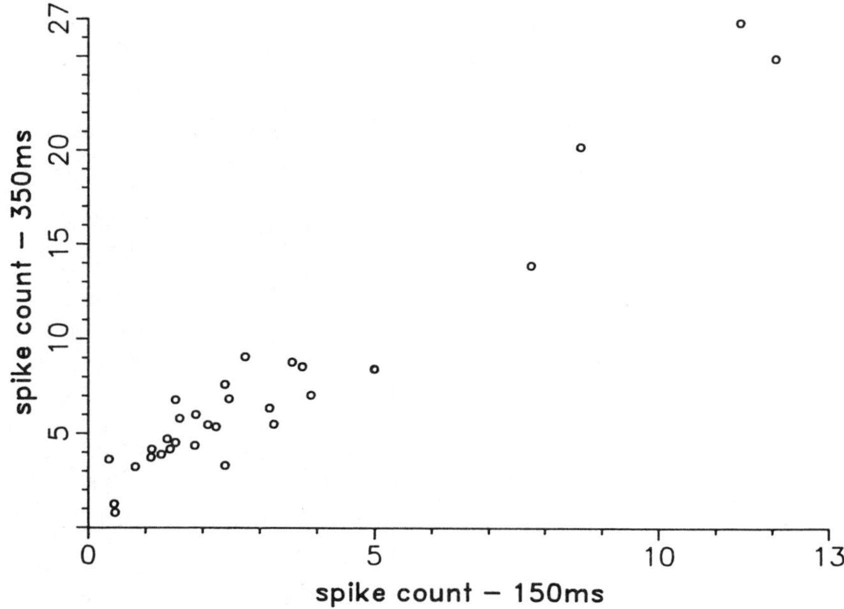

FIG. 3. Correlation of the number of spikes from 50 to 200 ms after stimulus onset with the number of spikes from 50 to 400 ms for all the tasks from 5 neurons. The responses were quantified during the period from 50 to 200 ms after stimulus onset for statistical analysis. This period was chosen because of the constraints imposed by the blink plus stimulus attention task. This figure indicates that the conclusions reached from the statistical tests were unlikely to be significantly different if a different period had been used for counting the spikes in the response. $r_{xy} = 0.97$.

4) THE BLINK-STIMULUS ATTENTION TASK (FIXATION POINT OFF DURING STIMULUS PRESENTATION, STIMULUS RELEVANT). This task combined the principles of the blink and stimulus attention tasks. Ideally, the monkey would have maintained eye position with no fixation point present while waiting for the stimulus to dim, but, in fact, the monkeys were not able to suppress a saccade to the bar of light under these conditions. On the other hand, the monkeys were able to maintain gaze after the bar of light appeared if the fixation point reappeared 200 ms later. Thus, for this task, unlike the blink task, the fixation point was turned on again 200 ms after the bar of light appeared, and 300–700 ms later the stimulus dimmed and then disappeared (together with the fixation point). As required by the experimental question being addressed, this procedure resulted in a period at the time of stimulus appearance during which the fixation point was off. These trials lasted 1,350–1,900 ms.

5) PATTERN DISCRIMINATION. Each of the tasks above consisted of one type of trial that was repeated in blocks of 15–20 trials each without interruption by other trial types. The discrimina-

TABLE 2. *Number of visually responsive units with significant (*P *< 0.05) differences between pairs of conditions*

	Blink-Fix Attn	Blink-Stim Attn	Fixation Attn	Stim Attn
Discrim (stim attn)	6	6	6	32
Blink-fix attn		0	3	60
Blink-stim attn			0	2
Fixation attn				0

For the 72 inferior temporal neurons responsive to visual stimulation each table entry gives the number of neurons that had a significant ($P < 0.05$, Kruskal-Wallis test) difference in the responses between the two conditions represented by the column-row intersection. These are ordered so that they differ with the condition in the left column, giving a greater response than the condition at the top of the column.

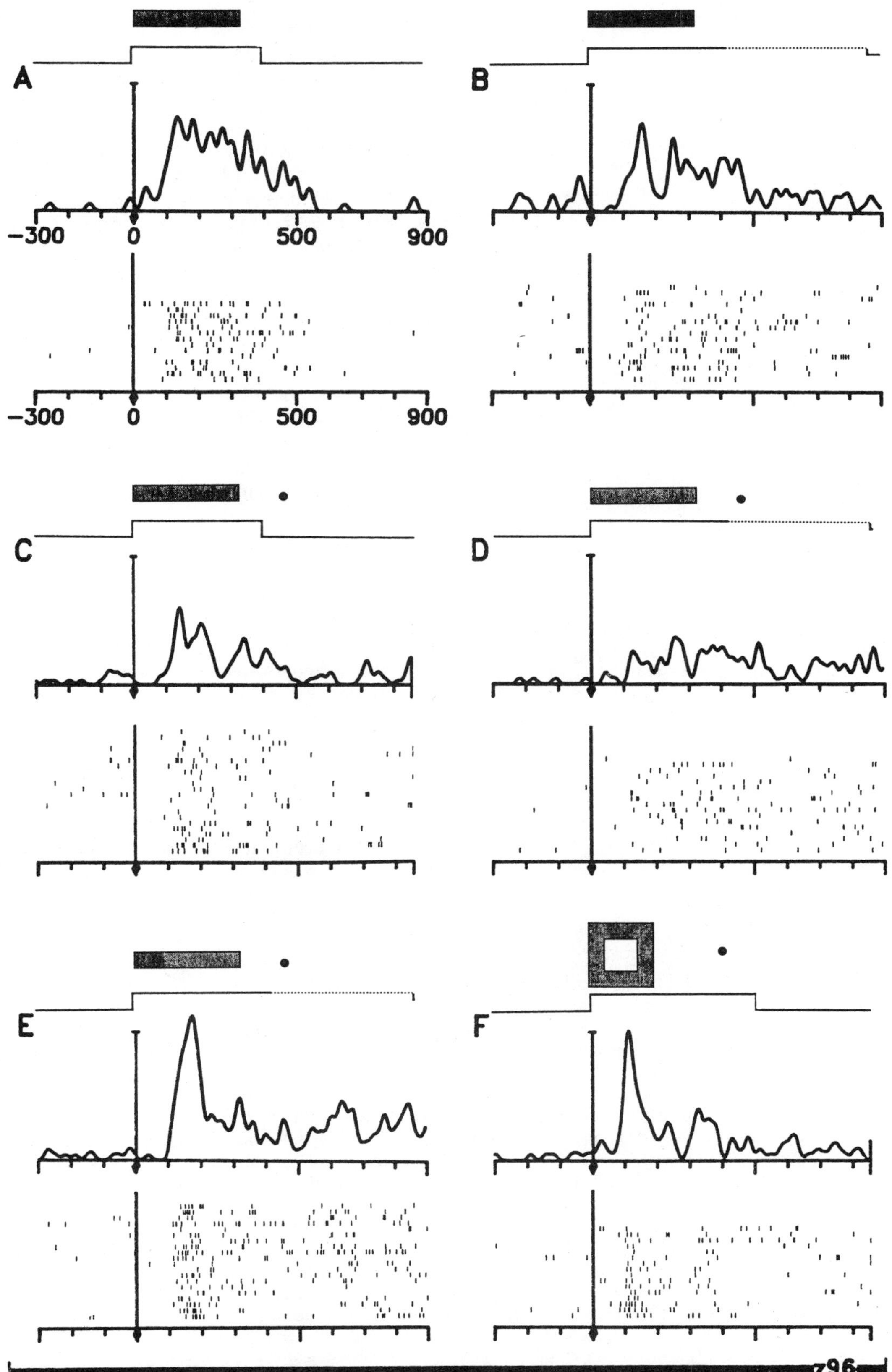

FIG. 4. Responses of one neuron in all tasks. Each panel consists, from the bottom up, of a raster, a spike density or histogram, a line indicating the presence or absence of the stimulus, a schematic illustration of the stimulus, and for those tasks in which the fixation point remained on during stimulus presentation, a *black dot* next to the

tion task consisted of two trial types mixed in an unpredictable order and presented for 15-20 trials each: one trial type was identical to the stimulus attention task as described above, and the other consisted of trials in which a different visual stimulus, namely, an outline square, appeared (Fig. 1*B*). On trials in which the outline square appeared the monkey was required to release the touch-sensitive plate within 500 ms. The outline square did not dim. This discrimination task required the monkey to choose the correct motor response, i.e., release the touch-sensitive plate immediately upon seeing the outline square or delay release of the plate on seeing the bar of light, releasing it only when the bar of light dimmed. The bar and outline square were matched for area of illumination and brightness. The longest possible duration for a trial with the outline square was 500 ms, although the monkey's reaction time in these trials was generally 250–320 ms.

During task changes the monkeys were prevented from working for 20–30 s. This delay was the only cue the monkey received to indicate the start of the new task. The monkeys adapted quickly to task changes and generally started the new tasks with zero to one error. Data from the first three trials after each task change were excluded from the analyses. There were not enough task changes during recording from any one neuron to make any reliable estimate of the dynamics of response adaptation by the neuron following task changes. After all the tasks were presented once, they were repeated if the neuron remained well isolated and the monkey continued to work. When a task was repeated, the data for that task were combined across repetitions for statistical analyses.

Single-unit recording

Both a chronic recording chamber and head-fixation device were attached to the skull, and a scleral magnetic search coil was implanted under Tenon's capsule using sterile surgical technique while the monkey was anesthetized with pentobarbital sodium (7, 14, 23). The recording cylinder was placed in the stereotaxic plane over IT cortex (AP + 16 mm, lateral 20 mm). The monkey was given a 2- to 3-wk recovery period, after which final training was undertaken. When behavioral performance was stable in all five tasks, single-unit recording was begun.

All recording was done by passing fine tungsten microelectrodes (Frederick Haer) through a 20-gauge guide tube whose tip was placed 5–8 mm from the tissue of interest. The electrodes were moved through the guide tube and positioned with a hydraulic microdrive. The shaft of the microelectrode was bent slightly so that it would exit the guide tube in a different direction on each penetration. The guide tube was removed and repositioned after each two to five penetrations. Single-unit action potentials (spikes) were isolated using a voltage level discriminator and converted to pulses when a voltage threshold was reached. The times of all events including spike occurrence were stored by the computer with a 1-ms time resolution.

During the last few days of the experiment, 5–10 μA of direct current were passed through the electrode for 60 s to produce marking lesions at the locations of a few recorded neurons. Three days after placement of the last electrolytic lesion the monkey was given a lethal dose of pentobarbital sodium and, after deep anesthesia was

---

FIG. 4, *cont.*
illustration of the stimulus (*C-F*). Each *line* of a raster shows the times of spike occurrence with *tick marks*. The most recent trial is at the *top*. The *vertical line* indicates the time of stimulus onset for both the rasters and spike density diagrams. The spike density is the average, at a 1-ms resolution, of the convolution of each raster line with a Gaussian pulse, $\sigma = 10$ ms. The height of the vertical line represents a probability of spike occurrence of 0.05/ms, or a rate of 50 spikes/s/trial. The *horizontal line* above the spike density rises at the time of stimulus onset, and falls at stimulus offset. A *dotted line* indicates a variable length period before the bar of light dimmed. The bar of light appeared for 400 ms and then disappeared during the blink and fixation tasks, Fig. 4, *A and C*, or appeared, remained bright for 400 ms plus some variable period lasting up to an additional 400 ms, and then dimmed as a behavioral cue, Fig. 4, *B, C*, and *E*. The stimulus that appeared is shown schematically at the *top* of each figure. The *black dot* next to the stimulus in Fig. 4, *C-F* indicates that the fixation point remained on during the period of stimulus presentation. The *heavy line* under Fig. 4, *E* and *F* indicates that these data came from the two trial types of the same task, the discrimination task. *A-D* are arranged so effects due to presence or absence of the fixation point can be seen through comparison of the data from the 2 tasks shown in a column, i.e., Fig. 4, *A* vs. *C* and 4, *B* vs. *D*, and effects due to the difference in attention to the stimulus can be seen through comparison of the data from the 2 tasks shown in a row, i.e., Fig. 4, *A* vs. *B*, and Fig. 4, *C* vs. *D*. The responses shown in Fig. 4, *A-D*, are also in descending order according to response strength. The strongest responses were during the blink-fixation attention task, 23.8 ± 3.8 (SE) ($n = 14$) spikes/s/trial, followed by the blink-stimulus attention, 14.9 ± 2.8 ($n = 17$), fixation attention, 12.4 ± 2.0 ($n = 22$) and stimulus attention tasks, 5.4 ± 1.3 ($n = 17$), (Fig. 4, *A, B, C*, and *D*), respectively. The difference in responses during the blink, Fig. 4*A*, and the stimulus attention task, Fig. 4*D*, were significant (see text). *E* and *F* show the responses from the two trial types used in the discrimination, stimulus attention and second pattern, respectively. The responses to the bar of light during the stimulus attention trials of the discrimination task, Fig. 4*E*, were nearly as strong as the responses during the blink task, 21.7 ± 3.2 spikes/s/trial. These responses were significantly different from the responses during the stimulus attention task, Fig. 4*D*. The responses to the outline square are shown in *F*.

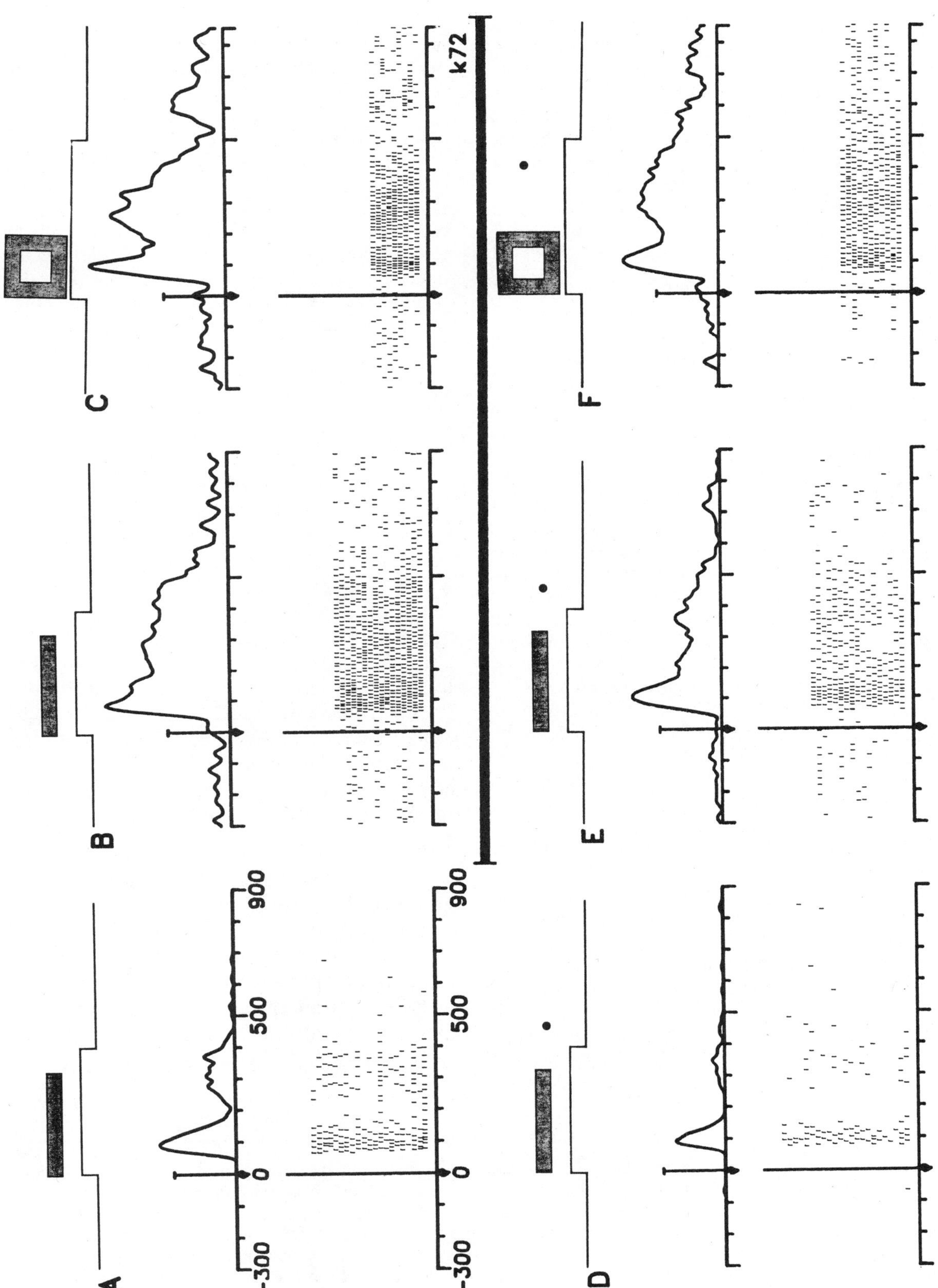
A
B
C
D
E
F
k72
−300
0
500
900

achieved, perfused through the left ventricle with saline followed by 10% formaldehyde. The microlesions were identified on cresyl violet-stained histological sections. They were found to lie within the cortex on both the lower bank of the superior temporal sulcus and the inferior surface of the temporal lobe. These sites were in the lateral middle third of the inferior temporal cortex, within the area demarcated as TE by Bonin and Bailey (3).

Data display and analysis

Single-unit data were first analyzed by inspection of rasters and spike density diagrams. The data in the raster diagrams were aligned on a common event, such as stimulus appearance, and were displayed on a trial-by-trial basis. Each row of dots in a raster represented the unit discharges from one behavioral trial. The sets of trials in each raster were also displayed as spike density diagrams. Spike density diagrams were created by convolution of each spike train with a Gaussian pulse (σ = 10 ms) and averaging the individual spike density functions at each millisecond. Spike density diagrams are similar to conventional histograms but they represent the data more accurately because they minimize binning artifacts (21). They are interpretable as the probability of spike occurrence at each millisecond in time.

Responses for all trial types are quantified by counting spike occurrence during a 150-ms period beginning 50 ms after stimulus onset. The 50-ms delay between the appearance of the bar of light and the start of the analysis period was used to take into account some of the neuronal response latency. The 150-ms counting period was chosen because of the constraints imposed by the blink-stimulus attention task. During that task, the desired combination of visual and behavioral conditions, that is, fixation point absent while the still fixating monkey waited for the bar of light to dim, lasted only 200 ms, after which the fixation point reappeared (Fig. 2). Figure 3 shows that the spike count during this short period, 150 ms, was representative of the responses during longer periods. The figure shows that the responses of five neurons quantified during both 150- and 350-ms periods starting at the same time were highly correlated (r_{xy} = 0.97).

The responses that occurred under different conditions were compared through use of the nonparametric Kruskal-Wallis test with multiple comparisons (15), the nonparametric analog of the F test. A nonparametric test was chosen because the variance of different groups was unlikely to be uniform, and the populations underlying the data sets were unlikely to have been normally distributed (21, 27). Data sets (rasters) were accepted as being significantly different when $P < 0.05$.

RESULTS

The activity of 110 single neurons was recorded from the middle one-third of the IT cortex, within area TE of Bonin and Bailey (3), of two rhesus monkeys. Four neurons seemed similar to the rapidly habituating neurons found previously by others (11, 20). These four responded only to the initial presentation of a bar of light in a block of trials. Seventy-two other neurons responded consistently to the appearance of a bar of light located 5-10° from the point of fixation. Of these, nine responded to the bar of light equally across all five tasks. The remaining 63 responded differentially to the bar of light across the five tasks (Table 1), and the following analyses are based on them.

Relative enhancement

For most of the differentially responsive neurons, the effect of pattern discrimination on the stimulus-elicited responses was to overcome the suppressive effects of *1*) the presence of a fixation point during the stimulus presentation and *2*) the requirement that the monkey attend to the peripherally located bar of light. The effects of these two

FIG. 5. Responses from a neuron that gave its greatest response during discrimination. *A*: blink-fixation attention task. *B*: blink-fixation attention trials during discrimination. *C*: blink-second pattern trials during discrimination. *D*: fixation attention task. *E*: fixation attention trials during discrimination. *F*: second pattern trials during discrimination. For most of the neurons the greatest response elicited by the stimulus occurred during the blink task. In this neuron the greatest response occured during the discrimination task, an example of absolute enhancement (see RESULTS). The responses from the discrimination task with blink-fixation trials substituted for stimulus attention trials (*B*) were stronger than the responses from the blink-fixation attention task (*A*). The responses in the *lower row* were taken from the tasks related to those in the *upper row*, except the fixation point remained on during stimulus presentation, i.e., the fixation attention task (*D*), and fixation attention trials in the discrimination task (*E*). *C* and *F* show the responses from the second pattern trials of the discrimination task. The responses were consistently stronger when the fixation point was absent (*upper row*). All markings are as defined for Fig. 4.

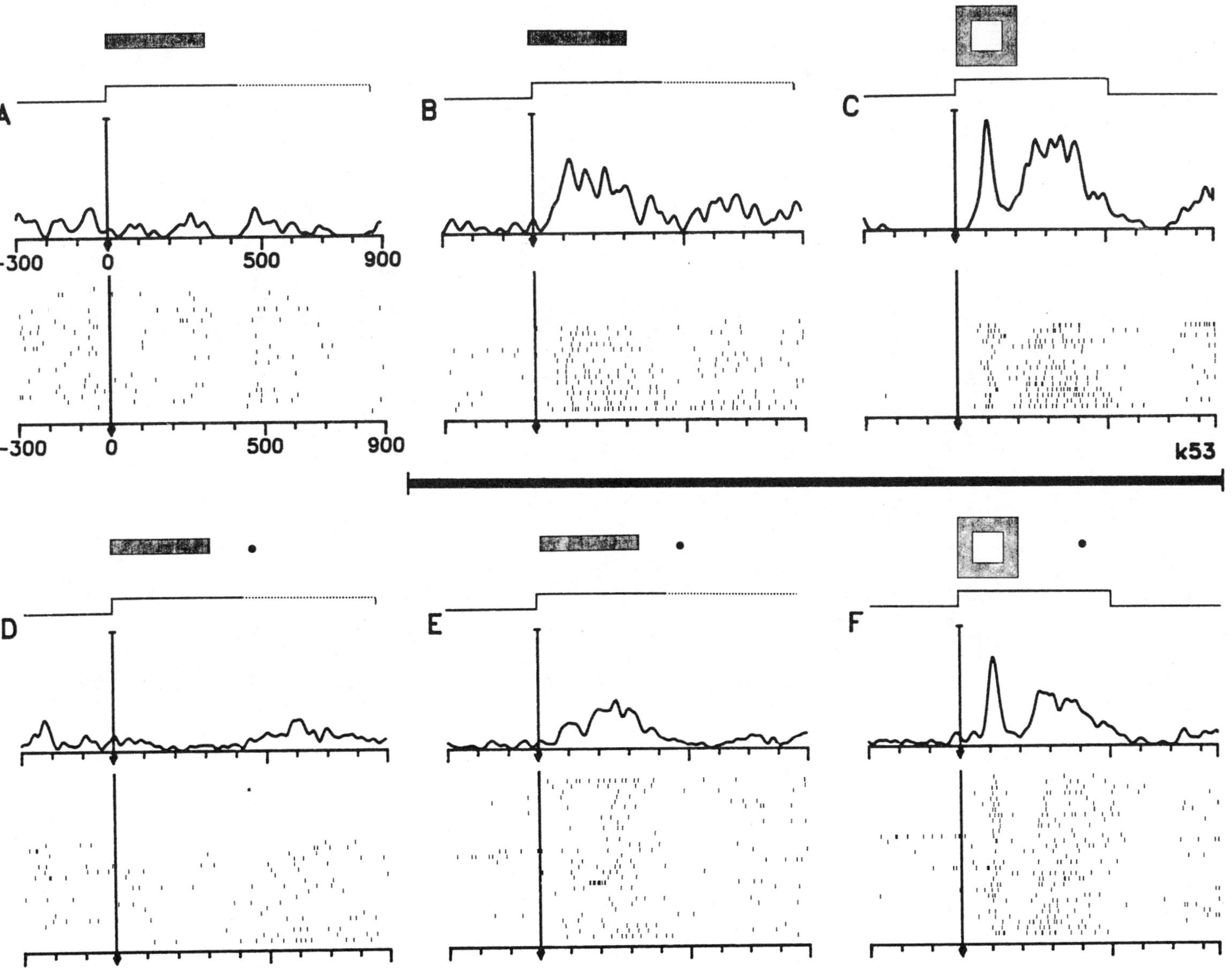
A
B
C
-300
0
500
900
-300
0
500
900
k53
D
E
F

factors were revealed by the four control tasks, which were arranged in a 2 × 2 design, as illustrated in the upper four panels of Fig. 4, *A-D*. The response suppression due to the presence of the fixation point can be seen through comparison of the first two panels in each column, i.e., blink-fixation attention versus fixation attention (Fig. 4, *A* vs. *C*) and blink-stimulus attention versus stimulus attention (Fig. 4, *B* vs. *D*). Similarly, the suppression due to the requirement that the monkey attend to the peripherally located bar of light can be seen through comparison of the two panels in each of the upper two rows, i.e., blink-fixation attention versus blink-stimulation attention (Fig. 4, *A* vs. *B*) and fixation attention versus stimulus attention (Fig. 4, *C* vs. *D*). Neither influence alone reached significance in this neuron, or in most others. However, in 60/63 neurons, when both influences were present the responses to the bar of light were significantly different from those when neither influence was present (e.g., responses in the stimulus attention task, Fig. 4*D*, vs. those in the blink-fixation attention task, Fig. 4*A*, were different, $P < 0.025$, Kruskal-Wallis $H = 15.4$, df = 4). Table 2 gives the number of neurons that showed significant differences across all pairs of conditions.

Also illustrated in Fig. 4 is the influence of pattern discrimination on the stimulus-elicited responses. This influence can be seen by comparing Fig. 4*E* (stimulus-attention trials of the pattern discrimination task) to Fig. 4*D* (stimulus-attention task). The visual and motor demands during these two tasks were identical, yet the responses were significantly stronger in the discrimination task than in the stimulus attention task ($P < 0.005$, $H = 22.86$, df = 4). The responses in the pattern discrimination task did not differ significantly from those in the other three tasks. A total of 26/63 neurons showed the same pattern of significant differences in the responses as those of the neuron illustrated in Fig. 4. For these 26 neurons the requirements of the discrimination task resulted in relative enhancement of their responses, i.e., discrimination overcame the combined effect of the two suppressive factors and raised the response strength in stimulus attention trials to equal, but not surpass, those seen in the blink-fixation attention task. The relative nature of the enhancement was also apparent when blink-fixation attention trials were substituted for stimulus-attention trials in the discrimination task; the responses to the bar of light were no stronger than the responses in the blink-fixation attention task itself, i.e., there was no enhancement.

Absolute enhancement

Three neurons showed absolute enhancement, i.e., their responses were enhanced whenever the bar of light was presented during discrimination without regard to the trial type. Indeed, these neurons had significantly stronger responses during blink-fixation attention trials in the discrimination task than during the blink-fixation attention task itself (Fig. 5, *B* vs. *A*). For these three neurons, the fixation point continued to exert a suppressive effect on the responses even during the discrimination task (Fig. 5, compare upper row panels with respective lower row panels).

Three neurons responded to the bar of light during pattern discrimination only (Fig. 6). A larger proportion of such neurons might have been present, but we usually searched for responsive neurons while the monkey performed the blink task because this ordinarily revealed the strongest response. It was only midway in the exploration of the second monkey that we began to test some apparently unresponsive neurons in the pattern discrimination task and found these three that responded only during dis-

FIG. 6. Neuron that responded to bar stimulus during discrimination only. Data from one of three neurons that showed a response to the bar of light only during the discrimination task. *A*: blink-stimulus attention task. *B*: blink-stimulus attention trials of pattern discrimination. *C*: blink-second pattern trials of the pattern discrimination (not used for comparisons). *D*: stimulus attention task. *E*: stimulus attention trials of pattern discrimination. *F*: second pattern trials of pattern discrimination (not used for comparisons). Discrimination task, *center column*. No response was seen to the bar stimulus in the stimulus attention tasks, *left column*, whereas a clear response occurred in response to the same stimulus in the same types of trials during the pattern discrimination. Again, the responses were stronger when the fixation point was absent, *upper row*.

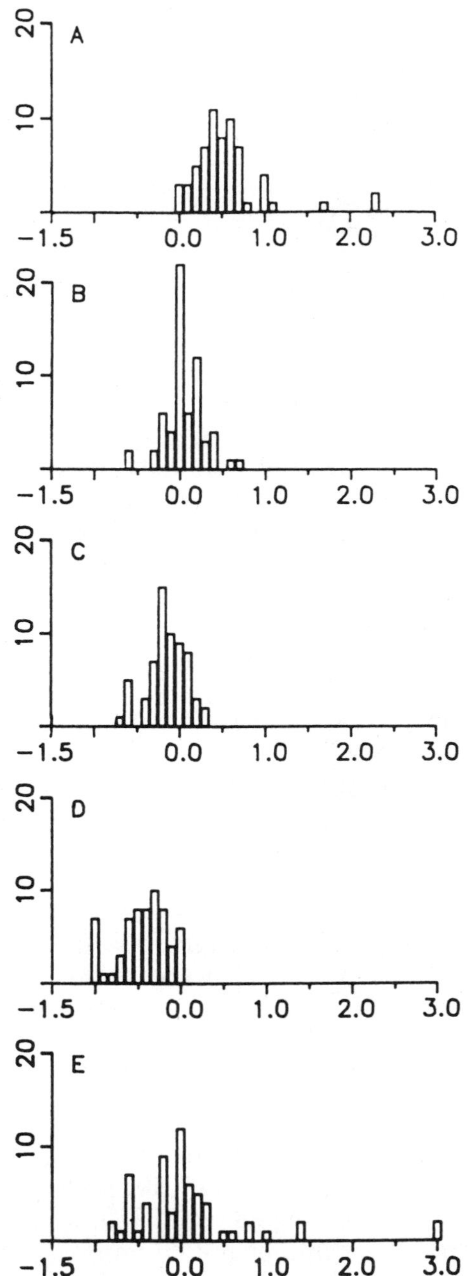

FIG. 7. Distributions of responses of 63 neurons to the bar of light during different behavioral tasks. The responses of each neuron to the bar of light during each task was transformed into a response ratio. The average response over the four control tasks, blink-fixation attention, blink-stimulus attention, fixation attention, and stimulus attention, was taken as the estimated expected response. For each task, the expected response was subtracted from the response to the bar of light during that task and the difference was divided by the expected response. This ratio then represented a normalized deviation from the expected response. $ratio_i = (R_i\text{-average})/\text{average}$, where R_i was the response during task i and $\text{average} = (R_{blink} + R_{blink+st\ attn} + R_{fixation} + R_{st\ attn})/4$. An entry was then made into each histogram for each neuron. *A*: blink-fixation task. *B*: blink-stimulus attention task. *C*: fixation attention task. *D*: stimulus attention task. *E*: pattern discrimination task (with stimulus attention trials).

crimination. All three neurons responded even more strongly to the outline square than to the bar of light in the pattern discrimination task, but since the outline square was not used in any other tasks, it is unknown whether responses to the square, like those to the bar of light, depended on the discrimination requirement. As with the three neurons described earlier in this section, the three that responded only during discrimination showed a noticeable suppressive effect when the fixation point was present. (Fig. 6, compare upper row panels with respective lower row panels.)

Population response

As already indicated, neither of the two suppressive factors alone had a significant effect on the strength of the responses of individual neurons (with two exceptions). However, each factor did have a significant effect when the relative strengths of the responses were grouped across all the neurons. The influence of the fixation point is seen through comparison of the response strength histograms of the blink-fixation attention task with those in the fixation attention task (Fig. 7, *A* vs. *C*, $P < 0.005$, $H = 50.34$, df = 4) and of the histograms of the blink-stimulus attention task with those in the stimulus attention task (Fig. 7, *B* vs. *D*, $P < 0.005$, $H = 34.44$, df = 4). The influence of the requirement that the monkey attend to the bar of light is seen through comparison of the histograms of the blink-fixation attention task with those of the blink-stimulus attention task (Fig. 7, *A* vs. *B*, $P < 0.005$, $H = 17.35$). The second comparison for this factor, fixation attention versus stimulus attention tasks (Fig. 7, *C* vs. *D*) fell short of significance ($P > 0.05$, $H = 8.64$). As expected, the effect of both suppressive factors combined was highly significant (Fig. 7, *A* vs. *D*, $P < 0.005$, $H = 100.68$).

Also as expected, the population response in the discrimination task showed significant enhancement over that in the stimulus attention task (Fig. 7, *E* vs. *D*, $P < 0.005$, $H =$

20.05) but fell significantly below that for the blink-fixation attention task (Fig. 7, *E* vs. *A*, $P < 0.05$, $H = 30.87$).

Lack of trial length influence

In anaesthetized monkeys, when a stimulus is presented repeatedly, some IT neurons show progressive response weakening when interstimulus intervals are short (6, 11, 20). During experiments using awake trained monkeys, IT neuronal responses to visual stimuli seemed stronger than in anesthetized monkeys (10), and gradual habituation has not been prominent (21, 23, 26). Nevertheless, responses in the tasks with short interstimulus intervals, e.g., stimulus attention task, could have been more susceptible to habituation than responses in tasks with longer interstimulus intervals, e.g., blink-stimulus attention task, and so could have led to some of the results reported here. Inspection of sequential trials in any single task did not reveal progressively decreasing response strengths (e.g., Fig. 4). However, the discrimination task consisted of two unpredictably mixed stimuli, the bar of light and the square of light, thereby giving rise to different interstimulus intervals between successive presentations of the bar of light. Stimulus attention trials were therefore tested to see whether the ones preceded by a stimulus attention trial formed a different group than those preceded by a pattern trial, and vice versa. The responses from 20/26 relatively enhanced neurons were tested, and none showed a significant dependence on the preceding trial type.

Influence of behavioral performance

Spitzer and Richmond (27) found that increased task difficulty was related to increased response strength in IT neurons. This suggests that increased attentiveness may lead to increased stimulus-elicited response strength. Since the different tasks in this study may not all have been equally difficult, this effect must be controlled to support the idea of function-dependent enhancement.

During the discrimination task the monkeys adopted a strategy that was biased toward more accurate performance of the stimulus attention trials than the trials with the second pattern (Table 3). The stimulus attention trials of the discrimination task were performed perfectly (100%), whereas the stimulus attention task was performed less well (91.4%). The trials with the second pattern were performed relatively poorly (84%), giving an overall performance level of 90.2%. This can be seen in Fig. 5: the rasters contain only successful trials, and there are more trials in the raster lines of Fig. 5*B* than in Fig. 5*C*.

TABLE 3. *Behavioral performance*

Task	Correct (%)	SE
Blink-fix attn	94.8	1.59
Blink-stim attn	90.0	2.84
Fixation attn	99.8	.20
Stim attn	91.4	1.36
Discrimination (total)	90.2	2.73
Pattern	84.0	4.27
Stim attn	100	0

The increased accuracy of the performance of the stimulus attention trials in the discrimination task compared with that in the stimulus attention task itself (100 vs. 91.5%) suggests that the monkeys put forth more effort in the discrimination task. This raises the possibility that the enhancement effect seen here during discrimination was due to increased attentiveness.

DISCUSSION

Ablation of inferior temporal cortex leads to a severe deficit in visual pattern discrimination (13). A previous study showed that attention to a stimulus mildly suppresses the responses of IT neurons (23). This study confirmed that result and also showed that responses to a stimulus could be enhanced when it was used in a pattern discrimination task. These results are consistent with the hypothesis that responses are enhanced when neurons are involved in a task for which that brain region is specialized.

Relative versus absolute enhancement

The enhanced neurons found here fell into two groups. For the larger group (57 neurons), responses seen during pattern discrimination were only enhanced relative to the suppressed responses (when the fixation point was present and attention to the stimulus without pattern discrimination was required). For the smaller group (6 neurons), enhancement was absolute, i.e., it occurred whenever pattern discrimination was required, even in the absence of the suppressive influences.

The difference between the two groups suggests enhancement may reflect two different mechanisms. The relative enhancement could be regarded as counteracting interference in the area from suppressive influences irrelevant to the behavioral task. The absolute enhancement was much larger and qualitatively different (cf. Fig. 5, *A* vs. *B* and *D* vs. *E*). Relative enhancement may help the ability to process visual stimulus features in the face of otherwise distracting and suppressive influences, whereas absolute enhancement may reflect the need to perform pattern discrimination.

Specific versus nonspecific enhancement

The enhancement seen in these IT neurons could have been specific for pattern discrimination or it could have been related to general arousal. Recent results have suggested that a relation exists between task difficulty and the stimulus-elicited response strength of IT neurons (27). In the experiments here, the monkeys were required to decide between two behavioral responses during the discrimination task. If the bar stimulus appeared, the correct response was to hold the touch plate until the bar dimmed. If the square stimulus appeared, the correct response was to release the touch plate immediately. If the monkeys were substantially more attentive in this task, then the increase in neuronal responsiveness might be a consequence of the increase in attentiveness and not the task. As the results showed, the performance level in the bar stimulus trials of the discrimination task did improve, implying that the monkeys put forth more effort in the discrimination task. This increased attentiveness might be a nonspecific cause of the enhancement.

If this increased attentiveness gave rise to the enhancement observed here, all of the neurons should have been enhanced, and there should have been only one type of enhancement. The enhancement actually observed had three characteristics that suggest that enhancement was specific. First, enhancement occurred only during pattern discrimination. Second, only 50% of the differentially responsive neurons showed enhancement. Third, neurons could show either of two types of enhancement, relative or absolute. Thus enhancement may arise from either specific or nonspecific mechanisms, or from a combination of both. New experiments would be required to differentiate among these possibilities.

Pattern discrimination and spatial attention

Results from recent psychophysical and neurophysiological experiments suggest that pattern discrimination is intimately related to spatial attention. When human subjects had to identify a unique stimulus within a field composed of a different stimulus repeated many times, their performance was progressively impaired as the number of repetitions of the second stimulus in the field increased (2). This result implies that a subject must find a stimulus to identify it. Thus spatial attention may be required for pattern discrimination. The neural mechanism underlying the relationship between pattern discrimination and spatial attention is not yet known.

Recent neurophysiological studies examined the influences of both pattern discrimination and spatial attention on neurons in IT cortex. Moran and Desimone (17) recently showed that the spatial focus of attention appeared to gate the stimulus-elicited responses of V4 and IT neurons during a pattern discrimination task. In the experiments here, the focus of spatial attention had a mild suppressive effect that was overcome by pattern discrimination. The combination of our results with the results of the above study suggests that the influence of spatial attention on IT neurons may be complex and depend upon whether a visual pattern discrimination task is also being performed.

A cortical subsystem for pattern vision

Based on their analysis of ablation effects on primate behavior, Ungerleider and Mishkin (28) proposed that there are two cortical visual pathways underlying discriminative abilities, one that emphasizes stimulus characteristics to facilitate pattern discriminations and memories, and the other that emphasizes spatial relationships between objects (16). The pattern subsystem consists of a chain of connections through ventral extrastriate visual areas terminating in inferior temporal cortex. The spatial subsystem consists of a chain of connections through more dorsal extrastriate areas terminating in posterior parietal cortex. The activity of neurons in these termination areas have shown signals that have been related to the functions revealed by ablations (1, 4, 5, 10, 11, 18, 19, 25, 26).

This hypothesis suggests that IT neuronal responses to identical stimuli would be different during pattern discrimination than during a task for which the retinal location of the stimulus is of primary importance. The results of the present study, where enhancement occurred only when pattern discrimination was required in addition to attention to the stimulus, support the existence of the pattern subsystem of the two cortical visual systems hypothesis.

ACKNOWLEDGMENTS

We thank Dr. Mortimer Mishkin for his support in every phase of these experiments and both him and Dr. Lance Optican for their help in the preparation of this manuscript. We also thank Dr. Michael Goldberg for his helpful comments during the preparation of this manuscript.

Present address of T. Sato: Tokyo Metropolitan Science Institute, Tokyo, Japan.

Address for reprint requests: B. J. Richmond, Laboratory of Neuropsychology, Bldg. 9, Rm. IN-107, National Institute of Mental Health, Bethesda, MD 20205.

REFERENCES

1. ANDERSON, R. A. AND MOUNTCASTLE, V. B. The influence of the angle of gaze upon the excitability of light-sensitive neurons of the posterior parietal cortex. *J. Neurosci.* 3: 532–548, 1983.
2. BERGEN, J. R. AND JULESZ, B. Parallel versus serial processing in rapid pattern discrimination. *Nature Lond.* 303: 696–698, 1983.
3. BONIN, G. VON AND BAILEY, P. *The Neocortex of Macaca mulatta.* Urbana, IL: Univ. of Illinois Press, 1947.
4. BUSHNELL, M. C., GOLDBERG, M. E., AND ROBINSON, D. L. Behavioral enhancement of visual responses in monkey cerebral cortex: I. Modulation in posterior parietal cortex related to selective visual attention. *J. Neurophysiol.* 46: 755–772, 1981.
5. DESIMONE, R., ALBRIGHT, T. D., GROSS, C. G., AND BRUCE, C. Stimulus-selective properties of inferior temporal neurons in the macaque. *J. Neurosci.* 4: 2051–2062, 1984.
6. DESIMONE, R. AND GROSS, C. G. Visual areas in the temporal cortex of the macaque. *Brain Res.* 178: 363–380, 1979.
7. EVARTS, E. V. Methods for recording activity of individual neurons in moving animals. In: *Methods in Medical Research,* edited by R. F. Rushmer. Chicago, IL: Year Book, 1966, p. 241–250.
8. GOLDBERG, M. E. AND BUSHNELL, M. C. Behavioral enhancement of visual responses in monkey cerebral cortex. II. Modulation in frontal eye fields specifically related to saccades. *J. Neurophysiol.* 46: 773–787, 1981.
9. GOLDBERG, M. E. AND WURTZ, R. H. Activity of superior colliculus in behaving monkey: II. The effect of attention on neuronal responses. *J. Neurophysiol.* 35: 560–574, 1972.
10. GROSS, C. G., BENDER, D. B., AND GERSTEIN, G. L. Activity of inferior temporal neurons in behaving monkeys. *Neuropsychologia* 17: 215–229, 1979.
11. GROSS, C. G., ROCHA-MIRANDA, C. E., AND BENDER, D. B. Visual properties of neurons in inferotemporal cortex of the macaque. *J. Neurophysiol.* 35: 96–111, 1972.
12. HAYS, A. V., RICHMOND, B. J., AND OPTICAN, L. M. A UNIX-based multiple process system for real-time data acquisition and control. *WESCON Conf. Proc.* 2: 1–10, 1982.
13. IWAI, E. AND MISHKIN, M. Further evidence on the locus of the visual area in the temporal lobe of the monkey. *Exp. Neurol.* 25: 585–594, 1969.
14. JUDGE, S. J., RICHMOND, B. J., AND CHU, F. C. Implantation of magnetic search coils for measurement of eye position: an improved method. *Vision Res.* 20: 535–538, 1980.
15. MILLER, JR., R. G. *Simultaneous Statistical Inference.* New York: McGraw-Hill, 1966.
16. MISHKIN, M., LEWIS, M. E., AND UNGERLEIDER, L. Equivalence of parieto-preoccipital subareas for visuospatial ability in monkeys. *Behav. Brain Res.* 6: 41–55, 1982.
17. MORAN, J. AND DESIMONE, R. Selective attention gates visual processing in the extrastriate cortex. *Science Wash. DC* 229: 782–784, 1985.
18. MOUNTCASTLE, V. B., ANDERSEN, R. A., AND MOTTER, B. C. The influence of attentive fixation upon the excitability of the light-sensitive neurons of the posterior parietal cortex. *J. Neurosci.* 1: 1218–1235, 1981.
19. PERRETT, D. I., ROLLS, E. T., AND CAAN, W. Visual neurons responsive to faces in the monkey temporal cortex. *Exp. Brain Res.* 47: 329–342, 1982.
20. POLLEN, D. A., NAGLER, M., DAUGMAN, J., KRONAUER, R., AND CAVANAUGH, P. Use of Gabor elementary functions to probe receptive field substructure of posterior inferotemporal neurons in the owl monkey. *Vision Res.* 24: 233–241, 1984.
21. RICHMOND, B. J., OPTICAN, L. M., PODELL, M.,

AND SPITZER, H. Temporal encoding of two-dimensional patterns by single units in primate inferior temporal cortex. I. Response characteristics. *J. Neurophysiol.* 57: 132–146, 1987.

22. RICHMOND, B. J. AND SATO, T. Visual responses of inferior temporal neurons are modified by attention to different stimulus dimensions. *Soc. Neurosci. Abstr.* 8: 812, 1982.
23. RICHMOND, B. J., WURTZ, R. H., AND SATO, T. Visual responses of inferior temporal neurons in the awake rhesus monkey. *J. Neurophysiol.* 50: 1415–1432, 1983.
24. ROBINSON, D. A. A method of measuring eye movement using a scleral search coil in a magnetic field. *IEEE Trans. Biomed. Eng. Electron.* 10: 137–145, 1963.
25. ROBINSON, D. L., GOLDBERG, M. E., AND STANTON, G. B. Parietal association cortex in the primate: sensory mechanisms and behavioral modulations. *J. Neurophysiol.* 41: 910–932, 1978.
26. SATO, T., KAWAMURA, T., AND IWAI, E. Responsiveness of inferotemporal single units to visual pattern stimuli in monkeys performing discrimination. *Exp. Brain Res.* 38: 313–319, 1980.
27. SPITZER, H. AND RICHMOND, B. J. Visual task difficulty correlates with neuronal activity in inferior temporal cortex. *Perception* 14: A13, 1985.
28. TOLHURST, D. J., MOVSHON, J. A., AND DEAN, A. F. The statistical reliability of signals in single neurons in cat and monkey visual cortex. *Vision Res.* 23: 775–785, 1983.
29. UNGERLEIDER, L. AND MISHKIN, M. Two cortical visual systems. In: *Analysis of Visual Behavior,* edited by D. J. Ingle, M. A. Goodale, and R. J. W. Mansfield. Cambridge, MA: MIT Press, 1982, p. 549–586.

26

J. Moran and R. Desimone

Selective attention gates visual processing in the extrastriate cortex

1985. *Science* 229: 782–784

Abstract

Single cells were recorded in the visual cortex of monkeys trained to attent to stimuli at one location in the visual field and ignore stimuli at another. When both locations were within the receptive field of a cell in prestriate area V4 or the inferior temporal cortex, the response to the unattended stimulus was dramatically reduced. Cells in the striate cortex were unaffected by attention. The filtering of irrelevant information from the receptive fields of extrastriate neurons may underlie the ability to identify and remember the properties of a particular object out of the many that may be represented on the retina.

Our retinas are constantly stimulated by a welter of shapes, colors, and textures. Since we are aware of only a small amount of this information at any one moment, most of it must be filtered out centrally. This filtering cannot easily be explained by the known properties of the visual system. In primates, the visual recognition of objects depends on the transmission of information from the striate cortex (V1) through prestriate areas into the inferior temporal (IT) cortex (*1*). At each successive stage along this pathway there is an increase in the size of the receptive fields; that is, neurons respond to stimuli throughout an increasingly large portion of the visual field. Within these large receptive fields will typically fall several different stimuli. Thus, paradoxically, more rather than less information appears to be processed by single neurons at each successive stage. How, then, does the visual system limit processing of unwanted stimuli? The results of our recording experiments on single neurons in the visual cortex of trained monkeys indicate that unwanted information is filtered from the receptive fields of neurons in the extrastriate cortex as a result of selective attention.

The general strategy of the experiment was as follows. After isolating a cell, we first determined its receptive field while the monkey fixated on a small target. On the basis of the cell's response to bars of various colors, orientations, and sizes, we determined which stimuli were effective in driving the cell and which were ineffective. Effective stimuli were then presented at one location in the receptive field concurrently with ineffective stimuli at a second location. The monkey was trained on a task that required it to attend to the stimuli at one location but ignore the stimuli at the other. After a block of 8 or 16 trials, the monkey was cued to switch its attention to the other location. Although the stimuli at the two locations remained the same, the locus of the animal's attention was repeatedly switched between the two locations. Since the identical sensory conditions were maintained in the two types of blocks, any difference in the response of the cell could be attributed to the effects of attention.

The task used to focus the animal's attention on a particular location was a modified version of a "match-to-sample" task. While the monkey held a bar and gazed at the fixation spot, a sample stimulus appeared briefly at one location followed about 500 msec later by a brief test stimulus at the same location. When the test stimulus was identical to the preceding sample, the animal was rewarded with a drop of water if it released the bar immediately, whereas when the test stimulus differed from the sample the animal was rewarded only if it delayed release for 700 msec. Stimuli were presented at the unattended location at the times of presentation of the sample and test stimuli, affording two opportunities to observe the effects of attention on each trial (*2*).

We recorded from 74 visually responsive cells in prestriate area V4 of two rhesus monkeys and found that the locus of the animal's attention in cell's receptive field had a dramatic effect on the cell's response (Fig. 1A). When an effective and an ineffective sensory stimulus were present in a cell's receptive field, and the animal attended to the effective stimulus, the cell responded well. When the animal attended to the ineffective stimulus, however, the response was greatly attenuated, even though the effective (but ignored) sensory stimulus was simultaneously present in the receptive field. Thus when there were two stimuli in the receptive field the response of the cell was determined by the properties of the attended stimulus.

To characterize the magnitude of the attenuation, an attenuation index (AI) was derived for each cell by dividing the response (minus baseline) to an effective stimulus when it was being ignored by the response to the same stimulus when it was being attended. For the large majority of cells in V4, the outcome of ignoring an effective sensory stimulus in the receptive field was to reduce the response by more than half (median AI, 0.36 for the sample stimulus and 0.33 for the test (Fig. 2A).

In the design described, the effective stimuli at one location in the receptive field always differed in some sensory quality, such as color, from the ineffective stim-

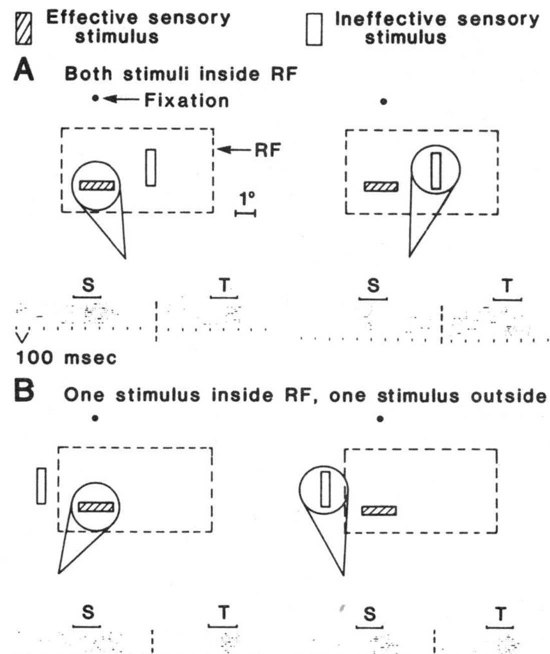

Figure 1. Effect of selective attention on the responses of a neuron in prestriate area V4. (A) Responses when the monkey attented to one location inside the receptive field (RF) and ignored another. At the attended location (circled), two stimuli (sample and test) were presented sequentially and the monkey responded differently depending on whether they were the same or different. Irrelevant stimuli were presented simultaneously with the sample and test but at a separate location in the receptive field. In the initial mapping of the receptive field, the cell responded well to horizontal and vertical red bars placed anywhere in the receptive field but not at all to green bars of any orientation. Horizontal or vertical red bars (effective sensory stimuli) were then placed at one location in the field and horizontal or vertical green bars (ineffective stimuli) at another. The responses shown are to horizontal red and vertical bars but are representative of the responses to the other stimulus pairings. When the animal attended to the location of the effective stimulus at the time of presentation of either the sample (S) or the test (T), the cell gave a good response (left), but when the animal attended to the location of the ineffective stimulus, the cell gave almost no response (right), even though the effective stimulus was present in its receptive field. Thus the response of the cell were determined by the attended stimulus. Because of the random delay between the sample and test stimulus presentations, the rasters were synchronized separately at the onsets of the sample and test stimuli (indicated by the vertical dashed lines). (B) Same stimuli as in (A), but the ineffective stimulus was placed outside the receptive field. The neuron responded similarly to the effective sensory stimulus, regardless of which location was attended.

uli at the other location. Thus attenuation of the response to an ignored stimulus could have been based on either its location or its sensory qualities. For example, for the cell described in the legend to Fig. 1, effective horizontal or vertical red bars were presented at one location while ineffective horizontal or vertical green bars were presented at the other. When the monkey attended to the green bars, the cell's response to the irrelevant red bars might have been attenuated because they were red or because they were at the wrong location. To test whether attenuation could be based on spatial location alone, for some cells we randomly intermixed the stimuli at the two locations so that, for example, red or green could appear at either spatial location on any trial.

When the locations of the effective and ineffective sensory stimuli were switched randomly, the responses of cells were still determined by the stimulus at the attended location. Cells responded well when the effective sensory stimulus appeared at the attended location and poorly when it appeared at the ignored location (median AI, 0.57 for the sample and test stimuli). Thus attenuation of irrelevant information can be based purely on spatial location.

When attention is directed to one of two stimuli in the receptive field of a V4 cell, the effect of the unattended stimulus is attenuated, almost as if the receptive field has contracted around the attended stimulus. What, then, would be the effect on the receptive field if attention were directed outside it? To answer this, for 112 visually responsive cells (including 51 in the original sample) we placed an effective sensory stimulus inside the receptive field and an ineffective stimulus outside (Fig. 1B). The cells gave a good response regardless of which stimulus was attended (Fig. 2B). Thus, when attention is directed outside a receptive field, the receptive field appears to be unaffected. Furthermore, since the firing rates of cells were the same regardless of whether attention was directed inside or outside the receptive field, we can conclude that attention does not serve to enhance responses to attended stimuli.

To test whether the attenuation of irrelevant information also occurs at the next stage of processing after V4, we recorded from 161 visually responsive neurons in the IT cortex. As in V4, when the animal attended to one stimulus inside the receptive field and ignore another, the response to the ignored stimulus was reduced. Unlike receptive fields in V4, which were typically 2° to 4° wide in the central visual field, those in the IT cortex were so large that the responses of cells could be influenced by attention to stimuli throughout at least the central 12° of both the contralateral and ipsilateral visual fields (the maximum distance that could be tested). The magnitude of the effect was some-

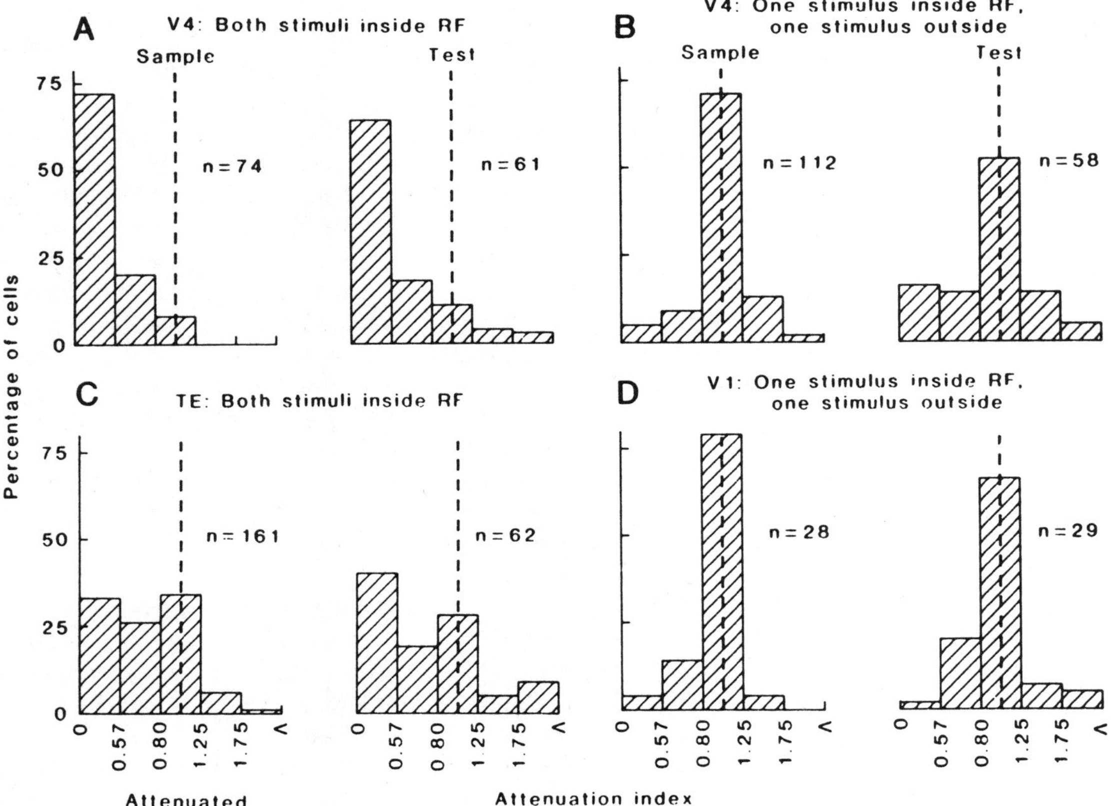

Figure 2. Comparison of effect of attention in area V4 (A and B), the IT cortex (C), and the striate cortex (V1) (D). An attention index (AI) for each cell was calculated by first subtracting its baseline firing rate from the responses to the sample and test stimuli. The responses to stimuli when ignored were then divided by responses to the same stimuli when attended. AI values less than 1 (dashed line) indicate that responses were reduced when a stimulus was ignored. The number of cells is indicated by *n*. For a few cells, irrelevant stimuli were paired only with the sample stimuli

what smaller than in V4 (Fig. 2C), possibly because IT neurons generally gave weaker, more variable responses than neurons in V4.

The results from area V4 and the IT cortex indicate that the filtering of irrelevant information is at least a two-stage process. In V4 only those cells whose receptive fields encompass both attended and unattended stimuli will fail to respond to unattended stimuli. In the IT cortex, where receptive fields may encompass the entire visual field, virtually no cells will respond well to unattended stimuli.

In contrast to area V4 and the IT cortex, there was no effect of attention in V1. When relevant and irrelevant stimuli were in a receptive field (typically 0.5° to 0.9° wide), the animal could not perform the task. When one stimulus was located inside the field and one just outside, the monkey was able to perform the task, but, as in V4 under this condition, attention had little or no effect on the cells (Fig. 2D).

Our results indicate that attention gates visual processing by filtering out irrelevant information from within the receptive fields of single extrastriate neurons. This role of attention is different from that demonstrated previously in the posterior parietal cortex (*3*), to our knowledge the only other cortical area in which spatially directed attention has been found to influence neural responses. In the posterior parietal cortex, some neurons show enhanced responses when an animal attends to a stimulus inside the neuron's receptive field compared to when the animal attends to a stimulus outside the field.

Since parietal neurons have large receptive fields with little or no selectivity for stimulus quality, these cells may play a role in directing attention to a spatial location (*4*), but by themselves do not provide information about the qualities of attended stimuli. By contrast, in area V4 and the IT cortex selective attention may allow the animal to identify and remember the properties of a particular stimulus out of the many that may be acting on the retina at any given moment. If so, then the attenuation of response to irrelevant stimuli found in V4 and the IT cortex may underlie the attenuated processing of irrelevant stimuli shown psychophysically in humans (*5*).

References and Notes

1. C. G. Gross in *Handbook of Sensory Physiology*, vol. 7, part 3, *Central Processing of Visual Information*, R. Jung, Ed. (Springer, Berlin, 1973), pp. 451–482; L. G. Ungerleider and M. Mishkin, in *Analysis of Visual Behavior*, D. J. Ingle, M. A. Goodale, R. J. W. Mansfield, Eds. (MIT Press, Cambridge, 1984), pp. 549–586; R. Desimone, S. J. Schein, J. Moran, L. G. Ungerleider, *Vision Res.* **25**, 441 (1985).

2. Both sample and test stimuli were presented for 200 msec, with a delay between them of 400 to 600 msec. The sample and test were randomly chosen on each trial from a set of two stimuli, and the irrelevant stimuli were chosen from a different set of two. If the animal attempted to perform the task on the basis of the irrelevant stimuli, its performance would be governed by chance. The performance of the animals was 94 percent correct. The cue to the animal to switch the locus of its attention was to delete the testtime stimulus from the previously relevant location for two trials. On the first of these trials, the animals' performance dropped to 65 percent correct and their reaction time increased by 90 msec, indicating that they had been ignoring the irrelevant stimuli. The neural responses on the two cue trials were not counted. The locus of attention was switched frequently enough to acheive a minimum of ten trials per stimulus configuration. Fixation was monitored by a magnetic search coil, and trials were aborted if the eyes deviated from the fixation target by more than 0.5°.

3. J. C. Lynch, V. B. Mountcastle, W. H. Talbot, T. C. T. Yin, *J. Neurophysiol.* **40**, 362 (1977); M. C. Bushnell *et al.*, *ibid.* **46**, 755 (1981).

4. M. I. Posner, J. A. Walker, F. J. Friedrich, R. D. Rafal, *J. Neurosci.* **4**, 1863 (1984).

5. D. E. Broadbent, *Acta Psychol.* **50**, 253 (1982); D. Kahneman and A. Ireisman, in *Varieties of Attention*, R. Parasuraman and D. R. Davies, Eds. (Academic Press, New York, 1984).

6. We thank M. Mishkin for his support in all phases of the study.

27

R. H. Wurtz, M. E. Goldberg, and D. L. Robinson

Behavioral modulation of visual responses in the monkey: Stimulus selection for attention and movement

1980. *Progress in Psychobiology and Physiological Psychology* 9: 43–83

I. Introduction

The visual system must be constantly bombarded by a changing pattern of retinal stimulation. An eye movement can occur as often as three times per second, and the pattern of stimulation in the more than a million optic nerve fibers (Ogden and Miller, 1966; Kupfer *et al.*, 1967) can therefore change as often. At some point in the brain there must be a selective reduction of this sensory barrage since only a fraction of it can actually be utilized within a given period of time. Perceptually, this selection seems reasonable since we usually attend to only one thing at a time. This selective attention was described by William James (1890) as "taking possession of the mind, in clear and vivid form, of one out of what seems several simultaneous possible objects or trains of thought. Focalization, concentration of consciousness are of its essence. It implies withdrawal from some things in order to deal effectively with others." The case for selection in preparation for movement is even more powerful. We cannot move our arm or eye in two directions at once; selection of which stimulus to follow is a necessity.

In a series of investigations of the primate visuomotor system we have described a physiological phenomenon that may well be related to selection processes. There are neurons in the visual system that yield enhanced responses to visual stimuli when those stimuli are relevant in some way to the animal's behavior. This article largely summarizes work on this visual enhancement phenomenon done in our respective laboratories. Several experimental strategies underlie our experiments. We concentrated on the visual system because the sensory transformations at successive levels in the brain have been better understood here than in any other sensory system. We have used extracellular recording rather than evoked potentials because issues of control and stimulus specificity are better handled at the level of a single cell, and at least certain ensemble inferences are possible from the study of adequate numbers of single neurons. We have used the rhesus monkey trained in a number of visuomotor tasks because it is easier to infer the bases of human behavior from phenomena studied in a subhuman primate. Finally, we have used a behaving animal because of a conviction that the neurophysiology of the central nervous system is the neurophysiology of behavior. The phenomenon that we have investigated could only have been described in a behaving animal since it represents the union of environmental and internal phenomena.

In outline we will discuss the visual enhancement effect in the brain areas shown in Fig. 1. First we will consider the superior colliculus where the selection effect was initially encountered, where the general methods were worked out, and where an hypothesis about the source of the effect can be most clearly argued. Then we will go from this midbrain visual pathway to consider the geniculostriate pathway, as well as the prestriate cortex. Two areas of association cortex will then be analyzed: the frontal eye fields of the frontal lobe and the posterior parietal region of the parietal lobe. Finally, we will evaluate the possible functional significance of the enhancement effect.

II. Superior Colliculus

The superior colliculus has long been identified with both a visual and a movement function (Adamük, 1870; Apter, 1945, 1946) and recent analyses of single cell activity in the colliculus have borne out these earlier suppositions. Single cell analyses in an awake, behaving monkey have indicated that the layers of this structure can be divided into at least two distinct groups as shown in Fig. 2 (Goldberg and Wurtz, 1972a; Wurtz and Goldberg, 1972a). The superficial layers comprise a thin surface layer of fibers, the stratum zonale, a cell layer, the stratum griseum superficiale, and a white layer, the stratum opticum. The input from the retina and striate cortex terminates in these layers (Wilson and Toyne, 1970; Lund, 1972; Hubel *et al.*, 1975). The stratum opticum in part is made up of retinal fibers which terminate near the dorsal surface of the stratum griseum superficiale as does a prominent projection from the striate cortex. Cells in these superficial layers respond to visual stimuli (Humphrey, 1968; Cynader and Berman, 1972; Marrocco and Li, 1977) and do not discharge before rapid (saccadic) eye movements (Schiller and Koerner, 1971; Goldberg and Wurtz, 1972a; Schiller *et al.*, 1974; Wurtz and Mohler, 1976a; Robinson and Wurtz, 1976).

The deep layers of the colliculus consist of alternating gray and white layers: the stratum griseum intermediale and stratum album intermediale, the stratum griseum profundum and the stratum album profundum (Kanaseki and Sprague, 1974). Cells in these layers may also have visual responses (Schiller and Koerner, 1971; Goldberg and Wurtz, 1972a: Cynader and Berman, 1972; Updyke, 1975; Mohler and Wurtz, 1976) but their salient feature is that they increase their rate of discharge before rapid or saccadic eye movements

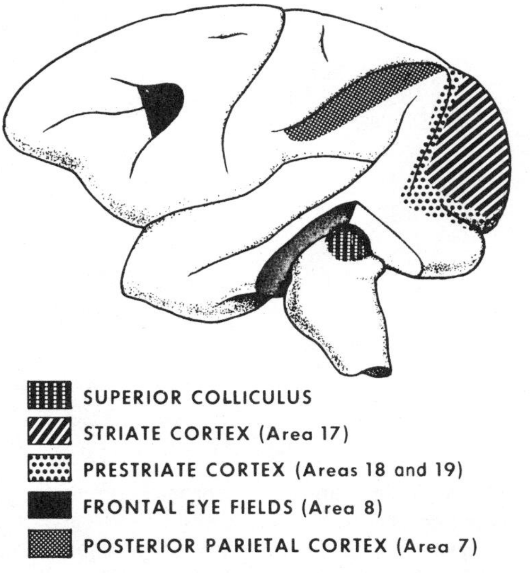

Figure 1. Shematic drawing of the lateral surface of the monkey brain showing regions which have been studied for the enhancement effect. The temporal lobe has been drawn as if a large section has been removed in order to expose the superior colliculus lying on the dorsal surface of the brainstem.

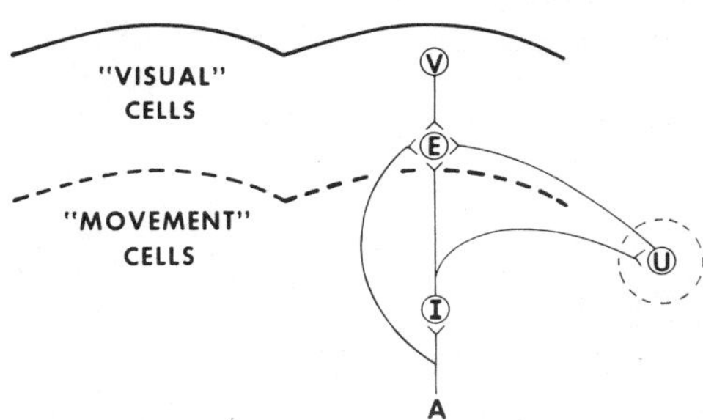

Figure 2. Schematic drawing of the organization of the superior colliculus and afferents to enhanced cells. The dorsal surface of the colliculus is represented by the solid curved line, and the dashed line parallel to the surface separates the superficial layers from the intermediate layers. Cells in the superficial layers respond to visual stimuli independent of eye movements ("visual cells"); cells in the intermediate layers discharge before eye movements regardless of the stimulus conditions ("movement cells"). Enhanced cells (E) most likely receive their visual inputs from the visual cells (V) in the dorsal parts of the colliculus. The afferent(s) which modulate the visual response to produce the enhancement could arise from: (1) the movement cells deep in the intermediate layers (I), (2) direct projections from or collaterals of those afferents (A) which drive the movement cells, or (3) cells in some unknown (U) nucleus outside of the colliculus which are driven by the movement cells.

(Goldberg and Wurtz, 1970; Wurtz and Goldberg, 1971, 1972a; Schiller and Koerner, 1971; Robinson and Jarvis, 1974; Mohler and Wurtz, 1976; Sparks *et al.*, 1976; Sparks, 1978). The cells discharging before eye movements do so regardless of whether the saccade is made in the light or in the dark.

Goldberg and Wurtz (1972b) in their studies on the superior colliculus were the first to notice the visual enhancement effect. They routinely determined the response of each cell encountered on a microelectrode penetration to both visual stimuli independent of eye movement and to eye movements alone. While they found that cells in the superficial layers did not discharge before eye movements in the dark, they noticed that the *visual* response of such cells to a spot of light that was the target for a saccade was more vigorous when the monkey repeatedly made an eye movement to the spot. They then systematically checked the visual response of cells in the superficial layers as well as how this response was modulated by the monkey's behavior.

A. Basic Observations and Methods

The behavioral methods used have been applied to other areas of the brain covered in later parts of this article and are worth setting forth clearly. The monkey first learned a task which required him to fixate on a spot of light (the fixation point) for several seconds in order to detect a brief dimming of the spot (Wurtz, 1969). Release of the bar by the monkey during the dimming period was rewarded by a drop of water. If the monkey looked away from the fixation spot, he missed the dimming and missed the reward. The monkey also learned to make a saccadic eye movement from one spot to another if the first fixation spot went out and another spot came on. The training thus provided periods when the eyes were not moving and periods when a particular saccade was repeatedly made to a visual target.

The single unit recording and head restraint techniques used were those developed for monkeys by Evarts (Evarts, 1966, 1968a). During experiments the receptive fields of superior colliculus cells were determined while the monkey fixated on the spot. An outline of such a receptive field is shown in Fig. 3 (top). Collicular fields are easily mapped by spots of light; slits or bars are effective but not required to activate collicular cells in the monkey (Schiller and Koerner, 1971; Goldberg and Wurtz, 1972a; Cynader and Berman, 1972; Schiller *et al.*, 1974; Marrocco and Li, 1977; Robinson and Wurtz, 1976) as they generally are for neurons in monkey striate cortex (Hubel and Wiesel, 1968).

In order to study the visual enhancement effect (Goldberg and Wurtz, 1972b; Wurtz and Goldberg,

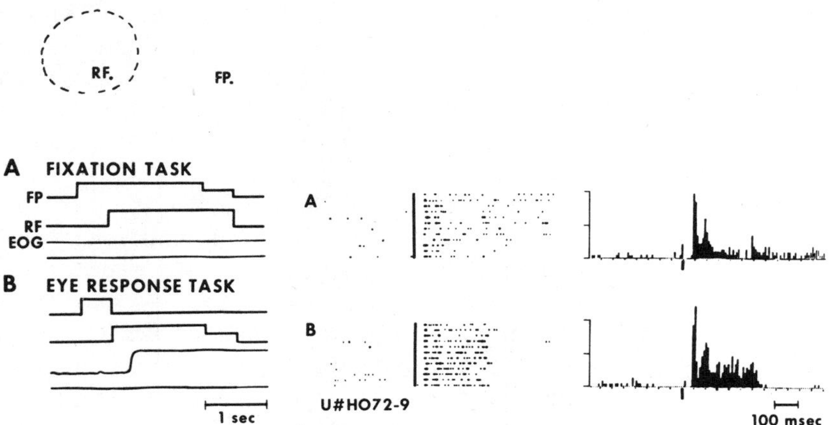

Figure 3. Schematic illustration of the enhancement paradigm (left) with representative data for a cell in the superior colliculus (right). The diagram on the upper left shows the location of the fixation point (FP), with the dashed circle outlining the extent of the excitatory central area of a visual receptive field (RF). The spot in the receptive field is the stimulus for experiment (A) and the saccade target for experiment (B). (A) (left) illustrates the time of onset of the fixation point in response to the monkey's bar press. After the onset of the fixation point, the monkey fixates it, as indicated by the representative horizontal (top) and vertical (bottom) electro-oculogram traces (EOG). The receptive field stimulus comes on 0.5 seconds later. In the experiment for (B) (left), the fixation point comes on after the monkey presses the bar and then goes off when the light in the receptive field comes on. The monkey makes a saccadic eye movement to fixate the saccade target as indicated by the deflection in the horizontal electro-oculogram trace. The data in (A) (right) show the consistent response of a superior colliculus cell to the spot of light in the receptive field while the monkey fixates. Data in (B) (right) show the enhanced response of this cell to the onset of the same stimulus when the monkey uses it as the target for a saccadic eye movement. Each dot represents an action potential, and each horizontal row of dots represents a single fixation trial for the monkey. The vertical line indicates the time of onset of the visual stimulus. Histograms sum the data in the adjacent dot pattern (raster). The divisions on the vertical scale indicate a discharge rate of 250 spikes/second/trial with 8 msec bin widths. The format and conventions described here will be used throughout this paper unless stated otherwise. After Wurtz and Mohler (1974).

1972c), one point within the field was picked and the response of the cell to a spot of light at that point was determined (as illustrated in Fig. 3A). During these trials the monkey need only look at the fixation point to obtain a reward; the receptive field stimulus was not related to the reward. Next, the conditions of the experiment were changed. Now, at the same time that the receptive field stimulus came on, the fixation point went off (Fig. 3B). The monkey knew from previous training that under this condition the spot of light in the receptive field would eventually dim and so he made a saccade to the receptive field stimulus in order to easily detect this dimming. On the first trial the on-response of the cell was not changed by the execution of the saccadic eye movement, but on subsequent trials it was: the response of the cell was more regular and more vigorous—an enhanced visual response. This enhancement in different cells took the form of a more vigorous on-response (an early enhancement), a more prolonged response (a late enhancement), or both effects. About half of the cells studied in the superficial layers showed one of these enhancement effects.

Note that the discharge of the cell is modified at the time that the monkey was presumably preparing to make the saccadic eye movement to the receptive field stimulus but before he actually made the saccade. Thus the retinal stimulation is identical in both fixation and saccade conditions. Since there is a reaction time of about 200 msec for the monkey to make the eye movement and since the visual response occurs with a latency of only 35–60 msec (Wurtz and Mohler, 1976a), the initial visual response of the cell is over well before the eye starts to move. Once this reaction time is over the monkey makes an eye movement and of course moves the stimulus off the receptive field of the cell. This terminates the analysis.

It must be emphasized that the cells showing visual enhancement do not discharge in relation to eye movement per se (Goldberg and Wurtz, 1972b; Wurtz and Mohler, 1976a). They do not discharge before spontaneous eye movements made in the dark; their discharge is synchronous with onset of the visual stimulus, not with onset of saccadic eye movements as is the case with movement related cells in deeper collicular layers. Thus the enhancement effect requires a visual stimulus and is a modulation of the visual response of the cell.

Following a series of saccades to the receptive field stimulus, the conditions of the experiment were returned to the original state as shown for another cell in Fig. 4. Now when the receptive field stimulus came on, the fixation point stayed on, and the monkey no longer made saccades to the receptive field stimulus (Fig. 4C). Over a number of trials, the response of the cell then returned to about the same level as in the

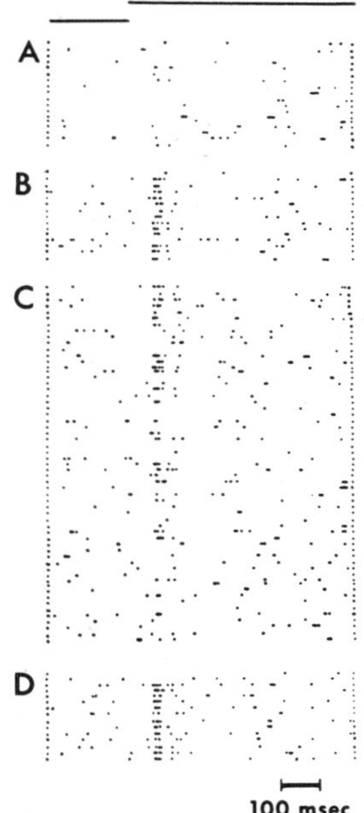

Figure 4. Habituation of the visual response and lack of habituation of the enhanced response. The indicator line at the top represents the time of onset of a spot of light in the receptive field. In (A), the monkey fixates and the spot of light in the receptive field elicits a very weak response. This activity is enhanced in (B) when the animal saccades to the stimulus; when the task is changed, this level of activity habituates over many trials in (C) after the monkey returns to the fixation task. The enhanced response is rapidly dishabituated in (D) and persists as the monkey returns to the saccade task. From Goldberg and Wurtz (1972b).

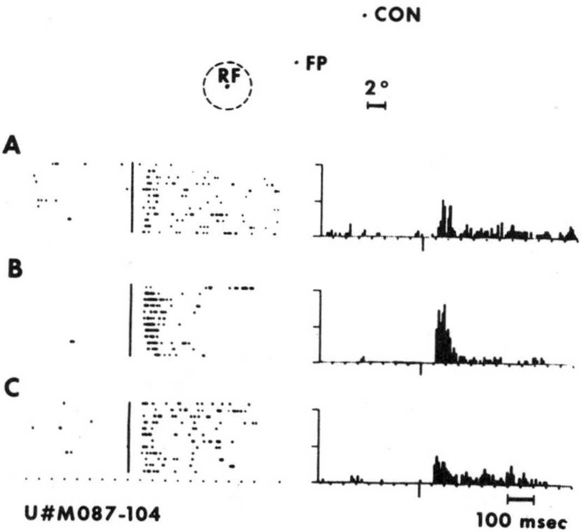

Figure 5. Control experiment for enhancement selectivity. (A) shows the discharge of a collicular neuron to a spot of light in the receptive field (RF) and a control spot (CON) in the ipsilateral visual field while the monkey looks at the fixation point (FP). (B) shows the enhanced response on those trials when the monkey makes a saccadic eye movement to the receptive field stimulus whereas (C) illustrates the lack of enhancement on the trials when the monkey saccades to the control stimulus. Since the stimulus conditions are the same in all three experiments, these data demonstrate that there is a selective facilitation associated with eye movements to the receptive field. From Wurtz and Mohler (1976a).

original state. If this series of declining responses was examined alone, a reasonable description would be that the response was "habituating"—a point we will consider more extensively in Section V, B.

These experiments show that use of the visual stimulus by the monkey produces an enhancement of the visual response of superior colliculus cells. In these experiments the visual stimulus remained the same when the monkey did and did not saccade to the stimulus. Only the use of the stimulus changed; the physical characteristics did not.

B. Spatial Selectivity

The experiments described so far implicitly assume that the enhanced visual response is due to the monkey's saccade to a visual stimulus rather than to some nonspecific modulation. In order to determine how selective the enhancement effect is, a control experiment for these nonspecific factors was carried out. In this experiment, as the fixation point went off, two spots of light came on and the monkey could saccade to either one of these stimuli (see Fig. 5).[1] One spot of light was in the receptive field as before; the other spot was located outside the receptive field as indicated by the lack of a visual response of the cell when that stimulus was presented alone. The monkey could make a series of saccades to either stimulus. When the monkey made saccades to the receptive field stimulus, the enhancement effect was clear (Fig. 5b). But when the saccades were made to the control stimulus, no such clear enhancement was seen (Fig. 5C) although a slight nonspecific effect was occasionally present. The enhancement effect was spatially selective; it was related to saccades made to the receptive field stimulus but not to those made to other areas. The enhanced visual response is therefore not related to some general alerting or arousal effect associated with making saccadic eye movements, since the enhancement is not present with all eye movements. For the same reason factors such as pupil dilation during saccades or a visual effect of the fixation light going off as the receptive field stimulus comes on cannot be producing the visual enhancement.

C. Hypothesis on Source of the Effect

A specific hypothesis has been developed by Wurtz and Mohler (1976a) to account for this enhancement effect in the superior colliculus. We shall present this hypothesis first and then consider how the characteristics of the enhancement effect fit it. While this discussion is the opposite of the actual sequence of experiments and analysis, it has the advantage of organizing the experimental results to point up both the strengths and weaknesses of the hypothesis.

The hypothesis starts from the fact that the superior colliculus can be divided into two functional parts as outlined in Fig. 2; their separation depends on whether the cells discharge to a visual stimulus or whether they discharge before an eye movement. The simplest explanation of the enhancement effect is that the cells in the intermediate and deep layers of the colliculus, which are the ones which discharge before eye movements, have a projection to those superficial layer cells which show an enhancement. In this hypothesis the enhancement of the visual response of the superficial layer cells results from a facilitation from the movement-related discharge of the deeper cells or a movement-related input to these cells.

Figure 2 shows schematically the organization of the cells showing visual enhancement and connections which might produce the enhancement. The enhanced cells are shown in the deeper part of the superficial layers, since the percentage of the enhanced cells was found to increase as one recorded deeper in the superficial layers (Wurtz and Mohler, 1976a). The visual input to these cells (labeled V in Fig. 2) might well come from superficial layer cells above the enhanced cells; the superficial layer cells in turn receive input from other more dorsal superficial layer cells or directly from retinal afferents. Input to enhanced cells from the visual areas of cortex also cannot be excluded (Schiller *et al.*, 1974). This sequence of visual input is suggested by increased latency for the visual response with increased depth (Wurtz and Mohler, 1976a), but such serial processing is not clearly established. The facilitation acting on these enhanced cells may come from the eye movement-related cells deep in the colliculus (labeled I in Fig. 2), from an external input (labeled A in Fig. 2) which might also project to the movement-related cells, or directly from some other unknown area of the brain (labeled U in Fig. 2). There are several possibilities for the afferents labeled A. One source is the nucleus parabigeminus, which is connected reciprocally with the superior colliculus (Graybiel, 1978b; Baleydier and Magnin, 1979). The intermediate gray layer of the superior colliculus projects to the nucleus parabigeminus, which in turn projects to the superficial layers of the colliculus. The parabigeminal nucleus may also receive eye movement-related information from the nucleus prepositus hypoglossi (Baleydier and Magnin, 1979). A second possible source of this input is the substantial nigra (Graybiel, 1978a), but eye movement-related activity has yet to be described here. Although the ventral lateral geniculate nucleus projects to the superficial layers of the colliculus in the cat (Edwards *et al.*, 1974), the saccade-related activity recorded in the monkey occurs after the saccade onset (Büttner and Fuchs, 1973) and therefore occurs too late to be a plausible candidate for the enhancement afferent. There are no established projections from deep layers to superficial layers within the superior colliculus. The essential point of the hypothesis is that the enhancement comes from a presaccadic discharge which produces facilitation within the superficial layers of the superior colliculus.

The facilitation of the visual input could logically be presynaptic or postsynaptic; no experimental evidence is currently available to distinguish between the two alternatives. For purposes of our analysis this is not a critical point, since the effect of the movement input is simply to change the effectiveness of the visual input.

In the following sections we will consider the relation of this hypothesis to experimental observations on the enhancement effect.

D. Temporal Characteristics

The basic argument that the visual enhancement is a result of eye movement-related activity rests on the temporal properties of the effect: the enhancement varies in relation to the time of onset of the eye movement. This conclusion is based on experiments done by Wurtz and Mohler (1976a). They first showed that the type of enhancement was modified by the time at which the eye movement occurred. Their experiments started from the observation that there are cells showing an early enhancement (the on-response was facilitated), a late enhancement (a prolongation of the on-response), or both (Goldberg and Wurtz, 1972b). By changing the time when the monkey made a saccade to the receptive field stimulus, Wurtz and Mohler (1976a) found that a late enhancement could be converted into an early enhancement and vice versa. Saccades made soon after the onset of the target were associated with early enhancement and later saccades were associated with late enhancement. Conversion of one type of enhancement to the other by changing the monkey's behavior indicates that these variations are due to the monkey's eye movements and do not reveal intrinsic differences among cells. The *type* of enhancement is dependent on the *time* of the eye movement relative to the onset of the stimulus target. This might explain why Goldberg and Wurtz (1972a) were unable to see any orderly relation of early and late enhancement with other characteristics of the cells.[2]

If shifting the onset of the saccade closer in time to the onset of the stimulus produces a potentiated on-response to the visual stimulus, shifting the saccade to a much later time might produce a later enhancement. Goldberg and Wurtz (1972b) tested this by leaving the receptive field stimulus on all the time; there was then no on-response remaining and only the disappearance of the fixation point signaled the monkey to make a saccade. In this situation they found that the on-going response of the cell to the receptive field stimulus was more vigorous just before the onset of the saccade—the ultimate in late enhancement.

Another experiment attempted to determine the time course of the enhancement effect (Wurtz and Mohler, 1976a). In this experiment the monkey made a saccade from the fixation point to a small target within the receptive field area. The experiment tested the response of the cell to a brief light stimulus (50 msec) flashed at various times before and after the signal to initiate the saccade. The goal of the experiment was to use this brief stimulus to test the change in excitability of the cell to stimuli applied progressively closer in time to the onset of the eye movement. If the enhancement effect were a result of input from movement-related activity, the excitability of the cell should change in close temporal relation to the eye movement. This was what happened. A typical result, shown in Fig. 6, indicates that the enhancement effect is present about 200 msec before the onset of the eye movement, becomes larger at the time of the eye movement, and is present even after the eye movement is over. The enhancement effect is therefore transient and synchronous with the eye movement. It is not a tonic process that is set by the monkey's readiness to respond and would be expected to act continuously between trials. This phasic development of the enhancement effect is consistent with the phasic discharge of the movement cells before each eye movement; had the enhancement been a tonic effect persisting between trials, it would have been difficult to relate to any other cells in the colliculus since none show such tonic discharge between trials.

That the enhanced visual response occurs several hundred milliseconds before the onset of the eye movement does, however, raise a potential problem. The cells deeper in the colliculus that discharge before eye movements seldom precede a spontaneous eye movement by more than 150 msec. If the response to a visual stimulus occurred in the colliculus 50 msec after stimulus onset, and the reaction time for a saccade to the target were 200 msec, the movement-related activity would barely overlap the visual activity in time. This may not be as much an embarrassment for the hypothesis as it might at first seem, since Mohler and Wurtz (1976) observed that many of the movement cells began to discharge in anticipation of the signal to make an eye movement (Fig. 7B). In cases where the monkey made eye movements to the same visual target on repeated trials, the onset of the eye movement and the discharge of the movement cells came earlier on successive trials. On many trials the movement cells actually started to discharge before the onset of the visual target. In this case the discharge of the movement cells started early enough to act on the visual input of cells in the superficial layer and facilitate the visual response of these cells.

This anticipatory effect in fact fits with a number of other observations on the enhancement effect. First, there is never a demonstrable enhancement of the on-response on the first trial when the monkey is required to make a saccade to the visual stimulus (Goldberg and Wurtz, 1972a; Wurtz and Mohler, 1976a). When Wurtz and Mohler (1976a) grouped together data from trials in which the monkey first made a saccade to the visual receptive field stimulus no enhancement of the on-response was apparent. Since the monkey cannot anticipate the requirement to make a saccade, there is probably no anticipatory activity by the movement cells, and they would not be expected to facilitate the visual response. However, there are occasional cases of late enhancement on these first trials and this could

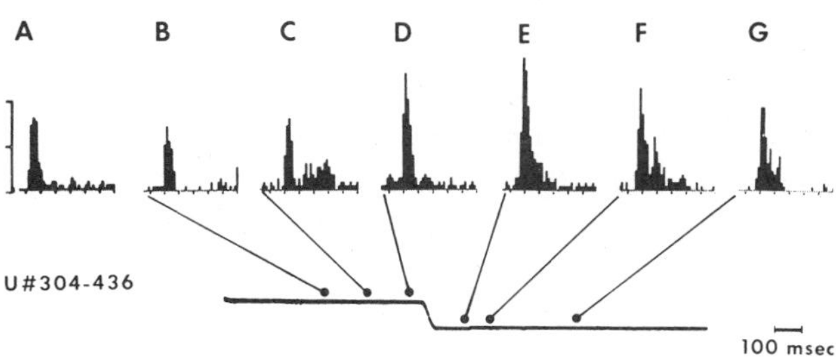

Figure 6. Transient time course of pre- and posteye movement enhancement. (A) shows the response of a superior colliculus neuron to a spot of light in its receptive field while the monkey fixates. (B) through (G) show the build-up and decay of the facilitated visual response when stimuli are flashed for 50 msec in the receptive field at times close to the time of the saccadic eye movement. From Wurtz and Mohler (1976a).

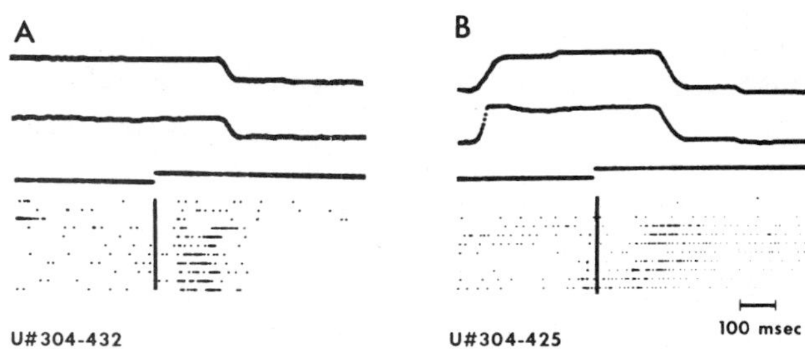

Figure 7. Sequential build-up of the enhancement effect (A) and progressive anticipation of the discharge of movement cell (B). The monkey fixated on the first three trials in both (A) and (B) and then started making saccades to the visual stimulus on the fourth trial. The vertical line in each dot pattern indicates the onset of the visual target (for the first three trials) and both the onset of the visual and offset of the fixation point in subsequent trials. The enhanced response of a superficial layer cell in (A) becomes progressively more vigorous on successive trials. Under similar conditions in (B), cells in the intermediate layers of the superior colliculus which discharge before eye movements become active progressively sooner and eventually precede the signal to make an eye movement. From Mohler and Wurtz (1976).

result from the start of movement cell discharge 150 msec before the onset of the eye movement.

The second observation in relation to anticipation is that visual enhancement of the on-response frequently becomes progressively better on successive trials when the monkey makes saccades to the visual stimulus (Fig. 7A). This could be due to the greater anticipation over a series of trials which is seen in movement cells in similar circumstances.

The final point is that the enhanced response was found to "habituate" over a number of trials after the monkey had stopped making saccades to the visual target (see Fig. 4C). This at first also seemed a problem for our hypothesis, which derived the enhancement effect from eye movement-related activity. This may not be a problem, however, since some movement cells continue to discharge as if the monkey were about to make an eye movement even though the monkey does not in fact make the saccade (Wurtz and Mohler, 1976a). If these cells discharged in such a manner after the end of a series of saccades to a visual stimulus, their continued facilitation of the visual cells would account for the prolongation of the enhancement effect beyond the end of the actual saccade trials. The gradual waning of the enhancement might result from the reduction of the number of movement cells discharging on successive trials.

This independence of discharge of the movement-related cells and the actual occurrence of the saccade has a parallel in the occasional independence of collicular cell discharge and the metrics of a saccade. The discharge of some collicular cells is the same before a 40° saccade as it is when the monkey instead makes two 20° saccades (Mohler and Wurtz, 1976); the cell discharge is the same whether a saccade is 20° or much less due to the modification of the eye movement by simultaneous occurrence of a head movement (Robinson and Jarvis, 1974). These examples probably represent a modification of eye movement control downstream from the superior colliculus, and in the present context serve to indicate that the collicular cells are not locked to the onset of a saccade.

What the temporal properties of the enhancement effect indicate is that it relates not so much to the monkey's eye movement but to the discharge of movement cells in anticipation of such a movement regardless of whether the movement actually occurs or not. The enhancement effect relates to a readiness to respond. The lack of a one-to-one relationship of the enhancement effect to the eye movement originally led Goldberg and Wurtz (1972b) to argue that the enhancement was independent of the saccades. Subsequent investigation of the characteristics of the movement cells deeper in the colliculus (summarized previously) has indicated that some of these cells also can be independent of the actual eye movement. The enhancement effect, as Goldberg and Wurtz (1972b) pointed out, *is* independent of the actual occurrence of eye movement, but we now realize that the discharge of some of the movement-related cells may also be independent.

E. Spatial Characteristics

The enhancement effect has been found to have several characteristics related to the spatial organization of the visual receptive field. We shall consider two questions and then see how the answers fit the hypothesis about the source of the enhancement.

To produce the enhancement effect the monkey must saccade to the receptive field stimulus. But need he saccade exactly to it? By having the monkey saccade to a small spot of light at varying distances from the effective receptive field stimulus, Wurtz and Mohler (1976a) answered this question: the enhanced response to the visual stimulus occurred even when the saccade target was outside but close to the receptive field. At target points farther from the receptive field, the enhancement disappeared.[3] In net, saccades near the receptive field produced an enhanced response; saccades remote from the field did not. A convenient description of this observation was that there was an "enhancement field," an area where saccades to any point produced a facilitated response to a stimulus in the center of the receptive field. This enhancement field was sometimes slightly larger than the visual receptive field, the area where spots of light alone produced a visual response.

The next question concerned the effect of the enhancement on receptive field size. Does a stimulus that produces no response from a cell when the monkey fixates produce a response when he makes a saccade to the visual stimulus? The answer to this question is that it does for some cells. But the maximum effect is a slight expansion of the receptive field of several degrees (Goldberg and Wurtz, 1972b; Wurtz and Mohler, 1976a) as indicated in Fig. 8.

The response of most superior colliculus cells to a spot of light falling in the central area of their receptive fields is probably the result of two antagonistic processes: an excitatory effect, concentrated in the central part of the receptive field, and an inhibitory or antagonistic effect spreading throughout the field, including a surrounding area. One possible mechanism underlying the expansion of the receptive field size might be a facilitation of the excitatory inputs to the cell; at the edge of the excitatory area of the field this increases the effectiveness of the stimulus just enough to lift the response above a background noise level and reveal a response to the stimulus. Another possibility might be a decrease in the strength of the suppressive surround

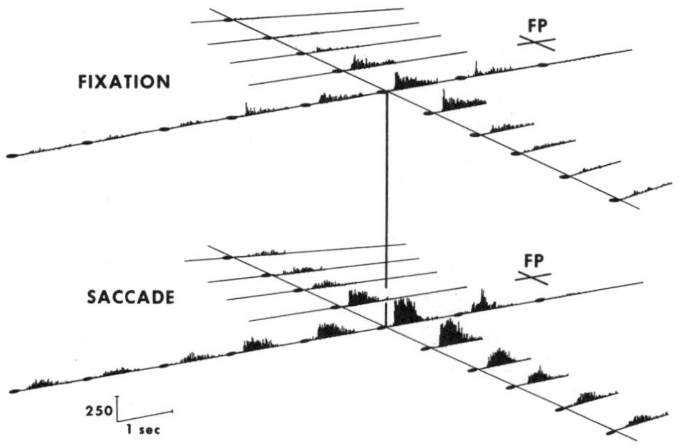

Figure 8. Expansion of the visual receptive field during the enhancement experiment. Histograms on the top show the response of a collicular neuron to spots of light falling on the tangent screen at the positions illustrated. The histograms on the bottom show the enhanced response to the corresponding spot of light when the monkey uses that stimulus as the target for a saccadic eye movement. FP, fixation point. From Wurtz and Mohler (1976a).

which would produce a similar effect. The experiments done so far do not allow an estimate of the relative contribution of these two mechanisms.

The major point, however, is that receptive field size is altered only slightly. The enhancement effect modifies the vigor of the response to a spot of light, but it does not alter significantly the indication by the cell that a point of light lies within the receptive field. In other words, the signal-to-noise ratio of the cell is improved but the meaning of the signal remains the same.

An effect which is similar to the spatial features of the enhancement effect has recently been demonstrated in the cat superior colliculus by Rizzolatti *et al.* (1974). They found that moving a stimulus in the visual field of the paralyzed cat remote from the visual receptive field of a colliculus cell produced a *decrease* in the response to a receptive field stimulus. They suggested that this remote inhibitory effect might be a result of the cat's readiness to respond or to shift its attention to another part of the visual field with a resultant loss of facilitation to the area of the visual field where the receptive field of the cell is located—an inverse of the enhancement effect.

Recent experiments by Richmond and Wurtz (1978) suggest that in the awake monkey, which can move its eyes, this remote inhibitory effect results from visual interactions of the two stimuli rather than from any shift in gaze or attention. During a series of experiments on visual masking, they noticed that a stimulus remote from the central receptive field area, flashed on 50 msec before the onset of a stimulus within the central excitatory area, was effective in reducing the response to that stimulus in the central excitatory area. As in the cat, the effect was a suppressive one: the remote stimulus alone did not alter the discharge rate of the cell; it only reduced the response to a stimulus falling within the central area of the receptive field. The reduction in response persisted when the remote stimulus was turned on several hundred milliseconds before the onset of the stimulus in the central part of the receptive field. The remote stimulus was effective even when it was at least 30° from the edge of the central area but in the same hemifield. However, when the remote stimulus was on the contralateral side of the visual field, it was only slightly effective. No saccades or shift of attention need be invoked in these experiments since the monkey fixated on the small central fixation point throughout the entire experiment. The characteristics of these visual interactions are similar to those observed by Rizzolatti *et al.* (1974) in the cat although other factors, such as the greater effect of a moving rather than a stationary remote stimulus, are not obvious in the monkey. However, the effects in cat and monkey are sufficiently similar to suggest that the effect in the cat, like that in the monkey, is a purely visual sensory interaction, not a shift in attention and not related to the enhancement effect which requires a saccadic eye movement toward the stimulus.

F. Specific Relation to Eye Movement

One of the key points in the analysis of the enhancement effect in the colliculus has been that it is related at least loosely to eye movements in both temporal and spatial properties. The temporal relationship between onset of the eye movement or preparation to move the eyes and the enhanced visual response supports this dependence of the enhancement on eye movement-related cells. A supplementary behavioral experiment also supports this view.

In this experiment (Wurtz and Mohler, 1976a), the monkey was trained for one set of trials to respond to a visual stimulus with a saccadic eye movement as in the previously described experiments *or* for another set of trials to indicate use of the stimulus by a hand movement instead of an eye movement. In this latter experiment, the monkey looked at the fixation point but learned that either the fixation point or the receptive field stimulus would dim and that release of the bar was required in either case to obtain a reward. The fixation point was small, the receptive field stimulus large, so that it was possible for the monkey to look at the fixation point and detect a dimming of the receptive field stimulus using peripheral vision. In addition, if the monkey made an eye movement during the fixation period, the trial was automatically terminated. This task forced the monkey not only to fixate but also to respond to a change in the receptive field stimulus with a hand rather than an eye movement. If the enhancement effect were related to use of the stimulus in a general way rather than in a way specifically related to eye movement, the visual cells should show enhancement in this task just as in the eye movement task. This was not the case; the enhancement in this task without eye movement was never as sharp and clear as with the eye movement. Therefore the enhancement seems to be more closely associated with preparation to make eye movements than to either make limb movements or possibly general use of the stimulus. Further details on the variations of the experiment and the limitations on interpretation are considered by Wurtz and Mohler (1976a).

If the enhancement effect, and indeed the function of the superior colliculus as a whole, is related to the initiation of eye movements, damage to the structure should produce a deficit at least in visually initiated and guided eye movements. This appears to be the case: following lesions placed in the superior colliculus, Wurtz and Goldberg (1972b) found an increased latency to make saccades, and Mohler and Wurtz (1977) found an additional tendency to make saccades somewhat shorter than required to reach a visual target.

III. Striate and Prestriate Cortices

Striate (area 17) and prestriate cortices (roughly areas 18 and 19 for the present discussion) have traditionally been thought to be involved in the detailed analysis of visual input. Area 17 receives a massive projection from the retina via the lateral geniculate nucleus (Wilson and Cragg, 1967; Hendrickson *et al.*, 1970; Garey and Powell, 1971; Hubel and Wiesel, 1972; Bunt *et al.*, 1975) and damage along this pathway leads to devastating visual deficits in primates (see Doty, 1973, for review; Weiskrantz, 1972; Mohler and Wurtz, 1977). Furthermore, neurons in striate and prestriate cortices are selective for the types of visual stimuli which excite them (Hubel and Wiesel, 1968; Wurtz, 1969; Dow and Gouras, 1973; Schiller *et al.*, 1976; Poggio and Fischer, 1977; Baizer *et al.*, 1977; Michael, 1978).

It was of interest to determine whether the visual enhancement effect seen in the superior colliculus is a general phenomenon found throughout the visual system or whether it might be restricted to the midbrain visual areas. Wurtz and Mohler (1976b) found that there is occasionally a facilitation of the visual response when monkeys made saccadic eye movements to a stimulus in the receptive field of a striate cortical neuron. However, this enhancement occurs in a smaller proportion of striate neurons than collicular cells and is never as intense as that found in the colliculus. In contrast to the rather homogeneous receptive field properties found in the colliculus, there are several different types of receptive fields for neurons in striate cortex; all types in striate cortex have this behavioral modulation of their visual response (Wurtz and Mohler, 1976b).

The facilitation in striate cortex is seen in association with many directions of eye movements: those into the receptive field as well as those to points distant from the receptive field (Wurtz and Mohler, 1976b) (Fig 9). The effect is therefore spatially nonselective. In addition, this modulation in striate cortex does not require an eye movement as does the collicular effect (Wurtz and Mohler, 1976a,b). If, while recording from a cell in striate cortex that shows this enhancement, the monkey is required to detect the dimming of a stimulus in the receptive field but not make an eye movement to it, the enhancement effect can still be demonstrated. Thus the enhancement in striate cortex is qualitatively different from that in the colliculus, being spatially nonselective and dissociable from the eye movement. It is also quantitatively different, occurring less frequently and less intensely than the selective enhancement in the superior colliculus.

One of the efferent pathways from the superficial layers of the colliculus in primates is to the inferior pulvinar (Myers, 1963; Harting *et al.*, 1973; Mathers, 1971; Benevento and Fallon, 1975; Partlow *et al.*, 1977; Raczkowski and Diamond, 1978) and then to areas 18

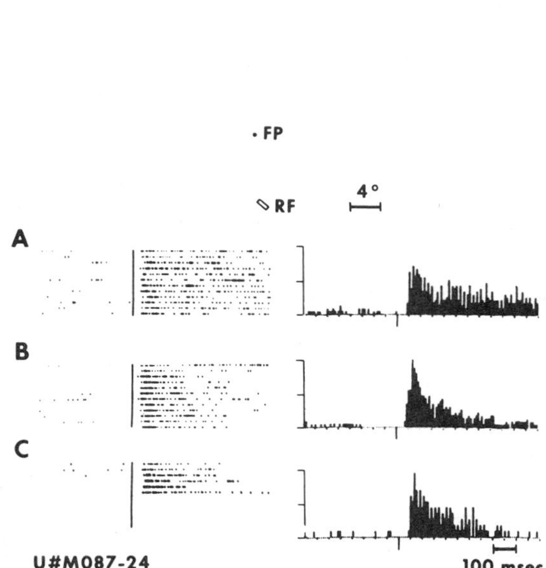

Figure 9. Nonselective enhancement for a cell in striate cortex. The drawing at the top shows the location of the receptive field (RF) and control (CON) stimuli which fell on the screen while the monkey fixated. (A) illustrates the response of a cell to these stimuli. (B) and (C) demonstrate the enhanced responses in the saccade condition whether the monkey saccades to the stimulus in the receptive field (B) or to the control stimulus (C). FP, fixation point. From Wurtz and Mohler (1976b).

and 19 (Glendenning *et al.*, 1975; Benevento and Rezak, 1976; Raczkowski and Diamond, 1978). Thus prestriate cortex may have inputs indirectly from the colliculus as well as directly from striate cortex (Kuypers *et al.*, 1965; Cragg, 1969; Zeki, 1975, 1978a,b), and it is of interest to know which of the types of enhancement, if any, occurs here. The visual properties of cells in areas 18 and 19 resemble those in striate cortex in most ways except for their increased size of the receptive fields (Baizer, 1976; Baizer *et al.*, 1977; Zeki, 1978a,b; Poggio and Fischer, 1977), and these visual properties are dependent on striate afferents (Schiller and Malpeli, 1977). For prestriate cells in the posterior bank of the lunate sulcus, enhancement is present and resembles that in striate cortex in that it is spatially nonselective, occurring with a wide variety of eye movements, and is seen with all cell types tested (Robinson *et al.*, in preparation). However, it occurs with greater frequency in prestriate cortex than in striate cortex.

Since the enhancement effects seen in areas 17, 18, and 19 are qualitatively and quantitatively different from that seen in the superior colliculus, it is unlikely that this cortical enhancement is derived from that seen in the superior colliculus. More likely it directly enters the geniculostriate system and may then be transmitted to areas 18 and 19.

We conclude that those parts of striate cortex and the prestriate cortex studied to date are well organized for the fine-grained analysis of the visual scene but poorly endowed for the evaluation of the behavioral context in which visual stimulation takes place. The only modulation observed in these areas appears to be a nonspecific one possibly related to alertness.

Initial experiments in the pulvinar nuclei of the thalamus have shown that the enhancement effect is present; here it is spatially nonselective but specific for eye movements (Keys and Robinson, 1979).

A major efferent of layer V of the striate cortex projects to the superficial layers of the superior colliculus (Hayaishi, 1969; Toyama *et al.*, 1969; Wilson and Toyne, 1970; Lund, 1972; Holländer, 1974; Palmer and Rosenquist, 1974; Lund *et al.*, 1975; Finlay *et al.*, 1976). Because the enhancement in striate cortex is so different from that seen in the colliculus, it seems unlikely that collicular enhancement is mediated through this corticotectal pathway, and this is in fact the case. Monkeys that have recovered from focal striate lesions have cells in the colliculus which show enhancement in the visual field representation corresponding to the damaged region of striate cortex (Wurtz and Mohler, 1976a). In fact, cells showing visual enhancement are slightly more frequent in the portions of the colliculus deprived of input from the ipsilateral striate cortex than in those areas with intact corticotectal afferents; such tectal cells contralateral to the striate lesion appear to be less frequent.

IV. Parietal and Frontal Association Cortices

Stimulation experiments in the nineteenth century implicated two areas of association cortex as being important in the generation of eye movements (see Wagman, 1964). These areas, the frontal eye fields (Brodmann's area 8) and the posterior parietal eye fields (Brodmann's area 7) have also been considered important in the neural processes underlying visual attention (Welch and Stuteville, 1958; Critchley, 1953; Mountcastle *et al.*, 1975; Lynch *et al.*, 1977; Robinson *et al.*, 1978). Recent work has shown that cells in both of these areas are visually responsive and that these responses are behaviorally modifiable (Mohler *et al.*, 1973; Wurtz and Mohler, 1976b; Goldberg and Robinson, 1977a,b; Yin and Mountcastle, 1977; Robinson *et al.*, 1978). However, there are striking differences between the kinds of behavioral modifiability found in these two association cortices.

A. Frontal Eye Fields

More recent stimulation experiments (Robinson and Fuchs, 1969) have indeed shown that electrical excitation of area 8 reliably induces saccadic eye movements in the unanesthetized monkey. Nonetheless, single cell recording studies did not confirm a role of frontal neurons in the generation of spontaneous eye movements. This is in contrast to primary motor cortex, area 4, where cells discharge reliably before limb movements (Evarts, 1968b). Bizzi (1968) showed that there was a small percentage of neurons in the frontal eye fields of the monkey that discharged in relation to saccades, but these cells discharged during and after the eye movements. Bizzi and Schiller (1970) described neurons discharging before head movement. Neither of these cell types could account for eye movements induced by stimulation.

Mohler *et al.* (1973) showed that roughly half of the cells they sampled in the frontal eye fields had visual responses with well-defined receptive fields. The receptive fields of the cells were large and were generally contralateral to the cerebral hemisphere containing the cells. The cells did not respond selectively to orientation or direction of movement. Like neurons in the superior colliculus, cells in the frontal eye fields were easily driven by small spots of light, but unlike collicular neurons they responded better to small spots within their excitatory regions than they did to larger spots which lay entirely within their excitatory regions. A major difference between these visual responses in the frontal eye fields and in superior colliculus was the latency of the visual response, 40–60 msec for the

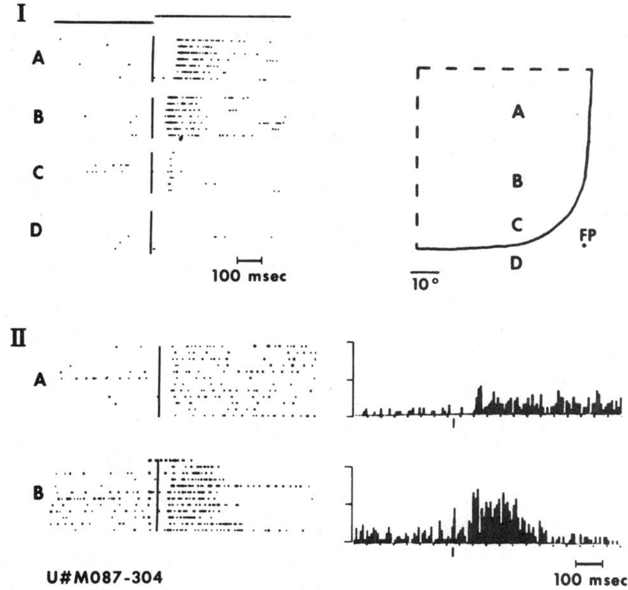

Figure 10. Visual receptive field (I) and enhanced response (II) for a cell in the frontal eye fields. The dot patterns in (I) show the discharge of a frontal eye field cell in response to a spot of light flashed on the tangent screen at the locations illustrated on the right. The solid line indicates the boundary determined for the receptive field; dashed lines are for indeterminant edges of the field. The lettered rasters (A–D) illustrate the cell's response to a spot of light in the correspondingly lettered location in the receptive field. FP, fixation point. Part (II) shows the response of another cell in area 8 to a spot of light in the fixation (A) and saccade (B conditions. From Mohler *et al.* (1973) and Wurtz and Mohler (1976b).

superior colliculus and 80–120 msec for frontal eye fields. Any serial relationship between these two areas must therefore be from superior colliculus to frontal cortex. Figure 10,I shows the visual response and receptive field outline of a neuron in the frontal eye fields of the monkey.

Half of these visually responsive neurons show enhancement when the stimulus in the receptive field is the target for an eye movement (Wurtz and Mohler, 1976b) (Fig. 10, II). The enhancement of the frontal eye fields is present only when the animal makes a saccade to the stimulus in the field and not when the animal makes a saccade to a stimulus outside the field. The enhancement is therefore spatially selective, like that found in the superior colliculus but unlike that found in the striate and prestriate cortices.

Since visually responsive frontal eye field neurons do not discharge before eye movements made spontaneously in the dark, any increased activity before visually guided eye movements must result from a modulation of a visual response. For the same reason, the enhancement cannot be the addition of a gaze-related discharge to a visual discharge. This is in contrast to those cells in the intermediate layers of the superior colliculus that do have such a dual visual- and movement-related discharge (Wurtz and Goldberg, 1972a).

Bushnell *et al.* (1978) have recently shown that neurons in area 8 display enhancement only when the monkey actually makes a saccadic eye movement to the stimulus. There is no enhancement when the monkey uses the stimulus as data for some other movement, such as the signal for a bar release or the target for a hand movement unassociated with an eye movement. These enhanced visual responses, occurring only when the animal intends to make a saccadic eye movement, may provide a retinal error signal for the generation of visually guided saccades. This retinal error signal may be the activity mimicked by the electrical stimulation which induces saccades from the frontal eye fields.

In summary, the frontal eye fields show a clear visual enhancement effect similar to that observed in the superior colliculus (spatially selective and specifically related to saccadic eye movements) but very different from that seen in striate and prestriate cortices (spatially nonselective and independent of saccadic eye movements). In addition, the type of visual stimulus required to activate cells is similar in frontal eye fields and superior colliculus but different from stimuli required to activate striate and prestriate cortical cells.

B. Posterior Parietal Cortex

Area 7 of the posterior parietal cortex is another visual area which may be linked to the eye movement process through the phenomenon of enhancement. Hyvärinen and Poranen (1974) described cells in area 7 of the awake rhesus monkey that discharged in association with eye movements. Using monkeys trained in an eye movement task, Mountcastle and his colleagues (Mountcastle *et al.*, 1975; Lynch *et al.*, 1977) described neurons that discharged in association with visually guided eye movements. Yin and Mountcastle (1977, 1978) described a small population of neurons in area 7 that responded to the onset of small light-emitting diodes, the response of some of which was enhanced when the animal made a saccade to the diode. Robinson *et al.* (1978) showed that every neuron they isolated in area 7 that discharged in association with some form of visually guided behavior could be driven by some visual stimulus independent of behavior. They proposed that all of the eye movement-related activity in area 7 could be explained as either passive visual responses or as behaviorally enhanced visual responses to stimuli falling in the receptive fields of the parietal cells, rather than as a movement signal independent of the sensory properties of the neurons. Figure 11 shows a neuron discharging before an eye movement, its time relationship to the eye movement, and its response to the stimulus in the absence of the eye movement (Fig. 11C). The response of the neuron is significantly en-

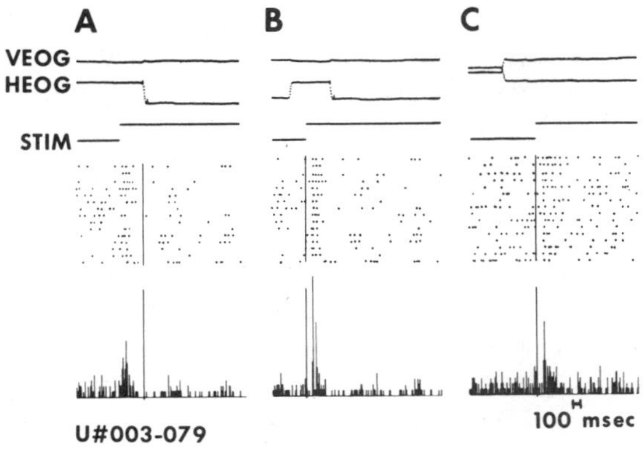

Figure 11. Enhanced response and synchrony of activity with target onset for a cell in posterior parietal cortex. Data in (A) show the activity of the cell aligned with the onset of the saccadic eye movement, whereas (B) illustrates the same activity aligned with the onset of the target to which the eye movement was made. (C) demonstrates the visual response of the same cell to the same stimulus while the monkey fixates throughout the trial. VEOG, vertical electrooculogram; HEOG, horizontal electrooculogram; STIM, stimulus or target onset. From Robinson *et al.* (1978).

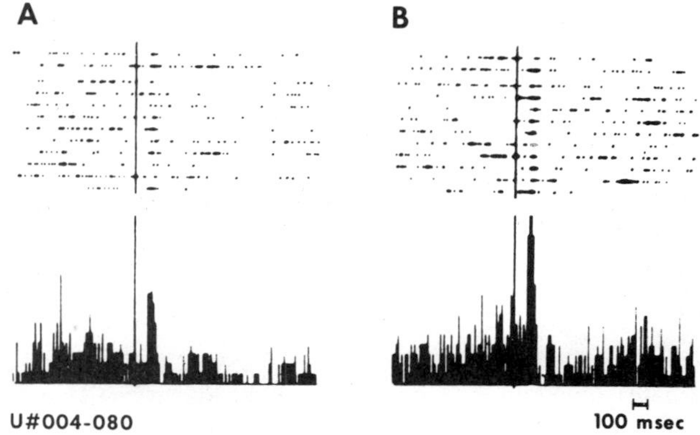

Figure 12. Enhancement elicited by attention without movement. Responses in (A) were produced by the onset of a visual stimulus presented while the monkey fixated. The enhanced discharge in (B) was present when the monkey was required to attend to the same stimulus but did not make an eye movement to fixate the light. From Bushnell, Goldberg, Land Robinson (unpublished data).

hanced when the animal makes a saccade to fixate the stimulus (Fig. 11B and C).

Parietal neurons also require the presence of the stimulus: if the animal makes the equivalent eye movement in total darkness, there is no change of the rate of discharge of the cell in relation to the eye movement (Mountcastle *et al.*, 1975; Lynch *et al.*, 1977; Robinson *et al.*, 1978). Therefore in area 7, too, the eye movement-related activity is a modulation of the visual response rather than an independent movement-related response.

Like the superior colliculus and the frontal eye fields, the enhancement in parietal cortex is spatially selective. A neuron that gives an enhanced response when a stimulus in its receptive field is a target for a saccade will not give an enhanced response when the animal makes a saccade to a target outside the receptive field (Robinson *et al.*, 1978).

Enhancement in posterior parietal cortex is very different from that in the colliculus and frontal eye fields in its independence of the motor aspects of the response to the stimulus. Bushnell *et al.* (1978) trained monkeys to respond to a peripheral stimulus but not to fixate it. As in experiments previously described, in each trial the animal was presented with two stimuli, a small central fixation point and a larger peripheral stimulus. Either one might dim in a given trial, and the animal learned to release the bar at the dimming of either. If the animal made an eye movement to fixate the peripheral stimulus, the trial was aborted. At the onset of the peripheral stimulus the animal did not know which stimulus might dim, and his response was the same regardless of which actually did dim. Since the animal released the bar whenever either stimulus dimmed, the investigators concluded that on each trial he was attending to the peripheral stimulus as well as to the fixation point. Those area 7 neurons that display presaccadic enhancement also show enhancement during a series of trials when the animal attends to but does not fixate the stimulus in the receptive field. Figure 12 compares the response of a neuron in area 7 in this no-saccade attention task to the response of the same neuron to the same stimulus during a series of trials in which the stimulus was irrelevant to the animal. There is a marked enhancement when the animal attends to the stimulus.

V. Functional Implications

In the monkey brain the intensity of the response of a neuron to a visual stimulus may depend not only on the physical characteristics of the stimulus but frequently on behavioral factors intrinsic to the animal. We have found that we can best understand the significance of this sensory modulation, the visual enhancement, by defining the set of behavioral circumstances under which it takes place. By correlating behavioral circumstances with neuronal responses we have shown that there are at least three different kinds of enhancement in the monkey visual system as summarized in Table I. The enhancement seen in the striate and prestriate cortices is spatially nonselective and response nonspecific. That seen in the superior colliculus and frontal eye fields is spatially selective and response specific. That seen in the posterior parietal cortex is spatially selective but response independent. We will argue that each of these types of enhancement might well have a different role to play in the sensory pro-

Table 1. Varieties of enhancement

Type	Brain location	Possible function
Spatially nonselective	Striate cortex, prestriate cortex, pulvinar	Arousal or alertness
Spatially selective response specific	Superior colliculus frontal eye fields	Initiation of movement
Spatially selective response independent	Parietal cortex	Selective attention

cesses underlying behavior. The enhancement that is both spatially and response nonspecific may well be related to alertness; that which is spatially selective and response specific may be more related to the initiation and guidance of specific movements; that which is spatially selective and independent of the specific motor response may well be participating in the neuronal mechanisms underlying attention.

A. Arousal and Alerting

The role of arousal in modifying behavior was stimulated by the work of Moruzzi and Magoun (1949) on the reticular formation of the brain-stem (see Lindsley, 1961; Magoun, 1958). These physiological studies in turn produced a surge of interest on the effects of activation or vigilance on a number of psychological factors including sensory processing (Duffy, 1962; Hebb, 1955). The nonselective enhancement effects seen in areas 17 and 18 have the characteristics one would expect of a general arousal process: the enhancement modifies the response to all adequate stimuli and is independent of the behavioral response made to the stimuli. It is therefore tempting to correlate spatially nonselective enhancement with arousal, but there is one problem: behavioral state extends over a large spectrum from deep sleep to the performance of a difficult task. We have studied the responses of these neurons only over a limited portion of this range—while the animal was performing intricate visuomotor tasks of varying degrees of difficulty. If the enhancement that we have seen is related to arousal then we have seen only a small fraction of its total range of modulation; had we studied the neurons when the animals were less alert we might have seen a more pronounced modulation of sensitivity.

The responsiveness of the monkey's visual pathway has been shown to change following stimulation of the midbrain reticular formation (Singer, 1977). Bartlett and Doty (1974a,b) showed that the responses of neurons in the striate cortex of the squirrel monkey are augmented by electrical stimulation of the mesencephalic reticular formation. This group had previously shown that stimulation of the same area can also facilitate the transmission of impulses through the lateral geniculate of the monkey (Doty *et al.*, 1974) and that the efficacy of the stimulalion is related to the animal's level of alertness (Bartlett *et al.*, 1973): reticular stimulation when the monkey was already alert had much less effect than when the animal was drowsy.

Posner has described a possible psychophysical counterpart of these physiological effects in his human performance experiments (Posner, 1975). He described alertness as the measure of receptivity of the organism to all external signals. Human subjects, for example, decrease their reaction time to a visual stimulus when the stimulus is preceded by a warning signal, and this more efficient processing is independent of the nature of the material to be processed. In the striate and prestriate cortices of the monkey, where the nonselective enhancement was the only effect seen, such enhancement could easily be a physiological representation of an alertness change: the brain becomes more receptive to all visual stimuli, not only those directly relevant to the task. When the animal is alert, it is more receptive to all stimuli, and its striate cortex is similarly more receptive throughout its entire retinotopic map.

B. Habituation

Enhancement also may be related to the phenomenon of habituation. If a stumulus is given repeatedly, the behavioral and physiological response to that stimulus wanes or habituates (see Humphrey, 1933, and Sokolov, 1960). This habituation occurs in most sensory systems when the stimuli are of no more than moderate strength and when the stimuli are given at regular intervals. There are remarkable similarities across species and experimental conditions in the habituation process (Thompson and Spencer, 1966).

In the visual system of mammals such habituation has been repeatedly observed, particularly in the superior colliculus (Horn and Hill, 1966; Horn, 1970), but we have seldom seen it in our analysis of the visual system of awake monkeys. One possible reason is that the responses that we study have already habituated to a stable state. This would not be surprising because the monkey has seen the same type of visual stimulus tens and frequently hundreds of times in the course of determining the receptive field of the neuron. Over the experimental lifetime of the animal he may well see similar stimuli hundreds of thousands of times, and although a neuron may respond to that stimulus a few times when the electrode is near, one can assume that the neuron has responded similarly when the electrode was in another group of cells. This situation in an awake animal may be profoundly different from an acute physiological experiment where the animal sees the experimental environment as a novel event, and the visual stimuli used to explore the responses on the neurons are truly new.

A habituated response recovers to original levels if no additional stimulation is given, or the habituated response may be dishabituated by presentation of a different stimulus (Thompson and Spencer, 1966). The dishabituation process and its relation to habituation have been studied intensively over the last 15 years, particularly in the flexor reflex of the cat (Spencer *et al.*, 1966) and frog (Groves and Thompson, 1970; Thompson and Glanzman, 1976) and in the gill withdrawal reflex of the aplysia (Castellucci and Kandel, 1974; Kandel, 1978). A salient point that has emerged from these lines of investigation is that dishabituation is a separate process superimposed upon habituation rather than a reversal of habituation. The dishabituation studied in the cat and frog spinal cord and the aplysia abdominal ganglion is a sensitization effect: a general change in responsiveness which could result from a number of different stimulus changes in the environment or motivational changes in the animal. If the factor producing the sensitization is removed, the response returns to its habituated level. It is the dishabituation process that might have a clear parallel in our experiments on the visual enhancement effects. The response of visual cells we study might ordinarily be habituated, and the enhancement effect might be a dishabituation of this habituated response (Goldberg and Wurtz, 1972b). The visual enhancement effect could be regarded as an example of this separate process which is superimposed upon an habituated response and increases the response of the cell to a stimulus.

In the places where the enhancement effect is nonselective (as in striate and prestriate cortices) the enhancement is similar to the sensitization effect, and this is in turn very similar to arousal. However, we have not studied enough of the aspects of nonspecific enhancement to make a detailed comparison between it and sensitization.

When the enhancement effect is specifically related to a particular movement (as in the superior colliculus and frontal eye fields), it is clearly different from sensitization. Our findings emphasize that in the central nervous system of the primate the dishabituation can be the result of a selective facilitation which acts on just one aspect of visual processing without modifying all of sensory processing as does sensitization.

This reversal of habituation may indicate one of the basic functions of the enhancement effect in those areas where it is selective. The brain cannot respond to all sensory stimuli in the same way all the time, and a mechanism must exist to select novel and important stimuli from the sensory environment. Habituation is one mechanism; it assumes that all novel stimuli are important. When a stimulus ceases to be novel it ceases to have a significant effect, and the response wanes, or habituates. The dishabituation produced by selective enhancement prevents an important stimulus from being lost and enables it to continue to have an effect on behavior.

C. Selective Attention

Along with initial reports of the visual enhancement effect in the superior colliculus, Goldberg and Wurtz (1972a,b) suggested that the effect might be related to a shift in visual attention. Denny-Brown (1962) and Sprague and Meikle (1965) had suggested earlier, on the basis of lesion experiments, that the superior colliculus might be related to attentional processes. Attention is a concept as old as psychology, and like most classical concepts in psychology has been defined nearly as frequently as it has been discussed. In order to discuss how physiological experiments might relate to this important concept, it is necessary to define what we mean by the term.

Attention has been frequently regarded as having at least two components. The first is an intensive (Berlyne, 1969) or alerting (Posner and Boies, 1971; Kahneman, 1973; Moray, 1969) component. This is essentially what we have considered as arousal or alerting and have compared to nonselective visual enhancement. The intensive effect is general and is probably a necessary condition for the second factor of attention to operate; selection of one stimulus from among many (James, 1890; Broadbent, 1958; Berlyne, 1969; Treisman, 1969; Berlyne, 1969; Kahneman, 1973; Moray, 1969; Posner and Boies, 1971). Selection can operate across sensory modalities or within modalities on the basis of the significance of a stimulus or its characteristics.[4]

We have dealt with the visual modality and with selection of spatial location within that modality. Enhancement of sensory response provides a possible mechanism for stimulus selection; neuronal activity induced by the important stimulus has more effect than neuronal activity induced by a less important stimulus. The enhancement is spatially specific in the superior colliculus, frontal eye fields, and parietal cortex, and these areas could therefore be logically involved in focusing attention on certain areas of the visual field.

In both the behavioral experiments of others and our own physiological experiments, selective attention is always indicated by the occurrence of a response to a stimulus, and this presents a difficulty with the measurement of attention. Man can contemplate an object in the environment or in his memory, select that object for analysis, and yet make no externally observable response related to the object. We know that we attend, but an observer need not know. The investigator performing behavioral or physiological experiments cannot rely on the "ineffable, effable, effanineffable"[5] process of attention, but rather on the occurrence of a response to the attended stimuli, from which he must reason backward that attention was there. In fact, some discussions of attention regard it as being closely related to response—Woodworth (1929) refers to an attentional response as in the case of a cat waiting by a mouse hole. This, in turn, is similar to the orienting response of Pavlovian conditioning (Pavlov, 1928). A problem arises when one confounds the response with the act of attention itself. Thus attention in man is well studied by measuring eye movement patterns (Yarbus, 1967) since it is the human style to look at what we attend.

Although visual attention is most often associated with movement, it can be dissociated from eye movement. For example, young monkeys never look at a dominant male, since eye contact is a threatening gesture, yet clearly they attend to the male (Perachio and Alexander, 1975). We therefore propose that although attention can be studied by looking at movements, particularly eye movements, true selective attention must be considered independent of the type of movement response.

In the posterior parietal cortex (area 7), Bushnell *et al.* (1978) found that visual responses are enhanced whenever the animal uses the stimulus in the receptive field for some behavior, regardless of the nature of the response. Thus the enhanced response will be seen if the animal makes an eye movement to the stimulus, reaches out to touch it, or merely knows that he may have to respond to it. We propose that these neurons have the properties one would expect to underly selective attention; they must be spatially selective and they must be independent of the movement the animal uses to respond to the stimulus. Posterior parietal cortex may well contain the neuronal substrate of visual attention in the form of its enhancement effect.

While we have postulated that the enhancement process in posterior parietal cortex participates in the mechanisms of selective attention, the enhancement effect in this area might in fact be derived from activity in other areas. The enhancement effect which is independent of particular movement might be summed from enhancements related to various movements. For example, the eye movement-related enhancement might come from enhanced visual input directly from the frontal eye fields or indirectly from the superior colliculus via the lateral posterior nucleus of the thalamus. Other enhancements may arise from the rich limbic connections of area 7 (Divac *et al.*, 1977; Stanton *et al.*, 1977; Mesulam *et al.*, 1977; Kasdon and Jacobson, 1978). This caution emphasizes that the sources of enhancement remain unexplored.

It is interesting that all of the areas studied where cells show spatially selective enhancement share the property of having visual responses that do not require very specific stimuli. The requirements for visual orientation and directional selectivity which are the hallmarks of striate (Hubel and Wiesel, 1968, 1977) and prestriate cortices (Zeki, 1975, 1978a,b; Baizer *et al.*, 1977) are not found in the superior colliculus and the frontal and parietal association cortices. This may indicate that pattern analysis is a function separate from the behavioral processes found outside of the geniculostriate system. These nongeniculostriate areas may only need to analyze the location of an object in space and its functional relevance but not the specific details of its visual properties.

An important practical point that emerges from this analysis is that in an awake animal it may not be possible to look at passive input alone and describe the function of a cell. For example, Robinson *et al.* (1978) showed that cells in area 7 respond more briskly to passively presented large, bright stimuli. However, it is difficult to argue that these cells, which also respond to small spots of light used as targets for eye movements, are in fact bigness and brightness detectors. Rather, it is likely that the animals cannot escape attending to distracting stimuli of this magnitude; therefore, in this seemingly passive situation, the animals are indeed attending to the stimulus. The behavioral modulation of the response may be unavoidable here and must be considered at each step in sensory processing to determine the extent of its effect. The awake, behaving animal offers the only opportunity to study this effect, but it also presents the hazard of being misled by it.

D. Initiation of Movement

The enhancement in the superior colliculus and the frontal cortex does not fit our requirement for selective attention because the selection occurs only when the stimulus is intimately linked to a specific motor act, an eye movement, and not when the stimulus is linked to other responses. If a stimulus is to be the target for an eye movement, it is convenient for that stimulus to have a greater effect on the motor system than equivalent stimuli that are not to be targets of eye movements. This has been well studied in the pyramidal motor system. For example, Evarts and Fromm (1977) demonstrated that brisk load perturbations are accurately represented in motor cortex only when the load perturbation is relevant to the movement. A similar situation may obtain in the visual system, where in both the superior colliculus and the frontal eye fields, neurons have markedly enhanced responses only when the visual stimulus is the target for a saccadic eye movement.

One of the persisting problems in analyzing sensorimotor behavior is the transition from stimulus input to movement output. The machinery for the generation of a saccadic eye movement of a given amplitude has been analyzed and modeled (Robinson, 1975), but where in the brain the visual to motor transition lies for the generation of visually guided saccades remains unknown. One possible transition might occur through the phenomenon of enhancement, where a premovement signal acts on a visual signal. Stimulation in the frontal eye fields and superior colliculus evokes eye movements; the effect of this stimulation may be to mimic an enhanced visual response and send such a compelling message to the gaze system that the stimulus of interest is placed on the fovea. Thus these enhancements might represent intermediate stages between visual input and oculomotor output. The anatomical connections of both the frontal eye fields and the superficial layers of the superior colliculus make this an excellent possibility. The former projects to regions in the intermediate layers of the superior colliculus including those layers that have cells discharging before eye movements (Kuypers and Lawrence, 1967; Astruc, 1971; Künzle *et al.*, 1976). The subtlety of the transition between an enhanced visual response and a visually triggered movement response in the superior colliculus (Wurtz and Mohler, 1976a) makes it likely that cells of the two sorts could share local circuit communications. The enhancement could then be the first stage in the definition of which object in the environment will be the target for the next saccadic eye movement.

VI. Conclusion

The apparent necessity for selection among the myriad stimulus inputs of the visual system at the behavioral level seems to have been confirmed by findings at the physiological level; there is, in fact, a selection operating at many different levels of the visual system, ranging from a primary afferent area, the superficial layers of the superior colliculus, to several "association" areas of cerebral cortex, areas 7 and 8. Selective enhancement may also be present in the auditory (Beaton and Miller, 1975; Hocherman *et al.*, 1976) and somatosensory systems (Hayes *et al.*, 1979) although these systems are just beginning to be investigated in detail for these nonsensory modulations.

We have suggested that enhancement may be a mechanism by which sensory association areas combine data from the external world and data from the internal organism to generate a signal for the organization of behavior. While we have suggested a number of functions for the various types of enhancement in different parts of the brain, experiments have not been done which show that an absence of this visual enhancement leads to a pronounced deficit at the behavioral level. However, recent psychophysical experiments in man (Singer *et al.*, 1977) have shown that a saccadic eye movement to a spot of light lowers the detection threshold for that spot of light. These authors suggest that this threshold change is a correlate of the enhancement effect; since it occurs in the absence of occipital cortex, it might be related to activity of the superior colliculus. Demonstration of the behavioral importance of enhancement is probably the most important experimental issue to be resolved.

Notes

1. This control experiment was in fact run in two different ways. Using the first method, both the control point and the receptive field stimulus came on for every trial, and *both* dimmed on every trial when they became the target for a saccade. This method had the advantage that the stimuli were exactly the same throughout on all trials but the disadvantage that the monkey was free to saccade to one or the other at will. Trials on which the monkey made a saccade to the receptive field stimulus were identified from the eye movement records and the raster lines of these trials grouped together. However, since the enhancement effect tends to build up over several successive saccade trials, this method tended to minimize the enhancement effect. In the second method both the receptive field stimulus and the control point came on but only *one* dimmed. This made the reward conditions somewhat different between blocks of trials, but required the monkey to make a series of saccades to one target or the other and potentiated the serial effects of enhancement. The enhancement effect is associated with the onset of the stimulus and the dimming occurred seconds later. The first method was used by Goldberg and Wurtz (1972b) and the latter by Wurtz and Mohler (1976a); both methods yielded comparable results.

2. The signal to initiate a saccade to a target is actually the fixation point going off. By turning it off before or after the onset of the visual target, the initiation of the saccade could be shifted in time nearer to or farther from the stimulus onset. This paradigm works only within a limited time period. If the fixation light is turned off too long before the stimulus target comes on, the monkey will make a saccade to another point in the visual field of his own choosing before the target point comes on. If the fixation point is turned off too close in time to the onset of the target light, the monkey will not recognize the light as such and will again saccade to a point of his choosing. Why some cells show predominantly earlier enhancement while others show only later enhancement when the monkey controls the timing of his saccades is not entirely resolved by these experiments. One possibility is that the monkey shifts the time at which he initiates saccades at different times during an experimental day and therefore produces early enhancement at some times and late enhancement at others. An alternative explanation might be a differing threshold for the facilitation effect so that the same level of facilitation produces earlier enhancement in some cells than in others.

3. An important point in this experiment is the control for the effect of the target spot alone. This spot might produce a visual response (even though it was selected to be as ineffective as possible) and this response might be enhanced; what might have been determined in this experiment was simply the addition of the enhanced response to the target spot to the response to the receptive field stimulus. To control for this, other trials were run to determine the response to the target spot alone when the monkey made saccades to the stimulus. Near the edge of the receptive field the response was negligible so that conclusions on "enhancement field" were uncontaminated by any response to the target spot. In the receptive field center it was frequently not possible to distinguish the enhancement response to the saccade target and the visual receptive field stimulus, and no detailed study within the receptive field was therefore attempted. In addition, once the two points were within a few degrees of one another, determination of which stimuli the saccade was directed toward became difficult since eye movements were recorded with an electrooculogram with a resolution limited to about one degree of visual angle.

4. An additional type of attention related to limited channel capacity is listed by Posner and Boies (1971). This type of attention is derived largely from reaction time interference studies which have indicated that the brain has a limited capacity to process sensory signals, and concentration on one set of tasks will increase the reaction time to a sporadically presented task using different sensory cues. In our physiological experiments, this channel capacity limitation probably is not distinguishable from a selection process, and for the purposes of our discussion this can be regarded as a type of selection. Other authors have identified as many as six types of attention (Moray, 1969), but for purposes of physiological comparison most of these can be subsumed under the rubric of selection.

5. T. S. Eliot (1952) dealt with this issue in his marsupial analysis of carnivores:

The name that no human research can discover—
  But THE CAT HIMSELF KNOWS, and will never confess.
When you notice a cat in profound meditation,
  The reason, I tell you, is always the same:
His mind is engaged in a rapt contemplation
  Of the thought, of the thought, of the thought of his name:
    His ineffable effable
    Effanineffable
Deep and inscrutable singular Name.

References

Adamük, E. (1870). Ueber die innervation der augenbewegungen. *Zeitschrift für Medizinische Wissenschaft* **8**, 65.

Apter, J. T. (1945). Projection of the retina on superior colliculus of cats. *Journal of Neurophysiology* **8**, 123–134.

Apter, J. T. (1946). Eye movements following strychninization of the superior colliculus of cats. *Journal of Neurophysiology* **9**, 73–86.

Astruc, J. (1971). Cortifugal connections of area 8 (frontal eye field) in *Mocaca mulatta. Brain Research* **33**, 241–256.

Baizer, J. S (1976). Receptive fields in areas 18 and 19 of the awake, behaving monkey. *Neuroscience Abstracts* **2**, 1101.

Baizer, J. S., Robinson, D. L., and Dow, B. M. (1977). Visual responses of area 18 neurons in awake, behaving monkey. *Journal of Neurophysiology* **40**, 1024–1037.

Baleydier, C., and Magnin, M. (1979). Afferent and efferent connections of the parabigeminal nucleus in cat revealed by retrograde axonal transport of horseradish peroxidase. *Brain Research* **161**, 187–198.

Bartlett, J. R., and Doty, R. W., Sr. (1974a). Response of units in striate cortex of squirrel monkeys to visual and electrical stimuli. *Journal of Neurophysiology* **37**, 621–641.

Bartlett, J. R., and Doty, R. W., Sr. (1974b). Influence of mesencephalic stimulation on unit activity in striate cortex of squirrel monkeys. *Journal of Neurophysiology* **37**, 642–652.

Bartlett, J. R., Doty, R. W., Pecci-Saavedra, J., and Wilson, P. D. (1973). Mesencephalic control of lateral geniculate nucleus in primates. III. Modifications with state of alertness. *Experimental Brain Research* **18**, 214–224.

Beaton, R., and Miller, J. M. (1975). Single cell activity in the auditory cortex of the unanesthetized, behaving monkey: Correlation with stimulus controlled behavior. *Brain Research* **100**, 543–562.

Benevento, L. A., and Fallon, J. H. (1975). The ascending projections of the superior colliculus in the rhesus monkey (*Macaca mulatta*). *Journal of Comparative Neurology* **160**, 339–362.

Benevento, L. A., and Rezak, M. (1976). The cortical projections of the inferior pulvinar and adjacent lateral pulvinar in the rhesus monkey (*Macoca mulatta*): An autoradiographic study. *Brain Research* **108**, 1–24.

Berlyne, D. E. (1969). The development of the concept of attention in psychology. *In* "Attention in Neurophysiology" (C. R. Evans and T. B. Mulholland, eds.), pp. 1–26. Appleton-Century-Crofts, New York.

Bizzi, E. (1968). Discharge of frontal eye field neurons during saccadic and following eye movements in unanesthetized monkeys. *Experimental Brain Research* **6**, 69–80.

Bizzi, E., and Schiller, P. H. (1970). Single unit activity in the frontal eye fields of unanesthetized monkeys during eye and head movement. *Experimental Brain Research* **10**, 151–158.

Broadbent, D. E. (1958). "Perception and Communication." Pergamon, London.

Bunt, A. H., Hendrickson, A. E., Lund, J. S., Lund, R. D., and Fuchs, A. F. (1975). Monkey retinal ganglion cells: Morphometric analysis and tracing of axonal projections, with a consideration of the peroxidase technique. *Journal of Comparative Neurology* **164**, 265–285.

Bushnell, M. C., Robinson, D. L., and Goldberg, M. E. (1978). Dissociation of movement and attention: Neuronal correlates in posterior parietal cortex. *Neuroscience Abstract* **4**, 621.

Büttner, M., and Fuchs, A. F. (1973). Influence of saccadic eye movements and unit activity in Simian lateral geniculate and pregeniculate nuclei. *Journal of Neurophysiology* **36**, 127–141.

Castellucci, V., and Kandel, E. (1974). An invertebrate system for cellular study of habituation and sensitization. *In* "Habituation" (T. J. Tighe and R. N. Leaton, eds.), pp. 1–47. Erlbaum, Hillsdale, New Jersey.

Cragg, B. G. (1969). The topography of the afferent projections in the circumstriate visual cortex of the monkey studied by the Nauta method. *Vision Research* **9**, 733–747.

Critchley, M. (1953). "The Parietal Lobes." Arnold, London.

Cynader, M., and Berman, N. (1972). Receptive-field organization of monkey superior colliculus. *Journol of Neurophysiology* **35**, 187–201.

Denny-Brown, D. (1962). The midbrain and motor integration. *Proceedings Royal Society Medicine* **55**, 527–538.

Divac, I., LaVail, J. H., Rakic, P., and Winston, K. R. (1977). Heterogeneous afferents to the inferior parietal lobule of the rhesus monkey revealed by the retrograde transport method. *Brain Research* **123**, 197–207.

Doty, R. W. (1973). Ablation of visual areas in the central nervous system. *In* "Handbook of Sensory Physiology" (R. Jung, ed.), Vol VII/3B, pp. 483–541. Springer, Berlin.

Doty, R. W., Wilson, P. D., Bartlett, J. R., and Pecci-Saavedra, J. (1973). Mesencephalic control of lateral geniculate nucleus in primates. I. Electrophysiology. *Experimental Brain Research* **18**, 189–203.

Dow, B. M., and Gouras, P. (1973). Color and spatial specificity of single units in rhesus monkey foveal striate cortex. *Journal of Neurophysiology* **36**, 79–100.

Duffy, E. (1962). "Activation and Behavior." Wiley, New York.

Edwards, S. B., Rosenquist, A. C., and Palmer, L. A. (1974). An autoradiographic study of ventral lateral geniculate projections in the cat. *Brain Research* **72**, 282–287.

Eliot, T. S. (1952). The Naming of Cats. "The Complete Poems and Plays," p. 149. Harcourt Brace, New York.

Evarts, E. V. (1966). Methods for recording activity of individual neurons in moving animals. *In* "Methods in Medical Research" (R. F. Rushmer, ed.), Vol. II, pp. 241–250. Year Book, Chicago.

Evarts, E. V. (1968a). A technique for recording activity of subcortical neurons in moving animals. *Electroencephalography and Clinical Neurophysiology* **24**, 83–86.

Evarts, E. V. (1968b). Relation of pyramidal tract activity to force exerted during voluntary movement. *Journal of Neurophysiology* **31**, 14–27.

Evarts, E. V., and Fromm, C. (1977). Sensory responses in motor cortex neurons during precise motor control. *Neuroscience Letters* **5**, 267–272.

Finlay, B. L., Schiller, P. H., and Volman, S. F. (1976). Quantitative studies of single-cell properties in monkey striate cortex. IV. Corticotectal cells. *Journal of Neurophysiology* **39**, 1352–1361.

Garey, L. J., and Powell, T. P. S. (1971). An experimental study of the termination of the lateral geniculo-cortical pathway in the cat and monkey. *Proceedings of the Royal Society of London* **179**, 41–63.

Glendenning, K. K., Hall, J. A., Diamond, I. T., and Hall, W. C. (1975). The pulvinar nucleus of *Galago senegalensis. Journal of Comparative Neurology*, **161**, 419–457.

Goldberg, M. E., and Robinson, D. L. (1977a). Visual responses of neurons in monkey inferior parietal lobule: The physiologic substrate of attention and neglect. *Neurology* **27**, 350.

Goldberg, M. E., and Robinson, D. L. (1977b). Visual mechanisms underlying gaze: Function of the cerebral cortex. *In* "Control of Gaze by Brainstem Neurons. Developments in Neuroscience" (R. Baker and A. Berthoz, eds.). Elsevier North Holland, Amsterdam.

Goldberg, M. E., and Robinson, D. L. (1978). The superior colliculus. *In* "Handbook of Behavioral Neurobiology. Vol. 1. Sensory Integration" (R. B. Masterton, ed.), pp. 119–164. Plenum, New York.

Goldberg, M. E., and Wurtz, R. H. (1970). Effects of eye movement and stimulus on units in monkey superior colliculus. *Federation Proceedings* **29**, 453.

Goldberg, M. E., and Wurtz, R. H. (1972a). Activity of superior colliculus in behaving monkey. I. Visual receptive fields of single neurons. *Journal of Neurophysiology* **35**, 542–559.

Goldberg, M. E., and Wurtz, R. H. (1972b). Activity of superior colliculus in behaving monkey. II. Effect of attention on neuronal responses. *Journal of Neurophysiology* **35**, 560–574.

Graybiel, A. M. (1978a). Organization of the nigrotectal connection: An experimental tracer study in the cat. *Brain Research* **143**, 339–348.

Graybiel, A. M. (1978b). A satellite system of the superior colliculus: The parabigeminal nucleus and its projections to the superficial collicular layers. *Brain Research* **145**, 365–374.

Groves, P. M., and Thompson, R. F. (1970). Habituation: A dual process theory. *Psychological Review* **77**, 419–450.

Harting, J. K., Glendenning, K. K., Diamond, I. T., and Hall, W. C. (1973). Evolution of the primate visual system: Anterograde degeneration studies of the tecto pulvinar system. *American Journal of Physical Anthropology* **38**, 383–392.

Hayaishi, Y. (1969). Recurrent collateral inhibition of visual cortical cells projecting to superior colliculus in cats. *Vision Research* **9**, 1367–1380.

Hayes, R. L., Price, D. D., and Dubner, R. (1979). Behavioral and physiological studies of sensory coding and modulation of trigeminal nociceptive input. *Advances in Pain Research and Therapy* **3**, 219–243.

Hebb, D. O. (1955). Drives and the CNS. *Psychological Review* **62**, 243–254.

Hendrickson, A., Wilson, M. E., and Toyne, M. J. (1970). The distribution of optic nerve fibers in *Macaca mulatta. Brain Research* **23**, 425–427.

Hocherman, S., Benson, D. A., Goldstein, M. H., Jr., Heffner, H. E., and Heinz, R. D. (1976). Evoked activity in auditory cortex of monkeys performing a selective attention task. *Brain Research* **117**, 51–68.

Holländer, H. (1974). On the origin of the corticotectal projections in the cat. *Experimental Brain Research* **21**, 433–439.

Horn, G. (1970). Changes in neuronal activity and their relationship to behaviour. *In* "Short Term Changes in Neural Activity and Behavior" (G. Horn and R. A. Hinde, eds.), pp. 567–606. Cambridge University Press, Cambridge.

Horn, G., and Hill, R. M. (1966). Responsiveness to sensory stimulation of units in the superior colliculus and subjacent tectotegmental regions of the rabbit. *Experimental Neurology* **14**, 199–223.

Hubel, D. H., and Wiesel, T. N. (1968). Receptive fields and functional architecture of monkey striate cortex. *Journal of Physiology* **195**, 215–243.

Hubel, D. H., and Wiesel, T. N. (1972). Laminar and columnar distribution of geniculo cortical fibers in the macaque monkey. *Journal of Comparative Neurology* **146**, 421–450.

Hubel, D. H., and Wiesel, T. N. (1977). Functional architecture of macaque monkey visual cortex. *Proceedings of the Royal Society of London* **B 198**, 159.

Hubel, D. H., LeVay, S., and Wiesel, T. N. (1975). Mode of termination of retinotectal fibers in the macaque monkey: An autoradiography study. *Brain Research* **96**, 25–40.

Humphrey, G. (1933). "The Nature of Learning." Harcourt, New York.

Humphrey, N. K. (1968). Responses to visual stimuli of units in the superior colliculus of rats and monkeys. *Experimental Neurology* **20**, 312–340.

Hyvärinen, J., and Poranen, A. (1974). Function of the parietal associative area 7 as revealed from cellular discharges in alert monkeys. *Brain* **97**, 673–692.

James, W. (1890). "The Principles of Psychology." Holt, New York (reprinted, Dover, New York, 1950).

Kahneman, D. (1973). "Attention and Effort." Prentice Hall, New York.

Kanaseki, T., and Sprague, J. M. (1974). Anatomical organization of pretectal and tectal laminae in the cat. *Journal of Comparative Neurology* **158**, 319–337.

Kandel, E. R. (1978). "A Cell Biological Approach to Learning," Grass Lecture Monograph 1, Society for Neuroscience, Bethesda, Maryland.

Kasdon, D. L., and Jacobson, S. (1978). The thalamic afferents to the inferior parietal lobule of the rhesus monkey. *Journal of Comparative Neurology* **177**, 685–706.

Keys, W., and Robinson, D. L. (1979). Eye movement-dependent enhancement of visual responses in the pulvinar nucleus of the monkey. *Neuroscience Abstracts* **5**, 791.

Künzle, H., Akert, K., and Wurtz, R. H. (1976). Projection of area 8 (frontal eye field) to superior colliculus in the monkey. An autoradiographic study. *Brain Research* **117**, 487–492.

Kupfer, C., Chumbley, L., and Downer, J. de C. (1967). Quantitative histology of optic nerve, optic tract and lateral geniculate nucleus of man. *Journal of Anatomy* **101**, 393–401.

Kuypers, H. G. J. M., and Lawrence, D. G. (1967). Cortical projections to the red nucleus and the brain stem in the rhesus monkey. *Brain Research* **4**, 151–188.

Kuypers, H. G. J. M., Szwarcbart, M. K., Mishkin, M., and Rosvold, H. E. (1965). Occipitotemporal corticocortical connections in the rhesus monkey. *Experimental Neurology* **11**, 245–262.

Lindsley, D. B. (1961). The reticular activating system and perceptual integration. *In* "Electrical Stimulation of the Brain" (D. E. Sheer, ed.), pp. 331–349. University of Texas Press, Austin.

Lund, R. D. (1972). Synaptic patterns in the superficial layers of the superior colliculus of the monkey, *Macaca mulatta. Experimental Brain Research* **15**, 194–211.

Lund, J. S., Lund, R. D., Hendrickson, A. E., Bunt, A. H., and Fuchs, A. F. (1975). The origin of efferent pathways from the primary visual cortex. area 17, of the macaque monkey as shown by retrograde transport of horseradish peroxidase. *Journal of Comparative Neurology* **164**, 287–304.

Lynch, J. C., Mountcastle, V. B., Talbot, W. H., and Yin, T. C. T. (1977). Parietal lobe mechanisms for directed visual attention. *Journal of Neurophysiology* **40**, 362–389.

Magoun, H. W. (1958). "The Waking Brain." Thomas, Springfield, Illinois.

Marrocco, R. T., and Li, R. H. (1977). Monkey superior colliculus: Properties of single cells and their afferent inputs. *Journal of Neurophysiology* **40**, 844–860.

Mathers, L. H. (1971). Tectal projection to the posterior thalamus of the squirrel monkey. *Brain Research* **35**, 295–298.

Mesulam, M.-M., Van Hoesen, G. W., Pandya, D. N., and Geschwind, N. (1977). Limbic and sensory connections of the inferior parietal lobule (area PG) in the rhesus monkey: A study with a new method for horseradish peroxidase histochemistry. *Brain Research* **136**, 393–414.

Michael, C. R. (1978). Color vision mechanisms in monkey striate cortex: Dual opponent cells with concentric receptive fields. *Journal of Neurophysiology* **41**, 572–588.

Mohler, C. W., and Wurtz, R. H. (1976). Organization of monkey superior colliculus: Intermediate layer cells discharging before eye movements. *Journal of Neurophysiology* **39**, 722–744.

Mohler, C. W., and Wurtz, R. H. (1977). Role of striate cortex and superior colliculus in visual guidance of saccadic eye movements in monkeys. *Journal of Neurophysiology* **40**, 74–94.

Mohler, C. W., Goldberg, M. E., and Wurtz, R. H. (1973). Visual receptive fields of frontal eye field neurons. *Brain Research* **61**, 385–389.

Moray, N. (1969). "Attention. Selective Processes in Vision and Hearing." Hutchinson, London.

Moruzzi, G., and Magoun, H. W. (1949). Brain stem reticular formation and activation of the EEG. *Electroencephalography and Clinical Neurophysiology* **1**, 455–473.

Mountcastle, V. B., Lynch, J. C., Georgopoulos, A., Sakata, H., and Acuna, C. (1975). Posterior parietal association cortex of the monkey: Command functions for operations within extrapersonal space. *Journal of Neurophysiology* **38**, 871–908.

Myers, R. E. (1963). Projections of superior colliculus in monkey. *Anatomical Record* **145**, 264.

Ogden, T. E., and Miller, R. F. (1966). Studies of the optic nerve of the rhesus monkey: Nerve fiber spectrum and physiological properties. *Vision Research* **6**, 485–506.

Palmer, L. A., and Rosenquist, A. C. (1974). Visual receptive fields of single striate cortical units projecting to the superior colliculus in the cat. *Brain Research* **67**, 27–42.

Partlow, G. D., Colonnier, M., and Szabo, J. (1977). Thalamic projections of the superior colliculus in the rhesus monkey, *Macaca mulatta*. A light and electron microscopic study. *Journal of Comparative Neurology* **171**, 285–317.

Pavlov, I. P. (1928). "Lectures on Conditioned Reflexes." International Publishers, New York.

Perachio, A. A., and Alexander, M. (1975). The neural basis of aggression and sexual behavior in the rhesus monkey. *In* "The Rhesus Monkey. Vol. I. Anatomy and Physiology" (G. H. Bourne, ed.), pp. 381–409. Academic, New York.

Poggio, G. F., and Fischer, B. (1977). Binocular interaction and depth sensitivity in striate and prestriate cortex of behaving rhesus monkey. *Journal of Neurophysiology* **40**, 1392–1405.

Posner, M. I. (1975). Psychobiology of attention. *In* "Handbook of Psychobiology" (M. S. Gazzaniga and C. Blakemore, eds.), chap. 15, pp. 441–480. Academic Press, New York.

Posner, M. I., and Boies, S. J. (1971). Components of attention. *Psychological Review* **78**, 391–408.

Raczkowski, D., and Diamond, I. T. (1978). Cells of origin of several efferent pathways from the superior colliculus in *Galago senegalensis. Brain Research* **146**, 351–357.

Richmond, B. J., and Wurtz, R. H. (1978). Visual masking by remote stimuli in monkey superior colliculus. *Neuroscience Abstracts* **4**, 642.

Rizzolatti, G., Camarda, R., Grupp, L. A., and Pisa, M. (1974). Inhibitory effect of remote visual stimuli on visual responses of cat superior colliculus: spatial and temporal factors. *Journal of Neurophysiology* **37**, 1262–1275.

Robinson, D. A. (1975). Oculomotor control signals. *In* "Basic Mechanisms of Ocular Motility and Their Clinical Implications" (G. Lennerstrand and P. Bach-Y-Rita, eds.), pp. 337–374. Pergamon Press, Oxford.

Robinson, D. A. and Fuchs, A. F. (1969). Eye movements evoked by stimulation of frontal eye fields. *Journal of Neurophysiology* **32**, 637–648.

Robinson, D. L., and Goldberg, M. E. (1977). Visual properties of neurons in the parietal cortex of the awake monkey. *Investigative Ophthalmology and Visual Science* **16**, Supplement, 156.

Robinson, D. L., and Jarvis, C. D. (1974). Superior colliculus neurons studied during head and eye movements of the behaving monkey. *Journal of Neurophysiology* **37**, 533–540.

Robinson, D. L., and Wurtz, R. H. (1976). Use of an extraretinal signal by monkey superior colliculus neurons to distinguish real from self-induced stimulus movements. *Journal of Neurophysiology* **39**, 852–870.

Robinson, D. L., Goldberg, M. E., and Stanton, G. B. (1978). Parietal association cortex in the primate: Sensory mechanisms and behavioral modulations. *Journal of Neurophysiology* **41**, 910–932.

Robinson, D. L., Baizer, J. S., and Dow, B. M. Visual response enhancement in prestriate cortex (in preparation).

Schiller, P. H., and Koerner, F. (1971). Discharge characteristics of single units in superior colliculus of the alert rhesus monkey. *Journal of Neurophysiology* **34**, 920–936.

Schiller, P. H., and Malpeli, J. G. (1977). The effect of striate cortex cooling on area 18 cells in the monkey. *Brain Research* **126**, 366–375.

Schiller, P. H., Stryker, M., Cynader, M., and Berman, N. (1974). Response characteristics of single cells in the monkey superior colliculus following ablation or cooling of visual cortex. *Journal of Neurophysiology* **37**, 181–194.

Schiller, P. H., Finlay, B. L., and Volman, S. F. (1976). Quantitative studies of single cell properties in monkey striate cortex. I. Spatio-temporal organization of receptive fields. *Journal of Neurophysiology* **39**, 1288–1319.

Singer, W. (1977). Control of thalamic transmission by corticofugal and ascending reticular pathways in the visual system. *Physiological Review* **57**, 386–420.

Singer, W., Zihl, J., and Pöppel, E. (1977). Subcortical control of visual thresholds in humans: Evidence for modality specific and retinotopically organized mechanisms of selective attention. *Experimental Brain Research* **29**, 173–190.

Sokolov, E. N. (1960). Neuronal models and the orienting reflex. *In* "The Central Nervous System and Behavior" (M. A. B. Brazier, ed.), pp. 187–276. Josiah Macy, Jr. Foundation, New York.

Sparks, D. L. (1978). Functional properties of neurons in the monkey superior colliculus: coupling of neuronal activity and saccade onset. *Brain Research* **156**, 1–16.

Sparks, D. L., Holland, R., and Guthrie, B. L. (1976). Size and distribution of movement fields in the monkey superior colliculus. *Brain Research* **113**, 21–34.

Spencer, W. A. Thompson, R. F., and Neilson, D. R., Jr. (1966). Response decrement of the flexion reflex in the acute spinal cat and transient restoration by strong stimuli. *Journal of Neurophysiology* **29**, 221–239.

Sprague, J. M., and Meikle, T. H., Jr. (1965). The role of the superior colliculus in visually guided behavior. *Experimental Neurology* **11**, 115–146.

Stanton, G. B., Cruce, W. L. R., Goldberg, M. E., and Robinson, D. L. (1977). Some ipsilateral projections to areas PF and PG of the inferior parietal lobule in monkeys. *Neuroscience Letters* **6**, 243–250.

Thompson, R. F., and Glanzman, D. L. (1976). Neural and behavioral mechanisms of habituation and sensitization. *In* "Habituation" (T. J. Tighe and P. H. Leaton, eds.), pp. 49–93. Erlbaum, Hillsdale, N.J.

Thompson, R. F., and Spencer, W. A. (1966). Habituation: A model phenomenon for the study of neuronal substrates of behavior. *Psychological Review* **73**, 16–43.

Toyama, K., Matsunami, K., and Ohno, T. (1969). Antidromic identification of association, commissural and corticofugal efferent cells in cat visual cortex. *Brain Research* **14**, 513–517.

Treisman, A. M. (1969). Strategies and models of selective attention. *Psychological Review* **76**, 282–299.

Updyke, B. V. (1975). Characteristics of unit responses in superior colliculus of the Cebus monkey. *Journal of Neurophysiology* **37**, 896–909.

Wagman, I. H. (1964). Eye movements induced by electric stimulation of cerebrum in monkeys and their relationship to bodily movement. *In* "The Oculomotor System" (M. B. Bender, ed.), pp. 18–39. Harper and Row, New York.

Weiskrantz, L. (1972). Behavioral analysis of the monkey's visual system. *Proceedings of the Royal Society of London, Ser B.* **182**, 427–455.

Welch, K., and Stuteville, P. (1958). Experimental production of unilateral neglect in monkeys. *Brain* **81**, 341–347.

Wilson, M. E., and Cragg, B. G. (1967). Projections from the lateral geniculate nucleus in the cat and monkey. *Journal of Anatomy* **101**, 677–692.

Wilson, M. E., and Toyne, M. J. (1970). Retinotectal and corticotectal projections in *Macaca mulatta*. *Brain Research* **24**, 395–406.

Woodworth, R. S. (1929). "Psychology." Holt, New York.

Wurtz, R. H. (1969). Visual receptive fields of striate cortex neurons in awake monkeys. *Journal of Neurophysiology* **32**, 727–742.

Wurtz, R. H., and Albano, J. E. (1980). The primate superior colliculus. *Annual Review of Neuroscience* **3**, 189–226.

Wurtz, R. H., and Goldberg, M. E. (1971). Superior colliculus cell responses related to eye movements in awake monkeys. *Science* **171**, 82–84.

Wurtz, R. H., and Goldberg, M. E. (1972a). Activity of superior colliculus in behaving monkey. III. Cells discharging before eye movements. *Journal of Neurophysiology* **35**, 575–586.

Wurtz, R. H., and Goldberg, M. E. (1972b). Activity of superior colliculus in behaving monkey. IV. Effects of lesions on eye movements. *Journal of Neurophysiology* **35**, 587–596.

Wurtz, R. H., and Goldberg, M. E. (1972c). The primate superior colliculus and the shift of visual attention. *Investigative Ophthalmology* **11**, 441–449.

Wurtz, R. H., and Mohler, C. W. (1974). Selection of visual targets for the initiation of saccadic eye movements. *Brain Research* **71**, 209–214.

Wurtz, R. H., and Mohler, C. W. (1976a). Organization of monkey superior colliculus: Enhanced visual response of superficial layer cells. *Journal of Neurophysiology* **39**, 745–762.

Wurtz, R. H., and Mohler, C. W. (1976b). Enhancement of visual responses in monkey striate cortex and frontal eye fields. *Journal of Neurophysiology* **39**, 766–772.

Yarbus, A. L. (1967). "Eye Movements and Vision" (L. A. Riggs, trans.). Plenum, New York.

Yin, T. C. T., and Mountcastle, V. B. (1977). Visual input to the visuomotor mechanisms of the monkey's parietal lobe. *Science* **197**, 1381–1383.

Yin, T. C. T., and Mountcastle, V. B. (1978). Mechanisms of neural integration in the parietal lobe for visual attention. *Federation Proceedings* **37**, 2251–2257.

Zeki, S. M. (1975). The functional organization of projections from striate to prestriate visual cortex in the rhesus monkey. *Cold Spring Harbor Symposium on Quantitative Biology* **40**, 591–600.

Zeki, S. M. (1978a). The cortical projections of foveal striate cortex in the rhesus monkey. *Journal of Physiology* **277**, 227–244.

Zeki, S. M. (1978b). Uniformity and diversity of structure and function in rhesus monkey prestriate visual cortex. *Journal of Physiology* **277**, 273–290.

28
F. Crick
Function of the thalamic reticular complex: The searchlight hypothesis

1984. *Proceedings of the National Academy of Science USA* 81: 4586–4590

Abstract

It is suggested that in the brain the internal attentional searchlight, proposed by Treisman and others, is controlled by the reticular complex of the thalamus (including the closely related perigeniculate nucleus) and that the expression of the searchlight is the production of rapid bursts of firing in a subset of thalamic neurons. It is also suggested that the conjunctions produced by the attentional searchlight are mediated by rapidly modifiable synapses—here called Malsburg synapses—and especially by rapid bursts acting on them. The activation of Malsburg synapses is envisaged as producing transient cell assemblies, including "vertical" ones that temporarily unite neurons at different levels in the neural hierarchy.

This paper presents a set of speculative hypotheses concerning the functions of the thalamus and, in particular, the nucleus reticularis of the thalamus and the related perigeniculate nucleus. For ease of exposition I have drawn my examples mainly from the visual system of primates, but I expect the ideas to apply to all mammals and also to other systems such as the language system in man.

Visual System

It is now well established that in the early visual system of primates there are at least 10 distinct visual areas in the neocortex. [For a recent summary, see Van Essen and Maunsell (1).] If we include all areas whose main concern is with vision, there may be perhaps twice that number. To a good approximation, the early visual areas can be arranged in a branching hierarchy. Each of these areas has a crude "map" of (part of) the visual world. The first visual area (area 17, also called the striate cortex) on one side of the head maps one-half of the visual world in rather fine detail. Its cells can respond to relatively simple visual "features," such as orientation, spatial frequency, disparity (between the two eyes), etc. This particular area is a large one so that the connections between different parts of it are relatively local. Each part therefore responds mainly to the properties of a small local part of the visual field (2).

As one proceeds to areas higher in the hierarchy, the "mapping" becomes more diffuse. At the same time the neurons appear to respond to more complex features in the visual field. Different cortical areas specialize, to some extent, in different features, one responding mainly to motion, another more to color, etc. In the higher areas a neuron hardly knows where in the visual field the stimulus (such as a face) is arising, while the feature it responds to may be so complex that individual neurons are often difficult to characterize effectively (3, 4).

Thus, the different areas analyze the visual field in different ways. This is not, however, how we appear to see the world. Our inner visual picture of the external world has a unity. How then does the brain put together all of these different activities to produce a unified picture so that, for example, for any object the right color is associated with the right shape?

The Searchlight

The pioneer work of Treisman and her colleagues (5–8), supported more recently by the elegant experiments of Julesz (9–11), have revealed a remarkable fact. If only a very short space of time is available, especially in the presence of "distractors," the brain is unable to make these conjunctions reliably. For example, a human subject can rapidly spot an "*S*" mixed in with a randomly arranged set of green *X*s and brown *T*s—it "pops out" at him. His performance is also rapid for a blue letter mixed in with the same set. However, if he is asked to detect a green *T* (which requires that he recognize the *conjunction* of a chosen color with a chosen shape), he usually takes much more time. Moreover, the time needed increases linearly with the number of distractors (the green *X*s and brown *T*s) as if the mind were searching the letters *in series*, as if the brain had an internal attentional searchlight that moved around from one visual object to the next, with steps as fast as 70 msec in favorable cases. In this metaphor the searchlight is not supposed to light up part of a completely dark landscape but, like a searchlight at dusk, it intensifies part of a scene that is already visible to some extent.

If there is indeed a searchlight mechanism in the brain, how does it work and where is it located? To approach this problem we must study the general layout of the brain and, in particular, that of the neocortex and the thalamus. The essential facts we need at this stage are as follows.

The publication costs of this article were defrayed in part by page charge payment. This article must therefore be hereby marked "*advertisement*" in accordance with 18 U.S.C. §1734 solely to indicate this fact.

Thalamus

The thalamus is often divided into two parts: the dorsal thalamus, which is the main bulk of it, and the ventral thalamus. [For a general account of the thalamus, see the review by Jones (12).] For the moment when I speak of the thalamus I shall mean the dorsal thalamus.

Almost all input to the cortex, with the exception of the olfactory input, passes through the thalamus. For this reason it is sometimes called the gateway to the cortex. There are some exceptions—the diffuse projections from the brainstem, the projections from the claustrum, and also some projections from the amygdala and basal forebrain—that need not concern us here.

This generalization is not true for projections *from* the cortex, which do not need to pass through the thalamus. Nevertheless, for each projection *from* a region of the thalamus there is a corresponding reverse projection from that part the cortex to the corresponding region of the thalamus. In some cases at least this reverse projection has more axons than the forward projection.

Most of the neurons in the thalamus are relay cells—that is, they receive an input from outside the thalamus (for example, the lateral geniculate nucleus of the thalamus gets a major input from the retina) and project directly to the cortex. Their axons form type I synapses and therefore are probably excitatory. There is a minority of small neurons in the thalamus—their exact number is somewhat controversial—that appear to form type II synapses and are therefore probably inhibitory.

While on the face of it the thalamus appears to be a mere relay, this seems highly unlikely. Its size and its strategic position make it very probable that it has some more important function.

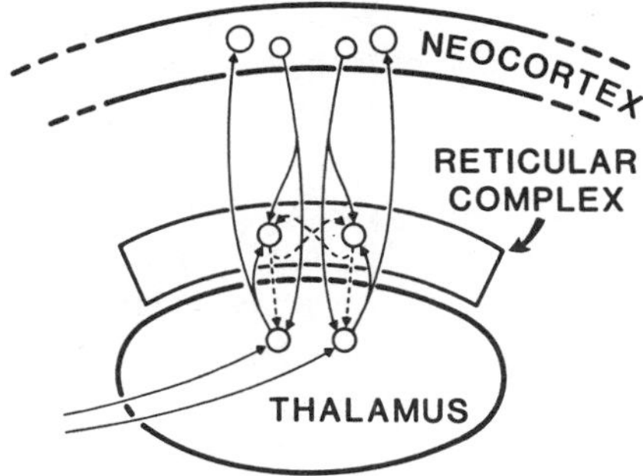

Figure 1. The main connections of the reticular complex, highly diagramatic and not at all to scale. Solid lines represent excitatory axons. Dashed lines show GABAergic (inhibitory) axons. Arrows represent synapses.

Reticular Complex

Much of the rest of the thalamus is often referred to as the ventral thalamus. This includes the reticular complex (part of which is often called the perigeniculate nucleus), the ventral lateral geniculate nucleus, and the zona incerta. In what follows I shall, for ease of exposition, use the term reticular complex to include the perigeniculate nucleus. Again, "thalamus" means the dorsal thalamus. Although much of the following information comes from the cat or the rat, there is no reason to think that it does not also apply to the primate thalamus.

The reticular complex is a thin sheet of neurons, in most places only a few cells thick, which partly surrounds the (dorsal) thalamus (13–32) (see Fig. 1). All axons from the thalamus to the cerebral cortex pass through it, as do all of the reverse projections from the cortex to the thalamus. The intralaminar nuclei of the thalamus, which project very strongly to the striatum, also send their axons through it, as may some of the axons from the globus pallidus that project back to the thalamus.

It is believed that many of the axons that pass in both directions through the reticular complex give off collaterals that make excitatory synaptic contacts in it (15, 18, 21, 29, 30). If the thalamus is the gateway to the cortex, the reticular complex might be described as the guardian of the gateway. Its exact function is unknown.

Not only is its position remarkable, but its structure is also unusual. It consists largely (if not entirely) of neurons whose dendrites often spread rather extensively in the plane of the nucleus (29). The size of these neurons is somewhat different in different parts of the complex (31). Their axons, which project to the thalamus, give off rather extensive collaterals that ramify, sometimes for long distances, within the sheet of the reticular complex (19, 29). This is in marked contrast with most of the nuclei of the thalamus, the principal cells of which have few, if any, collaterals either within each nucleus or between nuclei. The nuclei of the thalamus (with the exception of the intralaminar nuclei) keep themselves to themselves. The neurons of the reticular complex, on the other hand, appear to communicate extensively with each other. Moreover, it is characteristic of them that they fire in long bursts at a very rapid rate (25).

An even more remarkable property of reticular neurons concerns their output. Whereas all of the output neurons of the thalamus make type I synapses and appear to be excitatory, many (if not all) of the neurons in the reticular complex appear to be GABAergic (GABA = γ-aminobutyric acid) and thus almost certainly inhibitory (26–28). The excitation in the complex must come almost exclusively from the activity of the various axons passing through it.

Both the input and the output of the complex are arranged topographically (16, 29, 30, 32). It seems likely that if a particular group of axons going from the thalamus to the cortex passes through a small region of the reticular complex, the reverse projection probably passes through or near that same region. There may well be a rough map of the whole cortex on the reticular complex, though how precise this map may be is not known. It should be remembered, however, that the spread of the receiving dendrites of the reticular nucleus is quite large.

The projection of the reticular complex to the thalamus is also not random. Though any individual axon may spread fairly widely, there is a very crude topography in the arrangement. The projection from any one part of the reticular complex probably projects to that part of the thalamus from which it receives input as well as other neighboring parts. The exact nature of these various mappings would repay further study.

The neurons of the reticular complex project to the (dorsal) thalamus. The evidence suggests that they mainly contact the principal (relay) cells of the thalamus (22). What effect does the reticular input have on the behavior of the cells in the dorsal thalamus?

Obviously this is a crucial question. Let us consider two oversimplified but contrasting hypotheses. The first is that the main effect of the reticular complex is inhibitory. This would lead to the following general picture. The traffic passing through the reticular complex will produce excitation. Let us assume that one patch of the complex is more excited than the rest because of special activity in the thalamo-cortical pathways. The effect of this will be 2-fold. That region will tend to suppress somewhat the other parts of the reticular complex, because of the many inhibitory collaterals. It will also suppress the corresponding thalamic region. These two effects will damp down the thalamus in its most active region and have the opposite effect (since the inhibition from the reticular complex will be reduced there) on the remaining parts. The total effect will be to even out the activity of the thalamus. This is not a very exciting conclusion. The function of the reticular complex would be to act as an overall thermostat of thalamic activity, making the warm parts cooler and the cool parts warmer.

The second hypothesis is just the opposite. Let us assume that the effect of the reticular complex on the dorsal thalamus is mainly excitation in some form or other. Then we see that, once again, an active patch in the complex will tend to suppress many other parts of the complex. This time, however, the effect will be to heat up the warmer parts of the thalamus and cool down the cooler parts. We shall have positive feedback rather than negative feedback, so that "attention" will be focused on the most active thalamo-cortical regions.

How can GABAergic neurons produce some sort of excitatory effect on the relay cells of the thalamus? One possibility is that they might synapse only onto the local inhibitory neurons in the thalamus. By inhibiting these inhibitory cells they would thereby increase the effect of incoming excitation on the relay cells.

This is certainly possible but the anatomic evidence (22) suggests that in the main the neurons of the reticular complex project directly to the thalamic relay neurons. One would expect that this would inhibit these neurons. We must therefore ask if thalamic neurons show any unusual types of behavior.

Properties of Thalamic Neurons

The recent work of Llinás and Jahnsen (33–35) on thalamic slices from the guinea pig confirms that this is indeed the case. Their papers should be consulted for the detailed results, which are complicated, but, broadly, they show that all thalamic neurons display two relatively distinct modes of behavior. When the cell is near its normal resting potential (say, −60 mV) it responds to an injected current by firing (producing axonal spikes) at a fairly modest rate, usually between 25 and 100 spikes per second. The rate increases with the value of the current injected.

If, on the other hand, the negative potential of the membrane is increased somewhat (that is, if the cell is hyperpolarized) to, say, −70 mV, then a neuron responds to an injected current, after a short delay, with a spike or a *short fast burst of spikes*, firing briefly at rates nearer *300 spikes per second*. Moreover, the aftereffect of this burst is that, even though the injected current is maintained constant. the cell will not produce a further burst for a time of the order of 80–150 msec. Jahnsen and Llinás (34, 35), by means of many elegant controls, have shown that this behavior depends on a number of special ion channels, including a Ca^{2+}-dependent K^{+}-conductance.

Thus, it is at least possible that the effect of the GABAergic neurons of the reticular complex on the thalamic relay cells is to produce a brief burst of firing in response to incoming excitations. followed by a more prolonged inhibition. Whether this is actually the effect they produce in natural circumstances remains to be seen. since it is not easy to deduce this with certainty from the results of Jahnsen and Llinás on slices.

The Searchlight Hypothesis

What do we require of a searchlight? It should be able to sample the activity in the cortex and/or the thalamus and decide "where the action is." It should then be able to intensify the thalamic input to that region of the cortex, probably by making the active thalamic neurons in that region fire more rapidly than usual. It must then be able to turn off its beam, move to the next place demanding attention, and repeat the process.

It seems remarkable, to say the least, that the nature of the reticular complex and the behavior of the thalamic neurons fit this requirement so neatly. The extensive inhibitory collaterals in the reticular complex may allow it to select a small region that corresponds to the most active part of the thalamo-cortical maps. Its inhibitory output, by making more negative the membrane potential of the relevant thalamic neurons, could allow them to produce a very rapid, short burst and also effectively turns them off for 100 msec or so. This means that the reticular complex will no longer respond at that patch and its activity can thus move to the next most active patch. We are thus led to two plausible hypotheses:

(i) The searchlight is controlled by the reticular complex of the thalamus.

(ii) The expression of the searchlight is the production of rapid firing in a subset of active thalamic neurons.

So far I have lumped the perigeniculate nucleus (17–24) in with the reticular nucleus proper which adjoins it. It seems probable that the lateral geniculate nucleus (which in primates projects mainly to the first visual area of the cortex) sends collaterals of its output to the perigeniculate nucleus, while the rest of the dorsal thalamus sends collaterals to the reticular nucleus proper (20). This suggests that there may be at least two searchlights: one for the first visual area and another for all of the rest. Indeed, there may be several separate searchlights. Their number will depend in part on the range and strength of the inhibitory collaterals within the reticular complex. Clearly, much more needs to be known about both the neuroanatomy and the neurophysiology of the various parts of the reticular complex.

Malsburg Synapses

We must now ask: what could the searchlight usefully do? Treisman's results (5–8) suggest that what we want it to do is to form *temporary* "conjunctions" of neurons. One possibility is that the conjunction is expressed merely by the relevant neurons firing simultaneously, or at least in a highly correlated manner. In artificial intelligence the problem would be solved by "creating a line" between the units. There is no way that the searchlight can rapidly produce new dendrites, new axons, or even new axon terminals in the brain. The only plausible way to create a line in a short time is to strengthen an existing synapse in some way. This is the essence of the idea put forward in 1981 by von der Malsburg in a little known but very suggestive paper.* After describing the conjunction problem in general terms he proposed that a synapse could alter its synaptic weight (roughly speaking, the weight is the effect a presynaptic spike has on the potential at the axon hillock of the postsynaptic cell) on a fast time scale ("fractions of a second"). He proposed that when there was a strong correlation between presynaptic and postsynaptic activity, the strength of the synapse was temporarily increased—a dynamic version of Hebb's well-known rule (36)—and that with *un*correlated pre- and postsynaptic signals the strength would be temporarily decreased below its normal resting value.

Notice that we are not concerned here with *long-term* alterations in weight, as we would if we were considering learning, but very short-term *transient* alterations that would occur during the act of visual perception. The idea is not, however, limited to the visual system but is supposed to apply to all parts of the neocortex and possibly to other parts of the brain as well.

Most previous theoretical work on neural nets does not use this idea, though there are exceptions (37, 33). The usual convention is that while a net, or set of nets, is *performing*, the synaptic weights are kept constant. They are only allowed to alter when *learning* is being studied. Thus, von der Malsburg's idea represents a rather radical alteration to the usual assumptions. I propose that such (hypothetical) synapses be called Malsburg synapses. Notice that in the cortex the number of synapses exceeds the number of neurons by at least three orders of magnitude.

Let us then accept for the moment that Malsburg synapses are at least plausible. We are still a long way from knowing the exact rules for their behavior—How much can their strength be increased? What exactly determines this increase (or decrease) of strength? How rapidly can this happen? How does this temporary alteration decay?—to say nothing of the molecular mechanisms underlying such changes.

In spite of all of these uncertainties it seems not unreasonable to assume that the effect of the searchlight is to activate Malsburg synapses. We are thus led to a third hypothesis.

(iii) The conjunctions produced by the searchlight are mediated by Malsburg synapses, especially by rapid bursts acting on them.

We still have to explain exactly how activated Malsburg synapses form associations of neurons. This is discussed by von der Malsburg in his paper in some

* von der Malsburg, C. (1981) Internal Report 81-2 (Department of Neurobiology, Max-Planck-Institute for Biophysical Chemistry, Goettingen, F.R.G.).

detail but most readers may find his discussion hard to follow. His argument depends on the assumption that the system needs to have more than one such association active at about the same time. He describes at some length how correlations, acting on Malsburg synapses, can link cells into groups and thus form what he calls topological networks. What characterizes one such cell assembly is that the neurons in it fire "simultaneously," an idea that goes back to Hebb (36). von der Malsburg suggests that two kinds of signal patterns can exist in a topological network: waves running through the network or groups of cells switching synchronously between an active and a silent state. He next discusses how a set of cells rather than a single cell might form what he calls a "network element." Finally, after an elaborate development of this theme he broaches the "bandwidth problem." In simple terms, how can we avoid these various groups of cells interfering with each other?

Cell Assemblies

The cell assembly idea is a powerful one. Since a neuron can usually be made to fire by several different combinations of its inputs, the *significance* of its firing is necessarily ambiguous. It is thus a reasonable deduction that this ambiguity can be removed, at least in part, by the firing pattern of an *assembly* of cells. This arrangement is more economical than having many distinct neurons, each with very high specificity. This type of argument goes back to Young (39) in 1802.

There has been much theoretical work on what we may loosely describe as associative nets. The nets are usually considered to consist of neurons of a similar type, receiving input, in most cases, from similar sources and sending their output mainly to similar places. If we regard neurons (in, say, the visual system) as being arranged in some sort of hierarchy, then we can usefully refer to such an assembly as a *horizontal* assembly.

von der Malsburg's ideas, however, permit another type of assembly. In his theory a cell at a higher level is associated with one at a lower level (we are here ignoring the direction of the connection), and these, in turn, may be associated with those at a still lower level. (By "associated with" I mean that the cells fire approximately simultaneously.) For example, a cell at a higher level that signified the general idea "face" would be temporarily associated, by Malsburg synapses, with cells that signified the parts of the face, and, in turn, perhaps with their parts. Such an assembly might usefully be called a *vertical* assembly. It is these vertical assemblies that have to be constructed anew for each different visual scene, or for each sentence, etc. Without them it be a difficult job to unite the higher level concepts with their low level details in a rather short time. This idea is reminiscent of the K lines of Minsky.[†]

The idea of *transient* vertical assemblies is a very powerful one. It solves in one blow the combinational problem—that is, how the brain can respond to an almost unlimited number of distinct sentences, passages of music, visual scenes, etc. The solution is to use *temporary* combinations of a subset of a much more limited number of units (the 10^{12} or so neurons in the central nervous system), each new combination being brought into action as the circumstances demand and then largely discarded. Without this device the brain would either require vastly more neurons to do the job or its ability to perceive, think, and act would be very severely restricted. This is the thrust of von der Malsburg's arguments.

A somewhat similar set of ideas about simultaneous firing has been put forward by Abeles. His monograph (40) should be consulted for details. He proposes the concept of "synfire chains"—sets of cells, each set firing synchronously, connected in chains, which fire sequentially. He gives a plausible numerical argument, based mainly on anatomical connectivity, which suggests that to establish a functioning synfire chain only a few (perhaps five or so) synapses would be available at any one neuron. Since this is such a small number he deduces that the individual synapses must be strengthened (if these five synapses by themselves are to fire the cell) perhaps by a factor of 5 or so. However, he gives no indication as to how this strengthening might be done.

Abeles' argument stresses the importance to the system of the *exact time of firing* of each spike, rather than the *average* rate of firing, which is often taken to be the more relevant variable. This exact timing is also an important aspect of von der Malsburg's ideas. These arguments can also be supported by considering the probable values of the passive cable constants of cortical dendrites. Very rough estimates (for example, $\tau = 8$ msec, $X = \lambda/5$) suggest that inputs will not add satisfactorily unless they arrive within a few milliseconds of each other (see figure 3.18 in ref. 41).

Notice the idea that a cell assembly consists of neurons firing simultaneously (or at least in a highly correlated manner) is a very natural one, since this means that the impact of their joint firing on *other* neurons, elsewhere in the system, will be large. The content of the cell assembly—the "meaning" of all of the neurons so linked together—can in this way be impressed on the rest of the system in a manner that would not be possible if all of the neurons in it fired at random

[†] Minsky, M. (1979) Artificial Intelligence Memo No. 516 (Artificial Intelligence Laboratory, Massachusetts Institute of Technology, Cambridge, MA).

times, unless they were firing very rapidly indeed. Therefore, our fourth hypothesis follows.

(iv) Conjunctions are expressed by cell assemblies, especially assemblies of cells in different cortical regions.

It should not be assumed tnat cell assemblies can only be formed by the searchlight mechanism. Some important ones may well be laid down, or partly laid down, genetically (e.g., faces?) or be formed by prolonged learning (e.g., reading letters or words?).

It is clear that much further theoretical work is needed to develop these ideas and make them more precise. If the members of a vertical assembly fire approximately synchronously, exactly how regular and how close together in time do these firings have to be? Are there special pathways or devices to promote more simultaneous firing? Are dendritic spikes involved? How does one avoid confusion between different cell assemblies? Do neurons in *different* cell assemblies briefly inhibit each other, so that accidental synchrony is made more difficult? Etc.

The idea that the dorsal thalamus and the reticular complex are concerned with attention is not novel (19, 42, 43). What is novel (as far as I know) is the suggestion that they control and express the internal attentional searchlight proposed by Treisman (5–8), Julesz (9, 10), Posner (44, 45), and others. For this searchlight at least two features are required. The first is the rapid movement of the searchlight from place to place while the eyes remain in one position, as discussed above. There is, however, another aspect. The brain must know what it is searching *for* (the green *T* in the example given earlier) so that it may know when its hunt is successful. In other words, the brain must know *what* to attend to. That aspect, which may involve other cortical areas such as the frontal cortex, has not been discussed here. The basic searchlight mechanism may depend on several parts of the reticular complex, but these may be influenced by top-down pathways, or by other searchlights in other parts of the reticular complex, which may be partly controlled by which ideas are receiving attention. An important function of the reticular complex may be to limit the number of subjects the thalamus can pay attention to at any one time.

Experimental Tests

These will not be discussed here in detail. It suffices to say that many of the suggestions, such as the behavior of the dorsal thalamus and the reticular complex, are susceptible to fairly direct tests. The exact behavior of reticular neurons and thalamic neurons is difficult to predict with confidence, since they contain a number of very different ion channels. Experiments on slices should therefore be complemented by experiments on animals. Obviously, most of such experiments should be done on alert, behaving animals, if possible with natural stimuli. An animal under an anesthetic can hardly be expected to display all aspects of attention. Various psychophysical tests are also possible.

Other aspects of these ideas, such as the behavior of Malsburg synapses, may be more difficult to test in the immediate future. It seems more than likely that dendritic spines are involved, both the spines themselves and the synapses on them (46, 47).

The existence and the importance of rapid bursts of firing can also be tested. Such bursts, followed by a quiet interval, have been seen in neurons in the visual cortex of a curarized, unanesthetized and artificially respired cat when they respond to an optimal visual signal [see figure 1 in Morrell (48)]. It is unlikely that the two systems—the rapid-burst system and the slow-firing system—will be quite as distinct as implied here. In fact, as von der Malsburg has pointed out, one would expect them to interact.

Thus, all of these ideas, plausible though they may be, must be regarded at the moment as speculative until supported by much stronger experimental evidence. In spite of this, they appear as if they might begin to form a useful bridge between certain parts of cognitive psychology, on the one hand, and the world of neuroanatomy and neurophysiology on the other.

Note Added in Proof. Recent unpublished experimental work suggests that the reticular complex may produce bursts of firing in some thalamic neurons but merely an increase of firing rate in other others.

This work originated as a result of extensive discussions with Dr. Christopher Longuet-Higgins. I thank him and many other colleagues who have commented on the idea, in particular, Drs. Richard Anderson, Max Cowan, Simon LeVay, Don MacLeod, Graeme Mitchison, Tomaso Poggio, V. S. Ramachandran, Terrence Sejnowski, and Christoph von der Malsburg. This work has been supported by the J. W. Kieckhefer Foundation and the System Development Foundation.

Notes

1. Van Essen, D. C. & Maunsell, J. H. R. (1983) *Trends Neurosci.* **6**, 370–375.

2. Hubel, D. H. & Wiesel, T. H. (1977) *Proc. R. Soc. London Ser. B.* **198**, 1–59.

3. Bruce, C., Desimone, R. & Gross, C. G. (1981) *J. Neurophys.* **46**, 369–384.

4. Perrett, D. I., Rolls, E. T. & Caan, W. (1982) *Exp. Brain Res.* **47**, 329–342.

5. Treisman A. (1977) *Percept. Psychophys.* **22**, 1–11.

6. Treisman A. M. & Gelade. G. (1980) *Cognit. Psychol.* **12**, 97–136.

7. Treisman, A. & Schmidt, H. (1982) *Cognit. Psychol.* **14**, 107–141.

8. Treisman. A. (1983) in *Physical and Biological Processing of Images*, eds. Braddick. O. J. & Sleigh, A. C. (Springer, New York), pp. 316–325.

9. Julesz, B. (1980) *Philos. Trans. R. Soc. London Ser. B.* **290**, 83–94.

10. Julesz, B. (1981) *Nature (London)* **290**, 91–97.

11. Bergen, J. R. & Julesz, B. (1983) Nature *(London)* **303**, 696–698.

12. Jones, E. G. (1983) in *Chemical Neuroanatomy*, ed. Emson, P. C. (Raven. New York), pp. 257–293.

13. Sumitomo, I., Nakamura. M. & Iwama, K. (1976) *Exp. Neurol.* **51**, 110–123.

14. Dubin, M. W. & Cleland, B. G. (1977) *J. Neurophys.* **40**, 410–427.

15. Montero, V. M., Guillery, R. W. & Woolsey, C. N. (1977) *Brain Res.* **138**, 407–421.

16. Montero. V. M. and Scott, G. L. (1981) *Neuroscience* **6**, 2561–2577.

17. Ahlsén, G.. Lindström, S. & Sybirska, E. (1978) *Brain Res.* **156**, 106–109.

18. Ahlsén, G. & Lindström, S. (1982) *Brain Res.* **236**, 477–481.

19. Ahlsén, G. & Lindström, S. (1982) *Brain Res.* **236**, 482–486.

20. Ahlsén, G., Lindström, S. & Lo, F.-S. (1982) *Exp. Brain Res.* **46**, 118–126.

21. Ahlsén, G. & Lindström, S. (1983) *Acta Physiol. Scand.* **118**, 181–184.

22. Ohara. P. T., Sefton, A. J. & Lieberman, A. R. (1980) *Brain Res.* **197**, 503–506.

23. Hale, P. T., Sefton, A. J., Baur, L. A. & Cottee, L. J. (1982) *Exp. Brain Res.* **45**, 217–229.

24. Ide, L. S. (1982) *J. Comp. Neurol.* **210**, 317–334.

25. Schlag, J. & Waszak, M. (1971) *Exp. Neurol.* **32**, 79–97.

26. Houser, C. R., Vaughn, J. E., Barber, R. P. & Roberts, E. (1980) *Brain Res.* **200**, 341–354.

27. Oertel. W. H.. Graybiel, A. M., Mugnaini, E., Elde, R. P., Schmechel, D. E. & Kopin, I. J. (1983) *J. Neurosci.* **3**, 1322–1332.

28. Ohara, P. T., Lieberman. A. R., Hunt, S. P. & Wu, J.-Y. (1983) *Neuroscience* **8**, 189–211.

29. Scheibel. M. E. & Scheibel, A. B. (1966) *Brain Res.* **1**, 43–62.

30. Jones, E. G. (1975) *J. Comp. Neurol.* **162**, 285–308.

31. Scheibel, M. E. & Scheibel, A. B. (1972) *Exp. Neurol.* **34**, 316–322.

32. Minderhoud, J. M. (1971) *Exp. Brain Res.* **12**, 435–446.

33. Llinás, R. & Jahnsen, H. (1982) *Nature (London)* **297**, 406–408.

34. Jahnsen, H. & Llinás, R. (1984) *J. Physiol.* **349**, 205–226.

35. Jahnsen, H. & Llinás, R. (1984) *J. Physiol.* **349**, 227–247.

36. Hebb, D. O. (1949) *Organization of Behavior* (Wiley, New York).

37. Little W. A. & Shaw, G. L. (1975) *Behav. Biol.* **14**, 115–133.

38. Edelman, G. M. & Reeke, G. N. (1982) *Proc. Natl. Acad. Sci. USA* **79**, 2091–2095.

39. Young, T. (1802) *Philos. Trans.* 12–48.

40. Abeles, M. (1982) *Local Cortical Circuits: Studies of Brain Function* (Springer, New York), Vol. 6.

41. Jack, J. J. B., Noble, D. & Tsien, R. W. (1975) *Electric Current Flow in Excitable Cells* (Clarendon, Oxford).

42. Yingling. C. D. & Skinner. J. E. (1977) in *Attention, Voluntary Contraction and Event-Cerebral Potentials*, ed. Desmedt, J. E. (Karger, Basel, Switzerland), pp. 70–96.

43. Skinner, J. E. & Yingling, C. D. (1977) in *Attention, Voluntary Contraction and Event-Cerebral Potentials*, ed. Desmedt, J. E. (Karger, Basel, Switzerland), pp. 30–69.

44. Posner, M. I. (1982) *Am. Psychol.* **37**, 168–179.

45. Posner, M. I., Cohen, Y. & Rafal, R. D. (1982) *Philos. Trans. R. Soc. London Ser. B* **298**, 187–198.

46. Perkel, D. H. (1983) *J. Physiol. (Paris)* **78**, 695–699.

47. Koch, C. & Poggio, T. (1983) *Proc. R. Soc. London Ser. B.* **218**, 455–477.

48. Morrell. F. (1972) in *Brain and Human Behavior*, eds. Karczmar, A. G. & Eccles, J. C. (Springer, New York), pp. 259–289.

Addendum

Since this paper was written it has been pointed out by Steriade, Jones, and Llinas (*Thalamic Oscillations and Signalling*, 1990, John Wiley & Sons, New York, p. 312) that "... burst patterns specifically characterize the spontaneous and evoked activities of the thalamocortical neurons during EEG-synchronized sleep, and are virtually absent during wakefulness, the state in which the 'attentional searchlight' occurs." This part of my hypothesis must therefore be abandoned. Whether the hypothesis of double-negative feedback, suggested by Steriade, Domich, and Oakson (*J. Neurosci* 6: 68–81, 1986) applies to attention remains to be seen.

IV
Memory

Introduction to Part IV

The study of memory lies at the heart of cognitive neuroscience. Without memory, experience can have no lasting effects on an organism. For many years, researchers eschewed discussing memory, which involves the retention of information, and focused instead on learning, which involves the acquisition of information. This orientation was dictated in part by the behaviorist perspective that dominated psychology until the early 1960s. The behaviorists wanted to focus purely on what was observable, namely stimuli and responses, and not draw inferences about intervening variables. Although not without value, this approach faltered when faced with the complexity of stimulus/response relations—which proved much more easily understood if one posited an intervening system that stored and processed information.

The concept of a "representation" is inextricably bound to the concept of information storage. There are many ways of representing the same information, each of which makes explicit different facets of the data. And depending on how information is stored, different operations are more or less easy to perform. For instance, Marr (1982) pointed out that there are several ways of representing numbers, with Arabic numerals making it easy to extract powers of ten, binary digits making it easy to extract powers of 2, and small Roman numerals making it relatively easy to add because they encourage counting.

Anderson (1978) proved that any given set of behavioral data can always be explained by more than one theory. This result was disheartening to many researchers in experimental psychology because it meant that behavioral regularities alone could not implicate particular internal representations. Anderson noted that one way this indeterminancy could be resolved was by using knowledge of the anatomy and physiology of the brain to limit the possibilities.

Because of their behaviorist antecedents, many experimental psychologists initially were reluctant even to posit that internal representations might exist. Perhaps a residual consequence of these qualms is that cognitive scientists and researchers in AI rarely consider facts about the neural substrate of memory. In this section we present key articles that illustrate what has been learned about the neural bases of memory. We hope that this sampler is sufficient to demonstrate that enough is now known to begin in earnest to build a rigorous cognitive neuroscience of memory.

Our understanding of the neural mechanisms underlying memory has advanced by leaps and bounds because animal models are available. These models have been especially useful in the study of memory because they have allowed researchers to investigate memory at multiple levels of analysis—from the level of molecules to the level of the entire working brain.

In this part we have included papers that address two facets of memory. On the one hand, the physical state of the system must be altered if new information is to be stored; these processes occur at the level of molecular changes in individual neurons. On the other hand, in order to be stored and used effectively, many sorts of information must be coordinated and organized within an information-processing system.

Storage Mechanisms

The papers in the first section of this part address the processes that underlie our ability to store new information. This topic is particularly exciting not only because it is beginning to be understood at multiple levels of analysis but also because it is clear how these levels are related. A seminal clue regarding the physical basis of memory is described by Bliss and Lømo, who find that repeated stimulation of a neuron can produce *long-term potentiation* (LTP); after the stimulation, less stimulation subsequently is required to produce the same amount of activity. LTP is important because it illustrates how experience can change the connection strength between neurons. The concept of connection strength lies at the heart of contemporary conceptions of how neural networks learn; thus it is of interest that one aspect of these models may have a neural correlate. If so, then facts about the brain can have a direct bearing on such models.

The molecular basis of LTP is beginning to become clear, as is evident in the paper by Bekkers and Stevens. Donald Hebb (1949) speculated that neural networks may encode memory by increasing the strengths of the connections between neurons that are activated at the same time, and Bekkers and Stevens report a molecular mechanism that behaves similarly via a presynaptic mechanism. (At the same time Malinow and Tsien (1990) reported similar results and conclusions using similar techniques.) However, the *Hebb synapse* represents only one possible way in which neural networks could learn. Hawkins and Kandel describe a different mechanism that may underlie learning in a particular simple system, the molusc Aplysia. They show how relatively simple molecular events can produce a range of types of learning in this animal. These types of learning do not depend on simultaneous events in the "pre-synaptic" (sending) and "post-synaptic" (receiving) neurons but rather rest on neurochemical events within the sending neuron. The mechanisms underlying these simple types of learning may constitute components of a kind of processing "alphabet," which is utilized even in more complex animals.

Gluck and Thompson find that even simple systems of the sort studied by Kandel and his colleagues may be more complicated than meets the eye; their computational model of the phenomena described by Hawkins and Kandel points out the importance of actually building computer models that allow us to track dynamic interactions precisely. Many researchers were surprised by how difficult it is to understand intuitively how a handful of types of neurons would interact. Gluck and Thompson's work is a good example of the role of computer models in cognitive neuroscience; with their findings in hand, new experiments immediately come to mind.

Ambros-Ingerson, Granger, and Lynch show that the same kinds of principles that Gluck and Thompson use to model learning in the Aplysia also can provide a good account of olfactory learning in the rabbit. Ambros-Ingerson, Granger, and Lynch are able to provide a precise model that accounts for perceptual and learning phenomena within a single system; these findings suggest that similar principles of learning may govern how networks store information in different neural systems. If this is so, then differences among the systems may depend largely on the physical organization of the neurons and the patterns of inputs to and outputs from individual networks.

Barto and Jordan examine the basis of learning in neural network computer simulation models and offer an alternative to the popular back-propagation method (see

Kosslyn et al., Lehky and Sejnowski, and Zipser and Andersen). In many circumstances, the back-propagation method is not biologically plausible because it depends on a "teacher" that can adjust the connection strengths in the network when it produces incorrect outputs. Barto and Jordan's learning method has most of the advantages of back propagation but is more biologically plausible.

Memory Systems

In the second section of this part we present papers that illustrate how different brain structures coordinate various forms of memory within the context of a larger information-processing system. That is, "memory" is not a single entity but corresponds to a collection of separate mechanisms. Some of these mechanisms are modality specific and some are shared by multiple sensory modalities. Perhaps because the behaviorists assumed that there would be a single set of laws of learning, many experimental psychologists and researchers in AI have implictly assumed that there will be a single set of principles for memory. Even if the mechanisms of storage within individual neurons are the same, this does not imply that the networks store information according to the same principles. The same set of building materials can be used to construct many types of buildings, which have very different properties. Indeed, if structures used to store information often also perform other functions, it is possible that very different principles will govern how different types of information are stored. Research in the neural archtecture of memory suggests that such a supposition should be taken seriously.

As a first step, it is important to demonstrate that different types of information are stored differently. Three of the articles we have reprinted make a good case that perceptual structures also serve to store information. This is important in part because these structures accomplish two functions—encoding information on-line for recognition and storing information—hence properties of the memory function must be understood within the context of the perceptual function.

Specifically, Fuster and Jervey show that temporal lobe structures that are involved in encoding visual information during perception are also involved in storing that information; Miyashita and Chang extend this work, taking advantage of powerful ways of generating novel stimuli. Gnadt and Andersen push the theme that some forms of memory rely on perceptual structures one step further; they show that memory representations used to guide eye movements are represented at least in part in posterior parietal cortical areas that are used in motor control. Thus at least two different perceptual structures are involved in memory, one for storing information about object properties (such as shape and color) and one for storing information about location.

Memory representations in the brain clearly are used to guide a host of different sorts of processes, as illustrated by memory-related activity in temporal lobe structures used to encode objects during perception and in parietal lobe structures used in motor control. Indeed, Gnadt and Andersen's findings have a direct relation to the results reported by Funahashi, Bruce, and Goldman-Rakic. Funahashi et al. show that the dorsolateral prefrontal area contains a structure that codes the spatial locations of stimuli. This area (area 46) is very near the frontal eye fields (area 8), which play a critical role in executing planned sequences of eye movements. Area 46 is spatially organized and has precise and direct connections to the regions of the parietal lobe studied by Gnadt and Andersen. Hence it is possible that Gnadt and Andersen and Funahashi et al. are studying different facets of the same frontal-parietal system, which is used to represent locations of objects and then to direct eye movements to selected locations.

The articles noted so far have all focused on transient, short-term memories. Additional mechanisms exist to store information in what may be a near-permanent, long-term form. In a seminal paper, Mishkin draws on findings from animal models of memory to outline the architecture of the entire memory system, noting the possible role of the hippocampus and related structures in the context of a system of interacting components. One of the beauties of Mishkin's approach is that it explains how general-purpose mechanisms can encode all sorts of memories and yet different types of memory representations may nonetheless exist. His theory ties together multiple types of memory and perception, which is logical because much of the information we store is derived from our perceptions.

Squire presents a revision of Mishkin's picture of the system, which is based on more recent work that emphasizes the role of the entorhinal and related cortex in memory and de-emphasizes the role of the amygdala. The entorhinal cortex is interesting in part because this area receives input from all of the perceptual systems, and many of its neurons respond selectively to stimuli in multiple sensory modalities. Thus Squire's conception helps us to understand further how perceptually based memories are coordinated via a memory-encoding system that relies on medial temporal lobe structures.

Mishkin's and Squire's conceptions both stress the role of the hippocampus and related medial temporal lobe structures in storing new information. Thus it is not surprising that LTP was discovered in neurons taken from a medial temporal lobe structure, the dentate gyrus. Corkin shows that the medial temporal areas in the human brain are critical for encoding new information. She documents severe and lasting impairments in the ability to encode new memories in the patient H. M., who had his hippocampus, amygdala, and related medial temporal lobe structures surgically removed for the treatment of otherwise intractible epilepsy. This work is important in part because it serves as a bridge between the animal models and the human brain. Indeed, historically the direction of causality went the other way: findings with H. M. of the sort described by Corkin led Mishkin and others to develop the animal models, which now are leading to additional research with humans (for further discussion of this cross-fertilization, see Squire 1987).

Finally, the research described in papers by Corkin; Schacter; and Shimamura, Salmon, Squire, and Butters shows that memory for facts can be impaired quite independently of another kind of memory. Schacter contrasts these sorts of *explicit* memories, which can be accessed to guide multiple types of behavior and can rise to consciousness, with *implicit* memories, which are tied to specific contexts and cannot be accessed deliberately or detected except in special circumstances. This distinction seems to correspond roughly to the distinction between "cognitive" and "habit" memories drawn by Mishkin and to a distinction between "declarative" and "procedural" memory once offered by Squire.

Thus we not only have distinct types of memories for different perceptual modalities but also have different varieties of each type of memory. It seems possible that memory is an inherent feature of many different types of processes, either simply modulating input/output mapping (and hence being implicit) or being available to affect other processes. This idea is consistent with the way neural network computer simulations operate; in these models, memories consist of patterns of weights (which dictate the strengths) on the connections among units—which also determine how the network behaves when input arrives. Thus we should not be surprised to discover that there are many types of memory representations in the brain.

In short, the articles in this section provide a good picture of the emerging cognitive neuroscience conception of memory. Distinct functions are inferred on the basis of behavioral results in conjunction with information about properties of neural structures and computational systems that store information.

References

Anderson, J. R. 1978. Arguments concerning representations for mental imagery. *Psychological Review* 85: 249–277.

Hebb, D. O. 1949. *The Organization of Behavior*. New York: Wiley.

Marr, D. 1982. *Vision: A Computational Investigation into the Human Representation and Processing of Visual Information*. New York: W. H. Freeman.

Malinow, R., and R. Tsien. 1990. Presynaptic enhancement shown by whole-cell recordings of long-term potentiation in hippocampal slices. *Nature* 346: 177–180.

Squire, L. R. 1987. *Memory and Brain*. New York: Oxford University Press.

29

T. V. P. Bliss and T. Lømo

Long-lasting potentiation of synaptic transmission in the dentate area of the anaesthetized rabbit following stimulation of the perforant path

1973. *Journal of Physiology* 232: 331–356

Summary

1. The after-effects of repetitive stimulation oi the perforant path fibres to the dentate area of the hippocampal formation have been examined with extracellular micro-electrodes in rabbits anaesthetized with urethane.

2. In fifteen out of eighteen rabbits the population response recorded from granule cells in the dentate area to single perforant path volleys was potentiated for periods ranging from 30 min to 10 hr after one or more conditioning trains at 10–20/sec for 10–15 sec, or 100/sec for 3–4 sec.

3. The population response was analysed in terms of three parameters: the amplitude of the population excitatory post-synaptic potential (e.p.s.p.), signalling the depolarization of the granule cells, and the amplitude and latency of the population spike, signalling the discharge of the granule cells.

4. All three parameters were potentiated in 29% of the experiments; in other experiments in which long term changes occurred, potentiation was confined to one or two of the three parameters. A reduction in the latency of the population spike was the commonest sign of potentiation, occurring in 57% of all experiments. The amplitude of the population e.p.s.p. was increased in 43%, and of the population spike in 40%, of all experiments.

5. During conditioning at 10–20/sec there was massive potentiation of the population spike ('frequency potentiation'). The spike was suppressed during stimulation at 100/sec. Both frequencies produced long-term potentiation.

6. The results suggest that two independent mechanisms are responsible for long-lasting potentiation: (*a*) an increase in the efficiency of synaptic transmission at the perforant path synapses; (*b*) an increase in the excitability of the granule cell population.

Introduction

These experiments arose from an observation made during a study of the phenomenon of frequency potentiation in the dentate area of the hippocampal formation (Lømo, 1966). It was noticed that the response evoke in the dentate area by single test shocks to the afferent perforant pathway often remained potentiated for a considerable time after short periods of stimulation at 10–20/sec. In this paper we describe the effect in the anaesthetized rabbit. In the following paper (Bliss & Gardner-Medwin, 1973) it is shown to be present also in the unrestrained and unanaesthetized animal. Preliminary reports have been published (Bliss & Lømo, 1970; Bliss & Gardner-Medwin, 1971; Bliss, Gardner-Medwin & Lømo, 1973).

Methods

Preparation

The experiments were performed on eighteen adult rabbits. Both sexes were used. Anaesthesia was induced with a mixture of urethane (0.75 g/kg) and chloralose (40 mg/kg) given I.V., and maintained with urethane alone. The dorsal hippocampus was exposed bilaterally by removing the overlying cortex with a suction pipette. A small silver plate was sewn into the neck muscles to act as the indifferent electrode.

Electrodes and Equipment

Conventional NaCl-filled glass micro-electrodes with resistances of 1–3 MΩ were used for recording. Stimulating electrodes were constructed from electrolytically sharpened tungsten wire insulated with several coats of varnish. They were used in a monopolar tip-negative configuration to give constant voltage pulses with a duration of 0.1 msec and an amplitude of up to 100 V. The circuit was completed via a silver ball electrode positioned on a neighbouring cut muscle surface. The recording electrodes were connected through cathode followers to a.c. preamplifiers with 3 dB cut-off points at 4 Hz and 1 kHz. Evoked responses were displayed on an oscilloscope, either directly or after averaging, and photographed.

Anatomy

The hippocampal formation contains two curved interdigitating layers of cells, the pyramidal cells of regions CA_1 and CA_3, and the granule cells of the dentate area (Fig. 1*A*). It is with the perforant path input to the latter group of cells in the dorsal hippocampal formation that this paper is concerned. The thinly myelinated fibres of the perforant path arise from cells in the medial entorhinal area (Nafstad, 1967; Hjorth-Simonsen & Jeune, 1972) and ascend in the angular bundle in a rostromedial direction before fanning out to cross the subiculum and the hippocampal fissure. At this point some or all of the fibres bifurcate, one branch supplying the upper limb and the other the

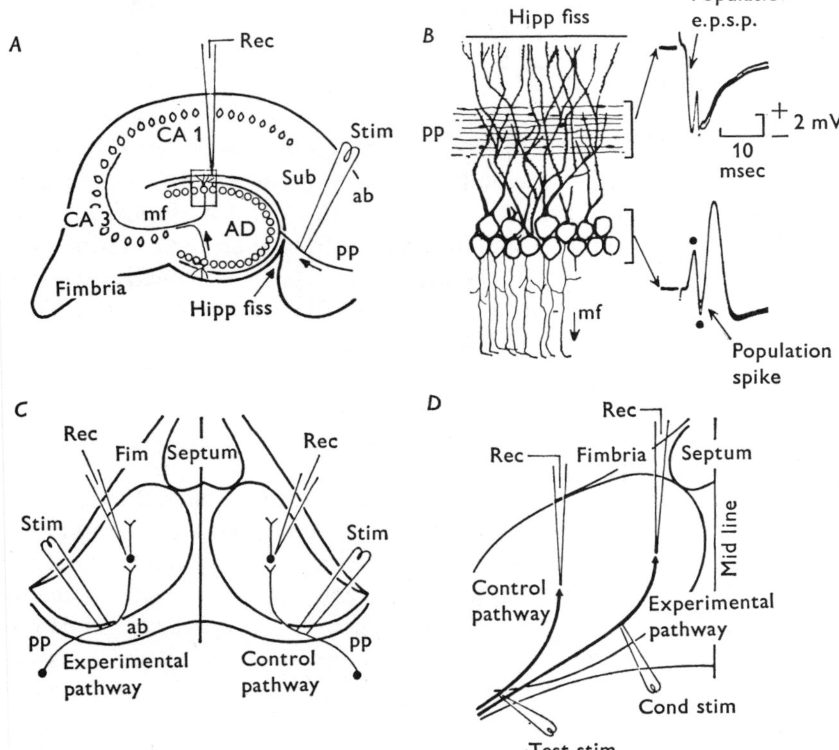

Figure 1. *A*, diagrammatic parasagittal section through the hippocampal formation, showing a stimulating electrode placed beneath the angular bundle (ab) to activate perforant path fibres (pp), and a recording micro-electrode in the molecular layer of the dentate area (AD). *B*, the region enclosed in the rectangle in *A* enlarged to show the apical dendritic field of the granule cells, with the perforant path fibres confined to the central one third of the field. The population responses evoked by a strong perforant path volley in the synaptic layer (upper trace) and in the cell body layer (lower trace) are displayed on the right. The spots (lower trace) mark the peaks between which the amplitude of the population spike was measured. *C*, arrangement of electrodes for experiments in which the control pathway was situated in the contralateral hippocampus. *D*, electrode arrangment for experiments in which both test and control pathways were on the same side.

Abbreviations: ab, angular bundle; AD, dentate area; CA_1, CA_3, pyramidal field CA_1 and CA_3; Fim, fimbria; hipp fiss, hippocampal fissure; mf, mossy fibreg; pp, perforant path.

lower limb of the dentate fascia. The fibres run in the molecular layer, which contains the apical dendrites of the granule cells (Fig. 1*B*). Here they make synaptic contacts of the *en passage* type with dendritic spines (Blackstad, 1958), each fibre making contact with many granule cells. The synapses are restricted to the middle third of the molecular layer, and account for nearly 40% of the total synaptic population in that region (Nafstad, 1967); the origin of the remainder is not known.

Population Potentials

Figure 1 *B* shows the population potentials recorded at two levels in the dentate area, following a strong perforant path volley. The upper trace was obtained with the recording electrode in the region of the perforant path synapses, i.e. in the middle third of the molecular layer. The two components of interest are the initial negative deflexion and the superimposed positive-going spike. If the recording electrode is advanced 150 μm into the cell body layer, all components of the potential become reversed (lower trace). This sequence of deflexions, and their reversal with depth, is explained in the following way. Activation of the perforant path synapses causes depolarization of the subjacent dendritic membrane, and extracellular current flows from the cell body layer towards the dendrites, resulting in a negative potential in the synaptic region, and a positive potential in the cell body region, relative to a distant electrode. This early synaptic potential is called the 'population e.p.s.p.' or, where there is no risk of confusion, simply the e.p.s.p., by analogy with the corresponding intracellular potential (Lømo, 1971*a*). The second component of the response, the 'population spike', is correlated in time and magnitude with unit discharges (Lømo, 1971*a*; Andersen, Bliss & Skrede, 1971*a*). It reflects the number of granule cells discharged, as well as the synchrony with which they fire, and is thus a measure of the over-all excitability of the granule cell population. The population spike is maximally negative in the cell body layer, where the current 'sink' of the spike generating mechanism is greatest.

The synaptic and spike potentials both reverse polarity at a depth intermediate between the granule cell bodies and the perforant path synapses and it is in this region that the potential profile is steepest. In contrast, the potential recorded in the cell body layer changes little, if at all, as the recording electrode is advanced into the hilus. This has an important practical application, since it means that potentials recorded in the hilus do not vary appreciably with slight brain movement.

Experimental Arrangement

The arrangement adopted at first is shown in Fig. 1*C*. The hippocampal formation was exposed bilaterally. A long sagittal cut was sometimes made to one side of the mid line to prevent commissural interaction between the two sides. Stimulating and recording electrodes, held in micromanipulators, were positioned in the perforant path and dentate area respectively, one pair on either side of the mid line.

The position and depth of each electrode was carefully adjusted so that maximal responses were obtained. Usually only one recording electrode was available on each side, and we preferred to place it just below the cell body layer, where the evoked potential was less affected by slight brain movements, rather than in the synaptie layer. The procedure followed was to move the recording electrode down to the reversal point for the synaptic potential, about 50 μm below the depth for maximal negativity. It was then advanced a further 150 μm from this easily identifiable reference point. The tip of the electrode was then 50 μm or so below the lower edge of the cell body layer.

Once the electrode positions were optimized on both sides, the routine testing of the excitability of each pathway began. Single shocks at a fixed strength, repeated at intervals of 2–3 sec, were given through each stimulating electrode. Superimposed single responses were photographed at regular intervals (usually every minute) together with averaged responses based on 20 or 30 consecutive single responses. A sequence of conditioning trains, each at intervals of 30 min or more, was given to one side only (the experimental pathway), the other side acting as a control for generalized excitability changes and gross movements of the brain. Throughout the course of an experiment frequent checks were made to ensure that the responses remained maximal, and appropriate minor adjustments of the electrodes were made if they were not. Adjustments of this sort were more frequently necessary when recording from the synaptic layer, but even there stable recordings for periods of an hour or more were not uncommon.

With the above arrangement the same stimulating electrode was used for both testing and conditioning, and the possibility of local changes at the site of stimulation leading to a larger number of fibres being stimulated by the standard test volley could not be excluded. In order to control for this contingency, we adopted in later experiments a rather different design. This exploited the fact that the perforant path fibres, as they ascend laterally from the entorhinal area, lie close together beneath the angular bundle, before fanning out to invest the dentate area of the dorsal hippocampal formation. A stimulating electrode placed in this lateral position will therefore monosynaptically excite granule cells over a wide area. Conversely, an electrode placed more medially and rostrally will excite only a narrow beam of cells (Lømo, 1971*a*; Andersen, Bliss & Skrede, 1971*b*), as indicated in Fig. 1*D*. Recording electrodes were placed in the dentate area at two points a few mm apart along the long axis of the hippocampus. Roughly equal responses could be obtained from both recording sites with the lateral stimulating electrode (Figs. 3*C* and 4*A*). A second stimulating electrode was then placed close to the more medial recording electrode and its position adjusted so that, with a suitable stimulus strength, a response was obtained at the medial, but not at the lateral recording site. Standard test shocks were given regularly throughout the experiment via the lateral stimulating electrode, while the medial electrode was used only to deliver the conditioning trains. With this ipsilateral arrangement, the effects of any generalized change in hippocampal excitability, or of gross brain movements, could be monitored with the control pathway, while any local changes at the site of the conditioning electrode would be unlikely to affect the distant test electrode.

Parameters of the Evoked Response

Three parameters of the evoked response were selected for analysis.

1. The amplitude of the population e.p.s.p., measured either as a negative potential in the synaptic layer, or as a positive potential in the cell body layer. Measurements were made at an arbitrarily chosen latency, fixed for each experiment and usually not more than 1 msec after onset to avoid distortion by the subsequent population spike.

2. The peak-to-peak amplitude of the population spike, recorded in the cell body layer, and measured between the initial peak positivity and peak negativity (spots, Fig. 1*B*, lower trace).

3. The latency of the population spike, taken as the time from the stimulus artifact to the initial peak positivity.

Results

Effects of Repetitive Stimulation

Stimulation of the perforant path at 10–15/sec for several seconds normally resulted in the following sequence of events.

1. A rapid build-up of the population spike during the conditioning train ('frequency potentiation'; Andersen, Holmqvist & Voorhoeve, 1966; Lømo, 1966).
2. A brief (1–2 sec) period of spike potentiation immediately after the conditioning train.
3. A phase of spike depression lasting from a few seconds to more than a minute.
4. A phase of potentiation, sometimes lasting for several hours, and in many cases involving synaptic as well as spike components of the response.

Although there was considerable variation in the degree and duration of these four phases in different preparations, the sequence as a whole was a characteristic feature of the experiments. An example is given in Fig. 2, which shows the effect of a conditioning train (15/sec for 15 sec) on the three parameters of the evoked response. During the train the spike amplitude increased greatly (Fig. 2*A*) and there was a corresponding decrease in latency (Fig. 2*B*). It was impossible to measure the population e.p.s.p. accurately during the conditioning train because of the distortion of the traces caused by the continuously moving film, and these values are therefore not plotted (Fig. 2*C*). There is, nevertheless, no doubt that the population e.p.s.p. was severely depressed during the latter part of the train, presumably owing to the profound depolarization of the granule cells which is associated with frequency potentiation (T. Lømo, unpublished observations). On this occasion the amplitude of the population spike began to rise steeply as soon as the conditioning train was initiated, reaching a maximal value after 10 sec. In other cases, the growth of the spike was delayed for several seconds, and was sometimes preceded by a brief period of depression. Within 1–2 sec after the end of the train, a marked depression of the spike occurred and its latency increased. The population e.p.s.p., on the other hand, began to recover from its depressed state almost immediately, and after about 15 sec passed into a supernormal or potentiated phase. The increase in the e.p.s.p. was associated with a gradual recovery and subsequent potentiation of the spike, and a concomitant fall in its latency. The potentiated values achieved after conditioning are plotted on a reduced time scale in Fig. 2. These levels were maintained for the rest of the experiment ($1\frac{1}{2}$ hr). Second and subsequent conditioning trains produced no further potentiation, in contrast to the steplike increases seen in some experiments (Figs. 4, 9).

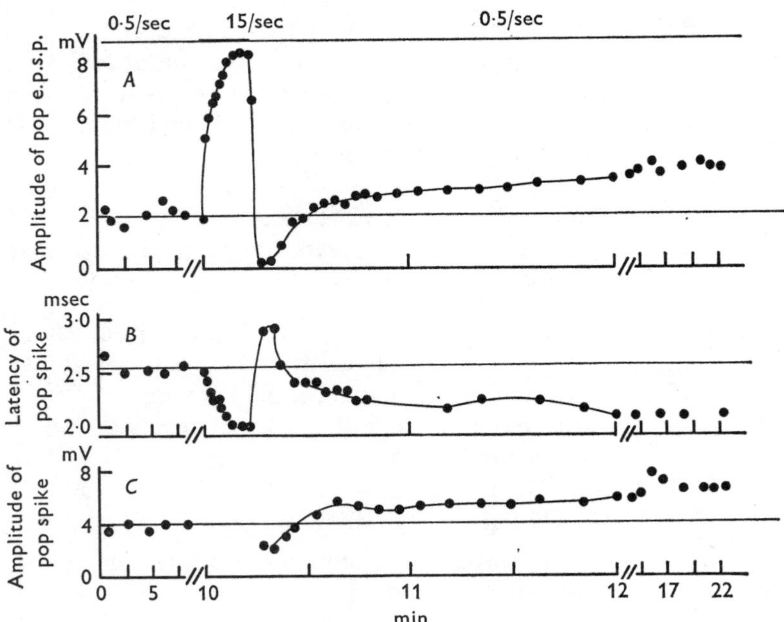

Figure 2. Frequency potentiation and the immediate after-effects of a conditioning train. The graphs show the changes produced in three parameters of the evoked response by increasing the rate at which the perforant path was stimulated from 0.5/sec to 15/sec for 15 sec. The points obtained during the conditioning train and the following 1 min 45 sec are shown on an expanded time scale. Note immediately after the train the brief period of spike potentiation followed by depression, and the subsequent maintained potentiation. The value of the population e.p.s.p. during the train could not be accurately measured from the film record and is not plotted.

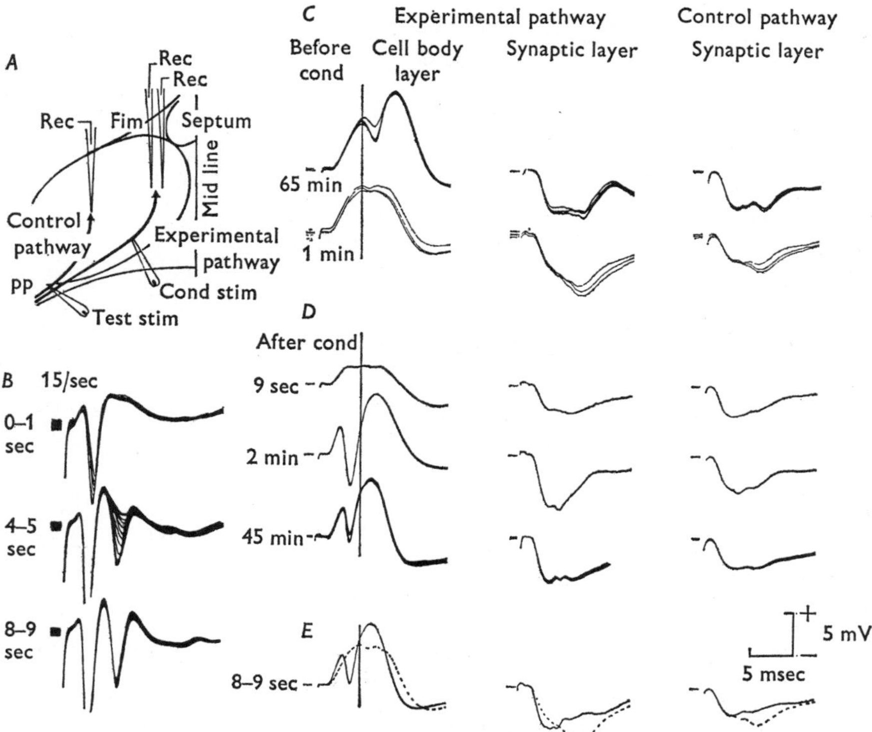

Figure 3. The effects of a conditioning train on the shape of the evoked response. *A*, arrangement of electrodes. Note the two recording electrodes in the experimental pathway, one in the synaptic layer, the other in the cell body layer. *B*, development of frequency potentiation recorded in the cell body layer during a conditioning train at 15/sec. The time from the beginning of the train is given on the left of each set of eight–twelve superimposed consecutive responses. *C, D*, evoked responses obtained at various times before (C) and after (D) the 15 sec conditioning train illustrated in *B*. Three potentials are shown in each case: the responses recorded in the cell body (left) and synaptic (centre) layers of the experimental pathway, and in the synaptic layer of the control pathway (right). For comparison, single responses obtained 1 min (stippled trace) and 45 min after conditioning have been superimposed in *E*. The vertical line in the left-hand column marks the pre-conditioning value of the latency of the population spike.

The form of the evoked potentials during each of the four phases listed above can be seen in Fig. 3, taken from a different experiment with electrode positions as in Fig. 3*A*. Fig. 3*B* shows superimposed responses from the cell body layer of the experimental pathway, recorded at the times indicated during a 15/sec train of stimuli delivered through the conditioning electrode. There is clear frequency potentiation, with an increase in spike amplitude, reduction in spike latency and development of a second spike. Before and after the conditioning train, test stimuli at 0.5/sec were delivered through the more laterally placed electrode. The responses evoked by these stimuli in the synaptic and cell body layers of the experimental pathway are shown in the first two columns of Fig. 3*C* and *D* (*C* before, and *D* after the conditioning train). The records in the third column are the responses evoked in the synaptic layer of the control pathway by the same test stimulus. In the 70 min control period preceding the first conditioning train, the size of the population spike evoked in the experimental pathway slowly declined (Fig. 3*C*). Immeditely after the train it was further depressed (Fig. 3*D* upper trace), but within 2 min, marked potentiation had developed, which was still clearly present 45 min after the train (Fig. 3*D*, experimental pathway, lower row). Again, potentiation took the form of an increase in the population spike, reduction in spike latency and a steeper rise of the population e.p.s.p. To show this more clearly, the responses immediately before (stippled trace) and 45 min after the train have been superimposed in Fig. 3*E*. The increase in the population e.p.s.p. was present not only in the synaptic layer where the active current sink is located, but was equally pronounced in the region of the passive source in the cell body layer. No similar potentiation occurred in the control pathway, where the slope of the early part of the population e.p.s.p. was the same after conditioning as it was before. In this experiment there was a decrease in the size of the late components of the response in both experimental and control pathways; a change in these later, presumably polysynaptic, components of the response was seen in several experiments (Fig. 4*B*).

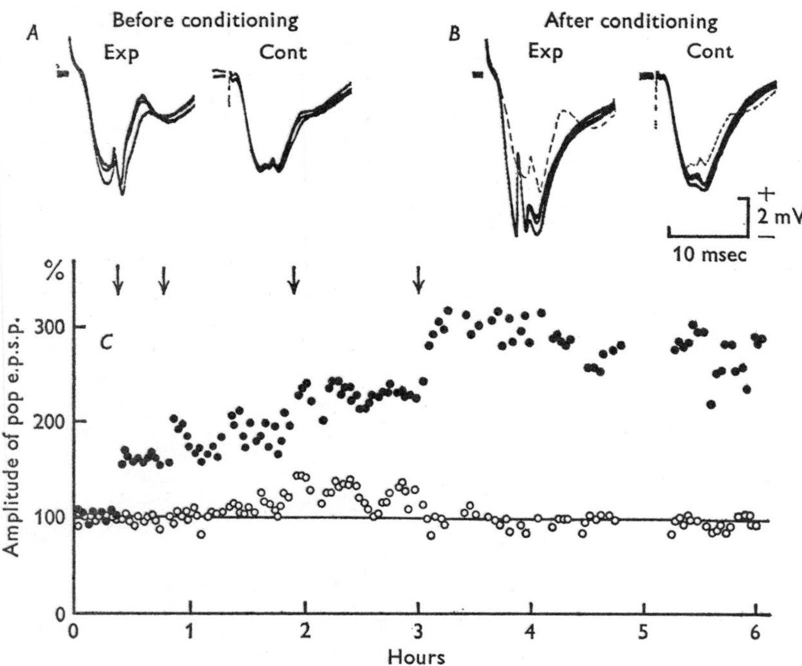

Figure 4. An experiment in which all three standard parameters of the evoked response were potentiated. Three superimposed responses obtained in the synpatic layer for both the experimental and control pathways are shown in *A* (before conditioning) and in *B* (2.5 hr after the fourth conditioning train). *C*, graph showing the amplitude of the population e.p.s.p. for the experimental pathway (filled circles) and the ipsilateral control pathway (open circles) as a function of time. Each point was obtained from the computed average of thirty responses by measuring the amplitude of the negative wave 1 msec after its onset. The values are plotted as percentages of the mean pre-conditioning value. Conditioning trains (15/sec for 10 sec) were given through a medially placed conditioning electrode at the times indicated by the arrows.

Long Lasting Potentiation
The potentiation which followed a conditioning train varied considerably in both duration and degree from experiment to experiment. If long-lasting potentiation is arbitrarily defined as potentiation lasting 30 min or more, then a positive result was obtained in fifteen out of eighteen animals. In most animals more than one pathway was conditioned. A total of twenty-four out of the thirty-five conditioned pathways showed long-lasting potentiation. Potentiation of all three parameters was observed in nine of the thirty-five conditioned pathways, although in some cases more than one conditioning train was needed to achieve this result. Considering the response parameters separately, a decrease in spike latency was the commonest form of facilitation (twenty pathways). The population e.p.s.p. was potentiated in fifteen pathways and the spike in fourteen pathways. A lack of correlation between e.p.s.p. and spike potentiation was a notable feature of several experiments and is discussed more fully below.

Potentiation of all Parameters An example of an experiment which involved potentiation of all three parameters is seen in Figs. 4 and 5. Four conditioning trains, each at 15/sec for 10 sec, were given at the times indicated by arrows. The amplitude of the e.p.s.p. for both the experimental (filled circles) and control pathway (open circles) is plotted in Fig. 4, while the amplitude and latency of the population spike for the experimental pathway are shown in Fig. 5. Each symbol in Fig. 4*C* represents thirty responses averaged over a period of 1.5 min. The first half minute after each train has not been included, so the initial post-activation depression is not seen. Each of the four conditioning trains resulted in a sudden increase in the population e.p.s.p., which reached a maximal level two to three minutes after each train and which then remained at that level until the next conditioning train was delivered. In several experiments the e.p.s.p. showed a gradual decline towards the preconditioned value over a period of one or more hours. In some of these cases a second conditioning train brought the e.p.s.p. size abruptly back to a new and higher value from which the decline was slower than before (see, for example, Fig. 9*C*). The experiment in Fig. 4 was continued beyond the 6 hr period illustrated. Six hr and 7.25 hr after the beginning of the experiment, fifth and sixth conditioning trains were given. These later trains had little further potentiating effect on the e.p.s.p., which started to decline about 8 hr after the beginning of the experiment. The three superimposed single responses shown in Fig. 4*A* (before conditioning) and in *B* (after conditioning, with the preconditioning responses indicated

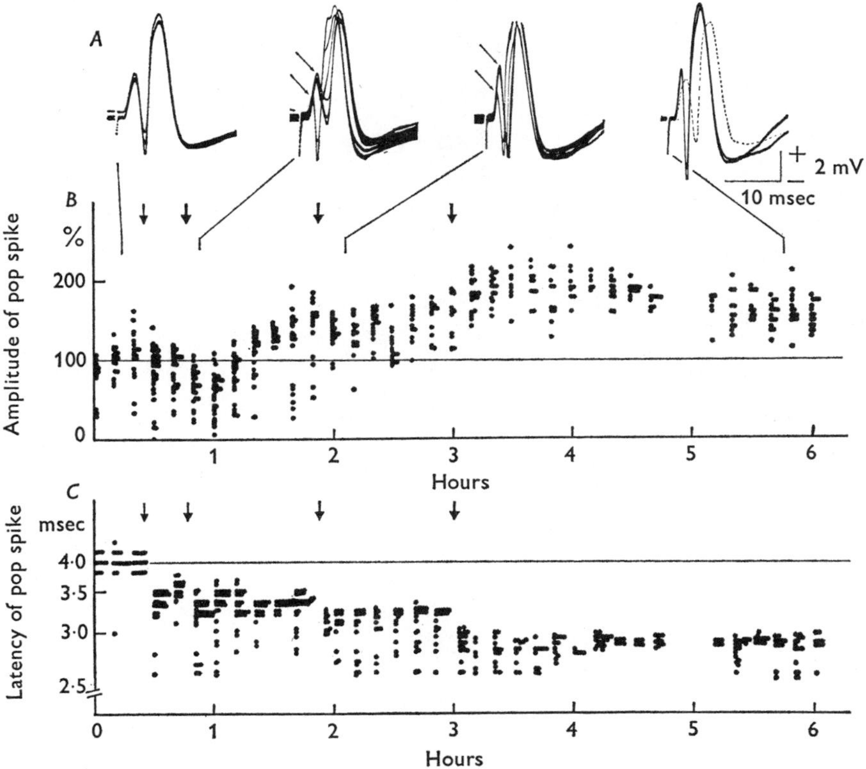

Figure 5. Potentiation of the population spike parameters in the experiment of Fig. 4. The Figure also illustrates the variability of the population spike. *A*, superimposed responses to several consecutive perforant path volleys, obtained at the four different times shown. Arrows indicate the two preferred latencies adopted by the population spike in the period between the second and fourth conditioning trains. The amplitude and latency of the population spike are plotted in *B* and *C* respectively, as functions of time. Each point was obtained from a single response, and each group of points represents a number (six to thirty) of consecutive responses.

by stippled traces) illustrate the potentiation in the experimental pathway and the lack of a similar effect on the early part of the response in the control pathway. It can safely be concluded that the effect on the population e.p.s.p. is restricted to the experimental pathway and is a direct result of the brief conditioning trains limited to this pathway. Potentiation of the population spike was marked by a fall in mean latency after each conditioning train and an increase in amplitude after the fourth train. In Fig. 5*A*, far right, the potentiated response obtained after 6 hr may be compared with that obtained before conditioning (stippled trace). Again (as in Figs. 3, 7 and 11), potentiation of the population e.p.s.p. can be seen not only in the synaptic layer (Fig. 4*A* and *B*) but also in the cell body layer, as an increase in the slope of the initial positive wave. In *B* the amplitude of a large number of individually measured population spikes, grouped at 10 min intervals, is displayed in order to show the considerable variability of this parameter. The mean amplitude of the population spike actually decreased after the first and the second conditioning train, in spite of the increase in the population e.p.s.p. (Fig. 4*C*). It was not until after the fourth train that the spike became clearly larger than it had been before conditioning.

The latency of the spike also varied, as can be seen both from the superimposed records of Fig. 5*A* and from the plot of individual latency measurements in Fig. 5*C*. Two separate phenomena underlie the latency changes observed in this and other experiments. One is the sudden reduction in latency which occurred after each conditioning train; the other is the tendency of the spike to jump, from one stimulus to the next, between an early and a late response as indicated by the arrows in Fig. 5*A*. These latency jumps were not associated with any corresponding change in the slope of the synaptic wave. Latency fluctuations were most marked after the first three trains in this experiment, but also occurred both before conditioning and after the fourth train when the spike as well as the population e.p.s.p. were maximally potentiated (Fig. 5*C*). The mean delay between the onset of the population e.p.s.p. and the early and late population spikes was 1.4 msec and 2.1 msec, respectively, before conditioning. After the fourth train these values had fallen to 0.9 msec and 1.3 msec. Thus, the onset of both types of spike was advanced with successive trains, while the time difference between them was reduced.

Stimulus-Response Relationships Additional information can be obtained by studying the changes which occurred in the stimulus–response curves after conditioning. In Fig. 6*A* and *B*, the amplitudes of the population e.p.s.p. and population spike in the experimental pathway have been plotted against the strength of the test stimulus for the same experiment as in Figs. 4 and 5. Filled circles show the relation before the first conditioning train, while the open circles give the same relation about 10 hr later (3 hr after the sixth and last conditioning train). The response was potentiated over the whole range of stimulus strengths, except near threshold. By this time (10 hr) the amplitude of the population e.p.s.p. evoked by a given stimulus in the control pathway was smaller than its preconditioning value (Fig. 6*C*), reflecting the gradual decline which set in after the eighth hour of the experiment; stimulus-response curves obtained at 7 hr in the control pathway were virtually identical to those obtained at the beginning of the experiment. A similar gradual decline of the e.p.s.p. occurred in the experimental pathway after the eighth hour. In spite of this the e.p.s.p. was still considerably potentiated at 10 hr (Fig. 6*A*) and remained potentiated for another 2 hr. In some experiments, as

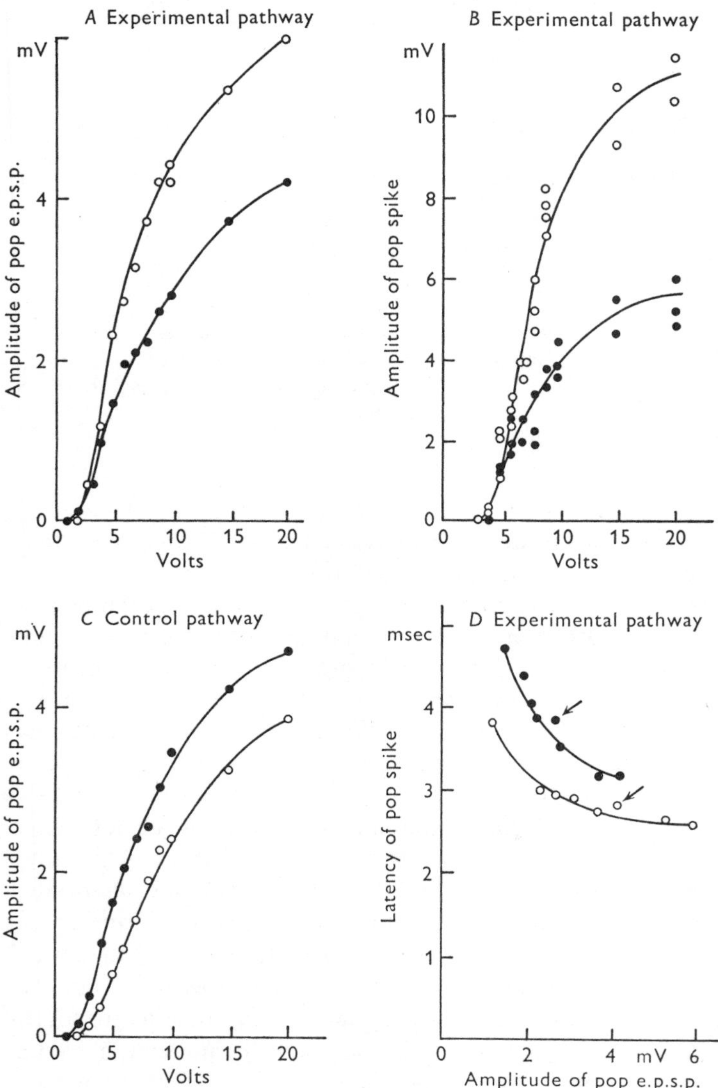

Figure 6. Effect of conditioning on stimulus–response curves. Same experiment as in Figs. 4 and 5. The two sets of points in *A* give the values of the population e.p.s.p. for the experimental pathway, as a function of stimulus strength before conditioning (filled circles), and almost 10 hr later (open circles) which was 3 hr after the last of six conditioning trains. Similar pairs of curves are plotted in *B* for the amplitude of the population spike (experimental pathway), and in *C* for the amplitude of the population e.p.s.p. (control pathway). In *D* the latency of the population spike has been plotted as a function of the amplitude of the population e.p.s.p. at the same times before (filled circles) and after (open circles) conditioning as in *A–C*. The arrows indicate the points obtained at the stimulus strength used for the standard test shocks given throughout the experiment.

here, a small increase in the voltage threshold for the e.p.s.p. was seen; in no case was there a decrease in threshold after conditioning.

In the majority of cases for which we have adequate data, the potentiation of the spike parameters could not be explained wholly in terms of potentiation of the e.p.s.p. In Fig. 6*D* the data from *A* and *B* have been replotted to show the latency of the population spike as a function of the e.p.s.p. amplitude, before and after conditioning. The two arrows point to values obtained at the normal test strength of 9 V. Before conditioning, an e.p.s.p. of 2.7 mV was associated with a spike latency of 3.9 msec, while after conditioning the same e.p.s.p. (obtained with a weaker stimulus) produced a spike with a latency of only 2.9 msec. There was thus a component of spike facilitation which could not be explained by e.p.s.p. potentiation alone.

Variability of the Population Spike The experiment displayed in Figs. 7 and 8 was chosen to illustrate the common observation that the population spike evoked by a constant test stimulus could vary markedly in amplitude, often from one response to the next (see also Fig. 5*B*). As with the variations in latency already described, these variations in amplitude were not accompanied by similar changes in the e.p.s.p. The variability tended to diminish as spike potentiation developed after conditioning. In Fig. 7, the spike amplitudes of over 30 consecutive responses obtained before and after conditioning (filled and open circles respectively) have been plotted against the amplitude of the population e.p.s.p. for each response (abscissa, Fig. 7*A*, *C* and *D*) and against spike latency (*B*). The increase in spike amplitude after conditioning was associated with an increase in the amplitude of the e.p.s.p., both in the synaptic layer (*A*) and in the cell body layer (*C*). The reduction in variability of spike amplitude, which occurred despite a slight increase in the range of e.p.s.p. values (*A*), is clearly brought out by this method of displaying individual responses. The range of values for spike amplitude in *A* was 1.0–9.0 mV before con-

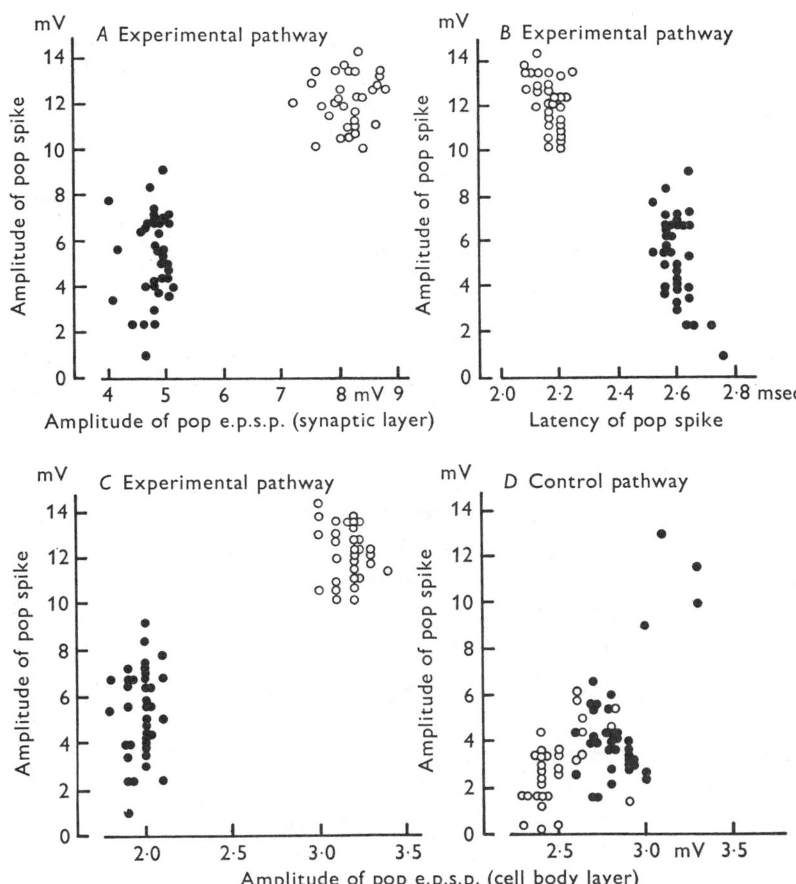

Figure 7. Effect of conditioning on the variability of the population spike. *A–C*, experimental pathway. The amplitude of the population spike of over thirty consecutive responses obtained before (filled circles) and after (open circles) conditioning, is plotted as a function of the amplitude of the population e.p.s.p. (synaptic layer in *A* and cell body layer in *C*), and of the latency of the population spike (*B*). A similar plot of the amplitude of the population spike as a function of the population e.p.s.p. (measured in the cell body layer) is shown in *D* for the control pathway.

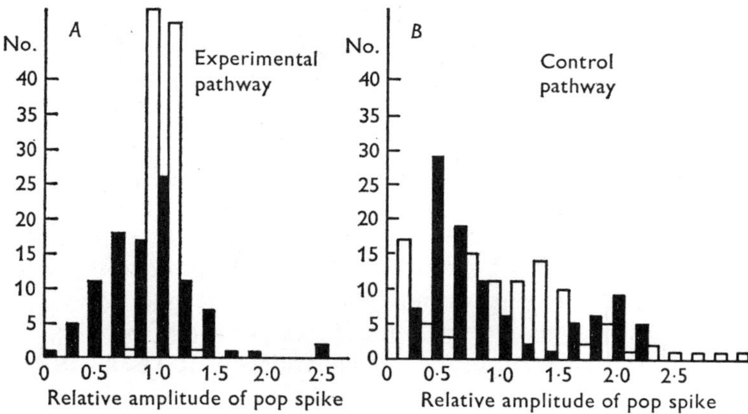

Figure 8. Histograms showing the amplitude distributions, expressed relative to the mean, of two sets of 100 consecutive population spikes, obtained before (filled bars) and 20–40 min after (open bars) a conditioning train to the experimental pathway. *A*, experimental pathway. *B*, control pathway. Same experiment as in Fig. 7.

ditioning, and 10.0–14.5 mV after conditioning. Expressed in terms of the dimensionless index, standard deviation/mean, the variability fell from 0.35 to 0.09. In the control pathway (*D*), the changes were restricted to a general reduction of both e.p.s.p. and spike amplitudes, with the disappearance after conditioning of the unusually large responses which in this experiment occasionally occurred, for unknown reasons, before conditioning.

The reduction in variability brought about by conditioning can also be seen in Fig. 8, taken from the same experiment. Two samples of one hundred consecutive responses, collected before and 20–40 min after a conditioning train, have been classified according to spike amplitude, expressed relative to the mean amplitude for each sample. The filled bars show the amplitude distribution before conditioning, for both experimental (*A*) and control (*B*) pathways. After conditioning, the amplitude distribution of the experimental pathway was much more sharply peaked (*A*, open bars), while that of the control pathway, although different in detail, was no less broad.

Potentiation of Spike Parameters without Corresponding Changes in the Population E.p.s.p. In the experiments described so far, conditioning resulted in a larger e.p.s.p. and a larger and earlier population spike. In some cases the spike facilitation was more than could be accounted for directly by the increase in the e.p.s.p. (Fig. 6*D*). Figs. 9 and 10 show that the spike was sometimes potentiated by conditioning trains which had little or no effect on the population e.p.s.p. In Fig. 9*C* the population spike of both the experimental (filled circles) and the contralateral control pathways (open circles) gradually declined in the 45 min before the first train was delivered to the experimental side. The first two trains were followed by a powerful but transitory potentiation of the population spike on the experimental side. With further trains, the time course of potentiation became progressively longer, until by the fourth train a stable plateau had been reached. No similar effects were seen on the control side. Averaged responses obtained before and after conditioning on the two sides are shown in Fig. 9*A*. In contrast to the steplike increase in spike size after each conditioning train (*C*), spike latency was not further reduced after the first train (*D*). The population e.p.s.p., measured in the cell body layer, increased slightly during the course of the experiment (*B*), but this increase was not clearly related to any of the conditioning trains.

A similar lack of correspondence between the population spike and population e.p.s.p. is seen in Fig. 10. In this case there was a sharp fall in latency, first on the left side (from 2.9 to 2.4 msec) and then on the right side, as each side received its first conditioning train. These shifts in latency can be seen in the superimposed averaged records shown in *B*. Conditioning had no obvious effect on the population e.p.s.p. (*B* and *E*) or the population spike (*B* and *F*), on either side. It is worth noting that a later experiment on a more lateral and previously unstimulated segment of the dentate area in the same animal produced potentiation of all three parameters (Fig. 2).

Conditioning with High Frequency Trains A question of some interest is whether long term potentiation depends on the ability of the conditioning train to discharge the granule cells. In order to reduce or eliminate firing of the granule cells during a conditioning train, the frequency was increased to 100/sec in three experiments. The duration of the train was reduced to 3–4 sec so that approximately the same number of stimuli was given. From field potential and single unit recordings it appears that granule cell discharges are usually abolished after the first shock in a train of stimuli at 100/sec. Furthermore, in two of the three

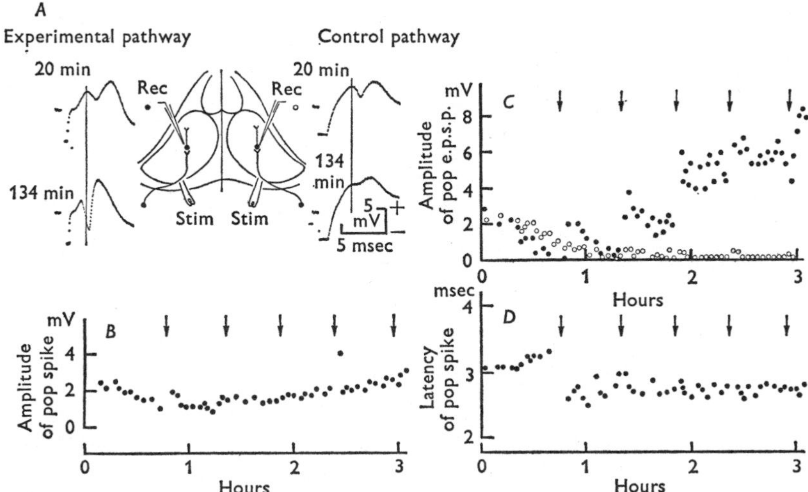

Figure 9. Potentiation of the population spike without potentiation of the population e.p.s.p. *A*, electrode arrangement. Sample average potentials for both experimental and control pathways before and after conditioning are shown. *B–D*, plots of the three standard parameters of the evoked response on the experimental side as functions of time. Conditioning trains (20/sec for 20 sec) were given at the times marked by arrows. In *C* the amplitude of the population spike is plotted for both experimental and control pathways (filled and open circles respectively).

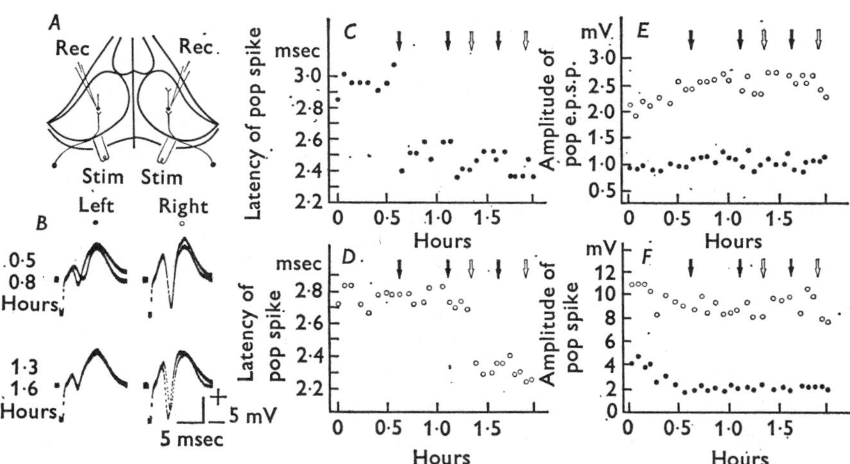

Figure 10. Decrease in the latency of the population spike, without change in the amplitude of the population spike or e.p.s.p. *A*, electrode arrangement. *B*, superimposed averages obtained before and after conditioning first the left-hand pathway (upper row) and later the right-hand pathway (lower row), showing that only the conditioned pathway was affected in each case. The times at which the averages were obtained is given on the left. *C–F*, plots of the time courses of the three standard parameters for both pathways. Conditioning trains (15/sec for 10 sec) were given either to the left side (filled arrows) or to the right side (open arrows) at the times indicated. *C*, *D*, latency of the population spike for the left-hand pathway (*C*) and the right-hand pathway (*D*). *E*, *F*, plots of the amplitude of the population e.p.s.p. measured in the cell body layer (*E*) and the amplitude of the population spike (*F*) for both left- and right-hand pathways (filled and open circles respectively).

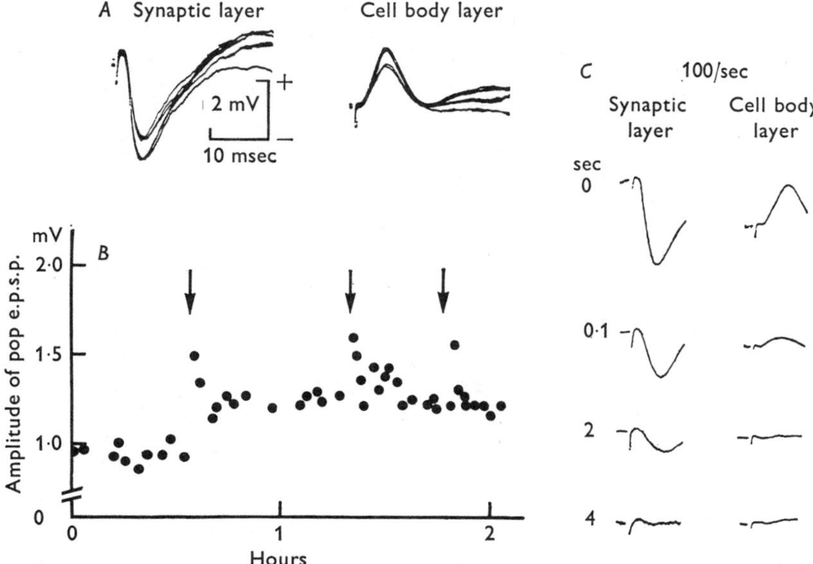

Figure 11. Long-lasting potentiation after conditioning at 100/sec. Synaptic potentials recorded in both the synaptic layer and in the cell body layer before conditioning and 45 min after the first conditioning train are superimposed in *A*. The time course of potentiation is plotted in *B*. The amplitude of the e.p.s.p. was measured 1.5 msec after the onset of the negativity in the synaptic layer. Conditioning trains at 100/sec for 4 sec were given at the times indicated. The absence of any population spike during the conditioning train can be seen from the sample responses in *C*, taken from both synaptic and cell body layers at the indicated times after the start of the conditioning train.

experiments of this type, a weak stimulus was used so that no population spike was evoked before or during the conditioning train. In spite of the absence of synchronous granule cell discharges, potentiation of the e.p.s.p. lasting an hour or more was obtained in all three experiments. The result of one of these experiments is shown in Fig. 11. The increase in slope and in the peak amplitude of the population e.p.s.p. after conditioning is apparent in the superimposed records in *A*, obtained from the synaptic and cell body layers just before and 45 min after the first of the three trains indicated in *B*. As in other experiments the e.p.s.p. potentiation was present both in the cell body and synaptic layers. The time course of the e.p.s.p. potentiation is plotted in *B*. Each train had an immediate effect which fell off within 10–20 min to the potentiated level set by the first conditioning train. Fig. 11*C* shows that no synchronous discharges of the granule cells occurred during the 100/sec train. Although extensive single unit recordings would be required to exclude the possibility of asynchronous spike discharges during the train, these results suggest that firing of the granule cells is not a requirement for long lasting potentiation of the e.p.s.p.

Duration of the After-Effect The longest after-effects we observed are illustrated in Fig. 12. The complete time course of the increase in amplitude of the population spike, for the experiment on Figs. 4–6, is shown in Fig. 12*A*. By the sixth conditioning train it was clear that no further increase could be induced. Thereafter, the spike remained undiminished until its sudden collapse nearly 7 hr later. By then the control responses had also declined markedly, suggesting that the overall condition of the preparation had deteriorated.

In another experiment (Fig. 12*B*), almost maximal potentiation of the population e.p.s.p. was reached after the second of four trains given alternately at 15/sec and 100/sec, the two later trains producing only transient further increases. Six to eight hr after the last train the amplitude began to fall off gradually, but was still well above its pre-conditioning value 10 hr after the last train.

Discussion

The amplitude of an evoked population potential depends on a number of factors, and it will be helpful to review these before considering the possible mechanisms which might be responsible for long-lasting potentiation.

As Rall & Shepherd (1968) have emphasized, the extracellular current which results from synchronous activation of a laminated cell population flows in a direction parallel to the long axes of the cells. From the point of view of the distribution of potential, whether actively or passively propagated, the situation resembles that of a nerve trunk in oil, and cable theory can be applied to extra- as well as intracellular potentials.

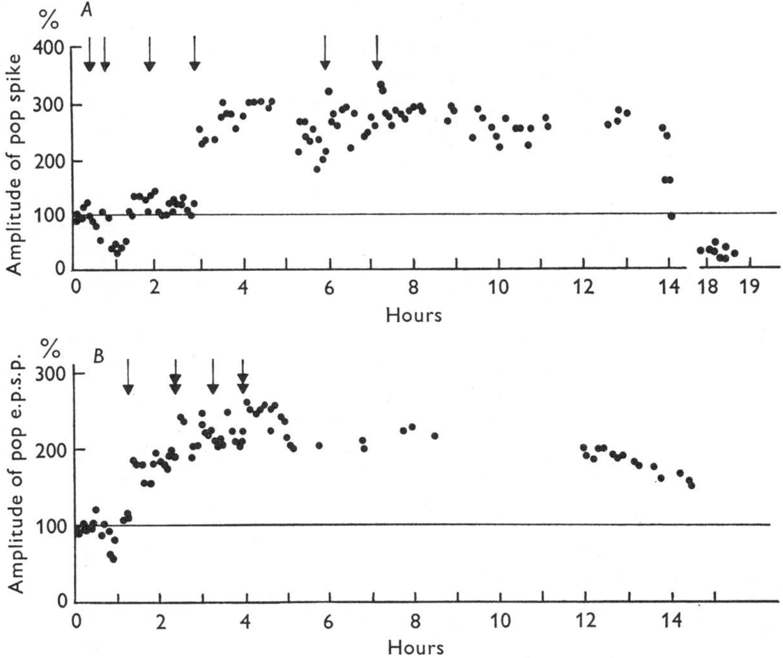

Figure 12. Two examples of potentiation lasting for many hours. *A*, the complete time course of the potentiation of the population spike for the experiment presented in Figs. 4–6. A total of six conditioning trains, each at 15/sec for 10 sec was given. *B*, the time course of e.p.s.p. potentiation in another experiment in which conditioning trains at 15/sec for 15 sec, and 100/sec for 3 sec were given alternately (single and double headed arrows respectively).

The amplitude of the extracellular potential, V_e, is related to the evoked membrane depolarization, ΔV_m, by the expression

$$V_e = \frac{r_e}{r_i + r_e} \Delta V_m + K, \tag{1}$$

where r_i and r_e are the resistances per unit length of the internal and external media respectively. K is a term containing constants of integration which need not be considered further in this context, providing, as was always the case, the amplitude of the potential was measured at the same depth and latency throughout the experiment.

The magnitude of the depolarization in the region of the perforant path synapses, $(\Delta V_m)pp$, will depend on the extent to which the conductance change $(\Delta g)pp$, evoked by the perforant path volley, short-circuits the membrane. There are two factors to consider—the magnitude of the evoked conductance change itself, and the effective membrane conductance, G_m, in the absence of perforant path activity. If there is no other afferent activity we may use the lumped, resistive equivalent circuit introduced by Fatt & Katz (1953) for the end-plate to write

$$(\Delta V_m)pp = \frac{(\Delta g)pp}{(\Delta g)pp + G_m} E, \tag{2}$$

where E is the difference between the resting membrane potential and the equilibrium potential for the perforant path transmitter. In cases where other afferent activity is present, eqn. (2) is no longer strictly applicable, but it remains true that any increase in G_m due to additional shunting conductances will result in a reduction in the evoked depolarization $(\Delta V_m)pp$ (see Ginsborg, 1967, p. 307 for a quantitative discussion of this point).

Thus, it is the magnitude of the evoked conductance change, relative to the effective conductance of the membrane, that determines the magnitude of the evoked synaptic potential, and both these factors must be taken into account when considering the mechanisms underlying potentiation.

The most likely causes of an increase in the amplitude of the synaptic response may now be summarized:

(1) an increase in the number of perforant path fibres activated by the test shock;

(2) an increase in the efficacy of the conditioned synapses;

(3) a decrease in the level of tonic afferent activity.

The first two possibilities would work by increasing $(\Delta g)pp$ in eqn. (2); the third by decreasing G_m.

The amplitude of the population spike reflects the number and synchrony of granule cell discharges (Andersen *et al.* 1971*a*). For a given synaptic input, the number of granule cells discharged will depend on the excitability of the population, and this could be controlled either by intrinsic factors, such as those which determine threshold, or by the extrinsic modulation of tonic excitatory and inhibitory afferent activity. Again, either mechanism might be available for long term modification. We now examine our results in the light of these various possibilities.

Evidence Against an Increase in the Size of the Perforant Path Volley

We were not able to detect a presynaptic compound action potential, and thus to obtain a direct measure of the size of the presynaptic volley. It is, however, unlikely that the number of perforant path fibres excited by the test volley increased significantly after conditioning, since there was no reduction in the threshold for evoking an e.p.s.p. after conditioning, and since the potentiated response could not be mimicked by increasing the size of the afferent volley with stronger shocks before conditioning. It seems evident from Fig. 6*A*, for example, that no pre-conditioning shock, however powerful, would have evoked an e.p.s.p. as large as those obtained with strong shocks after conditioning. Furthermore, after conditioning the magnitude of the spike parameters corresponding to a given synaptic input (i.e. to a given size of e.p.s.p.), were usually different from the values observed before conditioning: potentiation is thus not simply a question of moving up an 'input-output' curve (Fig. 6*D*), as would be expected under the hypothesis of a larger presynaptic volley. Finally, the evidence is conclusive that in some experiments potentiation of the population spike could not have been due to an increased perforant path volley, because there was in these cases no increase in the e.p.s.p. (Figs. 9 and 10).

Increased Synaptic Efficacy

The potentiation of the synaptic wave can in our view be most simply accounted for in terms of facilitated synaptic transmission. A similar conclusion was reached by Lømo (1971*b*) in his account of the brief facilitation of the e.p.s.p. which follows a single conditioning volley to the perforant path. Facilitation could take the form of an increase in the number of terminals invaded by the constant test volley, an increase in the amount of transmitter released per synapse, an increase in the sensitivity of the post-synaptic junctional membrane, or a reduction in the resistance of the narrow stem by which spines are attached to the parent dendrite (Rall, 1970). We have no evidence which could distinguish between these various possibilities.

Another possible mechanism for e.p.s.p. potentiation is a change in the level of tonic activity at other inputs. Such a change would affect the membrane conductance, which is one of the factors controlling the extracellular synpatic potential (eq. (2)). If, as a result of conditioning, there were a decline in tonic inhibitory activity to the same region of dendrites as that occupied by the perforant path synapses, the reduction in local shunting would lead to a larger e.p.s.p., both in the synaptic layer and at other levels. Furthermore, the reduction in inhibitory tone would lead to an over-all increase in excitability which would be reflected in the degree of spike potentiation. It seems unlikely, however, that the tonic inhibitory input to the region of the perforant path synapses which this scheme requires could be so powerful that its suppression would result in the doubling or even trebling of the e.p.s.p. seen in some experiments. The available physiological evidence suggests that inhibitory afferents to the granule cells terminate predominantly on the cell bodies and proximal dendrites (Andersen *et al.* 1966; Lømo, 1968). This conclusion is supported by recent anatomical observations on the distribution of axonal terminals with spheroidal and flattened vesicles in the dentate area (Gottlieb & Cowan, 1972).

Increase in Excitability of the Granule Cell Population

The likelihood that the granule cell population is subject to continuous fluctuations in excitability was strongly suggested in several experiments by the observation that large variations in the size and latency of the population spike could occur from one stimulus to the next, without any change in the e.p.s.p. (Figs. 5 and 7). Variations in the level of tonic afferent activity is the most probable explanation for these fluctuations.

The effect of conditioning seems to have been twofold. On the one hand, the variability of the spike, and hence of the presumed fluctuations in tonic activity, was frequently reduced; on the other, the mean level of tonic activity was shifted so that over-all the cell population became more excitable. We have no evidence for which pathways, whether intrinsic or extrahippocampal, might be responsible for this effect.

It is possible to find another explanation for experiments in which spike potentiation was greater than allowed for by e.p.s.p. potentiation alone. If the not unreasonable assumption is made that a substantial number of granule cells are so weakly excited by the unpotentiated perforant path input that they do not fire however strong a perforant path volley is given (see Lømo, 1971*a*), then the cells for which this were true would yield a population e.p.s.p. but no population spike. If the efficiency of the synapses increased above threshold as a result of conditioning then an increase in the population spike would be produced which could not have been mimicked before conditioning by an increase in stimulus strength. Whether or not a mechanism of this sort plays a role in spike potentiation is undecidable on the present evidence; it cannot, however, explain those experiments in which spike potentiation occurred in the absence of e.p.s.p. potentiation.

Changes in Synchrony of Activation

The extent to which increased synchrony of discharge is responsible for the increase in spike amplitude is difficult to estimate. Generally it seemed to be the case that where spike variation, or potentiation, was superposed on a stable e.p.s.p., there was little or no sign of increased synchrony, as estimated by the width of the spike at its base. In cases where there was substantial e.p.s.p. potentiation the correspondingly potentiated spike was usually narrower at its base, suggesting that the increase in amplitude in these cases was at least partly due to increased synchrony of discharge, resulting, presumably, from a more rapid approach to threshold (see, for example, Fig. 5*A*).

Variability of the Effect

A conspicuous feature of these experiments was the great variation in the degree of potentiation, both in different animals and in the same animal at different times and with different electrode positions (cf. Figs. 2 and 9 which are from the same animal). In three animals, no after-effect at all was seen, despite repeated conditioning trains. These differences cannot be explained as the result of differences in the perforant path input, since the monosynaptic e.p.s.p. was larger in some animals with little or no long-lasting potentiation than in others showing a marked effect.

Frequency Potentiation

Frequency potentiation was present in the great majority of experiments. It is not, however, a sufficient condition for potentiation, as shown by the three animals in which we failed to produce any after-effect; in each case, frequency potentiation was well developed. Nor is it a necessary condition; in three cases (two animals) there was clear-cut potentiation after conditioning trains at 10–14/sec in which frequency potentiation failed to develop. In another three cases (two animals) e.p.s.p. potentiation was recorded after conditioning at 100/sec (Fig. 11). These experiments show that the synaptic component of potentiation, at least, is not dependent on the massive synchronous firing of granule cells which takes place during frequency potentiation. Whether or not the same is true of the excitability component of spike potentiation is a question of some interest, but one which we are unable to answer on the available evidence.

The Critical Parameters for Conditioning

Potentiation occurred at all frequencies used for conditioning, i.e. 10–20/sec and 100/sec. The lower bound for producing an effect was greater than 0.5/sec, the rate used for testing. The number of stimuli during a train was normally 150–400. In one experiment a train at 5/sec for 4 sec produced an effect lasting 20 min, but we have not investigated systematically the minimum requirements for long-lasting potentiation, nor the relation between the size and duration of the after-effect and the number and frequency of the conditioning stimuli.

Significance of the Effect

The interest of these results derives both from the prolonged duration of the effect, and from the fact that an identifiable cortical pathway is involved. The perforant path is one of the main extrinsic inputs to the hippocampal formation, a region of the brain which has been much discussed in connexion with learning and memory (Douglas, 1967; Olds, 1972). Our experiments show that there exists at least one group of synapses in the hippocampus whose efficiency is influenced by activity which may have occurred several hours previously—a time scale long enough to be potentially useful for information storage. Whether or not the intact animal makes use in real life of a property which has been revealed by synchronous, repetitive volleys to a population of fibres the normal rate and pattern of activity along which are unknown, is another matter.

References

Andersen, P., Bliss, T. V. P. & Skrede, K. K. (1971*a*). Unit analysis of hippocampal population spikes. *Expl Brain Res.* **13**, 208–221.

Andersen, P., Bliss, T. V. P. & Skrede, K. K. (1971*b*). Lamellar organization of hippocampal excitatory pathways. *Expl Brain Res.* **13**, 222–238.

Andersen, P., Holmqvist, B. & Voorhoeve, P. E. (1966). Entorhinal activation of dentate granule cells. *Acta physiol. scand.* **66**, 448–460.

Blackstad, T. W. (1958). On the termination of some afferents to the hippocampus and fascia dentata. *Acta anat.* **35**, 202–214.

Bliss, T. V. P. & Gardner-Medwin, A. R. (1971). Long-lasting increases of synaptic influence in the unanaesthetized hippocampus. *J. Physiol.* **216**, 32–33 *P.*

Bliss, T. V. P. & Gardner-Medwin, A. R. (1973). Long lasting potentiation of synaptic transmission in the dentate area of the unanaesthetized rabbit following stimulation of the perforant path. *J. Physiol.* **232**, 357–374.

Bliss, T. V. P. & Lømo, T. (1970). Plasticity in a monosynaptic cortical pathway. *J. Physiol.* **207**, 61 *P.*

Bliss, T. V. P., Gardner-Medwin, A. R. & Lømo, T. (1973). Synaptic plasticity in the hippocampus. In *Macromolecules and Behaviour*, ed. Ansell, G. B. & Bradley, P. B., pp. 193–203. London: Macmillan.

Douglas, R. J. (1967). The hippocampus and behaviour. *Psychol. Bull.* **67**, 416–442.

Fatt, P. & Katz, B. (1953). The effect of inhibitory nerve impulses on a crustacean muscle fibre. *J. Physiol.* **121**, 374–389.

Ginsborg, B. L. (1967). Ion movements in junctional transmission. *Pharmac. Rev.* **19**, 289–316.

Gottlieb, D. I. & Cowan, W. M. (1972). On the distribution of axonal terminals containing spheroidal and flattened vesicles in the hippocampus and dentate gyrus of the rat and cat. *Z. Zellforsch. mikrosk. Anat.* **129**, 413–429.

Hjorth-Simonsen, A. & Jeune, B. (1972). Origin and termination of the hippocampal perforant path in the rat studied by silver impregnation. *J. comp. Neurol.* **144**, 215–232.

Lømo, T. (1966). Frequency potentiation of excitatory synaptic activity in the dentate area of the hippocampal formation. *Acta physiol. scand.* **68**, suppl. 277, 128.

Lømo, T. (1968). Nature and distribution of inhibition in a simple cortex (dentate area). *Acta physiol. scand.* **74**, 8–9*A*.

Lømo, T. (1971*a*). Patterns of activation in a monosynaptic cortical pathway: The perforant path input to the dentate area of the hippocampal formation. *Expl Brain Res.* **12**, 18–45.

Lømo, T. (1971*b*). Potentiation of monosynaptic EPSPs in the perforant path–granule cell synapse. *Expl Brain Res.* **12**, 46–63.

Nafstad, P. H. J. (1967). An electron microscope study on the termination of the perforant path fibres in the hippocampus and the fascia dentata. *Z. Zellforsch. mikrosk. Anat.* **76**, 532–542.

Olds, J. (1972). Learning and the hippocampus. *Rev. Can. Biol.* **31** (suppl.), 215–238.

Rall, W. (1970). Cable properties of dendrites and effects of synaptic location. In *Excitatory Synaptic Mechanisms*, ed. Andersen, P. & Jansen, J. K. S., pp. 175–187. Oslo: Universitetsforlaget.

Rall, W. & Shepherd, G. M. (1968). Theoretical reconstruction of field potentials and dendrodendritic synaptic interactions in olfactory bulb. *J. Neurophysiol.* **21**, 884–915.

J. M. Bekkers and C. F. Stevens

Presynaptic mechanism for long-term potentiation in the hippocampus

1990. *Nature* 346: 724–729

Experiments analysing the statistical properties of synaptic transmission, before and after the induction of long-term potentiation (LTP), suggest that expression of LTP largely arises in a presynaptic mechanism—an increased probability of transmitter release.

LONG-TERM potentiation (LTP) is a long-lasting use-dependent increase in the efficacy of excitatory synaptic transmission in the brain that is thought to underlie certain forms of learning and memory[1,2]. Although the trigger for LTP is generally agreed to occur in the postsynaptic cell[3–8], the site at which it is expressed is still disputed. Some authors have suggested that the mechanism of LTP is enhanced neurotransmitter release[9,10], others that it is increased postsynaptic sensitivity to transmitter[11,12], and still others that both may occur, perhaps in sequence[13]. Here we describe experiments analysing the statistical properties of synaptic transmission, before and after the induction of LTP, in both hippocampal cultures and patch-clamped slices.

Quantal analysis

Since the classic work of Del Castillo and Katz[14], the standard way to determine whether a phenomenon is pre- or postsynaptic has been to carry out a quantal analysis[15]. Such an analysis provides estimates of *a*, the amplitude of response to a single quantum of neurotransmitter, *p*, the probability of release, and *N*, the number of release sites. Synaptic transmission becomes more efficacious if *a*, *N*, or *p* is increased. In standard treatments, an increase in either *N* or *p* indicates a presynaptic mechanism, whereas a postsynaptic mechanism, such as greater receptor sensitivity, would produce an increase in *a*.

Quantal analysis has, however, proved difficult in the central nervous system for three main reasons. First, only rarely can one find a pair of cells that are monosynaptically connected[16]. The formalism for quantal analysis can be extended to include some situations in which more than one input to a neuron is stimulated, but such an extension is especially uncertain for classes of synapses where the Del Castillo and Katz statistical mechanism for release has not been confirmed. The second difficulty is that the characterization of the quantal event, the miniature excitatory postsynaptic current (m.e.p.s.c.), is uncertain both because spontaneous m.e.p.s.cs cannot usually be associated with a specific subset of the many synapses on a typical central neuron, and because cable filtering alters the amplitude and time course of m.e.p.s.cs that originate at a distance from the recording site[15,17]. Finally, the background noise in intracellular recording is frequently so large that m.e.p.s.cs are obscured[18,19].

We have circumvented these difficulties by studying neuronal connections in culture, where synaptically connected pairs of cells can be identified and where m.e.p.s.c. release can be evoked at defined locations so that the inherent properties of m.e.p.s.cs can be separated from cable filtering effects. M.e.p.s.cs at synapses in cultures of hippocampal neurons vary considerably in size, and the analysis of this variability has recently been extended in two ways[20]. First, m.e.p.s.c. amplitude fluctuations have been demonstrated to arise at single boutons (rather than reflecting the properties of a population of boutons); second, m.e.p.s.cs in hippocampal slices have been shown to exhibit about the same variability in size previously seen in culture[21]. An accurate quantal analysis of synaptic transmission in the hippocampus must take these properties of m.e.p.s.cs into account (see refs 22, 23).

Analysis in dissociated neurons

In a preliminary series of three experiments in culture, we used the nystatin perforated patch technique[24] to observe m.e.p.s.cs in a voltage-clamped neuron before and after briefly perfusing the bath with solution containing no Mg^{2+}. Such perfusion causes cells in the dish to fire spontaneous bursts of action potentials repeatedly and should have potentiated many synapses. Assuming LTP had been induced in a significant number of the neuron's synapses, we should have observed an increase in the mean size of m.e.p.s.cs if expression of LTP is postsynaptic. No detectable change in m.e.p.s.c. size was found up to 96 min after the induction of massive activity in the culture, suggesting that expression of LTP is not postsynaptic. The difficulty with this experiment was, of course, that we could not be sure that the synapses whose m.e.p.s.cs we recorded had undergone LTP. Therefore, we turned to a more conventional protocol.

At the outset we failed to observe LTP in 42 neuron pairs when standard whole cell recording methods were used[25], and therefore suspected that some critical cytoplasmic factor was being washed out of the cells. Accordingly, all our later experiments used the nystatin perforated patch technique to record from both pre- and postsynaptic neurons.

Figure 1 shows an experiment in which an action potential was repetitively fired (at 0.1 Hz) in one neuron, and the resulting synaptic current was recorded under voltage clamp in a neighbouring neuron (panel *a*). Panel *b* plots the amplitude of the current as a function of time during the experiment. For the first series of stimuli (before the arrow) the mean peak conductance was 1.62 nS, the standard deviation was 1.04 nS and on 8 out of 97 occasions the presynaptic action potential failed to evoke a postsynaptic response. At the arrow the bathing medium containing 10 mM Mg^{2+} (to prevent any possible potentiation during the test stimulation) was exchanged for one with no added Mg^{2+}, the postsynaptic neuron was switched from voltage clamp to current clamp, and the presynaptic neuron was tetanized three times for 2 s at 20 Hz. After this stimulation, the bathing solution with 10 mM Mg^{2+} was reintroduced, postsynaptic voltage clamp was re-established, and the 0.1 Hz stimulation of the presynaptic cell resumed. Following the tetanic stimulation, the mean synaptic current amplitude was 3.43 nS, the standard deviation 0.97 nS, and no failures in transmission occurred in 128 trials. The potentiation factor *f* in this case was $(3.43/1.62) = 2.1$. The amplitude histograms for pre- and post-tetanus synaptic current are shown in Fig. 2.

The following results argue in favour of the phenomenon in Fig. 1 being LTP. (1) The potentiation was long-lasting. For example, the e.p.s.c. in Fig. 1 was still at the same, elevated level 60 min after the tetanus. In two other cells the roughly threefold potentiation lasted for 80 and 90 min, respectively (at which point the cells were lost). (2) Potentiation could only be induced in a low Mg^{2+} concentration, as expected from the triggering characteristics of LTP[7,8]. (3) Potentiation was not an

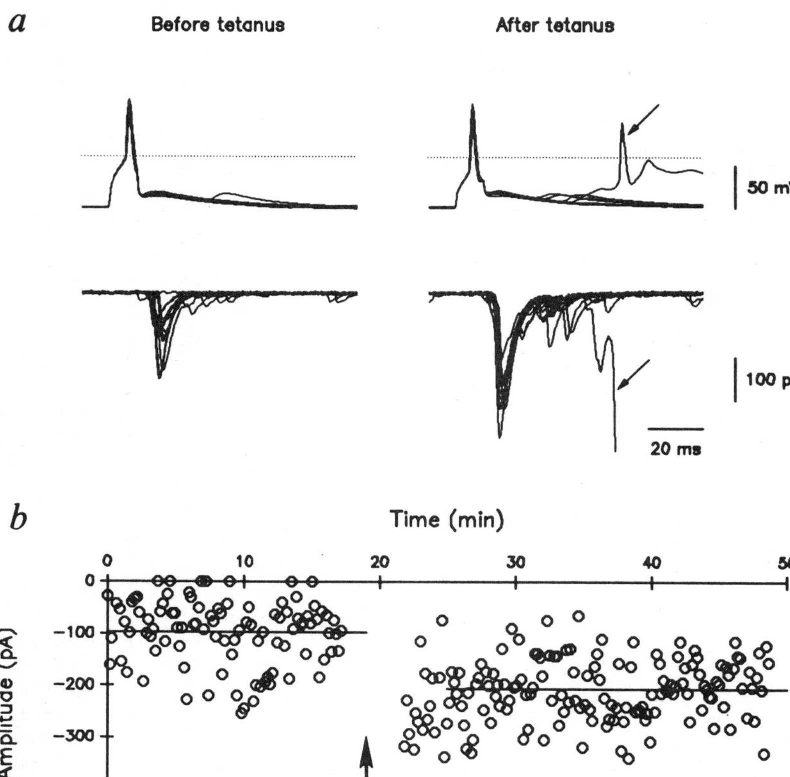

FIG. 1 Long-term potentiation of excitatory synaptic transmission between a pair of rat hippocampal neurons in dissociated cell culture. *a*, Superimposed action potentials recorded in the presynaptic cell (upper traces) and corresponding e.p.s.cs recorded simultaneously in the postsynaptic cell (lower traces). Left-hand panels were recorded shortly before, right-hand panels about 10 min after, a series of three 2-s tetani at 20 Hz separated by 30 s, performed with the postsynaptic cell in current clamp. All pre- and post-tetanus recordings were made with 10 mM Mg^{2+} solution (see below) in the bath; the tetani were delivered after briefly changing to a bath solution lacking Mg^{2+}. Action potentials were fired by injecting into the presynaptic cell a 10-ms 1 nA current step at 0.1 Hz. The presynaptic cell's resting membrane potential was near −60 mV; the postsynaptic cell was voltage clamped at −60 mV. Arrows in the right-hand panels indicate spontaneous polysynaptic activity that was recorded simultaneously in both cells (the current trace, lower panel, goes off-scale). Such activity was much more frequent after tetanus. Calibration bars refer to both right- and left-hand panels. The dotted lines in the upper panels indicate 0 mV. *b*, Plot of peak e.p.s.c. amplitude as a function of time for the same experiment as in *a*. The arrow indicates the time at which the sequence of tetani was applied. Immediately before this the bath was changed to a 0 mM Mg^{2+} solution, and then immediately afterward back to the control 10 mM Mg^{2+} solution. The straight lines through the data points represent the mean amplitudes over the time windows indicated by the horizontal positions of the lines.

METHODS. Pyramidal neurons from fields CA1 and CA3 of the hippocampi of newborn Long Evans rat pups were maintained in dissociated cell culture as previously described[21], except that 50 μM D-APV (D-2-amino-5-phosphonovaleric acid) was added to the culture medium after about a week to block possible potentiation due to spontaneous firing. For electrophysiology, the bath solution comprised (in mM) NaCl (137), KCl (5), $CaCl_2$ (3), $MgCl_2$ (10 or 0), D-glucose (10), HEPES-NaOH buffer (5), pH 7.3, osmolarity adjusted to 310 mOsm with sorbitol, to which was added 1 μM glycine, 1 μM strychnine and 100 μM picrotoxin. The tips of the patch electrodes were filled with a solution comprising (in mM) $KMeSO_4$ (150), KCl (5), EGTA (10), HEPES-KOH buffer (10), pH 7.2, and electrodes were back-filled with the same solution plus 100 μg ml^{-1} nystatin, diluted from a stock of 20 mg nystatin per ml of DMSO. Patch electrodes were Sylgarded and polished and had resistances of 1–3 MΩ with these solutions. After obtaining GΩ seals on a pair of cells, test pulses were applied until the access resistances stabilized (typically 30–50 min after forming the seals); access was checked for constancy throughout the experiment. Recordings were made with an Axopatch 1A, filter setting 1 kHz. The bath was perfused at about 1 ml min^{-1} (bath volume 1 ml). Electrode offset potentials were within 2 mV at the end of the experiment. All measurements were made at room temperature (23–25 °C).

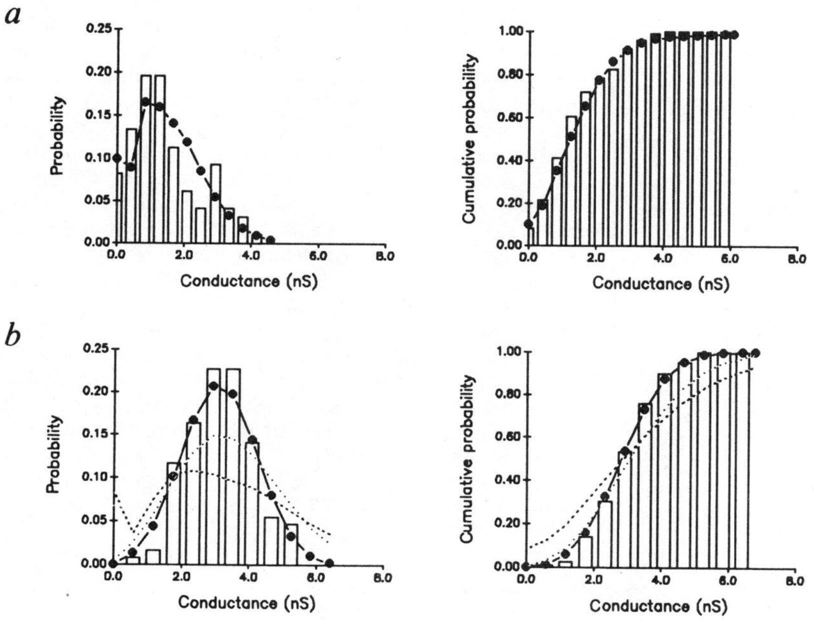

FIG. 2 Frequency histograms of e.p.s.c. conductance before and after inducing LTP are best fitted by assuming that LTP expression originates in an increase in release probability, *p*. *a*, Control (pre-tetanus) histograms. *b*, Post-tetanus histograms. (Same experiment as in Fig. 1.) In both *a* and *b* the right panel is the normalized cumulative histogram of the histogram in the left panel. In *a* the filled circles represent a binomial distribution fitted as described in the text. In *b* the filled circles were calculated from the distribution in *a* assuming that only *p* is scaled by the potentiation factor *f*, with no free parameters. The dotted line and the broken line were calculated assuming that the parameters *N* and *a*, respectively, are scaled by *f*.

artefact due to changing recording conditions. For example, the presynaptic action potential remained constant (Fig. 1*a*), and the bath was perfused at a continuous rate, preventing changes in the concentrations of possible modulatory substances[26].

Long-lasting potentiation was seen in 4 cell pairs out of 13 stable, connected pairs studied with the perforated patch technique. However, even in experiments in which the evoked e.p.s.c. was not potentiated, the above protocol usually caused a long-lasting increase in the general polysynaptic activity of cells in the culture. An example of this is visible in Fig. 1*a*, after tetanus (arrows). This is probably due to the potentiation of synapses other than those between the cell pair under study, and may arise in heterogeneity in the ability of synapses to support LTP[21].

Our strategy was to carry out a quantal analysis of the pre-tetanus responses then to test, without estimating additional parameters, three alternative mechanisms for the potentiation by predicting the amplitude histogram obtained after potentiation had developed. The potentiated response in Fig. 1 could be due to $f = 2.1$-fold scaling of N (the number of release sites), p (the quantal release probability) or a (the mean quantal size); as each of these factors enters the equation for the synaptic current size histograms in a different way, scaling each makes different predictions about the shape of the histograms. Thus we may determine which of the alternative theories best accounts for the data.

The probability of observing a synaptic current of a particular amplitude describing the amplitude histogram is given by the binomial distribution[14] suitably modified to take account of the observed variability in the m.e.p.s.c. size[20]. If a is taken to be the average value for the quantal size in culture (0.8 nS), the pre-tetanus binomial parameters N and p can be estimated from the standard equations for the mean $m = 1.62$ nS and variance $v = 1.073$ nS^2 of the amplitude histogram (Fig. 2*a*):

$$m = aNp$$

$$v = a^2Np(1-p) + a^2Npc_m^2.$$

The second term gives the contribution to the overall variance of fluctuations in the m.e.p.s.c. size; the coefficient of variation of m.e.p.s.cs is c_m and has an average value of 0.5 in culture and 0.42 in slices[20]. Solving these equations yields $N = 4.8$, $p = 0.42$. As N should be an integer, N was constrained to be 5 (rather than the calculated 4.8) and p was set to 0.37 (instead of 0.42).

The predicted and observed pre-tetanus histograms are shown superimposed in Fig. 2*a*; they are not significantly different at the 0.2 level (χ^2 goodness-of-fit test); that is, worse fits would occur by chance more than one time in five even if the histograms were generated by the same underlying mechanism. Although we could not in these experiments collect sufficient quantities of pre-tetanus data to carry out a very accurate quantal analysis, the fit exhibited in Fig. 2*a* confirms our previous conclusion[21] that the Del Castillo and Katz formalism, with the m.e.p.s.c. variability included, accounts for the observed amplitude histogram.

Figure 2*b* shows the result of assuming that the mechanism of LTP is an f-fold increase in the release probability p, with N and a unchanged; the predicted histogram that results is superimposed on the observed post-tetanus amplitude histogram. The predicted and observed histograms are not significantly different at $P < 0.2$. The two other alternative mechanisms, an f-fold increase in N or in a make predictions that differ from the observed histograms at $P < 0.05$ and 0.01 levels of significance, respectively (dotted and broken lines in Fig. 2*b*).

A convenient way to compare predicted and observed histograms uses the coefficient of variation (and its squared value h)

$$c = \sqrt{h} = \sqrt{v}/m$$

introduced in this context by Del Castillo and Katz[14], and modified here to take account of m.e.p.s.c. variability:

$$h(N, p) = (1 + c_m^2 - p)/(Np). \quad (1)$$

Note that a cancels in the right-hand side of this equation, so

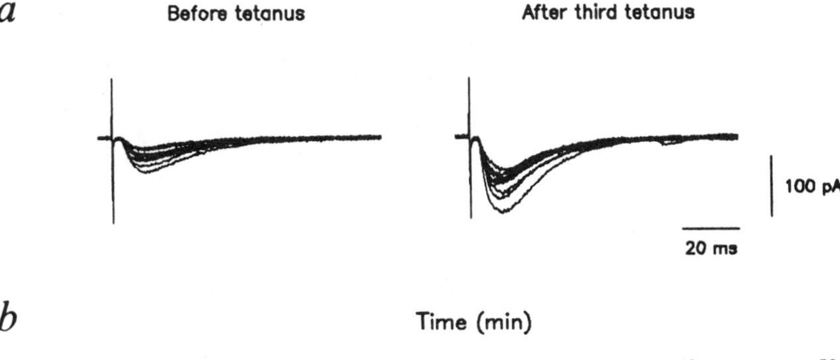

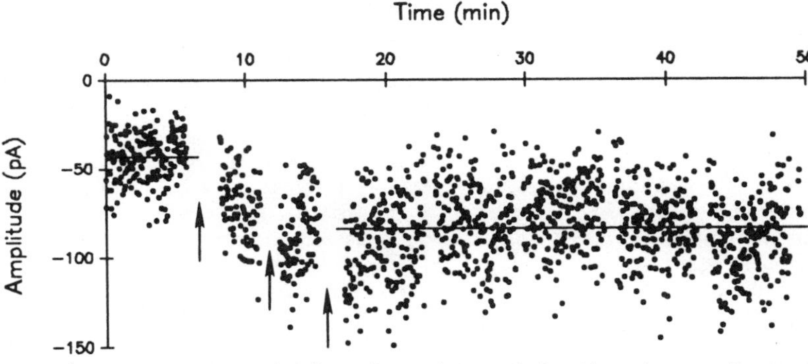

FIG. 3 Long-term potentiation of excitatory synaptic transmission in a patch-clamped hippocampal slice. *a*, Superimposed e.p.s.cs, elicited by stimulation of the Schaffer collateral pathway at 0.5 Hz, recorded from a cell in area CA1 before (left) and after (right) tetanus-induced LTP. The neuron was whole-cell voltage-clamped at the soma at −70 mV. Calibration bars refer to both panels. *b*, Plot of the amplitudes of evoked e.p.s.cs as a function of time during the experiment. At each arrow the patch amplifier was switched to current clamp mode and two 200-ms 100 Hz tetani were delivered 5 s apart. The amplifier was then returned to voltage clamp mode and testing resumed. The straight lines through the data points represent the mean amplitudes over the time windows indicated by the horizontal positions of the lines.

METHODS. Transverse slices (300–400 μm) were cut from the hippocampi of 14–21-day-old Long Evans rats using a vibratome, submerged and continuously perfused at 1–2 ml min^{-1} with oxygenated Krebs solution comprising (in mM) NaCl (120), KCl (3), $MgCl_2$ (1.2), $CaCl_2$ (2.5), $NaHCO_3$ (23), NaH_2PO_4 (1.2), D-glucose (11), to which 100 μM picrotoxin was added. Patch electrodes contained (in mM) Cs-methylsulphate (120), CsCl (5), EGTA (0.5), $MgCl_2$ (2), Mg-ATP (2), sorbitol (10), HEPES-CsOH buffer (10), pH 7.3. Gigaohm seals were obtained with unpolished electrodes (resistances 3–5 MΩ) on the somas of cells in region CA1 and recordings made in the whole-cell with an Axopatch 1A, filter setting 2 kHz. A monopolar stimulating electrode (35 μm diameter teflon-coated Pt-Ir wire) was positioned 200–300 μm away in *stratum radiatum* and the stimulus intensity set just above the level that gave mostly failures of synaptic transmission; this setting was subsequently left unchanged throughout the experiment. The stimulus duration for low frequency stimulation was 100 μs; for tetani it was 200 μs. Electrode offset potentials were within 2 mV at the end of the experiment. Experiments were performed at room temperature (23–25 °C).

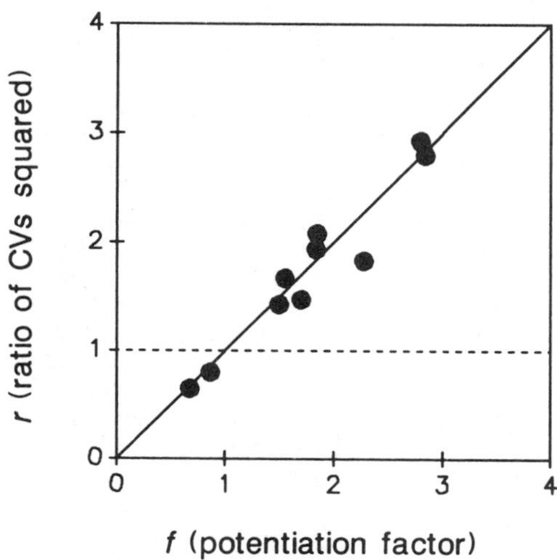

FIG. 4 A plot of r against f (defined in the text) for 10 different slice LTP experiments is best fitted by a model that locates the expression of LTP in the presynaptic terminal. The diagonal line is the prediction of a Poisson scheme in which LTP is expressed presynaptically, the horizontal line the prediction for postsynaptic expression. The two points for which f is less than unity were obtained from experiments in which 100 μM D-APV was present during the tetanus, and a long-lasting depression resulted.

that the value of h is not altered by a potentiation mechanism that operates through increases in a. According to this equation, if a increased f-fold, $h(N, p) = 0.48$ (the pre-tetanus value), whereas $h(fN, p) = 0.23$, and $h(N, fp) = 0.12$. The observed value for h in this experiment was 0.08. This supports the above conclusion that LTP in culture involves an increase in p rather than in N or a. The same conclusion was reached in full quantal analyses of three other cell pairs in culture that displayed long-lasting potentiation.

Because the potentiation just described is enduring, and requires activation of synapses under conditions that permit calcium influx through the NMDA (N-methyl-D-aspartate) receptor channels, it is like LTP[7,8]. LTP is, however, normally studied in relatively intact hippocampal circuits, not dissociated cultures, so one cannot be sure that the mechanism discussed above operates in the same way as actual LTP. For this reason, we experimented with whole-cell clamped neurons in hippocampal slices, where the properties of LTP are well known.

Experiments like those just described, in which one records with the perforated patch technique from defined cell pairs, are difficult in the slice as one can only rarely find monosynaptic connections[16]. Accordingly, we used the conventional whole cell ruptured patch technique to record from single postsynaptic pyramidal neurons while repetitively exciting axons of the Schaffer collateral pathway with a small extracellular stimulating electrode[27,28]. An example is shown in Fig. 3. Panel a shows superimposed e.p.s.cs recorded while voltage clamping the neuron at −70 mV, measured before and after tetanus. Panel b plots the e.p.s.c. amplitude as a function of time during the experiment. Tetani were delivered at each of the arrows in Fig. 3b while maintaining the cell in current clamp. This protocol induced a long-lasting potentiation of the e.p.s.c.; the mean control amplitude was 43.3 pA, and the mean following three series of tetani was 83.8 pA.

In the above experiment the stimulus level was set just above the threshold for synaptic transmission. We knew, however, that multiple axonal inputs onto the postsynaptic cell were being stimulated. This situation complicates the quantal analysis[15]

Analysis in hippocampal slices

We have taken two approaches to extending our analysis to the hippocampal slice. First, we have used a procedure, described below, that takes account of the possible nonuniformity of the stimulated inputs to a neuron. Second, we have simply applied the standard equations of quantal analysis, and have relied upon goodness-of-fit tests to determine if the application of these equations is valid. These approaches are described in turn.

The first approach is best described by presenting a graph that plots a quantity r as a function of the factor f by which the mean e.p.s.c. size is potentiated. The quantity r, like f, is determined directly from the experimental data and is defined as the ratio

$$r = h/h_p$$

where h (defined earlier in equation (1)) is the squared value of the coefficient of variation before a tetanus and h_p is the corresponding quantity in the potentiated slice. In the limiting case where p is small (the Poisson limit), r is, according to equation (1), equal to f if the mechanism of LTP is an f-fold change in either N or p (presynaptic mechanism) and equal to 1 if LTP results from a scaling of a (postsynaptic mechanism). Figure 4 shows such an r/f plot for 10 slice experiments and unambiguously accords with the predictions of the presynaptic mechanism. Note that in two cases f was less than unity; in these experiments the tetanus was applied with 100 μM D-APV in the bath, which resulted in a long-lasting depression.

The r/f plot can be generalized to many situations with multiple inputs to a neuron in which a standard quantal analysis is not applicable. It can be shown in these cases that points will fall on or to the left of the diagonal ($r = f$) if the LTP mechanism is presynaptic (an increase in either N or p), and will fall on a horizontal line ($r = 1$), or between that line and the diagonal, if the mechanism is postsynaptic (an increase in a). However, analysis reveals a special case for which the r/f plot does not correctly distinguish between a pre- and postsynaptic mechanism for LTP. Suppose that individual postsynaptic membranes could exist in only two states, 'on' and 'off'; for an 'off' synapse release of a quantum of neurotransmitter would result in essentially no response, and for an 'on' synapse, each quantum would give a standard-sized response. The mechanism of LTP in this model would be the postsynaptic switching (for example, by increasing the sensitivity of receptors in the postsynaptic membrane) from 'off' to 'on'. Such a switch would appear in our analysis to be an increase in N, and thus to be presynaptic, whereas in fact the site of LTP expression would be postsynaptic. From our slice experiments alone we would not be able to distinguish between the presynaptic mechanism and this particular postsynaptic mechanism. The observations in culture, however, are not consistent with the postsynaptic mechanism because LTP there resulted from an increase in the release probability p, not N.

We conclude that our observations in slices, like those in culture, are consistent with the expression of LTP being primarily presynaptic. Because points fall along the diagonal, indicating that release is described by the Poisson limit, we cannot here, as we could in some of the experiments on neuron pairs in culture, distinguish between effects on N and p.

An alternative way to test our conclusion is to carry out a full quantal analysis of transmission in these slice experiments: if the mechanism is indeed presynaptic and the quantal parameters sufficiently constant to give data points that fall along the diagonal in the r/f plots, then the distribution of synaptic current sizes should be well described by the standard equations of quantal analysis, and one should be able to predict the distribution of potentiated synaptic current sizes with the quantal parameters obtained from the unpotentiated distribution. If the conclusion is incorrect, then the observed distribution of synaptic current sizes should be a sum of Poisson distributions, and may not, in general, be adequately described by a single Poisson distribution.

Figure 5a shows a slice experiment in which the postsynaptic response for a small stimulus is plotted as a function of time

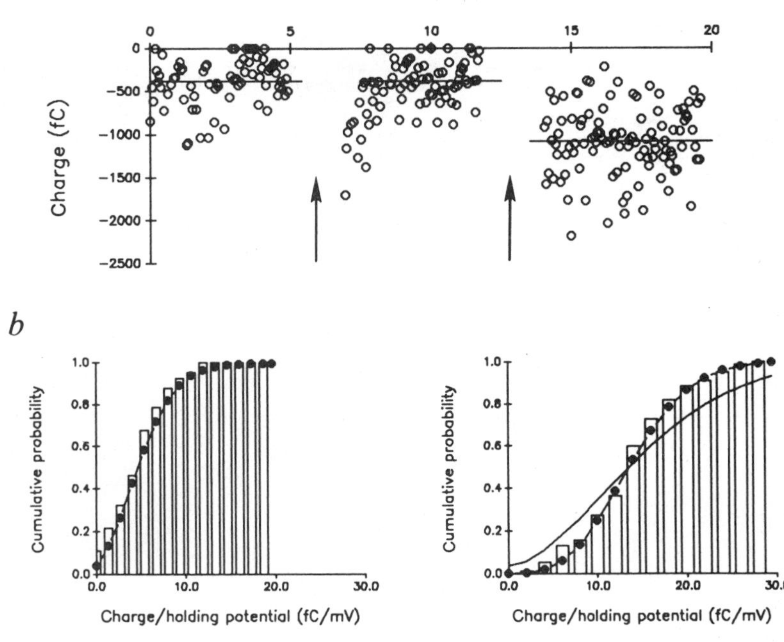

FIG. 5 Histograms of e.p.s.c. size in the slice are best fitted by a Poisson model in which LTP expression originates in a (presynaptic) increase in the mean quantal content, *Np*. *a*, Plot of the charge carried by evoked e.p.s.cs as a function of time during the experiment. Charge was calculated by integrating individual e.p.s.cs over an 80–90-ms time window starting at the foot of the e.p.s.c. Test stimuli were delivered at 0.5 Hz while voltage clamping the soma at −70 mV. At the first arrow, three trains of 200-ms 100 Hz tetani were delivered at 5-s intervals while still voltage clamping the soma at −70 mV. At the second arrow the same tetanus protocol was applied while the voltage clamping at −20 mV. The straight lines through the data points represent the mean amplitudes over the time windows indicated by the horizontal positions of the lines. *b*, Cumulative probability histograms derived from the data in *a* before (left) and after (right) inducing LTP. Note that the charge carried by the e.p.s.cs has been normalized by dividing by the holding potential (−70 mV). The filled circles on the left are a fit of the Poisson distribution to the experimental histogram. The filled circles on the right were calculated from the Poisson distribution assuming that LTP scales only *Np* by *f*, with no free parameters. The solid curve on the right is the prediction of a Poisson distribution assuming that only parameter *a* is scaled by *f*.

during the experiment. Note that charge, rather than amplitude, is measured because the former is a quantity less affected by cable attenuation in the dendrites[17,29]. At the point indicated by the first arrow, the inputs to the cell were stimulated repetitively but the postsynaptic neuron was maintained by the voltage clamp at −70 mV; the response did not potentiate after this procedure, as expected for LTP[3–6]. At the second arrow, the cell's inputs were again stimulated while the cell was held at −20 mV, a value that should maximize calcium influx through the NMDA receptor channels and produce LTP[7,8]. The mean response after this tetanus was potentiated by a factor $f = 2.84$. This particular experiment was chosen for illustration of the full quantal analysis because failures were apparent in the control records, which provides an additional check on the validity of the fitted parameters.

Figure 5*b* shows the histogram of observed synaptic responses for this experiment with superimposed predictions of the Poisson distribution, using appropriate values for *a* and *Np* estimated from the mean and variance of the raw data, and again taking into account the measured variance in m.e.p.s.c. size[20]. A χ^2 goodness-of-fit test detects no difference between these distributions at the 0.2 significance level. The quantal size estimated by the ratio variance/mean for this experiment is 2.1 fC mV^{-1} before (and after) the tetanus. For six experiments, the average quantal size was 1.35 ± 0.37 fC mV^{-1} before the tetanus and 1.41 ± 0.28 fC mV^{-1} in the potentiated slice (mean ± s.d.). These estimates should be compared with the mean value for *a* directly determined in slices of 1.5 fC mV^{-1} with a standard deviation of 0.5 fC mV^{-1} (ref. 20). The value for *a* estimated from the histogram is thus within the range of quantal sizes determined independently.

If the pre-tetanus value for *Np* is multiplied by *f*, the predicted histogram, superimposed on the experimental one after potentiation, is shown in Fig. 5*c*. Again the χ^2 goodness-of-fit test detects no difference between the observed and predicted histograms at the 0.2 significance level. If *a*, rather than *Np*, is multiplied by *f*, the predicted and observed histograms differ at the 0.01 significance level, so the differences are statistically different (Fig. 5*c*, smooth curve). Similar results were found in four other slice experiments in which we carried out full quantal analyses. We conclude that the potentiation mechanism is presynaptic, and that either *N* or *p* increases following the tetanus.

The longest LTP observed in our slice experiments is 98 min, and our conclusions hold up to that time. We cannot, however, exclude the possibility that slower developing phases of LTP use some different mechanism. Because our experiments were done at room temperature (23–25 °C), and we do not know the temperature coefficients of the various possible phases of LTP, we cannot even place limits of the validity of our conclusions for the hippocampus at body temperature. From just after the tetanus up to 1 h after, only a single phase of LTP was apparent in our experiments, and the statistical properties of the postsynaptic response were essentially invariant.

Discussion

Our conclusion is that the mechanism of LTP is presynaptic rather than postsynaptic, and probably involves *p* instead of *N*. We have not, however, attempted to place specific limits on the extent to which intermediate cases, in which two or three of the quantal parameters are affected by LTP, might hold. Specifically, we cannot exclude the possibility that some small fraction of LTP is postsynaptic, or that both *N* and *p* increase with the *p* effect predominating. Because the potentiation factor *f* enters squared if the LTP mechanism is postsynaptic and linearly if it is presynaptic, a large contribution from the postsynaptic site can be excluded. *N* as well as *p* could be affected significantly, and we would not be able to detect this.

Our conclusion that the expression of LTP is, under the conditions of our experiment, mainly presynaptic, directs attention to mechanisms whereby retrograde signals from the postsynaptic cell cause enhanced presynaptic release of neurotransmitter[13,30,31].

Note added in proof: Our observations and conclusions are in accord with those reported by R. Malinow and R. W. Tsien[32]. □

1. Bliss, T. V. P. & Lomo, T. *J. Physiol., Lond.* **232**, 331–356 (1973).
2. Bliss, T. V. P. & Lynch, M. in *Long-Term Potentiation: From Biophysics to Behavior* (eds Landfield, P. W. & Deadwyler, S. A.) 3–72 (Liss, New York, 1988).
3. Wigstrom, H., Gustafsson, B., Huang, Y.-Y. & Abraham, W. C. *Acta physiol. scand.* **126**, 317–319 (1986).
4. Kelso, S. R., Ganong, A. H. & Brown, T. H. *Proc. natn. Acad. Sci. U.S.A.* **83**, 5326–5330 (1986).
5. Malinow, R. & Miller, J. P. *Nature* **320**, 529–530 (1986).
6. Sastry, B. R., Goh, J. W. & Auyeung, A. *Science* **232**, 988–990 (1986).

7. Collingridge, G. L. & Bliss, T. V. P. *Trends Neurosci.* **10,** 288–293 (1987).
8. Gustafsson, B. & Wigstrom, H. *Trends Neurosci.* **11,** 156–162 (1988).
9. Skrede, K. K. & Malthe-Sorenssen, D. *Brain Res.* **208,** 436–441 (1981).
10. Dolphin, A. C., Errington, M. L. & Bliss, T. V. P. *Nature* **297,** 496–498 (1982).
11. Muller, D., Joly, M. & Lynch, G. *Science* **242,** 1694–1697 (1988).
12. Kauer, J. A., Malenka, R. C. & Nicoll, R. A. *Neuron* **1,** 911–917 (1988).
13. Davies, S. N., Lester, R. A. J., Reymann, K. G. & Collingridge, G. L. *Nature* **338,** 500–503 (1989).
14. Del Castillo, J. & Katz, B. *J. Physiol., Lond.* **124,** 560–573 (1954).
15. Redman, S. J. *Physiol. Rev.* **70,** 165–198 (1990).
16. Sayer, R. J., Redman, S. J. & Andersen, P. *J. Neurosci.* **9,** 840–850 (1989).
17. Rall, W. & Segev, I. in *Voltage and Patch Clamping with Microelectrodes* (eds T. G. Smith *et al.*) 191–215 (American Physiological Society, Bethesda, 1985).
18. Brown, T. H., Wong, R. K. S. & Prince, D. A. *Brain Res.* **174,** 194–199 (1979).
19. Yamamoto, C. *Expl Brain Res.* **46,** 170–176 (1982).
20. Bekkers, J. M., Richerson, G. B. & Stevens, C. F. *Proc. natn. Acad. Sci. U.S.A.* **87,** 5359–5362 (1990).
21. Bekkers, J. M. & Stevens, C. F. *Nature* **341,** 230–233 (1989).
22. Voronin, L. L. in *Synaptic Plasticity in the Hippocampus* (eds Haas, H. L. & Buzsaki, G.) 27–30 (Springer, Berlin, 1988).
23. Foster, T. C. & McNaughton, B. L. *Soc. Neurosci. Abstr.* **15,** 775 (1989).
24. Horn, R. & Marty, A. *J. gen. Physiol.* **92,** 145–159 (1988).
25. Hamill, O. P. *et al. Pflugers Arch.* **391,** 85–100 (1981).
26. Forsythe, I. D., Westbrook, G. L. & Mayer, M. L. *J. Neurosci.* **8,** 3733–3741 (1988).
27. Edwards, F. A., Konnerth, A., Sakmann, B. & Takahashi, T. *Pflugers Arch.* **414,** 600–612 (1989).
28. Blanton, M. G., Lo Turco, J. J. & Kriegstein, A. R. *J. Neurosci. Meth.* **30,** 203–210 (1989).
29. Bekkers, J. M. & Stevens, C. F. *Progr. Brain Res.* **83,** 37–45 (Elsevier, Amsterdam, 1990).
30. Piomelli, D. *et al. Nature* **328,** 38–43 (1987).
31. Williams, J. H., Errington, M. L., Lynch, M. A. & Bliss, T. V. P. *Nature* **341,** 739–742 (1989).
32. Manilow, R. & Tsien, R. W. *Nature* **346,** 177–180 (1990).

ACKNOWLEDGEMENTS. We thank Drs L. Chavez-Noriega and G. Richerson for their suggestions on the slice technique. This work was supported by the Howard Hughes Medical Institute and the NIH (C.F.S.).

31

R. D. Hawkins and E. R. Kandel

Is there a cell-biological alphabet for simple forms of learning?

1984. *Psychological Review* 91: 375–391

Recent studies indicate that the cellular mechanism underlying classical conditioning of the *Aplysia* siphon withdrawal reflex is an extension of the mechanism underlying sensitization. This finding suggests that the mechanisms of yet higher forms of learning may similarly be based on the mechanisms of these simple forms of learning. We illustrate this hypothesis by showing how several higher order features of classical conditioning, including generalization, extinction, second-order conditioning, blocking, and the effect of contingency, can be accounted for by combinations of the cellular processes that underlie habituation, sensitization, and classical conditioning in *Aplysia*.

Learning has traditionally been divided into two major categories: associative learning, which includes classical and operant conditioning, and nonassociative learning, which includes habituation and sensitization (see Hilgard & Marquis, 1940; Mackintosh, 1974). A central problem in the study of learning has been to discover how these different forms of learning are related to one another. Specifically, is each form of learning governed by a fundamentally different mechanism, or are they governed by variations on a common mechanism? During the past two decades there has been substantial progress in identifying the cellular mechanisms for habituation, sensitization, and conditioning in simple vertebrate systems and in higher invertebrates such as *Aplysia, Drosophila, Hermissenda,* locust, and crayfish (Alkon, 1979; Byers, Davis, & Kiger, 1981; Castellucci, Pinsker, Kupfermann, & Kandel, 1970; Crow & Alkon, 1980; Duerr & Quinn, 1982; Hawkins, Abrams, Carew, & Kandel, 1983; Hoyle, 1979; Kandel & Schwartz, 1982; Krasne, 1969; Spencer, Thompson, & Nielson, 1966; Zucker, 1972). On the basis of these studies, one can begin to specify several common mechanistic features in these different forms of learning. These general features can be summarized as follows:

1. Elementary aspects of learning are not diffusely distributed in the brain but can be localized to the activity of specific nerve cells.
2. Learning produces alterations in the membrane properties and in the synaptic connections of those cells.
3. The changes in synaptic connections so far encountered have not involved formation of totally new synaptic contacts. Rather, they are achieved by modulating the amount of chemical transmitter released by presynaptic terminals of neurons.
4. In several instances the molecular mechanisms of learning involve intracellular second messengers and modulation of specific ion channels.

Moreover, recent results in both *Aplysia* and *Drosophila* indicate that the molecular mechanism of conditioning, an associative form of learning, is an elaboration of the same molecular mechanism involved in sensitization, a nonassociative form of learning (Duerr & Quinn, 1982; Hawkins et al., 1983). The finding that unifying cell-biological principles may underlie both nonassociative and associative forms of learning raises another question: Do

Preparation of this article was supported in part by grants from the National Institute of Mental Health (MH26212), National Institute of General Medical Services (GM-32099), and Office of Naval Research (83-K-0166).

We are grateful to Tom Abrams, Tom Carew, Greg Clark, Ruth Colwill, Robert Rescorla, and Alan Wagner for their comments on an earlier draft of this article, to Kathrin Hilten and Louise Katz for preparing the figures, and to Harriet Ayers and Charlotte Alexander for preparing the manuscript.

Requests for reprints should be sent to Robert D. Hawkins, Center for Neurobiology and Behavior, College of Physicians & Surgeons, Columbia University, 722 West 168th Street, New York, New York 10032.

the mechanisms so far encountered represent the beginning of an elementary cellular alphabet of learning? That is, can these units be combined to yield progressively more complex learning processes? In this article we suggest that such an alphabet exists and that certain higher order forms of learning generally associated with cognition can be explained in cellular–connectionistic terms by combinations of a few relatively simple types of neuronal processes.

A particularly interesting focus for exploring a possible cellular alphabet for learning is the analysis of higher order features of classical conditioning. These features provide an important bridge between the experimental study of conditioning, which has been largely carried out in animals, and cognitive psychology, which until recently has been primarily concerned with human mentation. Furthermore, some of these higher order features (second-order conditioning, blocking, and an unconditioned stimulus [US] preexposure effect) have been shown to occur in conditioning of a terrestrial mollusc, *Limax maximus* (Sahley, Rudy, & Gelperin, 1981), and recent experiments suggest that another feature (the effect of contingency) occurs in *Aplysia* (Hawkins, Carew, & Kandel, 1983). It therefore may be possible to apply a cellular analysis to these aspects of conditioning in invertebrates.

Our purpose in this brief theoretical review is to illustrate that several higher order features of classical conditioning can be derived from our current understanding of the cellular mechanisms of habituation, sensitization, and classical conditioning. Studies by Kamin, Rescorla, Wagner, Mackintosh, and others have shown that these higher order features of conditioning appear to involve cognition in the sense that the animal's behavior depends on a comparison of current sensory input with an internal representation of the world (Dickinson & Mackintosh, 1978; Kamin, 1969; Rescorla, 1978; Wagner, 1978). Our goal is thus to suggest how cognitive psychology may begin to converge with neurobiology to yield a new perspective in the study of learning. The perspective we suggest is similar in some ways to that of Hull (1943), who attempted 40 years ago to explain a variety of complex forms of learning in terms of principles derived from simpler forms of learning. Our perspective differs from that of Hull, however, in that his system was based on postulates inferred from behavior, whereas our approach is based on directly observable cellular processes. We believe that a cell-biological approach to the rules of learning may be more fruitful, because it attempts to explain higher level phenomena (behavior) in terms of more basic phenomena (cell biology) and thus avoids some of the circularity inherent in a purely behavioral approach. Our approach also differs from that of theoreticians who have attempted to explain behavioral phenomena in terms of hypothetical neural elements (e.g., Hebb, 1949; Rosenblatt, 1962; Sutton & Barto, 1981) in that we have based our thinking on known neural mechanisms.

To illustrate these points, we divide this article into two parts. In the first part, which is empirical, we briefly review research on the cellular mechanisms of two forms of nonassociative learning and one form of associative learning in *Aplysia,* and suggest how these mechanisms form the outline of a cellular alphabet of learning. In the second part, which is theoretical, we show how this alphabet might be used to account for several higher order features of classical conditioning in *Aplysia* and in other animals. Although these proposals are speculative and may not turn out to be correct, we hope that they will at least provide a useful framework for further investigations into the neuronal basis of learning.

Three Forms of Learning in *Aplysia* Have Common Cellular Features

Studies of learning in *Aplysia* have focused on the defensive withdrawal reflexes of the external organs of the mantle cavity. In *Aplysia* and in other molluscs, the mantle cavity, a respiratory chamber housing the gill, is covered by a protective sheet, the mantle shelf, which terminates in a fleshy spout, the siphon. When the siphon or mantle shelf is stimulated by touch, the siphon, mantle shelf, and gill all contract vigorously and withdraw into the mantle cavity. This reflex is analogous to vertebrate defensive escape and withdrawal responses, which can be modified by experience. Unlike vertebrate withdrawal reflexes, however, the *Aplysia* withdrawal reflex is partly monosynaptic—siphon sensory neurons syn-

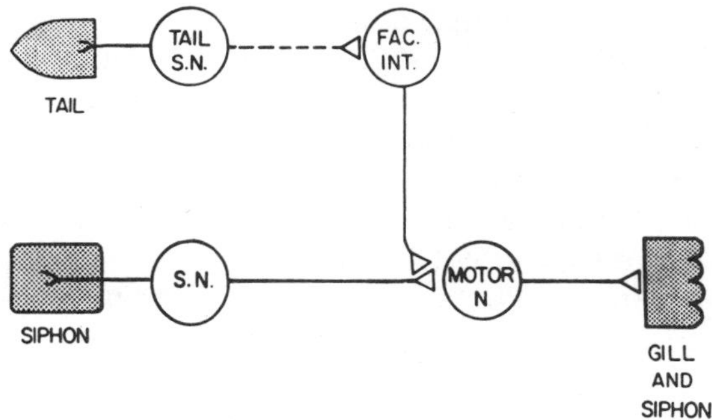

Figure 1. Partial neuronal circuit for the *Aplysia* gill- and siphon-withdrawal reflex and its modification by tail stimulation. (Mechanosensory neurons [S.N.] from the siphon make direct excitatory synaptic connections onto gill and siphon motor neurons. Tail sensory neurons excite facilitator interneurons, which produce presynaptic facilitation of the siphon sensory neurons. Tail stimulation also produces excitation of gill and siphon motor neurons through pathways not shown in Figure 1.)

apse directly on gill and siphon motor neurons (Figure 1). Nonetheless, this simple reflex can be modified by two forms of nonassociative learning, habituation and sensitization, as well as by a form of associative learning, classical conditioning.

Habituation

In habituation, perhaps the simplest form of learning, an animal learns to ignore a weak stimulus that is repeatedly presented when the consequences of the stimulus are neither noxious nor rewarding. Thus, an *Aplysia* initially responds to a tactile stimulus to the siphon by briskly withdrawing its gill and siphon. But with repeated exposure to the stimulus, the animal exhibits reflex responses that are reduced to a fraction of their initial value. Habituation can last from minutes to weeks, depending on the number and pattern of stimulations (Carew, Pinsker, & Kandel, 1972; Pinsker, Kupfermann, Castellucci, & Kandel, 1970).

At the cellular level, the short-term (minutes to hours) form of habituation involves a depression of transmitter release at the synapses that the siphon sensory neurons make on gill and siphon motor neurons and interneurons (Castellucci & Kandel, 1974; Castellucci et al., 1970). This depression involves, at least in part, a decrease in the amount of Ca^{++} that flows into the terminals of the sensory neurons with each action potential (Figure 2, Part A). Because Ca^{++} influx determines how much transmitter is released, a decrease in Ca^{++} influx results in decreased release (Klein, Shapiro, & Kandel, 1980). Long-term habituation appears to involve changes at the same locus, because it is accompanied by a decrease in the number and size of active zones (specialized areas where transmitter is released) at sensory neuron synapses (Bailey & Chen, 1983).

Sensitization

Sensitization is a somewhat more complex form of nonassociative learning in which an animal learns to strengthen its defensive reflexes and to respond vigorously to a variety of previously weak or neutral stimuli after it has been exposed to a potentially threatening or noxious stimulus. Thus, if a noxious sensitizing stimulus is presented to the neck or tail, the siphon- and gill-withdrawal reflexes are enhanced, as are inking, walking, and other defensive behaviors (Pinsker et al., 1970; Walters, Carew, & Kandel, 1981). This enhancement persists from minutes to weeks depending on the number and intensity of the sensitizing stimuli (Pinsker, Hening, Carew, & Kandel, 1973). Sensitization not only enhances normal (naive) reflex responses, but it enhances previously habituated reflex responses. On the cellular level, dishabituation of a previously habituated response by a noxious stimulus has been shown to be a special case of sensitization (Carew, Castellucci, & Kandel, 1971; Spencer et al., 1966).

The short-term (minutes to hours) form of sensitization involves the same cellular locus as habituation, the synapses that the sensory neurons make on their central target cells, and again the learning process involves an alteration in transmitter release—in this case an enhancement in the amount released (Castellucci & Kandel, 1976; Castellucci et al., 1970). But sensitization uses more complex molecular machinery. This machinery has at least five steps (see Figures 1 and 2, Part B): (a) Stimulating the tail activates a group of facilitator neurons that synapse on or near the terminals of the sensory neurons and act there to enhance transmitter release. This process is called *presynaptic facilitation.* (b) The transmitter released by the facilitator neurons, which is presumed to be serotonin or a related amine, activates an adenylate cyclase that increases the level of free cyclic AMP in the terminals of the sensory neurons. (c) Elevation of free cyclic AMP, in turn, activates a second enzyme, a cAMP-dependent protein kinase. (d) The kinase acts by means of protein phosphorylation to close a particular type of K^+ channel and thereby decreases the total number of K^+ channels that are open during the action potential. (e) A decrease in K^+ current leads to broadening of subsequent action potentials, which allows a greater amount of Ca^{++} to flow into the terminal and thus enhances transmitter release (Bailey, Hawkins, & Chen, 1983; Bernier, Castellucci, Kandel, & Schwartz, 1982; Castellucci, Nairn, Greengard, Schwartz, & Kandel, 1982; Hawkins, 1981a, 1981b; Hawkins, Castellucci, & Kandel, 1981b; Kandel & Schwartz, 1982; Kistler, Hawkins, Koester, Kandel, & Schwartz, 1983; Klein & Kandel, 1980; Siegelbaum, Camardo, & Kandel, 1982). Long-term sensitization appears to involve changes at the same locus, because it is accompanied by an increase in the number and size of active zones at sensory neuron synapses (Bailey & Chen, 1983). Kandel and Schwartz (1982) speculate that an increase in cAMP levels may trigger these long-term changes in the sensory neurons in parallel with the short-term changes.

Classical Conditioning

Classical conditioning resembles sensitization in that the response to a stimulus to one pathway is enhanced by activity in another. Typically, in classical conditioning an initially weak or ineffective conditioned stimulus (CS) becomes highly effective in producing a be-

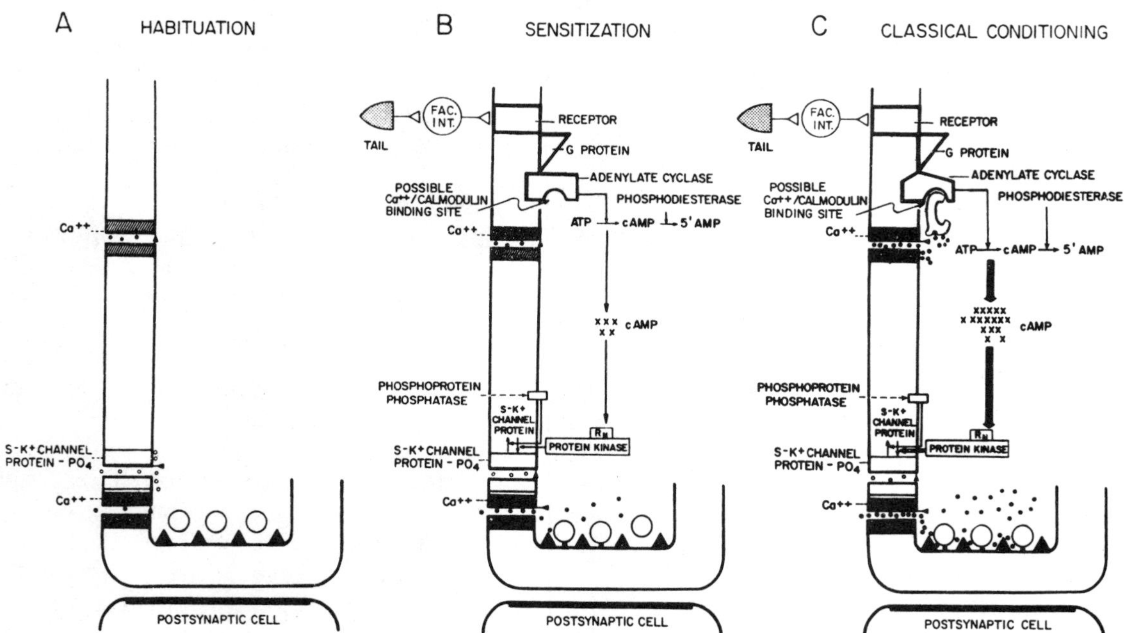

Figure 2. Cellular mechanisms of habituation, sensitization, and classical conditioning of the *Aplysia* gill- and siphon-withdrawal reflex. *Part A.* Habituation. (Repeated stimulation of a siphon sensory neuron, the presynaptic cell in the figure, produces prolonged inactivation of Ca^{++} channels in that neuron [represented by the closed gates], leading to a decrease in Ca^{++} influx during each action potential and decreased transmitter release.) *Part B.* Sensitization. (Stimulation of the tail produces prolonged inactivation of K^+ channels in the siphon sensory neuron through a sequence of steps involving cAMP and protein phosphorylation [see the text for details]. Closing these K^+ channels produces broadening of subsequent action potentials, which in turn produces an increase in Ca^{++} influx and increased transmitter release.) *Part C.* Classical conditioning. (Tail stimulation produces amplified facilitation of transmitter release from the siphon sensory neuron if the tail stimulation is preceded by action potentials in the sensory neuron. This effect may be due to priming of the adenyl cyclase by Ca^{++} that enters the sensory neuron during the action potentials, so that the cyclase produces more cAMP when it is activated by the tail stimulation.)

havioral response after it has been paired temporally with a strong US.[1] Often a reflex can be modified by both sensitization and classical conditioning. In such cases, the response enhancement produced by classical conditioning (paired presentation of the CS and US) is greater and/or lasts longer than the enhancement produced by sensitization (presentation of the US alone). Moreover, whereas the consequences of sensitization are broad and affect defensive responses to a range of stimuli, the effects of classical conditioning are specific and enhance only responses to stimuli that are paired with the US.

In conditioning of the *Aplysia* withdrawal response, the US is a strong shock to the tail that produces a powerful set of defensive responses; the CS is a weak stimulus to the siphon that produces a feeble response. After repeated pairing of the CS and US, the CS becomes more effective and elicits a strong gill- and siphon-withdrawal reflex. Enhancement of this reflex is acquired within 15 trials, is retained for days, extinguishes with repeated presentation of the CS alone, and recovers with rest (Carew, Walters, & Kandel, 1981). The siphon-withdrawal reflex can also be differentially conditioned using stimuli to the siphon and mantle shelf as the discriminative stimuli. Animals in which a CS^+ to the siphon has been paired with a tail shock and a CS^- to the mantle has been presented unpaired with the tail shock, show a greater response to siphon than to mantle stimulation when tested after training. The converse is true when a stimulus to the mantle has been paired, and one to the siphon has been presented unpaired with the tail shock. Using this differential procedure, we have found that a single training trial is sufficient to produce significant learning, and that the learning becomes progressively more robust with more training trials (Carew, Hawkins, & Kandel, 1983).

In many instances of conditioning in vertebrates, learning depends critically on the time between presentation of the CS and US, or the interstimulus interval (ISI). To examine the temporal specificity of conditioning of the withdrawal reflex, we varied the ISI in different groups of animals (Hawkins, Carew, & Kandel, 1983). Significant conditioning occurred when the onset of the CS preceded the onset of the US by 0.5 s, and marginally significant conditioning resulted when the interval between the CS and the US was extended to 1.0 s. In contrast, no significant learning occurred when the CS preceded the US by 2 or more s, when the two stimuli were simultaneous, or, in backward conditioning, when US onset preceded the CS by 0.5 or more s. Thus, conditioning in *Aplysia* resembles conditioning in vertebrates in having a steep ISI function, with optimal learning when the CS precedes the US by approximately 0.5 s (e.g., Gormezano, 1972).

What cellular processes give classical conditioning this characteristic temporal specificity? We have found that classical conditioning of the withdrawal reflex involves a pairing-specific enhancement of presynaptic facilitation (Hawkins et al., 1983). In classical conditioning, because the CS precedes the US, the sensory neurons of the CS pathway are set into activity and fire action potentials just before the facilitator neurons of the US pathway become active. Using a reduced preparation, we have found that if action potentials are generated in a sensory neuron just before the US is delivered, the US produces substantially more facilitation of the synaptic potential from the sensory neuron to a motor neuron than if the US is not paired with activity in the sensory neuron. Pairing spike activity in a sensory neuron with the US also produces greater broadening of the action potential in the sensory neuron than does unpaired stimulation, indicating that the enhancement of facilitation occurs presynaptically. Thus, at least some aspects of the mechanism for the temporal specificity of classical conditioning occur within

[1] We do not distinguish between the appearance of new responses and the strengthening of preexisting responses because we think this difference is not fundamental. Rather, we believe that the neural connections for most or all possible stimulus–response associations are prewired, and training merely alters the strengths of those connections, in some cases bringing the response from below threshold to above threshold. Support for this view comes from experiments in which neural activity is recorded in various regions of the brain during conditioning. For example, at the beginning of an eye-blink-conditioning experiment there is usually no overt response to the auditory conditioned stimulus, but there is a detectable response in the motor nucleus controlling eye blink (e.g., Cegavske, Patterson, & Thompson, 1979). Training strengthens this preexisting neural response until it is above threshold for producing an observable behavioral response.

the sensory neuron itself. We have called this type of enhancement *activity-dependent amplification of presynaptic facilitation* (Hawkins et al., 1983). Similar cellular results have been obtained independently by Walters and Byrne (1983), who have found activity-dependent synaptic facilitation in identified sensory neurons that innervate the tail of *Aplysia*. By contrast, Carew, Hawkins, Abrams, and Kandel (in press) have found that a different type of synaptic plasticity first postulated by Hebb (1949), which has often been thought to underlie learning, does *not* occur at the sensory neuron–motor neuron synapses in the siphon-withdrawal circuit.

These experiments indicate that a mechanism of classical conditioning of the withdrawal reflex is an elaboration of the mechanism of sensitization of the reflex: presynaptic facilitation caused by an increase in action potential duration and Ca^{++} influx in the sensory neurons. The pairing specificity characteristic of classical conditioning results because the presynaptic facilitation is augmented or amplified by temporally paired spike activity in the sensory neurons. We do not yet know which aspect of the action potential in a sensory neuron interacts with the process of presynaptic facilitation to amplify it, nor which step in the biochemical cascade leading to presynaptic facilitation is sensitive to the action potential. As a working hypothesis, Hawkins et al. (1983) proposed that the influx of Ca^{++} with each action potential provides the signal for activity and that it interacts with the serotonin-sensitive adenylate cyclase in the terminals of the sensory neuron so that the cyclase produces more cAMP in response to serotonin (Figure 2, Part C). Recent experiments have supported this hypothesis. Thus, brief application of serotonin to the sensory cells can substitute for tail shock as the US in the cellular experiments, and Ca^{++} must be present in the external medium for paired spike activity to enhance the effect of the serotonin (Abrams, Carew, Hawkins, & Kandel, 1983). Furthermore, serotonin produces a greater increase in cAMP levels in siphon sensory cells if it is preceded by spike activity in the sensory cells than if it is not (Kandel et al., 1983; see also Ocorr, Walters, & Byrne, 1983, for a similar result in *Aplysia* tail sensory neurons).

Is There a Cellular Alphabet for Learning?

The finding that the molecular mechanism of conditioning of the withdrawal reflex appears to be an extension of the mechanism of sensitization suggests two hypotheses about the mechanisms of yet higher forms of learning. These hypotheses assume that learning is not a unitary process, but a family of related processes that range from habituation to insight learning, with conditioning occupying an intermediate position. First, we propose that higher forms of learning may utilize the mechanisms of lower forms of learning as a general rule, and second, we speculate that this may occur because the mechanisms of higher forms of learning have evolved from those of lower forms of learning. It is easy to imagine how the cellular mechanism of conditioning in *Aplysia* might have evolved from the mechanism of sensitization. For example, a small change in the adenyl cyclase might have made it sensitive to Ca^{++} that enters the cell during an action potential, thus giving rise to the activity dependence of facilitation. This example suggests that the mechanisms of yet higher forms of learning may similarly have evolved from the mechanism of conditioning. Higher forms of learning may also use the mechanisms of lower forms of learning within an individual animal. Thus, whereas single neurons may possess only a few fundamental types of plasticity which are used in all forms of learning, combining the neurons in large numbers with specific synaptic connections (as occurs for example in mammalian cortex) may produce the much more subtle and varied processes required for more advanced types of learning.

We illustrate this idea at an elementary level by showing how some of the higher order features of classical conditioning might be generated by small systems of neurons utilizing known types of synaptic plasticity. For the most part, our proposals are simply attempts to translate into neuronal terms ideas that have been proposed at an abstract level by experimental psychologists. In this, we are particularly indebted to the theories of conditioning of Rescorla and Wagner. As an exercise, we have arbitrarily restricted ourselves to the use of physiological processes and neuronal connections that are known to occur in the neural circuit underlying the *Aplysia* gill- and siphon-withdrawal reflex. We should emphasize, however, that some of the higher order behavioral phenomena discussed have not yet been tested in *Aplysia*. Our arguments on these points are therefore entirely speculative and are simply meant to illustrate an initial approach to the problem of relating cognitive processes to neuronal events.

Several Higher Order Features of Classical Conditioning Can Be Derived From the Cellular Mechanisms of Simpler Forms of Learning

Classical conditioning has two attractive features that account for its central role in the analysis of learning. The first is that in acquiring a conditioned response, an animal learns a fundamental relationship about the environment: that the CS predicts and may appear to cause the US. Second, classical conditioning is accompanied by several higher order effects. Some of these were first described by Pavlov and the early students of associative learning; others have more recently been described by Kamin, Rescorla, Wagner, and others who have been interested in the cognitive or information-processing aspects of learning. According to this cognitive view, the animal builds an image of the external world, compares the image of the world with reality—with the view of the world as validated by current sensory information—and then modifies its behavior accordingly.

In light of the evidence for a cellular relationship between habituation, sensitization, and classical conditioning, it becomes interesting to examine the possibility that a general cellular alphabet exists for a wide variety of learning processes. Can combinations of the elementary mechanisms used in habituation, sensitization, and conditioning account for additional higher order aspects of associative learning without requiring additional cellular mechanisms? Here we consider five higher order features: (a) stimulus specificity and generalization, (b) extinction and spontaneous recovery, (c) second-order conditioning, (d) blocking, and (e) degeneration of learning by intermittent presentation of US alone or US preexposure. The explanations that we propose for these phenomena are not meant to be exclusive. Rather, we wish only to indicate how simple cellular processes such as synaptic depression and facilitation can be used in different combinatorial ways to contribute to these higher order features of behavior.

Stimulus Specificity and Generalization

Animals learn to respond to the conditioned stimulus and not to other irrelevant stimuli. Activity-dependent enhancement of presynaptic facilitation readily confers this stimulus specificity (Figure 3): Only those sensory neurons that are active preceding the US undergo the amplified form of presynaptic facilitation, and thus only the response to the paired conditioned stimulus is selectively enhanced (see also Carew et al., 1983; Hawkins et al., 1983).

Stimulus specificity is not generally complete, however. After conditioning, animals respond to stimuli other than the conditioned stimulus, and the strength of their response depends on the degree of similarity between the test stimulus and the conditioned stimulus. We suggest two cellular explanations for stimulus generalization. The first is sensitization: An aversive unconditioned stimulus produces some enhancement of defensive responses to *all* stimuli, whether they are paired with it or not. This enhancement is simply greater for the paired stimuli. The second explanation (which is basically similar to those proposed by Atkinson & Estes, 1963, and Bush & Mosteller, 1951) is that there will be some overlap in the sensory neurons and interneurons excited by different stimuli. Thus, conditioning of one stimulus produces amplified presynaptic facilitation of some (but not all) of the neurons that are excited by a second stimulus, and therefore produces partial enhancement of the response to the second stimulus. The greater the similarity between the stimuli, the more overlap there is in the neurons they excite, and consequently, the more generalization. This mechanism can account for a wider range of generalization if activity-dependent amplification of presynaptic facilitation occurs not only at sensory neurons but also at interneurons. We believe that this is likely to be true, because we have no reason to think that the sensory neurons are unique in this regard.

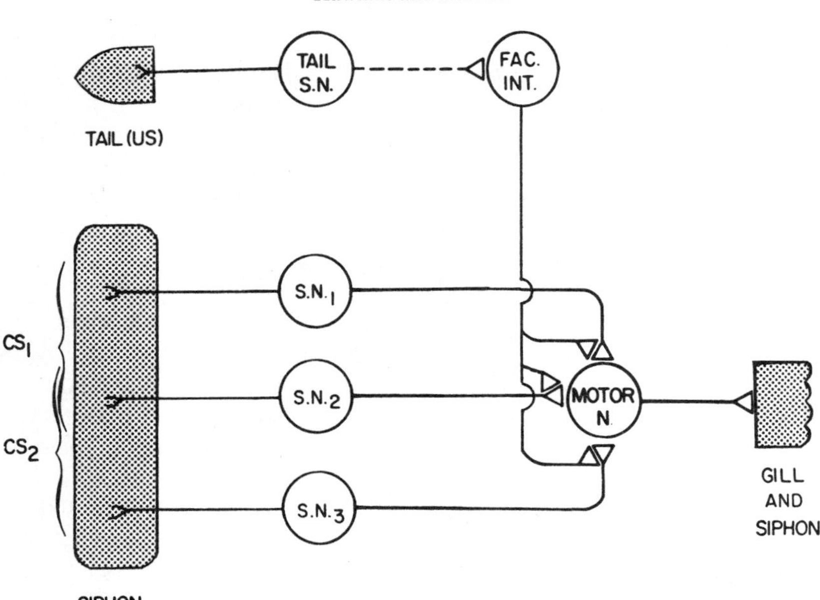

Figure 3. Proposed cellular mechanisms of stimulus specificity and generalization. (CS_1 excites siphon sensory neurons 1 and 2, and CS_2 excites neurons 2 and 3. Only those sensory neurons that are active preceding the US undergo the amplified form of presynaptic facilitation. Thus, conditioning of CS_1 produces partial, but not complete, generalization to CS_2.)

Extinction and Spontaneous Recovery

The conditioned response can be eliminated by extinction: If the CS is presented repeatedly without reinforcement by the US, the response to the CS gradually diminishes and eventually disappears. Extinction, however, does not return an animal to its naive state. A number of experimental procedures can restore or reinstate an animal's response to the conditioned stimulus. For example, if the CS is not presented for some time following extinction, the animal's response to the CS recovers, either partially or completely, thereby indicating that the animal remembers the original training.

We suggest that extinction and spontaneous recovery represent, at least in part, an interaction between habituation and classical conditioning. Thus, after the CS pathway has been classically conditioned, it can still undergo habituation due to synaptic depression of the input from the CS to the motor neurons. Because habituation has a different neuronal mechanism than does classical conditioning, its time course could be dramatically different. For example, if the CS is presented only a few times during extinction, the habituation produced would wear off rapidly. As a result, as the habituation (extinction) faded, learning would again become manifest (spontaneous recovery) in the response of the CS pathway (Figure 4).

Another procedure that reverses the effects of extinction is the presentation of a strong extraneous stimulus. Pavlov (1927) referred to this phenomenon as disinhibition, because he thought that extinction was due to inhibition that the extraneous stimulus removed. Because the characteristics of disinhibiting stimuli are

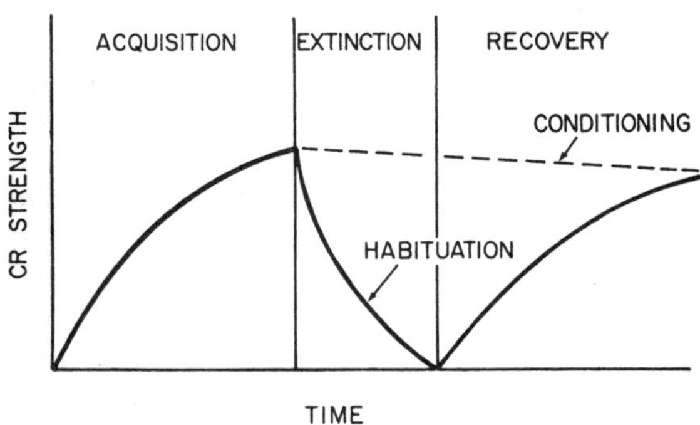

Figure 4. Proposed cellular mechanisms of extinction and spontaneous recovery. (Repeated presentation of the conditioned stimulus [CS] during extinction produces habituation of the response to that CS, and the response recovers with rest. These processes are superimposed on the memory for the conditioning, the dashed line.)

similar to those of sensitizing stimuli, however, we would argue that disinhibition is simply due to sensitization, as has been shown for dishabituation (Carew et al., 1971; Groves & Thompson, 1970; Spencer et al., 1966). There are several other parallels between extinction and habituation. For example, both processes generally occur faster with a shorter ITI, and both occur more rapidly if the training is repeated after a period of rest (Pavlov, 1927; Thompson & Spencer, 1966). These similarities support the idea that extinction has the same neuronal mechanism as habituation, which in *Aplysia* is synaptic depression.

Second-Order Conditioning

Second-order conditioning is the process whereby events that formerly did not reinforce behavior become reinforcing. In the first stage of a second-order conditioning experiment, an effective US is used to reinforce and thereby strengthen the response to an initially ineffective CS_1 by pairing the two stimuli (CS_1–US). After such pairing, CS_1 itself can now serve as a reinforcing stimulus to strengthen the response to a new conditioned stimulus, CS_2, if those two stimuli are paired (CS_2–CS_1). Second-order conditioning is thought to be ubiquitous in everyday life and to bridge the gap between laboratory experiments and complex natural behavior, which often does not have obvious reinforcers. Second-order conditioning also illustrates the interchangeability of the CS and the US, because the same stimulus can serve as either a CS or a US in a conditioning experiment.

Before considering a possible cellular mechanism of second-order conditioning, we must introduce three additional features of the neural circuitry of *Aplysia* that we believe may be general and that are important for the arguments that follow (Figure 5). First, in addition to the US, many CS inputs excite the

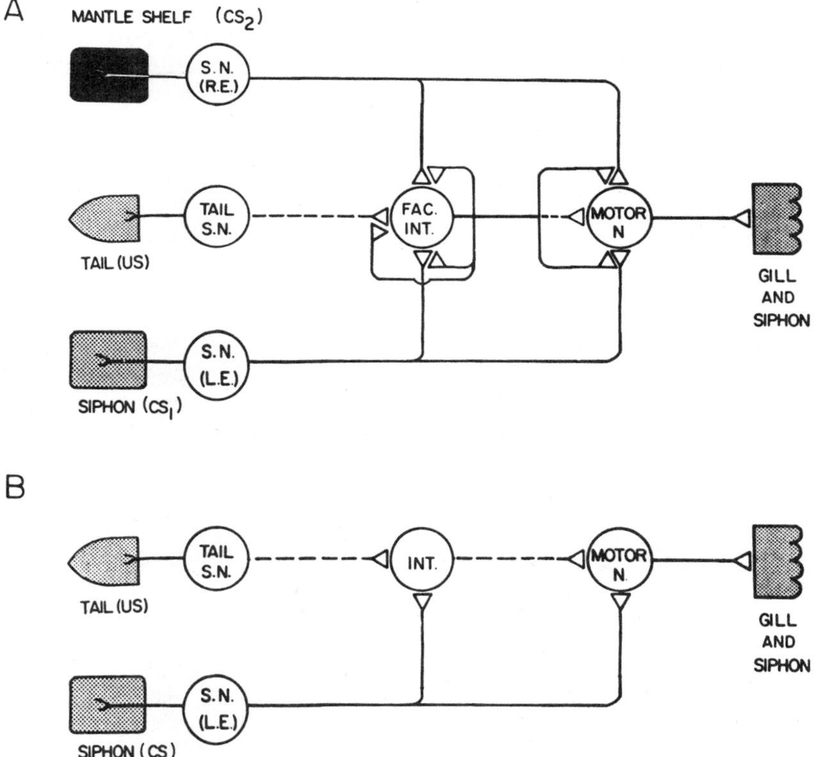

Figure 5. More complete neuronal circuit for the gill- and siphon-withdrawal reflex and its modification by tail stimulation. *Part A.* Circuit for differential conditioning of responses to stimulation of the siphon and mantle shelf. (The siphon is innervated by the LE cluster of sensory neurons and the mantle is innervated by the RE cluster.) *Part B.* Simplified version of Part A, illustrating possible neural representations of S–R and S–S learning (see the text).

facilitator neurons. Thus, the facilitator neurons may be thought of as a local arousal system (for earlier discussion of this point see Hawkins & Advocat, 1977; Kandel, 1978). Second, the facilitator neurons produce facilitation not only at the synapses from the sensory neurons to the motor neurons but also at the synapses from the sensory neurons to many interneurons, *including the synapses from the sensory neurons to the facilitator neurons themselves.* This fact has the interesting consequence that the sensory–facilitator synapses (unlike the sensory–motor synapses) should act like Hebb synapses. That is, firing a sensory neuron just before firing the facilitator should produce selective strengthening of the synapse from that sensory neuron to the facilitator (compared to other inputs onto the facilitator) because of activity-dependent enhancement of the facilitation. Third, the facilitator neurons also excite gill and siphon motor neurons, either directly or indirectly (Hawkins, Castellucci, & Kandel, 1981a).

Figure 5, Part A, illustrates how our model of conditioning could account for second-order effects. Once a particular pathway, for example, the siphon, is paired repeatedly with an unconditioned stimulus (to the tail), the CS pathway from the siphon becomes effective in producing a much stronger gill contraction. Moreover, activity-dependent enhancement of presynaptic facilitation occurs not only at the sensory–motor synapse but also at the sensory–facilitator synapse, increasing the ability of the CS to excite the facilitator neurons. As a result, the CS pathway now, in effect, becomes a potential US pathway, and CS_1 from the siphon might be able to serve as a US for conditioning of responses to stimulation of other sites such as the mantle (CS_2).

Second-order conditioning thus demonstrates that, in addition to changing the ability of a stimulus to produce a motor response, learning also changes the ability of the stimulus to gain access to some of the internal processing machinery over which the US previously had predominant control. This aspect of our neuronal model also suggests a possible reconciliation of two competing theories of learning. On the one hand, Guthrie (1935), Hull (1943), and others have proposed that an association is formed between the conditioned stimulus and the response (S–R) in classical conditioning. On the other hand, theorists such as Tolman (1932) have proposed that associations are formed between the experimental stimuli (S–S). This S–S viewpoint seems closer to Pavlov's (1927) idea that the conditioned stimulus comes to substitute for the unconditioned stimulus, and thereby produces a response similar to the unconditioned response. Figure 5, Part B, which is a simplified version of Figure 5, Part A, shows that our model incorporates extremely simple neural representations of each of these theories. Thus, changes at the sensory–motor synapses in Figure 5 are obviously consistent with S–R theories, whereas changes at the sensory–interneuron synapses are consistent with S–S theories, because those changes can be thought of as the process by which one stimulus (the CS) comes to substitute for another (the US) in the animal's internal processing machinery. This argument may seem more plausible if the interneuron in Figure 5, Part B is considered as a sensory interneuron, so that the CS comes to produce perceptions in some sense similar to those produced by the US.[2]

Our simple neuronal model therefore suggests that any instance of learning produces both S–R and S–S types of neuronal changes, with the type expressed perhaps depending on the experimental circumstances. For example, Rescorla and his colleagues have found that habituating the US following second-order conditioning decreases the response to CS_1, but habituating either the US or CS_1 does not decrease the response to CS_2 (Rescorla, 1973). Rescorla has interpreted these results as showing that first-order conditioning is predominantly S–S (that is, CS_1 is associated with the US, which in turn is associated with the response), whereas second-order conditioning is predominately S–R (that is, CS_2 is associated

[2] The interneuron in Figure 5 can be considered as a sensory interneuron, motor interneuron, or facilitator neuron. In the neuronal circuit for a more complex behavior these functions would presumably be distributed between different interneurons, so that the single interneuron in Figure 5 can be thought of as representing many different interneurons in a more complex circuit. In this case, we are considering it as a sensory interneuron in the US pathway and assuming that firing of that interneuron corresponds to the perception or recollection of some aspect of the US.

directly with the response). The circuit shown in Figure 5 could provide a neuronal explanation for Rescorla's results given two additional assumptions: first, that the interneuron has a discrete threshold for firing, and second, that habituation of the US is accompanied by depression at the interneuron–motor neuron synapse. We also suppose that following second-order conditioning the synaptic strengths of the sensory neurons for CS_1 are greater than those for CS_2, so that CS_1 is strong enough to fire the interneuron but CS_2 is not. CS_1 therefore excites the motor neuron both directly and via the interneuron, whereas CS_2 acts only directly. Under these circumstances habituation of the US decreases the indirect component of the response to CS_1 (due to depression at the interneuron–motor neuron synapse) but does not affect the response to CS_2. Similarly, habituation of CS_1 has no effect on the response to CS_2. This argument is essentially a neuronal version of Rescorla's suggestion that the response to CS_1 has an S–S component, whereas the response to CS_2 is purely S–R.

Blocking

Experimental psychologists have shown that animals learn not only about the temporal pairing or contiguity of stimuli, but also about their correlation or contingency—that is, how well one stimulus predicts another (e.g., Kamin, 1969; Rescorla, 1968). The cellular mechanism we have described for classical conditioning of the *Aplysia* siphon-withdrawal reflex (Hawkins et al., 1983) can account for learning about contiguity, but it cannot directly account for learning about predictability. We suggest that the circuitry shown in Figure 5 might also explain a class of learning phenomena having to do with the predictability of the stimuli, including blocking, overshadowing, and the effect of contingency. We illustrate this point by using blocking as an example. In the first stage of a blocking experiment, CS_1 is conditioned as usual. In the second stage, a second CS (CS_2) is added to CS_1 and the compound stimulus CS_1CS_2 is paired with the US. Generally, there is little conditioning of CS_2, although controls show that good conditioning of CS_2 is obtained if CS_1 is omitted or if CS_1 was not previously conditioned. A cognitive explanation that has been proposed is that an animal forms expectations about the world, compares current input with those expectations, and learns only when something unpredicted happens (Kamin, 1969). Because CS_1 comes to predict the US in the first stage of training, in the second stage the compound CS_1CS_2 is not followed by anything unexpected and, therefore, little conditioning occurs. Rescorla and Wagner (1972) have formalized this explanation by suggesting that the strength of conditioning is proportional to the difference between the strength of the CS and that of the US. They expressed this relationship in the following equation: $\Delta V_i = K(\lambda - \Sigma V_i)$, where V_i is the associative strength of element *i*, ΔV_i is the change in that strength on a given trial, K is a constant, and λ is the maximum strength attainable with the US being used. At the beginning of the first stage of training, the strength of CS_1 (V_1) is small, $\lambda - V_1$ is large, and the increment in the strength of CS_1 (ΔV_1) on each trial is large. As training progresses, V_1 becomes larger, ΔV_1 becomes smaller, and V_1 gradually approaches λ. When the second stage of training starts, the strength of CS_2 (V_2) is small, but the sum of V_1 and V_2 (ΣV_i) is nearly equal to λ, so there is little further change in the strengths of either CS_1 or CS_2.

A possible cellular embodiment of this proposal requires an additional assumption, which is that the output of the facilitator neurons decreases when they are stimulated continuously. This mechanism is similar to one that has recently been proposed on theoretical grounds by Wagner (1981), who suggests that activity in the US node in a memory network puts that node in a refractory state for a transient period. (This could occur in *Aplysia* for two reasons: The facilitator neurons undergo accommodation and receive recurrent inhibition, both of which tend to make the facilitators fire only at the onset of a sustained stimulus—Hawkins et al., 1981a and unpublished.) Thus, as the synapses from CS_1 to the facilitator neurons become progressively strengthened during the first stage of training, the facilitator neurons fire more during CS_1 and consequently less during the US (due to the accommodation and recurrent inhibition caused by the firing during CS_1—see Figure 6). This process reaches an assymptote when the firing during CS_1 is strong enough to prevent firing during the US.[3] Thus, when training with the compound stimulus CS_1CS_2 starts in the second stage of training, CS_2 is not followed by firing in the facilitator neurons, and therefore CS_2 does not become conditioned. Firing of the facilitator neurons at the *onset* of CS_2 does not produce amplified facilitation because that process requires a delay between CS onset and the onset of facilitation.

As Rescorla and Wagner (1972) point out, a similar explanation would apply if the same two types of trials (CS_1–US and CS_1CS_2–US) were alternated or intermixed, instead of being presented in two stages of training. According to the model we have described, early in training both CS_1 and CS_2 would gain in associative strength, but CS_1 would gain faster because it is paired with the US more frequently. This process would continue until the combined strength of CS_1 and CS_2 equaled the strength of the US. At that point the compound stimulus CS_1CS_2 would cause enough accommodation and recurrent inhibition in the facilitator neurons to prevent firing during the US, and no further conditioning would occur on the compound (CS_1CS_2–US) trials. In fact, CS_2 would then tend to undergo extinction, and the response to CS_2 would decline to some low level. CS_1 would also undergo extinction on the compound trials, but it would continue to be conditioned on the CS_1–US trials and would gain in strength until its strength equaled that of the US.

These examples illustrate that our model incorporates in very rudimentary forms the notions of predictability and internal representation. The predicted effect of CS_1 is represented internally as the strength of the synapse from CS_1 to the facilitator neuron. The actual consequences of CS_1 are compared to this prediction through the operations of accommodation and recurrent inhibition, which in effect subtract the strength of CS_1 from the strength of the US that follows it. When these

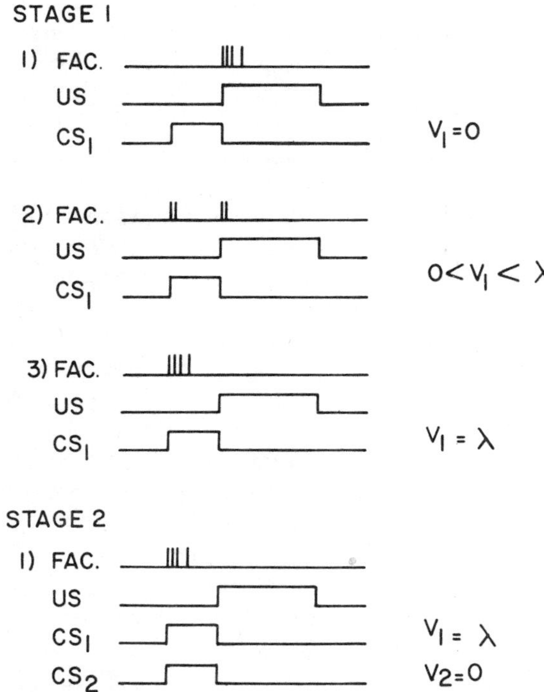

Figure 6. Proposed cellular mechanism of blocking. (As conditioning of CS_1 proceeds [Stage 1, Trials 1, 2, and 3] the facilitator neurons fire more during the conditioned stimulus [CS] period. This firing produces accommodation and recurrent inhibition, which reduce firing during the US period. When compound conditioning starts [Stage 2], CS_2 is not followed by firing of the facilitator neurons and therefore does not become conditioned.)

[3] This is a simplification. Like the Rescorla-Wagner model, our model suggests that the strength of conditioning approaches an assymptote because the US becomes progressively less effective. Unlike Rescorla and Wagner, however, we do not predict that the assymptote of conditioning is reached when the strength of the CS equals the strength of the US, but rather at a somewhat lower level. This is because our model includes synaptic depression as well as facilitation. In this respect, it is similar to the model of habituation of Groves and Thompson (1970), who proposed that presentation of any stimulus tends to elicit two competing processes: facilitation of that stimulus pathway via excitation of facilitator neurons, and depression of that stimulus pathway through a homosynaptic mechanism. The net result depends on the balance of the two processes. As Groves and Thompson (1970) point out, this two-process model can explain why repeated presentation of the same stimulus sometimes produces sensitization rather than habituation (see Hawkins et al., 1981b for a similar argument based on the circuit shown in Figure 5, Part A). We have attempted to extend this type of model to classical conditioning. Thus, we propose that on trials early in training, facilitation of the CS pathway caused by firing of the facilitator neurons is greater than depression of the CS pathway caused by firing of the sensory neurons, and therefore the reflex is strengthened. With continued training, the facilitation becomes progressively weaker, and the assymptote of acquisition is reached when the facilitation and depression are equal. During extinction, the facilitator neurons fire even less on each trial than they did at the assymptote of acquisition (because they are excited only by the CS, whereas during acquisition they are excited by both the CS and the US), and therefore depression predominates until a new equilibrium is reached.

two strengths become equal, CS_1 can be said to fully predict the US, which thus loses its reinforcing power, and no further learning occurs. This subtraction process has the additional benefit of setting an upper limit on a positive feedback circuit, thus circumventing a number of theoretical problems that have plagued Hebb-type models.

Degeneration of Learning by Intermittent Presentations of the US Alone or US Preexposure

In classical conditioning, animals do not simply learn that the CS precedes the US (contiguity), but they also learn the contingency or correlation between the CS and US; that is, they learn how well one event predicts another. Thus, if unannounced USs occur between pairing trials, the ability of the CS to predict the US is reduced and learning degenerates. In the limit, if the probability of unannounced USs is the same as the probability of announced (paired) USs so that there is zero contingency, animals do not learn to associate the CS and US despite the fact that they are paired many times (Rescorla, 1968).

Rescorla and Wagner (1972) proposed that this effect could be explained by an extension of the argument they advanced for blocking, simply by including in the analysis the stimuli that are always present in the experimental situation (the background stimuli). Thus, a zero-contingency experiment can be considered as a blocking experiment in which CS background–US trials are intermixed with background–US trials. By the same argument that is outlined above, this would prevent conditioning to the experimental CS. Our cellular version of this argument requires that the conditioned background stimuli be capable of causing continuous excitation of the facilitator neurons, making them unresponsive to the US. Such continuous excitation of the facilitator neurons might be the neural representation of a state of conditioned anxiety.

Our neuronal explanation for blocking involves a rather short-term decrease in the output of the facilitator neurons during and following excitation of those neurons. The idea that the CS and US are interchangeable suggests a second explanation of the effect of contingency, which involves a long-term decrease in the input to the facilitator neurons. Just as the CS pathway habituates with repeated presentations during extinction, so also might the US pathway undergo habituation with repeated presentations of the US. In a zero-contingency experiment, the unannounced US presentations would cause habituation to the US input, which would make the US less effective on the CS–US trials. If this effect was strong enough, it would more than compensate for the extra sensitization of the CS pathway caused by the unannounced US presentations. Figure 7 illustrates how this might work in an experiment in which animals receive either five trials of normal differential conditioning, or the same five trials plus five unpredicted US presentations. In this hypothetical example

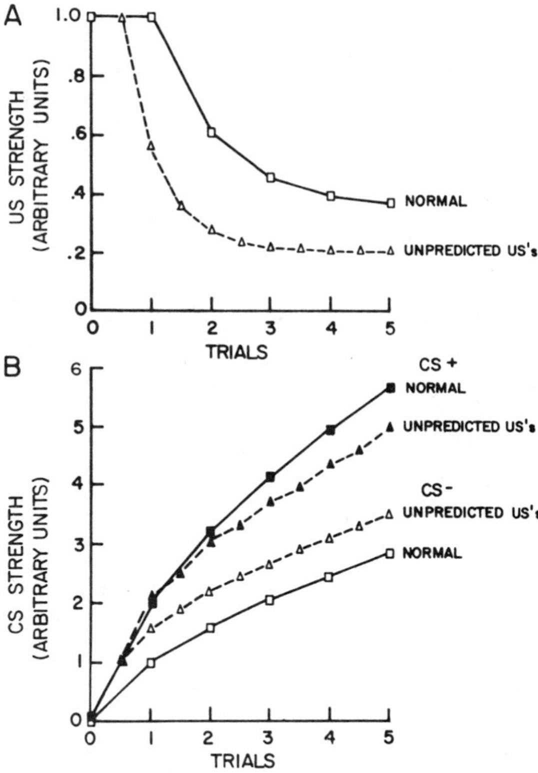

Figure 7. Proposed cellular mechanism of degeneration of learning by intermittent presentation of the unconditioned stimulus (US). *Part A.* US strength on each trial in a hypothetical experiment described in the text. (The US strength is assumed to decrease by 50% with each US presentation and to recover with a time constant of 20 min.) *Part B.* Conditioned stimulus (CS) strength on each trial in the same hypothetical experiment. (The CS is assumed to increase in strength by an amount proportional to the US strength when the US is presented alone, and by twice that amount when the US is paired with the CS.)

the addition of unpredicted USs would not only cause a decrease in the difference between the strengths of the CS^+ and CS^-, but would also cause a decrease in the absolute strength of the CS^+. Results similar to those shown in Figure 7, Part B, have recently been obtained in *Aplysia* in an experiment with this design (Hawkins, Carew, & Kandel, 1983).

We have suggested two alternate explanations for degeneration of conditioning by presentation of unannounced USs: conditioning of background stimuli (based on our neuronal version of the Rescorla-Wagner model) and habituation of the US input. It may be possible to test these alternatives by performing an experiment in which the additional USs are signaled by a second CS (that is, alternating CS_1–US and CS_2–US trials). The Rescorla-Wagner model predicts that conditioning of CS_1 in this case should be nearly the same as that produced by simple CS_1–US training, whereas the US habituation model predicts that conditioning of CS_1 should be reduced (unless pairing with a CS somehow prevents habituation of the US).

Learning can be impaired by unannounced presentations of the US *before* paired training begins as well as by unannounced USs during training. This treatment, which is called *US preexposure,* is thought to reduce the surprising or novel properties of the US and thus to reduce its effectiveness as a reinforcer. The neuronal mechanism of US preexposure could be the same as either (or both) of the mechanisms proposed above for degeneration of learning by unannounced presentations of the US during training, that is, either conditioning of background stimuli or habituation of the US input. The example of US habituation shown in Figure 7 includes one US preexposure, that contributes significantly to the net effect of the unannounced US presentations in that example.

Conclusion

The approach we have presented here attempts to explain a number of higher order features of learning by combinations of the cellular mechanisms used in simple forms of learning. In particular, we have tried to provide neuronal versions of the Rescorla and Wagner models of conditioning so as to explain some of the phenomena those models address, including bocking and the effect of contingency. A basic feature of the Rescorla and Wagner models is that learning depends on the degree to which the US is surprising or unpredicted. In our neuronal model we propose that the concepts of predictability and surprise can be related to the more elementary concepts of habituation and sensitization, because the neuronal mechanism for predictability may be the same as that for habituation (synaptic depression or accommodation), and the neuronal mechanism for surprise may be the same as that for sensitization (conventional or activity-dependent presynaptic facilitation). Combinations of these mechanisms might also explain other learning phenomena that we have not discussed here including overshadowing, latent inhibition and the effects of partial reinforcement, intertrial interval, CS strength, and US strength.

The model we describe differs from the Rescorla and Wagner models in an important way: It does not provide for negative learning in a way that is symmetrical with positive learning. Rather, our model depends on synaptic depression for negative learning. Thus, it is basically a two-process model, with the two processes being facilitation and depression. We believe that depression can adequately account for negative learning, although we realize that in many cases the predictions of a competing process model like ours are not obvious and that quantitative simulations are necessary. Our model cannot, however, account for learned inhibition—the actual reversal of sign of the effect of the CS—because the lowest depression can go is zero. Thus our model provides no insight into conditioned inhibition and related learning phenomena. This is not because we have any quarrel with those phenomena, but rather because we have restricted ourselves to the *Aplysia* circuitry shown in Figure 5, which does not include any inhibitory neurons. We do not yet know whether conditioned inhibition occurs in conditioning of the *Aplysia* withdrawal reflex, but if it does occur, we assume it could be modeled by the addition of inhibitory elements to the circuit shown in Figure 5.[4] Like the Rescorla-Wagner

[4] Figure 5 shows the minimal neuronal circuit necessary to account for differential conditioning of the gill- and

model, our model also has little to say about many other phenomena in the learning literature such as sensory preconditioning and the exact nature of the conditioned response.

In conclusion, we would emphasize the speculative nature of these proposals. First, although we have used cellular processes and patterns of neuronal connections known to occur in *Aplysia,* not all of the behavioral phenomena we have discussed have yet been demonstrated in *Aplysia.* Conditioning of the gill- and siphon-withdrawal reflex of *Aplysia* shows stimulus specificity, extinction, recovery, and the effect of contingency. Second-order conditioning, blocking, and US preexposure have not been tested in *Aplysia* (although they have been demonstrated in another mollusc, *Limax maximus*). Thus, there is no compelling reason to think that cellular processes that have been observed in *Aplysia* are relevant to all of these behavioral phenomena. Second, we do not provide any data suggesting that higher order features of conditioning must necessarily emerge from the basic cellular mechanisms of more elementary forms of learning. Nor would we argue that participation of the cellular mechanisms that we have outlined here in higher order features of conditioning would provide evidence for their role in yet more sophisticated types of learning. We would only argue that available evidence suggests that classical conditioning and sensitization are not fundamentally different, as is frequently thought, but rather the cellular mechanism of conditioning appears to be an elaboration of the mechanism of sensitization. We have attempted to extend this argument by suggesting that there may be a cellular alphabet of learning and that surprisingly complex forms of learning might be generated from combinations of this alphabet of simple cellular mechanisms. Most important, however, the hypotheses we have described should be testable on the neuronal level in several invertebrates. These tests should in turn indicate the degree to which the notions we have proposed here are useful.

---

siphon-withdrawal reflex and is not complete. Several known interneurons, including one inhibitory interneuron have been omitted, and many other interneurons have probably not yet been discovered. For a more complete description of the known neuronal circuit, see Hawkins et al. (1981a).

References

Abrams, T. W., Carew, T. J., Hawkins, R. D., & Kandel, E. R. (1983). Aspects of the cellular mechanism of temporal specificity in conditioning in *Aplysia:* Preliminary evidence for Ca^{2+} influx as a signal of activity. *Society for Neuroscience Abstracts, 9,* 168.

Alkon, D. L. (1979). Voltage-dependent calcium and potassium ion conductances: A contingency mechanism for an associative learning model. *Science, 205,* 810–816.

Atkinson, R. C., & Estes, W. K. (1963). Stimulus sampling theory. In R. D. Luce, R. R. Bush, & E. Galanter (Eds.), *Handbook of mathematical psychology* (Vol. 2, pp. 121–268). New York: Wiley.

Bailey, C. H., & Chen, M. (1983). Morphological basis of long-term habituation and sensitization in *Aplysia. Science, 220,* 91–93.

Bailey, C. H., Hawkins, R. D., & Chen, M. (1983). Uptake of [^{3}H] serotonin in the abdominal ganglion of *Aplysia californica:* Further studies on the morphological and biochemical basis of presynaptic facilitation. *Brain Research, 272,* 71–81.

Bernier, L., Castellucci, V. F., Kandel, E. R., & Schwartz, J. H. (1982). Facilitatory transmitter causes a selective and prolonged increase in adenosine 3′:5′-monophosphate in sensory neurons mediating the gill and siphon withdrawal reflex in *Aplysia. Journal of Neuroscience, 2,* 1682–1691.

Bush, R. R., & Mosteller, F. (1951). A model for stimulus generalization and discrimination. *Psychological Review, 58,* 413–423.

Byers, D., Davis, R. L., & Kiger, J. A. (1981). Defect in cyclic AMP phosphodiesterase due to the dunce mutation of learning in *Drosophila melanogaster. Nature (London), 289,* 79–81.

Carew, T. J., Castellucci, V. F., & Kandel, E. R. (1971). An analysis of dishabituation and sensitization of the gill-withdrawal reflex in *Aplysia. International Journal of Neuroscience, 2,* 79–98.

Carew, T. J., Hawkins, R. D., Abrams, T. W., & Kandel, E. R. (in press). A test of Hebb's postulate at identified synapses which mediate classical conditioning in *Aplysia. Journal of Neuroscience.*

Carew, T. J., Hawkins, R. D., & Kandel, E. R. (1983). Differential classical conditioning of a defensive withdrawal reflex in *Aplysia californica. Science, 219,* 397–400.

Carew, T. J., Pinsker, H. M., & Kandel, E. R. (1972). Long-term habituation of a defensive withdrawal reflex in *Aplysia. Science, 175,* 451–454.

Carew, T. J., Walters, E. T., & Kandel, E. R. (1981). Classical conditioning in a simple withdrawal reflex in *Aplysia californica. Journal of Neuroscience, 1,* 1426–1437.

Castellucci, V. F., & Kandel, E. R. (1974). A quantal analysis of the synaptic depression underlying habituation of the gill-withdrawal reflex in *Aplysia. Proceedings of the National Academy of Sciences of the U.S.A., 71,* 5004–5008.

Castellucci, V., & Kandel, E. R. (1976). Presynaptic facilitation as a mechanism for behavioral sensitization in *Aplysia. Science, 194,* 1176–1178.

Castellucci, V. F., Nairn, A., Greengard, P., Schwartz, J. H., & Kandel, E. R. (1982). Inhibitor of adenosine 3′:5′-monophosphate-dependent protein kinase blocks presynaptic facilitation in *Aplysia. Journal of Neuroscience, 2,* 1673–1681.

Castellucci, V., Pinsker, H., Kupfermann, I., & Kandel, E. R. (1970). Neuronal mechanisms of habituation and dishabituation of the gill-withdrawal reflex in *Aplysia. Science, 167,* 1745–1748.

Cegavske, C. F., Patterson, M. M., & Thompson, R. F. (1979). Neuronal unit activity in the abducens nucleus during classical conditioning of the nictitating membrane response in the rabbit (*Oryctolagus cuniculus*). *Journal of Comparative and Physiological Psychology, 93,* 595–609.

Crow, T.J., & Alkon, D. L. (1980). Associative behavioral modification in *Hermissenda:* Cellular correlates. *Science, 209,* 412–414.

Dickinson, A., & Mackintosh, N. J. (1978). Classical conditioning in animals. *Annual Review of Psychology, 29,* 587–612.

Duerr, J. S., & Quinn, W. G. (1982). Three *Drosophila* mutants that block associative learning also affect habituation and sensitization. *Proceedings of the National Academy of Sciences of the U.S.A., 79,* 3646–3650.

Gormezano, I. (1972). Investigations of defense and reward conditioning in the rabbit. In A. H. Black & W. F. Prokasy (Eds.), *Classical conditioning II: Current research and theory* (pp. 151–181). New York: Appleton-Century-Crofts.

Groves, P. M., & Thompson, R. F. (1970). Habituation: A dual-process theory. *Psychological Review, 77,* 419–450.

Guthrie, E. R. (1935). *The psychology of learning.* New York: Harper.

Hawkins, R. D. (1981a). Identified facilitating neurons are excited by cutaneous stimuli used in sensitization and classical conditioning of *Aplysia. Society for Neuroscience Abstracts, 7,* 354.

Hawkins, R. D. (1981b). Interneurons involved in mediation and modulation of gill-withdrawal reflex in *Aplysia.* III. Identified facilitating neurons increase Ca^{2+} current in sensory neurons. *Journal of Neurophysiology, 45,* 327–339.

Hawkins, R. D., Abrams, T. W., Carew, T. J., & Kandel, E. R. (1983). A cellular mechanism of classical conditioning in *Aplysia:* Activity-dependent amplification of presynaptic facilitation. *Science, 219,* 400–405.

Hawkins, R. D., & Advocat, C. (1977). Effects of behavioral state on the gill-withdrawal reflex in *Aplysia californica. Neuroscience Symposia, 3,* 16–32.

Hawkins, R. D., Carew, T. J., & Kandel, E. R. (1983). Effects of interstimulus interval and contingency on classical conditioning in *Aplysia. Society for Neuroscience Abstracts, 9,* 168.

Hawkins, R. D., Castellucci, V. F., & Kandel, E. R. (1981a). Interneurons involved in mediation and modulation of gill-withdrawal reflex in *Aplysia.* I. Identification and characterization. *Journal of Neurophysiology, 45,* 304–314.

Hawkins, R. D., Castellucci, V. F., & Kandel, E. R. (1981b). Interneurons involved in mediation and modulation of gill-withdrawal reflex in *Aplysia.* II. Identified neurons produce heterosynaptic facilitation contributing to behavioral sensitization. *Journal of Neurophysiology, 45,* 315–326.

Hebb, D. O. (1949). *The organization of behavior.* New York: Wiley.

Hilgard, E. R., & Marquis, D. G. (1940). *Conditioning and learning.* New York: Appleton-Century-Crofts.

Hoyle, G. (1979). Instrumental conditioning of the leg lift in the locust. *Neuroscience Research Program Bulletin, 17,* 577–586.

Hull, C. L. (1943). *Principles of behavior.* New York: Appleton-Century-Crofts.

Kamin, L. J. (1969). Predictability, surprise, attention and conditioning. In B. A. Campbell & R. M. Church (Eds.), *Punishment and aversive behavior* (pp. 279–296). New York: Appleton-Century-Crofts.

Kandel, E. R. (1978). *A cell-biological approach to learning.* Bethesda, MD: Society for Neuroscience.

Kandel, E. R., Abrams, T., Bernier, L., Carew, T. J., Hawkins, R. D., & Schwartz, J. A. (1983). Classical conditioning and sensitization share aspects of the same molecular cascade in *Aplysia. Cold Spring Harbor Symposia on Quantitative Biology, 48,* 821–830.

Kandel, E. R., & Schwartz, J. H. (1982). Molecular biology of learning: Modulation of transmitter release. *Science, 218,* 433–443.

Kistler, H. B. Jr., Hawkins, R. D., Koester, J., Kandel, E. R., & Schwartz, J. H. (1983). Immunocytochemical studies of neurons producing presynaptic facilitation in the abdominal ganglion of *Aplysia californica. Society for Neuroscience Abstracts, 9,* 915.

Klein, M., & Kandel, E. R. (1980). Mechanism of calcium current modulation underlying presynaptic facilitation and behavioral sensitization in *Aplysia. Proceedings of the National Academy of Sciences of the U.S.A., 77,* 6912–6916.

Klein, M., Shapiro, E., & Kandel, E. R. (1980). Synaptic plasticity and the modulation of the Ca^{++} current. *Journal of Experimental Biology, 89,* 117–157.

Krasne, F. B. (1969). Excitation and habituation of the crayfish escape reflex: The depolarization response in lateral giant fibers of the isolated abdomen. *Journal of Experimental Biology, 50,* 29–46.

Mackintosh, N. J. (1974). *The psychology of animal learning.* New York: Academic Press.

Ocorr, K. A., Walters, E. T., & Byrne, J. H. (1983). Associative conditioning analog in *Aplysia* tail sensory neurons selectively increases cAMP content. *Society for Neuroscience Abstracts, 9,* 169.

Pavlov, I. P. (1927). *Conditioned reflexes.* (G. V. Anrep, Trans.). London: Oxford University Press.

Pinsker, H. M., Hening, W. A., Carew, T. J., & Kandel, E. R. (1973). Long-term sensitization of a defensive withdrawal reflex in *Aplysia. Science, 182,* 1039–1042.

Pinsker, H. M., Kupfermann, I., Castellucci, V., & Kandel, E. R. (1970). Habituation and dishabituation of the gill-withdrawal reflex in *Aplysia. Science, 167,* 1740–1742.

Rescorla, R. A. (1968). Probability of shock in the presence and absence of CS in fear conditioning. *Journal of Comparative and Physiological Psychology, 66,* 1–5.

Rescorla, R. A. (1973). Second-order conditioning: Implications for theories of learning. In F. J. McGuigan & D. B. Hulse (Eds.), *Contemporary approaches to conditioning and learning.* Washington, DC: V. H. Winston.

Rescorla, R. A. (1978). Some implications of a cognitive perspective on Pavlovian conditioning. In S. H. Hulse, H. Fowler & W. Honig (Eds.), *Cognitive processes in animal behavior* (pp. 15–50). Hillsdale, NJ: Erlbaum.

Rescorla, R. A., & Wagner, A. R. (1972). A theory of Pavlovian conditioning: Variations in the effectiveness of reinforcement and nonreinforcement. In A. H. Black & W. F. Prokasy (Eds.), *Classical conditioning II: Current research and theory* (pp. 64–99). New York: Appleton-Century-Crofts.

Rosenblatt, F. (1962). *Principles of neurodynamics: Perceptrons and the theory of brain mechanisms.* Washington, DC: Spartan Books.

Sahley, C., Rudy, J. W., & Gelperin, A. (1981). An analysis of associative learning in a terrestrial mollusc. I. Higher-order conditioning, blocking, and a transient US pre-exposure effect. *Journal of Comparative Physiology, 144,* 1–8.

Siegelbaum, S. A., Camardo, J. S., & Kandel, E. R. (1982). Serotonin and cyclic AMP close single K^+ channels in *Aplysia* sensory neurons. *Nature, 299,* 413–417.

Spencer, W. A., Thompson, R. F., & Nielson, D. R., Jr. (1966). Decrement of ventral root electrotonus and intracellularly recorded PSPs produced by iterated cutaneous afferent volleys. *Journal of Neurophysiology, 29,* 253–273.

Sutton, R. S., & Barto, A. G. (1981). Toward a modern theory of adaptive networks: Expectation and prediction. *Psychological Review, 88,* 135–170.

Thompson, R. F., & Spencer, W. A. (1966). Habituation: A model phenomenon for the study of neuronal substrates of behavior. *Psychological Review, 173,* 16–43.

Tolman, E. C. (1932). *Purposive behavior in animals and men.* New York: Century.

Wagner, A. R. (1978). Expectancies and the priming of STM. In S. H. Hulse, H. Fowler, & W. Honig (Eds.), *Cognitive processes in animal behavior* (pp. 177–209). Hillsdale, NJ: Erlbaum.

Wagner, A. R. (1981). SOP: A model of automatic memory processing in animal behavior. In N. E. Spear & R. R. Miller (Eds.), *Information processing in animals: Memory mechanisms* (pp. 5–47). Hillsdale, NJ: Erlbaum.

Walters, E. T., & Byrne, J. H. (1983). Associative conditioning of single neurons suggests a cellular mechanism for learning. *Science, 219,* 405–408.

Walters, E. T., Carew, T. J., & Kandel, E. R. (1981). Associative learning in *Aplysia:* Evidence for conditioned fear in an invertebrate. *Science, 211,* 504–506.

Zucker, R. S. (1972). Crayfish escape behavior and central synapses. II. Physiological mechanisms underlying behavioral habituation. *Journal of Neurophysiology, 35,* 621–637.

M. A. Gluck and R. F. Thompson

Modeling the neural substrates of associative learning and memory: A computational approach

1987. *Psychological Review* 94: 176–191

We develop a computational model of the neural substrates of elementary associative learning, using the neural circuits known to govern classical conditioning of the gill-withdrawal response of *Aplysia*. Building upon the theoretical efforts of Hawkins and Kandel (1984), we use this model to demonstrate that several higher order features of classical conditioning could be elaborations of the known cellular mechanisms for simple associative learning. Indeed, the current circuit model robustly exhibits many of the basic phenomena of classical conditioning. The model, however, requires a further assumption (regarding the form of the acquisition function) to predict asymptotic blocking and contingency learning. In addition, if extinction is mediated by the nonassociative mechanism of habituation—rather than the associative process postulated by Rescorla and Wagner (1972)—then we argue that additional mechanisms must be specified to resolve a conflict between acquisition and maintenance of learned associations. We suggest several possible extensions to the circuit model at both the cellular and molecular levels that are consistent with the known *Aplysia* physiology and that could, in principle, generate classical conditioning behavior.

Significant progress has been made in recent years in identifying and characterizing neuronal substrates of learning and memory, due in large part to the model biological system approach developed initially by Pavlov (1927) and by Lashley (1929). Lashley (1950) states the essence of the approach most simply in the following passage: "In experiments extending over the past thirty years, I have been trying to trace conditioned reflex paths through the brain or to find the locus of specific memory traces" (p. 455). The basic approach is to select an organism capable of exhibiting behavioral phenomena of learning and memory and whose nervous system possesses properties that make neurobiological analysis feasible (Alkon, 1980; Chang & Gelperin, 1980; Cohen, 1980; Goldman-Rakic, 1984; Hawkins & Kandel, 1984; Ito, 1982; Kandel & Spencer, 1968; Kandel, 1976; Mishkin, 1978; Sahley, Rudy, & Gelperin, 1981; Squire, 1982; Thompson et al., 1976; Thompson et al., 1984; Thompson & Spencer, 1966; Tsukahara, 1981; Woody, 1982). A chief advantage of model systems is that the facts gained from biological and behavioral investigations for a particular preparation are cumulative and tend to have synergistic effects on theory development and research (Thompson, 1986; Thompson, Donegan, & Lavond, in press).

Each approach and model preparation has particular advantages. The value of certain invertebrate preparations as model systems results from the fact that certain behavioral functions are controlled by ganglia containing relatively small numbers of large, identifiable cells, cells that can be consistently identified across individuals of the species (Alkon, 1980; Davis & Gillette, 1978; Hoyle, 1980; Kandel, 1976; Krasne, 1969). Knowing the architecture of the system—the essential neural circuits—means the neurons exhibiting plasticity can be identified and studied. With intact vertebrate model biological systems, these goals are more difficult to attain, but here, too, recent progress has been substantial (Cohen, 1980; Goldman-Rakic, 1984; Kapp, Gallagher, Applegate, & Frysinger, 1982; Mishkin, 1978; Schneiderman, McCabe, Haselton, & Ellenberger, in press; Squire & Zola-Morgan, 1983; Thompson, 1986; Thompson et al., in press).

A critical feature of the model biological system approach is circuit analysis, which involves tracing the neuronal pathways and systems that generate the learned response. The essential memory trace circuit for a given instance of associative learning may be defined as the necessary and sufficient circuitry for the particular instance of learning and memory, from sensory neurons to motor neurons. The memory trace itself, the essential neuronal plasticity that codes the learned response, is presumably contained within some subset of the essential memory trace circuit.

When an essential memory trace circuit has been defined in sufficient detail as a biological system, it becomes necessary to determine if the circuit will in fact generate the phenomena of

This research was supported by Office of Naval Research Grant N00014-83K-0238, a grant from the Sloan Foundation to R. F. Thompson, and a National Science Foundation Fellowship to M. A. Gluck.

We are indebted to many people who helped us with this article: to Nelson Donegan for many incisive and helpful comments on earlier drafts and for sharing with us his invaluable insights into animal learning theory; to Andrew Barto, Richard Granger, Robert Hawkins, Eric Kandel, Joseph Steinmetz, and Richard Sutton for their comments and suggestions on an earlier draft; and to Gordon Bower, Gregory Clark, Leon Cooper, Michael Foy, Stephen Kosslyn, Michael Mauk, Mortimer Mishkin, Misha Pavel, and Terry Sejnowski for stimulating discussions and valuable commentary. The assistance of Katie Albiston, Doug Jones, Niels Mayer, Patrick McQuillan, and Audrey Weinland is also gratefully acknowledged.

Correspondence concerning this article should be addressed to Mark A. Gluck, Department of Psychology, Stanford University, Building 420, Stanford, California 94305.

learning and memory that it is presumed to model. Even in elementary circuits, it is not always evident what the outcome of a given set of stimulus and training conditions will be at a qualitative–logical level of analysis. It would seem necessary to develop a quantitative computational model of the model biological circuit to determine more precisely what in fact the circuit can do. We report here our efforts to develop a computational model of the circuitry in *Aplysia* that exhibits elementary associative learning as identified by Kandel and associates (Carew, Hawkins, Abrams, & Kandel, 1984; Carew, Hawkins, & Kandel, 1983; Carew, Pinsker, & Kandel, 1972; Carew, Walters, & Kandel, 1981; Hawkins, 1981; Hawkins, Abrams, Carew, & Kandel, 1983; Hawkins, Castellucci, & Kandel, 1981; Kandel & Schwartz, 1982; Pinsker, Kupfermann, Castellucci, & Kandel, 1970; Walters & Byrne, 1983).

Classical Conditioning in *Aplysia*

The basic reflex studied in *Aplysia* is withdrawal of the siphon, mantle shelf, and gill to tactile stimulation of the siphon or mantle shelf. This withdrawal reflex is partly monosynaptic and can be obtained in a reduced preparation of the abdominal ganglion with sensory and motor neurons. Thus, siphon sensory neurons synapse directly on gill and siphon motor neurons and repeated activation of the sensory neurons results in habituation of the motor neuron response (Castellucci, Pinsker, Kupfermann, & Kandel, 1970). The mechanism is synaptic depression, a presynaptic process involving a decrease in transmitter release as result of repeated activation. This appears due in turn to a decreased Ca^{++} influx in the sensory neuron terminals (Klein, Shapiro, & Kandel, 1980). Sensitization, an increase in the motor neuron response to stimulation, is produced by stronger stimulation of the neck or tail (Pinsker et al., 1970).

As in the spinal flexion reflex (Thompson & Spencer, 1966), sensitization is a superimposed increase in excitability independent of habituation, in other words, dishabituation is an instance of sensitization. In *Aplysia,* sensitization is a result of a presynaptic action of interneurons on the sensory neuron terminals that results in an increased Ca^{++} influx, which is believed to be a result of activation of a cAMP-dependent protein kinase (Bernier, Castellucci, Kandel, & Schwartz, 1982; Castellucci, Nairn, Greengard, Schwartz, & Kandel, 1982; Hawkins et al., 1981; Kandel & Schwartz, 1982).

If weak stimulation of the sensory nerves (the Conditioned Stimulus, hereinafter referred to as CS) is followed by strong shock to the tail (the Unconditioned Stimulus, hereinafter referred to as US), the synaptic potential of the motor neurons to the CS is facilitated. Further, the action potential in the sensory neurons is broadened, indicating a presynaptic effect, which has been termed a pairing-specific enhancement of presynaptic facilitation (Hawkins, Abrams, Carew, & Kandel, 1983). If repeated paired trials are given, this enhancement increases above the level produced by US sensitization alone, yielding a basic phenomenon of classical conditioning, an associatively induced increase in response of motor neurons to the CS. This conditioning depends critically on the time between presentation of the CS and the US, as noted above.

The tail-shock US pathway involves interneurons that are thought to exert presynaptic action on the sensory nerve terminals. Hawkins and Kandel (1984) propose that the phenomena of conditioning in *Aplysia* result from the interplay of habituation and sensitization (in much the same way as Groves and Thompson (1970) suggested that the two processes interact) together with a third process, namely pairing specific enhancement of the excitability of the CS terminals. The mechanism is thought to be an action of the sensitization process on the CS terminal excitability temporally dependent on the occurrence of an action potential in the CS terminal, which could be characterized as a Hebb synapse (Hebb, 1949) on a terminal rather than on a neuron soma or dendrites.

Hawkins and Kandel (1984) suggest that the existence of unifying cell-biological principles underlying nonassociative and associative learning may suggest the beginnings of a "cell-biological alphabet" for learning, in which the basic units may be combined to form progressively more complex learning processes. In particular, they hypothesized that several higher order features of classical conditioning may be derivable from our understanding of the cellular mechanisms for associative learning in *Aplysia.* Our primary goal in this article is to provide a quantitative analysis of this alphabet hypothesis. We develop here a computational model of *Aplysia* circuitry and use it to test Hawkins and Kandel's specific hypotheses regarding possible mechanisms for differential conditioning, second-order conditioning, blocking, and contingency learning.

A long-term goal of our work is to develop quantitative computational models of the more complex learning and memory circuits in the mammalian brain (see Thompson, Berger, & Madden, 1983; Thompson, 1986; Thompson et al., in press). We use the *Aplysia* circuit in our initial work, in part as a heuristic to select an appropriate level of computational analysis, and because it is simpler and more fully characterized at a neurobiological level.

Parallel–Associative Network Models

In developing a computational model of the *Aplysia* circuit, we draw heavily on previous work in cognitive psychology and artificial intelligence on models of parallel-associative networks, often referred to as "connectionist models" (cf. Feldman & Ballard, 1982). Despite differences in terminology, goals, and methodology, these models all have in common the assumption that complex information processes can be generated by networks of simple nodes that pass, in parallel, a form of excitation from node to node. These models have gained increasing usage in recent years as a framework for modeling complex cognitive behaviors including visual recognition (Anderson, 1977; Anderson & Hinton, 1981; Anderson, Silverstein, Ritz, & Jones, 1977; Hinton & Anderson, 1981), the effects of context on letter perception (McClelland, 1979; McClelland & Rumelhart, 1981), and the representation of concepts by patterns of distributed activation (Rumelhart & McClelland, 1986). The aspect of our network modeling approach that is perhaps new and distinctive is the use of actual neuronal circuits, to the extent they are known, to provide the structure of the associative network. The network is constrained by the actual connections of an identifiable neuronal circuit.

Of particular relevance to our own efforts is the work of Sutton and Barto (1981) who describe a neural-like adaptive ele-

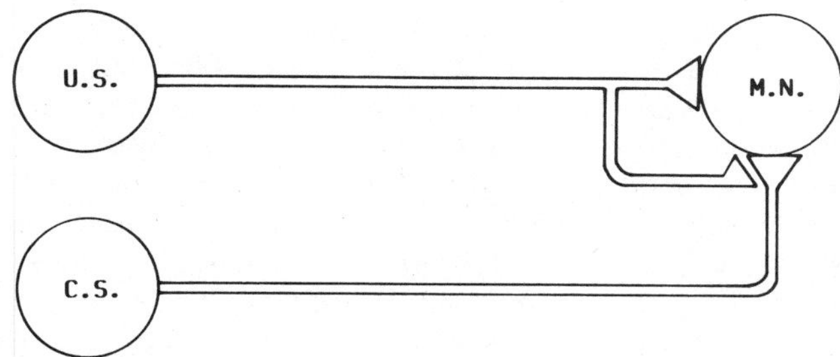

Figure 1. The basic circuit (Stage 1), composed of two sensory neurons (a conditioned stimulus, CS, and an unconditioned stimulus, US) and one motor neuron (MN).

ment more closely in accord with the animal learning literature than previous network models. As an extension of Rescorla and Wagner's (1972) trial-level model for associative learning, the Sutton–Barto model encodes the temporal dynamics of classical conditioning that are not captured by the Rescorla–Wagner model. In addition to providing a more detailed model of the real-time aspects of classical conditioning in animals, their element overcomes many of the stability and saturation problems encountered by network models. Though their model was designed to explain the same behavioral data as ours and used a similar computational framework, Sutton and Barto (1981) made no attempt to develop networks based on specific neural circuits nor was their adaptive element designed to behave in the manner of any identifiable neuron. To the extent that there are significant differences between our models, we might expect these differences to derive from the additional constraints of the relevant biological data.

Computational Model of *Aplysia* Circuit

We begin by describing a simple model of the circuit, including only the critical sensory and motor neurons for associative learning. After implementing this, and understanding what behavioral phenomena it does and does not account for, we add complexity, constrained by the neurobiological data.

The preliminary model consists of three neurons and three synapses, as represented in Figure 1. The neurons include a (to be) conditioned stimulus (the CS neuron), an unconditioned stimulus (the US neuron), and a motor neuron (the MN). One fiber originates at the conditioned stimulus and terminates as a synapse on the motor neuron (the CS→MN synapse). Two fibers originate at the unconditioned stimulus; one terminates as a synapse on the motor neuron (the US→MN synapse) and the other terminates as a synapse on the CS→MN synapse (the US→[CS→MN] synapse). The activations of both the CS and US sensory neurons are specified as input to the model. The primary output from the model is the activation of the MN in response to CS events and the CS→MN synaptic strength.

To implement the model on a digital computer, we adopt the convention of representing time as a series of discrete cycles of arbitrarily short duration. The activation of a neuron during cycle t is represented by $A(t)$ and is interpreted as the probability that the neuron will fire during that cycle. The state of a neuron, $S(t)$, is a binary number indicating whether or not the neuron fired during cycle t:

$$S(t) = \begin{cases} 1 & \text{with probability } A(t) \\ 0 & \text{otherwise.} \end{cases} \tag{1}$$

Synapses are similarly represented by both a continuous value and a discrete state: Each synapse has a strength, $V(t)$, that is interpreted as the probability that an action potential generated by the presynpatic neuron will be passed postsynaptically. The state of a synapse, $P(t)$, is a binary value indicating whether or not an action potential was passed postsynaptically during cycle t:

$$P(t) = \begin{cases} S(t) & \text{with probability } V(t) \\ 0 & \text{otherwise.} \end{cases} \tag{2}$$

Combining previous Equations 1 and 2 yields

$$P(t) = \begin{cases} 1 & \text{with probability } A(t)V(t) \\ 0 & \text{otherwise.} \end{cases} \tag{3}$$

The probability that a neuron transmits an action potential postsynaptically is the product of its activation level and its synaptic strength.

Pairing-Specific Enhancement of Sensitization

Sensitization occurs at the CS→MN synapse according to

$$\Delta V_{CS}(t) = \begin{cases} \beta_1[1 - V_{CS}(t)] & \text{with probability } \Phi(t) \\ 0 & \text{otherwise,} \end{cases} \tag{4}$$

where β_1 is a parameter governing the rate of sensitization and $\Phi(t)$ encodes the temporal specificity of conditioning as described below.[1] Like the Rescorla–Wagner (1972) model and the Sutton–Barto (1981) model, our model generates a negatively accelerating exponential function for the acquisition of the learned association. Kandel and Hawkins (1984) did not specify the form of the acquisition function in their model.

In our view, the effect of the interstimulus onset interval on conditionability is perhaps the most fundamental property of basic associative learning. The interval over which conditioning occurs varies widely in different preparations and paradigms, being minutes to hours for taste aversion, seconds to minutes for autonomic responses, and milliseconds to seconds for most skeletal muscle responses (see, e.g., Black & Prokasy, 1972; Hilgard & Bower, 1975). But regardless of the duration of the interval, there appears to be a relatively rapid rise and a slower decay of the conditionability function, as Clark Hull emphasized many years ago (Hull, 1943). In *Aplysia,* no learning occurs when the US precedes the CS or when the the two are presented simultaneously; optimal conditioning occurs when the CS precedes the US by .5 s and marginally significant conditioning occurs when the interstimulus interval is extended to 1 s (Hawkins, Carew, & Kandel, 1983).

To encode the temporal specificity of classical conditioning in *Aplysia,* it is necessary that the CS synaptic terminal have the potential to be modified in a pairing-specific manner that peaks some time after the synapse receives a pulse. The time course of this potential determines the possible interstimulus

[1] We use capital Roman letters for variables, capital Greek letters for functions, and lowercase Greek letters for fixed parameters.

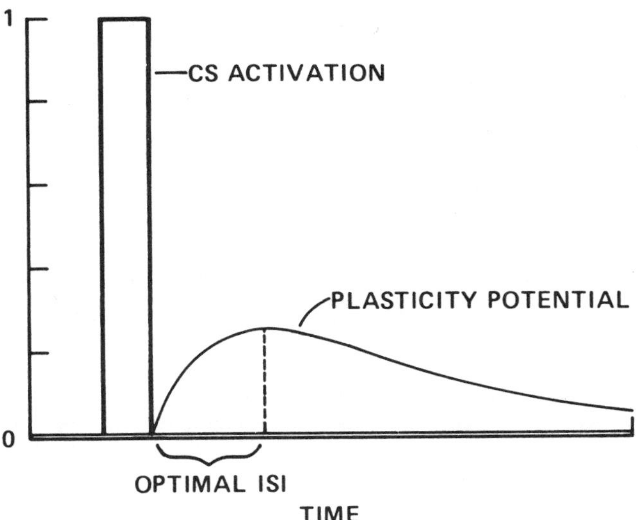

Figure 2. Time course of plasticity potential following a CS pulse with optimal interstimulus interval (ISI) indicated.

intervals (ISI). At this stage of model development we assume only that some mechanism must encode the temporal information and that this information must be present at the site of plasticity. The existence of this information is assumed without specifying the chemical or biological source. The temporal specificity of conditioning is governed in the model by $\Phi(t)$, the pairing-specific sensitization potential, which determines the degree to which US activity sensitizes the CS synapse. If an action potential is passed from the US neuron to the CS→MN synapse via the US→[CS→MN] synapse, then $\Phi(t)$ modulates the amount of sensitization as described above. $\Phi(t)$ is computed as

$$\Phi(t) = T(t)[1 - T(t)], \tag{5}$$

where $T(t)$ is a hidden variable whose default value is 0 but which jumps to 1 when a CS action potential is generated (i.e., $S_{CS}(t) = 1$) and then decays exponentially back to its default value according to

$$\Delta T = -\theta T, \tag{6}$$

where $\Delta T = T(t + 1) - T(t)$ and θ determines the rate at which T decays to 0. Like the eligibility traces of Sutton and Barto's (1981) adaptive element model, $\Phi(t)$ acts as a temporal trace at the site of plasticity for encoding the previous occurrence of a CS. This formulation of $\Phi(t)$ as the product of an exponentially decaying function, $T(t)$), and an exponentially rising function, $(1 - T(t))$, produces a temporal specificity that conforms to the behavioral data: Conditionability rises quickly, peaks shortly after the CS event (i.e., when $T(t) = .5$ and $\Phi(t) = .25$), and then slowly decreases (see Figure 2). Presentation of the CS and US simultaneously does not produce effective conditioning because onset of the CS event sets $T(t) = 1$ and therefore the conditionability, $\Phi(t) = 0$.

As noted above, this process can be measured in the *Aplysia* circuit and is termed a "pairing-specific enhancement." More generally, such a process, in combination with a process of plasticity, must be postulated to account for the powerful effect of the interstimulus interval on conditionability (see above and Black & Prokasy, 1972). A more complete computational model of the mechanism for classical conditioning in *Aplysia* would need to include the details of the time course of the molecular processes that mediate this temporal specificity. In the final section of this article we discuss some recent progress in this direction by Gingrich and Byrne (1985).

Habituation

To model habituation, we extend the Groves–Thompson model to the neuronal level: Each time the CS synapse passes a pulse to the motor neuron, its strength decreases according to

$$\Delta V_{CS}(t) = \begin{cases} -\beta_2 V_{CS}(t) & \text{if } P_{CS}(t) = 1 \\ 0 & \text{otherwise,} \end{cases} \tag{7}$$

where β_2 governs the rate of habituation.

Neuronal Firing

The firing rates of the sensory neurons constitute the input to the model. The firing rate of the motor neuron changes according to

$$\Delta A_{MN}(t) = \begin{cases} \delta_1[1 - A_{MN}(t)] & \text{if } (P_{CS}(t) = 1) \text{ or } (P_{US}(t) = 1) \\ -\delta_2 A_{MN}(t) & \text{otherwise,} \end{cases} \tag{8}$$

where δ_1 and δ_2 are the activation growth and decay rate parameters, respectively. The model as presently described has five free parameters: the neuronal activation increment and decrement rates (δ_1 and δ_2) the synaptic sensitization and habituation rates (β_1 and β_2), and a plasticity parameter, θ, that determines the time course of the ISI.

Associative Learning

At this level of detail, the circuit model is capable of producing the most basic associative learning phenomena exhibited by *Aplysia*. When a CS and US are paired with an appropriate interstimulus interval, pairing-specific learning occurs at the CS→MN synapse. The behavior of the model is shown in Figure 3A.[2] Initially the US produces a large amount of activity in the motor neuron compared to the small amount produced by the CS. After repeated presentations of the CS preceding the US, the motor-neuron response produced by the CS increases significantly. This change in the circuit's behavior can also be seen in the increased strength of the CS→MN synapse. Follow-

[2] In all the simulations of classical conditioning paradigms, we varied the full range of parameters in order to test the robustness of the phenomena and their sensitivity to parameter changes. All the basic associative conditioning phenomena were exceedingly robust across manipulations of the parameter values; changes in parameter values affected the rate and strength of conditioning and the duration of the optimal ISI but not the essential conditioning phenomena we sought to model. Parameters for the simulations shown in this article were set so as to generate a sample of conditioning in a sufficiently short number of trials to allow the complete protocol of the simulation to be shown in one figure.

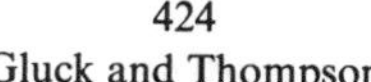

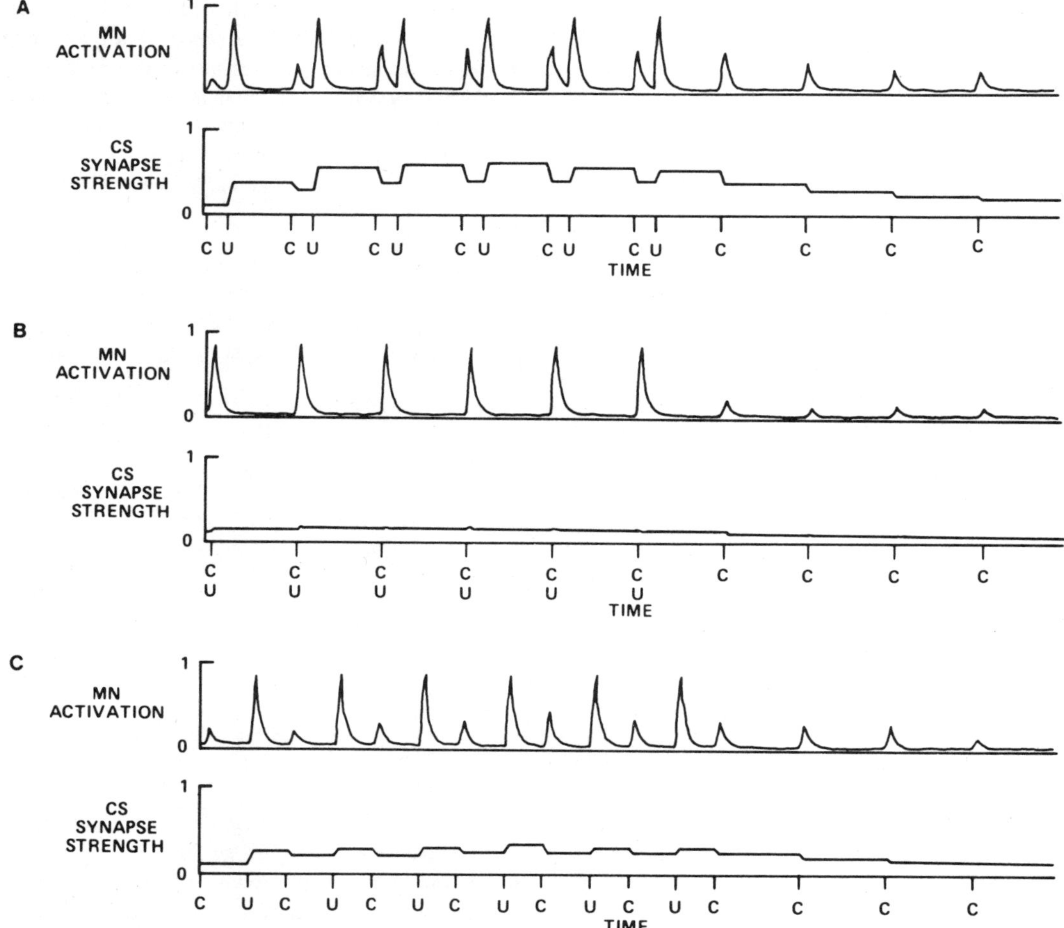

Figure 3. Stage 1 simulation of simple classical conditioning under three conditions: (a) optimal ISI produces maximal conditioning, (b) simultaneous presentation of CS and US (e.g., ISI = 0) produces essentially no conditioning, and (c) ISI much greater than optimal produces relatively small amount of conditioning. (For each of the three conditions, the time course of motor-neuron (MN) activation and the CS synaptic strength are shown. The CS (C) and US (U) pulses are indicated along the bottom of the graphs.)

ing this, repeated presentations of the CS alone habituates the CS→MN synapse strength with the consequence that motor-neuron activity during presentation of the CS returns to its initial state. This extinction is mediated by the nonassociative process of habituation that occurs during CS presentations (Carew et al., 1972; Castellucci & Kandel, 1974).

No learning occurs in *Aplysia* when the CS and US are presented simultaneously (Hawkins et al., 1983). The model's behavior under this training paradigm is shown in Figure 3B. No learning occurs because the sensitization potential, $\Phi(t)$, is at 0 when the US fires, inhibiting pairing-specific sensitization. Figure 3C shows simulated conditioning with an ISI longer than optimal; some learning occurs, but less than with an optimal ISI.

This preliminary model omits many components of the full *Aplysia* circuitry, including interneurons and many of the fine-grained details of the molecular processes of nonassociative and associative sensitization as identified and characterized by Kandel and colleagues. This model is presented only as a first approximation of the *Aplysia* circuitry, detailed at a level of description comparable with the connectionist models used in cognitive psychology and artificial intelligence.

By beginning with this simple network model and evolving it as necessary to account for the relevant behavioral data, we hope to come to a greater understanding of the computational roles played by the different circuit components and neurobiological processes in mediating higher order features of conditioning. In the remainder of this article we describe our attempt to instantiate Hawkins and Kandel's (1984) hypothetical elaborations of this basic circuitry to see if they will, in fact, account for (a) differential conditioning, (b) second-order conditioning, and (c) blocking and contingency learning.

Differential Conditioning

In differential conditioning an animal learns to respond specifically to one reinforced stimulus and not to another nonreinforced stimulus. Only those sensory neurons that are active

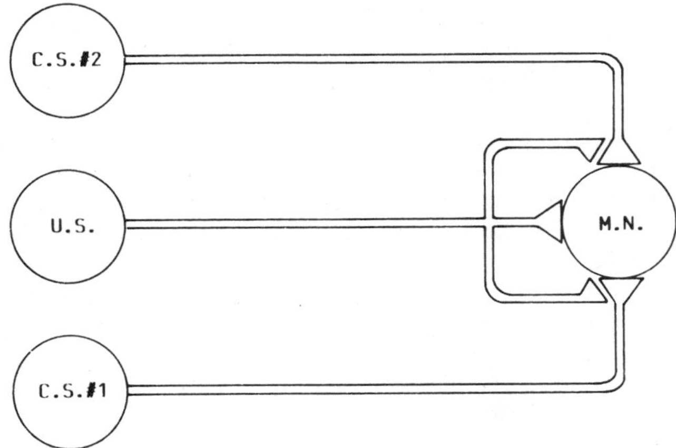

Figure 4. Stage 2 circuit with second CS added. (Both CS1 and CS2 are identically connected to the MN.)

prior to presentation of the US receive enhanced presynaptic facilitation. In *Aplysia,* a CS$^+$ is presented to the siphon paired with a US whereas an unpaired CS$-$ is presented to the mantle, or vice versa (Carew et al., 1983; Hawkins et al., 1983). To model this phenomena, it is necessary to include a second sensory neuron, CS2, connected to the motor neuron in a fashion similar to the other sensory neuron, CS1 (see Figure 4).

Successful differential conditioning using this model circuit is shown in Figure 5A. Activity in the CS1 neuron is paired consistently with the US, and activity in the CS2 neuron occurs randomly. This training procedure results in strong enhancement of the CS1→MN synapse (and thus in the ability of the CS1 neuron to generate activity in the motor neuron). Only mild nonassociative sensitization is produced in the CS2 synapse (Castellucci & Kandel, 1976; Pinsker et al., 1970).

Second-Order Conditioning

In second-order conditioning, a CS1 association is first trained via pairing with the US. After training, the CS1 can serve as a reinforcing stimulus to condition a new stimulus, CS2. For second-order conditioning to occur, the source of associative training could not logically be the US synapse or the CS1 could never gain the ability to sensitize the CS2. The results of Carew et al. (1984) implicate a presynaptic process. Hawkins and Kandel (1984) suggest that a facilitator interneuron plays the role of a local arousal system in second-order conditioning and serves as an intermediary between the sensory neuron (both CS and US) and the motor neuron. The facilitator interneuron produces facilitation not only at the sensory neuron synapses but also at the synapses from the facilitator neuron to itself. As shown in Figure 6 we include this interneuron in the model as an intermediary stage between the sensory and motor neurons. The same equations that were previously described for governing motor neuron activation and sensory to motor neuron synapses also govern the interneuron activation and the sensory to interneuron and interneuron to motor neuron synapses. The facilitator interneuron acts as the single source of sensitization enhancement for the synapses of the sensory neurons and the interneuron. One implication of this is that, unlike the CS synapses that terminate on the motor neuron, the CS synapses that terminate on the facilitator interneuron act as Hebb (1949) synapses, because firing of the CS neuron prior to firing of the facilitator interneuron enhances the ability of the CS neuron to activate the interneuron (Hawkins & Kandel, 1984, p. 384).

With the addition of the facilitator interneuron, the model successfully produces second-order conditioning (see Figure 7). The CS1 is paired with the US until an asymptotic level of conditioning is reached. Following this, the CS2 is paired with the CS1 and the US is omitted. Because the CS1 has now acquired the ability to act as a source of pairing-specific enhancement of sensitization, conditioning occurs at the CS2 synapses via the interneuron, and the CS1 synapse strength slowly extinguishes as a result of habituation and nonreinforcement.

Blocking

A class of behavioral phenomena exists that indicates animals learn not just the temporal contiguity of stimuli but also their predictive or informational value. Hawkins and Kandel (1984)

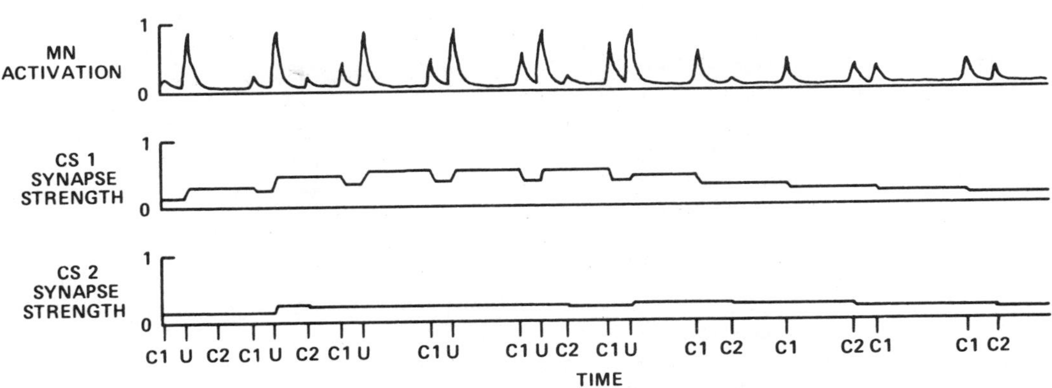

Figure 5. Stage 2 simulation of differential conditioning of the CS1 and CS2. (Three graphs are shown: The time course of motor-neuron (MN) activation and the synaptic strengths of CS1 and CS2. The CS1, CS2, and US pulses are indicated along the bottom by C1, C2, and U, respectively.)

A

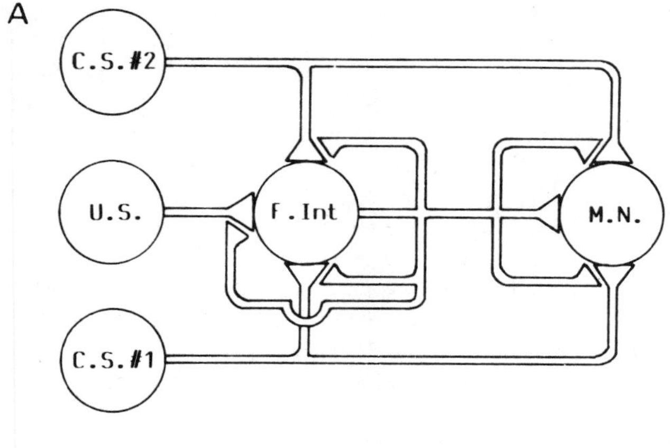

B

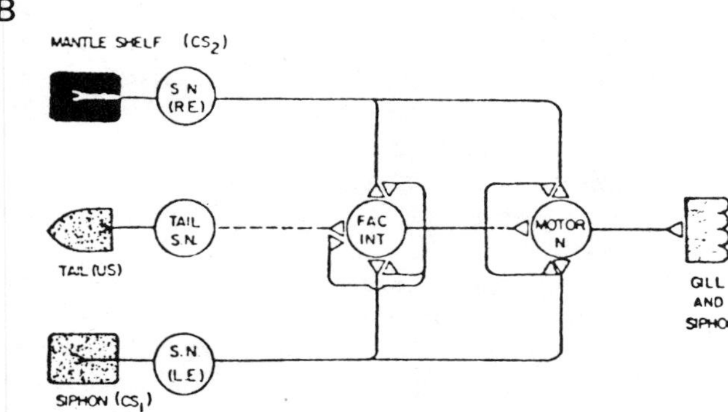

Figure 6. (a) Stage 3 circuit model with facilitator interneuron (F. Int) added; (b) *Aplysia* circuit (from Hawkins & Kandel, 1984). (The sensory neurons (S.N.) from the siphon and mantel shelf are the CS1 and CS2 input lines. The sensory neuron at the tail is the US. The output of the motor neuron excites the gill and siphon withdrawal reflex.)

proposed an elaboration of their basic cellular model that they suggest could account for these higher order features. They illustrate this hypothetical mechanism using blocking, whereby an animal learns not only about the contiguity of stimuli but also about their predictive contingency: If a CS1 is conditioned to predict the US, then the addition of a second stimulus, CS2, presented simultaneously with CS1, results in attenuated conditioning to the CS2 alone. A form of blocking has recently been reported for a behavioral response in intact *Aplysia,* but the magnitude of the effect was not described (Colwill, 1985).

In cognitive terms, this phenomena is described as a lack of association strength accruing to a stimulus that provides no new predictive power (Kamin, 1969). In the Rescorla–Wagner model of classical conditioning, this is formalized as

$$\Delta V_j = \alpha_j \beta_1 (\lambda - \sum V_i) \tag{9}$$

where ΔV_j is the change in the association strength between a stimulus element j and the US, α_j is the salience of the CS element, β_1 is a parameter governing the rate of learning during US presentation, λ is the maximum possible association strength associated with the US, and ΣV_i is the sum of the association strengths between the CS stimulus elements occurring on that trial and the US. In the initial phase of training, CS1 is paired with the US until V_1 approaches λ. In the compound (CS1 + CS2→US) phase of training, CS2 will acquire little associative strength since pretraining on CS1 results in ($\lambda - \Sigma V_i \approx 0$). To demonstrate blocking, however, it is not necessary that there be an absence of conditioning to CS2; this is only one extreme case that satisfies the definition. More generally, blocking is observed when responding to CS2 is less for subjects who have had pretraining on CS1 than for subjects not pretrained on CS1.

Hawkins and Kandel (1984) suggest that the interneuron may implement the ($\lambda - \Sigma V_i$) component of the Rescorla–Wagner algorithm in the following way: After being activated by the CS1, the interneuron undergoes a refractory period—caused perhaps by accommodation and recurrent inhibition—that persists throughout the presentation of the US. They speculate that this could mediate the blocking effect if the firing of the interneuron by the CS1, and its resulting inhibition, attenuated the sensitization that accrues to the CS2. Activation of the interneuron during the compound CS1 + CS2 stimulus occurs outside of the window of eligibility for ΔV_{CS2} and the interneuron is refractory during US stimulation, preventing interneuron activation at a time favorable to pairing-specific modification of the synaptic strength of CS2.

In modeling the refractory period of the interneuron we are concerned only with the resultant firing behavior and not the mechanisms for accommodation and recurrent inhibition. We introduce here an additional variable, R_{FI}, which represents the degree to which firing of the facilitator interneuron is inhibited. When the activation level of the facilitator interneuron exceeds a predetermined threshold, R_{FI} is set to 1. R_{FI} then decays slowly back to 0. In the computational model, R_{FI} affects the interneuron by probabilistically governing the growth of interneuron activation in the following manner:

$$\Delta A_{FI}(t) = \begin{cases} \delta_1[1 - A_{FI}(t)] & \text{with probability } (1 - R_{FI}) \text{ if } [P_{CS}(t) = 1] \text{ or } [P_{US}(t) = 1] \\ -\delta_2 A_{FI}(t) & \text{otherwise,} \end{cases} \tag{10}$$

where δ_1 is the rate parameter for activation increase and $\Delta A_{FI}(t)$ is the change in $A_{FI}(t)$, the current activation level of facilitator interneuron. As long as R_{FI} is near 1, the interneuron will be inhibited from firing. To produce the appropriate blocking behavior the decay rate of R_{FI} must be set so that the refractory period of the interneuron is longer than the possible interstimulus interval.

In the Hawkins and Kandel model, associative activation produces a graded refractoriness in the interneuron proportional to the strength of associative activation. A single behavioral trial is characterized in our model by multiple cycles of the simulation. Our model produces a somewhat continuous effect of associative strength on the degree of refractoriness that is proportional to the degree of overlap between interneuron activity and CS eligibility.

The implementation of a refractory period for the interneuron longer than the acceptable ISI necessitates the explicit inclusion of a direct US→MN connection (see Figure 8) in order to get an appropriate unconditioned response to the US. Although these pathways exist, they are often not represented in less ex-

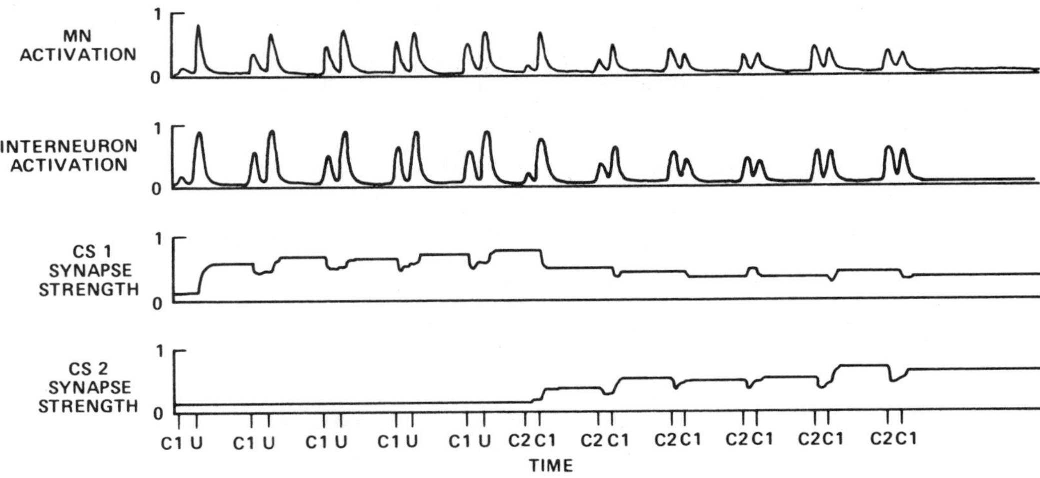

Figure 7. Stage 3 simulation of successful second-order conditioning of CS2 to CS1, showing the time course of the motor-neuron (MN) activation, the interneuron activation, and the CS1 and CS2 synaptic strengths. (The CS1, CS2, and US pulses are indicated along the bottom by, C1, C2, and U, respectively.)

plicit models of the circuitry for learning and memory. As shown in Figure 9, the addition of the implementation of this refractory behavior still allows for normal conditioning and second-order conditioning.

However, contrary to expectations, this circuit model failed to produce asymptotic blocking. Across variations of all the relevant parameters the asymptotic levels of conditioning after extended compound training were identical for CS1 and CS2 and indistinguishable from the levels attained without pretraining to the CS1.

However, as suggested by Nelson Donegan (personal communication, March 19, 1986) the model is capable of a short-term preasymptotic form of blocking. Figure 10A shows a trial-by-trial analysis of the changes in activation levels and synaptic strengths for a simulated blocking experiment using the same parameter setting that produced the successful second-order conditioning shown in Figure 9. In this simulation both CS and US events were 5 cycles long and the interstimulus interval was 30 cycles, an interval optimally favorable to associative learning

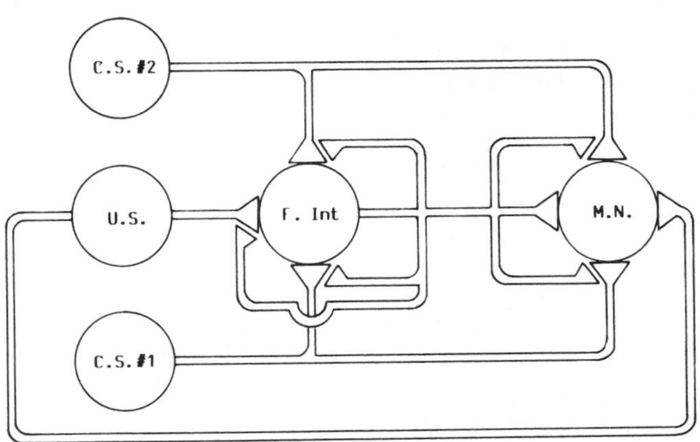

Figure 8. Stage 4 circuit with direct US→MN pathway.

given the time course of eligibility (as determined by θ). The rate of synaptic sensitization is $\beta_1 = .4$ and the rate of habituation is $\beta_2 = .05$, parameter settings that in previous simulations were sufficient to produce second-order conditioning.

After eight CS1→US trials, the CS1 synaptic strength reached an asymptotic level. During this period both the interneuron and motor neuron responses to CS1 increased considerably. Hawkins and Kandel suggest that as training to the CS1 reaches asymptote, activity in the interneuron during US presentation will disappear. Although the interneuron response during US presentation does decrease significantly during training, it cannot be entirely eliminated. If the associative strength of the CS stimulus were strong enough to entirely eliminate the interneuron response during US presentation, there would be no source of pairing-specific sensitization for the CS terminals. This would be an inherently unstable state because the nonassociative process of habituation would drive down the CS associative strength until enough interneuron activity occurred during the eligibility period for CS synapse modification (i.e., during US presentation) to offset the habituation. Thus, total refractoriness of the interneuron is not consistent with the basic mechanisms for strength revision. Interneuron activity during the US presentation does not entirely disappear, but rather decreases to a level where it is just sufficient to offset the effects of habituation. This can be seen in both the simulation of second-order conditioning shown in Figure 9 and in the simulation shown in Figure 10.

Following pretraining to the CS1 stimulus, 12 compound CS1 + CS2→US trials were presented. As is clear from the time course of CS2 synaptic strength, the CS2 synapse gains considerable associative strength; the important comparison, however, is with the time course of CS2 synaptic strength during compound training without pretraining to CS1 (shown in Figure 10 as a dashed line). Although these two curves reach the same asymptotic levels after extended compound training, there is an initial preasymptotic period in which the CS2 strength is below that found without pretraining to the CS1.

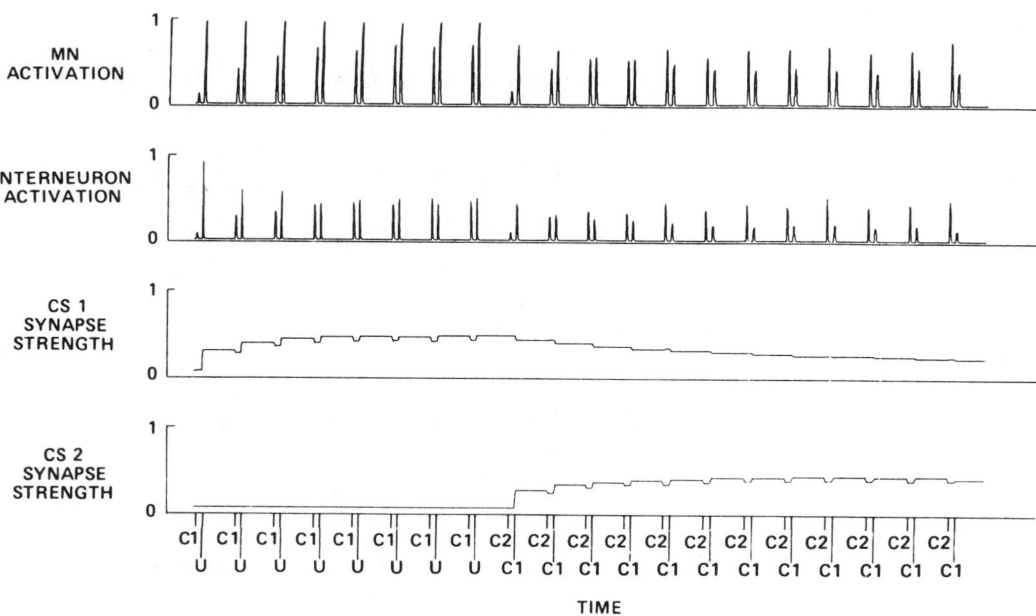

Figure 9. Successful second-order conditioning with refractory interneuron. (Eight CS1–US pairings are followed by 12 CS2–CS1 pairings. Note that at asymptotic CS1 conditioning (Trial 8), interneuron activity is attenuated but not eliminated during US presentation. This graph shows only the first half of the paradigm in which the decreasing strength of the CS1 association is still strong enough to maintain the CS2 association. Repeated pairings of CS2–CS1 would eventually habituate the CS1 association and, in turn, the CS2 association. Parameter settings: sensitization rate (β_1) = .4, habituation rate (β_2) = .05, ISI factor (θ) = .15, neuron activation increment and decrement (δ_1, δ_2) = .8 and .6. Initial synaptic strength settings: $V_{US} = 1$, $V_{CS_1} = V_{CS_2} = .05$. Figure shows average values of variables for 100 repetitions of paradigm.)

Thus, initial compound trials do produce a limited form of blocking. Because pretraining to CS1 attenuates interneuron activity during the eligibility period, the change in associative strength available to the CS2 (as measured by interneuron activity) is significantly less on the first trial than if there had been no pretraining to CS1, in much the same way that Hawkins and Kandel (1984) suggest. By the second trial, the CS2 has acquired some associative strength because of interneuron activity during the first trial. Because there is now less interneuron activity during the US presentation because of the combined effects of the compound stimuli, the CS1 strength decreases slightly. The CS2 strength, however, rises because (a) the absolute effect of habituation is smaller for a weak association than for a strong association, the rate of habituation being proportional to the absolute level of associative strength (Groves & Thompson, 1970); and (b) the sensitizing effect of the interneuron is greater for a weak association than for a strong association because of the negatively accelerated growth function for strength revision. This rise in the CS2 strength along with the slight decay in the CS1 strength continues until the associative strengths of the two stimulus elements are equal and stable: The combined effect of the stimulus elements decreases the level of interneuron activity until its sensitizing ability just counteracts the effects of habituation. With extended training on the compound stimulus, the effect of pretraining to the CS1 diminishes and disappears asymptotically. As is apparent from the simulation results, there is no difference in the CS2 synapse strengths between those subjects who were pretrained to the CS1 and those who were not.

The magnitude of this preasymptotic blocking is dependent on the relative strengths of the sensitization and habituation parameters: As shown in Figure 10B, when the sensitization rate is decreased (relative to the previous simulation), the absolute difference between the pretrained and nonpretrained conditions is less on any given trial. However, the total number of trials on which there is a significant difference between the two conditions is increased, in other words, it takes longer to reach the equilibrium point.

The failure of our computational model to produce the asymptotic blocking does not make a convincing case that the real circuit is unable to produce this behavior, nor does it make a strong argument that any formal model consistent with the model proposed by Hawkins and Kandel (1984) will be unable to produce blocking. Rather it only supports the weak claim that this particular form of the model does not robustly predict asymptotic blocking in that there exist interpretations of the model that do not produce this behavior.

Circuitry Models and Behavioral Learning Algorithms

In suggesting neuronal mechanisms for higher order features of classical conditioning, Hawkins and Kandel (1984) were guided by an attempt to identify possible neuronal-level correlates of Rescorla and Wagner's (1972) behavioral model of clas-

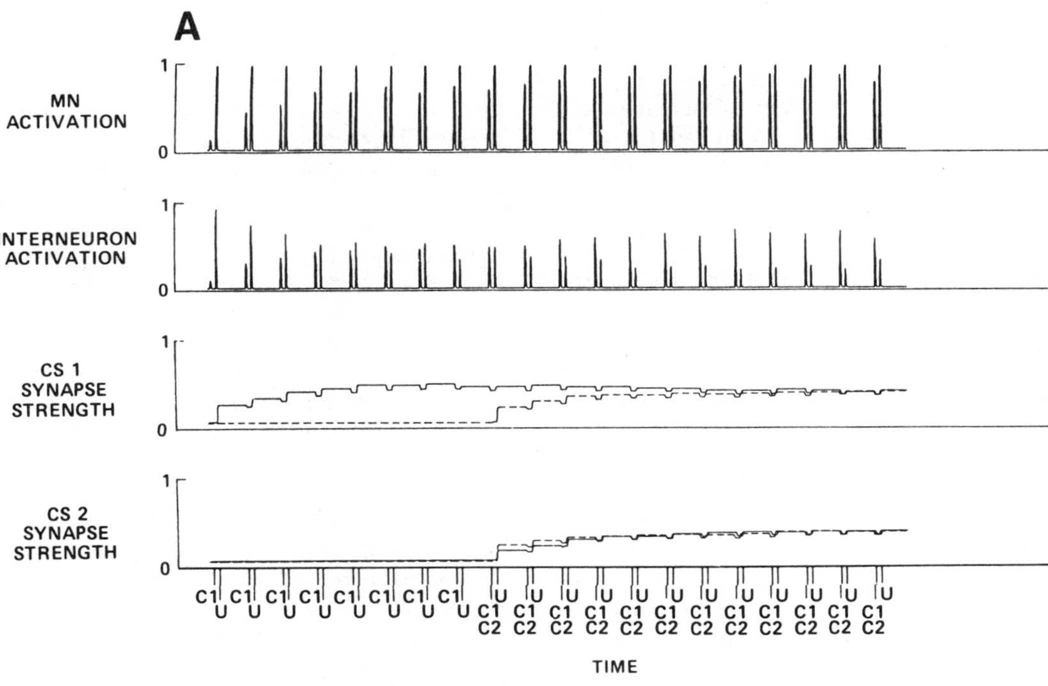

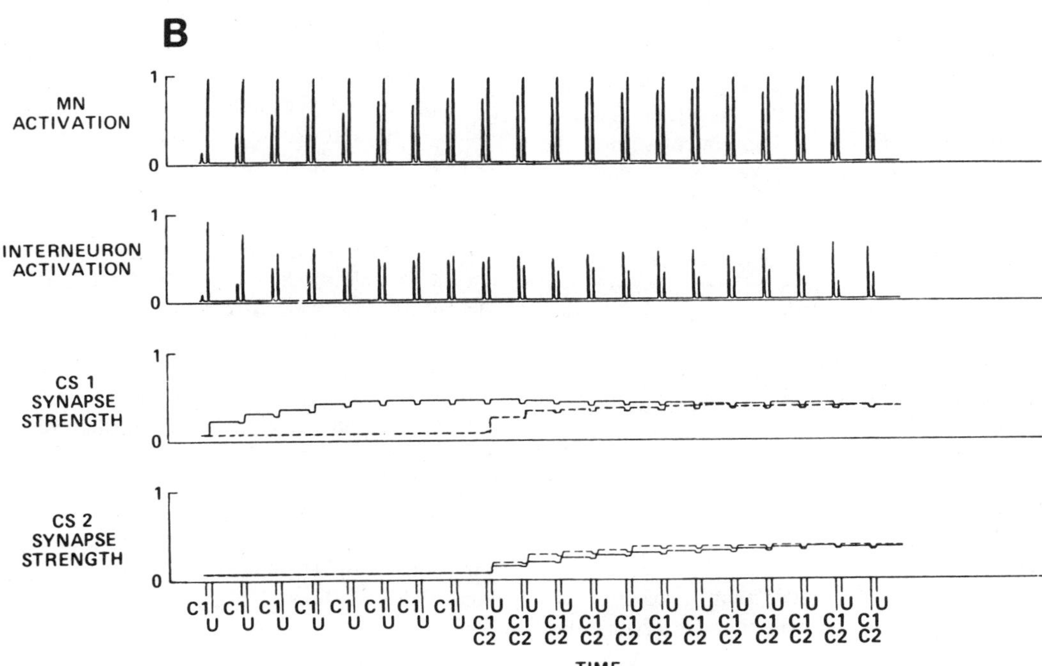

Figure 10. (a) Pre-asymptotic blocking with refractory interneuron. The solid lines graph the MN activation, interneuron activation, and CS1 and CS2 synapse strengths for 8 CS1–US pairings followed by 12 compound CS1/CS2–US pairings. The dashed lines show the CS1 and CS2 synaptic strengths from the simulated control experiment in which the 12 compound pairings were not preceded by CS1 pretraining. With the same parameter settings used in Figure 9, conditioning to the CS2 is attenuated on the first few trials but difference disappears after a few trials with no significant asymptotic difference between the pretrained and nonpretrained conditions. (b) Decreasing the sensitization rate (β_1) to .3 from .4 decreases the magnitude of the blocking effect on the first trial but increases the number of trials before the pretrained and nonpretrained conditions asymptote at the same level.

sical conditioning. The Rescorla–Wagner model does, however, predict blocking; it was proposed because previous simpler models of associative learning could not account for blocking. To the extent that the emergent behavior of the circuit-level model (Hawkins & Kandel, 1984) differs from both the behavior of the learning algorithm that inspired it (Rescorla & Wagner, 1972) and the target animal behavior, it might be fruitful to examine more closely the relationship between these two models.

Hawkins and Kandel's (1984) model of the *Aplysia* circuitry and the Rescorla–Wagner behavioral model differ primarily regarding the mechanisms for negative learning: The Rescorla–Wagner model posits two associative processes by which association strengths can be weakened, whereas the Hawkins–Kandel model posits one nonassociative process for the weakening of association strengths. In the Rescorla–Wagner model, the presentation of a spurious CS (i.e., not followed by a US) changes the association strength of a CS element, *j*, according to

$$\Delta V_j = -\alpha_j \beta_2 \sum V_i \tag{11}$$

where α_j is as before, β_2 is a parameter governing the rate of extinction and ΣV_i is the sum of the association strengths of the CS stimuli. One nonintuitive prediction of the Rescorla–Wagner model is that negative learning can occur during a positive CS–US presentation if the sum of the association strengths between the CS and US elements is greater than the maximum association strength available for the US (i.e., $\Sigma V_i > \lambda$). Kamin and Gaioni (1974) confirmed this by demonstrating that the novel compounding of two independently trained CS stimulus elements produces an overexpectancy effect resulting in a decrement of associative strength for the component stimuli. In summary, the Rescorla–Wagner model posits that decreases in associative strength always occur as the result of an associative process both on positive (i.e., US present) and negative trials. In contrast, the Hawkins–Kandel model of the *Aplysia* circuitry proposes that all decreases in association strength are mediated by the nonassociative process of habituation. As Hawkins and Kandel note (1984, p. 386), their model in this regard is more closely in accord with the Groves–Thompson (1970) model of habituation and sensitization than with the Rescorla–Wagner model. Adapting the Groves–Thompson behavioral model of habituation to the neuronal level, we have modeled habituation as

$$\Delta V_j = -\beta_2 V_j, \tag{12}$$

where the notation is as before.

The Rescorla–Wagner model predicts that an asymptotic level of conditioning to a CS element will be reached when the sum of the CS elements equals the maximum level of conditioning available for the US (i.e., λ). As Hawkins and Kandel note, their model differs in this regard in that the asymptotic level of conditioning is predicted to occur when there is an equilibrium between the associative process of pairing-specific enhancement of sensitization and the nonassociative process of habituation (Hawkins & Kandel, 1984, p. 386). Actually, the ability of a conditioned CS element to inhibit interneuron firing during US presentation provides an additional source of modulation for the growth of the CS synaptic strength. The asymptotic level of conditioning will occur in the *Aplysia* model when three interacting processes are in equilibrium: (a) habituation, (b) sensitization of the CS synapses via the facilitator interneuron, and (c) attenuation of pairing-specific sensitization of the CS synapses due to inhibition of facilitator interneuron activity by the conditioning of the CS synapses.

What is the implication of this for the blocking paradigm? For blocking to occur, there should be an attenuation of conditioning to the CS2 due to prior training to the CS1. According to the Hawkins and Kandel hypothesis, this should occur because the presentation of the previously conditioned CS1 stimulus will inhibit the interneuron from firing during the US presentation, eliminating the necessary source for pairing-specific learning. As we have seen in the simulations, however, it is necessary that there be some activity in the facilitator interneuron in order to maintain an equilibrium between pairing-specific enhancement of sensitization, which occurs during US presentations, and habituation, which occurs during CS presentations. If the maintenance of a conditioned response in *Aplysia* depends on an equilibrium between pairing-specific sensitization enhancement and habituation, then a process that eliminates or attenuates the source of pairing-specific sensitization will clearly change the equilibrium point. As a tentative hypothesis we suggest that the reason our quantitative simulation of their model circuit does not generate asymptotic blocking is that there is a conflict between the need to maintain interneuron firing during US presentation in order to maintain a learned association and the need to inhibit the interneuron from firing during the US presentation in order to resist the acquisition of a new association.

It appears that the conflict between acquisition and maintenance is attributable to the difference between the associative algorithm for extinction proposed by Rescorla and Wagner (1972) and the nonassociative circuitry mechanism proposed by Hawkins and Kandel (1984); this explains why the Rescorla–Wagner model—and Sutton and Barto's (1981) temporal extension of this model—both avoid the conflict. If the basic mechanisms for associative learning in *Aplysia*—an associative process for sensitization enhancement and a nonassociative process for habituation—are in fact the building blocks for classical conditioning, then we suggest that additional mechanisms must be identified and characterized that allow the circuit to functionally distinguish between acquisition and maintenance, that is, to give the circuit a way of differentially affecting novel and pretrained stimuli in a manner consistent with the behavioral data. In a speculative vein, we consider here two classes of extensions to the Hawkins–Kandel model, consistent with the known *Aplysia* physiology, which might produce blocking.

Single-Interneuron Models

If both retention and acquisition are governed by the same interneuron, as Hawkins and Kandel (1984) suggest, then the activity of this interneuron during US presentation must be sufficient to maintain the CS1 association but insufficient to acquire the CS2 association. The interneuron cannot be totally turned off (or the CS1 association would extinguish) nor can it be left entirely on or there would be no blocking of the CS2 association. This implies that if a single facilitator interneuron mediates both the acquisition of new conditioned pathways and the maintenance of previously learned pathways, then it must settle at an intermediate level of firing (i.e., less than for an unpredicted US). Furthermore, this activity must have a differential effect on the CS1 and the CS2; in other words, it must maintain the learned CS1 associations but resist in the acquisition of the new CS2 association. Because activity in the CS1 and CS2 neurons will be the same, the differential effect of the activity in the interneuron must be attributable to the different strengths of the CS1 and CS2 synapses. More precisely, the activity in the facilitator interneuron during the US presentation must be sufficient to maintain the stronger CS1 association but insufficient to strengthen the weaker CS2 association.

Within this single-interneuron framework, we consider one possible modification to the model of synaptic plasticity that would make it easier to maintain an old association than to acquire a new association. As discussed earlier, our model of the learning mechanisms for positive synaptic weight change follows the models of Rescorla and Wagner (1972) and Sutton and Barto (1981) in using a negatively accelerated acquisition function. Learning in these models is faster and easier for a novel association than for an existing association: The opposite of what we suggest is necessary to mediate blocking with a single source of sensitization. Because any learning curve must eventually be negatively accelerated to reach an asymptote, the critical issue is what happens during the early stages of learning. Negatively accelerated growth in the Rescorla–Wagner model is not behaviorally unrealistic: The model tracks associative strengths, not behavior. It is assumed that additional assumptions are necessary to map associative strengths to behavioral measures such as response probability or response strength. For example, a recent extension to the Rescorla–Wagner model (Frey & Sears, 1978) incorporates a mapping of the negatively accelerated growth of associative strength to a more behaviorally realistic S-shaped ogive learning curve that at first is positively accelerated (cf. Mackintosh, 1974). The initial positively accelerated learning curve could be implemented at the neuronal level by making the rate of sensitization (conditional on the temporal trace)

$$\Delta V_j = \beta_1[V_j(1 - V_j)], \tag{13}$$

rather than using the negatively accelerated rule given in Equation 4. A precondition for using this learning function, however, is that V_j may approach but never equal 0. The motivation for using this learning rule would be to make learning more difficult for a novel stimulus element than for a previously trained stimulus element. If the interneuron is only slightly active during US presentation, this might be sufficient to maintain a learned association but insufficient to acquire a novel association. We incorporated this rule within the model, and the resulting successful simulated blocking behavior is shown in Figure 11. Initial presentation of a single CS1 stimulus causes small bursts of activity in the interneuron and motor neuron relative to the more significant effects on these two neurons from presentation of the US. Repeated pairings of the CS1 and US result in a significantly increased asymptotic level of CS1 synaptic strength along with increased responsiveness of the motor neuron to the CS1 stimulus. The interneuron, which previously fired during US presentations, now fires primarily during CS1 presentations with significantly attentuated firing during the US. Following this, repeated compound trials, CS1 + CS2 → US, produce no significant change in the CS2 synapse strength, a clear case of blocking.

Multiple Interneuron Model

Though Hawkins and Kandel (1984) limited themselves to considering the possible functional significance of a single interneuron, many other interneurons exist that could in principle contribute to higher order features of classical conditioning, including at least four interneurons that receive excitatory input from the sensory neurons and two inhibitory interneurons (Hawkins et al., 1981). It seems reasonable, therefore, to ask what functional properties an additional interneuron might possess that would contribute to resolving the acquisition/maintenance conflict? We may speculate here about one possible mechanism: If a second interneuron does not go into a refractory period and sensitizes the CS synapses proportional to the current learned association, this might counteract the effect of the habituation of an already learned association but have little or no effect on an unlearned association. We implemented this in our model by adding an additional interneuron, FI_2, which is connected just like the original interneuron, FI_1, which provides an additional source of pairing-specific enhancement of presynaptic facilitation according to

$$\Delta V_{CS}(t) = \begin{cases} \beta_1[V_{CS}(t)] & \text{with probability } \Phi(t) \\ 0 & \text{otherwise,} \end{cases} \tag{14}$$

where Φ and β_1 are defined as before.

We implemented this additional interneuron and the behavior of the circuit in a blocking paradigm is shown in Figure 12. The circuit clearly generates an extreme case of blocking. We note that the asymptotic level of conditioning accruing to the CS1 is significantly higher in this model than in the previous model (without the additional interneuron); however, without further comparisons of these two models in a variety of additional behavioral paradigms, it is unclear that this is of any theoretical interest.

Contingency Learning

As discussed earlier, blocking is just one example of a class of behavioral phenomena, including overshadowing and the effect of US-alone trials, in which animals learn about the contingency or informational value of stimuli (Prokasy, 1965; Rescorla, 1968) rather than simply their contiguity or co-occurrence (Hull, 1943; Spence, 1956). The importance of the Rescorla–Wagner model is that it posits a single process that accounts for the role of these informational variables in addition to predicting a wide range of additional effects, especially those dealing with the learning of inhibitory associations. Similarly, Hawkins and Kandel (1984) propose that their hypothetical mechanism for blocking might also account for the degradation of learning due to intermittent presentation of US alone. Extending the arguments of Rescorla and Wagner (1972) to the neuronal level, they suggest that if context is viewed as an additional CS, then the presentation of US-alone trials would serve to increase the context→US association and, via the interneuron refractory mechanisms, attenuate the CS association. Thus,

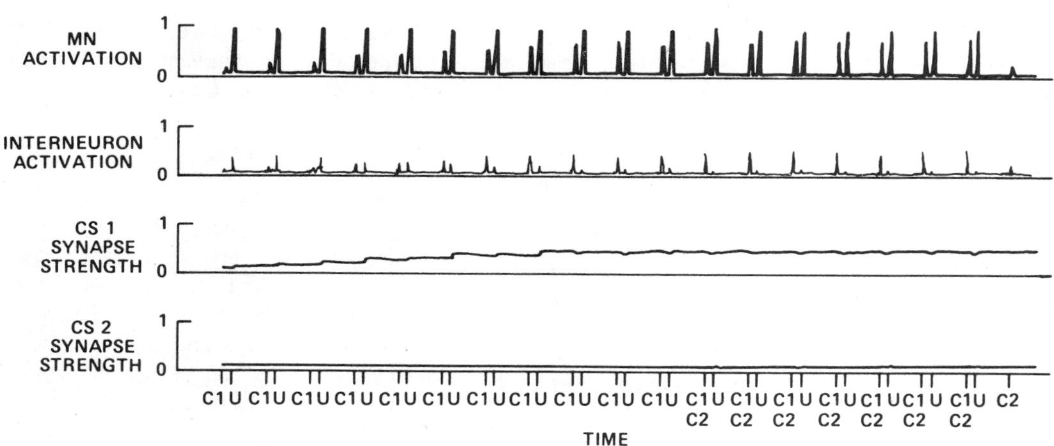

Figure 11. Successful blocking with new S-shaped learning function. (The degree to which a CS synapse can be strengthened is proportional to the strength × (1 − strength). The refractory state is interpreted as 1 minus the probability that the interneuron can fire. Thus, when the refractory state is high, the interneuron cannot fire. As the refractory state decays toward 0, the interneuron is again able to be fired.)

whether or not the circuit model can mediate blocking has important implications for a wider range of behavioral phenomena.

Summary and Conclusions

Our computational model of the *Aplysia* circuit suggests that several of the higher order features of classical conditioning do, as Hawkins and Kandel (1984) suggest, follow as natural elaborations of identified cellular mechanisms for associative and nonassociative learning. In particular we have provided quantitative support for their models of acquisition, extinction, differential conditioning, and second-order conditioning. In doing this, we found that we did not need to concern ourselves with the biophysical properties of neurons (e.g., ionic membrane properties), fine-grained temporal properties and mechanisms of neurotransmitter release, or the kinetics of transmitter–receptor interactions. Rather, the models suggested by Hawkins and Kandel (1984) for differential and second-order conditioning appear to be robust at a cellular level of description, a level comparable to that used by most cognitive-level connectionist models. Quantitative simulations of their models for blocking and contingency learning suggest, however, that it is necessary to assume a particular form of acquisition function (S-shaped) to robustly predict these higher order features of classical conditioning. We have speculated on two possible classes of extensions to the model, consistent with the known *Aplysia* physiology, that could in principle generate blocking behavior. The critical functional feature of these models is that they provide a mechanism for distinguishing between acquisition and maintenance of learned responses. If a single interneuron does mediate blocking and contingency learning, then we suggest that the rate of synaptic sensitization will be a critical factor. To test the plausibility of this model will necessitate modeling the sensitization process with far greater detail than we have attempted here. Recent computational models of the sub-

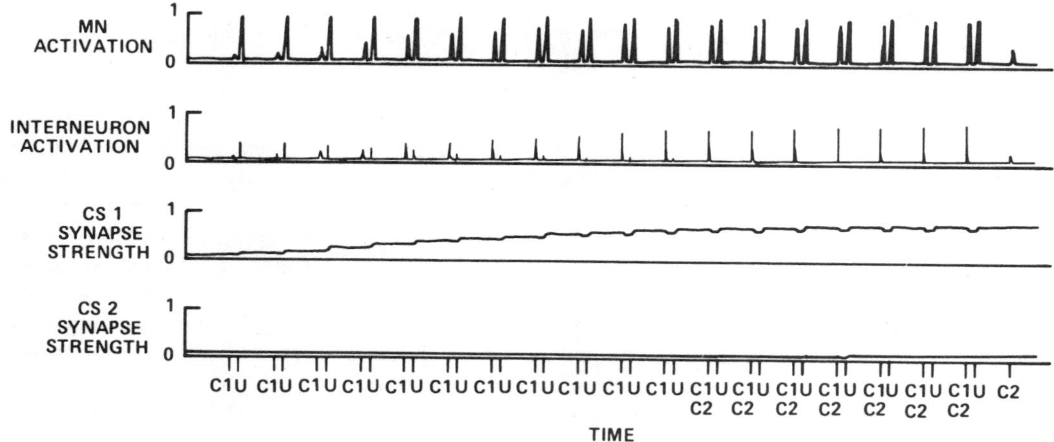

Figure 12. Successful and strong blocking with additional interneuron mediating retention added to previous circuit model.

cellular mollecular processes mediating associative and nonassociative sensitization in *Aplysia* (Gingrich & Byrne, 1985) may provide the necessary constraints to determine if in fact a single-interneuron model for classical conditioning in *Aplysia* is tenable. If other interneurons are indicated as being critical to contingency learning in *Aplysia,* then we speculate that there may exist interneurons whose function is to maintain learned associations but that have little or no effect on the acquisition of new associations.

Similarities to Mammalian Circuitry

The *Aplysia* circuit has certain similarities to the more hypothetical neuronal circuit defined in the mammalian spinal cord that subserves habituation and sensitization of spinal flexion reflexes (Groves & Thompson, 1970; Spencer, Thompson, & Neilson, 1966; Thompson & Spencer, 1966). In both, there is a direct circuit from CS afferents to motor neurons, monosynaptic in *Aplysia* and polysynaptic in the spinal cord, which exhibits habituation with repetitive activation. Strong stimulation of afferents induces sensitization of the response to CS via interneuron actions. In both systems, habituation appears due to a process of synaptic depression, and sensitization is a separate and independent superimposed increase in excitability. In *Aplysia,* sensitization appears due to a process of presynaptic facilitation (Castellucci & Kandel, 1976; Castellucci, Pinsker, Kupfermann, & Kandel, 1970; Kandel, 1976). In the spinal cord, it is not known whether presynaptic facilitation is involved in sensitization; postsynaptic increases in motor-neuron excitability do typically accompany sensitization (Spencer et al., 1966; Thompson & Spencer, 1966).

Both circuits are capable of elementary associative learning (Beggs, Steinmetz, Romano, & Patterson, 1983; Carew et al., 1983; Carew et al., 1981; Durkovic, 1975; Fitzgerald & Thompson, 1967; Patterson, 1975; Patterson, 1976; Patterson, Cegavske, & Thompson, 1973; Patterson, Steinmetz, Beggs, & Romano, 1982). In *Aplysia,* this appears to be a result of a persisting and pairing-specific sensitization-like presynaptic process (Carew et al., 1983; Hawkins & Kandel, 1984; Kandel, Abrams, Bernier, Carew, Hawkins, & Schwartz, 1983); in the spinal cord, the associative process is not yet understood at the synaptic level.

There is also a close correspondence between the properties of classical conditioning in the spinal mammal and those of the classically conditioned gill-withdrawal reflex in *Aplysia:* In both, the initial small response to the CS increases in amplitude as a result of pairing. They are true instances of associative learning in that the increase with pairing is significantly greater than any increase that may occur with unpaired control stimulation. The effect of the interstimulus onset interval on the degree of learning is evident in both preparations and essentially identical to that in classical conditioning of skeletal muscle responses in intact mammals (Gormezano, 1972). No learning occurs with backward pairings (US onset preceding CS onset) or with simultaneous CS–US onset, and the best learning occurs with a CS–US onset interval of about ¼–½ s (Hawkins et al., 1983; Patterson, 1975, 1980). Because *Aplysia* and spinal conditioning exhibit such strikingly parallel phenomena, it is at least possible that the underlying mechanisms of plasticity may be similar, perhaps the most basic or elementary form of associative learning. In any event, as noted above, the circuits and the associative learning they exhibit have many similar properties.

Levels of Analysis in Modeling Learning and Memory

In understanding a complex information-processing system, Marr (1982) described three distinct but interrelated levels of explanation: the level of the computation performed, the level of the algorithm for this computation, and the level of the physical mechanisms that implement this algorithm. In the domain of the neurobiology of learning and memory, the work of Kamin (1969), Rescorla (1968), and Wagner (1969) provided an important constraint on what is being computed in classical conditioning by demonstrating that it is contingency, and not merely contiguity, that determines the association strengths which develop between a CS and a US (see also Granger & Schlimmer, 1986). Various algorithms have since been proposed (e.g., Donegan & Wagner, in press; Rescorla & Wagner, 1972; Wagner, 1981) to describe the iterative trial-by-trial changes in association strengths by which animals learn to respond according to these contingencies. In attempting to identify neuronal correlates of the Rescorla–Wagner learning model, Hawkins and Kandel (1984) have taken a formidable step in attempting to bridge the gap between algorithmic-level models of classical conditioning and implementation-level models of the underlying neurophysiology. The particular advantage of formulating these models within a similar computational framework is that it allows researchers to test more precisely, at a quantitative level, whether the models are both computing the same target behavior.

Our analyses illustrate the complexities that arise in trying to understand a circuit involving only four neurons that generates phenomena of associative learning. If the functioning of this simple circuit is not evident at a qualitative level, then the more complex circuits that code, store, and retrieve memories in the mammalian brain will certainly require quantitative modeling.

References

Alkon, D. L. (1980). Membrane depolarization accumulates during acquisition of an associative behavioral change. *Science, 210,* 1375–1376.

Anderson, J. A. (1977). Neural models with cognitive implications. In D. Laberge & S. J. Samuels (Eds.), *Basic processes in reading: Perception and comprehension* (pp. 27–90). Hillsdale, NJ: Erlbaum.

Anderson, J. A., & Hinton, G. E. (1981). Models of information processing in the brain. In G. E. Hinton & J. A. Anderson (Eds.), *Parallel models of associative memory* (pp. 9–48). Hillsdale, NJ: Erlbaum.

Anderson, J. A., Silverstein, J. W., Ritz, S. A., & Jones, R. S. (1977). Distinctive features, categorical perception, and probability learning: Some applications of a neural model. *Psychological Review, 84,* 413–451.

Beggs, A. L., Steinmetz, J. E., Romano, A. G., & Patterson, M. M. (1983). Extinction and retention of a classically conditioned flexor nerve response in acute spinal cat. *Behavioral Neuroscience, 97,* 530–540.

Bernier, L., Castellucci, V. F., Kandel, E. R., & Schwartz, J. H. (1982). Facilitatory transmitter causes a selective and prolonged increase in adenosine 3:5 monophosphate in sensory neurons mediating the gill and siphon withdrawal reflex in Aplysia. *Journal of Neuroscience, 2,* 1682–1691.

Black, A. H., & Prokasy, W. F. (1972). *Classical conditioning II: Current research and theory.* New York: Appleton-Century-Crofts.

Carew, T. J., Hawkins, R. D., Abrams, T. W., & Kandel, E. R. (1984). A test of Hebb's postulate at identified synapses which mediate classical conditioning in *Aplysia. Journal of Neuroscience, 4,* 1217–1224.

Carew, T. J., Hawkins, R. D., & Kandel, E. R. (1983). Differential classical conditioning of a defensive withdrawal reflex in Aplysia californica. *Science, 219,* 397–400.

Carew, T. J., Pinsker, H. M., & Kandel, E. R. (1972). Longterm habituation of a defensive withdrawal reflex in Aplysia. *Science, 175,* 451–454.

Carew, T. J., Walters, E. T., & Kandel, E. R. (1981). Classical conditioning in a simple withdrawal reflex in Aplysia californica. *Journal of Neuroscience, 1,* 1426–1437.

Castellucci, V. F., & Kandel, E. R. (1974). A quantal analysis of the synaptic depression underlying habituation of the gill-withdrawal reflex in Aplysia. *Proceedings of the National Academy of Sciences, 71,* 5004–5008.

Castellucci, V. F., & Kandel, E. R. (1976). Presynaptic facilitation as a mechanism for behavioral sensitization in Aplysia. *Science, 194,* 1176–1178.

Castellucci, V. F., Nairn, A., Greengard, P., Schwartz, J. H., & Kandel, E. R. (1982). Inhibitor of adenosine 3:5-monophosphate-dependent protein kinase blocks presynaptic facilitation in Aplysia. *Journal of Neuroscience, 2,* 1673–1681.

Castellucci, V. F., Pinsker, H., Kupfermann, I., & Kandel, E. F. (1970). Neuronal mechanisms of habituation and dishabituation of the gill-withdrawal reflex in Aplysia. *Science, 167,* 1745–1748.

Chang, J. J., & Gelperin, A. (1980). Rapid taste aversion learning by an isolated molluscan central nervous system. *Proceedings of the National Academy of Sciences, 77,* 6204.

Cohen, D. H. (1980). The functional neuroanatomy of a conditioned response. In R. F. Thompson, L. H. Hicks, & V. B. Shvyrkov (Eds.), *Neural mechanisms of goal-directed behavior and learning* (pp. 283–302). New York: Academic Press.

Colwill, R. W. (1985). Context conditioning in Aplysia Californica. *Society for Neuroscience Abstracts, 11,* 796.

Davis, W. J., & Gillette, R. (1978). Neural correlates of behavioral plasticity in command neurons of Pleurobranchaea. *Science, 199,* 801–804.

Donegan, N. H., & Wagner, A. R. (in press). Conditioned dimunition and facilitation of the UCR: A sometimes-opponent-process interpretation. In I. Gormexano, W. Prokasy, & R. Thompson (Eds.), *Classical conditioning II: Behavioral, neurophysiological, and neurochemical studies in the rabbit.* Hillsdale, NJ: Erlbaum.

Durkovic, R. G. (1975). Classical conditioning, sensitization, and habituation of the flexion reflex of the spinal cat. *Physiology and Behavior, 14,* 297.

Feldman, J. A., & Ballard, D. H. (1982). Connectionist models and their properties. *Cognitive Science, 6,* 205–254.

Fitzgerald, L. A., & Thompson, R. F. (1967). Classical conditioning of the hindlimb flexion reflex in the acute spinal cat. *Psychonomic Science, 9,* 511–512.

Frey, P. W., & Sears, R. J. (1978). Model of conditioning incorporating the Rescorla–Wagner associative axiom, a dynamic attention process, and a catastrophe rule. *Psychological Review, 85,* 321–340.

Gingrich, K. J., & Byrne, J. H. (1985). Simulation of synaptic depression, posttetanic potentiation, and presynaptic facilitation of synaptic potentials from sensory neurons mediating gill-withdrawal reflex in Aplysia. *Journal of Neuroscience, 53,* 652–669.

Goldman-Rakic, P. (1984). The frontal lobes: Uncharted provinces of the brain. *Trends in Neurosciences, 7,* 425–429.

Gormezano, I. (1972). Investigations of defense and reward conditioning in the rabbit. In A. H. Black & W. F. Prokasy (Eds.), *Classical conditioning II: Current research and theory* (pp. 151–181). New York: Appleton-Century-Crofts.

Granger, R. H., & Schlimmer, J. C. (1986). The computation of contingency in classical conditioning. In G. H. Bower (Ed.), *The psychology of learning and motivation* (Vol. 20, pp. 137–192). New York: Academic Press.

Groves, P. M., & Thompson, R. F. (1970). Habituation: A dual-process theory. *Psychological Review, 77,* 419–450.

Hawkins, R. D. (1981). Interneurons involved in mediation and modulation of gill-withdrawal reflex in Aplysia. III. Identified facilitating neurons increase Ca2+ current in sensory neurons. *Journal of Neurophysiology, 45,* 327–339.

Hawkins, R. D., Abrams, T. W., Carew, T. J., & Kandel, E. R. (1983). A cellular mechanism of classical conditioning in Aplysia: Activity-dependent amplification of presynaptic facilitation. *Science, 219,* 400–404.

Hawkins, R. D., Carew, T. J., & Kandel, E. R. (1983). Effects of interstimulus interval and contingency on classical conditioning in Aplysia. *Society for Neurophysiology Abstracts, 9,* 168.

Hawkins, R. D., Castellucci, V. F., & Kandel, E. R. (1981). Interneurons involved in mediation and modulation of gill-withdrawal reflex in Aplysia. I. Identification and characterization. *Journal of Neurophysiology, 45,* 304–314.

Hawkins, R. D., & Kandel, E. R. (1984). Is there a cell-biological alphabet for simple forms of learning? *Psychological Review, 91,* 376–391.

Hebb, D. (1949). *Organization of behavior.* New York: Wiley.

Hilgard, E. R., & Bower, G. H. (1975). *Theories of learning.* Englewood Cliffs, NJ: Prentice-Hall.

Hinton, G. E., & Anderson, J. A. (1981). *Parallel models of associative memory.* Hillsdale, NJ: Erlbaum.

Hoyle, G. (1980). Learning, using natural reinforcements, in insect preparations that permit cellular neuronal analysis. *Journal of Neurobiology, 11,* 323–354.

Hull, C. L. (1943). *Principles of behavior.* New York: Appleton-Century-Crofts.

Ito, M. (1982). Cerebellar control of the vestibulo-ocular reflex around the flocculus hypothesis. *Annual Review of Neuroscience, 5,* 275–296.

Kamin, L. J. (1969). Predictability, surprise, attention and conditioning. In B. A. Campbell & R. M. Church (Eds.), *Punishment and aversive behavior* (pp. 279–296). New York: Appleton-Century-Crofts.

Kamin, L. J., & Gaioni, S. J. (1974). Compound conditioned emotional response conditioning with differentially salient elements in rats. *Journal of Comparative Physiological Psychology, 87,* 591–597.

Kandel, E. R. (1976). *Cellular basis of behavior: An introduction to behavioral neurobiology.* San Francisco, CA: Freeman.

Kandel, E. R., Abrams, T., Bernier, L., Carew, T. J., Hawkins, R. D., & Schwartz, J. A. (1983). Classical conditioning and sensitization share aspects of the same molecular cascade in Aplysia. *Cold Spring Harbor Symposium on Quantitative Biology, 48,* 821–830.

Kandel, E. R., & Schwartz, J. H. (1982). Molecular biology of learning: Modulation of transmitter release. *Science, 218,* 433–443.

Kandel, E. R., & Spencer, W. A. (1968). Cellular neurophysiological approaches in the study of learning. *Physiological Reviews, 58,* 65–134.

Kapp, B. S., Gallagher, M., Applegate, C. D., & Frysinger, R. C. (1982). The amygdala central nucleus: Contributions to conditioned cardiovascular responding during aversive Pavlovian conditioning in the rabbit. In C. D. Woody (Ed.), *Conditioning: Representation of involved neural functions* (pp. 581–600). New York: Plenum Press.

Klein, M., Shapiro, E., & Kandel, E. R. (1980). Synaptic plasticity and the modulation of the Ca^{++} current. *Journal of Experimental Biology, 89,* 117–157.

Krasne, F. B. (1969). Excitation and habituation of the crayfish escape reflex: The depolarizating response in lateral giant fibers of the isolated abdomen. *Journal of Experimental Biology, 50,* 29–46.

Lashley, K. S. (1929). *Brain mechanisms and intelligence.* Chicago: University of Chicago Press.

Lashley, K. S. (1950). In search of the engram. *Symposium of the Society for Experimental Biology, 4,* 454–482.

Mackintosh, N. J. (1974). *The psychology of animal learning.* New York: Academic Press.

Marr, D. (1982). *Vision: A computational investigation into the human representation and processing of visual information.* San Francisco, CA: Freeman.

McClelland, J. L. (1979). On the time relations of mental processes: An examination of systems of processes in cascade. *Psychological Review, 86,* 287–328.

McClelland, J. L., & Rumelhart, D. E. (1981). An interactive activation model of context effects in letter perception: Part 1. An account of basic findings. *Psychological Review, 88,* 375–407.

Mishkin, M. (1978). Memory in monkeys severely impaired by combined but not separate removal of amygdala and hippocampus. *Nature, 273,* 297–298.

Patterson, M. M. (1975). Effects of forward and backward classical conditioning procedures on a spinal cat hindlimb flexor nerve response. *Physiological Psychology, 3,* 86–91.

Patterson, M. M. (1976). Mechanisms of classical conditioning and fixation in spinal mammals. In A. H. Riesen & R. F. Thompson (Eds.), *Advances in psychobiology* (pp. 381–436). New York: Wiley.

Patterson, M. M., Cegavske, C. F., & Thompson, R. F. (1973). Effects of a classical conditioning paradigm on hindlimb flexor nerve response in immobilized spinal cat. *Journal of Comparative & Physiological Psychology, 84,* 88–97.

Patterson, M. M. (1980). Mechanisms of classical conditioning of spinal reflexes. In R. F. Thompson, L. H. Hicks, & V. B. Shvyrkov (Eds.), *Neural mechanisms of goal-directed behavior and learning* (pp. 263–272). New York: Academic Press.

Patterson, M. M., Steinmetz, J. E., Beggs, A. L., & Romano, A. G. (1982). Associative processes in spinal reflexes. In C. D. Woody (Ed.), *Conditioning: Representation of involved neural functions* (pp. 637–650). New York: Plenum.

Pavlov, I. (1927). *Conditioned reflexes.* London: Oxford University Press.

Pinsker, H. M., Kupfermann, I., Castellucci, V., & Kandel, E. R. (1970). Habituation and dishabituation of the gill-withdrawal reflex in Aplysia. *Science, 167,* 1740–1742.

Prokasy, W. F. (1965). Classical eyelid conditioning: Experimental operations, task demands, and response shaping. In W. F. Prokasy (Ed.), *Classical conditioning* (pp. 208–225). New York: Appleton-Century-Crofts.

Rescorla, R. A. (1968). Probability of shock in the presence and absence of CS in fear conditioning. *Journal of Comparative and Physiological Psychology, 66,* 1–5.

Rescorla, R. A., & Wagner, A. R. (1972). A theory of Pavlovian conditioning: Variations in the effectiveness of reinforcement and non-reinforcement. In A. H. Black & W. F. Prokasy (Eds.), *Classical conditioning II: Current research and theory* (pp. 64–99). New York: Appleton-Century-Crofts.

Rumelhart, D. E., & McClelland, J. L. (1986). *Parallel distributed processing: Explorations in the microstructure of cognition, Vol. 1: Foundations.* Cambridge, MA: Bradford Books/MIT Press.

Sahley, C. L., Rudy, J. W., & Gelperin, A. (1981). An analysis of associative learning in the terrestrial mollusk. I: Higher-order conditioning, blocking, and a US-preexposure effect. *Journal of Comparative Physiology, 144,* 1–8.

Schneiderman, N., McCabe, P. M., Haselton, J. R., & Ellenberger, H. H. (in press). Neurobiological bases of conditioned bradycardia. In I. Gormezzano, W. F. Prokasy, & R. F. Thompson (Eds.), *Classical conditioning III: Behavioral, neurophysiological, and neurochemical studies in the rabbit.* Hillsdale, NJ: Erlbaum.

Spence, K. W. (1956). *Behavior theory and conditioning.* New Haven, CT: Yale University Press.

Spencer, W. A., Thompson, R. F., & Neilson, D. R., Jr. (1966). Decrement of ventral root electronic and intracellularly recorded PSPs produced by iterated cutaneous afferent volleys. *Journal of Neurophysiology, 29,* 253–274.

Squire, L. R. (1982). The neurophysiology of human memory. *Annual Review of Neuroscience, 5,* 241–273.

Squire, L. R., & Zola-Morgan, S. (1983). The neurology of memory: The case for correspondence between the findings for man and nonhuman primate. In J. A. Deutsch (Ed.), *The physiological basis of memory* (2nd ed., pp. 199–268). New York: Academic Press.

Sutton, R. S., & Barto, A. G. (1981). Toward a modern theory of adaptive networks: Expectation and prediction. *Psychological Review, 88,* 135–170.

Thompson, R. F. (1986). The neurobiology of learning and memory. *Science, 233,* 941–947.

Thompson, R. F., Berger, T. W., Cegavske, C. F., Patterson, M. M., Roemer, R. A., Teyler, T. J., & Young, R. A. (1976). The search for the engram. *American Psychologist, 31,* 209–227.

Thompson, R. F., Berger, T. W., & Madden, J. (1983). Cellular processes of learning and memory in the mammalian CNS. *Annual Review of Neuroscience, 6,* 447–491.

Thompson, R. F., Clark, G. A., Donegan, N. H., Lavond, D. G., Madden, J. IV, Mamounas, L. A., Mauk, M. D., & McCormick, D. A. (1984). Neuronal substrates of basic associative learning. In L. Squire & N. Butters (Eds.), *Neuropsychology of memory* (pp. 424–442). New York: Guilford Press.

Thompson, R. F., Donegan, N. H., & Lavond, D. G. (in press). *The psychobiology of learning and memory.* New York: Wiley.

Thompson, R. F., & Spencer, W. A. (1966). Habituation: A model phenomenon for the study of neuronal substrates of behavior. *Psychological Review, 173,* 16–43.

Tsukahara, N. (1981). Synaptic plasticity in the mammalian central nervous system. *Annual Review of Neuroscience, 4,* 351–379.

Wagner, A. R. (1969). Stimulus selection and a modified continuity theory. In G. Bower & J. Spence (Eds.), *The psychology of learning and motivation* (Vol. 3, pp. 1–41). New York: Academic Press.

Wagner, A. R. (1981). SOP: A model of automatic memory processing in animal behavior. In N. Spear & G. Miller (Eds.), *Information processing in animals: Memory mechanisms* (pp. 5–47). Hillsdale, NJ: Erlbaum.

Walters, E. T., & Byrne, J. H. (1983). Associative conditioning of single sensory neurons suggests a cellular mechanism for learning. *Science, 219,* 404–407.

Woody, C. D. (1982). *Conditioning: Representation of involved neural function.* New York: Plenum Press.

33

J. Ambros-Ingerson, R. Granger, and G. Lynch

Simulation of paleocortex performs hierarchical clustering

1990. *Science* 247: 1344–1348

Abstract

Simulations were performed of layers I and II of olfactory paleocortex, as connected to its primary input structure, olfactory bulb. Induction of synaptic long-term potentiation by means of repetitive sampling of inputs caused the simulation to organize encodings of learned cues into a hierarchical memory that uncovered statistical relationships in the cue environment, corresponding to the performance of hierarchical clustering by the biological network. Simplification led to characterization of those parts of the network responsible for the mechanism, resulting in a novel, efficient algorithm for hierarchical clustering. The hypothesis is put forward that these cortico-bulbar networks and circuitry of similar design in other brain regions contain computational elements sufficient to construct perceptual hierarchies for use in recognizing environmental cues.

How various properties of memory might emerge from design features of circuits in cerebral cortex is a major problem area for neural network research (*1*, *2*). In previous studies, we addressed this in models of the superficial layers of the olfactory cortex (*3*) by incorporating several of the characteristics of the synaptic long-term potentiation (LTP) effect (*4*). Implementation of a repetitive sampling feature meant to represent the cyclic sniffing behavior of mammals (*5*) produced a system that exhibited a kind of dual encoding of learned cues: early cycles (sniffs) generated response patterns that were common to a subset of cues that resembled each other, whereas later responses were specific to an individual member of the subset. This could mean that the cortical model simply constructs two types of representations (category and individual) or that it discovers hierarchical structure in the cue world and stores memory in this highly structured form. Human subjects in perceptual studies robustly recognize objects first at categorical levels and subsequently at successively subordinate levels (*6*), suggesting the presence of structured memories that are organized and searched hierarchically during recognition. Here we show that the olfactory cortex–olfactory bulb model, during learning, generates a multilevel hierarchical memory that uncovers statistical relationships inherent in collections of learned cues, and, during retrieval, sequentially traverses this hierarchical recognition memory. Moreover, simplification of the network results in an algorithm that provides a novel and efficient solution to the computationally difficult problem of hierarchical clustering.

The elements and circuitry simulated are shown in Fig. 1. Two networks, bulb and cortex, consisting of distinct architectures and physiologies, are extensively connected by both feedforward and feedback projections (*7*). The entire system works in synchrony with a 4- to 7-Hz (theta) sampling pattern that is characteristic of small mammals (*5*). Bulb mitral cells (those neurons innervated by the peripheral receptors and that project to cortex) receive inputs presented repetitively for brief periods. Inputs to the cortical network arise from the resultant synchronous bursting in a subset of mitral cells, yielding cyclic activity in relatively discrete "operation cycles" time-locked to the sampling rhythm. Sparse random connectivity in the simulation selectively activates those cortical cells whose dendrites are most connected to the input lines that are active. Learning increments active synapses on sufficiently depolarized cells via a rule based on LTP (*3*), which has been shown to produce a measurable increment in synaptic strength during even a single 50-ms burst of activity (*4*), that is, within a single operation cycle in the model. Learning requires only a few training trials per cue, as in rapid olfactory learning in mammals (*8*). Input lines shared across many similar input cues, and thus participating in many learning episodes, will strengthen their target synapses more than lines that participate in relatively fewer episodes. The result is that cortical dendrites (which can be viewed as vectors being moved by synaptic learning) become increasingly well tuned to those inputs containing the shared subset; that is, those inputs that are sufficiently similar to constitute members of a cluster. We have shown that this circuit will generate cell-firing responses that group learned cues by similarity. For a given threshold of input similarity among a set of cues, outputs are identical for all of the cues, whereas below that similarity threshold, outputs are much less similar than corresponding inputs (*3*). This form of unsupervised learning (*9*, *10*) is to be distinguished from supervised learning, in which categorization information is provided to the learner.

Feedback from cortex to the bulb inhibitory layer in the model (Fig. 1) is trained by means of a correlational rule during an earlier "developmental" period via a Hebb rule coarsely correlating activity in cortex with activity in bulb. The feedback then selectively inhibits the mitral cells in those bulb patches (Fig. 1) that are most responsible for the cortical output response, via

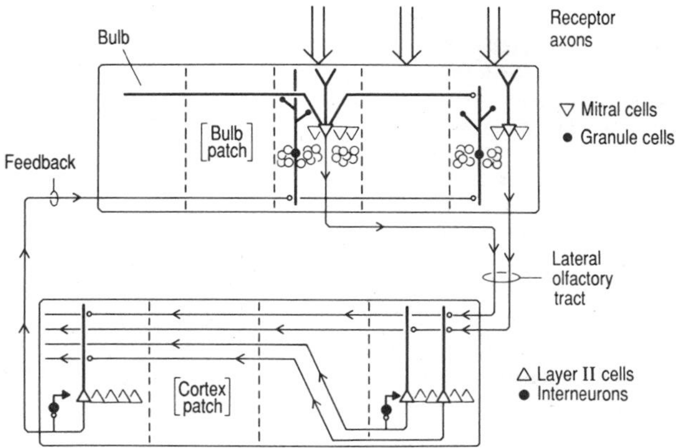

Figure 1. Anatomical architecture of the bulbar-cortical simulation. The bulb simulation contains 400 projection (mitral) units (simulated neurons), divided into 40 separate groups, each of which receives an input from one group of peripheral receptor axons (*22*). The intensity of an input is reflected in the number of cells within the appropriate group (or groups in the case of multicomponent cues) that it activates. The (excitatory) mitral projection cells in bulb have been shown to have extremely long oblique dendrites that form dendrodendritic contacts with a dense granule cell inhibitory network (*22*). We adopt an assumption made by others (*12*) that this excitatory-inhibitory arrangement serves to normalize the output of the bulb (that is, the total number of mitral cells that are activated is reasonably constant across cues with different intensities and compositions). The inhibitory neurons (granule and probably periglomerular) are represented in the model by a single layer of cells and are innervated by randomly organized excitatory feedback from cortex. The strength of the simulated feedback contacts is set during a "development" period in which hundreds of cues are presented and the strength of feedback synapses allowed to vary according to a correlational (Hebb) rule. The mitral cells of bulb project sparsely and nontropographically to the outermost layer of olfactory cortex via the LOT, both biologically (*7*) and in the simulation. The cortex is simulated as a layer of 1000 excitatory layer II cells that are assumed in the model to be arranged into patches of 20 cells each by the radial axonal arborizations of local (feedback) inhibitory interneurons. The modeled neurons sum the voltages from their active synaptic inputs and require different amounts of depolarization for discharges, bursts of discharges, and for induction of synaptic change via LTP. A more detailed simulation of individual patches has shown that active cells that trigger inhibitory interneurons can suppress firing by other cells in a patch; because of this, typically only one or two cells in a patch will discharge in response to bulbar inputs, making each patch into a competitive (or modified winners-take-all) arrangement of the type discussed by many authors (*9*, *10*). Such an arrangement is assumed in the present simulation. Each cortical cell receives input from the LOT and from a feedforward associational system generated by the cortical neurons themselves, in both cortex (*7*, *23*) and the simulation. The operating rules for the model are based on physiological data reported in the literature (*5*, *24*).

relatively long-lasting inhibition that has been shown to exist in olfactory bulb (*11*). Resulting renormalization of bulb activity (*12*) maintains the total number of firing mitral cells at a roughly constant level. This renormalization thus recruits additional mitral cells in remaining (uninhibited) bulb patches to fire to compensate for those selectively inhibited by the feedback. Thus, the pattern of mitral cell firing on the next operation cycle (roughly 200 ms later) is distinct spatially from the previous pattern. This in turn activates a distinct set of cortical cells. This sampling cycle (bulb activation → cortical activation → inhibitory feedback → renormalization) can be repeated until bulb is sufficiently inhibited to be largely quiescent. The sequence of cortical responses after the initial (first-sample) response becomes progressively more different for different cues (*3*), increasingly approximating a given cue, thus producing unique encodings for individuals.

Until now it had not been determined whether the network had the ability to discover secondary or intermediate structure in hierarchically organized input cues. Table 1 gives responses of the simulation after training to such a structured environment, one consisting of clusters subclusters within those clusters, and individuals within the subclusters. On its first cycle, network responses to members of a given cluster of input cues are nearly identical, thus grouping those cues together, whereas between-group overlap is extremely low. Second-cycle responses are nearly identical for members of subclusters, but not for members of the containing clusters. Third-cycle network responses are nearly unique for each individual cue. The network thus discovers intermediate structure, exhibiting an ability corresponding to hierarchical clustering (*13*), which identifies multilevel statistical structure in novel data.

Empirical results of this type do not by themselves elucidate the mechanism by which the hierarchical clustering operation is accomplished. Of primary interest is the identification and characterization of the essential design features of the network underlying its hierarchical clustering ability. Analysis led to such a characterization, and controlled testing revealed that the resulting simplified formulation of the network provides a novel and efficient method of hierarchical clustering.

The simplified formulation of the cortex contains a weight matrix W [corresponding to the connections between the lateral olfactory tract (LOT) and piriform layer II cell dendrites] (Fig. 1), divided into H non-overlapping "winners-take-all" or "competitive" (*9*, *10*) subnets of cells, each competing to "win" within their subnet. Each (densely connected) subnet $S_i \in \{S_1, S_2, \ldots, S_H\}$ contains weight vectors $\mathbf{C}$ (that is, columns of W) such that $W = \bigcup_i S_i$ (*14*). Each subnet S_h corresponds to the network response at hierarchical level

Table 1. Overlaps among responding vectors in cortical-bulbar simulation to eight hierarchically organized input cue vectors. The input cues can be visualized as the hierarchical cluster dendrogram at the left side of the table (see the legend to Fig. 2b), breaking the input space into two superordinate clusters, which are divided into four intermediate subclusters (two subclusters in each cluster), which in turn are subdivided into eight individual cues (a to h), two individuals to a subcluster. Average Euclidean distance between the two cues in a subcluster is 1.9; between the means of the subclusters with a cluster is 2.6; and between the means of the two clusters is 3.2. Response overlaps are defined as follows: let $\zeta = \{\zeta_1, \zeta_2, \ldots, \zeta_k\}$ be the set of clusters at one level (superordinate, intermediate, or subordinate), where each cluster consists of a set of cues. For $\mathbf{X} \in \zeta_i$ let $R_h(\mathbf{X})$ be the set of cortical cells responding to **X** at operation cycle h. The average percent within-cluster overlap at level ζ for cycle h is:

$$\mathcal{W}_{\zeta,h} = \frac{100}{A|\zeta|} \sum_{\zeta_i \in \zeta} \left| \bigcap_{\mathbf{X} \in \zeta_i} R_h(\mathbf{X}) \right| \tag{5}$$

where A is the number of patches (assuming one winner per patch) and $|\zeta|$ is the cardinality of set ζ. Analogously, average percent between-cluster overlap is

$$\mathfrak{B}_{\zeta,h} = \frac{100}{A\binom{|\zeta|}{2}} \sum_{\substack{\zeta_i,\zeta_j \in \zeta \\ i<j}} \left[\sum_{\substack{\mathbf{X}_i \in \zeta_i \\ \mathbf{X}_j \in \zeta_j}} \frac{|R_h(\mathbf{X}_i) \cap R_h(\mathbf{X}_j)|}{|\zeta_i||\zeta_j|} \right] \tag{6}$$

First-cycle responses were nearly identical (average overlap among responses was 91%) for all objects within either of the two (superordinate) clusters, indicating simply membership of a cue in a cluster, whereas between-cluster overlap between the superordinate clusters (right-hand column) was extremely low (8% or less) for all trials. Second-cycle responses were very similar (average within-group overlap 88%) for subcluster members, but were distinct for other members of the containing cluster that were not members of the subcluster (average within-group overlap 31%). Third-cycle responses were distinct for each individual cue: little or no overlap exists among responses to individual members of clusters (0%) or subclusters (17%).

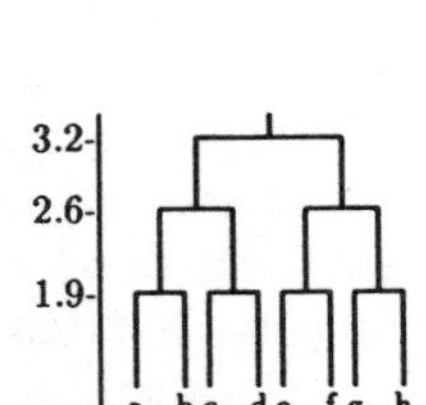

	$\mathcal{W}_{\zeta,h}$*			$\mathfrak{B}_{\zeta,h}$*
Cycle	Superordinate (clusters) (%)	Intermediate (subclusters) (%)	Subordinate (individuals) (%)	Superordinate (clusters) (%)
1	91	99	100	8
2	31	88	100	5
3	0	17	100	2

*$\mathcal{W}_{\zeta,h}$, Within-group overlap among all responses; $\mathfrak{B}_{\zeta,h}$, between-group overlap between superordinates.

h. The simplified bulb receives N-dimensional real-valued vectors (corresponding to frequency and spatial patterns of activation input to bulb) and passes these to cortex, relaxing the requirement in the biological model that inputs to cortex must be binary. The cortical network is thus trained on a set of N-dimensional real-valued vectors via an extension of a correlational (Hebbian) learning algorithm (a simplification of the LTP rules for synaptic modification). An input vector **X** is presented first to the highest subnet in the hierarchy, S_1. The column vectors (dendrites) **C** in this subnet that win the (winners-take-all) competition on **X** (corresponding to target cells that are most depolarized by this input) are identified. The synaptic contacts on these winning vectors are then trained, moving the vectors closer to **X** by an increment γ_c. Feedback from the just trained vectors then partially inhibits or "masks" the input. The remainder of the input is presented to the next lower subnet of cells in the hierarchy, until all hierarchical subnets $S_1, S_2, \ldots, S_H$ have been trained, over H operation cycles. At any given hierarchical level S_h, the **C**s in that subnet can be shown to converge to the means of the clusters of cues on which they are trained, as in related "competitive learning" algorithms (*3*, *9*, *10*). The feedback inhibition step enables vectors in W assigned to the subordinate hierarchical levels to converge to means of subclusters of the data, allowing secondary (and H-ary) structure to be identified (for H divisions of the weight matrix into subnets). Formally

Step 1. Do steps 2 to 5 for each input **X** to be learned.

Step 2. Do steps 3 to 5 for each hierarchical level $h \in \{1, 2, \ldots, H\}$.

Step 3. Identify winning cells (column vectors) in subnet S_h for input **X**: win $(\mathbf{X}, S_h)$.

Step 4. Train each of the winning cells $\mathbf{C} \in \text{win}(\mathbf{X}, S_h)$ identified in step 3: $\mathbf{C} \leftarrow \mathbf{C} + \gamma_c(\mathbf{X} - \mathbf{C})$.

Step 5. Subtract winners from input: $\mathbf{X} \leftarrow \mathbf{X} - \text{mean}[\text{win}(\mathbf{X}, S_h)]$.

where H is the depth of the hierarchy; $\text{win}(\mathbf{X}, S_h) = \{\mathbf{C} \in S_h\colon [\mathbf{X} \cdot \mathbf{C} = \max_{\mathbf{C}_i \in S_h}(\mathbf{X} \cdot \mathbf{C}_i)] \wedge \mathbf{X} \cdot \mathbf{C} > 0\}$ is the set of weight vectors within a subnet S_h that wins the competition on the input **X**; and γ_c is the learning rate (*15*).

To enable controlled testing of the ability of the simplified formulation to identify hierarchical struc-

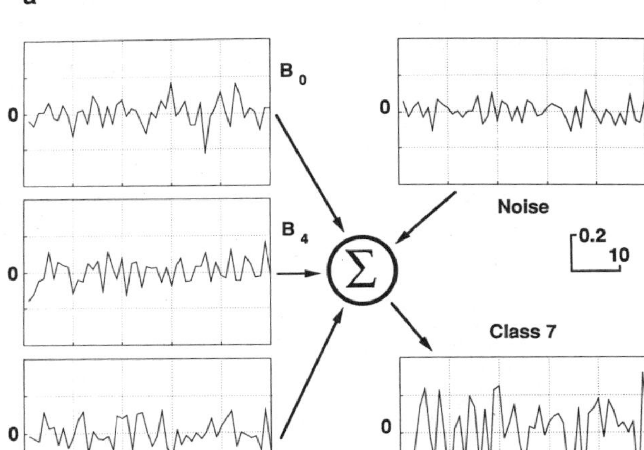

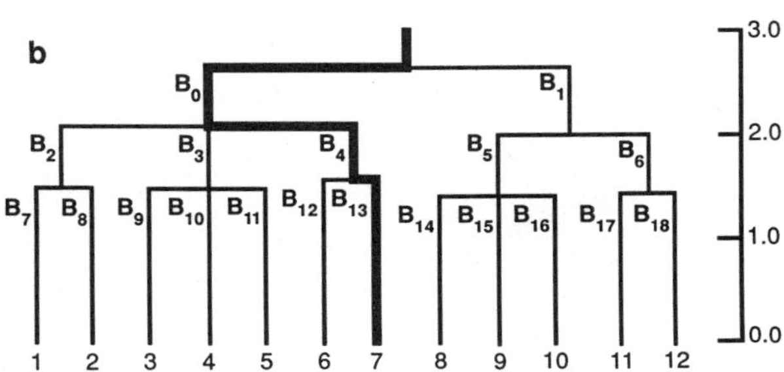

Figure 2. (**a**) A sample member of one group of a created hierarchy of cues. The 50-dimensional vector, an example of one group (class 7) of 12 [see (b)], is the sum of three orthogonal vectors plus a noise vector. Positions on the *x*-axes correspond to each of the 50 dimensions of the vectors; the *y*-axes denote the values of each of the dimensions. This particular vector sum corresponds to the end point of the path indicated by darkened lines in the hierarchical tree in (b). (**b**) A hierarchy of 50-dimensional real-valued vectors like the instance in (a), created such that they are naturally clustered at each of three levels, via an algorithm described in the text. Each vector is the sum of three orthogonal component vectors plus a noise vector. All vectors under node $\mathbf{B}_0$ contain the same initial component ($\mathbf{B}_0$); all under node $\mathbf{B}_1$ contain initial component $\mathbf{B}_1$; of the vectors under node $\mathbf{B}_0$, those under node $\mathbf{B}_3$ all contain initial component $\mathbf{B}_0$ and second component $\mathbf{B}_3$; and so on. The height of each node corresponds to the average distance among the means of the data below the node.

ture, we created cue environments with known hierarchical structure. The cues each consist of the sum of a sequence of orthogonal multidimensional vectors with noise, forming a hierarchy of subclusters within clusters:

$$\text{cue} = M + \sum_{i \in \text{path to cue}} (\mathbf{B}_i + K_i) \tag{1}$$

where each $\mathbf{B}_i$ is an orthogonal vector in the summation path to the cue (Fig. 2); M is noise and

$$K_i = N(\mu_i, \sigma_i)\frac{\mathbf{B}_i}{\|\mathbf{B}_i\|} \tag{2}$$

that is, each K_i is unidimensional Gaussian noise in the direction of component i. The result is a set of vector sums that correspond to groups of vectors that are naturally clustered at each of the i levels of the hierarchy (Fig. 2, a and b) (*16*).

The dendrograms produced by the simplified formulation (*17*) are shown in Fig. 3a. Single-level competitive learning partitions the input space in a piecewise linear fashion (*9*); for the present algorithm, the input space at level h is itself a partition generated at level $h - 1$ and is recursively subpartitioned in the same piecewise linear manner. Like most probabilistic algorithms, the one presented here can fail to identify the full hierarchical structure in some circumstances (for example, degenerate initial conditions, initial skew bias in the data); empirically however, failure tends to be graceful in that correct structure is identified, although intermediate structure may be either missed or interposed. The breadth of the categories created is dependent on the number and distribution of units in a subnet.

The simplified formulation of the network, besides representing selected characteristics of the interacting biological systems (olfactory bulb and cortex) in the larger simulation, can be treated as a proposed novel algorithm for hierarchical clustering. As such, its performance on structured data can be compared directly against standard algorithms in the hierarchical clustering literature (Fig. 3b). Moreover, the space and time complexity of the algorithm can be evaluated. The weight matrix W contains H layers or distinct sets (subnets) of units. For complete separability of n cues, the bottom of the hierarchy (S_H) must contain at least n units, so the complete hierarchy will contain roughly $b(b-1)^{-1}\, n$ units, organized into a tree consisting of $\log_b n$ hierarchical layers, where b is the average branching factor at each level. Thus the number of units required grows linearly with the number of cues to be learned: the space complexity of the algorithm is $O(nN)$, where N is the dimensionality of $\mathbf{X}$ [a function $g(n)$ is "order" $f(n)$—denoted $O(f(n))$—if for large n, $g(n) \leq kf(n)$ for some constant k].

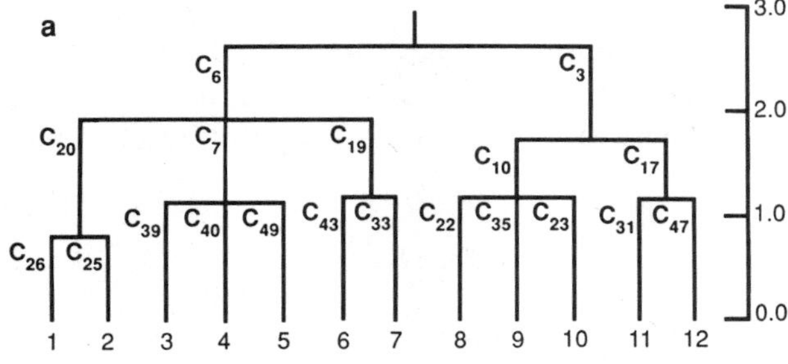

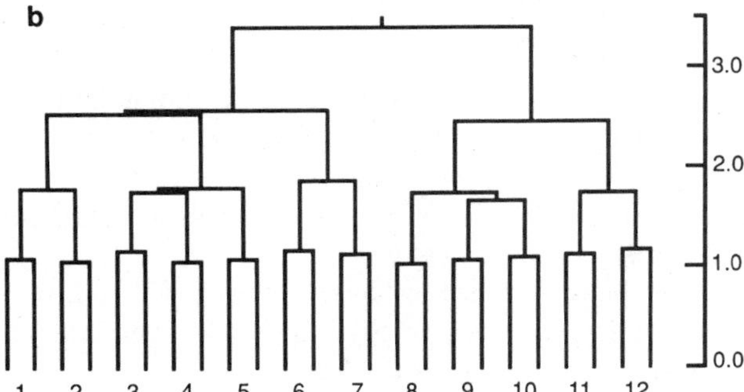

Figure 3. (**a**) Dendrogram structure created by simplified network after training. The network was trained on three passes over a training set consisting of a sample of 120 cues in random order (each of 12 categories represented by approximately ten instances). After training, the network was tested on a distinct testing set consisting of ten novel instances of each of the 12 categories, and a record was kept of which cells won on each cue presentation. Analysis of this record showed that cells become tuned to groups of cues that correspond to categories; cell responses are indicated in the dendrogram. For instance, cell $\mathbf{C}_6$ wins on the first sniff for all instances of cues from categories 1 through 7 and not on any other (that is, $\mathbf{C}_6$ wins if and only if the cue is from category 1 through 7); cell $\mathbf{C}_{19}$ wins on the second sniff for cues from categories 6 and 7 and no other; cell $\mathbf{C}_{33}$ wins on the third sniff if and only if the cue comes from category 7. The height of each node is given by the average Euclidean distance among the weight vectors represented by each cell at that level (for example, the average distance between weight vectors $\mathbf{C}_{39}$, $\mathbf{C}_{40}$, and $\mathbf{C}_{49}$ is 1.11). (**b**) Dendrogram created by agglomerative hierarchical clustering algorithm using Euclidean group–mean distance metric (*13*) on the same testing set data as in (a). Height of each node denotes distance between the two immediately subordinate constituents of the node.

The three time costs of the algorithm for each input vector **X** at level h are (i) summation of inputs on subnets S_h; (ii) computation of subnet winners **C**; and (iii) weight modifications on **C**. On a serial processor, after processing all levels (i) is $O(nN)$, (ii) is $O(n)$, and (iii) is $O(N \log n)$. Because of the inherent parallelism of the algorithm, on a suitable parallel processor, (i) is $O(\log N)$, (ii) is $O(\log n)$, and (iii) is constant. Thus training time per presentation, assuming $O(n)$ units in the net, is $O(nN)$ in serial and $O(\log n \cdot \log nN)$ in parallel. We have not determined analytically the number of instance presentations per cue required for convergence, though empirically a small number (~ 10) has sufficed (see legend to Fig. 3). Hence, we conjecture that training time to process a collection of n objects to convergence is $O(n^2 N)$ in serial and $O(n \cdot \log n \cdot \log nN)$ in parallel. The inherent parallelism and uniformity of the steps permits efficient hardware implementation (*18*).

The simplified network formulation aforementioned consists of specific operations of winning a competitive subnet, training winning vectors, and masking the input by the trained vectors. Admitting a range of different mechanisms for competition, training, and masking yields formulation of a general algorithm of which the simplified network is a special case.

Step 1. Do steps 2 to 5 for each input **X** to be learned.

Step 2. Do steps 3 to 5 for each hierarchical level $h \in \{1, 2, \ldots, H\}$.

Step 3. Identify winning cells (column vectors) in subnet S_h for input **X**.

Step 4. Train each winning cell identified in step 3.

Step 5. Mask structure identified by winners in step 3 from input **X** to produce remainder of input **X** for further processing.

The generalization bears some relation to algorithms identifying principal components of data (*19*, *20*); indeed, the algorithms set forth by Oja *et al.* and Sanger (*19*) can be cast as distinct special cases of the generalized formulation of the algorithm. We conjecture that the new general algorithm characterizes a class of repetitive sampling algorithms that successively approximate statistical aspects of data, including eigenvectors and clusters.

Our results provide an instance in which a novel and efficient alogrithm for a well-studied computational problem is developed from a simulation of a specific cortical network. Reflecting the system from which it is derived, the algorithm is inherently parallel and hence lends itself to efficient implementation in hardware. The present findings also point to the hypothesis that approximate hierarchical clustering will emerge as a fundamental property of memories based (at least in part) on LTP-like synaptic modifications in damped oscillatory networks of the type found in the bulbar-cortical system. The model is sufficiently detailed to make testable predictions at both behavioral and physiological levels (for example, different cortical cells should discharge over successive sampling cycles with progressively more selective tuning), but relevant experimental data is not yet available. Finally, the general architectural plan of the bulbar-cortical system finds parallels in certain aspects of thalamo-cortical relations [that is, secondary thalamic projection nuclei → superficial neocortex → deep layers of cortex → nucleus reticularis → projection nuclei (*21*)]. This similarity suggests a possible connection with attentional functions proposed for thalamocortical interactions (*2*), and raises the possibility that this biologically generated mechanism for hierarchical clustering may be a routine part of perceptual recognition memory behavior in animals and humans (*6*).

References and Notes

1. M. A. Gluck and R. F. Thompson, *Psychol. Rev.* **94** (2), 176 (1986): W. J. Freeman, *Mass Action in the Nervous System* (Academic Press, New York, 1975); L. B. Haberly and J. M. Bower, *Trends Neurosci.* **12**, 258 (1989); K. D. Miller, J. B. Keller, M. P. Stryker, *Science* **245**, 605 (1989): C. von der Malsburg and D. J. Wilshaw, *Exp. Brain Res. Suppl.* **1**, 463 (1976); G. M. Edelman and G. N. Reeke, Jr., *Proc. Natl. Acad. Sci. U.S.A.* **79**, 2091 (1982); M. F. Bear, L. N. Cooper, F. F. Ebner, *Science* **237**, 42 (1987); D. H. Ballard, G. E. Hinton, T. J. Sejnowski, *Nature* **306**, 21 (1983).

2. F. Crick, *Proc. Natl. Acad. Sci. U.S.A.* **81**, 4586 (1984).

3. R. Granger, J. Ambros-Ingerson, H. Henry, G. Lynch, in *Neural Information Processing Systems*, D. Anderson, Ed. (American Institute of Physics Press, New York, 1988); R. Granger, J. Ambros-Ingerson, G. Lynch, *J. Cog. Neurosci.* **1**, 61 (1989); G. Lynch and R. Granger, *Psychol. Learn. Motiv.* **23**, 205 (1989); R. Granger, J. Ambros-Ingerson, U. Staubli, G. Lynch, in *Neuroscience and Connectionist Theory*, M. A. Gluck and D. E. Rumelhart, Eds. (Erlbaum, Hillsdale, NJ, 1989); R. Granger, J. Ambros-Ingerson, P. Anton, G. Lynch, in *Connectionist Modeling and Brain Function: The Developing Interface*, S. J. Hanson and C. R. Olson, Eds. (MIT Press, Cambridge, MA, 1989).

4. G. Lynch, *Synapses, Circuits and the Beginnings of Memory* (MIT Press, Cambridge, 1986); J. Larson and G. Lynch, *Science* **232**, 985 (1986); *Brain Res.* **441**, 111 (1988); D. Muller, M. Joly, G. Lynch, *Science* **242**, 1694 (1988).

5. F. Macrides, *Behav. Biol.* **14**, 295 (1975); ———, H. Eichenbaum, B. Forbes, *J. Neurosci.* **2**, 1705 (1982); B. R. Komisaruk, *Neurosciences Research Program Bulletin* **11**, 376 (1973); D. v. Holst and H. Kolb, *J. Comp. Physiol.* **105**, 243 (1976).

6. I. Biederman, *Science* **177**, 77 (1972); M. C. Potter and B. A. Faulconer, *Nature* **253**, 437 (1975); A. M. Collins and E. F. Loftus, *Physiol. Rev.* **82**, 407 (1975); E. Rosch, C. B. Mervis, W. D. Gray, D. M. Johnson, P. Boyes-Braem, *Cog. Physiol.* **8**, 382 (1976); E. Rosch and B. B. Lloyd, *Cognition and Categorization* (Erlbaum, Hillsdale, NJ, 1978); E. E. Smith and D. L. Medin, *Categories and Concepts* (Harvard Univ. Press, Cambridge, MA, 1981); J. Hoffmann and C. Ziessler, *Z. Psychol.* **194**, 135 (1983); P. Jolicoeur, M. A. Gluck, S. M. Kosslyn, *Cog. Psychol.* **16**, 243 (1984); J. Corter, M. A. Gluck, G. H. Bower, *Proc. 10th Annu. Conf. Cog. Sci. Soc.* (Erlbaum, Hillsdale, NJ, 1988); M. A. Gluck and G. H. Bower, *J. Exper. Psych.* **117** (3), 227 (1988).

7. J. L. Price, *J. Comp. Neurol.* **150**, 87 (1973); L. B. Haberly and J. L. Price, *Brain Res.* **129**, 152 (1977); L. B. Haberly, *Chem. Senses* **10** (2), 219 (1985).

8. J. W. Jennings and L. H. Keefer, *Psychol. Reports* **24**, 3 (1969); B. M. Slotnick and H. M. Katz, *Science* **185**, 796 (1974); B. M. Slotnick and N. Kaneko, *ibid.* **214**, 91 (1981); H. Eichenbaum, A. Fagan, N. J. Cohen, *J. Neurosci.* **6**, 1876 (1986); U. Staubli, D. Fraser, R. Faraday, G. Lynch, *Behav. Neurosci.* **101**, 757 (1987).

9. S. Grossberg, *Biol. Cybernetics* **23**, 121 (1976); T. Kohonen, *Self-Organization and Associative Memory* (Springer-Verlag, New York, 1984).

10. C. von der Malsburg, *Kybernetik* **14**, 85 (1973); D. E. Rumelhart and D. Zipser, in *Parallel Distributed Processing*, D. Rumelhart and J. McClelland, Eds. (MIT Press, Cambridge, MA, 1986).

11. R. A. Nicoll, *Brain Res.* **14**, 157 (1969); K. Mori and G. M. Shepherd, *ibid.* **172**, 155 (1979); K. Mori, M. C. Nowycky, G. M. Shephard, *J. Physiol.* **314**, 311 (1981).

12. G. M. Shepherd, in *The Neurosciences: Second Study Program*, F. O. Schmitt, Ed. (Rockefeller Univ. Press, New York, 1970); G. M. Shepherd and R. K. Brayton, *Brain Res.* **175**, 377 (1979); J. S. Kauer, in *The Neurobiology of Taste and Smell*, T. E. Finger, Ed. (Wiley, New York, 1987).

13. Agglomerative (bottom-up) hierarchical clustering algorithms are of the following form: (i) calculate (or update) a distance matrix (all pairwise distances among cues); (ii) identify "closest" pair of cues in the data according to a chosen distance metric, and group those into a cluster; (iii) repeat steps (i) and (ii) using newly formed clusters in place of their members, until all elements are members of a cluster. Divisive (top-down) hierarchical clustering methods typically subdivide each cluster (initially a single one comprising all the data) into k subclusters for each hierarchical level (k is typically chosen by the user). This is done by iteratively attempting to locally optimize a given objective function (for example, mean-squared distance from cluster members to cluster mean) by refining an initial, often arbitrary, assignment of data points into k clusters [R. R. Sokal and P. H. A. Sneath, *Principles of Numerical Taxonomy* (Freeman, San Francisco, 1963); G. N. Lance and W. T. Williams, *Nature* **212**, 218 (1966); R. O. Duda and P. E. Hart, *Pattern Classification and Scene Analysis* (Wiley, New York, 1973); B. Everitt, *Cluster Analysis* (Wiley, New York, 1980)].

14. Each subnet S_h in the simplified formulation consists of those cells that respond at particular operation cycle h of the network. The subnet structure is constructed from the anatomical network via two steps: (i) the sparsely connected anatomical patches in the network are combined into a single network with dense connectivity; (ii) the cells in the single network are then divided into H subnets and the cells in each subnet are allowed to respond during only one prespecified operation cycle. That is, each subnet at level h contains only those cells that respond on operation cycle h; these correspond to the responses at hierarchical level h. Even without this simplification, the network still identifies hierarchical structure, as shown earlier (Table 1); the simplification enables formal distinction among cells responding to a given operation cycle, enabling a tractable algorithmic formulation.

15. The learning rate, γ_c, is chosen to satisfy $\gamma_c(t) \to 0$ and $\Sigma_t \gamma_c(t) = \infty$ where t is the number of times **C** has been trained [L. Ljung, *IEEE Trans. Autom. Control* **AC-22**, 551 (1977)].

16. Parameters are set as follows: $\mu_{0,1} = 1.6$; $\mu_{2,\ldots,6} = 1.3$; $\mu_{7,\ldots,18} = 1.0$; $\sigma_i = 0.1$, $\|\mathbf{B}_i\| = 1$, $i = 0,\ldots,18$; and M is uncorrelated Gaussian noise on each input line with $\mu = 0.0$ and $\sigma = 0.1$.

17. $H = 3$; $\gamma_c = 0.2t^{-1/2}$ (satisfying the specified constraints for γ); and the cardinalities of S_i's are set so that $|S_{i+1}| = b|S_i|$ is maintained as closely as possible (b, the average branching factor of the tree, is a small number in the range 2 to 5). We use $|S_1| = 7$, and $|S_2| = 14$, and $|S_3| = 29$. W was constructed by selecting pseudorandom vectors from a uniform distribution over the hypersphere of radius $r = 0.5$ [G. S. Watson, *Statistics on Spheres* (Wiley, New York, 1983)].

18. J. Bailey, D. Hammerstrom, J. Mates, M. Rudnick, in *An Introduction to Neural and Electronic Networks*, S. F. Zornetzer, J. L. Davis, C. Lau, Eds. (Academic Press, New York, 1989); D. Hammerstrom, in *Neural Information Processing Systems*, D. Anderson, Ed. (American Institute of Physics Press, New York, 1988).

19. E. Oja, *J. Math. Biol.* **15**, 276 (1982); ——— and J. Karhunen, *J. Math. Anal. Appl.* **106**, 69 (1985); T. D. Sanger, *Neural Network* **2**, 459 (1989).

20. R. Linsker, *Proc. Natl. Acad. Sci U.S.A.* **83**, 7508 (1986); *ibid.*, p. 8390; *ibid.*, p. 8779; *ibid.*, p. 8783; *IEEE Computer* **21**, 105 (1988).

21. M. E. Scheibel and A. B. Scheibel, *Brain Res.* **1**, 43 (1966); E. G. Jones, *J. Comp. Neurol.* **162**, 285 (1975); M. Herkenham, in *Cerebral*

Cortex, E. Jones and A. Peters, Eds. (Plenum, New York, 1986), vol. 5, pp. 403–445.

22. G. M. Shepherd, *Physiol. Rev.* **52**, 864 (1972); F. R. Sharp *et al.*, *J. Neurophysiol.* **40**, 800 (1977); K. Mori, *Prog. Neurobiology* **29**, 275 (1987).

23. J. E. Schwob and J. L. Price, *Brain Res.* **151**, 369 (1978).

24. W. J. Freeman and W. Schneider, *Psychophysiology* **19**, 44 (1978); L. B. Haberly and J. M. Bower, *J. Neurophysiol.* **51**, 90 (1984); G. Tseng and L. B. Haberly, *ibid.* **59**, 1352 (1988); F. Roman, U. Staubli, G. Lynch, *Brain Res.* **418**, 221 (1987).

25. We thank J. W. Whitson, Jr., and P. Antón for their assistance with this research. We also thank the helpful comments of the reviewers of this paper. Supported in part by the Office of Naval Research under grants N00014-89-J-1255 and N00014-89-J-3179.

A. G. Barto and M. I. Jordan

Gradient following without back-propagation in layered networks

1987. *Proceedings of the IEEE First Annual International Conference on Neural Networks* 2: 629–636

Abstract

We describe a method for solving nonlinear supervised learning tasks by multilayer feed-forward networks. It estimates the performance gradient without back-propagating error information by using the *Associative Reward-Penalty*, or A_{R-P}, algorithm that has been the subject of previous papers [2, 3, 4, 5]. We introduce a variant of the A_{R-P} algorithm, called the S-model A_{R-P}, for learning with real-valued reinforcement, and we introduce a method, called "batching", for increasing the learning efficiency of A_{R-P} networks. We describe simulation experiments using the task of learning symmetry axes to compare the variants of the A_{R-P} network method as well as the back-propagation method of Rumelhart, Hinton, and Williams [11].

Introduction

Methods relying on gradient following have long been central in the study of adaptive systems.[1]. A major problem in extending gradient following methods for single neuron-like adaptive units to networks of these units is the problem of computing the gradient of a global performance measure in a way that can be implemented using information locally available to each unit. The Boltzmann learning procedure [1] does this by taking advantage of equilibrium properties of symmetric stochastic networks, and the error back-propagation methods developed by Parker [10], Le Cun [6], and Rumelhart, Hinton, and Williams [11] do this by recursively computing the gradient through back-propagating error information. We have developed a method that differs from all of these. Instead of relying on a back-propagation process, it works by broadcasting a measure of global performance (a scalar reinforcement or payoff signal) to all the hidden units in the network. By correlating variations in its own activity with resultant variations in this signal, each unit can estimate the partial derivative of the performance measure with respect to its own activity. It is then a simple matter for each unit to estimate the partial derivative of this measure with respect to each of its weights. Weight changes can therefore be made according to an estimate of the gradient of the global network performance measure. By determining gradient *estimates* rather than the exact gradient,[2] the method dispenses with the more complicated back-propagation computation. The cost of this estimation method is learning speed in terms of the number of stimulus presentations compared to the back-propagation method, but the method may be more amenable to parallel implementation and may be more plausible from a biological perspective.

We call the learning algorithm used by the units in our approach the *Associative Reward-Penalty*, or A_{R-P}, algorithm [3, 4], and we call the networks A_{R-P} networks. This algorithm combines aspects of stochastic approximation methods as applied to supervised learning tasks [7] with aspects of stochastic learning automata [9]. In studying units of this type, we have been influenced by the hypothesis of Klopf [8] that neurons are self-interested adaptive units. Networks of these units can be thought of as "teams" of learning automata, a perspective discussed in Refs. [2, 3, 5].

In this paper, we describe a method by which the A_{R-P} algorithm can be applied to supervised learning tasks where nonlinear associative mappings are to be learned by a multilayer network. This method is a special case of more general uses of the A_{R-P} algorithm. We introduce a variant of the A_{R-P} algorithm, called the S-model A_{R-P}, that is capable of learning with real-valued reinforcement, and we introduce a method, which we call "batching", for increasing the learning efficiency of A_{R-P} networks. We describe simulation experiments using the task of learning symmetry axes [12] to compare the variants of the A_{R-P} network method as well as the back-propagation method of Rumelhart et al. [11]. Finally, we discuss the various methods in terms of computational efficiency and biological plausibility.

Estimating a Gradient

To gain an understanding of the principle behind the method we are proposing for gradient following without back-propagation, suppose a given unit in the interior of a layered network (i.e., a "hidden unit") can vary its output around its current value while the outputs of all of the other units remain fixed. By correlating the variation in its output with the consequences of this variation on the performance measure, the unit can determine the derivative of the measure with respect to its output at the current point in weight space. From this the unit can easily determine the performance measure's derivative with respect to its weights, and so can alter them appropriately. Suppose each unit in turn does this with the other units' outputs fixed. If a unit's new weights are not put into place until all the units have varied their outputs, the result will be a step in weight space according to the gradient of the performance measure.

This process might work but has obvious shortcomings since some outside agency would have to orchestrate the process, and it would be quite slow. But what if all the units could vary their outputs *simultaneously* and observe the consequences to achieve the same result? This could be made to work if the units independently influenced the performance measure, but it is difficult to see how it could be done if these influences are not independent, which is the only case of real interest. It turns out, however, that it is possible for interacting units to simultaneously vary their outputs to obtain an *estimate* of the appropriate derivatives. This is essentially what happens in the method based on the A_{R-P} learning rule that we describe here.

It is important to understand that in this method, it is the units' activity that is "jittered" so that an estimate of the partial derivatives of the performance measure with respect to unit activity can be estimated. The gradient with respect to the weights, which is the information ultimately needed to change the weights, is in effect computed from the estimates of these partial derivatives. The method does not directly jitter the weights to estimate the gradient with respect to the weights. This could be done but would be much slower due to the fact that knowledge that is available, namely, knowledge of how a unit's weight influence that unit's activity, would not be used.[3]

Two Types of Learning Tasks

There are several variants of A_{R-P} networks depending on the type of learning task to be accomplished. One type of task is the *supervised-learning task* to which Boltzmann learning, back-propagation, and most other network learning methods are applicable. The training procedure consists of presenting the network with input patterns together with the desired network responses to those inputs. In some formulations, error vectors are presented to the network that are the differences between the actual and desired network output patterns. In any case, desired network responses must be known for a set of training inputs.

Another type of learning task is the *associative reinforcement learning task* discussed in Refs. [3, 4]. In this case the training procedure consists of a sequence of trials in each of which the network is presented with an input pattern, produces a response, and is then is fed back a *scalar* value that provides a measure how "good" a response the network made to that input pattern. The object is to maximize this goodness measure, which can be thought of as a reinforcement or payoff value. It is not necessary to assume that reinforcement is determined by an agency external to the learning system. Indeed, the more interesting cases probably involve reinforcement computed by adaptive evaluation mechanisms within the learning system. Because a reinforcement value may measure the degree of match between the network's output pattern and a desired output, any supervised learning task can be transformed into an associative reinforcement learning task. However, it may not be possible to transform an associative reinforcement learning task into a supervised learning task. The reinforcement may be determined without knowledge of a desired network output. An example of this is when the reinforcement evaluates the *consequences* of the network's activity, on some other system—desired consequences may be known but not what network outputs cause them.

Because we are interested in comparing the A_{R-P} method with back-propagation, we are concerned with supervised learning in this paper. Back-propagation, by itself, is not applicable to associative reinforcement learning tasks. The A_{R-P} learning method, on the other hand, was designed for associative reinforcement learning. How can we apply such a method to supervised learning tasks? Perhaps the most straightforward way to do this would simply be to use a (decreasing) function of the sum of the squared errors of the network's output units as the scalar reinforcement. However, by collapsing the error vector to a scalar, a lot of information is discarded that can be used by the network's output units. Instead, we let the network's output units learn exactly as they would in a back-propagation network and use a function of the sum of their squared errors as reinforcement for the rest of the network's elements. Thus, although the network as a whole faces a supervised learning task, the interior part of the network (the network of hidden units) faces an associative reinforcement learning task.

A_{R-P} Networks for Supervised Learning

In this paper we discuss only nonrecurrent networks, that is, networks with acyclic interconnection structures. In addition to strictly layered networks, this case includes any feed-forward architecture. Following the usual practice, we distinguish between *input* units, which are clamped at values specified by sources external to the network, *output* units, whose activities are available to outside systems, and *hidden* units, which communicate only with other units in the network. We also assume that there is a permanantly active "true unit" providing input to every unit of the network so that each unit has an adjustable bias.

Let x_i denote the output of unit i and let $v_i = \sum_j w_{ij} x_j$ denote its *net input*, where the x_j are the outputs of the units that provide input to unit i, and w_{ij} is the connection weight from unit j to unit i. The network's output units are deterministic logistic units identical to those used in the Rumelhart et al. back-propagation method [11]; that is, if unit i is an output unit,

$$x_i = f(v_i) = 1/(1 + e^{-v_i}). \tag{1}$$

The input/output behavior of the hidden units, however, is identical to that of Boltzmann units [1]. If unit i is a hidden unit,

$$x_i = \begin{cases} 1, & \text{with probability } f(v_i); \\ 0, & \text{with probability } 1 - f(v_i). \end{cases} \tag{2}$$

This is a special case of the stochastic input/output behavior of general A_{R-P} units [4].

All of the units in the network therefore use the logistic function, f, in determining their outputs, but this function directly gives the output value for a real-valued deterministic output unit, whereas it gives the probability of firing for a binary stochastic hidden unit. Note that the *expected* output of hidden unit i is $f(v_i)$, which is the value a deterministic logistic unit produces directly.[4] It is convenient to denote the activity pattern over the output units by $(y_1, \ldots, y_N)$, where there are N output units (so that y_i is just a relabeling of some x_k).

The goal of the supervised learning process is to minimize the expected value, over a set of training input patterns, of a measure of the error between the actual network output and a desired output for each input pattern. As is usual, this measure of network error for any given input pattern is

$$\varepsilon = \frac{1}{N}\sum_{i=1}^{N} (y_i^* - y_i)^2, \tag{3}$$

where y_i is the response of output unit i to the input pattern, and $y_i^* \in [0, 1]$ is the desired response of unit i supplied by the "teacher".

The first step in the training process is to compute the network output for a given input. This is done by clamping the input units to the input pattern and successively computing the outputs of the remaining layers (using Eqs. 1 and 2). The weights of the output units are updated exactly as in the error back-propagation method of Rumelhart et al. [11]. That is, if w_{ij} is a weight of output unit i, then

$$\Delta w_{ij} = \rho(y_i^* - y_i)f'(v_i)x_j, \tag{4}$$

where $f'(v_i) = f(v_i)(1 - f(v_i)) = y_i(1 - y_i)$ is the derivative of the logistic function f evaluated at v_i, and ρ is a constant determining the step size. Consequently, the weights of the output units change so as to move down the gradient of the network's error (Eq. 3) for this particular training step. Note, however, that unlike the error back-propagation method, this error for a given input pattern is a random variable due to the randomness of the hidden units.

We now describe how the weights of the hidden units are updated. Instead of back-propagating error information, we broadcast the same reinforcement signal to all of the hidden units. The weight-update rule of the hidden units depends on what values the reinforcement signal can take. We consider two cases, each of which depend on ε, the average squared error over the output units for the current trial. Note that $0 \leq \varepsilon \leq 1$.

In the first case, the reinforcement signal, denoted r, probabilistically takes on one of two values:

$$r = \begin{cases} 1, & \text{with probability } 1 - \varepsilon; \\ 0, & \text{with probability } \varepsilon. \end{cases}$$

One can think of $r = 1$ as "success" and $r = 0$ as "failure". Thus, the better the match between the network's output pattern and the desired pattern, the higher the probability that the hidden units will receive the signal "success". Given a reinforcement value, each hidden unit i updates its weights according to the following equation:

$$\Delta w_{ij} = \begin{cases} \rho[x_i - f(v_i)]x_j, & \text{if } r = 1; \\ \lambda\rho[1 - x_i - f(v_i)]x_j, & \text{if } r = 0; \end{cases} \tag{5}$$

where $0 \leq \lambda \leq 1$ and $\rho > 0$. According to Eq. 5, when $r = 1$ ("success"), w_{ij} changes so that $f(v_i)$, the probability of the unit emitting 1 in the presence of the current input pattern (and patterns similar to it), moves toward the action that was chosen, x_i. This means that the probability of choosing *that same action* in similar circumstances increases (because if $x_i = 1$, then $f(v_i)$, the probability of emitting 1, increases, and if $x_i = 0$, then $1 - f(v_i)$, the probability of emitting 0, increases because $f(v_i)$ decreases). When $r = 0$ ("failure"), on the other hand, w_{ij} changes so that the probability of choosing *the other action* in similar circumstances increases (because $1 - x_i$ is the action *not* chosen). Note that the parameter λ in Eq. 5 determines the degee of asymmetry in the magnitude of the weight change for the "success" and "failure" cases. The weight update rule given by Eq. 5, is a special case of the A_{R-P} learning rule that has been discussed extensively in Refs. [2, 3, 4, 5]. It is most closely related to the "selective bootstrap" method presented by Widrow, Gupta, and Maitra [13].

The task of the hidden units is made more difficult that it needs to be by using the probabilistic binary reinforcement just described. A more informative reinforcement signal is simply the real-valued signal $r = 1 - \varepsilon$. Larger values of r correspond to better matches between the network's output pattern and the desired pattern. In this case, the hidden units update their weights according to the following equation:

$$\Delta w_{ij} = \rho[r(x_i - f(v_i)) + \lambda(1 - r)(1 - x_i - f(v_i))]x_j. \tag{6}$$

This equation is applicable whenever $0 \leq r \leq 1$, as is true here. It linearly proportions the weight changes between the extreme cases handled by Eq. 5 (which can be seen to be a special case of Eq. 6 obtained in the case of binary reinforcement). We call this the "S-model A_{R-P}" rule after similar usage in the theory of stochastic learning automata [9]. The learning rule for the case of binary reinforcement (Eq. 5) is called the "P-model A_{R-P}" rule.

The A_{R-P} network learning procedure for a supervised learning task is summarized as follows. The input units are clamped to a training input pattern. The output of the network is computed in a forward pass using the stochastic rule (Eq. 2) for the hidden units and the deterministic rule (Eq. 1) for the output units. An error is determined for each output unit based on the desired output pattern, and the weights of the output units are updated as in the back-propagation method (Eq. 4). A scalar reinforcement value is broadcast uniformly to all of the hidden units, which update their weights according to either the P-model or S-model A_{R-P} rule (Eq. 5 or 6) depending on whether the reinforcement is binary or real-valued. This process is repeated for each pattern in the training set until the desired level of performance is achieved.

Some Theory

Williams [14, 15] has proved the following fact about arbitrary nonrecurrent networks of P-model A_{R-P} units in associative reinforcement learning tasks where a global reinforcement signal is broadcast to all the units. If the units' outputs are determined using the logistic distribution according to Eq. 2, and if the parameter λ in Eq. 5 is zero for each unit[5], then the expected change of *any* weight in the network is proportional to the partial derivative of the expected network reinforcement with respect to that weight; that is, for any weight w_{ij} in the network:

$$E\{\Delta w_{ij}|W\} = k\frac{\partial E\{r|W\}}{\partial w_{ij}}, \tag{7}$$

where W is the matrix of the current network weights, r is the network reinforcement, and k is a positive scalar.[6]

According to this result, the weights change according to an *unbiased estimate of the gradient of the expected global reinforcement as a function of the weights.* On any particular trial, the step in weight space actually taken may or may not amount to an improvement, but the average update direction will be in the correct direction. Moreover, the expected reinforcement is a natural performance measure because even if reinforcement is a deterministic function of the network's output (as it is in the supervised tasks considered here), it is a random function of the weights since the hidden units are stochastic. The most remarkable thing about this result is that it does not depend on how the reinforcement signal is determined as a function of the network output.

Applied to the network learning method for supervised tasks that is our major concern here, this result implies that on each trial, the expected trajectory of the weight vector of the hidden units in weight space is down the gradient of the expected network error, ε, as a function of the weights. This is true for both the P-model and S-model A_{R-P} learning rules because the expected reinforcement for the P-model equals the reinforcement for the S-model. Thus, in a probabilistic sense, the A_{R-P} method for supervised learning tasks does something similar to what a back-propagation method does.

For several reasons, however, the situation is a bit more complicated than this. First, the A_{R-P} method does not provide an exact probabilistic approximation to what is accomplished by the back-propagation method. The function whose gradient is estimated by the A_{R-P} method, the expectation of ε, is a *different* function of the network's weights than the function whose gradient is followed by the back-propagation method of Rumelhart et al. [11]. A second complication is that gradient-following in a probabilistic sense, even if the gradient estimate is unbiased, does not guarantee that the process converges in any strong sense to an extremal value. The variance of the estimate may be so large that satisfactory performance is never achieved, or the variance may even grow without bound. Given the less than total understanding we currently have of the stochastic process generated by the A_{R-P} network method, we have to resort to our experience with simulation experiments and to our better understanding of a single A_{R-P} element.

We have found that when we run simulations of A_{R-P} networks with the parameter λ in Eq. 5 or 6 set to zero as required to obtain Williams' result (Eq. 7), the process tends to converge to suboptimal weights. When we set λ to a small non-zero value, however, the process appears always to avoid these local minima. We do not as yet understand the role of λ in the case of networks. The convergence theorem proved by Barto and Anandan [4], shows how λ influences the asymptotic result of learning by a *single* P-model A_{R-P} unit if its input patterns are linearly independent and the parameter ρ decreases over trials.[7] In this case, setting λ non-zero removes absorbing states from the stochastic process, and a similar thing appears to happen in the case of networks. Although the network learning process with $\lambda \neq 0$ is a kind of stochastic approximation method, it appears to be more complicated than the standard methods. Additional research is required before we can make rigorous statements about network convergence.

The Batched A_{R-P} Method

The fact that an unbiased estimate of a performance gradient is followed by an A_{R-P} network suggests that making more observations at each iteration of the learning process may improve performance by improving the gradient estimate. This is a method for accelerating convergence that has been studied for more standard stochastic approximation algorithms [7]. As the number of observations per step increases, performance should approach that obtained with deterministic gradient-following algorithms while the network retains its simple character in that all the A_{R-P} units still receive the same scalar signal. To investigate this possibility, we considered a modification of the A_{R-P} network learning procedure described above. The modification consists of allowing the weight updating sequence to take place several times during the presentation of a single input pattern. The weight changes induced by these updates are accumulated in a temporary location, and only at the end of the stimulus presentation are the accumulated weight changes added to the actual weights. Geometrically, this procedure amounts to obtaining several sample vectors at a given point in weight space, and taking a step that is the resultant of the sample vectors. We call this procedure the "batched" A_{R-P} method.

Simulation Results

The symmetry task introduced by Sejnowski, Kienker, and Hinton [12] involves learning to detect symmetry axes in binary patterns on a four-by-four grid. In one version of the task, the network has three output units, and must categorize the input as having either horizontal, vertical, or diagonal symmetry (only one of the two possible diagonal axes is used). We also studied a simpler task with a single output unit, in which the network must discriminate between horizontal or non-horizontal symmetry. For either version of the task, our networks had sixteen input units, corresponding to the four-by-four grid, and twelve hidden units. There was full connectivity between layers, yielding a total of 243 modifiable weights and biases in the case with three output units, and 217 modifiable weights and biases in the case with one output unit.

In comparing variants of the A_{R-P} method, it is important to separate two factors that contribute to the speed of convergence: the *direction* of steps in weight space and the *magnitude* of the steps. As our interest was in the former, we controlled for the latter by the choice of learning rates. Thus, in the batched presentation method, the learning rate ρ associated with each sample step was chosen so that the resultant step was of the same average magnitude as the steps taken in the non-batched case. In particular, when ten samples were taken per stimulus presentation in the batched case, we found that a value of $\rho = 0.078$ was needed so that the magnitudes would match when a value of $\rho = 0.5$ was used in the non-batched case. The fact that the ratio of these values is less than ten shows that the sample vectors tended to point in different directions and cancel to a certain degree, which is necessary if the batching is to have any effect. We used $\lambda = .01$ in all the simulations.

We conducted experiments with P-model and S-model hidden units, both with and without batching. Ten replications were performed in each condition, with the dependent measure being the number of stimulus presentations needed until the sum of squared error averaged over fifty consecutive trials became less than 0.05. It is important to note that the batching method must perform more computation per stimulus presentation than the non-batching method, although the two methods take steps of equal magnitude in weight space. Thus, the dependent measure reflects the number of steps taken rather than the amount of computation. The results for the single output task are shown in Table 1. As can be seen, the batching decreased the number of steps by a factor of five. Note also that the networks with S-model hidden units learned in fewer steps than the networks with P-model hidden units. Learning in the fewest number of steps was obtained with batching and S-model hidden units, yielding learning to criterion in 4,234 stimulus presentations. By way of comparison, we found that with the back-propagation method the task was learned in 2,787 presentations when we used a learning rate of 0.5 and a momentum term of 0.9. (With no momentum, back-propagation required 12,267 trials.)

In the task with three output units, back-propagation learned in 4,528 presentations. Table 2 shows the

Table 1. Average number of stimulus presentations until criterion in the one output symmetry task

	P-model	S-model
Non-batched	34,336	25,696
Batched	6,146	4,234

Table 2. Average number of stimulus presentations until criterion in the three output symmetry task

	P-model	S-model
Non-batched	687,420	442,904
Batched	38,899	36,268

results for the A_{R-P} methods. Batching and the S-model algorithm were even more effective in decreasing the number of steps required for this more difficult task. Indeed, batching decreased the required number of steps by a factor of 18. That this factor more than compensates for the 10 cycles of the sampling process suggests that as well as being of theoretical interest, the batching method can be useful in practice for decreasing processing time for a given learning task.

Discussion

The A_{R-P} network method we have described requires performance information to be sent back to the hidden units, but it does not require a complex error propagation process. Because the performance gradient is estimated for each input pattern instead of being computed exactly, learning takes more trials than it does using the back-propagation algorithm. This speed disadvantage is especially apparent when the network has multiple output units. Collapsing the network error vector into a scalar reinforcement value loses information that is preserved in the back-propagation method. Despite this speed penalty, the A_{R-P} network method may have certain kinds of advantages over back-propagation methods. Because of its simplicity, it may be easier to implement in hardware and may be more plausible from a biological perspective. There is no shortage of neurally plausible mechanisms to broadcast reinforcement to a large number of units.

Our results with the batched A_{R-P} method show that it is possible to obtain increasingly accurate estimates of a gradient by repeated sampling for each input vector. There are both practical and biological implications of this result. In some learning domain, for example, it may be costly to obtain stimulus items but not costly to update the network and obtain evaluations. In such a domain, the batching procedure would be a natural way to speed learning. From a biological point of view, the batched approach emphasizes the point that the agent evaluating the output of a network need only be external to the network, not necessarily external to the organism. If some internal agent has sufficient knowledge to be able to evaluate actions, in particular if the agent constitutes a model of the environment, then it would be possible to improve learning performance by using the batched method without going through the environment.

In addition to the batched method, there are other ways that learning rate might be improved that have not yet been investigated, some of which have been suggested by Williams' [15]. For example, we regard the process of broadcasting global reinforcement to the hidden units as the simplest possible way to evaluate their performance. More sophisticated credit-assignment mechanisms will involve the adaptive computation of local reinforcement as knowledge of the causal structure of the network accumulates. The method described in this paper may be seen as the case to which more sophisticated methods will revert in the absence of this kind of knowledge.

Notes

1. This research was supported by the Air Force Office of Scientific Research, Bolling AFB, through grant AFOSR-87-0030. We wish to thank Ron Williams for providing essential theoretical insight underlying the method presented here.

2. More precisely, most back-propagation methods exactly compute a *sample* gradient for each input pattern, which is an estimate for the overall gradient of the performance measure over all the input patterns. Our method estimates the sample gradients too. Parker's [10] "direct propagation" method also estimates the sample gradients but uses a method different from the one we are proposing.

3. Introducing variation directly into the weights would amount applying a Kiefer-Wolfowitz style stochastic approximation procedure, whereas the A_{R-P} method combines aspects of both Kiefer-Wolfowitz and Robbins-Munro procedures [7].

4. It is not the case, however, that the expected activity of the *network* of hidden units is given by a corresponding network of deterministic logistic units. The expected activity does not propagate from unit to unit in the same way that activation does in the deterministic case. Consequently, a network of deterministic logistic units does not provide an exact "mean field theory" for the network of stochastic units.

5. We call units with $\lambda = 0$ A_{R-I} units, for *Associative Reward-Inaction* units: upon penalty, no weight changes occur.

6. This result can be seen to hold also for the S-model A_{R-P} learning rule presented above (Eq. 6) if it is noted that if $\lambda = 0$, the S-model is a special case of Williams' "restricted REINFORCE" algorithm for which he shows the general result.

7. This theorem extends to the case of an S-model A_{R-P} unit by noting that $E\{\Delta w_{ij} | W\}$ is the same for P and S-model A_{R-P} units.

References

[1] D. H. Ackley, G. E. Hinton, and T. J. Sejnowski. A learning algorithm for Boltzmann machines. *Cognitive Science*, 9: 147–169, 1985.

[2] A. G. Barto. Game-theoretic cooperativity in networks of self-interested units. In J. S. Denker, editor, *Neural Networks for Computing*, American Institute of Physics, New York, 1986.

[3] A. G. Barto. Learning by statistical cooperation of self-interested neuron-like computing elements. *Human Neurobiology*, 4: 229–256, 1985.

[4] A. G. Barto and P. Anandan. Pattern recognizing stochastic learning automata. *IEEE Transactions on Systems, Man, and Cybernetics*, 15: 360–375, 1985.

[5] A. G. Barto, P. Anandan, and C. W. Anderson. Cooperativity in networks of pattern recognizing stochastic learning automata. In K. S. Narendra, editor, *Adaptive and Learning Systems: Theory and Applications*, Plenum, New York, 1986.

[6] Y. Le Cun. Une procedure d'apprentissage pour reseau a sequil assymetrique [A learning procedure for assymetric threshold network]. *Proceedings of Cognitiva*, 85: 599–604, 1985.

[7] R. L. Kasyap, C. C. Blaydon, and K. S. Fu. Stochastic approximation. In J. M. Mendel and K. S. Fu, editors, *Adaptive, Learning, and Pattern Recognition Systems*, Academic Press, New York, 1970.

[8] A. H. Klopf. *The Hedonistic Neuron: A Theory of Memory, Learning, and Intelligence*. Hemishere, Washington, D.C., 1982.

[9] K. S. Narendra and M. A. L. Thathachar. Learning automata—A survey. *IEEE Transactions on Systems, Man, and Cybernetics*, 4: 323–334, 1974.

[10] D. B. Parker. *Learning Logic*. Technical Report TR-47, Massachusetts Institute of Technology, 1985.

[11] D. E. Rumelhart, G. E. Hinton, and R. J. Williams. Learning internal representations by error propagation. In D. E. Rumelhart and J. L. McClelland, editors, *Parallel Distributed Processing: Explorations in the Microstructure of Cognition, vol. 1: Foundations*, Bradford Books/MIT Press, Cambridge, MA, 1986.

[12] T. J. Sejnowski, P. K. Kienker, and G. E. Hinton. Learning symmetry groups with hidden units: Beyond the perceptron. Submitted to Physica D.

[13] B. Widrow, N. K. Gupta, and S. Maitra. Punish/reward: Learning with a critic in adaptive threshold systems. *IEEE Transactions on Systems, Man, and Cybernetics*, 5: 455–465, 1973.

[14] R. J. Williams. *Reinforcement Learning in Connectionist Networks: A Mathematical Analysis*. Technical Report ICS 8605, Institute for Cognitive Science, University of California at San Diego, La Jolla, CA, 1986.

[15] R. J. Williams. *Reinforcement-Learning Connectionist Systems*. Technical Report NU-CCS-87-3, College of Computer Science, Northeastern University, 360 Huntington Avenue, Boston, MA, 1987.

35

J. M. Fuster and J. P. Jervey

Neuronal firing in the inferotemporal cortex of the monkey in a visual memory task

1982. *Journal of Neuroscience* 2: 361–375

Abstract

The objective of this study was to elucidate the functional role of neurons in the inferotemporal cortex of the primate. Single unit activity was recorded with microelectrodes in monkeys performing a visual delayed matching-to-sample task. On each trial, the animal was exposed briefly to a color—the sample—and, after a period of delay, had to select the same color among two or four colors simultaneously presented. Thus, correct performance of the task required perception, retention, and recognition of the sample color for every trial. A large number of inferotemporal units were seen to react to the stimuli with changes of firing frequency. Many units showed color-dependent reactions, suggesting their involvement in perception and discrimination of colors. A substantial contingent of cells showed increased, sustained, and in some cases, color-dependent discharge during the delay which was not necessarily preceded or succeeded by firing changes in sample or match periods. It is proposed that those cells were engaged in temporary retention of the sample stimulus. Since most of the inferotemporal units examined showed firing changes in more than one period of a trial, they appeared to be involved in more than one of the operations required by the task. Thus, the data do not support a clear-cut topographic separation of visual functions within the inferotemporal cortex. However, neurons that appear to participate in visual memory, either exclusively or in addition to other functions, are concentrated in the cortex of the lower bank of the superior temporal sulcus.

In primates, it has been well demonstrated that the inferior temporal cortex takes part in higher visual functions (see review by Gross, 1973). That cortical region (area TE of Von Bonin and Bailey, 1947) receives input from the peristriate cortex (Jones and Powell, 1970; Rocha-Miranda et al., 1975; Seltzer and Pandya, 1978; Desimone et al., 1980). Inferotemporal (IT) cortex neurons have relatively large visual receptive fields, almost invariably including the fovea, and show selective reactions to such stimulus features as size, shape, contrast, and color (Gross et al., 1972; Desimone and Gross, 1979; Sato et al., 1980). It has long been known that monkeys with IT lesions show a deficit in performance of visual discrimination tasks (Chow, 1951; Cowey and Gross, 1970; Dean, 1976; Moss et al., 1981). Such a deficit does not seem attributable to a disruption of the sensory aspects of vision but rather of the ability to form and retain associations of visual stimuli with each other and with reinforcement (Gross, 1973).

The present study investigates the activity of the monkey's IT neurons during the performance of a delayed matching-to-sample task. The purpose of the investigation was to determine which facets of visual function IT neurons subserve. That behavioral task is exceptionally well suited for the purpose, because every delayed matching trial requires from the animal the perception, temporary retention, and recognition of a discrete item of visual information. These operations are conveniently bracketed in time, thereby allowing assessment of neuron participation in each of them separately. The rationale for our study is supported by evidence that both permanent and reversible IT lesions cause deficits in delayed matching performance (Kovner and Stamm, 1972; Delacour, 1977; Sahgal and Iversen, 1978; Fuster et al., 1981).

Other studies in monkeys performing visual discrimination tasks (Braitman and Wilson, 1976; Ridley et al., 1977; Gross et al., 1979; Sato et al., 1980; Mikami and

This work was supported by Grant BNS 76-16984 from the National Science Foundation and Grant AA-3513 from the National Institute of Alcohol Abuse and Alcoholism. J. M. F. is the recipient of Research Scientist Award MH 25082 from the National Institute of Mental Health. We wish to thank R. Bauer, W. Bergerson, M. Dunst, L. Holifield, J. Kruse, R. Lindsay, B. Lubell, G. Mount, D. Riley, J. Romano, R. Smith, and J. Thomas for their valuable help in various aspects of this research.

Kubota, 1980) have demonstrated the feature-dependent reactivity of IT units to the stimuli controlling performance. Furthermore, the reactions of some of the units described in those studies appear to some degree related to such factors as attention and relevance of the stimulus. The present study not only confirms and extends those findings but indicates that neurons in certain parts of IT cortex are most probably engaged in retention of visual information.

Materials and Methods

Subjects. Seven male macaques (*Macaca mulatta*) were used in this study. Their weight ranged between 6 and 9 kg. They were housed in individual cages and maintained on an *ad libitum* diet of chow and, periodically, some fruit. Fluid intake was limited (no water for the 24 hr preceding a testing session).

Behavior. The animals were trained to perform a delayed matching-to-sample (DMS) task with colored stimuli. In the testing apparatus, the subject sat in a primate chair facing a white panel with translucent stimulus-response buttons (each 2.5 cm in diameter). A trial began with the presentation of the sample, a colored light, in a centrally located button (Fig. 1). The animal turned it off by pressing the button. After a delay, two or four colors, one of them that of the sample, appeared simultaneously in a horizontal row of buttons under the sample button. Pressing the button with the sample color induced automatic delivery of fruit juice (about 1 ml) to the animal's mouth by way of a metal spigot. Choice of any other color terminated the trial without reward. The sample color and its position in the choice buttons were changed at random from trial to trial. Thus, for a correct response, the animal had to perceive the sample and retain it through the delay. The length of the delay was varied during both training and testing, but for unit recording, it was ordinarily set between 16 and 20 sec.

Two of the subjects were trained to perform the task with two colors, red and green, as sample and choice colors. Five others were trained with red, yellow, green, and blue. The color of the buttons was achieved by rear projection of white light through Cinemoid color filters. Intensity and wavelength were measured by means of a Pritchard Spectra photometer. The sample stimulus, whatever the color, had a luminance of 13.5 cd/m^2 (±0.1 log unit) and subtended 8° of visual field. The dominant λ was 620 nm for red, 590 nm for yellow, 530 nm for green, and 480 nm for blue.

It took 3 to 6 months to train an animal to an asymptotic level of performance. Having reached that level, most animals made only occasional errors on trials with a 16- to 20-sec delay.

Surgery. Upon completion of behavioral training, the animals were submitted to surgery, under Nembutal anesthesia, for implantation of recording gear. Hollow stainless steel pedestals for a microelectrode positioner were implanted in temporal bone over IT cortex. One of the animals was fitted with periorbital Ag/AgCl eye movement recording electrodes (Bond and Ho, 1970). Threaded metal sleeves were embedded in cement, over the skull, for eventual fixation of the head during recording.

Recording. Recording was initiated between 2 and 4 weeks after full recovery from surgery. Before the start of recording sessions, the experimental animal was habituated to behavioral testing with its head fixed. In preparation for a recording session, a hydraulic positioner (Fuster, 1961) with a metal microelectrode was attached to an implanted pedestal for remotely controlled penetration of IT cortex during behavioral testing. Either tungsten or platinum/iridium microelectrodes were used in these experiments, with impedance, at 1000 cps, ranging between 0.7 and 3.0 megohms. Input from a microelectrode was led to a capacity-coupled amplifier with matching input impedance and monitored acoustically and with an oscilloscope. Ordinarily, the animal was submitted to a series of DMS trials with short delays (6 to 10 sec), while the microelectrode was advanced slowly in search of single unit activity. As soon as the extracellularly recorded spikes from a single unit were picked up, the movement of the microelectrode was halted and its depth was noted on the micrometric scale of the hydraulic system controlling its advance. The possible relationships then were explored between the firing frequency of the unit and the events of the task. Only those units that showed an apparent correlation, however minor, between firing and one or more events of the trial sequence were selected for recording. As it turned out, the great majority of IT units encountered with the microelectrode fulfilled that broad criterion and were characterized by us as "responsive." After ascertaining the responsiveness, isolation, and stability of a unit, recording was initiated with a multichannel (Ampex FR-1200) tape recorder and the animal was subjected to a series of DMS trials with 16- to 20-sec delays. Recorded on one channel was the output of a Schmitt trigger

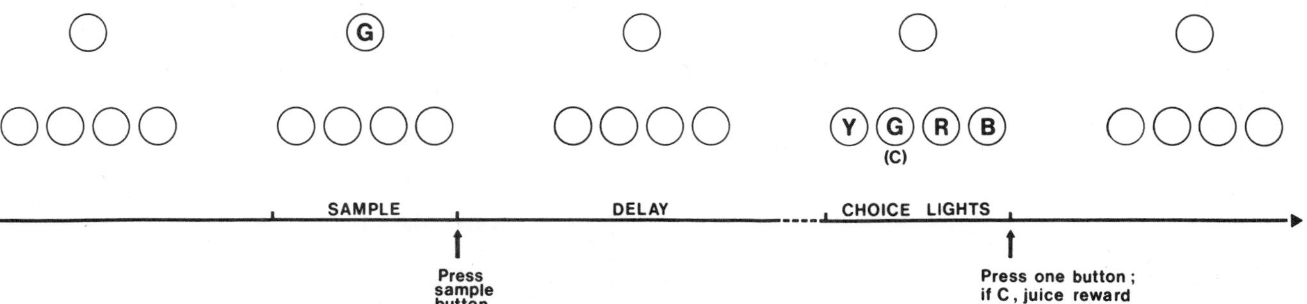

Figure 1. Sequence of events in a delayed matching-to-sample trial (with a green sample light). *G*, Green; *Y*, yellow; *R*, red; *B*, blue; *C*, correct choice light.

transforming the unit spikes into standard pulses (0.5 msec, 1 V) for subsequent computer analysis of spike frequency. Two other channels were used for the DC-recorded and amplified vertical and horizontal eye movements. A fourth channel was used for recording a digital code to mark the initiation of trials and DC voltage changes marking the events within them (i.e., onset and offset of the sample light, onset and offset of the choice lights, and juice delivery after correct response trials).

During recording from a given cell, successive trials were presented at intervals of about 50 sec for as long as the unit record remained stable and until data from sufficient trials were collected for analysis. The number of trials varied somewhat from unit to unit, depending on the stability of the record and the frequency and variability of firing. Practically all units analyzed were recorded through at least five trials with each of the sample stimuli of the task. On completion of recording from a given unit, microelectrode advancement was resumed in search of another. Ordinarily, activity from one to three units was recorded in any given session. A session usually lasted about 3 hr, and during this time, the animal consumed 100 to 200 ml of fruit juice.

Histology. Upon termination of experiments, small lesions were made in brain tissue at various locations by passing current (100 μA, 15 sec) through small electrodes introduced with the micropositioner. The electrolytic lesions were to serve as reference marks for reconstructing the position of the units recorded. The animals were sacrificed with an overdose of Nembutal and the brain was extracted, fixed in formalin, and coronally cut (80 μm), and the sections were stained by a Nissl method. The stained sections were photographed and the estimated location of all of the registered cells was marked in enlarged (×10) pictures.

Analysis. All analysis was done off-line by means of a MINC-11 computer system with graphic capability. The analysis of a single unit's activity proceeded through the following steps: (*1*) digital conversion of the unit's impulses and the event code with real time reference; (*2*) average frequency histograms of the unit's activity, time-locked with sample onset, for all trials with each of the sample colors; (*3*) statistical analysis of firing frequency changes as a function of sample color and trial epoch (sample period, delay period) using as a base line reference the firing of the unit during the 16 sec preceding each trial. Differences from the base line for each of those variables were submitted to t tests using the intertrial variance for computing the error term. The results of this analysis were used for characterizing the reactions of each unit to the events of a DMS trial.

For a few experiments, the electro-oculogram (EOG) was digitized and plotted to determine ocular fixation on DMS stimuli. The EOG was accurate within 5°. Graphic displays of cell discharge were generated using the start of fixation as a reference.

Results

Data base. The majority of cells selected for study were situated in area TE (Von Bonin and Bailey, 1947), comprising the cortex of the inferior temporal convexity (middle and inferior temporal gyri) and the cortex lining the lower bank of the superior temporal sulcus (Fig. 2). A smaller proportion of the units investigated were situated in the cortex of the upper bank of that sulcus (area TA) and, therefore, not in IT cortex proper; here, they will be generally referred to as "upper bank cells." In addition, cells in deeper structures, such as the caudate nucleus and the hippocampus, also were isolated and studied, but these cells will not be dealt with here. Table I summarizes the data base of the present study. As the table shows, all animals contributed substantially to the sample of IT units, but practically all upper bank units were contributed by one animal.

Spontaneous activity. As previously found in other regions of mammalian cortex (Fuster et al., 1965; Rosenkilde et al., 1981), the spontaneous firing frequency of cells in IT cortex was found to be, on the average, relatively low (median: 3.92 spikes/sec). The distribution of the cells by spontaneous rate shows a wide range of frequencies and marked skewness (Fig. 3). It should be noted that our sample does not include an indeterminate number of very slow units that were unresponsive to the stimuli of the behavioral task and, therefore, did not meet the selection criterion.

Also widely variable were the patterns of spontaneous discharge. Some cells fired continuously and relatively fast, while others showed slow and irregular sequences of spike bursts. In general, cells spontaneously firing continuous streams of spikes were more apt to react to the task stimuli than those firing slowly and in bursts.

Reactions to the sample stimulus. Most cells showed an excitatory reaction to the sample stimulus opening a trial (Table II). The reaction might be brisk or sluggish, but in either case, its latency after stimulus onset was relatively long, over 70 msec. Some cells—more commonly those in the upper bank than those in IT cortex—showed inhibitory reactions to the sample. The duration of the deviation from spontaneous firing varied considerably among cells. In some units, it was confined to the sample period, whereas in others, it extended into the subsequent delay period.

Complex reactions, including both excitation and inhibition, were relatively rare. In such cases, the first component of the reaction determined our typification of the cell. Also rare was the cell that exhibited both on and off reactions to the sample stimulus. However, it was not uncommon for a cell to first show firing deviation from the base line immediately following the termination of the sample presentation, at the beginning of the delay.

In spite of some intertrial variability, any cell could be readily classified into two broad categories, differential or nondifferential, depending on whether it showed statistically different reactions to different sample stimuli. Sample differential cells were found to be much more common in IT cortex than in the cortex of the upper bank (Table II).

Differential cells could be of three types. The most common were characterized by excitatory reactions of different magnitude to different colors. Other units showed reactions to at least one color and none to another, and still others, definitely a minority, showed reciprocal reactions, that is, excitation to one color and inhibition to another. Figure 4 shows an example of the first type. The cell reacts with different degrees of exci-

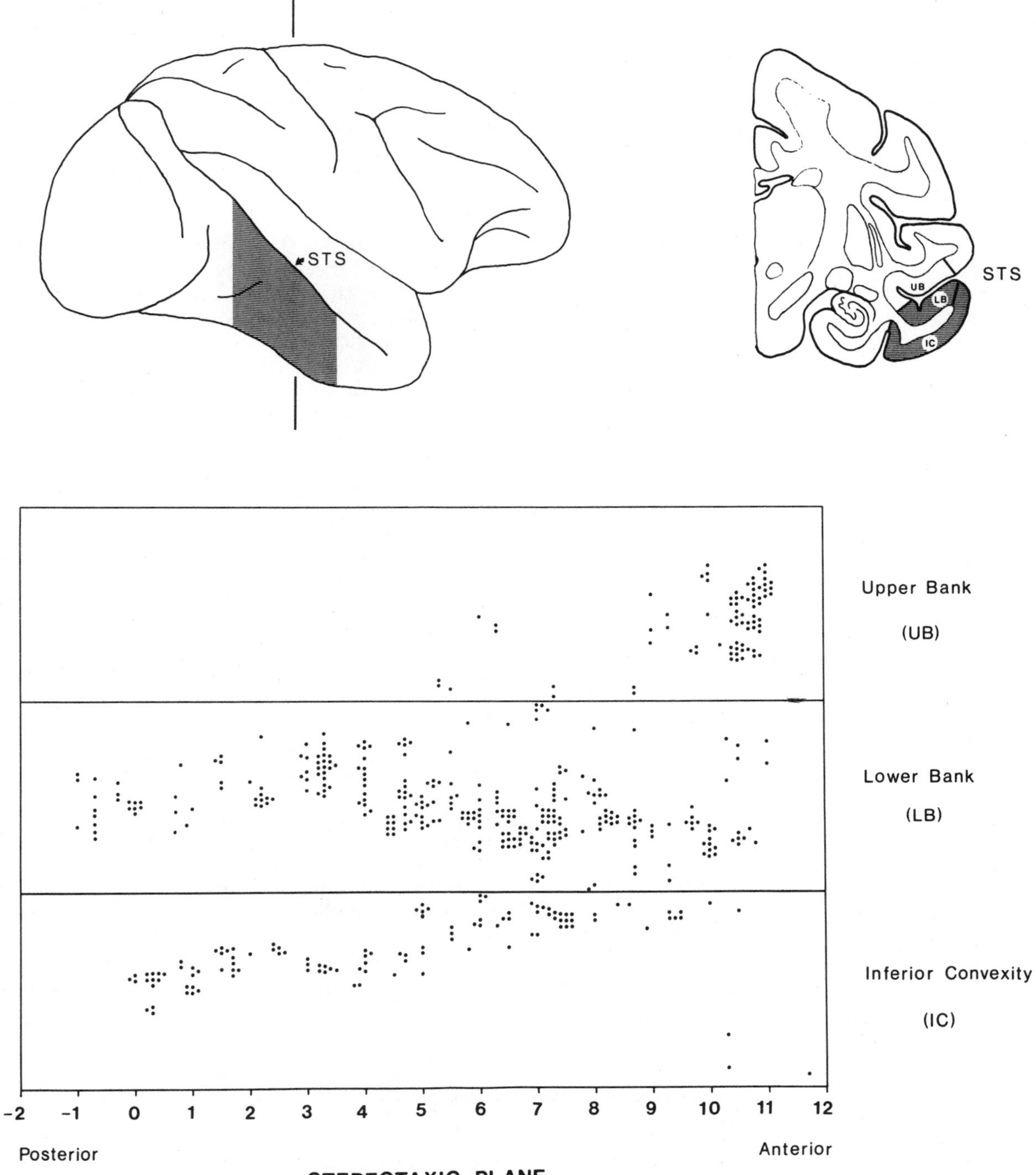

Figure 2. Above, Lateral view and cross-section of the monkey's brain; *shading* indicates the IT cortical region from which single unit records were obtained. The scatter plot *below* shows, in a highly schematic diagram of unfolded cortex, the relative position of all of the units constituting the data base of the present study. *STS,* Superior temporal sulcus.

tation to the four colored samples. Cells tested in four-color DMS, such as that one, frequently showed that the response to yellow, whether excitatory or inhibitory, was more similar in magnitude to the response to red than that to blue or green. Conversely, blue and green responses tended to be more similar to one another than to yellow or red responses. Thus, depending on which pair of colors elicited the highest excitatory response, a cell could be characterized as a "warm" or "cold color" cell. Figure 5 displays the reactions to the sample of a cold color cell.

Green and red were the two colors tested on all animals and units. In the area of IT cortex explored, the proportion of cells predominantly activated by the green sample

TABLE I
Data base

Monkey	Side	Penetrations	Units: Inferior Convexity	Lower Bank	Upper Bank	Total
DMS-5	Right	15	5	19	0	24
DMS-7	Right	11	4	8	3	15
	Left	39	19	68	0	87
DMS-9	Right	51	2	8	62	72
	Left	9	3	6	0	9
DMS-11	Right	20	1	25	0	26
	Left	20	28	1	0	29
DMS-15	Right	18	13	15	0	28
	Left	22	12	16	0	28
DMS-17	Right	32	6	44	4	54
	Left	14	0	11	7	18
DMS-21	Right	38	8	45	3	56
	Left	35	18	32	0	50
		—	—	—	—	—
Total		324	119	298	79	496

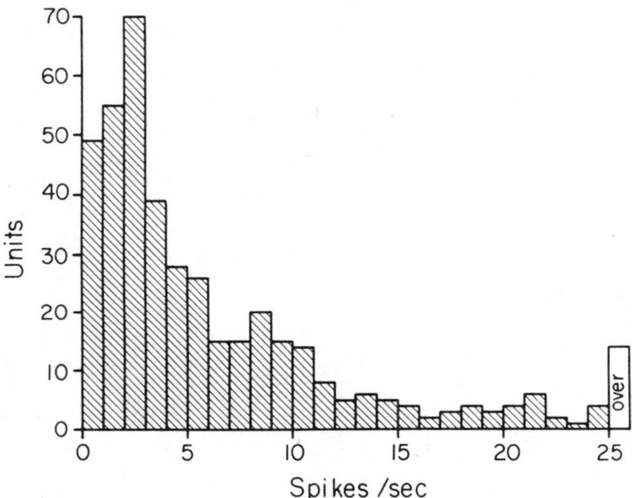

Figure 3. Ranked distribution of the IT units according to the frequency of spontaneous discharge.

was comparable overall to that of cells predominantly activated by the red sample (13 versus 14%), although the two proportions varied somewhat for different subareas.

Activity during the delay. More than half of all cells exhibited different frequency of firing during the delay than during the intertrial base line period. About one-third of those in IT cortex showed elevated delay discharge, whereas one-fifth showed depressed delay discharge (Table III). The rest showed either no changes or reciprocal deviations of delay discharge, that is, excitation or inhibition depending on the color of the sample. The ratio of delay-excited to delay-inhibited cells was just about reversed in the upper bank cortex, where the latter were more common than the former and where virtually no delay differential cells were observed.

In general, IT cell activity deviated more from the base line early in the delay than later in that period. Both delay excitation and inhibition tended to diminish in the course of the delay. Some units, however, showed the opposite trend, that is, an enhanced deviation from base line firing frequency as the delay progressed. In any event, the important point is that a large proportion of IT cells manifested persistent deviation from the base line until the very end of the commonly used delays (16 to 20 sec).

During the delay, 10% of the IT cells showed differential firing, in other words, a different level of activity depending on the color of the sample for the trial. In most instances, the difference was merely of degree: a cell was significantly more activated or inhibited after one color than after another. However, in some, the difference was one of direction (reciprocal): excitation after one color and inhibition after another.

Some units carried over into the delay the differential firing that they exhibited during the sample period (Fig. 6). However, differential sample activity was not a necessary condition for differentiation during the delay. A cell might show nondifferential reactions or no reaction at all to sample presentation yet show differential firing during the ensuing delay (Fig. 7). Differential activity generally terminated with the end of the trial (Figs. 6, 7, and 8).

Reactions to the choice stimuli. On presentation of the choice lights, at the end of the delay, IT units tended to react in a manner similar to their reaction to the sample. Thus, excitation and inhibition at the sample were followed, respectively, by excitation and inhibition on appearance of the choice lights for the color match, although the reactions to the two events often differed considerably in degree: some units showed little reaction to the sample and much to the choice lights (Fig. 8), while in others, the opposite was true.

The general similarity of reactivity to sample and choice lights applies also to color differentiation. Thus, the selective reactions shown by some units at the sample were observable again at the choice, even though now the sample color was not presented alone but in combi-

TABLE II
Reaction to sample stimulus

All units were classified by their reactions to red and green sample stimuli. Percentages are in parentheses.

Type	Units: Inferior Convexity	Lower Bank	Upper Bank	Total
Nondifferential				
No change	5 (4)	39 (13)	3 (4)	47
Excitation	47 (39)	117 (39)	41 (52)	205
Inhibition	24 (20)	62 (21)	24 (31)	110
Differential				
Excitation	35 (30)	73 (25)	5 (6)	113
Inhibition	3 (3)	4 (1)	1 (1)	8
Reciprocal[a]	5 (4)	3 (1)	5 (6)	13
Total	119 (100)	298 (100)	79 (100)	496

[a] Excitation by one color and inhibition by the other.

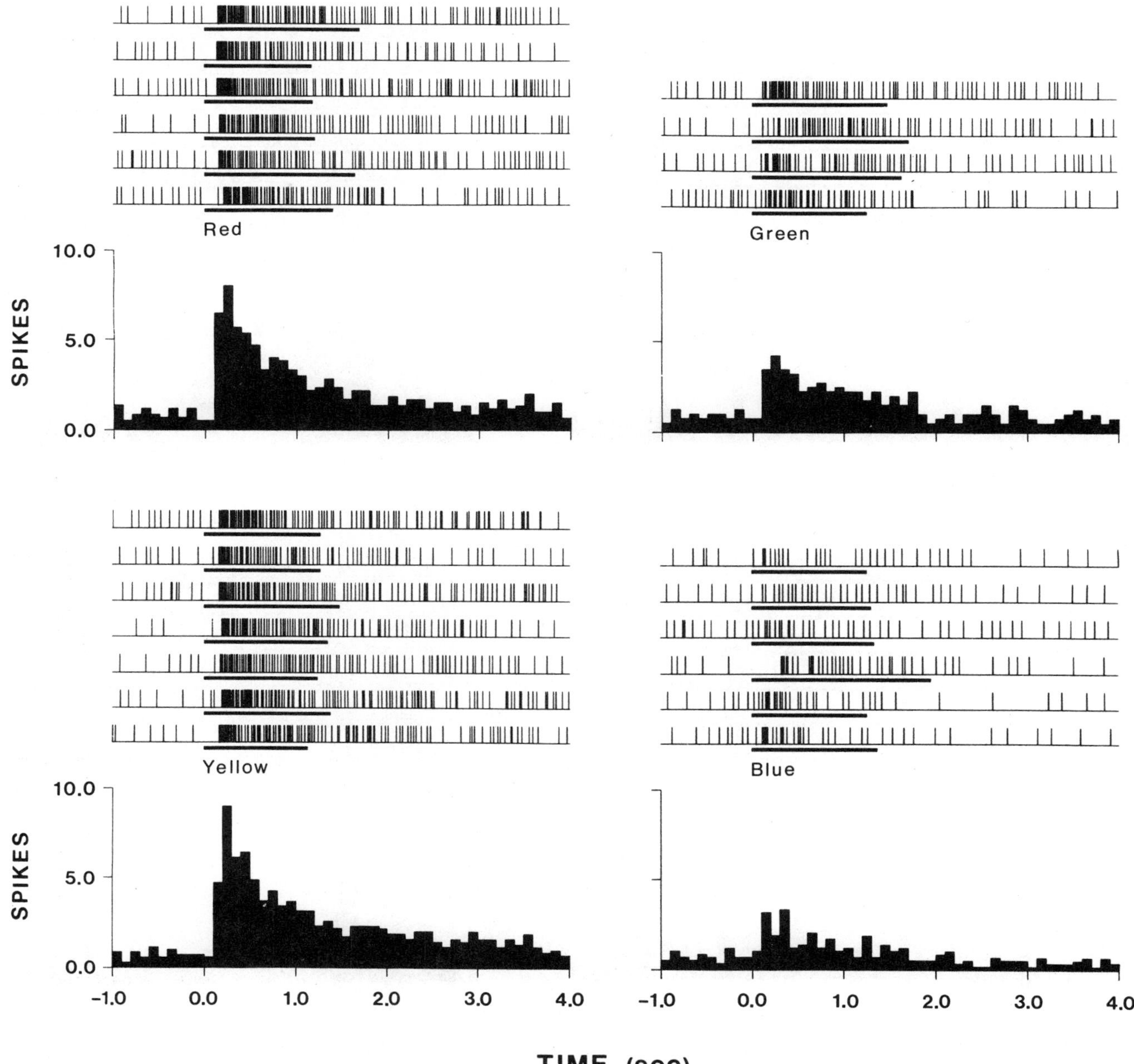

Figure 4. Graphic display of the firing of an IT cell during the sample period (*horizontal bars*) of DMS trials. Each histogram (time-locked with sample onset) represents the average frequency for the individual records above it, which are grouped by sample color. Bin width, 100 msec. The unit shows a preferential reaction to red and yellow.

nation with one or three other colors. For example, if a unit showed a greater excitatory response to the yellow sample than to any other sample, the unit had a tendency to show a greater excitatory response to the presentation of the four choice lights on trials in which yellow was the color of the sample than on trials in which it was not (Fig. 6).

In other words, cell reactions to the sample were, in some respects, "matched" by comparable reactions to the array of choice lights. One simple explanation is that the animal, just before the choice, foveated the sample color for the trial more intently or for a longer time than the other colors by it. However, analysis of the activity of a few selected units in relation to eye movement revealed that foveation of the sample color was not the only factor accounting for differential reactions to the choice lights. Indeed, as the unit in Figure 9 illustrates, the response to the sample color, in some cases, appeared to begin before fixation of the eyes on the button that displayed that color, as if anticipating it.

After the choice, cell activity, as a rule, returned promptly to the base line. This was more remarkable in units that exhibited protracted deviations from that base line during the entirety of the delay or large reactions to

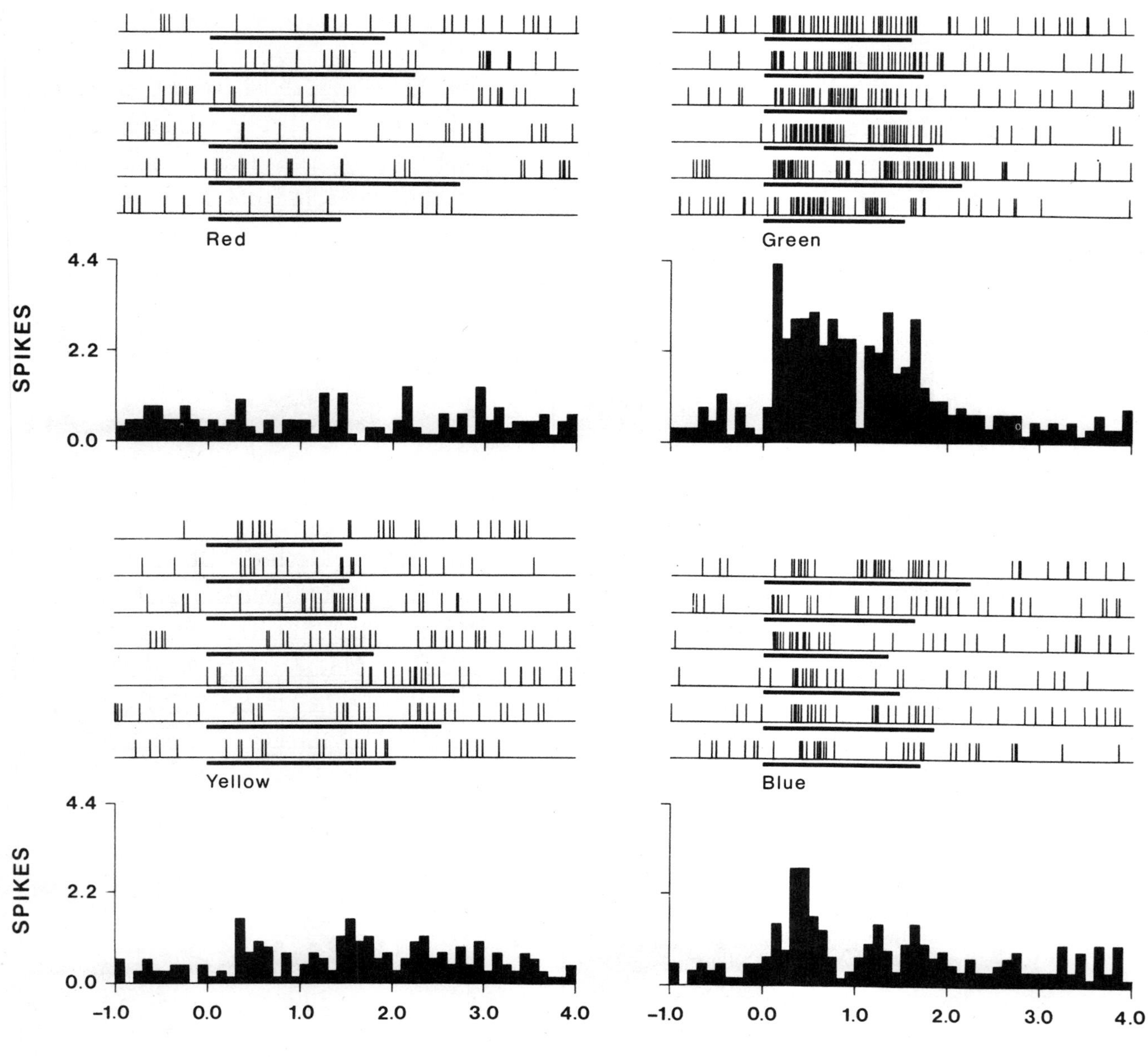

Figure 5. Sample period activity of an IT cell reacting markedly to the green sample and also, though less, to the blue sample.

the choice lights; in many cases, those deviations were of greater magnitude than those to the sample (Figs. 6, 7, and 8).

Relations to performance. In spite of the relatively long delays interposed between the sample and match, the animals committed few errors. Consequently, the appropriate comparison of unit activity between correct and incorrect response trials was usually difficult and rarely revealed statistically significant differences. Nevertheless, during the recording of certain IT units that could be held and tested through an exceptionally long series of trials, a subtle but unmistakable attenuation of cell reactions was observed periodically in correct as well as incorrect response trials. That attenuation, to judge from concomitant increases in behavioral reaction time and incidence of errors, could best be ascribed to lapses of attention or motivation.

Subtle correlations between IT unit activity and performance also could be detected by careful consideration of peculiarities in the behavior of individual monkeys. One animal, for example, showed a tendency to confuse red and yellow in DMS performance; his errors might be attributed to proactive interference (Wilson et al., 1972), since most of them occurred in red sample trials succeeding yellow sample trials or vice versa. In any event, that tendency to confuse red and yellow was reflected by relatively low unit differentiation of those two colors, as compared to green and blue, in the sample and delay

TABLE III
Activity during the delay
All units were classified by their differences of activity (with respect to intertrial base line) after red and green sample stimuli. Percentages are in parentheses.

Type	Units			
	Inferior Convexity	Lower Bank	Upper Bank	Total
Nondifferential				
No change	67 (56)	118 (39)	39 (49)	224
Excitation	25 (21)	88 (30)	11 (14)	124
Inhibition	21 (18)	57 (19)	28 (36)	106
Differential				
Excitation	4 (3)	25 (8)	1 (1)	30
Inhibition	1 (1)	8 (3)	0 (0)	9
Reciprocal[a]	1 (1)	2 (1)	0 (0)	3
Total	119 (100)	298 (100)	79 (100)	496

[a] Excitation after one color and inhibition after the other.

periods. By contrast, units in approximately the same region in another animal that rarely confused red and yellow showed marked red-yellow differentiation.

Topographic distribution. Cells showing similar responses to the sample colors or similar forms of color-related delay activity were often found in close vicinity of each other. On advancing the microelectrode some 50 to 150 μm after completing the recording of a unit, it was not unusual to encounter another unit with like properties; nor was it unusual to find similar units along the same path of penetration, and at the same depth, on separate recording sessions. These observations suggest that cells of common properties were clustered together. However, because of such factors as the difficulty of ensuring orthogonal penetration of the cortex and the limitations of accuracy in the reconstruction of unit positions (particularly in sulcal cortex), it was not possible to determine precisely the shape and size of the apparent clusters of functionally similar cells.

Nonetheless, at a coarser anatomical level, it was possible to determine that some of the general types of units encountered in our study were not distributed uniformly in IT cortex (Tables II and III). Sample-activated cells, differential or not, were about evenly distributed throughout IT cortex, while delay-activated cells were more common in the cortex of the lower bank of the superior temporal sulcus than in that of the IT convexity ($\chi^2 = 6.14$; $p < 0.02$). Also more common in the lower bank were delay differential cells ($\chi^2 = 3.59$; $p < 0.06$). Figure 10 schematically illustrates the topographic distribution of delay-activated cells and delay differential cells.

Discussion

Color was only one of several attributes of the sample stimulus appearing before the animal at the start of the trial. Other features of that stimulus were its size, its brightness, and the temporal and spatial contrast that it produced in the display panel. In order to test the role of color, those other parameters were made equal for all trials. However, it may be that many of the IT units investigated responded to one or more of those other physical features, which here by design were kept constant from trial to trial and which other experiments have shown to activate IT units (Gross et al., 1972; Desimone and Gross, 1979; Sato et al., 1980). There may lie the explanation for the high proportion of nondifferential (color-independent) sample-activated cells in IT cortex.

Moreover, it is possible that a large number of IT cells were activated not only by physical characteristics of the sample but by internal input deriving from its meaning—i.e., association with reward—in the context of the task, another property of that stimulus that may be assumed to be constant across trials and samples. Both behavioral significance and situational variables have been seen to modify the response of IT cells to a visual stimulus (Braitman and Wilson, 1976; Rolls et al., 1977; Gross et al., 1979; Mikami and Kubota, 1980). The modulating role of attention in IT unit responses is examined in another study using a variant of the DMS task (Fuster and Jervey, 1981).

Whatever the role of meaning and attention or visual features other than color in the reaction of IT cells, it is clear that color determined the magnitude and, in some cases, direction (excitation or inhibition) of some reactions. Since color was also the critical factor determining the choices of the animal and their outcome, it is reasonable to conclude that sample differential cells probably took part in the perception and discrimination of the colors guiding the task.

The most salient finding of this study is the presence of a large number of IT cells that exhibited marked deviations from base line firing during the intratrial delay. Among such cells, the most remarkable were those that showed color-dependent activity after the sample color had disappeared.

At least three interpretations of the sustained activation of IT units during the relatively long delay period that followed the sample should be considered. One is that it is a form of sensory afterdischarge elicited by the sample in the geniculostriate system and propagated to IT cortex. Brief visual stimuli, in the acute preparation, have been noted to elicit exceptionally long reactions in some IT units (Gross et al., 1977; C. G. Gross, personal communication). However, the concept of afterdischarge cannot easily be applied to delay activations following little or no reaction to the sample or developing in the course of the delay. Another possible explanation is that, in the interval between the sample presentation and match, the animal was under increased alertness and, in that state, nonspecific input of subcortical origin was responsible for the increased general activity of cortical cells. Such an explanation is inconsistent with the scarcity of delay activation and prevalence of delay inhibition in a cortical area outside of the IT region, namely, the upper bank of the superior temporal sulcus. A third possibility, which cannot be entirely dismissed even in the absence of supporting behavioral or EOG evidence, is that the animals attended more to "background" stimuli during the delay than during the intertrial interval,

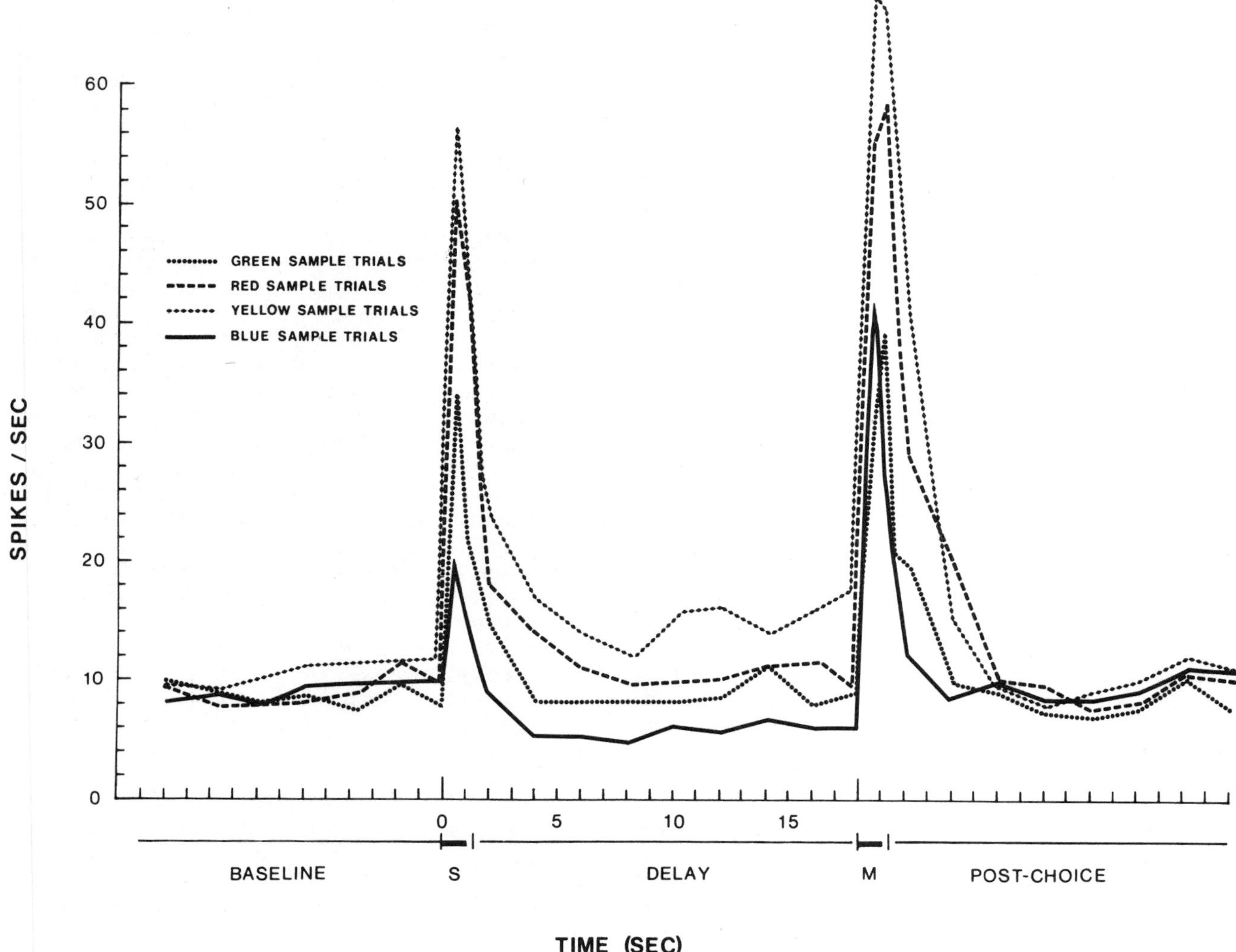

Figure 6. The average firing frequency of a cell (the same cell as in Fig. 4) through the entire length of the DMS trials. Sample (*S*) and match (*M*) periods are marked by *horizontal bars* under the time base. Note the color-related ranking of firing frequencies in sample and match periods as well as during the delay.

and thus, some of the neurons were more active during the delay. In any case, all three interpretations are inadequate for differential delay activation, that is, for color-dependent elevation of firing after the sample.

A plausible view of delay activation is that the cells exhibiting it are involved in short term retention. A few points can be adduced in support of this proposition. First, the activation occurs during that time span which, for correct performance, the animal must bridge with mnemonic retention of the sample. Second, the relationships between delay-activity and performance, however few and difficult to substantiate statistically, point to the functional significance of that activity for sample retention. Third, there is the striking contrast between delay and post-trial discharge: activation, as a rule, terminated with the trial and did not resume after the choice, even though, at the time just preceding the choice, the animal again had to foveate the sample color for correct response (a point also against the afterdischarge hypothesis). Thus, with the termination of the need to remember the sample, elevated firing likewise came to an end.

On grounds similar to those for sample reactions, it is reasonable to suppose that nondifferential delay-activated cells were involved in the retention of stimulus features that were constant for all samples and trials. Furthermore, it is possible that they also were subject to internal input related to motivation or expectancy of reward. However, in addition to such external and internal factors which our experiments were not designed to sort out, it is evident that the color of the sample determined the activity of some cells during the subsequent delay. Those may have been neurons engaged in temporary memory of color.

Caution is necessary, however, in ascribing to any cell a color-specific memory function. For one thing, the number of tested hues was very limited. Therefore, even units whose firing was clearly and preferentially elevated after a given color could not be assumed to specialize

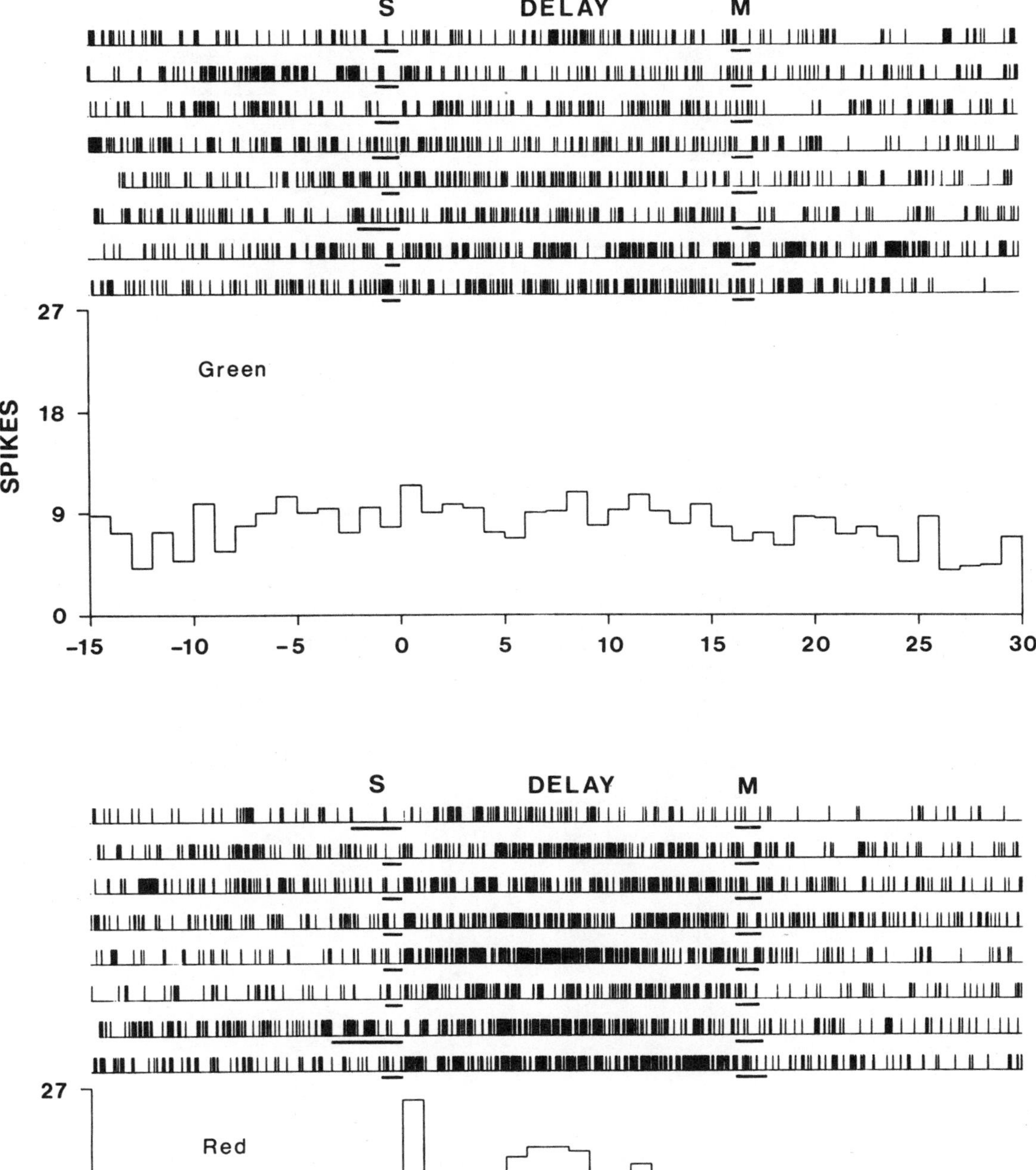

Figure 7. Discharge of a delay differential IT cell during green and red sample trials (*S*, sample; *M*, match). Frequency histograms are time-locked with the offset of the sample. Note the activation during the delay of the red sample trials.

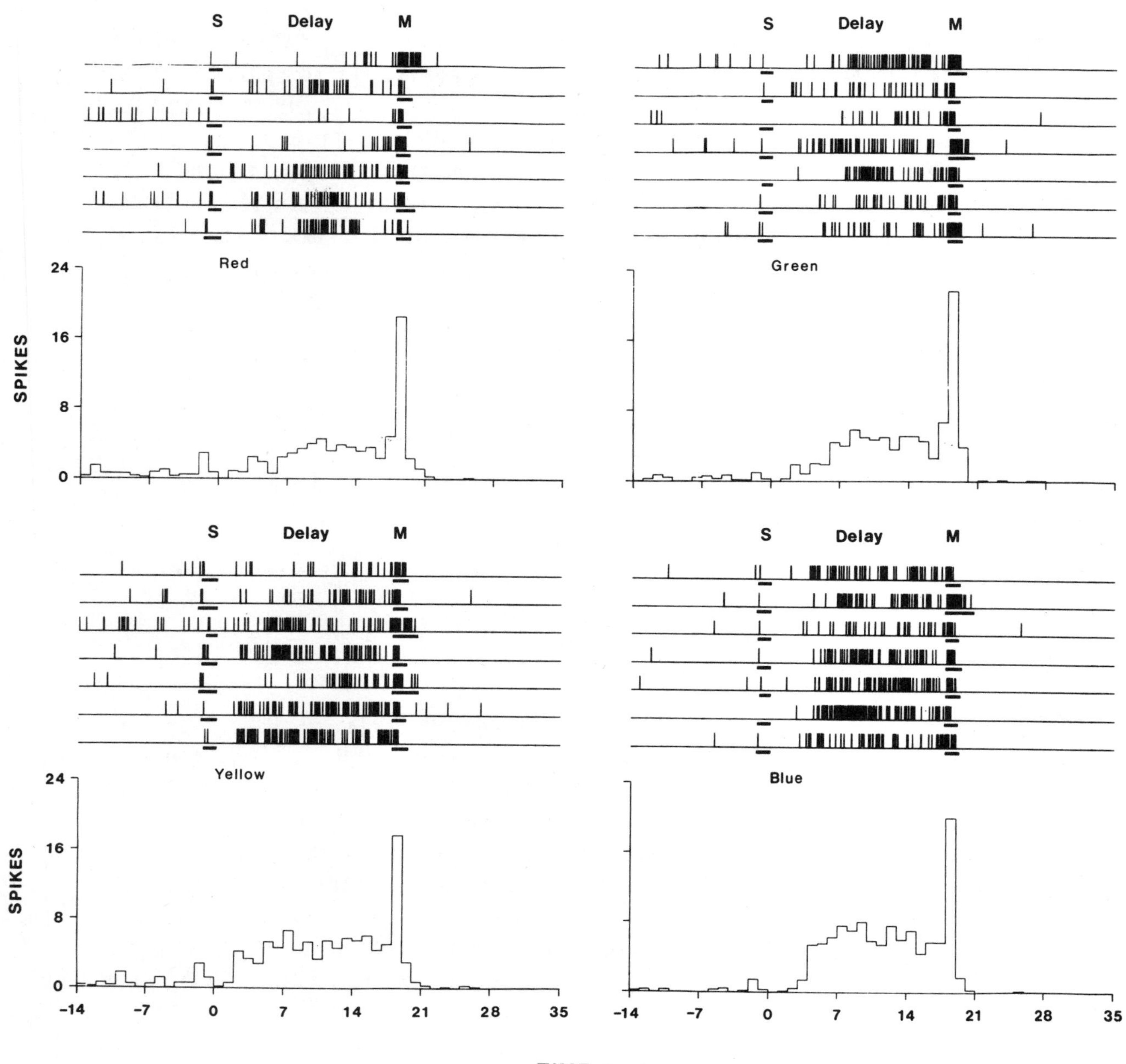

Figure 8. Delay-activated IT unit exhibiting minor reactions to the sample (*S*) and large reactions to the choice (*M*, match) lights.

exclusively in coding or retaining that color. At most, such units can be presumed to participate more than others in the representation and memory of that color and perhaps other features of the sample stimulus as well. That stimulus, by virtue of its various attributes, may be supposed to activate a large pool of IT cells. Subsets of neurons in that pool (e.g., delay differential units) may be especially attuned to a sample color while also reacting to properties deriving from the animal's experience in the task. In other words, even cells that appear engaged in categorical memory of color may be activated by context and therefore may participate in associative memory. In fact, the reaction to color itself may be entirely determined by context (Fuster and Jervey, 1981). This takes us to the logical question: how much of what we see is "pre-wired" and how much is a product of learning? The question could only be answered definitively by recording from the same IT units throughout the learning of the task, which is technically impractical.

The importance of context is underscored by the finding that some units responded more to the sample color when presented alone than as one of the choice colors or vice versa. In this respect, our results are in accord with those obtained by Gross et al. (1979) and Mikami and Kubota (1980) using a task (Konorski task) somewhat

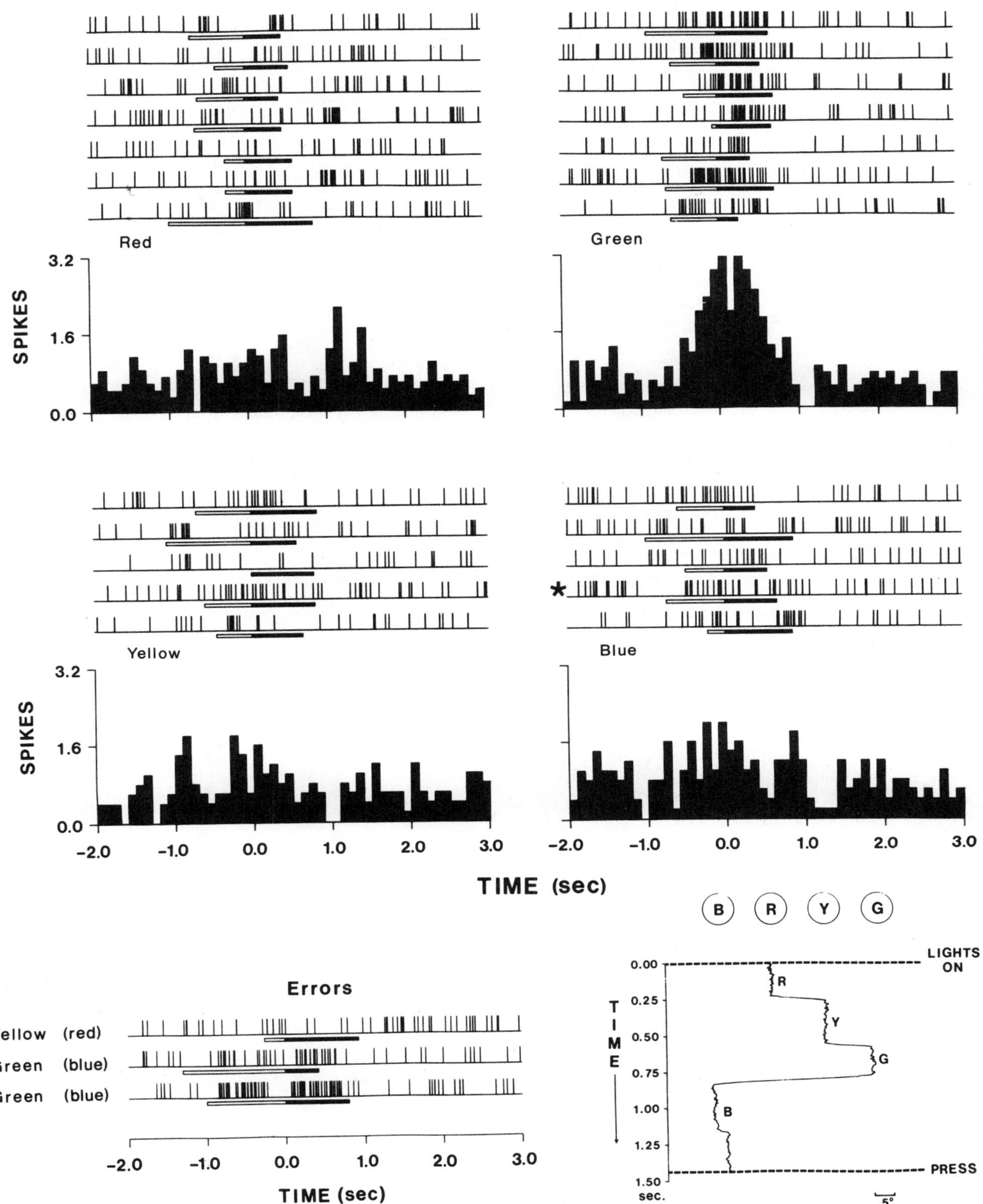

Figure 9. The activity of a cell in the matching period, that is, during exposure to the choice lights (*horizontal bars*). Histograms are time-locked with ocular fixation on the chosen color (marked by the transition from *open* to *black bar* under the individual records). Note the accelerated firing before and during foveation of the green choice light in trials with the green sample. *Lower left*, record excerpts from three trials ending in the incorrect choice (the chosen colors are indicated at *left*; *in parentheses*, the correct sample colors are given). The *inset* in the *lower right corner* shows the horizontal EOG during the matching period of the trial marked above with an *asterisk*. Capital letters indicate the colors of the buttons and the record of ocular fixation of each of them (*B*, blue; *R*, red; *Y*, yellow; *G*, green). Note that, in that trial, the animal scanned all four buttons before pressing the blue one.

Delay Excitation

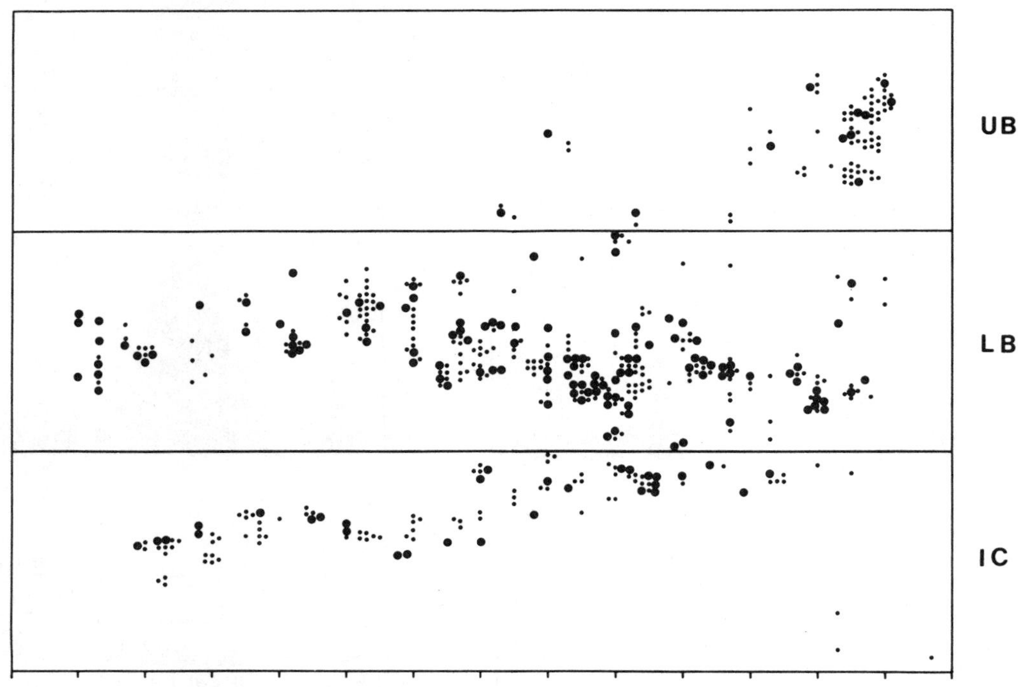

Differential Delay Activity

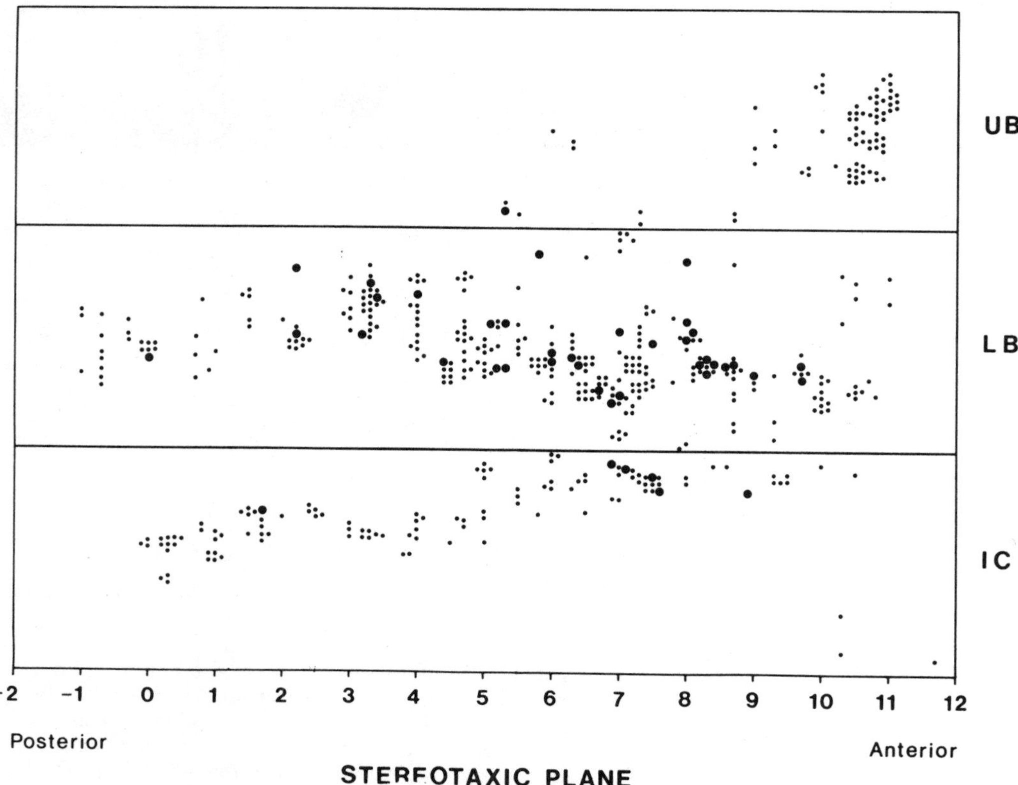

Figure 10. Scatter plots of units showing (*above*) delay activation (both differential and nondifferential) and (*below*) delay differential activity only. The two-unit categories are indicated by *larger dots* against the background display of all of the units investigated in the study. *IC*, Inferior convexity; *LB*, lower bank; *UB*, upper bank.

similar to ours. They noted different unit reactions to one and the same colored stimulus depending on whether it appeared as the sample or as a stimulus for matching. Neither of those studies, however, provided clear evidence of color-dependent delay activity, perhaps because of the relative brevity of the delays utilized. Another reason may be that both studies were concerned primarily with the cortex of the IT convexity.

Comparing IT units with prefrontal units in the same task (Rosenkilde et al., 1981; J. M. Fuster, R. H. Bauer, and J. P. Jervey, manuscript in preparation), some general differences become apparent: (*1*) spontaneous activity is somewhat higher in IT cortex than in prefrontal cortex; (*2*) more differentiation of colors is found in IT cortex, both in terms of the number of color-dependent units and the magnitude of firing frequency differences; and (*3*) more post-trial firing changes are seen among prefrontal units than among IT units.

The apparent involvement of IT neurons in visual DMS is fully consistent with observations that, in man (Milner, 1968) and other primates (Stepień et al., 1960; Buffery, 1967; Kovner and Stamm, 1972; Delacour, 1977; Fuster et al., 1981), the functional integrity of the IT cortex is important for the performance of short term memory tasks. Our results are also consistent with those of circumscribed ablations of temporal cortex (Mishkin, 1972; Wilson et al., 1972; Sahgal and Iversen, 1978), leading to the inference that "anterior" IT cortex, which is the cortical region chiefly explored in this study, is especially important for some aspect of visual memory. (Functionally and anatomically, what has been called "posterior IT cortex" is not IT cortex proper but foveal prestriate cortex; Dean, 1976.) However, inasmuch as delay-activated and delay differential units were found more frequently in the cortex of the lower bank than in that of the convexity, our results suggest a functional dissociation of these two parts of IT cortex that lesion studies have not heretofore revealed. If our interpretation of the behavior of those units is correct, our findings may be viewed as pointing to a substantial involvement of sulcal cortex in visual retention. Thus, under conditions such as those of the present experiments, visual information may be analyzed first in the convexity cortex and then provisionally deposited in the cortex of the superior temporal sulcus. At any rate, the suggested progression of processing from convexity to ventral bank of the sulcus follows the direction of demonstrated anatomical pathways (Seltzer and Pandya, 1978; Desimone et al., 1980).

In conclusion, IT neuron populations seem to participate in three major operations required from the monkey in a delayed matching trial: the acquisition, the retention, and the retrieval of visual information. A clear topographic separation of these operations is not possible because many units appear to participate in more than one of them. However, units that mainly or exclusively participate in short term retention seem to be concentrated in the lower bank of the superior temporal sulcus.

The cortical mechanisms at play in the short term memory trial may be essential for the formation of long term memory and, in this respect, the role of IT cortex in visual short term memory may be at the foundation of its well recognized importance for the learning of visual discriminations. Future research should help us understand how those mechanisms, which are reflected in the behavior of IT units, help the organism establish permanent representations of the visual world.

References

Bond, H. W., and P. Ho (1970) Solid miniature silver-silver chloride electrodes for chronic implantation. Electroenceph-alogr. Clin. Neurophysiol. *28:* 206–208.

Braitman, D. J., and W. A. Wilson (1976) Unit activity in the inferotemporal cortex of rhesus monkey during the performance of visual discrimination tasks. Soc. Neurosci. Abstr. *2:* 1068.

Buffery, A. W. H. (1967) Learning and memory in baboons with bilateral lesions of frontal or inferotemporal cortex. Nature *214:* 1054–1056.

Chow, K. L. (1951) Effects of partial extirpation of posterior association cortex on visually mediated behavior in monkeys. Comp. Psychol. Monogr. *20:* 187–217.

Cowey, A., and C. G. Gross (1970) Effects of foveal prestriate and inferotemporal lesions on visual discrimination by rhesus monkeys. Exp. Brain Res. *11:* 128–144.

Dean, P. (1976) Effects of inferotemporal lesions on the behavior of monkeys. Psychol. Bull. *83:* 41–71.

Delacour, J. (1977) Cortex inférotemporal et mémoire visuelle à court terme chez le singe. Nouvelles données. Exp. Brain Res. *28:* 301–310.

Desimone, R., and C. G. Gross (1979) Visual areas in the temporal cortex of the macaque. Brain Res. *178:* 363–380.

Desimone, R., J. Fleming, and C. G. Gross (1980) Prestriate afferents to inferior temporal cortex: An HRP study. Brain Res. *184:* 41–55.

Fuster, J. M. (1961) Excitation and inhibition of neuronal firing in visual cortex by reticular stimulation. Science *133:* 2011–2012.

Fuster, J. M., and J. P. Jervey (1981) Inferotemporal neurons distinguish and retain behaviorally relevant features of visual stimuli. Science *212:* 952–955.

Fuster, J. M., A. Herz, and O. D. Creutzfeldt (1965) Interval analysis of cell discharge in spontaneous and optically modulated activity in the visual system. Arch. Ital. Biol. *103:* 159–177.

Fuster, J. M., R. H. Bauer, and J. P. Jervey (1981) Effects of cooling inferotemporal cortex on performance of visual memory tasks. Exp. Neurol. *71:* 398–409.

Gross, C. G. (1973) Inferotemporal cortex and vision. In *Progress in Physiological Psychology*, E. Stellar and J. M. Sprague, eds., Vol. 5, pp. 77–123, Academic Press, New York.

Gross, C. G., C. E. Rocha-Miranda, and D. B. Bender (1972) Visual properties of neurons in inferotemporal cortex of the macaque. J. Neurophysiol. *35:* 96–111.

Gross, C. G., D. B. Bender, and M. Mishkin (1977) Contributions of the corpus callosum and the anterior commissure to visual activation of inferior temporal neurons. Brain Res. *131:* 227–239.

Gross, C. G., D. B. Bender, and G. L. Gerstein (1979) Activity of inferior temporal neurons in behaving monkeys. Neuropsychologia *17:* 215–229.

Jones, E. G., and T. P. S. Powell (1970) An anatomical study of converging sensory pathways within the cerebral cortex of the monkey. Brain *93:* 793–820.

Kovner, R., and J. S. Stamm (1972) Disruption of short-term visual memory by electrical stimulation of inferotemporal cortex in the monkey. J. Comp. Physiol. Psychol. *81:* 163–172.

Mikami, A., and K. Kubota (1980) Inferotemporal neuron activities and color discrimination with delay. Brain Res. *182:* 65–78.

Milner, B. (1968) Visual recognition and recall after right temporal-lobe excision in man. Neuropsychologia *6:* 191–209.

Mishkin, M. (1972) Cortical visual areas and their interactions. In *Brain and Human Behavior*, A. G. Karczmar and J. C. Eccles, eds., pp. 187–208, Springer, New York.

Moss, M., H. Mahut, and S. Zola-Morgan (1981) Concurrent discrimination learning of monkeys after hippocampal, entorhinal, or fornix lesions. J. Neurosci. *1:* 227–240.

Ridley, R. M., N. S. Hester, and G. Ettlinger (1977) Stimulus- and response-dependent units from the occipital and temporal lobes of the unanaesthetized monkey performing learnt visual tasks. Exp. Brain Res. *27:* 539–552.

Rocha-Miranda, C. E., D. B. Bender, C. G. Gross, and M. Mishkin (1975) Visual activation of neurons in inferotemporal cortex depends on striate cortex and forebrain commissures. J. Neurophysiol. *38:* 475–491.

Rolls, E. T., S. J. Judge, and M. K. Sanghera (1977) Activity of neurones in the inferotemporal cortex of the alert monkey. Brain Res. *130:* 229–238.

Rosenkilde, C. E., R. H. Bauer, and J. M. Fuster (1981) Single cell activity in ventral prefrontal cortex of behaving monkeys. Brain Res. *209:* 375–394.

Sahgal, A., and S. D. Iversen (1978) Categorization and retrieval after selective inferotemporal lesions in monkeys. Brain Res. *146:* 341–350.

Sato, T., T. Kawamura, and E. Iwai (1980) Responsiveness of inferotemporal single units to visual pattern stimuli in monkeys performing discrimination. Exp. Brain Res. *38:* 313–319.

Seltzer, B., and D. N. Pandya (1978) Afferent cortical connections and architectonics of the superior temporal sulcus and surrounding cortex in the rhesus monkey. Brain Res. *149:* 1–24.

Stepień, L. S., J. P. Cordeau, and T. Rasmussen (1960) The effect of temporal lobe and hippocampal lesions on auditory and visual recent memory in monkeys. Brain *83:* 470–489.

Von Bonin, G., and P. Bailey (1947) *The Neocortex of Macaca mulatta*, University of Illinois Press, Urbana, IL.

Wilson, M., H. M. Kaufman, R. E. Zieler, and J. P. Lieb (1972) Visual identification and memory in monkeys with circumscribed inferotemporal lesions. J. Comp. Physiol. Psychol. *78:* 173–183.

36

Y. Miyashita and H. S. Chang

Neuronal correlate of pictorial short-term memory in the primate temporal cortex

1988. *Nature* 331: 68–70

It has been proposed that visual-memory traces are located in the temporal lobes of the cerebral cortex, as electric stimulation of this area in humans results in recall of imagery[1]. Lesions in this area also affect recognition of an object after a delay in both humans[2,3] and monkeys[4–7], indicating a role in short-term memory of images[8]. Single-unit recordings from the temporal cortex have shown that some neurons continue to fire when one of two or four colours are to be remembered temporarily[9]. But neuronal responses selective to specific complex objects[10–18], including hands[10,13] and faces[13,16,17], cease soon after the offset of stimulus presentation[10–18]. These results led to the question of whether any of these neurons could serve the memory of complex objects. We report here a group of shape-selective neurons in an anterior ventral part of the temporal cortex of monkeys that exhibited sustained activity during the delay period of a visual short-term memory task. The activity was highly selective for the pictorial information to be memorized and was independent of the physical attributes such as size, orientation, colour or position of the object. These observations show that the delay activity represents the short-term memory of the categorized percept of a picture.

In a trial of our visual short-term memory task, sample and match stimuli were successively presented on a video monitor, each for 0.2 s at a 16 s delay interval (Fig. 2*a*). The stimuli were newly selected for each trial among 100 computer-generated coloured fractal patterns (examples are shown in Fig. 1) and 100 pseudo-coloured images of scenery. Two monkeys (*Macaca fuscata*) were trained to memorize the sample stimulus and to decide whether the match stimulus was the same or different (see legend to Fig. 2). Extracellular spike discharges of 188 neurons were recorded from the anterior ventral part of the temporal cortex (Fig. 2*b*) of these monkeys with standard physiological techniques[19]. Recording of electro-oculographs revealed no systematic differences in eye position which could be related to differential neural responses described below.

Figure 2*c* shows reproducible stimulus-dependent discharges during the delay obtained in one cell for four different sample stimuli (Fig. 1*a–d*) (prominent in *a* and *b*, but virtually ineffective in *c* and *d*). A time course of the delay activity in Fig. 2*c*i is shown in Fig. 2*d*, as contrasted with those for six other ineffective stimuli (Fig. 1*c–h*). These histograms are representative of those accumulated with 57 other sample stimuli. Only two of the 64 tested stimuli (Fig. 2*e*) were followed by especially high delay activity (>10 impulses $\cdot$ s^{-1}), shown in Fig. 2*c*i and ii.

These delay activities do not represent mere sensory after-discharge[9,11] for the following reasons. First, the high rate of firing did not decline throughout the whole 16 s delay period (Fig. 2*d*). Second, firing frequency exhibited during the delay was not necessarily correlated with that during the stimulus presentation (Fig. 2*c* and *d*). Third, the delay activity in some neurons started after a latency of a few seconds following stimulus presentation (data not shown). Thus, it is concluded that the delay activity is not a passive continuation of the firing during the sensory stimulation, but represents a mnemonic activity to retain visual information.

Of the 188 neurons tested, 144 showed a correlation between firing and one or more events of the trials. Among the 144 cells, 95 showed a sustained increase or decrease of discharge frequency during the delay period, whereas the others fired only during stimulus presentation. In 77 of these 95 cells, the discharge frequency varied depending on sample stimuli, but the remaining 18 did not exhibit such selectivity. In many of the 77 selective cells, only a few pictures elicited a strong delay activation such as shown in Fig. 2*c* and *d*. It is notable that the optimal picture differed from cell to cell, and that the whole population of the optimal pictures for the 77 cells covered a substantial part of the repertory of 200 pictorial stimuli.

For further analysis of triggering features of the delay responses, sample pictures were manipulated in the following way (for example Fig. 1*i–l*): (1) stimulus size was reduced by half, (2) stimuli were rotated by 90° in a clockwise direction, (3) coloured stimuli were transformed into monochrome by referring to a pseudo-colour look-up table, and (4) stimulus position was changed on the video monitor (data not shown) (a 0.2 s stimulus presentation time is short enough to exclude the contribution of saccadic eye movement). Figure 3 shows responses of a neuron which consistently fired during the delay after one particular picture (shown in Fig. 1*i–l*) but not after others, irrespective of stimulus size (Fig. 3*a*ii and *b*ii), orientation (Fig. 3*a*iii and *b*iii), or colour (Fig. 3*a*iv and *b*iv). Similar tolerance of responses was observed in a majority of the tested delay neurons: to size in 16 out of 19 cells, to orientation in 5 out of 7 cells, to colour-monochrome in 15 out of 20 cells, and to position in 8 out of 13 cells. In other neurons, manipulation of the most effective stimulus reduced or abolished the delay discharge.

In the inferior temporal cortex, shape-selective neuronal discharges have been reported for Fourier descriptors[12], face[13,16,17], hands[10,13] or stimuli used in a discrimination task[14,15], although all of these were sensory responses evoked during presentation of stimulus. The relative selectivity of these sensory neurons remained invariant over changes of size, position, orientation or contrast[12–15,17]. The present delay responses could be derived through such sensory responses, inheriting from them the tolerance to such stimulus transformations. It is notable that, for the Fourier descriptor neurons[12], the absolute level of the response varied widely over changes in stimulus size, although this was not the case for many of the present neurons. This may suggest that the present neurons represent more abstract properties of objects (like shape percept) than do such sensory neurons.

In the colour-selective delay neurons previously described[9], time courses of sustained delay discharge were similar to those found in the present shape-selective delay neurons (compare Fig. 2*d* or Fig. 3*a* with Fig. 7 or Fig. 6 of ref. 9). The differential delay activity in the colour task was mainly found in the cortex of the lower bank of the superior temporal sulcus[9], lying more posteriorly and dorsally to the presently explored area, and the colour cells seemed to be scattered[9], whereas the present cells tended to group in smaller areas.

A majority of our shape-selective delay neurons were recorded in TE_{av}[20] (or TE_1-TE_2[21]) and some in TG_v[20] and in area 35. These areas are anatomically designated as the last link from the visual system to limbic memory systems[4,20,22,23]. Neurons in these areas were visually responsive with a large receptive field[24]. Impairment of the recognition memory task resulted from lesions including these areas[4–7], consistent with the presently-postulated mnemonic role of neurons in these areas.

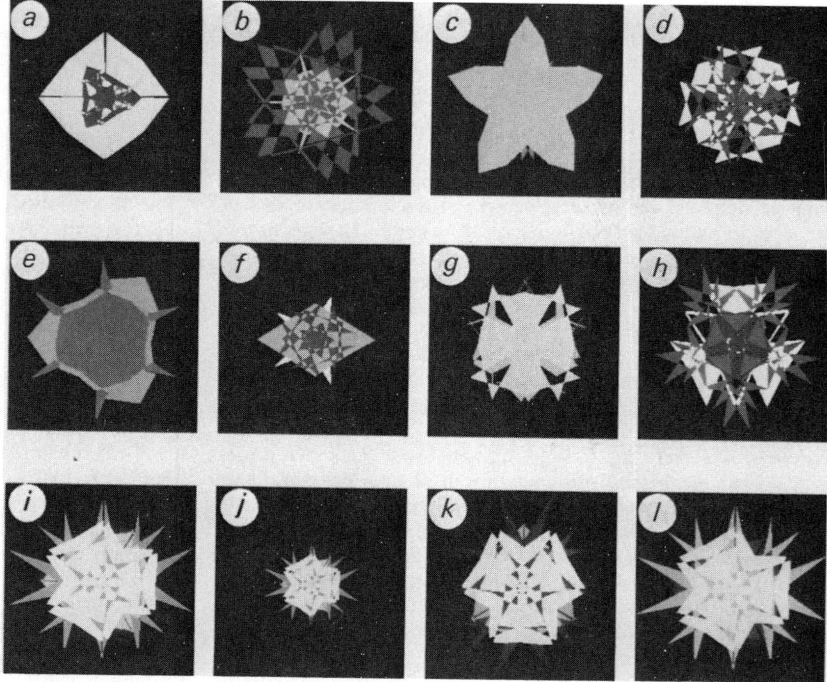

Fig. 1 Examples of coloured fractal patterns. *a–h*, Stimuli used in the trials of Figs 2*c* and *d*. Panels *i–l*, illustrate size reduction (*j*), rotation (*k*) and colour-monochrome transformation (*l*) of stimulus (*i*), as used in the test shown in Fig. 3.

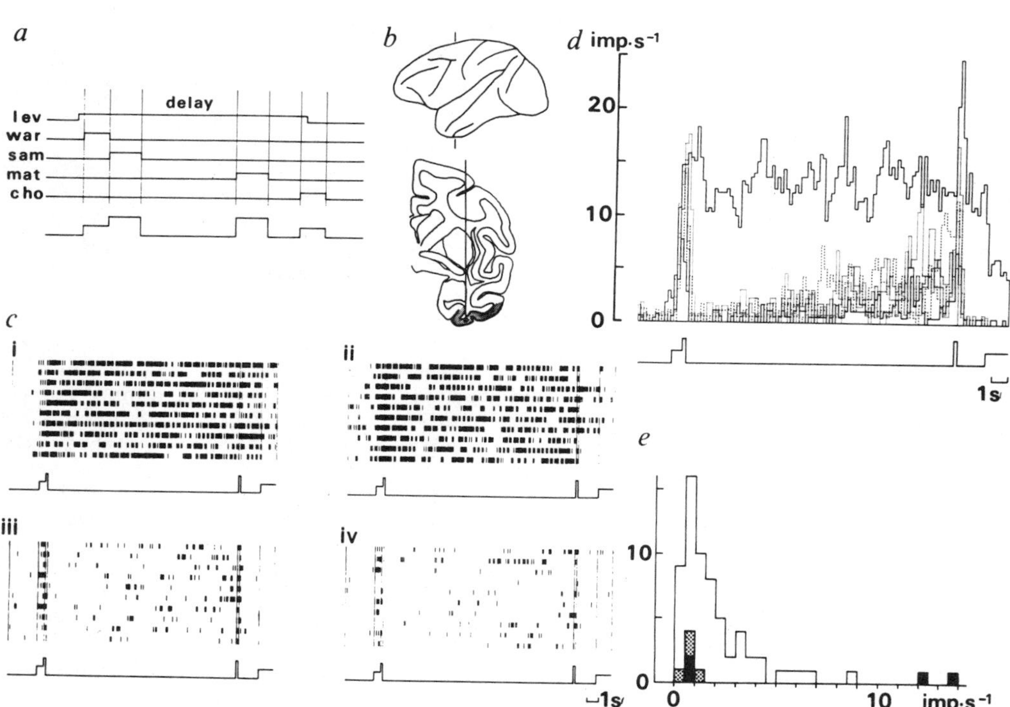

Fig. 2 Responses of a neuron in the anterior ventral temporal cortex in a visual short-term memory task. *a*, Sequence of events in a trial (Lev, lever press by the monkey; War, warning green image (0.5 s); Sam, sample stimulus (0.2 s); Mat, match stimulus (0.2 s) following a delay of 16 s; Cho, choice signal of white image). Lowest trace, the events-chart used in Fig. 2*c–d* and Fig. 3*a*. *b*, Location of recording sites. Top, a lateral view of a macaque brain. Bottom, a section indicated by a vertical line on the lateral view. The stippled area represents the range of recording sites. The vertical line and the dot at its end represent the microelectrode track and the position of the cell shown in Fig. 2*c–e*. *c*, Raster recordings of impulse discharge from a cell. i, Trials whose sample stimulus was as shown in Fig. 1*a*. ii, iii and iv, Obtained as in Fig. 1*b*, *c* and *d*, respectively. Trials of the same sample stimulus were originally separated by intervening trials of other sample stimuli, and these were sorted and collected by off-line computation. *d*, Spike-density histograms for the delay activity of Fig. 2*c*i and for those for six other ineffective stimuli (Fig. 1*c–h*). Seven to 16 trials were accumulated for each sample stimulus. Bin width, 200 ms. *e*, Distribution of average delay spike frequencies following 64 different sample pictures, with which more than four trials were tested. The same cell as in *c* and *d*. Ordinate, number of sample pictures used as stimuli. Closed columns, responses shown in Fig. 2*c*. The stippled columns, other responses included in Fig. 2*d*.

Method. Each sample picture was paired with a match stimulus that was identical and one that was not identical. For each trial, the identical or non-identical match stimulus was assigned randomly. If the match stimulus was different from the sample, the monkey had to release the lever and touch the video screen to obtain fruit juice. If the match stimulus was the same as the sample, the monkey had to keep pressing the lever until the choice signal was turned off. If the monkey released the lever before the choice signal, the trial was cancelled. The monkeys' decisions were 85–100% correct. Error trials were excluded from the analysis presented here. In training sessions and the search period stimuli were presented in a fixed sequence. In the recording session, a long sequence of trials using the entire repertory of stimuli was run repeatedly. When some pictures were found to elicit stronger responses than others, the relevant pictures were selected and shorter sequences run with fewer stimuli.

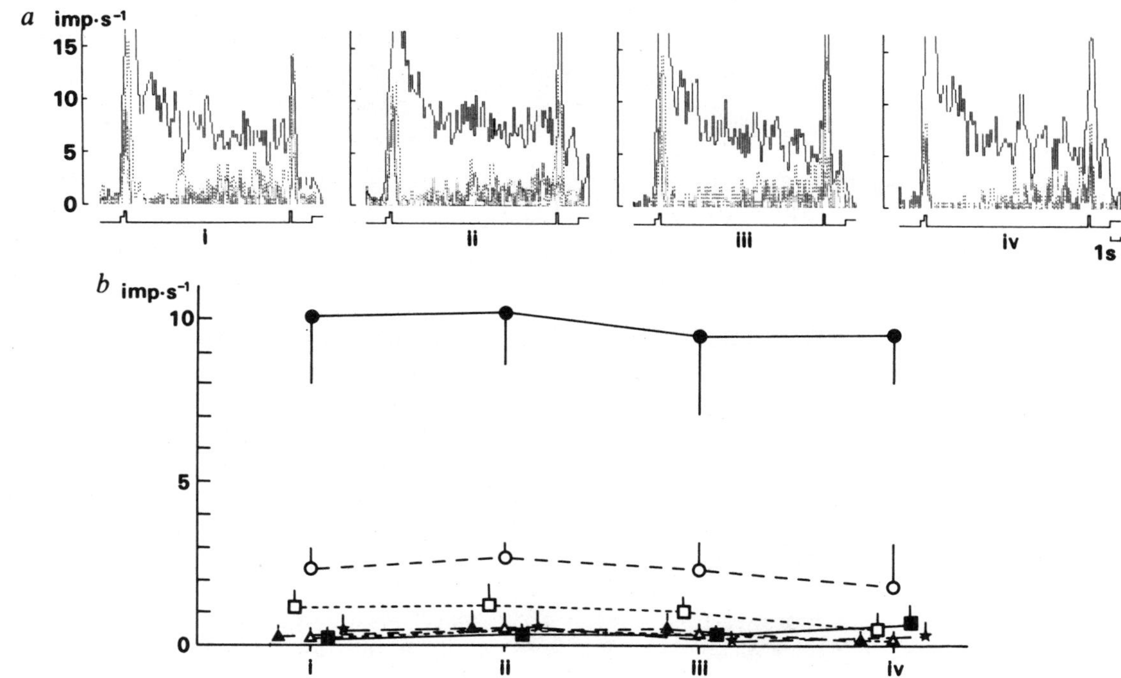

Fig. 3 Response invariance under stimulus transformation in size, orientation or colour. A different cell from that in Fig. 2. *a*, Histograms similar to that in Fig. 2*d*, but for five different sample pictures. i, Control responses. Note that the sample stimulus of Fig. 1*i* elicited the strongest delay activity in this cell. ii, iii and iv, Effects of stimulus size reduction by half (for example Fig. 1*j*), of stimulus rotation by 90° in a clockwise direction (for example Fig. 1*k*) and of colour-to-monochrome transformation (for example Fig. 1*l*). *b*, Average delay spike frequencies as a function of stimulus transformation (i, original; ii, size reduction; iii, rotation; iv, colour to monochrome). Responses to seven different sample pictures (including five shown in *a*) are plotted with different symbols. ●, Responses to stimuli of Fig. 1*i*–*l*. Error bars indicate standard deviations for 4–15 trials.

The present results suggest that pictorial short-term memory is coded by temporary activation of an ensemble of neurons in the region of the association cortex that processes visual information[4,9,25], rather than by neuronal activity in a brain area specialized for short-term memory. Although each neuron in the ensemble has highly abstract and selective coding features, representation of the memory of a picture seems to be distributed among a number of neurons. We need to know how the distributed information is decoded for subsequent decision processes[26].

We thank Professor Masao Ito for his encouragement.

1. Penfield, W. & Perot, P. *Brain* **86**, 595–697 (1963).
2. Kimura, D. *Arch. Neurol.* **8**, 48–55 (1963).
3. Milner, B. *Neuropsychologia* **6**, 191–209 (1968).
4. Mishkin, M. *Phil. Trans. R. Soc.* B **298**, 85–95 (1982).
5. Gaffan, D. & Weiskrantz, L. *Brain Res.* **196**, 373–386 (1980).
6. Sahgal, A., Hutchinson, R., Hughes, R. P. & Iverson, S. D. *Behav. Brain Res.* **8**, 361–373 (1983).
7. Fuster, J. M., Bauer, R. H. & Jervey, J. P. *Expl Neurol.* **71**, 398–409 (1981).
8. Warrington, E. K. & Shallice, T. *Quart. J. exp. Psychol.* **24**, 30–40 (1972).
9. Fuster, J. M. & Jervey, J. P. *J. Neurosci.* **3**, 361–375 (1982).
10. Gross, C. G., Rocha-Miranda, C. E. & Bender, D. B. *J. Neurophysiol.* **35**, 96–111 (1972).
11. Gross, C. G., Bender, D. B. & Mishkin, M. *Brain Res.* **131**, 227–239 (1977).
12. Schwartz, E. L., Desimone, R., Albright, T. D. & Gross, C. G. *Proc. natn. Acad. Sci. U.S.A.* **80**, 5776–5778 (1983).
13. Desimone, R., Albright, T. D., Gross, C. G. & Bruce, C. *J. Neurosci.* **4**, 2051–2062 (1984).
14. Sato, T., Kawamura, T. & Iwai, E. *Expl Brain Res.* **38**, 313–319 (1980).
15. Iwai, E. *Vision Res.* **25**, 425–439 (1985).
16. Perret, D. I., Rolls, E. T. & Caan, W. *Expl Brain Res.* **47**, 329–342 (1982).
17. Rolls, E. T. & Baylis, G. C. *Brain Res.* **65**, 38–48 (1986).
18. Baylis, G. C. & Rolls, E. T. *Expl Brain Res.* **65**, 614–622 (1987).
19. Miyashita, Y. & Nagao, S. *J. Physiol., Lond.* **351**, 251–262 (1984).
20. Turner, B. H., Mishkin, M. & Knapp, M. *J. comp. Neurol.* **191**, 515–543 (1980).
21. Seltzer, B. & Pandya, D. N. *Brain Res.* **149**, 1–24 (1978).
22. Herzog, A. G. & Van Hoesen, G. W. *Brain Res.* **115**, 57–69 (1976).
23. Van Hoesen, G. W. & Pandya, D. N. *Brain Res.* **95**, 1–24 (1975).
24. Desimone, R. & Gross, C. G. *Brain Res.* **178**, 363–380 (1979).
25. Anderson, J. R. *Cognitive Psychology and its Implications* (Freeman, San Francisco, 1980).
26. Coltheart, M. *Phil. Trans. R. Soc.* B **302**, 283–294 (1983).

J. W. Gnadt and R. A. Andersen

Memory related motor planning activity in posterior parietal cortex of macaque

1988. *Experimental Brain Research* 70: 216–220

Summary. Unit recording studies in the lateral bank of the intraparietal cortex (area LIP) have demonstrated a response property not previously reported in posterior cortex. Studies were performed in the Rhesus monkey during tasks which required saccadic eye movements to remembered target locations in the dark. Neurons were found which remained active during the time period for which the monkey had to withhold eye movements while remembering desired target locations. The activity of the cells was tuned for eye movements of specific direction and amplitude, and it was not necessary for a visual stimulus to fall within the response field. The responses appeared to represent a memory-related motor-planning signal encoding motor error. The relation of the activity to the behavior of the animal suggests that the response represents the intent to make eye movements of specific direction and amplitude.

Key words: Saccade – Parietal cortex – Memory – Monkey – Motor-planning – Oculomotor – Motor error – Intention

Introduction

The posterior parietal cortex of primates is involved in sensorimotor processing in both somatic and visual/oculomotor modalities (Critchley 1953, Mountcastle et al. 1975; Hyvärinen 1982; Lynch 1980; Andersen 1987). Recent studies in our lab have focused on the visual-motor properties of neurons in the lateral intraparietal area (LIP), a cortical field in the lateral bank of the intraparietal sulcus (Andersen et al. 1987; Gnadt et al. 1986). In the course of these studies we have unexpectedly discovered a response property not previously reported in posterior parietal cortex. These responses were triggered by visual stimuli and maintained their activity for several seconds during tasks which required the monkey to withhold planned eye movements. The activity of the neurons was modulated according to the direction and amplitude of the planned eye movement. Using tasks which temporally and spatially separate visual responses from motor responses, we have shown that the activity was related to the eye movements and can occur in the absence of visual stimuli falling within the response field. These neurons appear to hold in short-term memory the metrics of planned eye movements and thus represent the intention to make specific eye movements. The neurons appear to have similar properties to the 'quasi-visual' (QV) cells of the superior colliculus (Mays and Sparks 1980) and to some cells in the frontal eye fields (Bruce and Goldberg 1985) and prefrontal cortex near the principal sulcus (Goldman-Rakic 1987). The QV cells also had sustained activity to brief visual stimuli during delayed saccade trails, and did not require visual stimuli to fall within their response fields (Mays and Sparks 1980). The frontal cortex cells responded tonically to brief visual stimuli and were suggested to be involved in short-term visual and spatial memory (Bruce and Goldberg 1985; Goldman-Rakic 1987).

Methods

An adult male Rhesus monkey (7.5 kg) was trained to fixate and make eye movements to 0.4° light spots backprojected onto a tangent screen 57 cm in front of the animal. Experiments were performed in a completely dark room while the monkey was seated in a primate chair with the head fixed. Eye movements were monitored using the scleral search coil technique (Robinson 1963) and the monkey was given liquid reward for completing the correct sequence of eye movements, as described elsewhere (Andersen et al. 1987). Single unit extracellular recordings were made according to standard techniques using transdural penetrations with a hydraulically sealed microdrive mounted over the parietal cortex. Results were obtained from both hemispheres over a period of 10 months. Recording site locations were reconstructed by interpolation from microdrive coordinates (corrected for shrinkage) compared to histologically verified marking lesions made at known coordinates during the last two weeks of recording and to guide wires placed at the time of sacrifice. Estimates were corrected to conform to the histological sections according to landmarks obtained during recordings, such as transitions from somatosensory responses in area 5 on the medial bank of the intraparietal sulcus and the postcentral gyrus, and from transitions in activity levels and spike forms between gray matter and white matter. Penetrations were made into the dorsomedial extent of the lateral bank of the intraparietal sulcus (area LIP) and the adjacent anterior edge of the convexity of the inferior parietal lobule (area 7a).

The monkey was trained to make eye movements to the remembered location of a flashed visual stimulus, similar to the delayed saccade task of Hikosaka and Wurtz (1983). The monkey learned to fixate one spot of light while a second spot was flashed for 300 ms at an eccentric position. When the fixation spot extinguished 500 to 1600 ms later (pseudorandom presentation), the monkey would saccade to the remembered target location and fixate in the dark for an additional 500 ms. An important aspect of this tasks is that it temporally separates stimulus-related activity from movement-related activity. Movements were performed in complete darkness thus precluding artifactual visual stimulation during the movements. Additionally, this task is interesting because it necessitated the use of a memory-linked internal representation of visual or motor space. To test for visual responses to the offset of the fixation spot, the monkey was trained to maintain fixation of the fixation spot location for 500 ms while the spot extinguished and then reappeared.

Additionally, the double-saccade task first described by Hallett and Lightstone (1976) and later refined by Mays and Sparks (1980) was used to investigate the sensorimotor and the memory related properties of the cells. The monkey was trained to look from an extinguished fixation spot to a target position defined by a brief (60 ms) light flash and then to return to the original fixation position. Both eye movements were performed in complete darkness since the latency to the first eye movement was longer than the duration of the target light, and the target position for the second movement was the remembered location of the original fixation spot. The task was designed such that a visual stimulus never appeared in the response field of the neuron when the trajectory of the second eye movement corresponded to that cell's preferred direction of response.

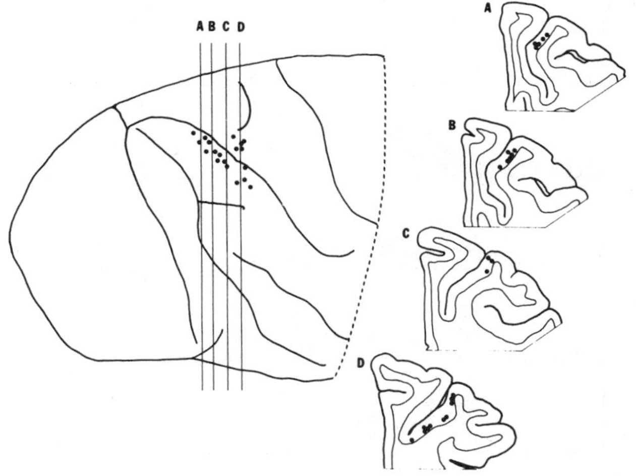

Fig. 1. Recording sites where intended movement cells were encountered. The panel to the left shows the entry points of the penetrations on a drawing of the lateral surface of the macaque brain. Penetrations from both hemispheres have been drawn onto this schematic view from the right hemisphere. Panels *A–D* show the locations of the recording sites along the lateral bank of the intraparietal sulcus in the representative coronal sections from the positions shown on the drawing to the left. Recording sites have been drawn onto or adjacent to lamina IV, at their estimated locations

Results

The following criteria were used to classify functional types according to their response in the task of making single saccades to remembered visual targets. Cells having a response to the visual cue, which was not sustained throughout the response delay period, were classified as *light sensitive*. Cells having a burst of activity slightly before, during, or slightly after the eye movement were classified as *saccade-related*. A third class of cells had sustained activity above background during the time period for which the monkey was required to remember the target position but withheld the eye movement. The sustained response of these cells was turned off by the eye movement. For reasons described below, these cells were classified as *intended movement cells*. The data base for this paper is taken from 141 cells recorded from 76 penetrations. Fifty nine cells (42%) were classified as light sensitive, 33 cells (23%) as saccade-related, 10 cells (7%) as light sensitive and saccade-related, and 24 (17%) as intended movement cells. Fifteen cells (11%) were modulated uniquely by gaze direction or other parameters. Twenty five of the 59 light sensitive cells exhibited stronger responses when tested with moving stimuli. Because this sustained responses property was an unexpected finding, systematic searching and testing was not performed until the later stages of the studies. In fact, if not tested explicitly, these cells could appear to be simply light sensitive cells by many routine criteria. They responded phasically and less vigorously to visual stimuli in blocks of visual probe trials that did not require eye movements. For this reason, the proportion of the intended movement cells out of the total is under-represented. This paper will discuss only this new functional class of cells, all of which were located on the lateral bank of the intraparietal

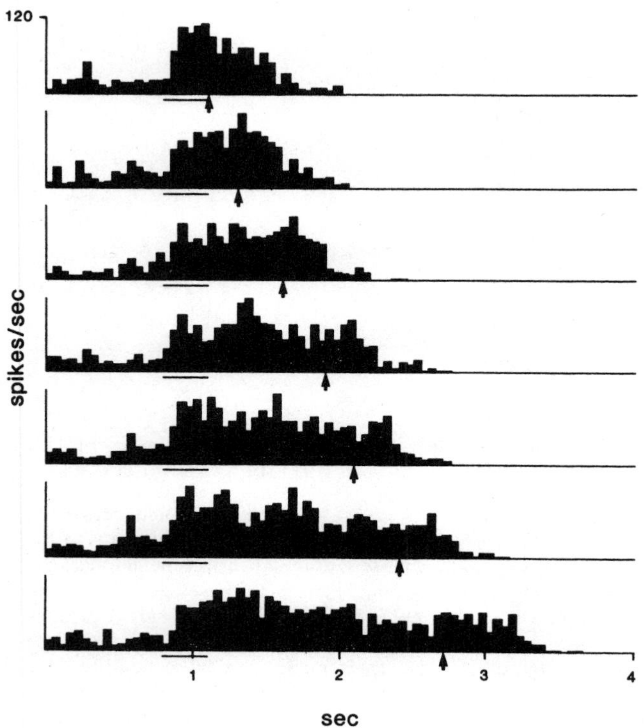

Fig. 2. Spike histograms of an intended movement cell during saccades to a remembered target location within the cell's motor field. Each histogram includes responses for 8–10 trials. Trials are grouped according to increasing response delay times from top to bottom. The horizontal bar below each histogram indicates the stimulus presentation. The arrow indicates the time at which the fixation spot was extinguished. Eye movements occurred from 150 to 400 ms following offset of the spot. Binwidths = 50 ms

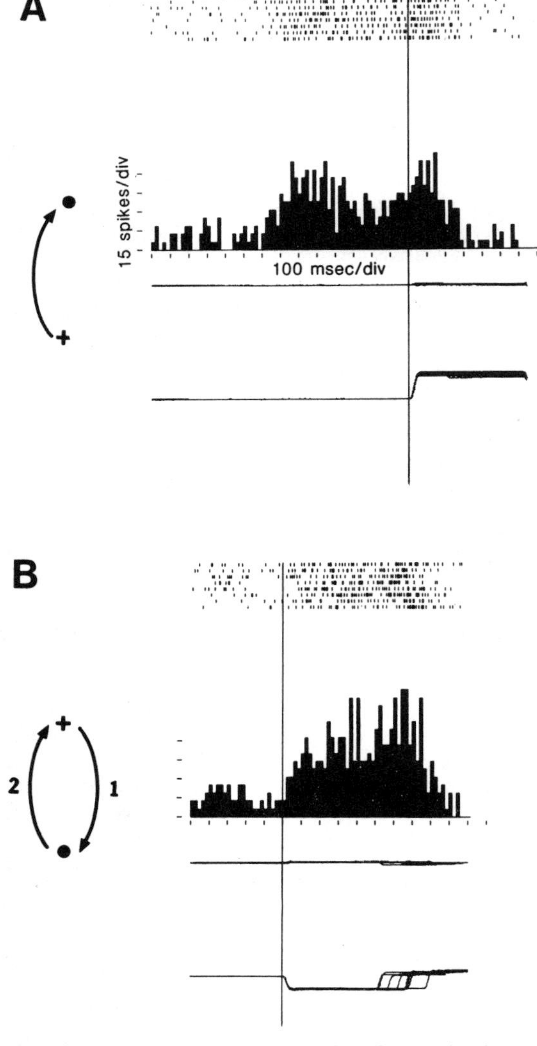

Fig. 3A, B. Motor planning properties of a sustained-response cell. **A** Eye movements straight up into the center of a cell's response field. Trials are aligned to the beginning of the saccade. **B** Double saccade trials with a movement first down then back up into the cell's motor field. Trials are aligned to the first movement. Each panel shows, from top to bottom, the spike rasters for 8 trials, the corresponding histogram with spike rate and time base (binwidths = 50 ms), and horizontal and vertical eye position traces for each trial

sulcus as determined by histological reconstruction of the penetrations (Fig. 1).

Figure 2 shows the response of one of these cells during eight different delay periods. The cell began to respond within 100 ms of the onset of a visual stimulus within its response field. It continued to discharge after the stimulus was extinguished until the eye movement was made, regardless of whether the movement occurred within a few hundred milliseconds or was withheld for more than one and one half seconds. Some of these cells also had either excitatory or inhibitory phasic responses associated with the visual stimulus (2 cells), the saccade (6 cells), or both (7 cells). The beginning of the saccade-related burst for a given cell could either precede or follow the eye movement within a range of 140 ms before to 100 ms after the beginning of the saccade (median = 50 ms before). Interestingly, the QV cells of superior colliculus also often continued to discharge beyond the end of the saccades (Mays and Sparks 1980). The activity during the response delay could be as high as 200–250 spikes/s, sometimes diminishing during the long delays.

The activities of the cells was tuned broadly according to the direction and amplitude of eye movements. Of the 24 cells, twelve were centered in the contralateral direction, eleven near the vertical meridian, and one in the ipsilateral direction. Due to their broad tuning, however, many cells included large portions of both hemifields. Cells having peak activity for 15° eye movements typically had response fields for 50% of peak response of about 90° in direction and 25° visual angle in amplitude. Response fields were smaller for cells tuned for shorter movements, particularly in the amplitude parameter.

Twelve of the 24 intended movement cells were tested in the double saccade task as shown in Fig. 3. This figure shows the response of an intended movement cell with a response field centered approximately 15° straight up. In Fig. 3a, saccades were made to a remembered target location 15° straight up. Trials have been aligned with the beginning of the saccade. The stimulus appeared approximately 800 ms (500 ms delay plus 200–400 ms saccade latency) prior to the beginning of the eye movement. This cell also had a phasic saccade-related burst of activity. Figure 3b shows the response of the same neuron for a sequence of two eye movements: first down to the location of the flashed light, then back up to the remembered location of the extinguished fixation point. The slight hypometria of the second saccades is well within the response field of the cell. Note that the activity of the neuron increased as soon as the monkey achieved the first target and was in a position to make the next saccade into the cell's motor field. The activity ceased after completion of the second movement. Because a visual stimulus never fell within the cell's response field, the activity represents the motor coordinates of direction and amplitude of the pending saccade and not the retinotopic location of a visual stimulus on the retinae.

The activity of this cell appeared to represent the intended trajectory of the impending saccade, holding in register the direction and amplitude until the eye movement was performed, but only for the next intended movement.

Discussion

We have shown that there is memory-linked activity in lateral bank of the intraparietal sulcus which is associated with saccadic eye movements of specific direction and amplitude. The activity can be dissociated from the visual stimuli which guide the eye movements. This observation indicates that the cells were not retaining the stimulus property of retinal position. Quantitative testing during limb or head movements was not performed. However, we have tested many cells in this cortical area for cutaneous receptive fields and for responses to passive movements of the limbs and have never observed somatosensory responses in association with these cells. Furthermore, this cortical field projects to other oculomotor structures, but not to somatomotor structures (Fries 1984; Asanuma et al. 1986; Lynch 1985; Petrides and Pandya 1984; Andersen et al. 1985), and, finally, stimulation in this area has been shown to produce saccadic eye movements (Shibutani et al. 1984). Therefore, these cells' activity appeared to be related to the pre-movement planning of saccades in a manner which we have chosen to describe as motor intention. The term motor intention, as we use it here, is meant to convey an association between the behavioral event (i.e. saccade) and the neural activity. It is not meant to suggest that this neural signal is necessary and sufficient to produce the eye movement. As has been argued for the QV activity of the superior colliculus (Mays and Sparks 1980), a motor error signal such as this must be combined with a 'trigger' signal to produce a saccade after decisions such as target selection have been made. Indeed, in the occasional trials in which the monkey failed to make the appropriate second eye movement into the cells' response field, the pre-saccadic activity was sporadic and not sustained. Furthermore, during spontaneous movements in the dark, the activities of the cells appeared to be only weakly correlated with the eye movements: occasionally bursting for wrong eye movements or for no movements and often not responding vigorously before appropriate saccades. Quantitative testing using behavioral paradigms which systematically control the behavioral significance and consequence of 'wrong' eye movements and 'spontaneous' eye movements will be necessary to characterize these relationships in detail.

The association of parietal cortex function with movement intention is not without precedent. Hyvärinen (1982) has suggested that the posterior parietal cortex may serve to integrate sensory and intentional factors, and the original 'command hypothesis' proposed by Mountcastle et al. (1975) also engendered some form of motor intention factors. Furthermore, Valenstein et al. (1982) have presented behavioral evidence that the characteristic hemineglect syndrome produced by parietal lesions can be explained as a deficit of movement intention rather than sensory neglect. These investigators trained monkeys to respond manually using the extremity contralateral to a stimulus cue. They found that parietotemporal lesions produced deficits related to reaching with the contralateral arm rather than to responding to the cue on the contralateral side of the body. The intended movement cells exhibit neural activity occurring early in the oculomotor planning process which corresponds to behaviorally defined intention. In terms of control system models, this response is a motor error signal of the impending saccade.

In order to make saccades to remembered target locations, the brain must be able to calculate an intended trajectory based on target position relative to current eye position, and must be able to use either proprioceptive feedback or efference copy of the eye movement to determine the new eye position at the completion of the movement (Helmholtz 1910; Sperry 1950; von Holst 1954). Note that the 'memory' of the target location could be held in sensory (retinal) coordinates until the time of making the movement or in pre-planned motor (trajectory) coordinates. Our data suggest that, at least for single eye movements, the remembered target locations are coded in area LIP as pre-planned motor trajectories by cells which are not sensory in the usual sense. It is not necessary for visual stimuli to fall within their response fields for the cells to become active.

Making two eye movements to two remembered target positions adds additional demands on the oculomotor system. Two general motor-planning strategies are possible. Either a series of two eye movements must be pre-planned or the system must be able to hold in some sort of spatial register the position of the second target, and must use the new eye position at the end of the first movement to calculate the trajectory of the second movement. Our data do not support the first hypothesis since the activity of these cells do not hold in register the movement trajectories during intervening movements.

The posterior parietal cortex of primates contains neural signals appropriate for the building of spatial maps of visual target space (Andersen et al. 1985), memory-linked motor-planning activity and possible corollary feedback activity of saccades (Andersen et al. 1987; Gnadt et al. 1986). These findings strongly argue that the parietal cortex is intimately involved in the guiding and motor planning of saccadic eye movements.

Acknowledgements. The authors would like to thank Drs. Gene Blatt and Ralph Siegel for their technical, theoretical and editorial input, Kris Trulock for the photography, Gwen Gnadt for her histological assistance, and Dr. Colin Bernstein for his consultation and optical evaluation of our primates' vision. This work was supported by NIH grant EY-05522 to RAA and National Research Service Award NS-081087 to JWG. RAA is the recipient of a McKnight Foundation Scholars Award and a Sloan Foundation Fellowship, and is a Clayton Foundation Investigator.

References

Andersen RA (1987) Inferior parietal lobule function in spatial perception and visuomotor integration. In: Mountcastle VB, Plum F, Geiger (eds) Handbook of physiology: the nervous system, Vol 5. American Physiological Society, Bethesda MD, pp 483–518

Andersen RA, Asanuma C, Cowan WM (1985) Callosal and prefrontal associational projecting cell populations in area 7a of the Macaque monkey: a study using retrogradely transported fluorescent dyes. J Comp Neurol 232: 443–455

Andersen RA, Essick GK, Siegel RM (1985) Encoding of spatial location by posterior parietal neurons. Science 230: 456–458

Andersen RA, Essick GK, Siegel RM (1987) Neurons of area 7 activated by both visual stimuli and oculomotor behavior. Exp Brain Res 67: 316–322

Asanuma C, Andersen RA, Cowan WM (1986) The thalamic relations of the caudal inferior parietal lobule and the lateral prefrontal cortex in monkeys: divergent cortical projections from cell clusters in the medial pulvinar nucleus. J Comp Neurol 241: 357–381

Bruce CJ, Goldberg ME (1985) Primate frontal eye fields. I. Single neurons discharging before saccades. J Neurophysiol 53: 603–635

Critchley M (1953) The parietal lobes. Hafner Publishing Co Inc, New York

Fries W (1984) Cortical projections to the superior colliculus in the macaque monkey: a retrograde study using horseradish peroxidase. J Comp Neurol 230: 55–76

Gnadt JW, Andersen RA, Blatt GJ (1986) Spatial, memory, and motor-planning properties of saccade-related activity in the lateral intraparietal area (LIP) of macaque. Soc Neurosci Abstr 12: 454

Goldman-Rakic PS (1987) Circuitry of primate prefrontal cortex and regulation of behavior by representational memory. In: Mountcastle VB, Plum F, Geiger (eds) Handbook of physiology: the nervous system, American Physiological Society, Bethesda MD, pp 373–417

Hallett PE, Lightstone AD (1976) Saccadic eye movements towards stimuli triggered by prior saccades. Vision Res 16: 99–106

von Helmholtz H (1910) Handbuch der physiologischen Optik. Translation by Southall JPC (1925), Helmholtz's treatise on physiological optics. Dover Publications, New York, Vol III, pp 242–247

Hikosaka O, Wurtz RH (1983) Visual and oculomotor functions of monkey substantia nigra pars reticulata. III. Memory-contingent visual and saccade responses. J Neurophysiol 49: 1268–1284

von Holst E (1954) Relations between the central nervous system and the peripheral organs. Br J Animal Behav 2: 89–94

Hyvärinen J (1982) The parietal cortex of monkey and man. Springer, Berlin Heidelberg New York

Lynch JC (1980) The functional organization of posterior parietal cortex. Behav Brain Sci 3: 485–534

Lynch JC, Graybiel AM, Lobeck LJ (1985) The differential projection of two cytoarchitectonic subregions of the inferior parietal lobule of macaque upon the deep layers of the superior colliculus. J Comp Neurol 235: 241–254

Mays LE, Sparks DL (1980) Dissociation of visual and saccade-related responses in superior colliculus neurons. J Neurophysiol 43: 207–231

Mountcastle VB, Lynch JC, Georgopoulos A, Sakata H, Acuna C (1975) Posterior parietal association cortex of the monkey: command functions for operations within extrapersonal space. J Neurophysiol 38: 871–908

Petrides M, Pandya DN (1984) Projection to the frontal cortex from the posterior parietal region in the rhesus monkey. J Comp Neurol 228: 105–116

Robinson DA (1963) A method of measuring eye movement using a scleral search coil in a magnetic field. IEEE Trans Bio-Med Electron 10: 137–145

Shibutani H, Sakata H, Hyvärinen J (1984) Saccades and blinking evoked by microstimulation of the posterior parietal association cortex of the monkey. Exp Brain Res 55: 1–8

Sperry RW (1950) Neural basis of the spontaneous optokinetic response produced by visual inversion. J Comp Physiol Psychol 43: 482–489

Valenstein E, Heilman KM, Watson RT, Van Den Abell T (1982) Nonsensory neglect from parietemporal lesions in monkeys. Neurology 32: 1198–1202

38

S. Funahashi, C. J. Bruce, and P. S. Goldman-Rakic

Mnemonic coding of visual space in the monkey's dorsolateral prefrontal cortex

1989. *Journal of Neurophysiology* 61: 331–349

SUMMARY AND CONCLUSIONS

1. An oculomotor delayed-response task was used to examine the spatial memory functions of neurons in primate prefrontal cortex. Monkeys were trained to fixate a central spot during a brief presentation (0.5 s) of a peripheral cue and throughout a subsequent delay period (1–6 s), and then, upon the extinction of the fixation target, to make a saccadic eye movement to where the cue had been presented. Cues were usually presented in one of eight different locations separated by 45°. This task thus requires monkeys to direct their gaze to the location of a remembered visual cue, controls the retinal coordinates of the visual cues, controls the monkey's oculomotor behavior during the delay period, and also allows precise measurement of the timing and direction of the relevant behavioral responses.

2. Recordings were obtained from 288 neurons in the prefrontal cortex within and surrounding the principal sulcus (PS) while monkeys performed this task. An additional 31 neurons in the frontal eye fields (FEF) region within and near the anterior bank of the arcuate sulcus were also studied.

3. Of the 288 PS neurons, 170 exhibited task-related activity during at least one phase of this task and, of these, 87 showed significant excitation or inhibition of activity during the delay period relative to activity during the intertrial interval.

4. Delay period activity was classified as *directional* for 79% of these 87 neurons in that significant responses only occurred following cues located over a certain range of visual field directions and were weak or absent for other cue directions. The remaining 21% were *omnidirectional,* i.e., showed comparable delay period activity for all visual field locations tested. Directional preferences, or lack thereof, were maintained across different delay intervals (1–6 s).

5. For 50 of the 87 PS neurons, activity during the delay period was significantly elevated above the neuron's spontaneous rate for at least one cue location; for the remaining 37 neurons only inhibitory delay period activity was seen. Nearly all (92%) neurons with excitatory delay period activity were directional and few (8%) were omnidirectional. Most (62%) neurons with purely inhibitory delay period activity were directional, but a substantial minority (38%) was omnidirectional.

6. Fifteen of the neurons with excitatory directional delay period activity also had significant inhibitory delay period activity for other cue directions. These inhibitory responses were usually strongest for, or centered about, cue directions roughly opposite those optimal for excitatory responses.

7. The distribution of preferred cue locations was examined across the population of PS neurons having directional delay period activity. All possible cue locations were represented (left, right, up, down, and obliques); however, preferred cue locations in the contralateral hemifield predominated.

8. Tuning curves were calculated by the Gaussian formula to determine the directional specificity of delay period activity. The mean tuning indices (T_d) of PS neurons were 26.8° for excitatory delay period activity and 43.5° for inhibitory delay period activity.

9. Delay period activity was examined on trials in which the monkey made large saccadic errors for cues in a neuron's preferred direction. Delay period activity was either truncated or absent altogether on such trials.

10. Of the 31 FEF neurons examined, 22 exhibited task-related activity: 17 had delay period activity and 10 showed directional delay period activity. The mean tuning index (T_d) of excitatory directional delay period activity in the FEF was 27.4°.

11. These results indicate that prefrontal neurons (both PS and FEF) possess information concerning the location of visual cues during the delay period of the oculomotor delayed-response task. This information appears to be in a labeled line code: different neurons code different cue locations and the same neuron repeatedly codes the same location. This mnemonic activity occurs during the 1- to 6-s delay interval—in the absence of any overt stimuli or movements—and it ceases upon the execution of the behavioral response. These results strengthen the evidence that the dorsolateral prefrontal cortex participates in the process of working or transient memory and further indicate that this area of the cortex contains a complete "memory" map of visual space.

INTRODUCTION

The role of the prefrontal cortex, particularly the principal sulcal (PS) region, in spatial memory has been strongly supported by lesion and developmental studies over the past two decades (17, 28, 57). Studies of single neuron activity in monkeys during performance of delayed-response tasks have also provided strong evidence of a prefrontal contribution to memory (4, 5, 15, 16, 20, 22, 37, 41, 42, 46, 50–53). Although many types of neural activity have been found in the prefrontal cortex, neurons that show sustained activity during the delay period are particularly relevant to the issue of mnemonic processing. Usually these neurons increase their discharge rates following the brief cue presentation and continue firing tonically during the delay period until the response is executed (5, 15, 20, 22, 52, 53). Such delay activity is often "directional" (44, 50–52) i.e., dependent on the left-right location of the cue or response, with some neurons responding only in conjunction with "left" trials and others only with "right" trials. Because experimental lesions of the dorsolateral prefrontal cortex profoundly affect the ability of monkeys to perform spatial delayed-response tasks correctly (17, 28), this delay activity has been assumed to be the cellular expression of a mnemonic code for the left-right direction of the cue or, equivalently, of the impending response (17, 18, 28).

In the present study we have explored further the properties of neural activity in the prefrontal cortex of monkeys performing delayed-response tasks. We sought to determine if prefrontal neurons were capable of accessing and maintaining activity reflecting the location of a target stimulus or motor response in any part of the visual field or if they were particularly tuned to left-right categorization. Further, we were interested in finding out if prefrontal neurons code stimuli in both the contralateral and ipsilateral visual fields equally well. To answer these questions, it was necessary to precisely control the retinotopic location of the cues, a requirement that has not been met in most previous studies. Accordingly, in the present study, we used an oculomotor analogue of the classical, manual delayed-response task, in which the monkeys were trained to maintain fixation during the cue presentation, and the visual cue could be presented at multiple locations around the visual field. This method allowed us to record the monkey's direction of gaze throughout the task, and consequently to know the precise retinotopic location of the peripheral visual cue. In addition, the fixation requirement during the delay period insured comparable behavior in this period on every trial and also made it difficult for the monkey to adopt postural rather than mnemonic strategies to perform the task. Similar oculomotor delay tasks have previously been used for neurophysiological experiments in the frontal eye fields (6), the posterior parietal cortex (30), the caudate nucleus (32), and the substantia nigra (33) as well as in the prefrontal cortex (37, 40). The present study, however, is the first to explore the full perimetry of visual space with this paradigm.

Preliminary results from this study have previously been presented in abstract form (15).

METHODS

Subjects

Three adult rhesus monkeys (*Macaca mulatta*, 3.2–5.3 kg, one male and two females) served as subjects. Prior to surgery and training they were adapted to a primate chair for 5–10 days.

Surgical procedures

Monkeys were prepared for chronic single-neuron recording using aseptic surgical technique and barbiturate anesthesia (pentobarbital sodium, intravenous to effect). For the purpose of recording eye movements (see below), a search coil was placed under the conjunctiva in one eye using the technique of Judge et al. (38). To secure the implant, stainless steel bolts with flattened heads were run along slots in the skull with the bolt head under the skull. The bolts, a connector for the search coil, and a stainless steel receptacle for attaching the monkey's head to the primate chair were bound together with dental acrylic. Because dura exposed during the lengthy training period (usually 3–4 mo) would thicken and impede the passage of electrodes, a second surgery to install the recording cylinder was performed only after the monkey became proficient on the oculomotor delayed-response task. Trephine holes (20 mm diam.) were made over the prefrontal region and a stainless steel recording cylinder placed over the hole. Additional acrylic was applied to bond the recording cylinder to the existing implant. Monkeys were given systemic antibiotics, fruits, and ad lib water and chow for 5–8 days following each surgery.

Behavioral techniques

The monkey sat in the primate chair during the experiment and his head was fixed to the chair by the restraining receptacle. Recording and training sessions usually lasted 2–3 h. A program on the PDP-11/23 computer presented the visual stimuli, sampled the monkey's gaze coordinates as well as neuron activity, and delivered rewards.

Visual stimuli were presented on a monochrome CRT (19-in., RCA TC1119) subtending 48 × 38° in visual angle using a GRAPH-11 graphics card (Pacific Binary Systems). The fixation target was a small white spot (0.1° diam.), usually presented at the center of the CRT. The peripheral visual cues were filled white squares (0.7 × 0.7°).

Gaze coordinates were obtained with Robinson's search coil method (56). The field coil and associated electronic equipment were made by C-N-C Engineering, Seattle, WA. Details concerning the sampling and storage of the eye and neural signals are given below.

The monkeys were rewarded with drops (0.2 ml) of lightly sweetened water via an electronic metering pump (A741, Waltham). Water was not available in the home cage; instead the monkeys worked to satiety (150–250 ml) each day in the laboratory. They were given monkey chow immediately upon return to their home cages and their intake of chow and body weight were closely monitored.

Oculomotor delayed-response task

Figure 1 shows schematic drawings of the oculomotor delayed-response task. Figure 1*A* depicts the timing of presentation of the fixation target, peripheral cues, and reward. Figure 1*B* illustrates records of horizontal and vertical eye movements and single neuron activity on a typical trial of the oculomotor delayed-response task.

Following a 5-s intertrial interval (ITI), the fixation target appeared at the center of the CRT. The monkey looked at the fixation target and maintained fixation for 0.75 s (the fixation period), whereupon the visual cue was presented for 0.5 s (the cue period) at one of four or eight peripheral locations (13° eccentric-

A Oculomotor delayed-response task

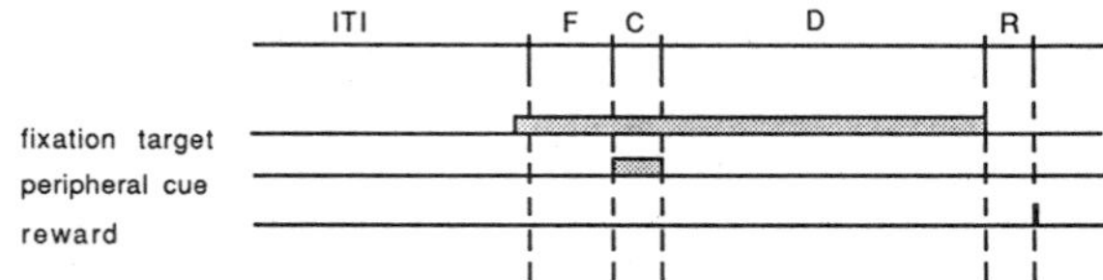

B An example of an oculomotor delayed-response trial

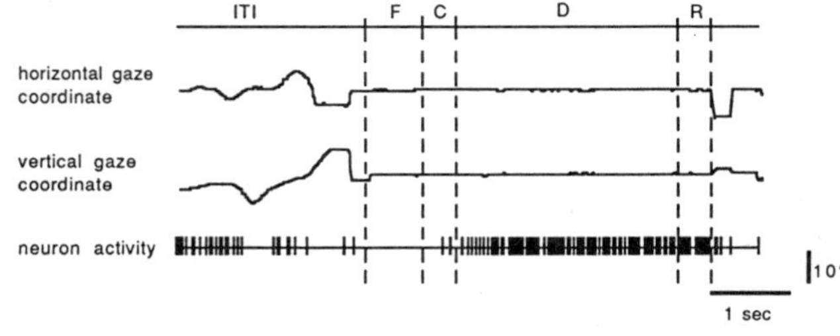

FIG. 1. *A*: temporal sequence of events in the oculomotor delayed-response task. *B*: eye movements and single neuron activity during an oculomotor delayed-response trial. ITI, intertrial interval; F, fixation period (0.75 s); C, cue period (0.5 s); D, delay period (3 s); R, response period (0.5 s).

ity). Stimulus location was randomized over trials so that the monkey could not predict where the cue would appear on any given trial. A crucial feature of the task was that the monkey had to maintain fixation throughout the cue period and also throughout the subsequent delay period. At the end of the delay period, the fixation target was extinguished; this was the "go" signal to make a saccade. If the monkeys made a saccadic eye movement within the next 0.5 s (the response period) to the location where the cue *had been* presented, they were rewarded with a drop of liquid. A correct response was defined as an eye movement that fell within a window (6° diam.) around the cue location.

We usually used one fixed delay interval (3 s) during recording, but longer delays (6 s) or combinations of two (3 and 6 s) or three (1.5, 3, and 6 s) different delays were sometimes used to examine activity across different delay intervals. Many of these neurons were also studied with other tasks (visual probe task, visually guided saccade task, etc.); these results will be presented in a future paper.

After analyzing the response properties of neurons, we sometimes employed microstimulation through the recording microelectrode to determine whether the recording site was in the frontal eye fields, based on the criteria of Bruce et al. (7).

Recording of single neuron activity

Single neuron activity was recorded with Parylene-coated tungsten microelectrodes (2–5 MΩ at 1 kHz, Micro Probe) that were advanced through the intact dura with a hydraulic microdrive (MO-95B, Narishige). Single neuron activity was amplified 10,000-fold by a differential amplifier (MDA-4, BAK). This signal passed through a low-pass filter to eliminate artifact from the search coil driver and then to a window discriminator (DIS-1, BAK) to isolate single neuron activity for the computer. We monitored both the raw activity signal and the window discriminator output simultaneously by an oscilloscope (5110, Tektronix) and an audio monitor. Usually one electrode track was explored each recording session. Electrode tracks were separated on a 1-mm grid.

For the microstimulation, trains of pulses were generated by a biphasic pulse generator (BPG-1, BAK). Each pulse was 0.2 ms in duration, stimulation frequency was 330 Hz, and the train duration was 70 ms. The pulse generator output was connected to a constant-current stimulus isolation unit (BSI-1, BAK). Current was monitored by the voltage drop across a 1-kΩ resistor in series between the output of the isolation unit and the microelectrode. Current tested ranged up to 200 μA.

Data acquisition

The on-line computer system, in addition to carrying out the behavioral paradigms, sampled neural and ocular signals and stored these data in relation to task events on magnetic media.

Voltages from the phase-sensitive detector representing the horizontal and vertical eye coordinates were digitized every 2 ms (500 Hz). These signals were also electronically differentiated to yield horizontal and vertical eye velocity. The velocity signals were also digitized and were used by the on-line computer program to identify each saccade that the monkey made via the algorithm of van Gisbergen et al. (25).

Two types of data storage files were stored. *Event buffer* files contained the time of every event that the computer had access to, including the time of each discriminated action potential, the time, duration, and amplitude of each saccade, and the time of events such as the appearance and disappearance of visual cues. Individual event buffer files usually contained 50–100 trials. *Analogue buffer* files contained multiple records (1–2-s epoches) of all of the analogue signals being sampled, together with the discriminated action potentials and a code representing progress through the task paradigm (see Fig. 1*B*).

Two types of computer-generated displays were monitored during the experiments. In one display, horizontal gaze, vertical gaze, and overall eye velocity were displayed as scrolling traces on a digital oscilloscope (1345A, Hewlett Packard). Discriminated neuron activity was scrolled below these traces and tics representing on-line saccade recognition were placed on the velocity trace. Superimposed on the scrolling display were two-dimensional representations of gaze, visual stimuli, and the fixation window. In the other display, rasters and histograms were viewed on the same oscilloscope to observe the overall neural data collection.

Data analysis

Using the stored event buffer files, we examined rasters and histograms of neuron activity for each cue location. These rasters and histograms were made with different alignment points including *1*) the onset of cue, *2*) the start of the delay period, *3*) the end of the delay period, *4*) the initiation of the saccadic eye movement during the response period, and *5*) the appearance of the fixation target. Rasters and histograms were examined on the digital oscilloscope and copies were made using a digital plotter (7470A, Hewlett-Packard).

Neural activity during the delay period was also analyzed quantitatively for all neurons recorded. The average discharge rate

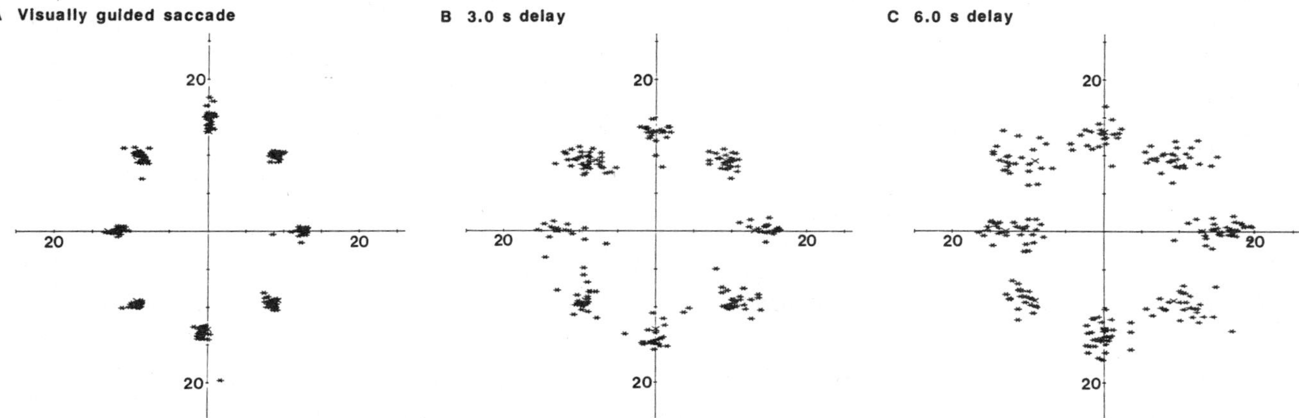

FIG. 2. The distribution of eye positions following the saccade in the visually guided saccade task (*A*), in the oculomotor delayed-response task with 3-s delay (*B*) and with 6-s delay (*C*). These plots contain both correct and incorrect trials (if any). All cue eccentricities were 13°.

during the delay period was calculated for each trial, and then overall mean discharge rates and standard deviations for each cue location were computed. We tested for significant delay period activity by comparing the mean discharge rate during the delay period for all trials having a given cue direction versus the mean discharge rate during the intertrial interval over all trials, using a two-tailed unpaired Student's t statistic and an alpha level of 0.05. Differences in delay period activity across different cue locations were evaluated using an analysis of variance (ANOVA).

Histological analysis

After 2–8 mo of nearly daily recording sessions the monkeys were killed with an overdose of pentobarbital sodium and perfused with saline followed by buffered Formalin. The brains were photographed. Frozen coronal sections were taken and stained with thionin.

Individual recording sites that had been marked with electrolytic lesions (20 μA, 10–15 s, tip negative) were identified. How-

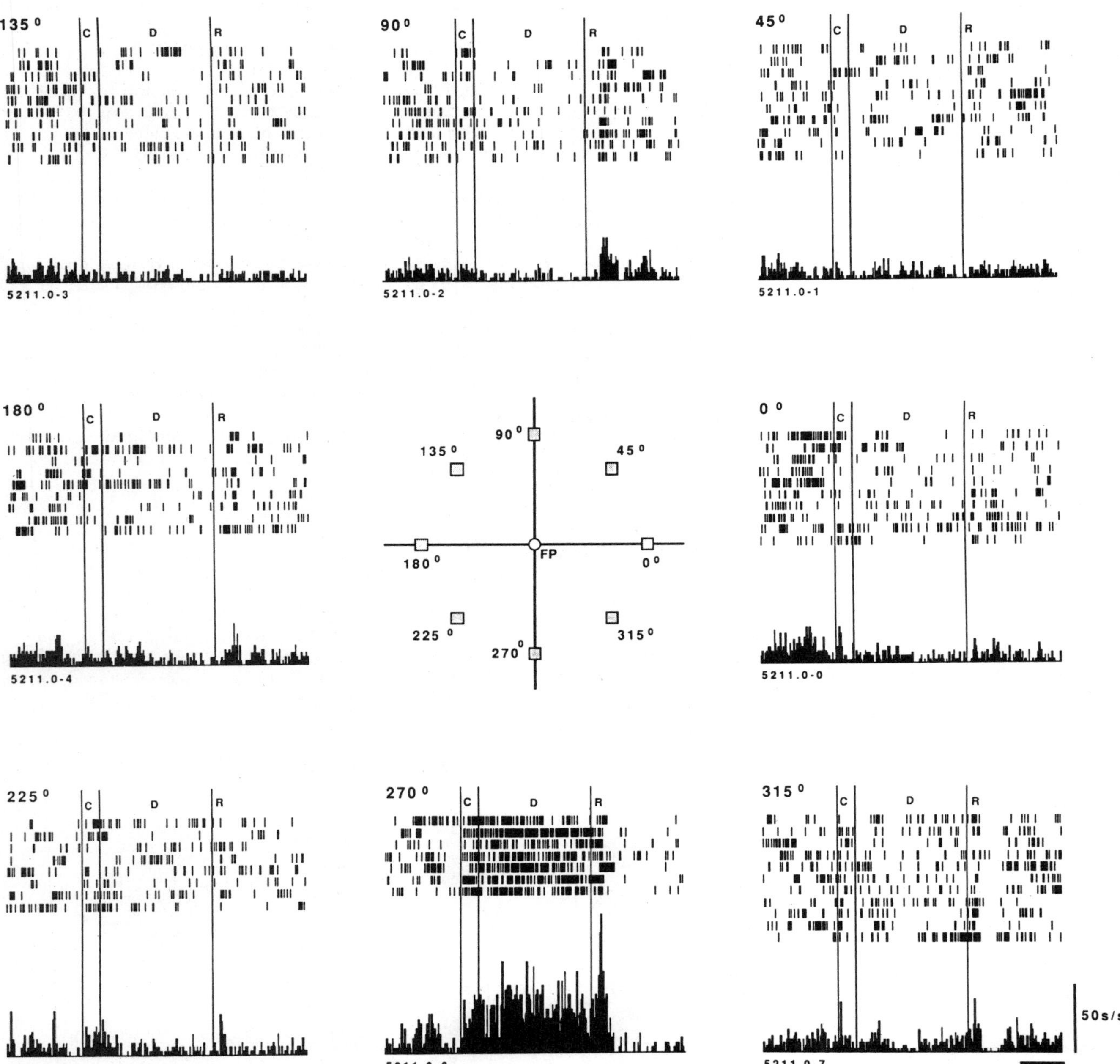

FIG. 3. Directional delay period activity of a principal sulcus neuron during the oculomotor delayed-response task. This neuron (5211, left hemisphere) had strongly directional delay period activity ($F = 48.35$; df = 7, 68; $P < 0.001$), responding only when the cue had been presented at the bottom (270°) location. It was suppressed during the delay when the cue was presented in the upper visual field, and in all 3 cases delay period activity was significantly below the ITI rate (45°, $t = 2.350$, df = 84, $P < 0.025$; 90°, $t = 3.451$, df = 85, $P < 0.001$; 135°, $t = 2.607$, df = 84, $P < 0.025$). Visual cues were randomly presented at 1 of the 8 locations indicated in the center diagram. All cue eccentricities were 13° and all delay periods were 3 s.

ever, the long duration of recording and large number of electrode penetrations precluded identification of most penetrations, and their locations in the brain were estimated from their microdrive coordinates.

RESULTS

Task performance

All monkeys performed the oculomotor delayed-response task proficiently and the percentage correct was usually 90% or better for all cue locations. Figure 2 shows the distribution of saccade end points of one monkey in a visually guided saccade task (Fig. 2*A*), and in the 3-s (Fig. 2*B*) and 6-s delay conditions (Fig. 2*C*) of the oculomotor delayed-response task. Although the distribution of saccade end points is wider in the delay task than in the visually guided saccade task, nearly all saccades end near the appropriate location, even with 6-s delays.

The mean latencies for saccadic eye movements in the response period were 216.4 ± 33.0 (SD) ms in the visually guided saccade task, 298.3 ± 34.4 ms in the 3-s delay task, and 293.0 ± 37.4 ms in the 6-s delay task. The difference in

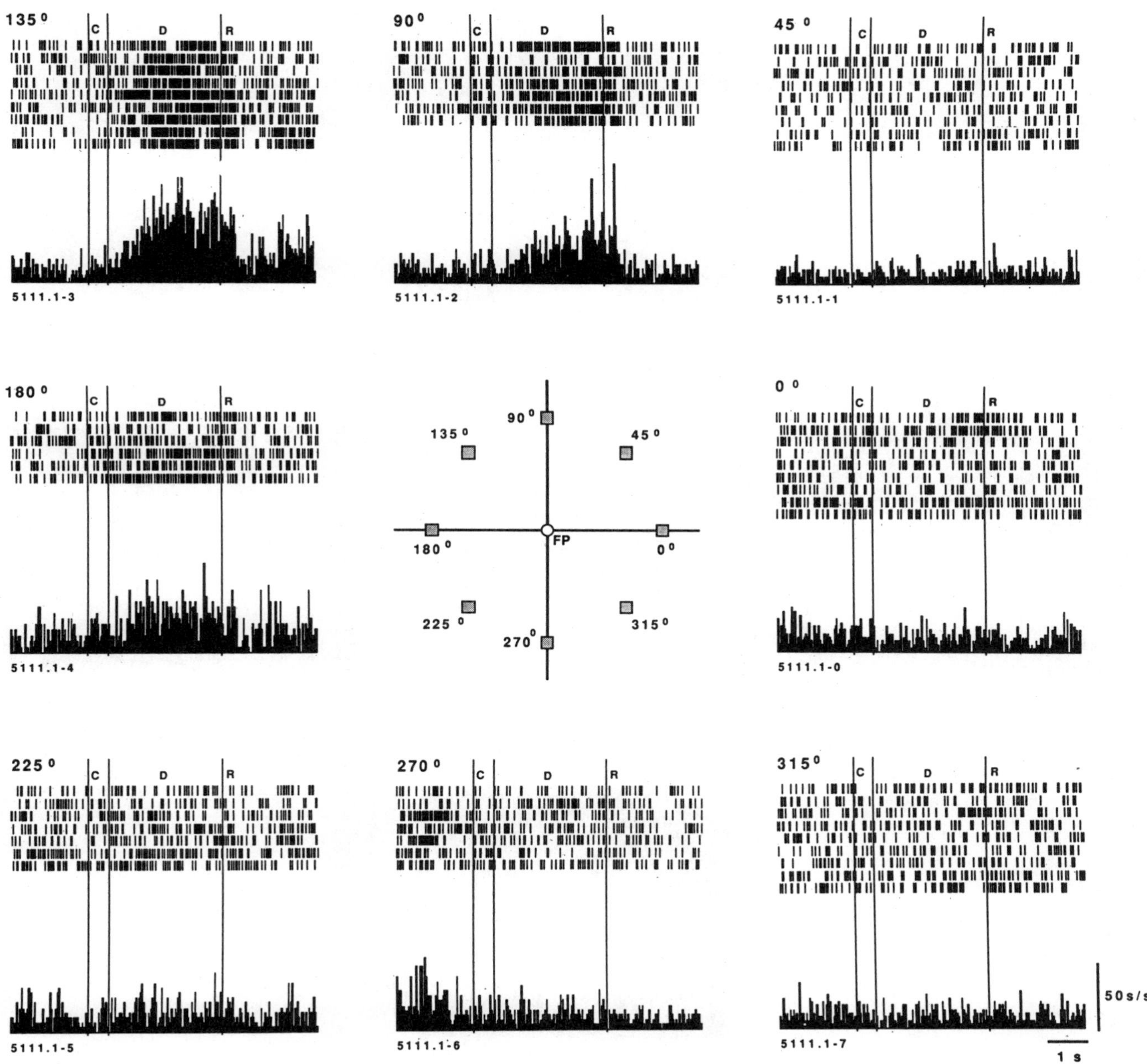

FIG. 4. Directional delay period activity of a principal sulcus neuron during the oculomotor delayed-response task. This neuron (5111, right hemisphere) exhibited directional delay period activity ($F = 25.23$; df = 7, 56; $P < 0.001$), responding only when the cue had been presented at locations in the upper quadrant of the contralateral visual field (90, 135, and 180°). The strongest delay period activity occurred at the 135° location. Visual cues were randomly presented at 1 of the 8 locations indicated in the center diagram. All cue eccentricities were 13° and all delay periods were 3 s.

mean latency between the visually guided saccade task and each of the delay tasks was statistically significant (3-s delay: $t = 25.93$, df = 454, $P < 0.001$; 6-s delay: $t = 24.08$, df = 493, $P < 0.001$), whereas that between the 3-s and the 6-s delay tasks was not significant ($t = 1.60$, df = 477, $P > 0.05$).

The mean duration of saccadic eye movements was 46.2 ± 8.5 (SD) ms in the visually guided saccade task, 44.9 ± 7.6 ms in the 3-s delay task, and 46.2 ± 8.2 ms in the 6-s delay task. There were no significant differences in mean saccade duration among the three tasks (ANOVA, $F = 1.982$; df = 2, 706; $P > 0.1$).

Neural data base

We recorded from 319 neurons in the prefrontal cortex of three rhesus monkeys while they performed the oculomotor delayed-response task. As discussed in detail below, 288 of these neurons were from cortex within and surrounding the caudal half of the principal sulcus. We term these PS (principal sulcus) neurons and most of this report concerns their activity. The other 31 neurons were located within and near the anterior bank of the arcuate sulcus and were classified as frontal eye field (FEF) neurons. At some sites this FEF classification was confirmed by low microstimulation thresholds (<50 μA) for the elicitation of sac-

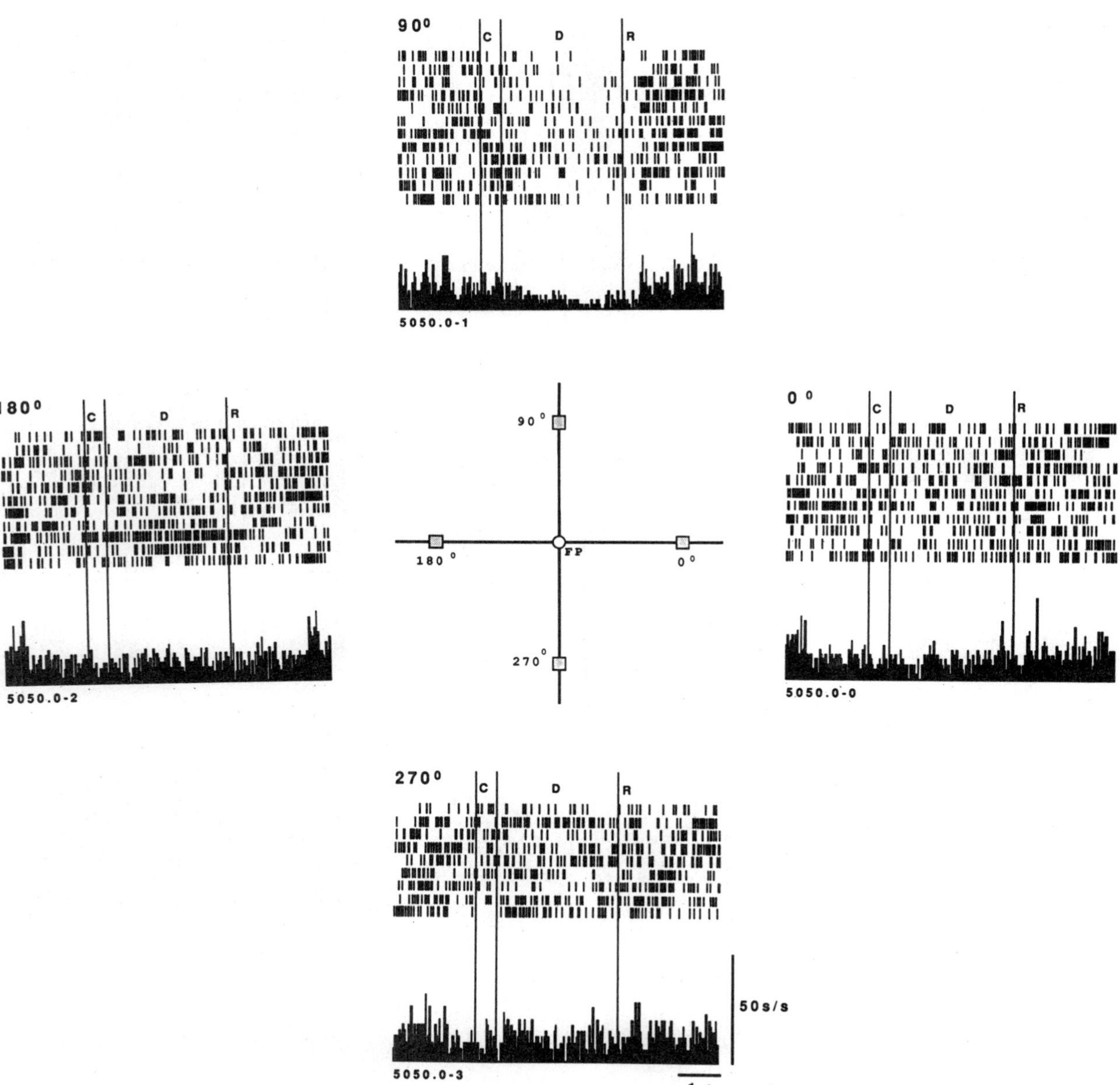

FIG. 5. Directional delay period activity of a principal sulcus neuron. This neuron (5050, right hemisphere) showed tonic inhibitory delay period activity only when the cue was presented at 90° ($F = 4.870$; df = 3, 39; $P < 0.025$). Visual cues were randomly presented at 1 of the 4 locations indicated in the center diagram. All cue eccentricities were 13° and all delay periods were 3 s.

cadic eye movements. Data concerning these 31 FEF neurons is separately presented at the end of the RESULTS.

Of the 288 PS neurons thoroughly analyzed, most (170 neurons, 59% of total sample) had task-related activity in that their average discharge rate during at least one phase of the delayed-response task differed significantly ($P < 0.05$, t test) from their ITI (InterTrial Interval) rate. Of these 170 neurons, 87 neurons (30% of total sample, 51% of total task-related neurons) had significant *delay period* activity. For 33 (38%) of these neurons the delay period activity was the only significant task-related activity, but most (54 neurons, 62%) also had significant activity in the task segments immediately preceding or following the delay period (delay and cue periods: 11 neurons, 13%; delay and response periods: 32 neurons, 36%; delay, cue, and response periods: 11 neurons, 13%). The remaining 83 task-related neurons exhibited significant activity only in the cue period (n = 12), only in the response period (n = 55), in both cue and response periods (n = 10), or at reward presentation (n = 6).

Directional specificity of delay period activity

Most PS neurons with delay period activity showed a significant increase or decrease in this activity relative to their base-line discharge rate only when the cue had been

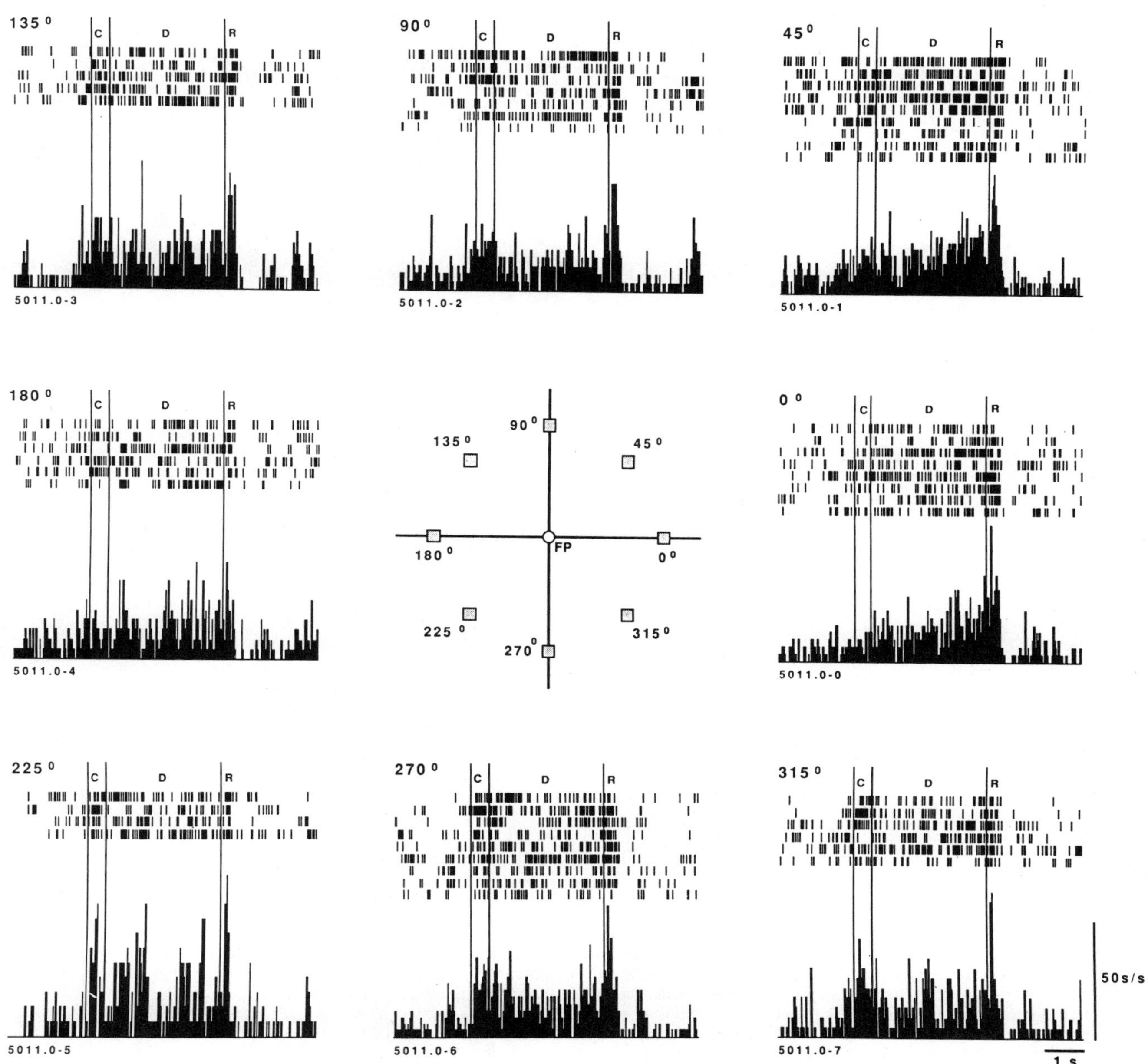

FIG. 6. Omnidirectional delay period activity of a principal sulcus neuron. This neuron (5011, right hemisphere) showed tonic excitatory delay period activity independent of cue location (F = 0.63; df = 7, 46; P > 0.1). Visual cues were randomly presented at 1 of the 8 locations indicated in the center diagram. All cue eccentricities were 13° and all delay periods were 3 s.

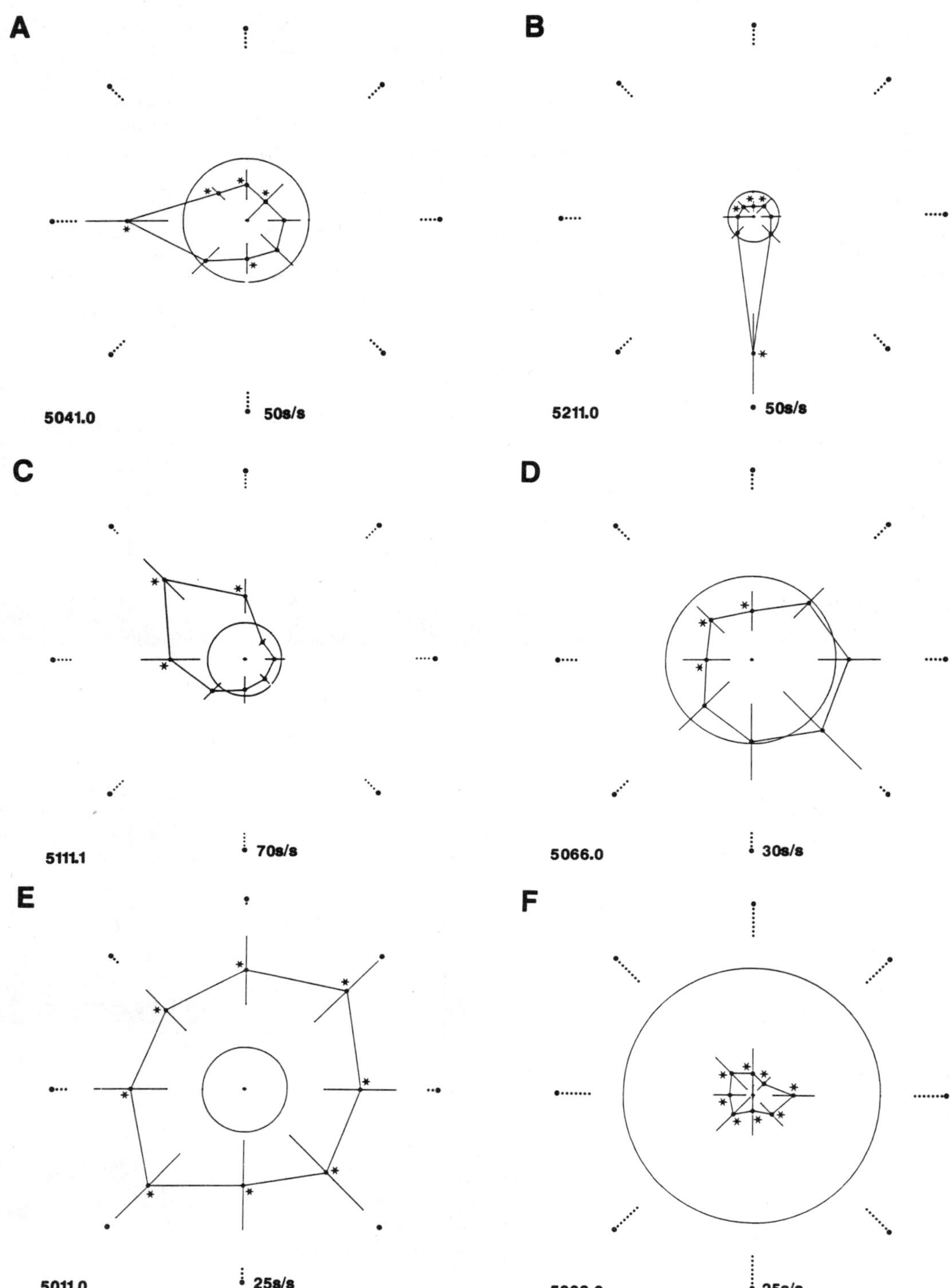

FIG. 7. Directional tuning of 6 principal sulcus neurons with delay period activity. In each radial plot, the neuron's average discharge rate during the delay period for each cue location is depicted by the radial eccentricity of the plot in that direction, the standard deviation of this rate is depicted by the radial line, and the neuron's average ITI discharge rate is the radius of the circle. Asterisks (*) indicate cue directions with statistically significant (*t* test, $P < 0.05$) differences between delay period activity and the ITI rate. *A* and *B*: 2 principal sulcus neurons (*A*: 5041, right hemisphere; *B*: 5211, left hemisphere) with very specific directional delay period activity (*A*, $F = 10.12$; df = 7, 54; $P < 0.001$; *B*, $F = 48.35$; df = 7, 68; $P < 0.001$). They have a significant elevation of delay period activity for only 1 direction. Notice that there is significant inhibition of delay period activity for cue directions roughly opposite the excitatory directions. *C* and *D*: 2 principal sulcus neurons (*C*: 5111, right hemisphere; *D*: 5066, right hemisphere) with directional, but broadly tuned, delay period activity (*C*, $F = 25.23$; df = 7, 56; $P < 0.001$; *D*, $F = 3.80$; df = 7, 71; $P < 0.005$). Notice that for *C* the responses are excitatory relative to the ITI rate whereas for *D* the only significant responses are inhibitory. *E* and *F*: 2 principal sulcus neurons (*E*: 5011, right hemisphere; *F*: 5008, right hemisphere) with omnidirectional delay period activity (*E*, $F = 0.63$; df = 7, 46; $P > 0.1$; *F*, $F = 1.26$; df = 7, 65; $P > 0.1$). One of these is excitatory (*E*) and the other inhibitory (*F*).

presented at one or a few among the 4 or 8 locations tested. Of the 87 PS neurons with delay period activity, 69 (79%) were *directional*, i.e., a statistically significant difference ($P < 0.05$) in delay period discharge rates across different cue locations.

Figure 3 shows directional activity in a PS neuron tested with eight cue locations. Strong tonic excitatory activation appeared throughout the delay period only when the cue was presented at the downward (270°) location. This response began ~100 ms after the cue presentation and ceased 130 ms after the initiation of the saccadic eye movement. Moreover, activity during the delay period was suppressed relative to the ITI discharge rate for the three cue locations in the upper (opposite) visual field (45°, t = 2.350, df = 84, $P < 0.025$; 90°, t = 3.451, df = 85, $P < 0.001$; 135°, t = 2.607, df = 84, $P < 0.025$). This phenomenon of an excitation of delay period activity for one set of cue locations and an inhibition of delay period activity for other directions is discussed further below.

Figure 4 shows another PS neuron with directional activity that exhibited broader tuning than the neuron shown in Fig. 3. The delay period activity was significantly elevated for the three locations that span the upper quadrant of the contralateral visual field (90, 135, and 180°), with the highest rate on 135° trials. The activity ceased abruptly 170 ms after the initiation of the saccadic eye movement. For the three cues spanning the opposite quadrant (lower ipsilateral, 270, 315, and 0°) this neuron's activity was depressed below its ITI rate (see also Fig. 7*C*), although this depression was not statistically significant for any individual direction.

Neurons with only inhibitory activity during the delay period could also be directional. The neuron shown in Fig. 5 was suppressed during the delay period only when the cue had been presented at the upper location (90°, t = 6.036, df = 53, $P < 0.001$); there was no significant change in activity during the delay period for the three other cue locations tested.

The remaining 18 neurons (21%) with significant delay period activity were classified as *omnidirectional* because they responded similarly during the delay period regardless of cue locations and the ANOVA criterion for directional selectivity was not met. Figure 6 shows an example of a PS neuron with omnidirectional delay period activity. The tonic excitatory delay period responses for all locations was significantly above the ITI rate by individual t test and the slight differences between locations were not statistically significant.

To more concisely show directional specificity of directional delay period activity, we constructed polar plots that depict the delay period discharge rate of a neuron as a function of polar direction by plotting discharge rate as a function of polar eccentricity. The base-line (ITI) rate of the neuron is shown on the plots by the radius of a circle, the standard deviations of the delay period discharge for each direction are shown by *radial bars*, and statistically significant departures from the ITI rate are indicated by *asterisks*. Figure 7, *B*, *C*, and *E*, show polar plots for the narrowly tuned, broadly tuned, and omnidirectional

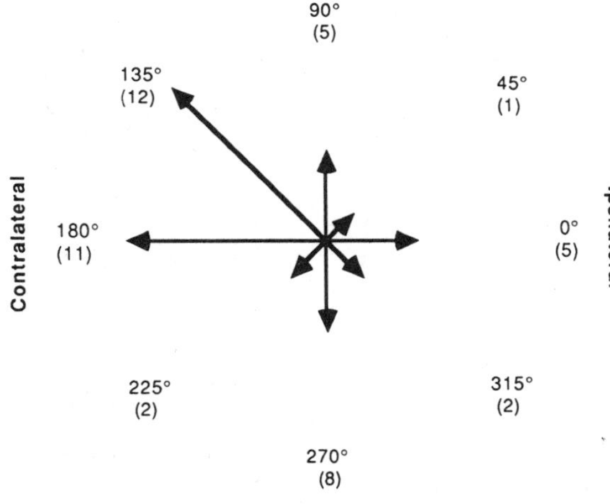

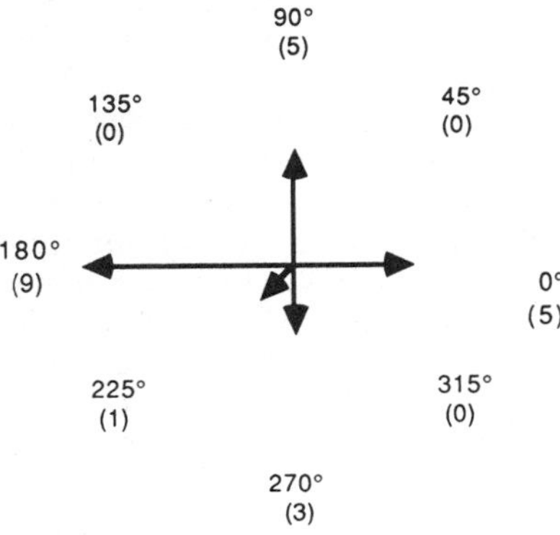

FIG. 8. Distribution of the preferred directions for delay period activity of principal sulcus neurons tested with the oculomotor delayed-response task. Length of radial lines is proportional to the number of cells for which that cue direction gave the best delay period response; the cell counts are also given beneath the directions. Preferred directions were normalized by a right-hemisphere convention: the preferred direction of each left hemisphere neuron was mirror reversed across the vertical meridian. *Top:* this plot summarizes the preferred directions for the 46 neurons having excitatory directional delay period activity. *Bottom:* this plot summarizes the preferred directions for the 23 neurons having inhibitory directional delay period activity. Note that 15 of the 46 neurons in the *top* plot also had significant inhibitory delay period activity, usually for cue directions roughly opposite their best excitatory direction. The best inhibitory direction for these neurons are not plotted in the *bottom* part, and hence the neuron populations comprising the *top* and *bottom* plots are mutually exclusive. The overall preference in both plots for directions along the horizontal and vertical meridians, as opposed to oblique directions, is an artifact because many neurons were only tested for four cue directions (left, right, up, and down) and not for oblique directions.

TABLE 1. *Response type of directional and omnidirectional delay period activity of principal sulcus neurons*

Response type	Directional	Omnidirectional	Total
Excitation	46	4	50
Inhibition	23	14	37
Total	69	18	87

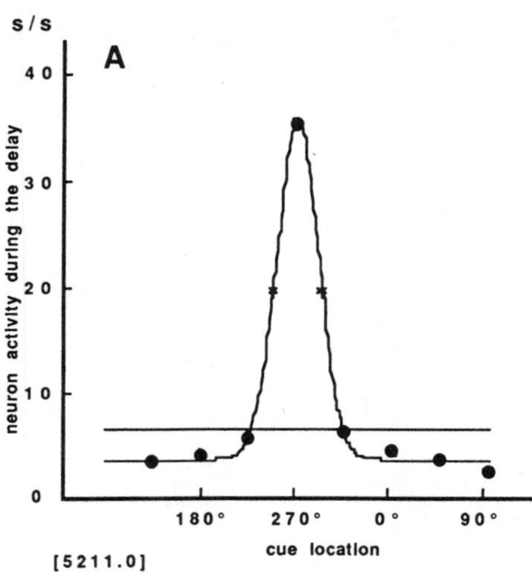

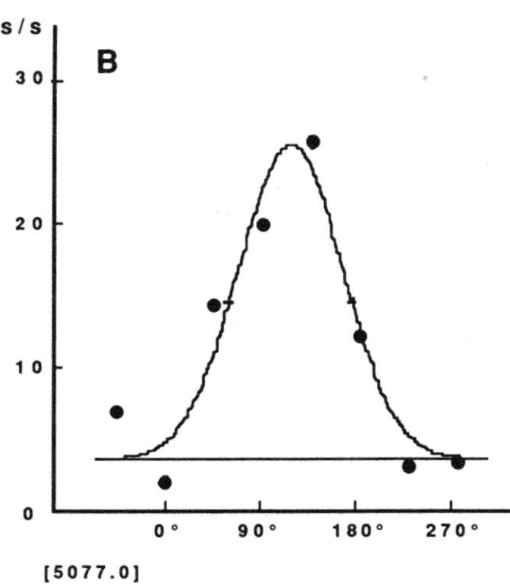

FIG. 9. Directional tuning of delay period activity for 2 principal sulcus neurons. Plots show discharge rate during the delay period for the 8 different cue directions, with a Gaussian function fit to the data. *A* (5211, left hemisphere) shows narrowly tuned directional activity (T_d = 19.7°, preferred cue direction = 270°) and *B* (5077, right hemisphere) shows broadly tuned directional activity (T_d = 48.4°, preferred cue direction = 135°).

neurons whose histograms were illustrated in the previous three figures (Fig. 3, Fig. 4, and Fig. 6, respectively), whereas Fig. 7, *A*, *D*, and *F*, show three additional examples: another PS neuron with narrowly tuned directional delay period activity is shown in Fig. 7*A*. For this PS neuron, the preferred cue direction was leftward (180°), whereas for most other cue directions, the discharge rate during the delay period was suppressed below base line. A neuron with directional delay period activity that was suppressed below base line when the to-be-remembered cues were in the upper-left quadrant of the visual field is shown in Fig. 7*D*. Finally, Fig. 7*F* shows a neuron with omnidirectional inhibition of delay period activity: comparable inhibition occurred for all eight cue locations.

Excitatory and inhibitory delay period activity

As evident from the polar plots in Fig. 7, we observed instances of both elevation and depression of delay period activity relative to a neuron's base-line rate. To further understand the relation between the "sign" of this activity and directional specificity, we classified each neuron as having either excitatory or inhibitory delay period activity by the statistical criteria previously described. A neuron was classified as excitatory (or inhibitory) if delay period rate for any cue direction was significantly elevated (or *only* reduced) relative to the neuron's ITI.

Table 1 shows the incidence of neurons for the different combinations of delay period response sign and directionality. As is evident from examining the Table, neurons having excitatory delay period activity were more likely to be directional (92%) than neurons with solely inhibitory responses (62%). Furthermore, we observed that directional tuning for inhibitory delay period activity was usually broader than that for excitatory directional activity.

The phenomenon of a single neuron having both an elevation of delay period activity for one set of directions and depression of delay period activity for another set was frequently encountered. Usually the best cue directions for

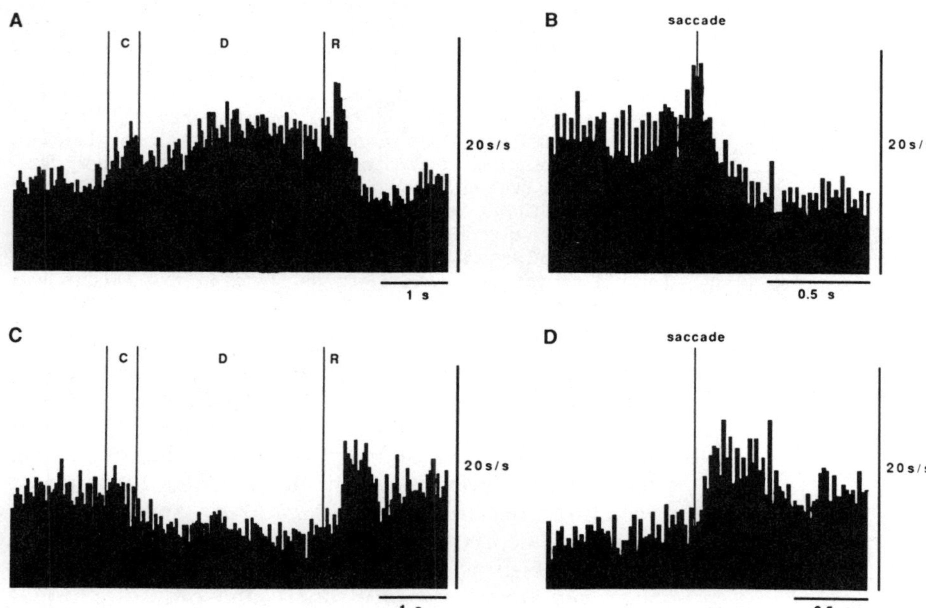

FIG. 10. The time course of excitatory and inhibitory delay period activity. These histograms sum neural activity at the preferred cue direction for all 46 principal sulcus neurons with excitatory directional delay period activity (*A, B*) and all 23 principal sulcus neurons with inhibitory directional delay period activity (*C, D*). *A* and *C* were aligned at the cue presentation; *B* and *D* were aligned at the initiation of the saccadic eye movements. All delay periods were 3 s.

eliciting inhibitory responses were opposite to the best directions for eliciting excitatory responses. For 15 neurons the criteria of having a statistically significant elevation of delay period activity for at least one direction *and* a statistically significant inhibition of activity for at least one other direction was met. However, several other neurons, such as the ones illustrated in Figs. 4 and 7*C*, had delay period discharge rates below base line for one or more directions that did not meet our statistical criteria yet seemed genuine because the inhibition was present for two or more adjacent directions opposite to the excitatory direction.

Distribution of preferred directions

To determine the distribution of directional preferences of delay period activity, we used the largest t statistic to classify the preferred direction of each neuron as the cue location where it showed the most prominent excitation or inhibition. For analytical and graphic purposes, the preferred directions of left-hemisphere neurons were transformed into mirror-image directions, as if all neurons were recorded from the right hemisphere. Among the 69 PS neurons with directional delay period activity, 30 were studied in the 4-cue condition and 39 were studied in the 8-cue condition. As shown in Fig. 8, the majority of neurons with excitatory directional delay period activity had preferred directions on the side contralateral to the hemisphere recorded from. This contralateral bias was statistically significant by a chi-square test ($\chi^2 = 8.758$, df = 1, $P < 0.01$). There was no statistical significance in the directional preference of inhibitory directional delay period activity ($\chi^2 = 1.667$, df = 1, $P > 0.1$), although most inhibitory directions were also contralateral.

Tuning of directional delay period activity

To determine the directional specificity of delay period activity, tuning curves were estimated using the Gaussian function

$$f(d) = B + R * e^{-1/2((d-D)/T_d)^2}$$

where $f(d)$ is discharge frequency, d is cue direction, and the remaining terms are constants: B is the discharge rate during the ITI, D is the best direction, R indexes delay period response strength, and T_d indexes tuning with respect to cue direction. The function was implemented by fixing B at the average background discharge rate, and then iteratively converging to the best least-squares solution for R, D, and T_d. This Gaussian approach has previously been used to describe visual receptive fields and presaccadic movement fields in the FEF (6).

We applied this Gaussian formula to all 69 PS neurons that exhibited directional delay period activity. However, we omitted 42 PS neurons because 30 PS neurons were only studied with 4 cue directions and the Gaussian fits to 8 data points for 12 PS cells were poor. The remaining 27 PS neurons had good fits based on 8 cue locations. Figure 9 shows the tuning curves obtained for two of these PS neurons, one with narrowly tuned excitatory delay period activity (T_d = 19.7°, Fig. 9*A*) and another with broadly tuned excitatory delay period activity (T_d = 48.4°, Fig. 9*B*). Excitatory delay period activity tended to have narrower tuning than inhibitory delay period activity. The mean tuning index (T_d) was 26.8 ± 14.2° (SD) (n = 22) for neurons with significant excitatory delay period activity versus 48.2 ± 43.5° (n = 5) for neurons with only inhibitory delay period activity. These means are not significantly different (t = 1.985; df = 25; $0.05 < P < 0.1$) proba-

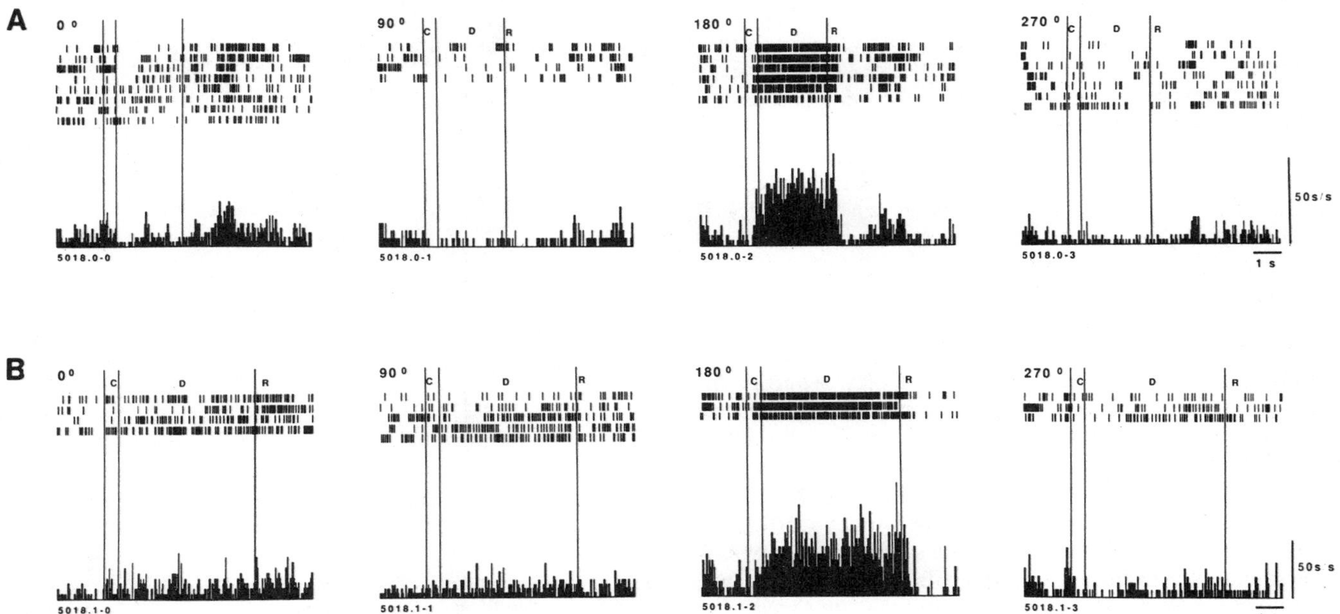

FIG. 11. Directional delay period activity of a principal sulcus neuron (5018, right hemisphere) for 2 different delay durations (3-s delay in *A* and 6-s delay in *B*), examined sequentially (3 s first, then 6 s). For each set of histograms the visual cues were presented randomly at 1 of 4 locations indicated (0° = right, 90° = up, 180° = left, and 270° = down). All cue eccentricities were 13°.

bly because of the small number of inhibitory neurons that could be fit and the large SD of inhibitory tunings.

Time course of delay period activity

To further characterize the overall activity of PS neurons during the oculomotor delayed-response task, we made histograms that summed activity across our sample of neurons, selecting for each neuron the trials with cues in that neuron's preferred direction. Figure 10 shows these composite histograms. Neurons with excitatory (n = 46) and inhibitory (n = 23) directional delay period activity were summed separately to prevent these activities from canceling each other. The left pair of histograms (Fig. 10, *A* and *C*) depict excitatory and inhibitory composite activities during the 3-s delay period, as well as during the fixation, cue, and response periods, and part of the ITI. For the excitatory composite histogram the overall delay period activity was 13.9 spikes/s, in comparison to 7.6 s/s during the first 1.5 s of the histogram (the ITI and fixation interval). For the inhibitory composite histogram the overall delay period discharge rate was 4.5 s/s, in comparison to 8.1 s/s during the ITI and fixation interval. Thus PS neurons with typical excitatory directional activity discharge at approximately twice their base-line rate during the delay period, whereas PS neurons with typical inhibitory directional activity discharge at approximately one-half their base-line rate.

The composite histograms also indicate the time course of PS neuron activity during the delay period. Although individual neurons have a variety of temporal changes during the delay period, these composite histograms indicate that overall PS neuron activity is well-maintained during a 3-s delay. In fact, there is an increase in discharge rate over the 3-s delay period in the excitatory composite histogram (12.4, 14.9, and 14.5 s/s in the first, second, and third second, respectively) and a decrease in the inhibitory composite histogram (4.8, 4.7, and 3.9 s/s).

A phasic response is evident during the 0.5-s cue period in the excitatory composite histogram (Fig. 10*A*). The earliest indication of this response begins ~70 ms following cue onset (all latencies were estimated using a cumulative histogram of the same data, which is not shown); but individual neurons had a wide variety of latencies, and many did not respond at all during the cue period. It should be noted that many PS neurons having strong visual responses, but lacking delay period activity, were not included in these composite histograms.

Finally, the composite histograms depict a phasic increase in activity during the response period for both the excitatory and inhibitory activity. The latency of this activity is 180 ms following the disappearance of the fixation target for the excitatory activity and 300 ms for the inhibitory activity. Since the typical saccade latency during the oculomotor delayed-response task is ~290 ms, it would appear that the excitatory burst leads the saccade in the excitatory composite histogram but follows the saccade in the inhibitory composite histogram. Histograms aligned at the saccade initiation (Fig. 10, *B* and *D*) support this interpretation: the additional burst of activity in the excitatory composite begins ~30 ms prior to the saccade initiation and ends ~40 ms after the saccade initiation (Fig. 10*B*). In contrast, the increased discharge in the inhibitory composite begins ~40 ms following the saccade initiation (which is approximately at the saccade termination) and continues for ~0.5 s (Fig. 10*D*).

Effects of different delay durations

Eighteen PS neurons that exhibited directional delay period activity were tested either with two (3 and 6 s) or three (1.5, 3, and 6 s) different delay durations. The monkeys had little difficulty with any of these delay times and maintained a high level (>80%) of correct performance at all delays tested.

Varying the delay length over this range of values had little effect on delay period activity. In particular, the directional preference was unchanged and the duration of excitation or inhibition expanded with longer delays. For example, Fig. 11*A* shows a neuron with tonic excitation during a 3-s delay period only when the cue was presented at the 180° location. Figure 11*B* shows the same neuron's

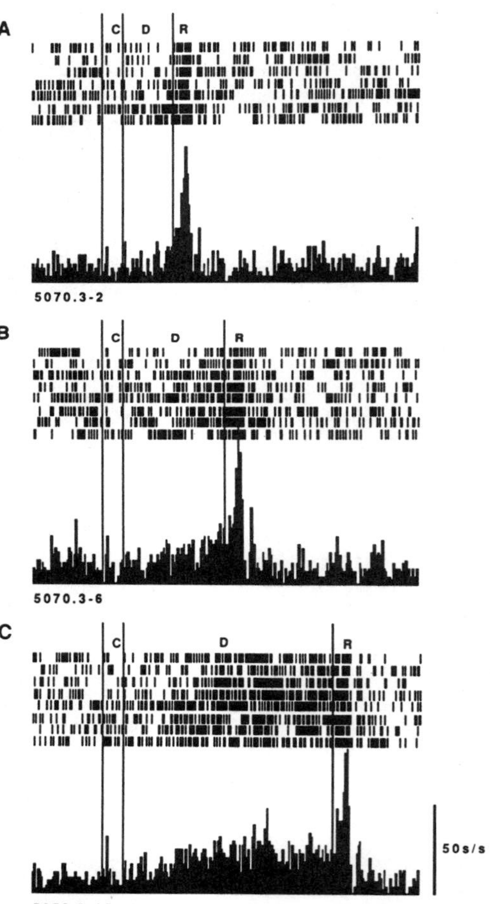

FIG. 12. Directional delay period activity of a principal sulcus neuron (5070, right hemisphere) for three different delay durations (1.5-s delay in *A*, 3-s delay in *B*, and 6-s delay in *C*). The data are from an experiment with 12 different types of trials: 1.5-, 3-, and 6-s delay durations crossed with 4 visual cue locations (0° = right, 90° = up, 180° = left, and 270° = down). All cue eccentricities were 13°. Only the 3 histograms from the preferred direction (180° location) are shown.

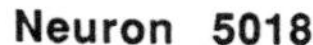

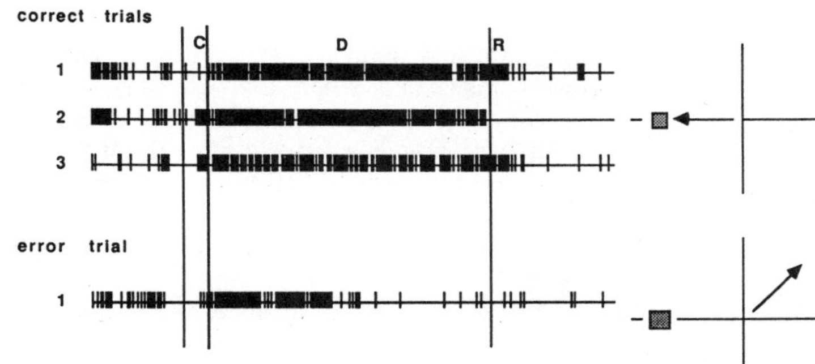

Neuron 5111

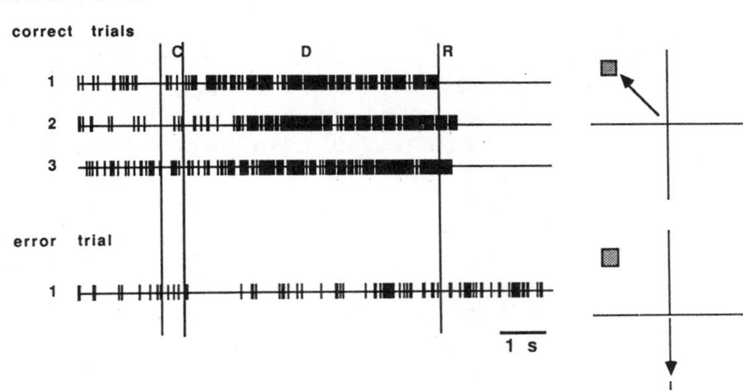

FIG. 13. Discharges of 2 principal sulcus neurons with directional delay period activity during correct performance of the oculomotor delayed-response task and during trials with errors. For each trial depicted, discharge traces are shown on the left and cue locations and saccade directions are shown on the right. *Top:* this neuron's (5018, right hemisphere) strongest delay period activity was associated with leftward cue presentations. On the error trial, its discharge ceased about midway through the delay period. *Bottom:* this neuron's (5111, right hemisphere) strongest delay period activity was associated with cue presentations in the upper-left visual field. On the error trial, its discharge in the delay period was absent.

activity during the delayed-response task with a 6-s delay. The tonic excitation still appeared only when the cue was presented at 180° and was maintained during the entire 6-s delay period. With both delays, the tonic excitation ceased at the initiation of the response. Eight other PS neurons with tonic delay period activity were similarly tested with different delay durations; all showed similar results, that is, the response expanded to fill the entire delay.

Figure 12 shows another PS neuron tested across different delay durations. In this case, four cue locations (0, 90, 180, and 270°) at three different delay durations (1.5, 3, and 6 s) were randomly intermixed. The rasters and histograms in Fig. 12 show neural activity during three different delay durations for cues presented at 180°, the preferred direction for this neuron. Notice that the activity in the first 1.5 s of the delay is very similar in all three conditions, that is little or no change in activity relative to the preceding fixation interval. Furthermore, the activity in the next 1.5 s of the delay period is the same in the 3-s and 6-s delay conditions, both showing a gradual rise in activity. This result was obtained in six other PS neurons that increased discharge rate during the delay. Likewise, two PS neurons with gradually decreasing discharge rates during the delay showed analogous patterning of activity when the delay duration was changed.

Directional delay period activity in error trials

Analysis of activity in error trials often aids the interpretation of delay period activity (5, 53, 54, 58, 64–66). Therefore, we examined the activity when the monkeys made errors on trials with the preferred cue direction for the neuron being studied. For this analysis, failure to saccade and misdirected saccades (i.e., ending outside the window) were counted as errors; however, nearly all errors were misdirected saccades. Premature saccades made during the delay period did not count as errors. Of 69 PS neurons

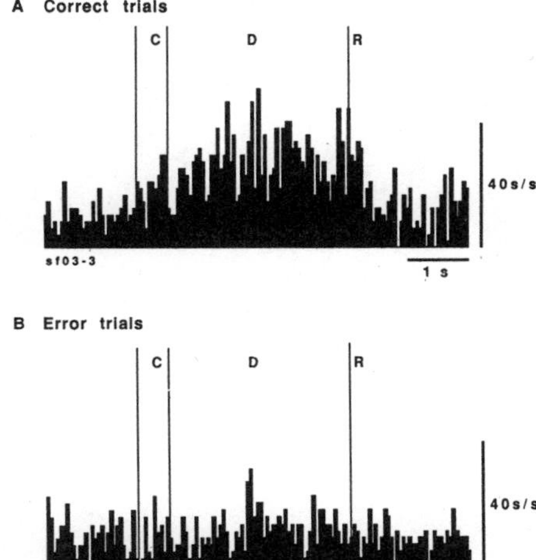

FIG. 14. Comparison of delay period activity for correct trials with activity for error trials. The first correct trial and the first error trial were taken from each of the 9 principal sulcus neurons that had excitatory directional delay period activity and for which the monkey made at least 1 error on a trial in the neuron's preferred direction. The *top* histogram sums the 9 correct trials and the *bottom* histogram sums the 9 error trials.

exhibited directional delay period activity, only 13 PS neurons (9 excitatory and 4 inhibitory) had one or more such error trials. Nevertheless, these data indicate that the responses of PS neurons during the delay period were significantly weaker on trials where the monkey made an error during the response period.

Figure 13 shows examples of neural activity in both correct and error trials for two neurons with directional delay period activity. The neuron shown at the top of the figure had its strongest delay period activity with leftward (180°) cue presentations. For trials on which the monkey's eventual saccade was to this location the neuron responded tonically throughout the delay period. However, on the one trial in which an error was made (saccade to upper right) the neuron's discharge ceased about midway through the delay period. The neuron at the bottom of Fig. 13 showed a similar pattern except that its delay period activity was absent altogether on the one trial in which an error was made.

To examine the error data as a whole we summed the first error trial (usually the only one) across the nine excitatory neurons with an error trial in the neuron's preferred direction. This histogram was compared to a histogram composed of the first correct trial (from the same event buffer) of these nine neurons at their preferred direction. Figure 14 shows these two histograms. The delay period activity on the correct trials was significantly greater than activity on the error trials by a paired t test ($t = 2.76$, df = 8, $P < 0.025$).

Directional and omnidirectional delay period activity in the frontal eye fields

Of the 319 examined neurons, 31 were recorded from the frontal eye fields (FEF), where low- (<50 μA) and intermediate-threshold (between 50 and 100 μA) microstimulation generated saccadic eye movements (7). Of these 31 neurons, 22 showed task-related activity during the oculomotor delayed-response task, with 17 (54.8%) having significant responses during the delay period (10 excitatory and 7 inhibitory).

Of these 17 FEF neurons, 10 exhibited directional delay period activity. Figure 15 provides an example of a neuron with a preferred direction at 90°; this FEF neuron showed tonic excitation during the delay period (see Fig. 15*B*) and also exhibited presaccadic excitation at the time of response when the monkey made saccadic eye movements to the cue location which was the neuron's preferred direction for delay period activity (see Fig. 15*C*). Like some PS neurons, the delay period activity was suppressed when the cue was presented at roughly opposite directions to its preferred direction (135, 180, and 225°).

Of the 10 FEF neurons with directional delay period activity, 5 had preferred directions into the contralateral hemifield, 4 preferred upward directions, and 1 preferred ipsilaterally directed stimuli. The mean tuning index (T_d) was 27.4 ± 20.0° ($n = 7$) for FEF neurons with excitatory directional delay period activity. The three FEF neurons with inhibitory directional delay period activity were very broadly tuned.

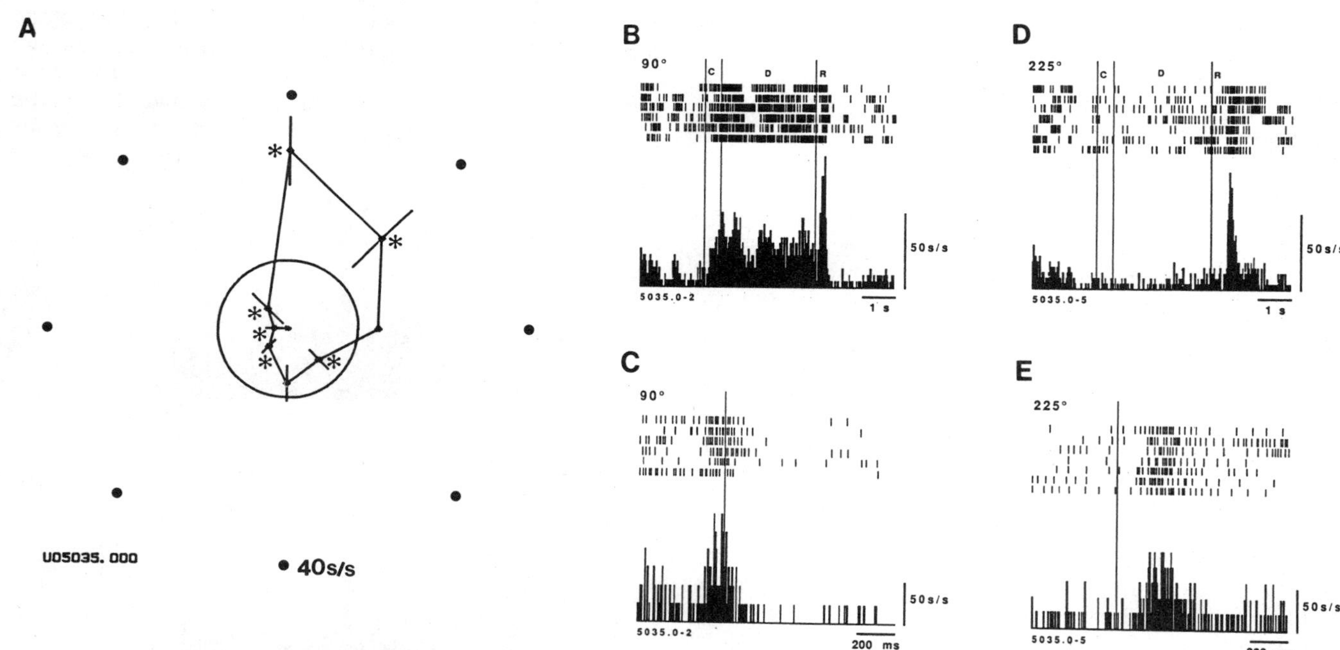

FIG. 15. Directional delay period activity ($F = 29.582$; df = 7, 33; $P < 0.001$) of a frontal eye fields neuron. This neuron (5035, right hemisphere) had significant tonic excitatory delay period activity only when the cue was presented at the 45 and 90° locations and was suppressed during the delay when the cue was presented at roughly opposite locations (135°, $t = 2.647$, df = 43, $P < 0.025$; 180°, $t = 3.158$, df = 42, $P < 0.005$; 225°, $t = 3.759$, df = 46, $P < 0.001$). Visual cues were presented randomly at 1 of the 8 locations. All cue eccentricities were 13° and all delay durations were 3 s. *A*: radial plot showing the directional tuning of delay period activity. *B* and *D*: neuron's delay period activity on the 90° trial and the 225° trial, respectively. *C* and *E*: activity aligned at the start of saccadic eye movements at the response period on the 90° trial and the 225° trial, respectively. Note that this neuron had presaccadic activity for 90° saccades and postsaccadic activity for 225° saccades.

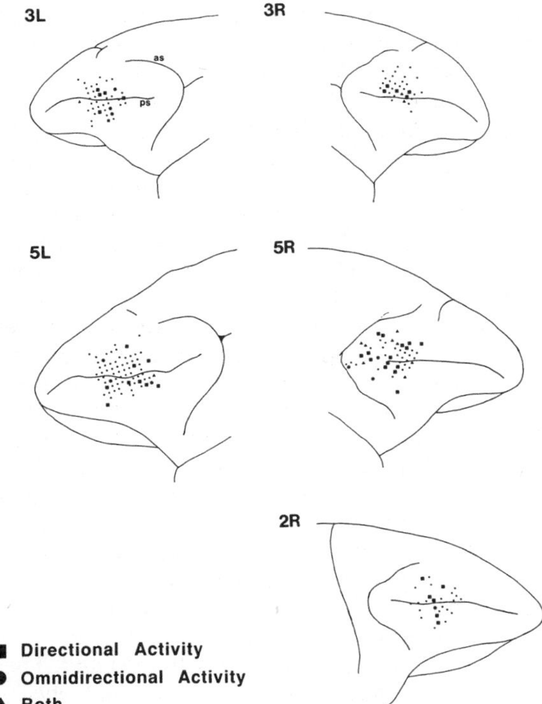

FIG. 16. Tracings of the dorsolateral prefrontal cortex showing the location of electrode penetrations for the 3 monkeys (*monkeys 2, 3,* and *5*) studied. The perspective of the tracings is approximately normal to the dorsolateral prefrontal cortical surface, roughly midway between standard lateral and dorsal views. Locations of neurons with directional delay period activity (●), omnidirectional delay period activity (■), and locations where both types of activity were found (▲). *Small dots* indicate surface locations of electrode penetrations where neurons with delay period activity were not found. PS, principal sulcus; AS, arcuate sulcus.

Cortical distribution of neurons with directional and omnidirectional delay period activity in the prefrontal cortex

Recording sites in each hemisphere were located on reconstructions of the dorsolateral prefrontal region. Most electrode penetrations were in the dorsal and ventral banks of the medial and posterior part of the principal sulcus and also in the surrounding regions of the principal sulcus [Walker's area 46 (63)]; however, in one hemisphere nine penetrations were made in the prearcuate region bordering the anterior bank of the arcuate sulcus where the frontal eye fields are located.

Figure 16 illustrates the location of all penetrations and also shows the location of neurons with directional and omnidirectional delay period activity in each of five hemispheres studied. We were unable to discern any clear localization or clustering of neurons with directional delay period activity and neurons with omnidirectional delay period activity.

DISCUSSION

Memory fields of prefrontal neurons

Prefrontal neurons with directionally selective delay period activity were first described in conjunction with the classical manual version of the delayed-response task (50) and a related task, spatial delayed alternation (51, 52). Prefrontal neurons in previous studies were characterized as directionally selective because their delay period activity was specific for the left- *or* right-of-center locations of the cues or the left *or* right direction of the manual response (50–52). Similar selective delay period activity has been observed in prefrontal neurons during performance of delayed discrimination (22, 47, 58) and conditional response (64) tasks. Although the overall percentage of neurons with directionally selective delay period activity in previous studies of the prefrontal cortex was small [i.e., 6% of total "task-related" neurons in Niki (50); 13% in Niki (51); 19% in Niki and Watanabe (53); 10% in Fuster et al. (22)], these neurons are nevertheless reflective of central mnemonic processes guiding the correct choice at the end of delay (18, 28, 50).

The present study differs from previous recording efforts in that we employed fixation and perimetry in order to extend the analysis of delay-related activity beyond the traditional two-choice (left and right) paradigms (5, 16, 20, 22, 37, 40–42, 45, 50, 53, 54, 58, 67). We found that the delay period activity of prefrontal neurons codes the spatial coordinates of visual cues during a delayed-response task and thus provides a mnemonic code for direction over the full perimetry of visual space, not for left-right direction alone. Each neuron with directional delay period activity had a "mnemonic" receptive field: only when the cue was presented in that field did the neuron show excitation or inhibition during the subsequent delay period. Moreover, directional delay period activity expanded when the delay was lengthened and faltered on occasional trials when errors were made. Therefore, we propose that this area of the visual field be termed the *memory field* of the neuron analogous to the receptive fields of visual neurons or the movement fields of oculomotor neurons. Memory fields may be the cellular expression of a working memory process (3) that allows mnemonic information to guide behavior.

The mechanisms by which a memory field is constructed are not known at present. It is highly relevant that the caudal prefrontal areas around the principal sulcus and prearcuate cortex are heavily interconnected with the posterior parietal cortex (2, 9, 11, 35, 36, 55, 59), which is a major center for processing of spatial vision (1, 49). Our recent anatomic studies of the posterior parietal cortex (10) indicate that visuotopic information may be transmitted to posterior parietal areas from a recently described visual area on the medial surface of the occipital lobe (area PO) which receives a direct input from the striate cortex (12) and where neurons are responsive to peripheral stimuli (13). The posterior parietal cortex also receives afferents from the superior temporal sulcus, from area MT, from the inferotemporal cortex, and from other prestriate areas (10). Thus we speculate that prefrontal neurons may access visuotopic information via the parietoprefrontal pathway, although that information may be also available from other cortical and subcortical sources.

Delay period activity has been reported for neurons in several cortical or subcortical structures during performance of delayed-response tasks, as well as in prefrontal cortical areas. These cortical and subcortical structures include the posterior parietal cortex (5, 30, 39), the inferotemporal cortex (23, 24), the cingulate cortex (54), the basal ganglia (32, 33), the mediodorsal nucleus of the thalamus (21), and the hippocampus (67). Interestingly, almost all of these structures are reciprocally connected with the prefrontal cortex (17, 29, 62). These data are compatible with the idea that the mnemonic information in the prefrontal cortex reflected by neurons with directional delay period activity may be a result of the neural interaction among these cortical and subcortical structures (28, 29) and that many of these structures may be part of a distributed network of cortical and subcortical structures dedicated to spatially guided behavior (29, 61).

Laterality of memory fields

Previous studies of prefrontal cortex in delay tasks have not emphasized the laterality (left or right, contralateral versus ipsilateral) of neuronal activity. In contrast, our study found a predominance of neurons preferring contralateral cues for their delay period activation. Among the 69 PS neurons with directional delay period activity, one half (49.3%) had memory fields centered in the visual field contralateral to the hemisphere where the neurons were located, only 17.4% had ipsilateral memory fields, and 17.4 and 15.9% had memory fields in upward and downward directions, respectively. This result indicates that, although the population of neurons in each hemisphere may be capable of coding cues over the entire visual field, the prefrontal neurons within each hemisphere code mainly contralateral locations. Accordingly, these results provide evidence that memory for spatial location is lateralized, with memories for locations in the right visual field coded mainly in the left hemisphere and memories for left field locations coded in the right hemisphere.

This physiological evidence of lateralization of spatial memory is supported by results from lesion studies. Fuster and Alexander (19) observed a higher proportion of errors to the contralateral side in monkeys with unilateral cryogenic depression of the dorsolateral prefrontal cortex. In a study using the oculomotor delayed-response task (15), we found that monkeys with a unilateral surgical ablation in the principal sulcus had marked difficulty making correct saccadic eye movements to remembered visual targets which had been presented in the visual field contralateral to the lesioned hemisphere and only mild or no difficulty making saccades to remembered targets which had been presented in the ipsilateral visual field. A similar result was obtained by Deng et al. for a unilateral lesion of the frontal eye fields on a task requiring memory over a 100-ms time interval (14). Because the monkeys with unilateral prefrontal lesions made normal saccadic eye movements to targets in both fields when their eye movements were visually guided, the difficulty of making saccades to remembered targets in the oculomotor delayed-response task seems to reflect a mnemonic deficit, which we have termed a "mnemonic hemianopia" (15) or "mnemonic scotoma."

Incidence and specificity of delay period activity

More research is still needed to know if the principal sulcus region has one population of neurons with delay period activity specific for the oculomotor delayed-response task and a separate population specific for manual types of delay tasks. We saw no indication of an anatomic subregion of the prefrontal cortex particularly dense in neurons with directional delay period activity for the oculomotor task, and our sampling area largely overlapped with the regions where neurons with directional activity on manual types of delay tasks have been found (16, 22, 50, 51, 53). Thus it is possible that the same region of the prefrontal cortex codes mnemonic representations across different types of delay tasks, and may even generalize across both sensory (visual versus auditory) and response (hand versus eye) modality. Some evidence favors such a type of generalized coding by individual prefrontal neurons, primarily the relatively high incidence of neurons with directional delay period activity during the oculomotor task (40.5% of total "task-related" neurons) obtained in the present study. If there were separate populations of prefrontal neurons for mnemonic representations in conjunction with eye movements and hand movements, then both populations would be active during the conventional, manual types of delayed-response tasks because primates invariably first direct their gaze with a saccade to stimuli that are to be touched or grasped with the hand. Therefore, previous studies should have found an even higher proportion of prefrontal neurons with delay period activity than we found with the oculomotor delay task. In fact, the reverse is the case, with 6–19% being the incidence of directional delay neurons from previous studies using the manual task, as reviewed earlier. Thus it is possible that the same prefrontal neurons code delay period representations for both oculomotor and manual response systems. On the other hand, there is no anatomic evidence in primates that would indicate that single neurons in the prefrontal cortex have axon collaterals to both eye- and hand-movement centers. Therefore, the question of "supramodal" neurons in the prefrontal cortex must remain open for future evaluation.

The higher proportion of prefrontal neurons with directional delay period activity may be explained by two other differences between our study and most previous ones. First, our use of four or eight cue locations increases the number of responsive neurons relative to studies employing only two (left and right) cue locations; many of our neurons with directional delay period activity responded best to cues above or below the fixation point (see Figs. 3 and 4) and would have been classified as nondirectional or nonresponsive if only the histograms for the left and right cue locations are considered. Another important reason is that other observers seem reluctant to attend to inhibitory responses; however, neurons with *only* inhibitory responses account for nearly one-half of our sample of neurons with significant delay period activity and slightly over one-third of the population of directional delay period neurons.

Inhibitory delay period activity

Inhibitory delay period activity was much more prevalent than previous studies have indicated. Nearly one-half of the neurons with significant delay period activity were solely inhibitory. Inhibitory responses were less likely to be directional than excitatory ones; even so, nearly one-third of the directional responses were classified as directional because of selective inhibitory responses in the delay period. In addition, some neurons with excitatory delay period activity for particular cue locations had inhibitory activity for other cue locations, usually such inhibition being strongest for, or centered about, cue directions opposite to those optimal for excitatory responses.

These inhibitory responses may have several functions. First, neurons with inhibitory omnidirectional delay period activity comprised 16% of all the PS cells with significant delay period activity. We suggest that a tonic reduction in activity over this prefrontal pathway during the delay period may help the monkey suppress all saccadic eye movements for the duration of the delay period. There is an intense projection from the prefrontal cortex to the intermediate and deeper layers of the superior colliculus, the collicular zones responsible for saccadic eye movements (27, 48). A tonic reduction in activity over this pathway may provide a mechanism whereby the prefrontal cortex can prevent inappropriate saccades; patients with frontal lobe lesions have difficulty withholding responses to salient sensory stimuli (31). Another role for the inhibitory delay period activity is suggested by the neurons with inhibitory activity for directions opposite the excitatory cues. For these neurons inhibitory activity may be sharpening the spatial tuning of excitatory delay period activity. Opposing patterns of activity are reminiscent of the complex response patterns of neurons in sensory and motor centers that respond with excitation to one parameter of stimulation but are inhibited by the opposite or complementary stimulation, e.g., the opponent vector organization of parietal neurons, the color opponency of visual cortical neurons, and the reciprocal activation of motor cortex neurons by extension and flection. Our findings indicate that mnemonic coding is organized on a common physiological principle.

Comparison between the principal sulcal area and the frontal eye fields

We recorded neurons with memory fields from both the principal sulcal (PS) region [Walker's area 46 (63)] and from the frontal eye fields (FEF) region in and near the anterior bank of the arcuate sulcus. Although the number of FEF neurons sampled was small, several had directional delay period activity similar to that of PS neurons and the tuning of directional delay period activity was comparable (mean T_d = 26.8° in PS and 27.4° in FEF). Furthermore, the directional tuning of delay period activity in PS is comparable to the directional tuning of presaccadic movement fields in FEF (mean T_d of visuomovement neurons = 31.3° [1], Ref. 6).

Bruce and Goldberg (6) reported that many FEF neurons, particularly those having either tonic visual activity or visuomovement activity, responded throughout a 1-s delay period preceding saccades into their visual or movement field. Our FEF results are in general agree with that report and our PS results indicate that many prefrontal neurons anterior to the FEF behave similarly in the context of the delayed-saccade task.

The primary pathway of mnemonic information pertinent to saccadic eye movements in the frontal lobe may be from the PS to the FEF. We suggested in the previous section that PS neurons could code mnemonic representations of previous stimuli and impending responses across different delayed-response tasks. The FEF may construct appropriate saccadic commands based on these inputs from the PS region. Other cortex, such as the supplementary motor area, may fabricate hand movements based on similar PS inputs, with the context of the task potentiating one or both of these motor-specific cortical zones. Indeed, Goldberg and Bushnell (26) found that FEF visual activity was only enhanced in the context of eye movements, but Bushnell et al. (8) found that the visual activity on the surface of the inferior parietal lobule, which projects to the PS region, was enhanced in the context of both eye and hand movements. On the other hand, the PS and FEF regions also could function independently with respect to the delayed-saccade task. Both areas receive visual inputs from the temporal and parietal cortices (17, 62) and both have direct projections to the superior colliculus (27, 34, 43, 48) as well as indirect projections there via the corticostriatal system (60, 61). The actual circuit for memory guided behavior is probably complex, and at present, we can only postulate that the PS region handles delay information for both saccades and for arm movements whereas the FEF are specific for eye movements.

Oculomotor delayed-response task

We used an oculomotor delayed-response task to examine the functions of the primate prefrontal cortex, whereas most information about previous studies of spatial delayed-response have been conducted in a Wisconsin General Test Apparatus (WGTA), in which freely moving monkeys reach through the bars of a small cage to retrieve a food reward manually after an imposed delay. Testing in a WGTA precludes precise experimental control over the animal's regard of visual stimuli as well as its behavior during the delay period. In neurophysiological experiments using behaving monkeys, modified versions of the WGTA-based task, such as two-choice (left and right) paradigms, have been used. Although the monkey's head is fixed and stimulus presentations and response movements are more controlled in this situation, the monkey's behavior during the delay period, especially its eye movements, have still not been controlled. The question could be raised as to whether, under these testing conditions, a monkey really needs memory to perform correctly, because he could maintain an ocular or postural orientation to the appropriate response key throughout the delay period. Obviously, if a monkey looked at the prospective response window continuously during this period, he would not need to remember the correct cue location. Although investigators have sometimes recorded electrooculographic data during task performance (21, 22, 37, 40, 65, 66), they

[1] All T_d estimates of Bruce and Goldberg (6) are inflated by a factor of 1.4142 because of a program error discovered while completing the present study. Thus their average T_d of 44.2° for visuomovement neurons should be 31.3°.

have not usually continuously monitored or controlled eye movements during the collection of single neuron activity.

In this respect, the oculomotor delayed-response paradigm that we used has several advantages. First, the monkey's behavior can be controlled more precisely during the performance of the delayed-response task. Because the monkey must maintain fixation of the center spot of light during the delay period, and as there is no clue available during this period to indicate the direction of the correct response, the monkey is required to use working memory to achieve a high level performance. Second, this paradigm allows the use of multiple cue locations in the monkey's visual field in order to more rigorously test whether directionally selective activity of prefrontal neurons reflects coding of specific spatial information rather than just a general preparatory set. Finally, recording eye position during the delay as well as the latency, direction, and amplitude of the eye movement at the time of response allows a more accurate analysis of correlations between prefrontal single neuron activity and behavior. Thus the oculomotor delayed-response task may be a powerful tool for analyzing the mnemonic functions of the prefrontal cortex in both neurophysiological and ablation experiments.

The authors thank L. Ladewig and S. Morgenstern for surgical assistance and animal preparation, J. Coburn and M. Pappy for histological assistance, and J. Musco for photography. The authors are also grateful to D. Burman, M. Chaffee, T. Preuss, T. Sawaguchi, and F. Wilson for reading an earlier draft and providing constructive comments.

This work was supported by National Institute of Mental Health Grants MH-38546 and MH-00298 to P. S. Goldman-Rakic, National Eye Institute Grant EY-04740 to C. J. Bruce, and by Jacob Javits Center for Excellence in Neuroscience Grant NS-22807.

REFERENCES

1. Andersen, R. A. Inferior parietal lobule function in spatial perception and visuomotor integration. In: *Handbook of Physiology. The Nervous System.* Bethesda, MD: Am. Physiol. Soc., 1987, vol. V, p. 483–518.
2. Andersen, R. A., Asanuma, C., and Cowan, W. M. Callosal and prefrontal associational projecting cell populations in area 7A of the macaque monkey: a study using retrogradely transported fluorescent dyes. *J. Comp. Neurol.* 232: 443–455, 1985.
3. Baddeley, A. D. Working memory. *Philos. Trans. R. Soc. Lond. B Biol. Sci.* 302: 311–324, 1983.
4. Batuev, A. S., Orlov, A. A., and Pirogov, A. A. Short-term spatiotemporal memory and cortical unit reactions in the monkey. *Acta Physiol. Acad. Sci. Hung.* 58: 207–216, 1981.
5. Batuev, A. S., Shaefer, V. I., and Orlov, A. A. Comparative characteristics of unit activity in the prefrontal and parietal areas during delayed performance in monkeys. *Behav. Brain Res.* 16: 57–70, 1985.
6. Bruce, C. J. and Goldberg, M. E. Primate frontal eye fields. I. Single neurons discharging before saccades. *J. Neurophysiol.* 53: 606–635, 1985.
7. Bruce, C. J., Goldberg, M. E., Bushnell, M. C., and Stanton, G. B. Primate frontal eye fields. II. Physiological and anatomical correlates of electrically evoked eye movements. *J. Neurophysiol.* 54: 714–734, 1985.
8. Bushnell, M. C., Goldberg, M. E., and Robinson, D. L. Behavioral enhancement of visual responses in monkey cerebral cortex. I. Modulation in posterior parietal cortex related to selective visual attention. *J. Neurophysiol.* 46: 755–772, 1981.
9. Cavada, C. and Goldman-Rakic, P. S. Parieto-prefrontal connections in the monkey: topographic distribution within the prefrontal cortex of sectors connected with the lateral and medial posterior parietal cortex. *Soc. Neurosci. Abstr.* 11: 323, 1985.
10. Cavada, C. and Goldman-Rakic, P. S. Subdivisions of area 7 in the rhesus monkey exhibit selective patterns of connectivity with limbic, visual and somatosensory cortical areas. *Soc. Neurosci. Abstr.* 12: 262, 1986.
11. Chavis, D. A. and Pandya, D. N. Further observations on corticofrontal connections in the rhesus monkey. *Brain Res.* 117: 369–386, 1976.
12. Colby, C. L., Gattass, R., Olson, C. R., and Gross, C. G. Topographic organization of cortical afferents to extrastriate visual area PO in the macaque: a dual tracer study. *J. Comp. Neurol.* 269: 392–413, 1988.
13. Covey, E., Gattass, R., and Gross, C. G. A new visual area in the parieto-occipital sulcus of the macaque. *Soc. Neurosci. Abstr.* 8: 681, 1982.
14. Deng, S.-Y., Goldberg, M. E., Segraves, M. A., Ungerleider, L. G., and Mishkin, M. The effect of unilateral ablation of the frontal eye fields on saccadic performance in the monkey. In: *Adaptive Processes in Visual and Oculomotor Systems,* edited by E. L. Keller and D. S. Zee. New York: Pergamon, 1987, p. 201–208.
15. Funahashi, S., Bruce, C. J., and Goldman-Rakic, P. S. Perimetry of spatial memory representation in primate prefrontal cortex: evidence for mnemonic hemianopia. *Soc. Neurosci. Abstr.* 12: 554, 1986.
16. Fuster, J. M. Unit activity in prefrontal cortex during delayed-response performance: neuronal correlates of transient memory. *J. Neurophysiol.* 36: 61–78, 1973.
17. Fuster, J. M. *The Prefrontal Cortex.* New York: Raven, 1980.
18. Fuster, J. M. The prefrontal cortex and temporal integration. In: *Cerebral Cortex,* edited by A. Peters and E. G. Jones. New York: Plenum, 1985, vol. 4, p. 151–177.
19. Fuster, J. M. and Alexander, G. E. Delayed response deficit by cryogenic depression of frontal cortex. *Brain Res.* 20: 85–90, 1970.
20. Fuster, J. M. and Alexander, G. E. Neuron activity related to short-term memory. *Science Wash. DC* 173: 652–654, 1971.
21. Fuster, J. M. and Alexander, G. E. Firing changes in cells of the nucleus medialis dorsalis associated with delayed response behavior. *Brain Res.* 61: 79–91, 1973.
22. Fuster, J. M., Bauer, R. H., and Jervey, J. P. Cellular discharge in the dorsolateral prefrontal cortex of the monkey in cognitive tasks. *Exp. Neurol.* 77: 679–694, 1982.
23. Fuster, J. M., Bauer, R. H., and Jervey, J. P. Functional interactions between inferotemporal and prefrontal cortex in a cognitive task. *Brain Res.* 330: 299–307, 1985.
24. Fuster, J. M. and Jervey, J. P. Neuronal firing in the inferotemporal cortex of the monkey in a visual memory task. *J. Neurosci.* 2: 361–375, 1982.
25. van Gisbergen, J. A. M., Robinson, D. A., and Gielen, S. A quantitative analysis of generation of saccadic eye movements by burst neurons. *J. Neurophysiol.* 45: 417–442, 1981.
26. Goldberg, M. E. and Bushnell, M. C. Behavioral enhancement of visual responses in monkey cerebral cortex. II. Modulation in frontal eye fields specifically related to saccades. *J. Neurophysiol.* 46: 773–787, 1981.
27. Goldman, P. S. and Nauta, W. J. H. Autoradiographic demonstration of a projection from prefrontal association cortex to the superior colliculus in the rhesus monkey. *Brain Res.* 116: 145–149, 1976.
28. Goldman-Rakic, P. S. Circuitry of primate prefrontal cortex and regulation of behavior by representational memory. In: *Handbook of Physiology. The Nervous System.* Bethesda, MD: Am. Physiol. Soc., 1987, vol. V, p. 373–417.
29. Goldman-Rakic, P. S. Topography of cognition: paralleled distributed networks in primate association cortex. *Ann. Rev. Neurosci.* 11: 137–156, 1988.
30. Gnadt, J. W. and Andersen, R. A. Memory related motor planning activity in posterior parietal cortex of macaque. *Exp. Brain Res.* 70: 216–220, 1988.
31. Guitton, D., Buchtel, H. A., and Douglas, R. M. Frontal lobe lesions in man cause difficulties in suppressing reflexive glances and in generating goal-directed saccades. *Exp. Brain Res.* 58: 455–472, 1985.
32. Hikosaka, O. and Sakamoto, M. Cell activity in monkey caudate nucleus preceding saccadic eye movements. *Exp. Brain Res.* 63: 659–662, 1986.
33. Hikosaka, O. and Wurtz, R. H. Visual and oculomotor functions

of monkey substantia nigra pars reticulata. III. Memory-contingent visual and saccade responses. *J. Neurophysiol.* 49: 1268–1284, 1983.

34. Huerta, M. F., Krubitzer, L. A., and Kaas, J. H. Frontal eye field as defined by intracortical microstimulation in squirrel monkeys, owl monkeys, and macaque monkeys. I. Subcortical connections. *J. Comp. Neurol.* 253: 415–439, 1986.
35. Jacobson, S. and Trojanowski, J. Q. Prefrontal granular cortex of the rhesus monkey. I. Intrahemispheric cortical afferent. *Brain Res.* 132: 209–233, 1977.
36. Jones, E. G. and Powell, T. P. S. An anatomical study of converging sensory pathways within the cerebral cortex of the monkey. *Brain* 93: 793–820, 1970.
37. Joseph, J. P. and Barone, P. Prefrontal unit activity during a delayed oculomotor task in the monkey. *Exp. Brain Res.* 67: 460–468, 1987.
38. Judge, S. J., Richmond, B. J., and Chu, F. C. Implantation of magnetic search coils for measurement of eye position: an improved method. *Vision Res.* 20: 535–538, 1980.
39. Koch, K. W. and Fuster, J. M. Single unit activity in the parietal cortex of the primate during a haptic delayed matching-to-sample task. *Soc. Neurosci. Abstr.* 11: 1275, 1985.
40. Kojima, S. Prefrontal unit activity in the monkey: relation to visual stimuli and movements. *Exp. Neurol.* 69: 110–123, 1980.
41. Kojima, S. and Goldman-Rakic, P. S. Delay-related activity of prefrontal neurons in rhesus monkeys performing delayed response. *Brain Res.* 248: 43–49, 1982.
42. Kojima, S. and Goldman-Rakic, P. S. Functional analysis of spatially discriminated neurons in prefrontal cortex of rhesus monkey. *Brain Res.* 291: 229–240, 1984.
43. Komatsu, H. and Suzuki, H. Projections from the functional subdivisions of the frontal eye field to the superior colliculus in the monkey. *Brain Res.* 327: 324–327, 1985.
44. Kubota, K. and Funahashi, S. Direction-specific activities of dorsolateral prefrontal and motor cortex pyramidal tract neurons during visual tracking. *J. Neurophysiol.* 47: 362–376, 1982.
45. Kubota, K., Iwamoto, T., and Suzuki, K. Visuokinetic activities of primate prefrontal neurons during delayed-response performance. *J. Neurophysiol.* 37: 1197–1212, 1974.
46. Kubota, K. and Niki, H. Prefrontal cortical unit activity and delayed alternation performance in monkeys. *J. Neurophysiol.* 34: 337–347, 1971.
47. Kubota, K., Tonoike, M., and Mikami, A. Neuronal activity in the monkey dorsolateral prefrontal cortex during a discrimination task with delay. *Brain Res.* 183: 29–42, 1980.
48. Leichnetz, G. R., Spencer, R. F., Hardy, S. G. P., and Astruc, J. The prefrontal corticotectal projection in the monkey: an anterograde and retrograde horseradish peroxidase study. *Neuroscience* 6: 1023–1041, 1981.
49. Mountcastle, V. B. The world around us: neural command functions for selective attention. *Neurosci. Res. Program Bull.* 14, *Suppl.*: 1–47, 1976.
50. Niki, H. Differential activity of prefrontal units during right and left delayed response trials. *Brain Res.* 70: 346–349, 1974.
51. Niki, H. Prefrontal unit activity during delayed alternation in the monkey. I. Relation to direction of response. *Brain Res.* 68: 185–196, 1974.
52. Niki, H. Prefrontal unit activity during delayed alternation in the monkey. II. Relation to absolute versus relative direction of response. *Brain Res.* 68: 197–204, 1974.
53. Niki, H. and Watanabe, M. Prefrontal unit activity and delayed response: relation to cue location versus direction of response. *Brain Res.* 105: 79–88, 1976.
54. Niki, H. and Watanabe, M. Cingulate unit activity and delayed response. *Brain Res.* 110: 381–386, 1976.
55. Petrides, M. and Pandya, D. N. Projections to the frontal cortex from the posterior parietal region in the rhesus monkey. *J. Comp. Neurol.* 228: 105–116, 1984.
56. Robinson, D. A. A method of measuring eye movement using a scleral search coil in a magnetic field. *IEEE Trans. Biomed. Eng.* 10: 137–145, 1963.
57. Rosenkilde, C. E. Functional heterogeneity of the prefrontal cortex in the monkey: a review. *Behav. Neurol. Biol.* 25: 301–345, 1979.
58. Rosenkilde, C. E., Bauer, R. H., and Fuster, J. M. Single cell activity in ventral prefrontal cortex of behaving monkeys. *Brain Res.* 209: 375–394, 1981.
59. Schwartz, M. L. and Goldman-Rakic, P. S. Callosal and intrahemispheric connectivity of the prefrontal association cortex in rhesus monkey: relation between intraparietal and principal sulcal cortex. *J. Comp. Neurol.* 226: 403–420, 1984.
60. Selemon, L. D. and Goldman-Rakic, P. S. Longitudinal topography and interdigitation of corticostriatal projections in the rhesus monkey. *J. Neurosci.* 5: 776–794, 1985.
61. Selemon, L. D. and Goldman-Rakic, P. S. Common cortical and subcortical target areas of the dorsolateral prefrontal and posterior parietal cortices in the rhesus monkey: evidence for a distributed neural network subserving spatially guided behavior. *J. Neurosci.* 8: 4049–4068, 1988.
62. Stuss, D. T. and Benson, D. F. *The Frontal Lobes.* New York: Raven, 1986.
63. Walker, A. E. A cytoarchitectural study of the prefrontal area of the macaque monkey. *J. Comp. Neurol.* 73: 59–86, 1940.
64. Watanabe, M. Prefrontal unit activity during delayed conditional discriminations in the monkey. *Brain Res.* 225: 51–65, 1981.
65. Watanabe, M. Prefrontal unit activity during delayed conditional Go/No-Go discrimination in the monkey. I. Relation to the stimulus. *Brain Res.* 382: 1–14, 1986.
66. Watanabe, M. Prefrontal unit activity during delayed conditional Go/No-Go discrimination in the monkey. II. Relation to Go and No-Go responses. *Brain Res.* 382: 15–27, 1986.
67. Watanabe, T. and Niki, H. Hippocampal unit activity and delayed response in the monkey. *Brain Res.* 325: 241–254, 1985.

39
M. Mishkin
A memory system in the monkey
1982. *Philosophical Transactions of the Royal Society of London* B298: 85–95

Abstract
A neural model is presented, based largely on evidence from studies in monkeys, postulating that coded representations of stimuli are stored in the higher-order sensory (i.e. association) areas of the cortex whenever stimulus activation of these areas also triggers a cortico-limbo-thalamo-cortical circuit. This circuit, which could act as either an imprinting or rehearsal mechanism, may actually consist of two parallel circuits, one involving the amygdala and the dorsomedial nucleus of the thalamus, and the other the hippocampus and the anterior nuclei. The stimulus representation stored in cortex by action of these circuits is seen as mediating three different memory processes: recognition, which occurs when the stored representation is reactivated via the original sensory pathway; recall, when it is reactivated via any other pathway; and association, when it activates other stored representations (sensory, affective, spatial, motor) via the outputs of the higher-order sensory areas to the relevant structures.

Introduction

How do we learn to recognize new stimuli? In particular, how do we often manage to do this after only a single, brief exposure? A reasonable guess for vision is that in the course of inspecting a new stimulus, such as a new object or face or scene, we automatically store a coded representation of it in visual association cortex; recognition occurs when this central representation is reactivated by the same stimulus on a later occasion. Evidence from studies on monkeys fits this scheme and suggests how such central representations could be formed.

In the act of perceiving a new visual stimulus, a unique constellation of prestriate outputs, representing a unique constellation of visual attributes such as size, colour, texture and shape converges on single inferior temporal neurons. This initial activation, constituting a novel perception, leaves a lasting effect after the inferior temporal neurons, in turn, trigger a cortico-limbo-thalamo-cortical circuit. Once triggered, this circuit acts as an automatic rehearsal or imprinting mechanism, strengthening the prestriate–temporal connections that participated in firing the circuit in the first place. As a result, many of the same inferior temporal neurons that were maximally activated by the stimulus initially are likely to be activated again whenever the same constellation of visual attributes (i.e. the same visual stimulus) reappears in the field; the neurons so reactivated may thus be viewed as the stored central representation for that stimulus. Once established, this central representation can enter into association with a variety of other stored central representations (sensory, affective, spatial, motor) and thereby arouse them or be aroused by them through associative recall, via the reciprocal connections of inferior temporal cortex with the relevant structures.

The neural events that have just been pictured are of course hypothetical. At the same time, they are conceived as taking place in parts of the brain that are now known to be important for visual recognition, and in a sequence that fits our current understanding of how the parts are connected. This hypothetical scheme thus provides a convenient framework for integrating a large amount of neurobehavioural information relevant to visual memory. The purpose of my paper will be to develop that evidence.

The Prestriate Complex

At the outset, it is important to make clear that inferior temporal cortex, in particular area TE in Bonin & Bailey's (1947) terminology (see figure 1), stands at the end of a long line of modality-specific visual areas that begins in the striate cortex, or area OC, and continues through the prestriate and posterior temporal areas, OB, OA, and TEO (Mishkin 1972). This ventrally directed chain of cortical visual areas appears to extract stimulus-quality information from the retinal input reaching the striate cortex (Ungerleider & Mishkin 1982), processing it for the purpose of identifying the visual stimulus and ultimately assigning it some meaning through mediation of area TE's connections with the limbic system, specifically the amygdaloid complex and the hippocampal formation (Jones & Mishkin 1972; Mishkin 1979; Spiegler & Mishkin 1981). How the visual system performs its perceptual feat is still almost totally unknown. But a major aspect of its operation is the distribution of the striate output to the numerous re-representations of the visual field located within the prestriate and posterior temporal areas (Allman 1977; Merzenich & Kaas 1980), perhaps for the purpose of submodality processing (Zeki 1978; Cowey 1981). Thus such object features as size, colour, texture and shape could be analysed separately within specific subdivisions of the region. The subdivision about which we know the most from a behavioural standpoint is area TEO, and the behavioural evidence regarding it supports the foregoing conjecture. That is, area TEO appears to be critical for shape perception (Yaginuma *et al.* 1982) in that its removal impairs

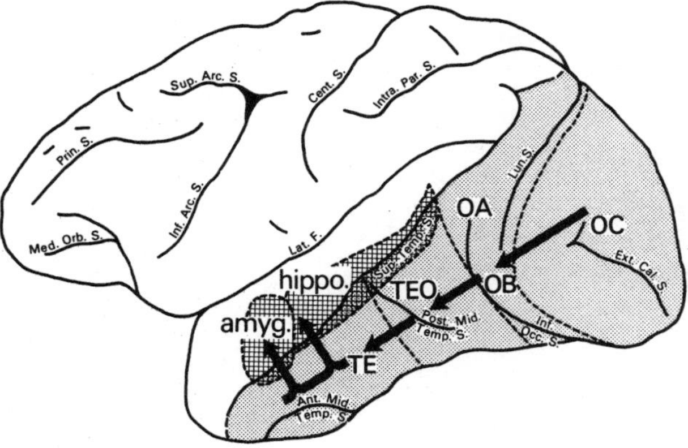

Figure 1. Flow of visual information from primary cortical area (OC) through secondary areas (OB, OA and TEO) to the highest-order visual area (TE), and from there into the medially located amygdaloid complex (amyg.) and hippocampal formation (hippo.). Cytoarchitectonic designations are those of Bonin & Bailey (1947). For clarity, the hippocampal formation is pictured slightly dorsal to its actual location.

the discrimination of two-dimensional patterns far more than does equivalent damage on either side of it, including even substantial damage to the striate cortex itself (Blake *et al.* 1977). At the same time, as will become clear shortly, the removal does not impair discrimination of an object's other, less complex, features, which it is therefore reasonable to assume are processed in other subdivisions of the prestriate complex and then relayed forward to area TE, bypassing TEO. According to the view being advanced here, the analysis of the several physical properties or dimensions of a visual object may proceed in parallel in the various subdivisions of the prestriate complex and perhaps even be completed within this tissue. But the synthesis of these several physical properties into a unique configuration representing the unique object may normally entail the funnelling of the outputs from the prestriate—posterior temporal region into area TE. It is this postulated convergence or integration of visual inputs in area TE that makes it particularly well suited to serve not only as the highest-order area for the perception of visual stimuli but also as the storehouse for their central representations.

Area TE

That area TE is important for some form of visual learning or memory has been known for decades (Mishkin 1954; Iwai & Mishkin 1968). But that the area is critical for visual recognition specifically was discovered only recently in a study that compared the effects of partial temporal-lobe lesions on a test of one-trial object recognition. Because the test is central to the development of the model, I shall describe it briefly. In this test (Mishkin & Delacour 1975), the monkey subject is shown a distinctive object over a central food-well, which it uncovers to obtain a concealed peanut. Ten seconds later the same object is paired with an equally distinctive novel object, each presented over a lateral well; but to find a peanut on this second occasion the monkey must avoid the familiar (previously baited) object and displace instead the unfamiliar one. The pair of objects is then discarded, not to appear again, and, 20 s later, the same procedure of single-object presentation followed by a choice trial is repeated with a new pair of objects. The procedure is repeated 20 times each day, each time with a new pair of objects, day after day, until the animal learns the principle of always selecting the novel object in the pair (i.e. delayed non-matching to sample), to a criterion of 90 correct choices in 100 trials. As it turns out, only a few days are needed to instil this principle of choosing the novel object, since it is one to which the naturally inquisitive monkey is already predisposed. Having not only learned the principle, but also, in the process, having demonstrated the ability to remember for at least 10 s something about the appearance of an object that was seen very briefly and only once before, trained animals were then given bilaterally symmetrical ablations of selected portions of the temporal lobe (Mishkin & Oubre 1977). Three animals each received complete removals of area TE, area TEO, the amygdaloid complex or the hippocampal formation, and three others were retained as unoperated controls. Two weeks after the operation the animals were retrained in the delayed non-matching principle, with the results indicated to the left of the curves in figure 2. No group required much more than about 100 trials on the average to relearn the task, except group TE, which required 1500 trials. In fact, each animal in group TE was given this amount of retraining, and yet not one fully reattained criterion within that time.

So specific and dramatic an impairment clearly indicates that the demands of the one-trial object recognition task approximate closely the functions of area TE. It was not yet clear, however, whether the impairment sustained by the TE group reflected a loss in recognition memory or whether it was due instead to a difficulty in relearning the delayed non-matching principle. To examine this question, once the animals had regained the principle, they were given a performance test (see Gaffan 1974) in which the delay between sample presentation and choice was increased in steps from 10 s to 2 min; after this, the number of objects to be remembered was also increased in steps from a single object to a list of ten objects. In this final condition, for example, each of the ten objects was presented in succession at 20 s intervals over the central well before each one was paired for choice with a different novel

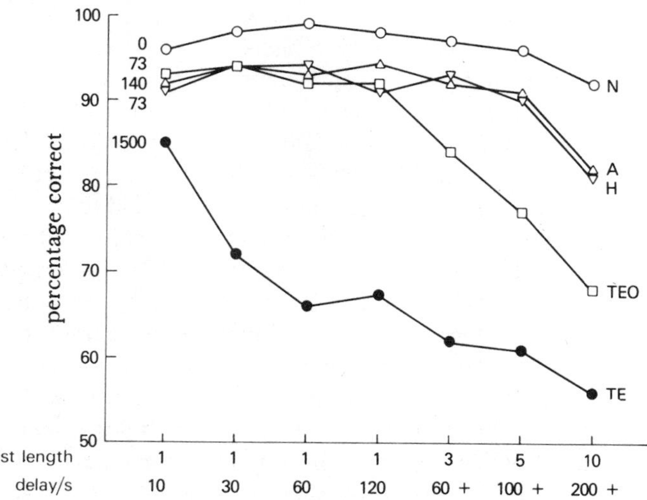

Figure 2. Average scores on the recognition performance test by groups with bilateral lesions of the amygdala (A), hippocampus and underlying fusiform–hippocampal gyrus (H), posterior temporal cortex (TEO), or anterior temporal cortex (TE), as well as a group of unoperated controls (N). Numerals to the left of the curves indicate the average number of trials to relearn the basic task, which entailed remembering a single object for 10 seconds, with the first point on the curve being the average final score achieved on this condition. Animals were tested on the six remaining conditions, involving gradually increasing delays and list lengths, for 1 week each.

object over the lateral wells. As the performance curves in figure 2 indicate, the normal animals maintained scores of better than 90% correct responses even under the last, most taxing, condition. Similarly, the animals with either amygdaloid or hippocampal lesions also maintained high levels of performance, showing only mild impairments relative to the unoperated controls. A different profile was exhibited by the animals in the TEO group, who performed as well as the best operated animals under conditions or increasing delay, but then dropped significantly below the others as the list lengths increased. This intensification of impairment on longer lists could reflect the specific disorder in shape perception that was attributed to TEO lesions. That is, an object's colour or size or texture might serve as an adequate mnemonic aid for recognition provided that this object alone had to be differentiated later from another. Consequently, a relatively intact perceptual ability along non-shape dimensions could account for the high level of performance shown by the TEO group on a list length of one, even with very long delays. When several objects in a list must be remembered and differentiated, however, then perhaps the unidimensional scales of colour, size and texture no longer serve as adequate mnemonic aids. Under these conditions, the highly variable attribute of shape may become a critical dimension, in which case a severe impairment in shape perception would account for the TEO group's sudden drop in scores during the second half of the performance test.

No such explanation, however, can account for the impairment shown by the animals with TE lesions, whose performance fell abruptly as soon as the delay between a single sample and choice was increased even slightly, and whose scores by the end of the performance test had fallen to chance. Animals with TE lesions are not markedly impaired in shape discrimination (Blake *et al.* 1977; Manning & Mishkin 1976), nor, for that matter, are they seriously impaired in discrimination along any particular dimension. Furthermore, they had already regained the non-matching principle to an average level of 85% correct responses at the end of retraining on the original condition. Their abrupt drop in performance with increasing delays, therefore, like their earlier difficulty in relearning the delayed non-matching principle with a single object and a 10 s delay, most probably reflects a severe recognition failure.

Amygdala and Hippocampus

According to the model being proposed here, the recognition failure after TE lesions is attributable to a loss of the neuronal network in which the central representations of visual stimuli are formed and stored. But the formation and storage process does not depend on the operation of the visual system alone. Despite the results from the study with partial temporal-lobe lesions described in the preceding section, there is substantial evidence now that the amygdala and hippocampus are in fact of crucial importance for the neural process underlying recognition. A clear demonstration of the role of these two structures in recognition memory, however, required removing them in combination

(Mishkin 1978). This demonstration grew out of a study of object–reward association, in which an attempt to exacerbate a deficit after amygdalectomy by addition of a hippocampal ablation proved to be extremely effective (Mishkin *et al.* 1982). When the severity of the associative memory impairment after the combined amygdalo-hippocampal removal was discovered, other animals with combined amygdalo-hippocampal ablation were tested for recognition memory, with equally dramatic results. Indeed, although these animals had less difficulty than those with TE lesions in relearning the basic delayed non-matching principle, their scores on the subsequent performance test with increasing delays and list lengths were, if anything, inferior to those of the animals with TE lesions. (The average scores of the two groups across the six conditions of the recognition performance test are compared in figure 4.) Partly on the basis of these findings of severe losses in both associative and recognition memory following the limbic lesion, as well as of a finding that the recognition loss extends beyond the visual modality (Murray & Mishkin 1981), it has been proposed (Mishkin *et al.* 1982) that amygdalo-hippocampal ablation in monkeys yields an animal model of the global amnesia that follows medial temporal-lobe surgery or pathology in clinical cases.

The ancillary evidence available in the animal model implies, however, that the participation of the limbic system in memory processes depends on its interaction with the neocortex, and specifically on the input it receives from the higher-order sensory areas, which for vision is area TE (Van Hoesen & Pandya 1975; Turner *et al.* 1980). To test this notion directly, a disconnection study was undertaken according to an experimental design that had been used previously (Mishkin 1966) to study the functional dependence of area TE on input from the striate cortex. In that earlier case, an inferior temporal lesion in one hemisphere was combined with an occipital lobectomy in the other, thereby leaving only a transcallosal pathway for visual information from the intact occipital lobe to reach the intact inferior temporal tissue on the opposite side. Transection of the splenium of the corpus callosum under these conditions rendered the intact inferior temporal cortex functionally inactive in visual learning and memory, owing to its isolation from visual input as demonstrated subsequently both in single-unit (Rocha-Miranda *et al.* 1975) and metabolic (Jarvis *et al.* 1978) studies. The special theoretical value of such a crossed-lesion disconnection experiment is that it permits the inference that the same functional dependency of one region upon another that has been demonstrated to exist between the hemispheres also exists within the hemispheres, where such dependency cannot be studied directly because of the inaccessibility of the intrahemispheric pathways.

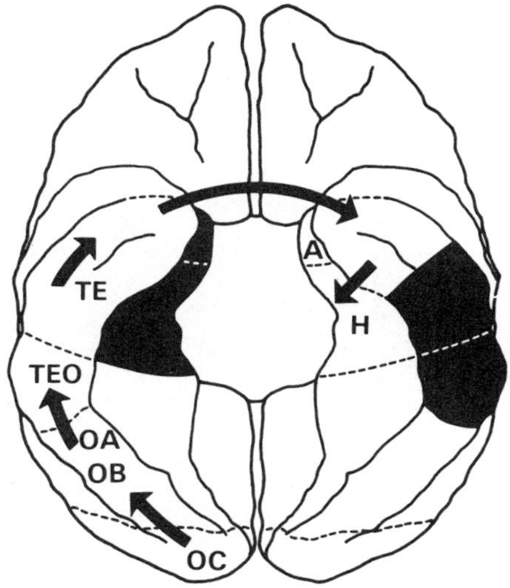

Figure 3. Surgical preparation for the crossed-lesion disconnection experiment, involving an amygdalo-hippocampal ablation in one hemisphere and an inferior temporal lesion in the other. Arrows on the left side of the illustration show information flow in the visually intact hemisphere, which then must cross in the anterior commissure to reach the intact amygdalo-hippocampal system on the opposite side. Animals were prepared with either these crossed lesions alone or with the crossed lesions combined with transection of the anterior commissure. Designations for cortical and limbic areas are the same as in figure 1.

Application of the crossed-lesion design to the study of cortico-limbic interaction led to the surgical preparation illustrated in figure 3. In this case, an inferior temporal lesion in one hemisphere (shown on the right) was combined with an amygdalo-hippocampal ablation in the other (shown on the left). As a result, visual information from the side with the intact visual system (areas labelled OC to TE) could reach the intact limbic system on the opposite side (areas labelled A and H) only through the anterior commissure (designated by the interhemispheric arrow). If limbic participation in visual memory requires this visual input, then transection of the anterior commissure should isolate the limbic system from vision and yield a recognition impairment equivalent to that produced by a bilateral limbic removal. To test the prediction, three animals each were given either crossed lesions alone, like those illustrated, or crossed lesions combined with anterior commissurotomy. All were trained on the recognition test in a manner identical to that described previously, with the result illustrated in figure 4. Those with crossed lesions alone obtained an average of better than 80% correct responses on the recognition performance test, a score that was about midway between the scores of the unoperated controls and the scores of the

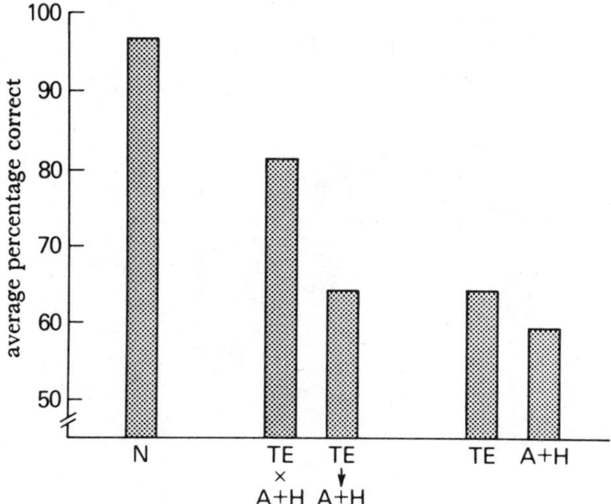

Figure 4. Average scores across the six conditions of the recognition performance test by the unoperated controls (N) on the left, and the animals with either bilateral inferior temporal (TE) or bilateral amygdalo-hippocampal (A + H) lesions on the right. In the middle are the scores of the two groups with crossed lesions described in figure 3, without (×) and with (↓) transection of the anterior commissure, respectively.

animals with either bilateral TE or bilateral limbic lesions. Thus, this extensive amount of damage to the visual-recognition system produced significant but incomplete impairment. By contrast, when the anterior commissure was transected in addition, the scores dropped to an average of less than 65%, or about the same as those of the groups with bilaterally symmetrical lesions. In short, it appears that the participation of the limbic system in visual memory does indeed depend on its receipt of visual input from area TE.

Medial Thalamus

Just as the visual system operating alone is insufficient to support visual recognition, so too is its interaction with the limbic system insufficient. It appears now that for stimulus recognition to occur, the limbic system must interact, in turn, with structures in the medial portion of the thalamus. The first evidence from animal work that diencephalic structures were critical for recognition memory came from studies on the effects of transections of the fornix (Gaffan 1974), the major hippocampo-diencephalic pathway. In the work in our own laboratory, by contrast, the recognition impairments that have been found to follow fornix transection alone are no more severe than those that were described above following hippocampectomy. As predicted by the effects of combined amygdalo-hippocampal ablations, however, transection of the fornix combined with amygdalectomy (see figure 5) produces a more striking impairment than either lesion by itself (Mishkin & Saunders 1979); and an equivalent combinatorial effect is produced by adding to a hippocampectomy a transection of the stria terminalis, a major amygdalo-diencephalic pathway. In both of these cases, the average scores on the recognition performance test after combined lesions were about 15% lower than those after any of the component lesions.

In considering which among the many diencephalic targets of the amygdala and hippocampus might be involved in the recognition memory process, an important clue was the clinical evidence that, in addition to the medial temporal region, a common site for the induction of amnesia by tissue destruction or pathology was the medial thalamus (Victor *et al.* 1971; McEntee *et al.* 1976). Since both the amygdala and the hippocampus project to this region—the amygdala to the magnocellular portion of the dorsomedial nucleus, and the hippocampus to the rostrally adjacent anterior nuclei—an attempt was made in three animals to ablate the region and to evaluate the effects on visual recognition. Preliminary results (Aggleton & Mishkin 1981; Mishkin & Aggleton 1981) indicate that, once again, recognition performance was severely disrupted, pointing to the critical participation of the medial thalamus as well in the recognition process.

The Recognition Memory Circuit

A diagrammatic summary of the circuit that has been implicated in visual recognition memory in these experiments is shown in figure 6. Severe lesion-induced memory losses have now been demonstrated at five different loci along the postulated pathway: (1) area TE, (2) the connections between area TE and the amygdalo-hippocampal complex, (3) the amygdalo-hippocampal complex itself, (4) the limbo-diencephalic pathways, and (5) limbic targets in the medial thalamus, including at least the medial parts of the dorsomedial and anterior nuclei. Whether or not still other structures belong to this system remains to be worked out; but one other structure, the midline thalamus, has been added as a potential relay for completion of the circuit, for reasons set out below.

As indicated at the outset, the recognition-memory model suggests that central representations of stimuli are formed and stored not within the limbic or thalamic portions of the circuit but rather within the highest levels of the cortical sensory processing areas. There are numerous arguments in favour of such a supposition, including one of parsimony—that organized percepts and perceptual memories are thereby localized in the same tissue—as well as one of capacity—that the storehouse for unique central representations within the primate sensory association cortex must be nearly limitless. But perhaps the strongest argument in favour

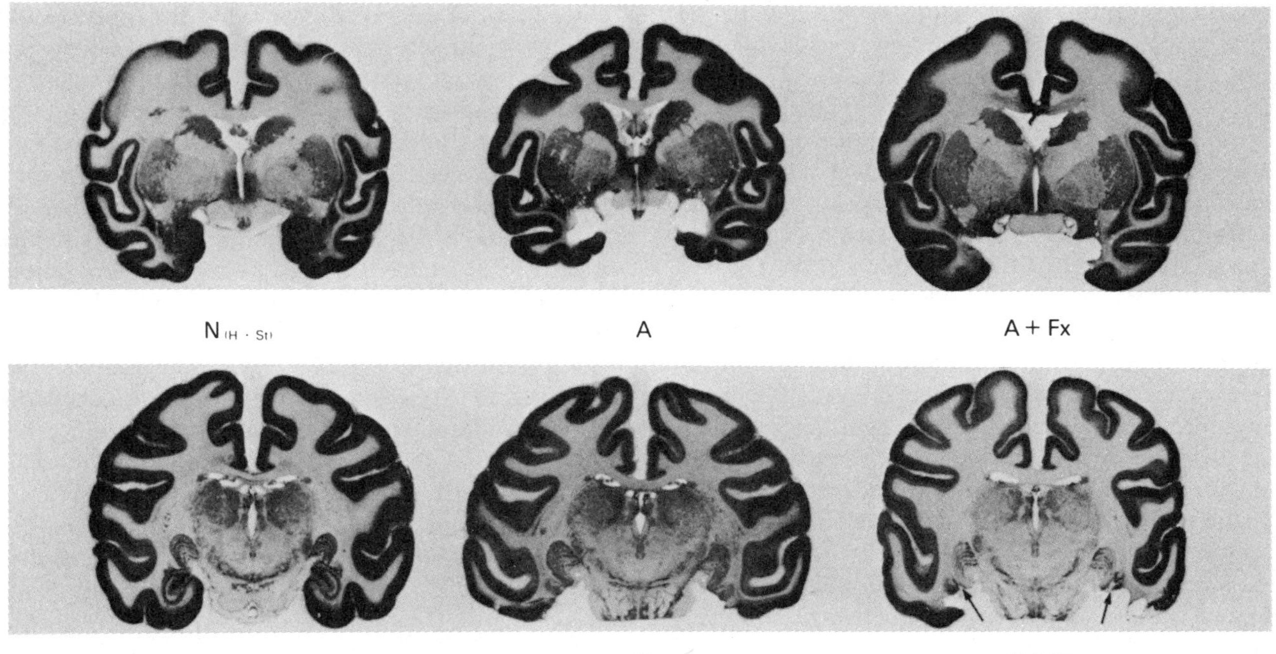

Figure 5. Frontal sections through the brains of animals with amygdalectomy alone (A), amygdalectomy plus fornix transection (A + Fx), hippocampectomy alone (H), or hippocampectomy plus transection of the stria terminalis (H + St). The stria terminalis transection is denoted by arrows. For comparison, a frontal section through a normal amygdala and fornix is shown from the brain of an animal with a hippocampectomy plus transection of the stria terminalis (N_{H+St}), and one through a normal hippocampus and stria terminalis is shown from the brain of an animal with an amygdalectomy plus fornix transection (N_{A+Fx}).

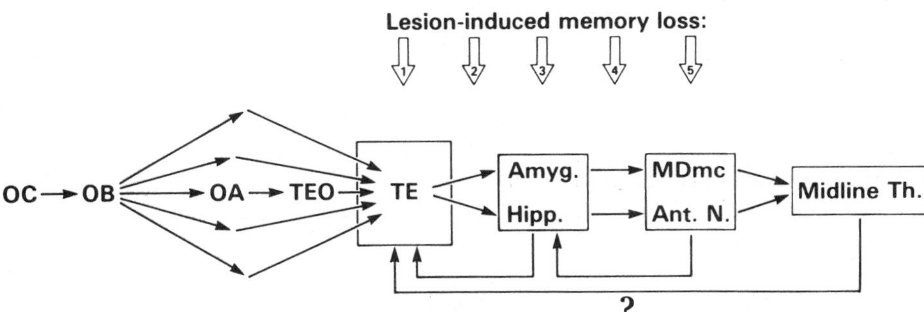

Figure 6. The postulated circuit for visual recognition memory. Visual information is distributed from area OC for submodality processing within the prestriate complex (areas OB, OA, and TEO) and is then reintegrated in area TE. The convergent inputs to area TE are stored as central representations of stimuli, provided that area TE activates either an amygdalo-thalamic or hippocampo-thalamic pathway, which then feeds back to strengthen the prestriate–TE synapses either through reciprocal connections or via a relay in the midline thalamus. Severe visual recognition losses have been induced by lesions at each of the five indicated loci. See text for further explanation. MDmc, magnocellular portion of the dorsomedial nucleus; Ant. N., anterior nuclei.

of this localization of the store is one that derives from the clinical syndrome of global amnesia following either medial temporal or medial thalamic injury. In this syndrome, the amnesia is mainly anterograde in nature, the patient being unable to lay down new memories of people, places, and events; old memories, on the other hand, except perhaps for those formed within a year or two of the cerebral injury, are ordinarily spared (Milner 1970; Cohen & Squire 1981). The conclusion seems inescapable that the older memories were stored upstream from both the limbic system and the medial thalamus, presumably within the cortical areas on which the limbic system and medial thalamus have the greatest influence. This conclusion fits exactly the proposed scheme for the establishment of central representations, which requires some feedback action by the subcortical portions of the system on the convergent prestriate–TE projections in order to close the automatic rehearsal or imprinting circuit. In the absence of any direct functional evidence regarding such feedback, two different but mutually compatible suggestions are offered in the summary diagram. One possibility simply entails reciprocal connections along the cortico-limbo-thalamic pathway, whereas the other postulates a role for diffuse cortical projections from the midline thalamic nuclei (Herkenham 1980) with which the medial thalamic nuclei may be connected.

Two further features of the proposed recognition memory circuit require comment. The first concerns the generalizability of the circuit to other sensory systems, through substitution of the cortical components of these other systems for those of the visual system. Since all the sensory modalities appear to be represented centrally by a hierarchical arrangement of primary, secondary and higher-order processing areas, and since the highest cortical level in each modality appears to project to both the amydala and the hippocampus (Van Hoesen & Pandya 1975; Turner *et al.* 1980), it is reasonable to suppose that the same circuit that mediates recognition memory in vision does so in the other sensory modalities as well, and perhaps according to the same basic set of principles.

Finally, at least some acknowledgement must be made of the unusual practice that has been followed here of treating the amygdala and the hippocampus as a single functional unit. In fact, from the standpoint of the recognition memory circuit, all of our experimental evidence so far does point to the nearly complete equivalence of these two structures, as well as of their projections to, and of their targets in, the medial thalamus. In short, with regard to the formation and storage of central representations of stimuli in association cortex, the parallel amygdalo-thalamic and hippocampo-thalamic systems appear to provide nearly complete substitutes for each other, such that the contribution of each to the recognition process becomes apparent only when both systems are damaged together. At the same time, reference was made earlier to other uses of stored central representations, specifically in the formation and recall of associations with the central representations of other stimuli and events, whether affective, spatial or motor. It is undoubtedly within this realm of associative as distinct from recognition memory that a clear separation between amygdaloid and hippocampal function will emerge.

I am indebted to Leon Dorsey for the testing of the animals and to Barbara Malamut and Ann Sutherland for help with the preparation of the manuscript.

References

Aggleton, J. P. & Mishkin, M. 1981 Recognition impairment after medial thalamic lesions in monkeys. *Soc. Neurosci. Abstr.* **7**, 236.

Allman, J. M. 1977 Evolution of the visual system in the early primates. *Prog. Psychobiol. Physiol. Psychol.* **7**, 1–53.

Blake, L., Jarvis, C. D. & Mishkin, M. 1977 Pattern discrimination thresholds after partial inferior temporal or lateral striate lesions in the monkey. *Brain Res.* **120**, 209–220.

Bonin, G. von & Bailey, P. 1947 *The neocortex of Macaca mulatta.* (163 pages.) Urbana: University of Illinois Press.

Cohen, N. J. & Squire, L. R. 1981 Retrograde amnesia and remote memory impairment. *Neuropsychologia* **19**, 337–356.

Cowey, A. 1981 Why are there so many visual areas? In *The organization of the cerebral cortex* (ed. F. O. Schmitt, F. G. Worden, G. Adelman & S. G. Dennis), pp. 395–413. Cambridge, Mass.: M.I.T. Press.

Gaffan, D. 1974 Recognition impaired and association intact in the memory of monkeys after transection of the fornix. *J. comp. Physiol. Psychol.* **86**, 1100–1109.

Herkenham, M. 1980 Laminar organization of thalamic projections to the rat neocortex. *Science, Wash.* **207**, 532–534.

Iwai, E. & Mishkin, M. 1968 Two visual foci in the temporal lobe of monkeys. In *Neurophysiological basis of learning and behavior* (ed. N. Yoshii & N. A. Buchwald), pp. 1–11. Osaka: Osaka Univ. Press.

Jarvis, C. D., Mishkin, M., Shinohara, M., Sakurada, O., Miyoaka, M. & Kennedy, C. 1978 Mapping the primate visual system with the (^{14}C)2-deoxyglucose technique. *Soc. Neurosci. Abstr.* **4**, 632.

Jones, B. & Mishkin, M 1972 Limbic lesions and the problem of stimulus–reinforcement associations. *Expl Neurol.* **36**, 362–377.

Manning, F. J. & Mishkin, M. 1976 Further evidence on dissociation of visual deficits following partial inferior temporal lesions in monkeys. *Soc. Neurosci. Abstr.* **2**, 1126.

McEntee, W. J., Biber, M. P., Perl, D. P. & Benson, D. F. 1976 Diencephalic amnesia: a reappraisal. *J. Neurol. Neurosurg. Psychiat.* **39**, 436–440.

Merzenich, M. M. & Kaas, J. H. 1980 Principles of organization of sensory-perceptual systems in mammals. *Prog. Psychobiol. Physiol. Psychol.* **9**, 1–42.

Milner, B. 1970 Memory and the medial temporal regions of the brain. In *Biology of memory* (ed. K. H. Pribram & D. E. Broadbent), pp. 29–50. New York: Academic Press.

Mishkin, M. 1954 Visual discrimination performance following partial ablations of the temporal lobe. II. Ventral surface *vs* hippocampus. *J. comp. Physiol. Psychol.* **47**, 187–193.

Mishkin, M. 1966 Visual mechanisms beyond the striate cortex. In *Frontiers of physiological psychology* (ed. R. Russell), pp. 93–119. New York: Academic Press.

Mishkin, M. 1972 Cortical visual areas and their interaction. In *The brain and human behavior* (ed. A. G. Karczmar & J. C. Eccles), pp. 187–208. New York: Springer-Verlag.

Mishkin, M. 1978 Memory in monkeys severly impaired by combined but not by separate removal of amygdala and hippocampus. *Nature, Lond.* **273**, 297–298

Mishkin, M. 1979 Analogous neural models for tactual and visual learning. *Neuropsychologia* **17**, 139–151.

Mishkin, M. & Aggleton, J. P. 1981 Multiple functional contributions of the amygdala in the monkey. In *The amygdaloid complex* (ed. M. Y. Ben-Ari), pp. 409–420. New York: Elsevier.

Mishkin, M. & Delacour, J. 1975 An analysis of short-term visual memory in the monkey. *J. exp. Psychol. Anim. Behav. Processes* **1**, 326–334.

Mishkin, M. & Oubre, J. L. 1977 Dissociation of deficits on visual memory tasks after inferior temporal and amygdala lesions in monkeys. *Soc. Neurosci. Abstr.* **2**, 1127.

Mishkin, M. & Saunders, R. C. 1979 Degree of memory impairment in monkeys related to amount of conjoint damage to amygdaloid and hippocampal systems. *Soc. Neurosci. Abstr.* **5**, 320.

Mishkin, M., Spiegler, B. J., Saunders, R. C. & Malamut, B. L. 1982 An animal model of global anmesia. In *Alzheimer's disease: A review of progress* (ed. S. Corkin, K. L. Davis, J. H. Growden, E. Usdin & R. J. Wurtman), pp. 235–247. New York: Raven Press.

Murray, E. A. & Mishkin, M. 1981 Role of the amygdala and hippocampus in tactual memory. *Soc. Neurosci. Abstr.* **7**, 237.

Rocha-Miranda, C. E., Bender, D. B., Gross, C. G. & Mishkin, M. 1975 Visual activation of neurons in inferotemporal cortex depends on striate cortex and the forebrain commissures. *J. Neurophysiol.* **38**, 475–491.

Spiegler, B. J. & Mishkin, M. 1981 Evidence for the sequential participation of inferior temporal cortex and amygdala in the acquisition of stimulus–reward associations. *Behav. Brain Res.* **3**, 303–317.

Turner, B. H., Mishkin, M. & Knapp, M. 1980 Organization of the amygdalopetal projections from modality-specific cortical association areas in the monkey. *J. comp. Neurol.* **191**, 515–543.

Ungerleider, L. G. & Mishkin, M. 1982 Two cortical visual systems. In *Analysis of visual behavior* (ed. D. J. Ingle, R. J. W. Mansfield & M. A. Goodale), pp. 549–586. Cambridge, Mass.: M.I.T. Press.

Van Hoesen, G. W. & Pandya, D. N. 1975 Some connections of the entorhinal (area 28) and perirhinal (area 35) cortices of the rhesus monkey. III. Efferent connections. *Brain Res.* **95**, 39–59.

Victor, M., Adams, R. D. & Collins, G. H. 1971 *The Wernicke–Korsakoff syndrome*. Oxford: Blackwell.

Yaginuma, S., Niihara, T. & Iwai, E. 1982 Further evidence on elevated discrimination limens for reduced patterns in monkeys with inferotemporal lesions. *Neuropsychologia*. (In the press.)

Zeki, S. M. 1978 Functional specialization in the cortex of the rhesus monkey. *Nature, Lond.* **274**, 423–428.

40

L. R. Squire

Mechanisms of memory

1989. In *Molecules to Models: Advances in Neuroscience*, edited by K. L. Kelner and D. E. Koshland. Washington, D.C.: American Association for the Advancement of Science

Most species are able to adapt in the face of events that occur during an individual lifetime. Experiences modify the nervous system, and as a result animals can learn and remember. One powerful strategy for understanding memory has been to study the molecular and cellular biology of plasticity in individual neurons and their synapses, where the changes that represent stored memory must ultimately be recorded (*1*). Indeed, behavioral experience directly modifies neuronal and synaptic morphology (*2*). Of course, the problem of memory involves not only the important issue of how synapses change, but also questions about the organization of memory in the brain. Where is memory stored? Is there one kind of memory or are there many? What brain processes or systems are involved in memory and what jobs do they do? In recent years, studies of complex vertebrate nervous systems, including studies in humans and other primates, have begun to answer these questions.

Memory Storage: Distributed or Localized?

The collection of neural changes representing memory is commonly known as the engram (*3*), and a major focus of contemporary work has been to identify and locate engrams in the brain. The brain is organized so that separate regions of neocortex simultaneously carry out computations on specific features or dimensions of the external world (for example, visual patterns, location, and movement). The view of memory that has emerged recently, although it still must be regarded as hypothesis, is that information storage is tied to the specific processing areas that are engaged during learning (*4, 5*). Memory is stored as changes in the same neural systems that ordinarily participate in perception, analysis, and processing of the information to be learned. For example, in the visual system, the inferotemporal cortex (area TE) is the last in a sequence of visual pattern-analyzing mechanisms that begins in the striate cortex (*6*). Cortical area TE has been proposed to be not only a higher order visual processing region, but also a repository of the visual memories that result from this processing (*4*).

The idea that information storage is localized in specific areas of the cortex differs from the well-known conclusion of Lashley's classic work (*7*) that memory is widely and equivalently distributed throughout large brain regions. In his most famous study, Lashley showed that, when rats relearned a maze problem after a cortical lesion, the number of trials required for relearning was proportional to the extent of the lesion and was unrelated to its location. Yet Lashley's results are consistent with the modern view if one supposes that the maze habit depends on many kinds of information (for example, visual, spatial, and olfactory) and that each kind of information is separately processed and localized. Indeed, the brain regions, or functional units, within which information is equivalently distributed may be very small (*5, 8*). Thus, memory is localized in the sense that particular brain systems represent specific aspects of each event (*9*), and it is distributed in the sense that many neural systems participate in representing a whole event.

The Neuropsychological-Neural Systems Approach

One useful strategy for learning about the neural organization of memory has been to study human memory pathology. In some patients with brain injury or disease, memory impairment occurs as a circumscribed disorder in the absence of other cognitive deficits. Careful study of these cases has led to a number of insights into how the brain accomplishes learning and memory (*10–12*). Moreover, animal models of human amnesia have recently been developed in the monkey (*4, 13*) and rat (*14*). Animal models make it possible to identify the specific neural structures that when damaged produce the syndrome, and they set the stage for more detailed biological studies.

It has been known for nearly 100 years that memory is impaired by bilateral damage to either of two brain regions—the medial aspect of the temporal lobe and the midline of the diencephalon. Damage to these areas makes it difficult to establish new memories (anterograde amnesia) as well as to retrieve some memories formed before the onset of amnesia (retrograde amnesia). General intellectual capacity is intact, as is immediate memory (for example, the ability to repeat correctly six or seven digits), language and social skills, personality, and memory for the remote past, especially childhood. Because amnesia can occur against a background of normal cognition, the severity of the condition is often underappreciated. For example, patient N.A. (an example of diencephalic amnesia) became amnesic in 1960 after an accident with a miniature fencing foil (*15*). Radiographic (CT) evidence identified damage in the left mediodorsal thalamic nucleus (*16*). More recent evidence from magnetic resonance imaging identified a larger diencephalic lesion involving thalamus and hypothalamus (*17*). This patient is a pleasant man with an agreeable sense of humor, who could join in any social activity without special notice. However, he would be unable to learn the names of his colleagues, or keep up with a developing conversation, or speak accurately about public events that have occurred since his injury. He has an intelligence quotient (IQ) of 124, can make accurate predictions of his own memory abilities (*18*), and has no noticeable impairment of higher cognitive functions except a severe verbal memory problem.

Medial temporal amnesia is best illustrated by the noted amnesic patient H.M. (*19*), who sustained a bilateral resection of the medial temporal lobes in 1953 in an effort to relieve severe epileptic seizures. Since that time, H.M. has exhibited profound anterograde amnesia, forgetting the events of daily life almost as fast as they occur. His defect in memory extends to both verbal and nonverbal material, and it involves information acquired through all sensory modalities. Other etiologies of diencephalic and medial temporal amnesia have also contributed useful information, including Korsakoff's syndrome (*20*), electroconvulsive therapy (*21*), anoxia and ischemia (*22*), and encephalitis (*23*).

Short-Term and Long-Term Memory

The study of amnesia has provided strong evidence for distinguishing between a capacity-limited immediate (sometimes called short-term) memory, which is intact in amnesia, and more long-lasting (long-term) memory, which is impaired (*10, 24*). Amnesic patients can keep a short list of numbers in mind for several minutes if they rehearse them and hold their attention to the task. The difficulty comes when the amount of material to be remembered exceeds what can be held in immediate memory or when recovery of even a small amount of material is attempted after an intervening period of distraction. Immediate memory is independent of the medial temporal and diencephalic regions damaged in amnesia. One possibility is that immediate memory is an intrinsic capacity of each cortical processing system (*25*). Thus, temporary information storage may occur within each brain area where stable changes in synaptic efficacy (long-term memory) can eventually develop. The capacity for long-term memory requires the integrity of the medial temporal and diencephalic regions, which must operate in conjunction with the assemblies of neurons that represent stored information.

Declarative and Nondeclarative Knowledge

In addition to a distinction between short-term and long-term memory functions, recent findings demonstrate a further distinction within the domain of long-term memory. The memory deficit in amnesia is narrower than previously thought in that not all kinds of learning and memory are affected. Amnesic patients (i) demonstrate intact learning and retention of certain motor, perceptual, and cognitive skills and (ii) exhibit intact priming effects: that is, their performance, like that of normal subjects, can be influenced by recent exposure to stimulus material. Both skill learning and priming effects can occur in amnesic patients without their conscious awareness of prior study sessions and without recognition, as measured by formal tests, of the previously presented stimulus material.

Skill learning has been studied in subjects being taught to read words that are mirror-reversed (Fig. 1) (*26*). For normal subjects, the ability to read mirror-reversed words improved gradually during 2 days of practice and was then maintained at a high level for more than a month. Skill learning in amnesia was studied in

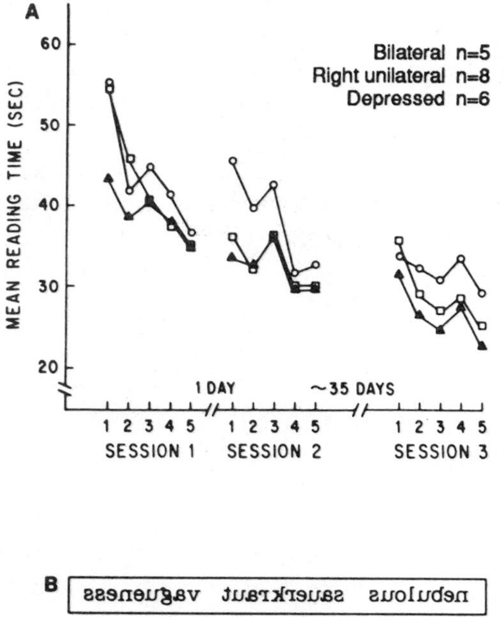

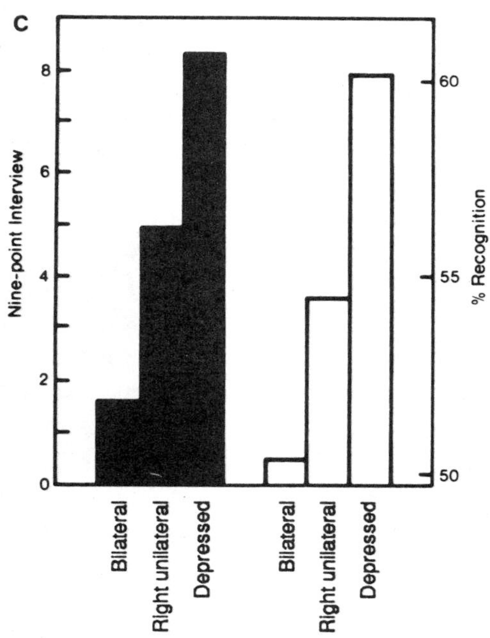

Fig. 1. Learning and retention of a mirror-reading skill despite amnesia for the learning experience (*26*). (**A**) Patients prescribed bilateral or right unilateral ECT and depressed patients not receiving ECT practiced mirror-reading during three sessions on three different days (three words per trial, 50 trials per session). The time required to read each word triad aloud during each block of ten trials provided the measure of mirror-reading skill. The first ECT of the prescribed series intervened between practice sessions 1 and 2. An average of seven ECT's and a total of 35 days intervened between practice sessions 2 and 3. (**B**) Sample word triad from the mirror-reading test. (**C**) At the beginning of session 3, subjects were tested for their recollection of the previous learning sessions (nine-point interview) and for their ability to recognize the words they had read (chance, 50%).

psychiatric patients whose memories were temporarily impaired as a result of a prescribed course of electroconvulsive therapy (ECT). Patients improved their mirror-reading skill at a normal rate and later retained the skill at a normal level (Fig. 1). Yet the same patients, unlike control subjects, could not recognize the words that they had read during the training sessions, and often they could not recall the training experience at all. Other kinds of amnesic patients also exhibit intact learning and retention of the mirror-reading skill (*27*).

Priming can be tested by presenting words and then providing the first three letters of the words as cues (*28*). The instructions determine the outcome (*29*). When subjects are instructed to use the three-letter fragments (each of which can form at least ten common words) as cues to retrieve recently presented words from memory, normal subjects perform better than amnesic patients. Amnesic patients perform normally only when subjects are directed away from the memory aspects of the task and are asked instead to complete each three-letter fragment to form the first word that comes to mind (Fig. 2).

Intact priming effects in amnesia can also be demonstrated in free association tests (*30*) and when recently presented words are cued by category names (*31*). For example, when the word *baby* had been presented, the probability was more than doubled that this word would later be elicited by instructions to free associate a single response to the word *child* (Fig. 2). In fact, priming effects in amnesia can be fully intact even when attempts to recall the words from memory fail altogether (*30*) and when multiple-choice recognition memory is no better than chance (*32*). Thus priming effects seem to be independent of the processes of recall and recognition memory. In the word-completion task, the words seem to "pop" into mind, yet

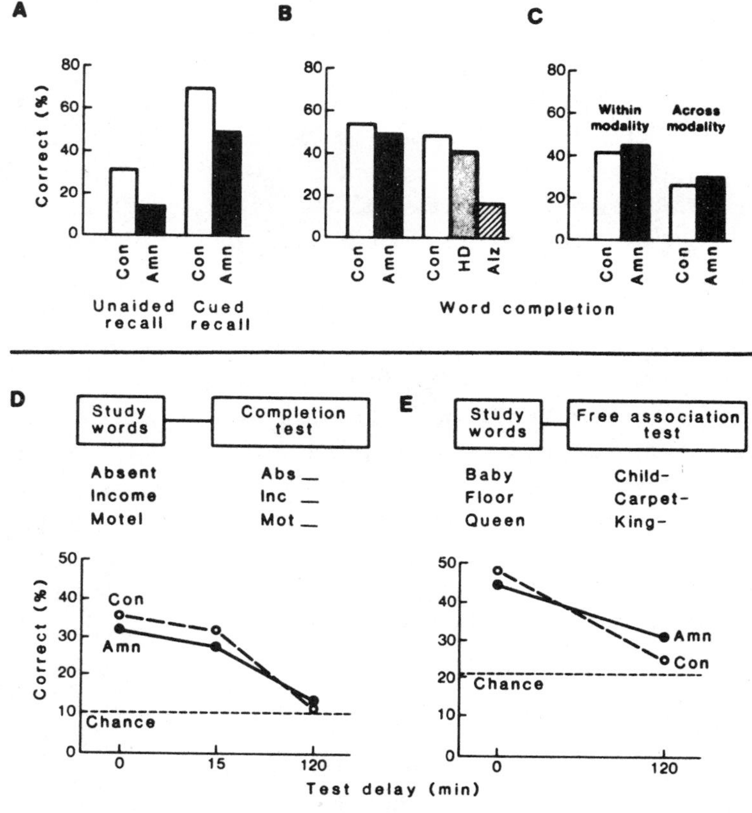

Fig. 2. Intact priming effects in amnesia (*29–31, 44*). Subjects studied words like those in (**D**) and (**E**) and then were tested in one of several ways. (**A**) Amnesic (Amn) patients were impaired at unaided recall and at cued recall, where the first three letters of the study words were given as cues. (**B**) Amnesic patients exhibited normal word completion effects (priming), where they completed each three-letter fragment with the first word that came to mind. Amnesic patients produced the study words as frequently as control (Con) subjects (chance, 10%). Patients with dementia resulting from Huntington's disease (HD) also exhibited intact priming effects, but priming effects were reduced in patients with dementia due to early-stage Alzheimer's disease (Alz). (**C**) When the study words and the three-letter fragments were presented in different sensory modalities (auditory-visual) rather than the same modality (visual-visual), priming effects were attenuated. (**D**) Priming effects were transient. (**E**) Amnesic patients exhibited normal free association (semantic priming) effects. (**B** and **E**) The amnesic patients were patients with Korsakoff's syndrome, $n = 7$ or 8; (**A**, **C**, and **D**) the amnesic patients were patients with Korsakoff's syndrome, $n = 7$ or 8, plus two cases of anoxic or ischemic amnesia. Control subjects, $n = 8$ to 20; Huntington's disease, $n = 8$; Alzheimer's disease, $n = 8$.

amnesic patients are unable to recognize them as familiar. Studies of normal subjects have also emphasized the differences between priming and standard recall and recognition tests (*33*).

These results suggest a distinction between at least two kinds of memory (*12, 34, 36*), a distinction that is reminiscent of earlier accounts in psychology and philosophy about how knowledge is represented (*35, 37*). The kind of memory that is impared in amnesia has been termed declarative memory. It is accessible to conscious awareness and includes the facts, episodes, lists, and routes of everyday life. It can be declared, that is, it can be brought to mind verbally as a proposition or nonverbally as an image. It includes both episodic memory (specific time-and-place events) and semantic memory (facts and general information gathered in the course of specific experiences) (*38, 39*). Declarative memory depends on the integrity of the neural systems damaged in amnesia as well as on the particular neural systems that store the information being learned.

In contrast, examples of intact learning in amnesia are implicit and accessible only through performance. The term "procedural" has been used to describe these intact abilities (*12, 34*). This term aptly applies to skill learning, but the similarities and differences between the various examples of preserved abilities are still poorly understood (e.g., skill learning and priming), so that it may be better to refer to them specifically (*40*). Indeed, the preserved abilities are collectively better described by a negative feature (they lack the characteristics of declarative knowledge, i.e., they are nondeclarative) than by any positive feature that can be identified at this time.

Nondeclarative memory seems to be embedded in specific procedures or stored as tunings, biases, or activations. In these cases, experience culminates in behavioral change without requiring conscious recollection of the learning episodes. Skill learning may depend on the participation of the extrapyramidal motor system (*41*). In priming, preexisting representations are activated (*42*), and the information that is acquired is implicit (*43*). Priming effects may depend exclusively on intact cortical representations because they are reduced in patients with dementia resulting from early stage Alzheimer's disease but not in anmesic patients with equivalently severe memory problems and not in patients with dementia resulting from Huntington's disease (*44*). The finding that skill learning and priming can be doubly dissociated (*45*) emphasizes the point that nondeclarative memory is heterogeneous.

Priming effects are distinct from declarative memory in two other important respects. (i) The information acquired by priming is fully accessible only through the same sensory modality in which material was presented initially (*31*). More complex information learned by amnesic patients may sometimes have this same feature; that is, it is inflexible, and the correct responses are accessible only if precisely the same stimuli that were used during learning are presented (*46*). (ii) Priming effects are short-lived in amnesic patients, declining to baseline in about 2 hours. When the task has only one common solution (for example, ***juice*** for ***jui--*** or ***assassin*** for ***a--a--in***), normal subjects exhibit word completion effects that last for days or weeks. However, amnesic patients exhibit such effects for only a few hours (*47*). It may be easy for normal subjects to use ordinary memory strategies in these circumstances. At the same time, it remains possible that priming could last longer under other conditions.

A number of considerations suggest that nondeclarative learning is phylogenetically old (*5*). It may have developed as a collection of encapsulated, special-purpose learning abilities (*48*). Memory was then realized as cumulative changes stored within the particular neural systems engaged during learning. By this view, some simple forms of associative learning, which occur in invertebrates (*49*) and are prominently developed in mammals (*50*), are examples of nondeclarative learning. These would be expected to be fully available to amnesic patients (*51*). In contrast, the capacity for declarative knowledge is phylogenetically recent, reaching its greatest development in mammals with the full elaboration of medial temporal structures, especially the hippocampal formation and associated cortical areas. This capacity allows an animal to record and access the particular encounters that led to behavioral change. The stored memory is flexible and accessible to all modalities.

The evidence thus supports the idea that the brain has organized its memory functions around fundamentally different information storage systems (Fig. 3). This notion necessarily accepts the concepts of conscious and unconscious memory as serious topics for experimental work. In most cases the same experience would engage both memory systems. For example, perception of a word transiently activates the preexisting assembly of neural elements whose conjoint activity corresponds to that perception. This activation subserves the priming effect, an unconscious process that temporarily facilitates processing of the same word and associated words. The same stimulus also establishes a longer lasting declarative, and conscious, memory that the word was seen, and seen at a particular time and place, through participation of the neural systems within the medial temporal and diencephalic regions.

Memory Consolidation and Retrograde Amnesia

Memory is not fixed at the moment of learning but continues to stabilize (or consolidate) with the passage of time. When this concept was first advanced in 1900 (*52*), strong support for it was found in the phenomenon of temporally graded retrograde amnesia (*53*). For example, when rats or mice are given electroconvulsive shock (ECS) after training, they later exhibit impaired memory for the training experience. As the interval between learning and ECS increases, the severity of retrograde amnesia decreases. In these studies, memory was usually susceptible to disruption from a few seconds to several minutes after initial learning (*54*). A number of treatments given shortly after learning, including drugs and hormones, can also influence the strength of memory (*55*). In contrast to these data from laboratory animals, clinical observations of human amnesia have suggested that temporally graded retrograde amnesia can have a much longer time scale (*56*). Thus, although the facts of retrograde amnesia support the idea that memory changes or consolidates after learning, it has been difficult to determine exactly what consolidation is or how long it lasts.

More recent findings have elaborated the concept of memory consolidation and brought the data from experimental animals and from humans into register. These findings suggest that memory consolidation is a dynamic feature of long-term, declarative memory. Consolidation can proceed for many years, during which time memory depends on the integrity of the neural systems that have been damaged in amnesic patients (*57, 58*). One relevant finding was that, in humans, temporal gradients of retrograde amnesia longer than 1 year could be

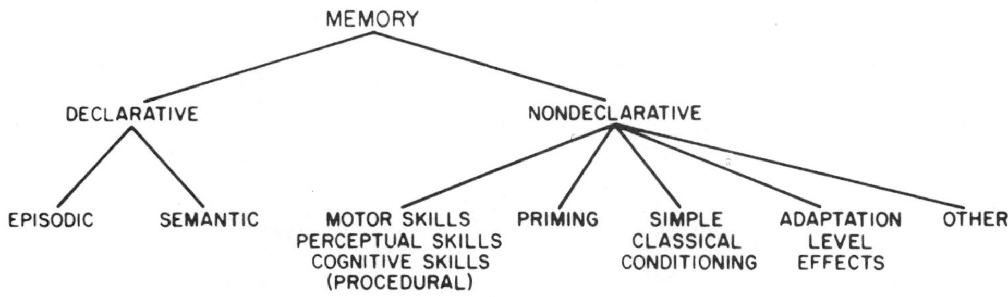

Fig. 3. A tentative taxonomy of memory. Declarative memory includes episodic and semantic memory (*38*), as well as the related terms, working and reference memory (*99*). Declarative memory can be retrieved explicitly as a proposition or image. Nondeclarative memory includes skills, priming effects, simple classical conditioning (*51*), adaptation-level effects (*100*), habituation, sensitization, and perceptual aftereffects, instances where what has been learned can be expressed only through performance.

substantiated with formal tests. Patients prescribed ECT were given a test about television programs that had been broadcast for only one season during the past 16 years. The use of popularity ratings and other criteria permitted the test to be designed so that past time periods could be sampled equivalently (*59*). Before ECT, patients exhibited a forgetting curve across the time period sampled by the test, performing best for recent time periods and worst for remote ones. One hour after the fifth treatment, at a time when verbal IQ was intact, memory was selectively impaired for programs that had broadcast 1 to 2 years previously. Memory for older programs was normal (*60*). Temporally limited retrograde amnesia after ECT has also been demonstrated with other remote memory tests (*61, 62*).

Continuity between studies in humans and in experimental animals was established by a study of retrograde amnesia in mice, which used multiple, spaced ECS to mimic the treatment associated with extensive retrograde amnesia in humans (Fig. 4). Four ECS treatments produced a graded impairment for one-trial passive avoidance learning that covered 1 to 3 weeks (*63*). Thus, in mice, memory for the one-trial experience persisted for at least 12 weeks, and memory grew resistant to disruption during the first few weeks after training. In humans, memory for television programs persisted for more than 16 years, and memory remained susceptible to disruption for a few years after initial learning. In both cases, retrograde amnesia covered a significant portion of the lifetime of the memory. Thus, initial acquisition of information was followed by two parallel events: gradual forgetting and gradually developing resistance to disruption of what remained.

These findings suggest that memory consolidation is neither an automatic process with a fixed lifetime nor a process that is determined entirely at the time of learning. Consolidation best refers to a hypothesized process of reorganization within representations of stored information, which continues as long as information is being forgotten. Memory is affected by rehearsal and by subsequent memory storage episodes. These events may influence the fate of recent, and unconsolidated, memories by remodeling the neural circuitry underlying the original representation or by establishing new representations. As time passes, some parts of the initial representation could be lost through forgetting, while other parts become more stable and coherent. In this sense, neural ensembles representing stored information could continually reorganize as they accommodate new information. The process of memory storage and consolidation may be competitive (*5*), in the same way that competition among axons occurs in the developing nervous system (*64*). Dynamic and presumably competitive changes have also been described in the representation of the hand in adult primate sensorimotor cortex after both deprivation and selective experience (*65*).

The processes of memory storage and consolidation can be related to the brain structures damaged in amnesia. In particular, remote memory tests have demonstrated that in some

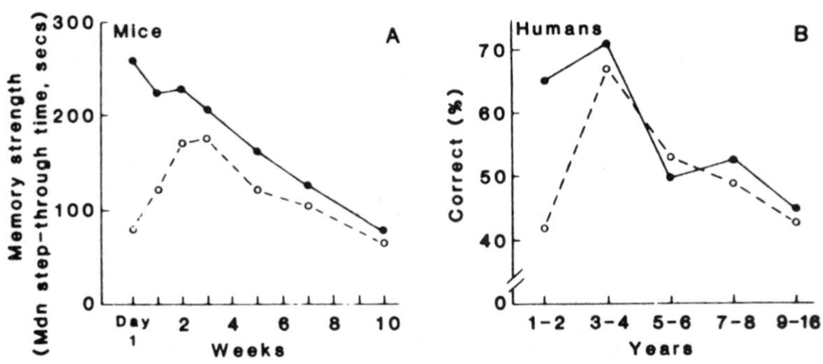

Fig. 4. Temporally limited retrograde amnesia in mice given ECS and in depressed psychiatric inpatients prescribed ECT (*60, 63*). (**A**) Mice were given a single training trial and then ECS or sham treatment (four treatments at hourly intervals) at one of seven times after training (1 to 70 days). Retention was always tested 2 weeks after ECS. (**B**) Patients were given a test about single-season television programs (from 1 to 16 years old) before the first and after the fifth in a prescribed course of bilateral ECT. In both cases, the abscissa shows the age of the memory at the time of treatment. Symbols: ●, normal forgetting; o, retrograde amnesia. Abbreviation: Mdn, median.

amnesic patients with medial temporal lesions retrograde amnesia is both extensive and temporally limited, affecting events that occurred during the years preceding the onset of amnesia. For example H.M., who has bilateral medial temporal lesions, exhibits amnesia extending from a few years to perhaps 11 years before his surgery in 1953 (*19, 66*). He can both produce well-formed autobiographical episodes and also recall information about public events that occurred before surgery. Other patients with medial temporal amnesia [for example, patient R.B. (*67*)], are reported to have no measurable retrograde amnesia, or perhaps 2 or 3 years of retrograde amnesia, despite marked anterograde amnesia. Still other patients with well-circumscribed amnesia exhibit retrograde amnesia covering 10–20 years (*58*). Finally, some patients exhibit prolonged and extensive retrograde amnesia without evidence of a temporal gradient (*23, 68*), but damage beyond the medial temporal region has either been demonstrated in these instances or can be reasonably presumed.

Because amnesic patients have access to many premorbid memories, even to the extent that the quality and detail of their recall cannot be distinguished from that of normal recall (*69*), the medial temporal region cannot be a permanent memory storage site. For the same reason, the deficit seen in amnesia cannot be a general impairment in retrieval. The medial temporal region would seem to do its job during the time of learning and during some or all of the lengthy period of consolidation. Thus, for a period after learning, the storage of declarative memory and its retrieval depend on an interaction between the neural systems damaged in amnesia and memory storage sites located elsewhere in the brain (*4, 5, 70*). This interaction is thought to maintain the organization of an ensemble of distant and distributed memory storage sites until the coherence of these sites has become an intrinsic property of the ensemble. If the interaction is disrupted, the ability to acquire new declarative memory is impaired, and recently acquired memories that have not fully consolidated become unavailable. After sufficient time has passed, at least some memories no longer require the participation of the medial temporal region.

Amnesic patients with diencephalic lesions also exhibit retrograde amnesia. For example, patients with Korsakoff's syndrome exhibit a severe impairment of remote memory that can spare older memories (*58*) or cover most of their adult lives (*62, 71*). One possibility is that amnesia is a unitary deficit affecting both the establishment of new memories and the retrieval of old ones and that the deficit is qualitatively the same reqardless of which part of the system is damaged, medial temporal or diencephalic (*72*). According to this view, the remote memory deficit observed in Korsakoff patients is correlated with and predicted by the severity of their anterograde amnesia. Another possibility is that some forms of remote memory impairment are dissociable from the remainder of the memory disorder (*73*) and that extensive, ungraded remote memory impairment is caused by additional neuropathology beyond that required to produce anterograde amnesia. This idea is supported by the near-zero correlation ($r = 0.04$) between anterograde amnesia and remote memory impairment in patients with Korsakoff's syndrome (*74*); by the finding that patient N.A., an example of diencephalic amnesia, has little remote memory impairment (*62, 69*); and by the finding that patient H.M. has better remote memory than Korsakoff patients, despite having a more profound anterograde amnesia (*66*). More data are needed to better understand the significance of extensive remote memory impairment. It seems reasonable to suppose that the typical Korsakoff patient has more widespread neuropathology than other amnesic patients. For example, even carefully selected study patients have frontal lobe atrophy (*75*). A list of cognitive deficits has accumulated in recent years—deficits that are particularly frequent in this patient group, and that are unrelated to the severity of anterograde amnesia. These include (i) failure to release from proactive interference (*76, 77*)—that is, the normal improvement in performance does not occur when subjects attempt to learn words belonging to a new category after attempting several word lists from another category; (ii) a disproportionately large impairment in making judgments about temporal order (*77*); (iii) impaired metamemory skills—that is, inability to monitor and predict one's own memory performance (*18, 78*); (iv) source amnesia in some Korsakoff patients (*39*)—that is, the successful recall of previously learned information without memory for when or where the information was acquired [also see (*79*)]. The question is whether severe and ungraded remote memory impairment should be added to this list.

Animal Models and the Neuroanatomy of Memory

Careful descriptions of amnesia have helped to define the particular memory function that is damaged and have led to other useful information about how memory is organized in the brain. Yet to understand how the brain actually accomplishes learning and memory, it is essential to identify the specific brain structures that when damaged produce amnesia. This information must then be guided by neuroanatomy to specify a functional brain system consisting of the identified structures and their connections. Clinicopathological material from amnesic patients has generally identified where damage must occur in the brain to produce amnesia: the medial temporal region, with emphasis on the hippocampus; and the midline diencephalic region, with emphasis on the mediodorsal thalamic nucleus and the mammillary nuclei. However, this information has not established precisely which structures and connections are important. Patients frequently have brain lesions in addition to those that cause amnesia. Moreover, patient material seldom includes both detailed neuropathological data and quantitative behavioral information.

Because of the recent development of an animal model of human amnesia in the monkey (*4, 13*), as well as the neuroanatomical information now available about the relevant brain regions in the monkey (*80*), these issues can now be studied systematically. Several behavioral tests of memory that are sensitive to human amnesia have been adapted for the monkey, and memory performance from different studies can be quantified and compared. At the same time, in other animal models progress has been made at identifying where in the brain memory is stored (*81*).

With regard to amnesia and the medial temporal region, interest has focused recently on both the hippocampus and the amygdala. The amygdaloid complex is linked directly and reciprocally to both sensory-specific and multimodal cortical association areas. Afferent and efferent cortical pathways also communicate with the hippocampal formation (*82*), albeit indirectly through polysensory adjacent regions including the perirhinal cortex and the parahippocampal gyrus. These extensive and widespread connections to the cortex are precisely what is needed if the medial temporal lobe is to have access to sites of information processing and memory storage.

Monkeys with bilateral lesions of the amygdala and hippocampal formation, which included perirhinal cortex and parahippocampal gyrus, exhibited severe memory impairment (Fig. 5). This lesion was intended to reproduce the surgical removal sustained by the amnesic patient H.M. As in human amnesia, the memory deficit in monkeys occurred in both visual and tactual modalities (*83*), and it was exacerbated by distracting the animals during the retention interval (*84*). Moreover, as in human amnesia, the same monkeys that were diagnosed as amnesic by these measures acquired perceptual-motor skills normally. They also learned normally skill-like cognitive tasks such as pattern discrimination learning, which, like motor skills, involve stimulus repetition and incremental learning over many trials (*85, 86*). Monkeys with lesions of the "temporal stem," a fiber system that lies superficial to the hippocampus, were not amnesic (*85, 87*). This fiber system links temporal neocortex with subcortical regions, and it had been proposed to be the critical structure damaged in medial temporal lobe amnesia (*88*).

Studies in monkeys have also evaluated the effects on memory of separate hippocampal lesions that included dentate gyrus, subicular cortex, most of the parahippocampal gyrus, and posterior entorhinal cortex (*83, 89–91*) (Fig. 5). Although hippocampal lesions produced a clear memory impairment, the impairment was still larger after the combined hippocampal-amygdaloid lesion. One possibility is that the larger memory impairment is due to amygdala damage (*83, 92*). Alternatively, recent evidence suggests that the larger impairment may result from damage to the cortical structures (anterior entorhinal and perirhinal cortex) that are damaged when the lesion is extended rostrally to include the amygdala (*93*). Thus, the severe memory impairment in monkeys and humans with medial temporal lesions might depend on damage to the hippocampal formation and adjacent, anatomically associated cortex, not on combined hippocampus-amygdala damage.

The anatomy of diencephalic amnesia has also been illuminated by recent studies. Bilateral medial thalamic lesions can cause moderately severe memory impairment (*94, 95*). Memory impairment can also occur following damage to other structures with strong anatomical connections to the medial temporal region and the medial thalamus, such as the mammillary nuclei (in this case perhaps only when additional thalamic damage is present (*96*), ventromedial frontal cortex (*97*), and basal forebrain (*98*). However, further studies are needed to quantify and compare the impairment that follows removal of these and other candidate structures. The amnesic syndrome is not an all-or-none phenomenon, and its severity can vary with the structure or combination of structures that are damaged.

Although animal studies are essential, they cannot illuminate the clinical significance of the observed memory impairments unless the severity of the impairments can be understood in terms of human memory dysfunction. For example, the hippocampus has long been linked to human memory impairment, though there have been few if any well-documented cases of amnesia with damage limited to this structure. Monkeys with hippocampal lesions do have a clear memory impairment. Would this correspond to a substantial memory impairment in humans or only a minor one?

Our laboratory recently obtained extensive clinicopathological information from a patient who developed amnesia at the age of 52 after an ischemic episode (*67*). Until his death 5 years later, he was tested extensively as part of our neuropsychological studies of memory and amnesia. He exhibited marked anterograde amnesia (Fig. 6), little if any retrograde amnesia, and no signs of cognitive impairment other

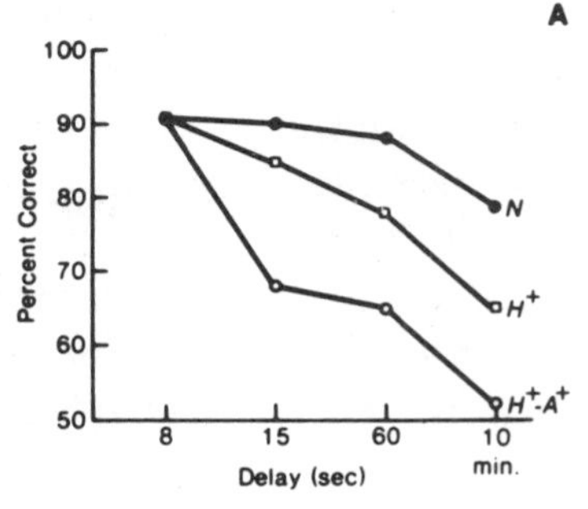

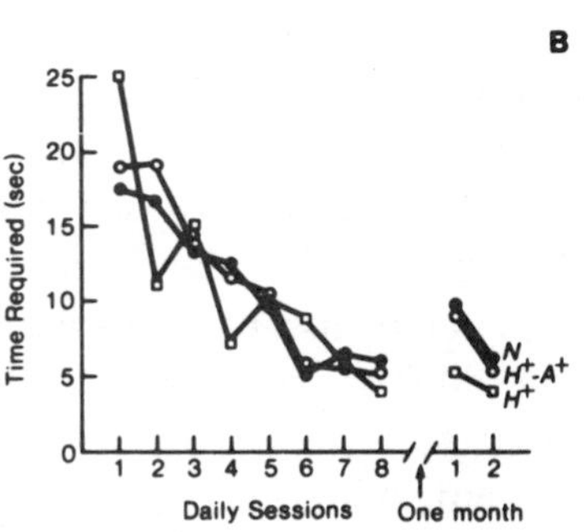

Fig. 5. Impaired recognition memory and intact skill learning in monkeys with medial temporal lesions (*85, 87, 89, 101*). (A) Eight normal (N) monkeys, eight with lesions of the hippocampus plus adjacent cortex (H^+) and four with lesions of hippocampus, amygdala, and adjacent cortex (H^+A^+) were tested on the trial-unique, delayed nonmatching-to-sample task (*102*), a test of recognition memory also failed by amnesic patients (*103*). To obtain a raisin reward, monkeys chose the novel one of two objects, the familiar one having been presented alone 8 seconds to 10 minutes previously. H^+ lesions impaired recognition memory, but conjoint H^+A^+ lesions produced a more severe impairment. Each data point is the average of 50–100 trials. (B) Three monkeys in each group learned to obtain a candy Lifesaver by maneuvering it along a metal rod and around a 90° bend. The rate of learning (six trials per session) was identical in the three groups, and retention was identical after a 1-month delay.

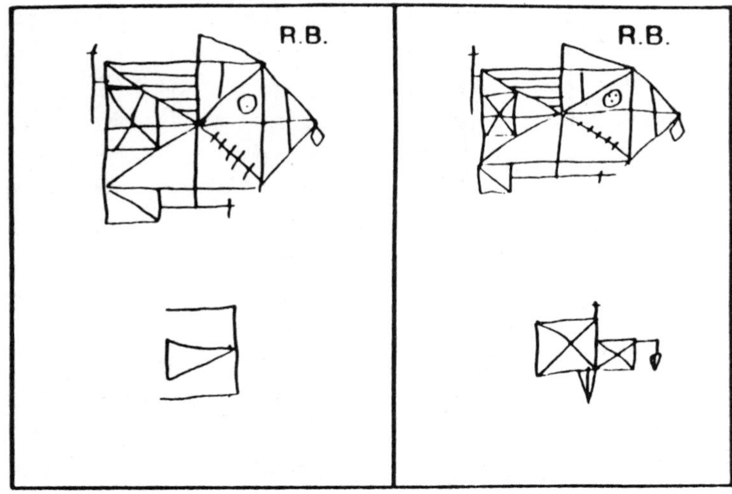

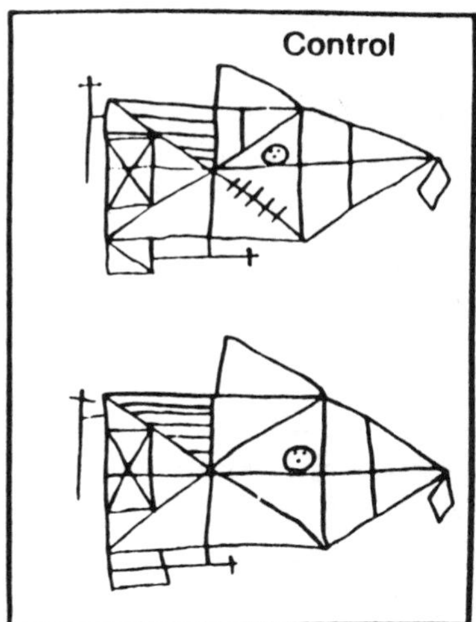

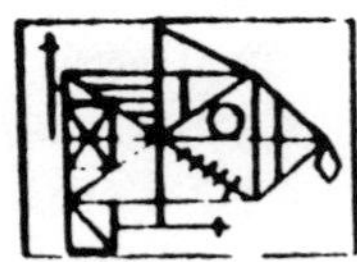

Fig. 6. Performance by amnesic patient R.B. on two separate administrations of the Rey-Osterreith complex figure test (*104*). R.B. was asked to copy the figure illustrated at left. Then 10 to 20 minutes later, without forewarning, he was asked to reproduce it from memory. (**A**) R.B.'s copy (top) and reproduction (bottom) 6 months after the onset of his amnesia. (**B**) His copy and reproduction 23 months after the onset of amnesia. (**C**) Copy and reproduction by a healthy control subject (*67*).

than memory. His score on the Wechsler Adult Intelligence Scale (WAIS) was 111, and his Wechsler Memory Scale (WMS) score was 91. In normal subjects the WMS score is equivalent to the WAIS IQ, and the difference between the two scores provides one index of the severity of memory impairment. Thorough histological examination revealed a circumscribed bilateral lesion of the CA1 field of the hippocampus that extended its full rostral-caudal length but not beyond (Fig. 7). Some additional minor pathology was found (for example, left globus pallidus, right postcentral gyrus, and patchy loss of cerebellar Purkinje cells), but the only damage that could be reasonably associated with the memory defect was the hippocampal lesion.

Although the lesion was spatially limited, it affected an estimated 4.6 million pyramidal cells and would be expected to have a profound impact on the function of the hippocampus. A lesion in the CA1 field interrupts the essentially unidirectional flow of information that begins at the dentate gyrus and ends in the subicular complex and entorhinal cortex. These structures are the main sources of output from the hippocampus to subcortical, limbic, and cortical structures. Thus, a CA1 lesion would significantly disrupt the interaction between the hippocampus and memory storage sites, an interaction presumed to be critical for the storage and consolidation of declarative memory.

Conclusion

In neuroscience, questions about memory have often been focused at the cellular and molecular level—for example, how do synapses change when memory is formed? In psychology, memory has often been studied as whole behavior, without reference to the brain, and as a problem of what computations learning and memory require. This article describes what can be learned from an intermediate, neuropsychological level of analysis, which focuses

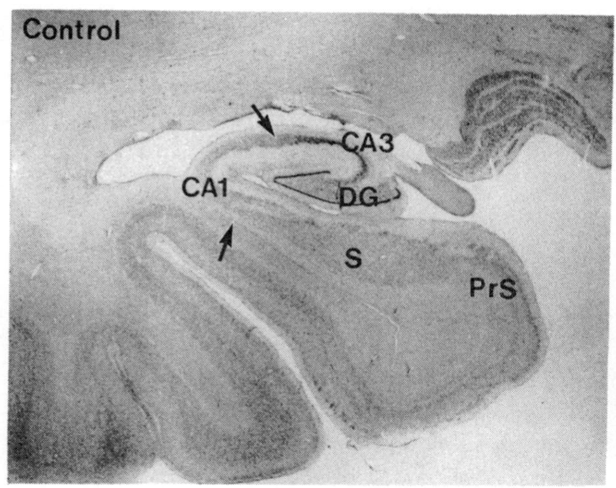

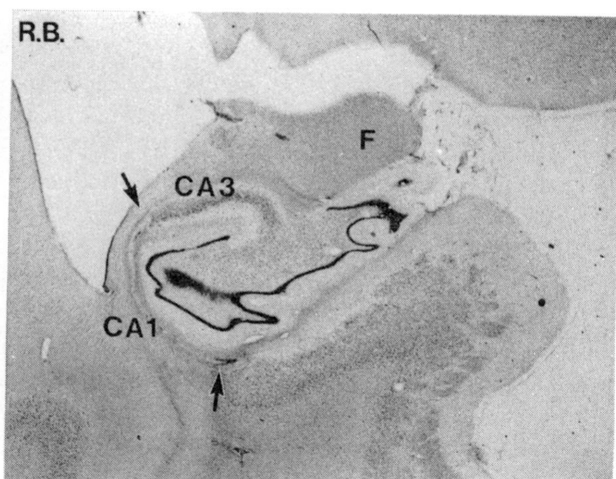

Fig. 7. Photomicrographs of thionin-stained, coronal sections through the hippocampal formation of a normal control brain (**left**) and patient R.B.'s brain (**right**). R.B. developed an amnesic syndrome in 1978 after an ischemic episode. He died in 1983 at the age of 57. Histological examination revealed a bilateral lesion involving the entire CA1 field of the hippocampus. In the control section, the two arrows indicate the limits of the CA1 field. In R.B.'s brain, the only pathology evident in the hippocampal formation was a complete loss of pyramidal cells from the CA1 field (between the arrows). The amygdala, mammillary nuclei, and mediodorsal thalamic nucleus were normal, and there was no other significant pathology that could reasonably account for the memory impairment. Abbreviations: PrS, presubiculum; S, subiculum; CA1 and CA3, fields of the hippocampus; DG, dentate gyrus; F, fimbria of the fornix. (*67*)

on the brain processes and brain systems involved in learning and memory. Study of animals with complex nervous systems, including humans and other primates, has led to a view of memory and the brain that should have considerable generality across vertebrate species, and certainly across all mammals. The ultimate goal is to be able to move across levels of analysis, from formal descriptions of cognition to underlying brain systems and finally to the neurons and cellular events within these systems. The problem of memory needs to be studied at all these levels, and should draw jointly on the disciplines of cognitive psychology, neuropsychology, and neurobiology.

References and Notes

1. E. R. Kandel and J. H. Schwartz, *Science* **218**, 433 (1982); G. Lynch and M. Baudry, *ibid.* **224**, 1057 (1984); J. P. Changeux and M. Konishi, Eds., *Neural and Molecular Mechanisms of Learning* (Springer-Verlag, Berlin, 1987).
2. M. R. Rosenzweig, in *Development and Evolution of Brain Size: Behavioral Implications*, M. E. Hahn, C. Jensen, B. Dudek, Eds. (Academic Press, New York, 1979), pp. 263–294; W. T. Greenough, in *Neurobiology of Learning and Memory*, G. Lynch, J. L. McGaugh, N. M. Weinberger, Eds. (Guilford, New York, 1984), pp. 470–478.
3. R. Semon, *die Mneme als erhaltendes Prinzip im Wechsel des organischen Geschehens* (Wilhelm Engelmann, Leipzig, 1904); D. L. Schacter, *Stranger Behind the Engram* (Erlbaum, Hillsdale, NJ, 1982).
4. M. Mishkin, *Philos. Trans. R. Soc. London Ser. B* **298**, 85 (1982).
5. L. R. Squire, in *Handbook of Physiology: The Nervous System*, J. M. Brookhart and V. B. Mountcastle, Eds. (American Physiological Society, Bethesda, MD, 1987); *Memory and Brain* (Oxford Univ. Press, New York, 1987).
6. C. G. Gross, in *Handbook of Sensory Physiology*, R. Jung, Ed. (Springer-Verlag, Berlin, 1973), pp. 451–452; A. Cowey, in *The Organization of the Cerebral Cortex*, F. O. Schmitt, F. G. Worden, G. Adelman, S. G. Dennis, Eds. (MIT Press, Cambridge, MA, 1981), pp. 395–413; W. Ungerleider and M. Mishkin, in *The Analysis of Visual Behavior*, D. J. Ingle, R. J. W. Mansfield, M. A. Goodale, Eds. (MIT Press, Cambridge, MA, 1982), pp. 549–586.
7. K. S. Lashley, *Brain Mechanisms and Intelligence: A Quantitative Study of Injuries to the Brain* (Univ. of Chicago Press, Chicago, 1929).

8. V. B. Mountcastle, in *The Neurosciences*, F. O. Schmitt and F. G. Worden, Eds. (MIT Press, Cambridge, MA, 1979), pp. 21–42.
9. M. Davis, D. S. Gendelman, M. D. Tischler, P. M. Gendelman, *J. Neurosci.* **2,** 791 (1982); R. F. Thompson, T. W. Berger, J. Madden, *Annu. Rev. Neurosci.* **6,** 447 (1983); D. H. Cohen, in *Memory Systems of the Brain*, N. M. Weinberger, J. L. McGaugh, G. Lynch, Eds. (Guilford, New York, 1985), pp. 27–48.
10. B. Milner, *Clin. Neurosurg.* **19,** 421 (1972); L. Weiskrantz, in *Philos. Trans. R. Soc. London* **298,** 97 (1982); L. S. Cermak, Ed., *Human Memory and Amnesia* (Erlbaum, Hillsdale, NJ, 1982); A. Mayes and P. Meudell, in *Memory in Animals and Humans*, A. Mayes, Ed. (Van Nostrand Reinhold, Berkshire, England, 1983), pp. 203–252.
11. W. Hirst, *Psychol. Bull.* **91,** 435 (1982); D. Schacter, in *Memory Systems of the Brain*, N. M. Weinberger, J. L. McGaugh, G. Lynch, Eds. (Guilford, New York, 1985), pp. 351–379.
12. L. R. Squire and N. J. Cohen, in *Neurobiology of Learning and Memory*, G. Lynch, J. L. McGaugh, N. M. Weinberger, Eds. (Guilford, New York, 1984), pp. 3–64.
13. L. R. Squire and S. Zola-Morgan, in *The Physiological Basis of Memory*, J. A. Deutsch, Ed. (Academic Press, New York, ed. 2, 1983); H. Mahut and M. Moss, in *Neuropsychology of Memory*, L. R. Squire and N. Butters, Eds. (Guilford, New York, 1984), pp. 297–315.
14. D. S. Olton, in *Neuropsychology of Memory*, L. R. Squire and N. Butters, Eds. (Guilford, New York, 1984), pp. 367–373; B. T. Volpe, W. A. Pulsinelli, J. Tribuna, H. P. Davis, *Stroke* **15,** 558 (1984); R. P. Kesner and B. V. DiMattia, in *Neuropsychology of Memory*, L. R. Squire and N. Butters, Eds. (Guilford, New York, 1984), pp. 385–398.
15. H. L. Teuber, B. Milner, H. G. Vaughan, *Neuropsychology* **6,** 267 (1968); P. I. Kaushall, M. Zetin, L. R. Squire, *J. Nerv. Ment. Dis.* **169,** 383 (1981).
16. L. R. Squire and R. Y. Moore, *Ann. Neurol.* **6,** 503 (1979).
17. L. R. Squire, D.G. Amaral, S. Zola-Morgan, M. Kritchevsky, G. Press, *Exp. Neurol.,* in press.
18. A. P. Shimamura and L. R. Squire, *J. Exp. Psychol. Learn. Mem. Cognit.* **12,** 452 (1986).
19. W. B. Scoville and B. Milner, *J. Neurol. Psychiatry* **20,** 11 (1957); S. Corkin, *Semin. Neurol.* **4,** 249 (1984).
20. N. Butters, *Semin. Neurol.* **4,** 226 (1984). M. Victor, R.D. Adams, G.H. Collins, *The Wernicke-Korsadoff Syndrome* (F.A. Davis, Philadelphia, 2nd Ed. 1989).
21. L. R. Squire, in *Basic Mechanisms of ECT*, B. Lerer, R. D. Weiner, R. H. Belmaker, Eds. (Libby, London, 1984), pp. 156–163.
22. B. T. Volpe and W. Hirst, *Arch. Neurol.* **40,** 436 (1983).
23. F. C. Rose and C. P. Symonds, *Brain* **83,** 195 (1960); L. S. Cermak and M. O'Connor, *Neuropsychologia* **21,** 213 (1983); A. R. Damasio, P. J. Eslinger, H. Damasio, G. W. Van Hoesen, S. Cornell, *Arch. Neurol.* **42,** 252 (1985).
24. A. D. Baddeley and E. K. Warrington, *J. Verb. Learn. Verb. Behav.* **9,** 176 (1970); R. C. Atkinson and R. M. Schiffrin, in *The Psychology of Learning and Motivation: Advances in Research and Theory*, K. W. Spence and J. T. Spence, Eds. (Academic Press, New York, 1968), vol. 2, pp. 89–195. This division between short-term and long-term memory expresses an idea at the level of neural systems, not at the level of neurons and synapses. Memory is first in a short-term store for a period of seconds to minutes, depending on rehearsal. The normal operation of the neural systems damaged in amnesia enables storage in and retrieval from long-term memory. The same terms have also been used in a different sense, at the level of single neurons, to describe the temporal sequence of synaptic change that leads to permanent memory.
25. S. Monsell, in *International Symposium on Attention and Performance*, H. Bouma and D. Bouwhuis, Eds. (Erlbaum, Hillsdale, NJ, 1984), vol. 10, pp. 327–350.
26. L. R. Squire, N. J. Cohen, J. A. Zouzounis, *Neuropsychologia* **22,** 145 (1984).
27. N. J. Cohen and L. R. Squire, *Science* **210,** 207 (1980); P. Nichelli, G. Bahmanian-Behbahani, M. Gentilini, A. Vecchi, *Brain* **111,** 1337 (1988).
28. E. K. Warrington and L. Weiskrantz, *Nature (London)* **228,** 628 (1988).
29. P. Graf, L. R. Squire, G. Mandler, *J. Exp. Psychol. Learn. Mem. Cognit.* **10,** 164 (1984).
30. A. P. Shimamura and L. R. Squire, *J. Exp. Psychol. Gen.* **113,** 556 (1984).
31. H. Gardner, F. Boller, J. Moreines, N. Butters, *Cortex* **9,** 165 (1973); P. Graf, A. P. Shimamura, L. R. Squire, *J. Exp. Psychol. Learn. Mem. Cognit.* **11,** 386 (1985).
32. L. R. Squire, A. P. Shimamura, P. Graf, *J. Exp. Psychol. Learn. Mem. Cognit.* **11,** 37 (1985).
33. E. Tulving, D. L. Schacter, H. A. Stark, *ibid.* **8,** 336 (1982); L. L. Jacoby and M. Dallas, *J.*

Exp. Psychol. Gen. **3,** 306 (1981); P. Graf, G. Mandler, P. E. Haden, *Science* **218,** 1243 (1982).

34. N.J. Cohen, thesis, University of California, San Diego (1981).
35. H. Bergson, *Matter and Memory* (Allen & Unwin, London, 1911); G. Ryle, *The Concept of Mind* (Hutchinson, San Francisco, 1949); J. S. Bruner, in *The Pathology of Memory,* G. A. Talland and N. C. Waugh, Eds. (Academic Press, New York, 1969), pp. 253–259.
36. L. R. Squire and S. Zola-Morgan, *Trends in Neurosci.* **11,** 125 (1988).
37. T. Winograd, in *Representation and Understanding: Studies in Cognitive Science*, D. Bobrow and A. Collins, Eds. (Academic Press, New York, 1975), pp. 185–210; J. R. Anderson, *Language, Memory, and Thought* (Erlbaum, Hillsdale, NJ, 1976).
38. E. Tulving, *Elements of Episodic Memory* (Clarendon, Oxford, 1983).
39. A. P. Shimamura and L. R. Squire, *J. Exp. Psychol. Learn. Mem. Cognit.* **13,** 464 (1987).
40. D. L. Schacter, *J. Exp. Psychol. Learn. Mem. Cognit.* **13,** 501 (1987).
41. M. Mishkin, B. Malamut, J. Bachevalier, in *Neurobiology of Learning and Memory*, G. Lynch, J. L. McGaugh, N. M. Weinberger, Eds. (Guilford, New York, 1984), pp. 65–77.
42. L. S. Cermak, N. Talbot, K. Chandler, L. R. Wolbarst, *Neuropsychologia* **23,** 615 (1985).
43. One kind of priming-like effect is reportedly based on the formation of new associations rather than on activation of preexisting representations (after presentation of window-reason, normal subjects show more word completion for window-rea– – – than for officer-rea– – –). This effect does not easily fit an exclusively declarative or nondeclarative classification [D. Schacter, in *Memory Systems of the Brain,* N. M. Weinberger, J. L. McGaugh, G. Lynch, Eds. (Guilford, New York, 1985, pp. 351–379). However, because amnesic patients exhibit markedly impaired priming in this paradigm (A. P. Shimamura and L. R. Squire, *J. Exp. Psychol. Learn. Mem. Cognit.,* in press), it appears that the effect depends importantly on declarative memory. For other possible examples of preserved learning in amnesic patients based on new associations, see M. Moscovitch, G. Winocur, and D. McLachlan, *J. Exp. Psychol. Gen.* **115,** 331 (1986) and M. McAndrews, E. Glisky, and D. Schacter, *Neuropsychologia,* **25,** 497 (1987).
44. A. P. Shimamura, D. Salmon, L. R. Squire, N. Butters, *Behav. Neurosci.* **101,** 347 (1987).
45. W. Heindel, D. Salmon, C. Shults, P. Walicke, N. Butters, *J. Neurosci.* **9,** 582 (1989).
46. E. L. Glisky, D. L. Schacter, E. Tulving, *Neuropsychologia* **24,** 313, (1986); but see A. P. Shimamura and L. R. Squire, *J. Exp. Psychol. Learn. Mem. Cognit.* **14,** 763 (1988).
47. L. R. Squire, A. P. Shimamura, P. Graf, *Neuropsychologia,* **25,** 195 (1987).
48. P. Rozin, *Prog. Psychobiol. Physiol. Psychol.* **6,** 245 (1976).
49. G. J. Mpistos and W. J. Davis, *Science* **180,** 317 (1973); T. J. Chang and A. Gelperin, *Proc. Natl. Acad. Sci. U.S.A.* **77,** 6204 (1980); C. Sahley, A. Gelperin, J. W. Rudy, *ibid.* **78,** 640 (1981); R. D. Hawkins, T. W. Abrams, T. J. Carew, E. R. Kandel, *Science* **219,** 400 (1983); D. L. Alkon, *ibid.* **226,** 1037 (1984).
50. N. J. Mackintosh, *Conditioning and Associative Learning* (Oxford Univ. Press, New York, 1983); R. A. Rescorla and A. R. Wagner, in *Classical Conditioning II: Current Research and Theory*, A. Black and W. Prokasy, Eds. (Appleton-Century-Crofts, New York, 1972), pp. 64–99.
51. L. Weiskrantz and E. K. Warrington, *Neuropsychologia* **17,** 187 (1979); I. Daum, S. Channon, A. Canavan, *J. Neurol., Neurosurg., Psychiatry,* **52,** 47, (1989); see N.J. Mackintosh [in *Memory Systems of the Brain,* N.M. Weinberger, J.L. McGaugh, G. Lynch, Eds. (Guilford, New York, 1985), pp. 335-350] for a discussion of how some classical conditioning paradigms can produce both declarative and procedural knowledge; see R.T. Ross, W.B. Orr, P.C. Holland, T.W. Berger [*Behav. Neurosci. 98,* 211 (1984) for examples of classical conditioning that are affected by hippocampal lesions.
52. G. E. Muller and A. Pilzecker, *Z. Psychol.* **1,** 1 (1900).
53. W. H. Burnham, *Am. J. Psychol.* **14,** 382 (1903).
54. J. L. McGaugh and M. J. Herz, *Memory Consolidation* (Albion, San Francisco, 1972); S. L. Chorover, in *Neural Mechanisms of Learning and Memory*, M. R. Rosenzweig and E. L. Bennett, Eds. (MIT Press, Cambridge, MA, 1974), pp. 561–582.
55. J. L. McGaugh, *Annu. Rev. Psychol.* **34,** 297 (1983); J.L. McGaugh, *Annu. Rev. Neurosci.* **12,** 255 (1989).
56. W. R. Russell and P. W. Nathan, *Brain* **69,** 280 (1946); J. Barbizet, *Human Memory and Its Pathology* (Freeman, San Francisco, 1970).
57. L. R. Squire, N. J. Cohen, L. Nadel, in *Memory Consolidation*, H. Weingartner and E. Parker,

Eds. (Erlbaum, Hillsdale, NJ, 1984), pp. 185–210.
58. L. R. Squire, F. Haist, A. P. Shimamura, *J. Neurosci.* **9,** 828 (1989).
59. L. R. Squire and P. C. Slater, *J. Exp. Psychol. Hum. Learn. Mem.* **104,** 50 (1975); L. R. Squire, *J. Exp. Psychol. Learn. Mem. Cognit.* **15,** 241 (1989).
60. L. R. Squire, P. C. Slater, P. M. Chace, *Science* **187,** 77 (1975).
61. L. R. Squire, P. M. Chace, P. C. Slater, *Nature (London)* **260,** 775 (1976); L. R. Squire and N. J. Cohen, *Behav. Neural Biol.* **25,** 115 (1979).
62. N. J. Cohen and L. R. Squire, *Neuropsychologia* **19,** 337 (1981).
63. L. R. Squire and C. W. Spanis, *Behav. Neurosci.* **98,** 345 (1984).
64. D. Purves and J. W. Lichtman, *Science* **210,** 153 (1980); T. Wiesel, *Nature (London)* **299,** 583 (1982).
65. W. M. Jenkins and M. M. Merzenich, *Soc. Neurosci. Abstr.* **10,** 665 (1984); M. M. Merzenich *et al.*, *Neuroscience* **10,** 639 (1983).
66. W. D. Marslen-Wilson and H.-L. Teuber, *Neuropsychologia* **13,** 353 (1975); H. J. Sagar, N. J. Cohen, S. Corkin, J. H. Growdon, *Ann. N.Y. Acad. Sci.* **444,** 533 (1985).
67. S. Zola-Morgan, L. R. Squire, D. G. Amaral, *J. Neurosci* **6,** 2950 (1986).
68. A. J. Parkin, *Cortex* **20,** 479 (1984).
69. S. Zola-Morgan, N. J. Cohen, L. R. Squire, *Neuropsychologia* **21,** 487 (1983); D. MacKinnon and L. R. Squire, *Psychobiol.*, in press.
70. E. Halgren, in *The Neuropsychology of Memory*, L. R. Squire and N. Butters, Eds. (Guilford, New York, 1984), pp. 165–182; G. W. Van Hoesen, *Trends Neurosci.* **5,** 345 (1982). L.R. Squire, A.P. Shimamura, D.G. Amaral, in *Neural Models of Plasticity,* J.H. Byrne and W.O. Berry, Eds. (Academic, San Diego, 1989), pp. 208-239.
71. M. S. Albert, N. Butters, J. Levin, *Arch. Neurol.* **36,** 211 (1979); P. R. Meudell, B. Northern, J. S. Snowden, D. Neary, *Neuropsychologia* **18,** 133 (1980); H. I. Sanders and E. K. Warrington, *Brain* **94,** 661 (1971); B. Seltzer and D. F. Benson, *Neurology* **24,** 527 (1974).
72. L. Weiskrantz, in *Memory Systems of the Brain*, N. M. Weinberger, J. L. McGaugh, G. Lynch, Eds. (Guilford, New York, 1985), pp. 380–415.
73. N. Butters, P. Miliotis, M. S. Albert, D. S. Sax, in *Advances in Clinical Neuropsychology*, G. Goldstein, Ed. (Plenum, New York, 1984), vol. 1, pp. 127–159; E. Goldberg *et al.*, *Science* 213, 1392 (1981); S. Zola-Morgan and L. R. Squire, in *Memory Systems of the Brain*, N. M. Weinberger, J. L. McGaugh, G. Lynch, Eds. (Guilford, New York, 1985), pp. 463–477.
74. A. P. Shimamura and L. R. Squire, *Behav. Neurosci.* **100,** 165 (1986).
75. A. P. Shimamura, T.L. Jernigan, L. R. Squire, *J. Neurosci.* **8,** 4400 (1988).
76. L. S. Cermak and J. Moreines, *Brain Lang.* **3,** 16 (1976); M. Moscovitch, in *Human Memory and Amnesia*, L. S. Cermak, Ed. (Erlbaum, Hillsdale, NJ, 1982), pp. 337–370.
77. L. R. Squire, *J. Exp. Psychol. Learn. Mem. Cognit.* **8,** 560 (1982).
78. J. S. Janowsky, A. P. Shimamura, L. R. Squire, *Psychobiology* **17,** 3 (1988).
79. D. L. Schacter, J. L. Harbluk, D. R. McLachlan, *J. Verb. Learn. Verb. Behav.* **23,** 593 (1984).
80. D. G. Amaral, in *Handbook of Physiology: The Nervous System*, J. M. Brookhart and V. B. Mountcastle, Eds. (American Physiological Society, Bethesda, MD, 1987); G. Van Hoesen, *Ann. N.Y. Acad. Sci.* **444,** 97 (1985).
81. R. F. Thompson, *Science* **233,** 941 (1986).
82. The term hippocampal formation, as used here, includes the dentate gyrus, the hippocampus proper, the fields of the subicular complex, and the entorhinal cortex.
83. M. Mishkin, *Nature (London)* **273,** 297 (1978); E. A. Murray and M. Mishkin, *J. Neurosci.* **4,** 2565 (1984).
84. S. Zola-Morgan and L. R. Squire, *Behav. Neurosci.* **99,** 22 (1985).
85. ______, *J. Neurosci.* **4,** 1072 (1984).
86. B. A. Malamut, R. C. Saunders, M. Mishkin, *Behav. Neurosci.* **98,** 759 (1984).
87. S. Zola-Morgan, L. R. Squire, M. Mishkin, *Science* **218,** 1337 (1982).
88. J. A. Horel, *Brain* **101,** 403 (1978).
89. S. Zola-Morgan and L. R. Squire, *Behav. Neurosci.* **100,** 155 (1986).
90. H. Mahut, S. Zola-Morgan, M. Moss, *J. Neurosci.* **2,** 1214 (1982).
91. L. R. Squire and S. Zola-Morgan, *Ann. N.Y. Acad. Sci.* **444,** 137 (1985).
92. E. A. Murray and M. Mishkin, *J. Neurosci.* **6,** 1991 (1986).
93. S. Zola-Morgan, L. R. Squire, D. G. Amaral, *J. Neurosci.* **9,** 1922 (1989); S. Zola-Morgan, L. R. Squire, D. G. Amaral, W. Suzuki, *J. Neurosci.*, in press.
94. J. P. Aggleton and M. Mishkin, *Exp. Brain Res.* **52,** 199 (1983).

95. _____, *Neuropsychologia* **21,** 189 (1983); S. Zola-Morgan and L. R. Squire, *Ann. Neurol.* **17,** 558 (1985); D. von Cramon, N. Hebel, U. Schuri, *Brain* **108,** 993 (1985).
96. W. G. P. Mair, E. K. Warrington, L. Weiskrantz, *Brain* **102,** 749 (1979); A. Mayes, P. Mendell, D. Mann, A. Pickering, *Cortex* **24,** 367 (1988). Monkeys with bilateral lesions limited to the medial mammillary nuclei had a small, negligible impairment on the delayed nonmatching-to-sample task [J. P. Aggleton and M. Mishkin, *Exp. Brain Res.* **58,** 190 (1985)]. One monkey with a sectioned mammillothalamic tract, plus damage to some midline thalamic nuclei, was moderately impaired (*94*). In another study, monkeys with fornix transection or mammillary nuclei lesions had only transient memory impairment that recovered during the months after surgery *(101)*.
97. J. Bachevalier and M. Mishkin, *Behav. Brain Res.* **20,** 249 (1986).
98. T. Aigner *et al., Soc. Neurosci. Abstr.* **10,** 386 (1984); A. R. Damasio, N. R. Graff-Radford, P. J. Eslinger, H. Damasio, N. Kassell, *Arch. Neurol.* **42,** 263 (1985).
99. D. S. Olton, J. T. Becker, G. E. Handelmann, *Behav. Brain Sci.* **2,** 313 (1979).
100. W. C. Benzing and L. R. Squire, *Behav. Neurosci.* **103,** 538 (1989).
101. S. Zola-Morgan, L. R. Squire, D.G. Amaral, *J. Neurosci.* **9,** 898 (1989).
102. M. Mishkin and J. Delacour, *J. Exp. Psychol. Anim. Behav. Proc.* **1,** 326 (1975).
103. L. R. Squire, S. Zola-Morgan, K. Chen, *Behav. Neurosci.* **102,** 210 (1988).
104. P. Osterrieth, *Arch. Psychol.* **30,** 306 (1944).
105. I thank D. Amaral, A. Shimamura, and S. Zola-Morgan for helpful discussion and comments on the manuscript. Supported by the Medical Research Service of the Veterans Administration and by the National Institute of Mental Health (MH24600).

41
S. Corkin
Lasting consequences of bilateral medial temporal lobectomy: Clinical course and experimental findings in H. M.
1984. *Seminars in Neurology* 4: 249–259

DEDICATED TO WILLIAM BEECHER SCOVILLE, M.D. 1906–1984

The attention that has been devoted to the patient H.M. in terms of number of hours of evaluation and amount of journal and book space probably exceeds that devoted to any other single case. This circumstance is due to the unusual purity and severity of his amnesic syndrome, to its well-documented anatomical substrate, to the relatively static nature of his condition, and to his being a willing and cooperative subject. This article provides an overview of the history, 31-year postoperative clinical course, and neuropsychologic findings in this 58-year-old man.

HISTORY

PREOPERATIVE CLINICAL COURSE

H.M. was born in 1926. He was the only child of working-class parents. The hospital birth was apparently normal, but no details of the procedure are available. His development was said to have been unremarkable until age 7 years when he was knocked down by a bicycle. (Note that H.M.'s age at the time of this injury was given as 9 in an earlier report;[1] the correction was made following a subsequent conversation with his mother.) He sustained a laceration in the left supraorbital region, and was unconscious for 5 minutes. It should be noted, too, that three first cousins on his father's side of the family had epilepsy. H.M. experienced his first minor seizure at age 10 years, and his first major seizure on his 16th birthday. He still remembers that he was riding in the car with his parents at the time of the latter event, but states that it was his 15th birthday. He dropped out of high school because the other boys teased him about his seizures. After a two-year interval, however, he entered a different high school and graduated in 1947, at age 21. In high school, he took the "practical" course, in preference to the "commercial" or "college" course, and states that he took as little mathematics as possible because he did not care for it. He was a member of the Science Club and was fond of guns, hunting and roller skating.

After high school, he worked on an assembly line and also held a job as a motor-winder until his seizures incapacitated him to the extent that he could no longer perform his duties. At that time, he was having on the average 10 petit mal seizures per day and 1 major seizure per week. Unsuccessful attempts had been made over a 10-year period to control these seizures with large doses of anticonvulsant medications, including Dilantin, phenobarbital, Tridione, and Mesantoin. The frequency and severity of the attacks ultimately led H.M. and his family to consider a brain operation. The proposal to do a radical experimental operation was discussed with them on several occasions before the decision to proceed was reached.

BRAIN OPERATION

In 1953, when H.M. was 27 years old, Dr. William Beecher Scoville performed a bilateral, medial temporal-lobe resection.[2] He approached the brain through two 1.5-inch supraorbital trephine holes. By inserting a flat brain spatula through each hole, he was able to elevate both frontal lobes, thereby exposing the tips of the temporal lobes. They in turn were retracted laterally in order to permit access to the medial surfaces, where electrocorticography was carried out in order to assess the activity of the uncus, amygdala, and hippocampus—structures that are often implicated in epilepsy. There was no clear-cut evidence of an epi-

From Corkin S, Lasting Consequences of Bilateral Medial Temporal Lobectomy: Clinical Course and Experimental Findings in H. M., in *Seminars in Neurology*, Volume 4, Number 2, New York, 1984. Thieme Medical Publishers, Inc. Reprinted by permission.

leptic focus in this region. An incision was then made that bisected the tips of the temporal lobes, and he resected the medial half of the tip of each temporal lobe. Next, Dr. Scoville removed by suction all of the gray and white matter medial to the temporal horns of the lateral ventricles, sparing the temporal neocortex almost entirely. The removal was bilateral, and it is said to have extended 8 cm back from the tips of the temporal lobes. It included the prepyriform gyrus, uncus, amygdala, hippocampus, and parahippocampal gyrus, and must have produced an interruption of some of the white matter leading to and from the temporal lobes (Fig. 1). H.M. was awake and talking during the operation.

Five pieces of excised brain tissue underwent gross neuropathologic study. Microscopic examination of three of them, taken from one uncus and both amygdalae, found them to be without inflammation or scarring.

POSTOPERATIVE CLINICAL COURSE

The operation reduced the frequency of H.M.'s major seizures to the point where now his attacks are infrequent, and he may be free of generalized convulsions for as long as a year. The minor seizures persist; they are atypical petit mal attacks that do not noticeably disturb him. His current seizure medications are Dilantin, 100 mg three times daily, and Mysoline, 250 mg three times daily. The reduction in seizure frequency is juxtaposed against the unexpected handicap produced by the resection: Since the time of his operation, H.M. has had a profound anterograde amnesia that is especially salient because his overall intelligence and neurologic status are relatively well-preserved. H.M.'s global amnesia has put marked limitations on his daily activities and accomplishments. Once the harmful effects of bilateral medial temporal lobectomy were recognized, Dr. Scoville campaigned widely against its use.[3]

Living Situation and Daily Activities

After his operation, H.M. returned home to live with his mother and father. His daily activities included accompanying his mother on errands, helping with household chores, mowing the grass, watching television, and doing crossword puzzles. His father, whom H.M. resembles both physically and in his gentle, passive nature, died in 1967. Beginning in that year, H.M. attended a rehabilitation workshop on a daily basis for about 10 years. There, he performed simple, repetitive tasks, went

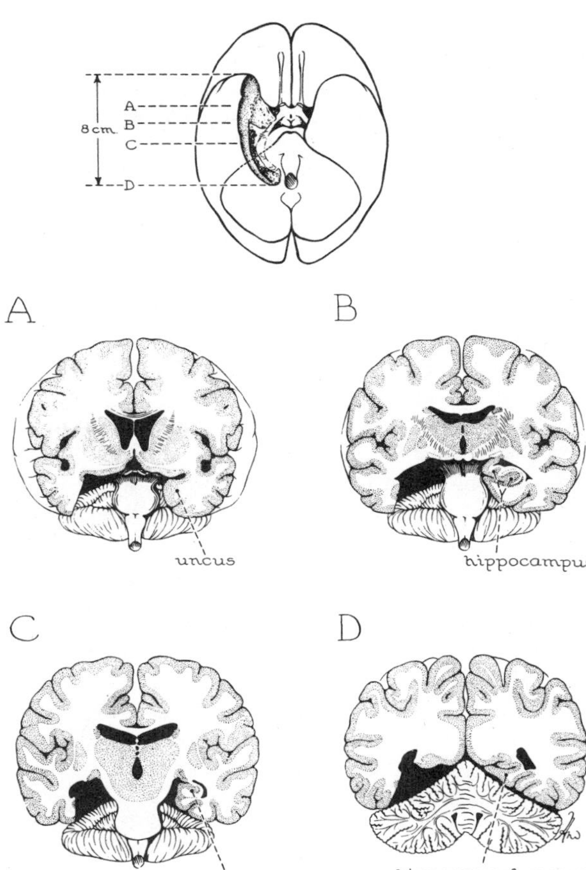

Figure 1. These cross-sections of human brain were prepared by Dr. Lamar Roberts to show the extent of H.M.'s resection. For didactic purposes, the resection is shown on the right side of the brain, and the intact structures on the left side of the brain, but note that the lesion is bilateral. At the top is a drawing of the base of the brain that shows where the cross-sections are taken from. Level A = uncus; level B = anterior hippocampus; the amygdala would be in a section between A and B, but is not shown; level C = more posterior hippocampus; level D = parahippocampal gyrus at the posterior limits of the resection (from Scoville and Milner, 1957).

on field trips, and also worked in this protective setting as a handyman. H.M. and his mother lived by themselves until 1974, when owing to his mother's advanced age, they went to live with a relative. Three years later, H.M.'s mother was admitted to a nursing home. Then, in 1980, because the relative who cared for him was terminally ill, H.M. moved to the nursing home where he currently resides (though not the one where his mother was living). His mother died in 1981 at age 94.

Currently, H.M. is assisted with his bath or shower, but dresses himself with the clothes that are laid out for him. He is reminded to shave, brush his teeth, and comb his hair. He spends much of his time doing difficult crossword puzzles and watching television. He also participates in the daily activities of the nursing home, such as poetry reading, crafts projects, games, and entertainment. His appetite is good, and he is reported to sleep well, but all-night electroencephalogram (EEG) recordings reveal that he wakes up often because of sleep apnea.

Motivation and Affect

One of H.M.'s most striking characteristics is that he rarely complains about anything. In 1968, his mother stated that "the trouble with H. is that he doesn't complain—ever. There could be something quite seriously wrong with him, but you would have to guess." At the nursing home, when H.M. is observed to be acting differently, the nurses question him by running through a list of possible complaints, such as toothache, headache, stomachache, until they hit upon the correct one. He will not spontaneously say, for example, "I have a headache," causing one to wonder whether he knows what is wrong. Similarly, he does not ask for food or beverages, and unless questioned, does not say that he is hungry, full, or tired. He sometimes asks to go to the bathroom, however. H.M. appears to be content at all times, and is always agreeable and cooperative to the point that if, for example, he is asked to sit in a particular place, he will do so indefinitely. The rare exceptions to this placid demeanor occur when H.M. is stressed. For example, during the time that H.M. and his mother lived with their relative, his mother's constant nagging would cause H.M. to become very angry. Occasionally, he would kick her in the shin or hit her with his glasses. More recently, another patient in the nursing home apparently liked to annoy H.M. by calling him names, criticizing him, and disturbing his Bingo card. Her behavior angered H.M. to the point that he would shake the sides of his bed and walk around in circles. As soon as he was distracted, his anger would dissipate immediately. Since this woman's discharge from the nursing home, H.M. has not had any such outbursts. He is described as even-tempered and well-behaved; he does not throw objects, swear, or hit. Moreover, his sense of humor is often evident, as it was the day that Dr. Harvey Sagar and H.M. walked out of a testing room into the hall, allowing the door to close behind them. Dr. Sagar commented to H.M., "I'm wondering whether I left my keys inside the room." H.M. replied, "At least you'll know where to find them!"

After H.M.'s father died, his mother believed that H.M. was depressed, and her concern for him motivated her to enroll him in the rehabilitation workshop mentioned above. When she died four years later, the staff at the nursing home where H.M. lives observed that his grief was mild. He told them what a nice woman she had been and that she had taken care of him all his life. He sometimes remembers that his parents are dead and mentions that he is all alone. His adjustment to all of the changes in his personal relationships and living situation has been smooth.

H.M. appears to have no interest in sexual relationships, as indicated by the absence of conversation on sexual topics and by his failure to seek sexual satisfaction. He does not flirt, he has never had a girlfriend, and he does not masturbate, as far as his caretakers have been able to determine. Hyposexuality is sometimes associated with temporal-lobe lesions, and thus it is tempting to speculate that H.M.'s sexual indifference is attributable to the brain operation; it may be due to other factors, however. Preoperative testing by a clinical psychologist, Dr. Liselotte K. Fisher, led her to conclude that H.M. had difficulty in his sexual adjustment. Moreover, anticonvulsant therapy produces elevated sex hormone binding globulin levels, which are associated with reduced plasma total testosterone, raised luteinizing hormone levels, and sexual dysfunction.[4] Thus, the sexual disorder may have been present before the operation, and it may be due at least in part to drug-induced hormonal abnormalities. Further study of sex hormone patterns is warranted in H.M.

PHYSICAL EXAMINATION

We have documentation of H.M.'s medical history since 1966; he has been free of major illnesses. Information relevant to his neurologic status is described below.

NEUROLOGIC EXAMINATION

During the postoperative years that we have followed H.M. his neurologic status has remained stable. Neurologic examination in 1984 revealed an ataxia of gait, polyneuropathy, and a left ulnar neuropathy. These signs are identical to those found in 1966, except for progression of the polyneuropathy since 1970 and the appearance of the ulnar neuropathy in 1977. The relative absence of neurologic deficit is surprising when one considers the nature and extent of the abnormal conditions that coexist in H.M.'s brain. In this man, six factors contribute to the total cerebral disorder: the long-standing neural abnormality that produced his frequent major and minor seizures; the lasting deleterious effects of repeated seizure activity; the effects of long-term use of anticonvulsant medications; the substantial loss of brain tissue due to bilateral medial temporal-lobe resection; the cortical and subcortical neuronal loss that normally occurs throughout life; and the chemical counterparts of the presumed morphologic changes.

LABORATORY TESTS

Urinalysis and routine blood tests show no consistent abnormality apart from a mild red cell macrocytosis, which is probably due to Dilantin therapy. The 1984 EKG tracing is within normal limits. In addition, urine testosterone, blood testosterone, free cortisol, and adrenocorticotropin levels measured in 1980 were all normal. These findings are of interest because there are numerous corticosterone receptors in the hippocampus, and this structure is involved in the control of glucocorticoid secretion,[5] and because the hippocampus sends extensive projections to the hypothalamus.[6]

A contrast-enhanced computed tomography (CT) scan was performed in 1984 on a GE 9800 scanner at the Massachusetts General Hospital. The use of this current generation scanner made it possible for the first time to visualize H.M.'s medial temporal-lobe lesions. Other evidence of the resection was dilation of the temporal horns of both lateral ventricles. Additional findings included cerebellar atrophy, possibly associated with long-term Dilantin treatment, and mild cortical atrophy, as is sometimes seen in a 58-year-old person (Fig. 2). These findings are in agreement with those obtained in 1978.

An EEG performed in 1978 showed a large amount of bilateral and diffuse seizure activity. The most prominent finding was that of wave and spike activity that was symmetrical and maximal in the frontal regions, and polyspike and wave activity in sleep. There was some slow activity in the temporal regions, which was greater on the left, but in that

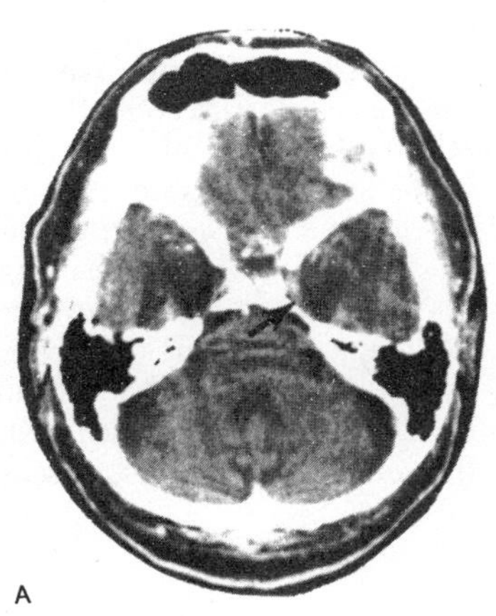

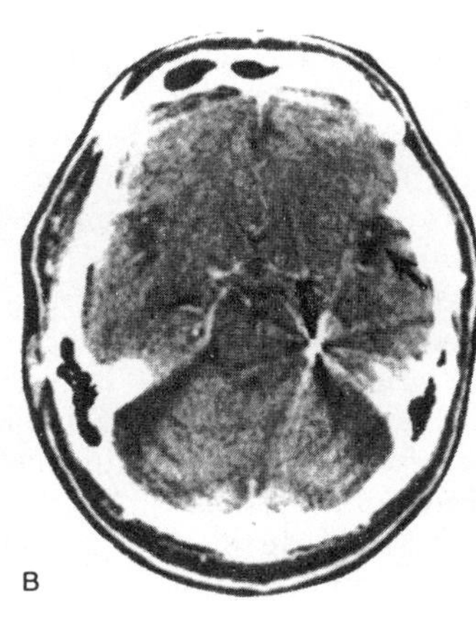

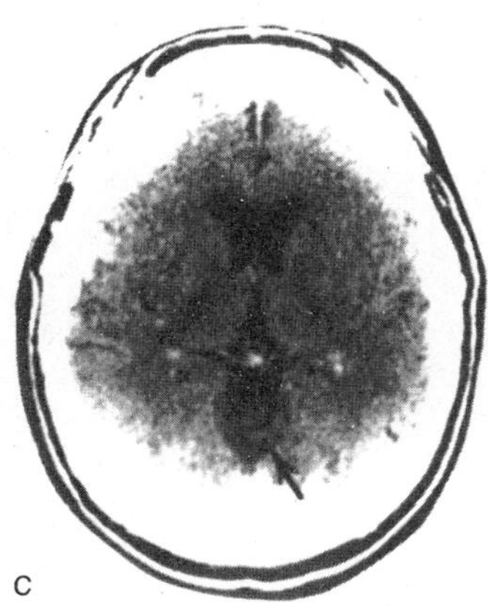

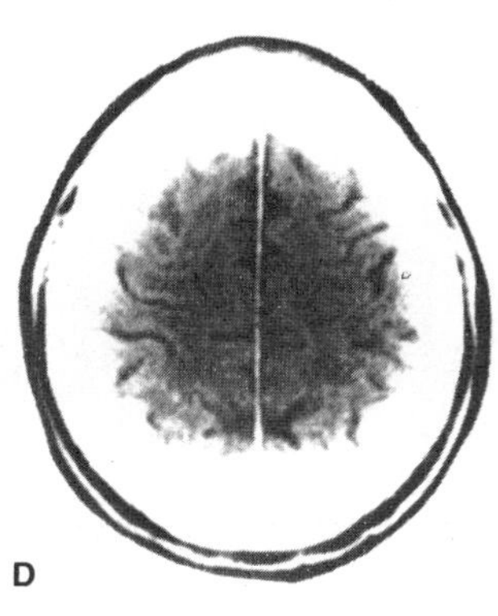

Figure 2. *A,* Areas of lower absorption value are observed bilaterally in the region of the medial aspects of the temporal lobes anteriorly. The changes are more prominent on the left side (arrow). These areas of low absorption value are consistent with partial volume averaging of tissue loss due to the surgical resection. *B,* Mild to moderate tissue loss is seen in the Sylvian cisterns anteriorly. An arrow denotes the enlarged Sylvian cistern on the left. These changes could be secondary to the surgical removal of tissue in the medial temporal lobes. The linear streaking more posteriorly is due to artifact from a surgical clip. *C,* The Sylvian cistern (arrow) is not well filled out by the superior cerebellar vermis, indicating atrophy of this structure. The cerebellum shows marked, diffuse atrophy. The ventricles are enlarged, consistent with the patient's age. *D,* The changes laterally, over the convexity, are consistent with the patient's age. The cortical sulci are prominent bilaterally, especially medially, in the interhemispheric fissure. Whether these changes reflect some secondary alteration in the region of the cingulate gyrus cannot be determined.

area only fragments of low amplitude spike activity were seen.

NEUROPSYCHOLOGIC EVALUATION

The information about H.M. described up to this point provides a background against which to consider the objective neuropsychologic test results. These findings serve two purposes: They illustrate the purity of H.M.'s amnesic syndrome, and they provide answers to a variety of questions about the organization of human memory systems. Now that H.M. is 58 years old, a new question has arisen: Will the aging process proceed normally in his brain, or will the symptoms of aging be accelerated in an already damaged structure? The experimental findings summarized here in brief have either been described in detail previously in separate research reports or will be the basis for future articles.

SENSORY AND SENSORIMOTOR FUNCTION

Visual field testing was carried out in 1966, 1970, and 1984 using the Tübingen perimeter.[7] H.M.'s visual fields are normal, as are most other visual functions tested, including prism adaptation (Held, unpublished data), masking and metacontrast (Schiller, unpublished data), and perception of spiral after-effects. The single exception is his contrast sensitivity function, which is slightly reduced for his age (Nissen and Corkin, unpublished data). Because he viewed the stimuli through the upper lens of his bifocals, and because the correction may not have been optimal, testing will be repeated with H.M. wearing full frame glasses with the proper correction.

H.M.'s performance on a series of olfactory tasks indicated a dissociation of function: He is able to detect weak odors compared with distilled-deionized water, to appreciate odor intensity, and to adapt normally to strong odors.[8] Discrimination, matching, and identification tasks, however, reveal that he is severely impaired in the perception of odor quality. This disorder is not surprising because the resection invaded primary olfactory cortex in the uncus, and because retraction of the frontal lobes during the operation might have damaged the orbitofrontal cortex, olfactory bulb, or olfactory tracts. Nevertheless, these structures must have been at least partially spared in order to support the residual olfactory capacities demonstrated in H.M.

Since 1962, we have documented H.M.'s peripheral neuropathy on his hands and forearms with quantitative measures of somatosensory function, including pressure sensitivity, two-point discrimination, point localization, position sense, thermal discrimination, and pain sensitivity.[9,10] On these tests, H.M. has mild to moderate deficits bilaterally, although his performance is variable and sometimes even falls within the normal range. His grip strength shows little fluctuation; in 1983, it was 70.3 pounds on the left, and 72.3 pounds on the right. H.M. appears to be right-handed, but he states that in second grade he was forced to switch his writing hand from left to right. On tests of repetitive finger tapping and visuomotor coordination,[11] H.M.'s scores for the two hands are comparable, and at the bottom of the normal range for his age. The exception is the Thurstone tapping test, in which his scores for the bimanual condition are markedly impaired; this abnormality is probably attributable at least in part to his cerebellar atrophy. His performance on a test of repetitive fine-finger movement[12] is asymmetric, with the left hand markedly inferior to the right, even on unimanual conditions. This finding suggests some interference with the primary motor cortex or other part of the pyramidal system, presumably in the right hemisphere.[13,14] The sensorimotor deficit revealed in the laboratory is also apparent in his daily activities. For example, the staff at the rehabilitation workshop noted some clumsiness in working with his hands, although the quality of his work was said to have been excellent.

OVERALL INTELLIGENCE

The Wechsler-Bellevue scale was administered to H.M. on seven occasions, including an examination the day before his operation by Dr. Liselotte K. Fisher (Table 1). Postoperative testing

Table 1. The Amnesic Patient H.M.: Wechsler Intelligence-Scale and Memory-Scale Results (1953–1983)

Date	Age	Test	Verbal IQ	Performance IQ	Full Scale IQ	Memory Quotient	Delayed Recall: Verbal (Deficit ≤ 11)	Delayed Recall: Nonverbal (Deficit ≤ 7)
Preop								
1953	27	W-B I	101	106	104	*	*	*
Postop								
1955	29	W-B I	107	114	112	67	*	*
1962	36	W-B II	109	125	118	64	1	0
1977	51	W-B I	107	126	118	74	5	0
1978	52	W-B II	91	104	98	63	1	0
1980	54	W-B II	97	108	104	64	1	0
1983	57	W-B II	97	115	108	64	0	0

*Not assessed

also included the Wechsler memory scale (WMS); the discrepancy between the memory quotient (MQ) and the full scale IQ rating provides a crude index of the severity of global amnesia, although marked IQ-MQ differences can occur for other reasons, such as severe verbal memory impairment. Overall IQ ratings have been consistently in the average range, whereas performance IQ ratings fall in the average to superior ranges. Individual subtest scores vary considerably: Preoperatively H.M.'s equivalent weighted score on the arithmetic subtest was 1, reflecting his dislike of mathematics; the postoperative arithmetic scores ranged from 4 to 7. Object assembly and digit symbol were both 7 preoperatively, but all other scores were above 10. On postoperative testing, the object assembly score has risen to 12 and 13, but the digit symbol scores remain low, perhaps reflecting the effects of medication. The full scale IQ ratings cover the average and bright normal ranges, and all are at least 35 points above the memory quotient, indicating an inferiority of memory function to overall intelligence. A more sensitive index of memory impairment, however, is performance on delayed recall of verbal (WMS logical memory and associate learning) and nonverbal (WMS visual reproduction) material.[15] On both tasks, H.M. is severely impaired on all occasions (see Table 1). More detailed studies of specific memory capacities are cited below.

A comparison of the 1977 and 1983 test results indicates that H.M.'s verbal IQ rating has dropped 10 points, his performance IQ rating 11 points, and his full scale IQ rating 10 points (see Table 1). In normal aging, IQ test performance is maintained until after age 70,[16] so that H.M.'s losses, though not dramatic, may reflect premature aging produced by his multiple neural abnormalities. The manifestation of this process could be a decrease in the number of neurons, in the number of receptor sites, or in the efficiency of the remaining neurons. Alternatively, transneuronal degeneration in the limbic system, a rare cause of progressive intellectual loss, could underlie H.M.'s slight deterioration.[17]

LANGUAGE CAPACITIES

H.M. is able to appreciate puns and linguistic ambiguities,[18] and although he does not usually initiate conversations himself, when someone begins a conversation with him, he talks readily and in general communicates effectively. Nevertheless, his language functions are now minimally impaired. Clinically, he has a slight anomia, but on the Boston naming test,[19] he scores in the normal range (Huff, unpublished data). Although he also achieves perfect scores on six subtests of the Minnesota test for differential diagnosis of aphasia—three reflecting receptive language capacities and three expressive language capacities—this test is relatively easy, and on more challenging language tests, he is less accurate. Thus, on the token test of language comprehension,[20] he achieves 34 of 36 and 32 of 36 correct on separate occasions (deficit≤33), and on the reporter's test of language production,[21] he succeeds on 19 of 26 and 23 of 26 items (deficit≤24). His spelling is poor, although this disorder may have antedated the brain operation. In addition, he is clearly impaired on tests of semantic and symbolic verbal fluency[11,22] (Nissen, unpublished data). Because other cognitive functions of the frontal lobes are preserved in H.M. (see later), it is believed that the fluency deficit is not related to frontal-lobe dysfunction, but rather reflects an alteration in more general cognitive capacities. Studies of language in aging and Alzheimer's disease reveal that performance on tests of verbal fluency is compromised early in the succession of cognitive changes.[23] H.M.'s mild language disorder, therefore, may be age-related. One of the issues of interest is the extent to which this deficit influences his performance on memory tests.[24]

SPATIAL AND PERCEPTUAL CAPACITIES

O'Keefe and Nadel[25] proposed a model of hippocampal function in which the hippocampus is concerned with context-dependent memory. They provided evidence that the hippocampal system develops objective spatial representations, and for the human hippocampus they postulated that an analogous mapping of linguistic information also occurs. We were initially resistant to this notion because of certain preserved spatial capacities in H.M., but a review of his performance on a wide range of spatial tests that do not rely heavily on memory function indicates that some spatial capacities are compromised, whereas others are not: Deficits are revealed on the hidden figures test,[11,26,27] visual locomotor mazes,[28] copy of the Rey-Osterrieth figure,[29] and the body scheme test.[28] He is similarly thwarted when given a floor plan of the MIT Clinical Research Center to use as a map and asked to walk the route from one room to another. In contrast, H.M.'s performance is exceptionally good on two other spatial tasks and two complex perceptual tasks, the block design subtest of the Wechsler-Bellevue scale, a modified version of Hebb's triangular blocks test,[29] the Mooney faces test,[30] and the McGill picture anomalies.[15] Moreover, his recognition of fragmented line drawings from the Gollin incomplete-pictures test is normal,[24,30] and he shows savings from one test session to the next: In 1962, 1980, 1982, and 1983, his respective error scores were 21, 16, 8, and 7. He is also able to draw an accurate floor plan of the house where he lived during the postoperative years from 1960 to 1974, showing all the rooms in their proper location. He believes that he still lives there and can recognize the floor plan, drawn by someone else, when it is presented with four foils. In the nursing home where he lives, he can find his way from the ground floor to his room, which is one flight up. These latter two instances of preserved spatial capacities occur in environments where H.M. has had thousands of learning trials, however. Because patients with right temporal-lobe lesions are often impaired on the complex spatial tasks that H.M. performs efficiently,[15,31,32] the distinction between the tests on which he succeeds and those on which he fails may reflect a contrasting specialization of the temporal neocortex and medial temporal-lobe structures, respectively.

FRONTAL-LOBE CAPACITIES

The constellation of symptoms observed in H.M. may be contrasted with that seen in patients with less pure amnesias due to ruptured anterior communicating artery aneurysm or to Korsakoff's syndrome; they show frontal-lobe dysfunctions that are believed to contribute to the memory impairment.[33–35] Specifically, they fail to show release from proactive interference, and are poor at judging the temporal order of events and at problem solving. Unlike these patients, H.M. shows preservation of the cognitive functions of the frontal lobes, aside from verbal fluency discussed above. Thus, on six of seven administrations of the Wisconsin card sorting test,[36] he has achieved more than three categories; on the seventh occasion, his Dilantin level was in the toxic range, and understandably he did not achieve any sorting categories. H.M. makes few perseverative errors, and he shows normal release from proactive interference (Cohen, unpublished data). Moreover, his test quotient on the Porteus maze test[37] has gone up from 110 in 1977 to 126 in 1983. The number of qualitative errors is abnormally high, but they are attributable to awkwardness in reorienting his hand, and not to a predilection for rule breaking.

SELECTIVE ATTENTION

Because of the importance of attention for the conscious remembering that takes place in conventional memory tests, it was important to determine whether H.M.'s memory impairment is accompanied by an attentional disorder. One way in which we probe for such a deficit is to ask whether detection of a stimulus is faster when it is in the expected position than when it is in the unexpected position. On a visual simple reaction time task,[38] H.M. responds more slowly than control subjects, but demonstrates normal effects of spatial and temporal expectancy, indicating that his selective attention is unaffected (Nissen and Corkin, unpublished data).

CLASSICAL CONDITIONING

Classical conditioning has been attempted only once with H.M., but without success because the unconditioned stimulus, a shock delivered to the right ankle, did not elicit the expected increase in galvanic skin response (Kimura, unpublished data). This kind of experiment should be pursued with H.M., however, using discrete striated muscle responses because of the reports that cerebellar lesions in animals permanently abolish classical conditioning of such responses with aversive unconditioned stimuli,[39] and because of the finding that the hippocampus plays a role in such conditioning.[40] H.M. does show an electrodermal response to white noise, which habituates during a testing session. In this paradigm, he shows savings several hours and one day later (Merker and Pastel, unpublished data).

RECENT-MEMORY CAPACITIES

Immediate Memory

A consistent finding with H.M. since 1955 has been the preservation of his immediate memory capacities. His digit span increased postoperatively, and since then his immediate memory span for both digits and block patterns has been borderline normal.[24,41] Nevertheless, his forward digit span was 6 through 1977, and dropped to 5 in each of four subsequent years, indicating a small deterioration of immediate memory function. Decay in short-term memory is normal, as measured by both recognition[42] and recall tasks[24] (see also Corsi). H.M.'s initial acquisition of complex visual stimuli, color photographs of scenes and objects from magazines, is also unimpaired (Grove, unpublished data). Thus, H.M. is able to register new information; his striking disability becomes apparent when his immediate memory span is exceeded, if only by a single item,[41,43] when distraction is introduced during retention intervals,[31] and with the mere lapse of time if the material cannot be rehearsed verbally.[44,45]

Long-Term Memory

A striking feature of H.M. is the stability of his symptoms during the 31 postoperative years. He still exhibits a profound anterograde amnesia, and does not know where he lives, who cares for him, or what he ate at his last meal. His guesses as to the current year may be off by as much as 43 years, and, when he does not stop to calculate it, he estimates his age to be 10 to 26 years less than it is. In 1982, he did not recognize a picture of himself that had been taken on his 40th birthday in 1966. Nevertheless, he has islands of remembering, such as knowing that an astronaut is someone who travels in outer space, that a public figure named Kennedy was assassinated, and that rock music is "that new kind of music we have." The following pieces of anecdotal evidence illustrate the severity of his anterograde amnesia and provide some examples of the information that he has been able to recall.

In July 1973, H.M. could not identify Watergate, John Dean, or San Clemente, in spite of the fact that he watched the news on television every night. He did not know who the President was, but when told that his name began with an "N," H.M. said "Nixon." When H.M. was asked whether he could tell the examiner anything about Skylab, he replied, "I think, uh, of a docking place in space." When asked how many people were in Skylab, he correctly said "three," but was not confident of his answer because he immediately added, "But then I had an argument with myself, then, was it three or five?" In response to the question, "What's it like to move around up there?" he said, "Well, they have weightlessness . . . I think of magnets to hold them on metal parts so they . . . won't float off away, and to hold them there so they can move around themselves and stay in one area, and they won't move away unvoluntarily (sic)." In 1980, he erroneously stated that a hippie is a dancer, that Howard Cosell does the news on television, and that Barbara Walters is a singer. However, he correctly said that "grass" could refer to drugs or marijuana, that Raymond Burr plays the part of a detective on television, and that Archie Bunker calls his son-in-law "Meathead." He is comfortable dealing with the products of new technology, such as computerized tests and portable radios with headphones. These anecdotes indicate that although H.M.'s fund of general knowledge is meager, it is not void.

The severity and pervasiveness of H.M.'s memory disorder have been documented repeatedly by his performance on a wide variety of neuropsychologic tests. For example, delayed recall is impaired whether the stimuli are stories, verbal paired associates, digit strings, new vocabulary words, drawings, nonverbal paired associates, block patterns, songs, common objects, or object locations[24,41,46] (Corkin and Sullivan, unpublished data; Cohen, Gabrieli, and Corkin, unpublished data). Further, H.M. does not benefit from the use of visual imagery in paired-associate learning,[47] and he is unable to learn the correct path from start to finish in both visual and tactual stylus mazes[48,49] unless the number of turns is within his immediate memory span.[30] H.M. is also impaired on continuous recognition of words, nonsense syllables, numbers, geometric drawings, and nonsense shapes,[50] and on forced-choice recognition of faces, houses, words, and tonal sequences (Corkin, unpublished data). Although the pattern of memory deficits in H.M. resembles that seen after unilateral temporal lobectomy coupled with hippocampectomy, the magnitude of H.M.'s losses are more marked than those typically seen after unilateral excisions.[51]

In the face of H.M.'s profound anterograde amnesia, it is impressive that certain classes of memory function are preserved. The first hint of a residual learning capacity was Milner's 1962 report that H.M.'s error and time scores on a mirror-drawing task decreased over three days of training, despite his being unaware that he had done the task before.[52] Later experiments provided further evidence of his ability to acquire new motor skills.[49,53] More recent studies make it clear, however, that the domain of preserved learning was formulated too narrowly as motor learning. Thus, H.M. can also acquire certain perceptual skills, such as reading of briefly presented words and mirror reading[54] (Cohen and Corkin, unpublished data), and the cognitive skills required to solve the Tower of Hanoi puzzle.[55,56] Other evidence of preserved learning is that H.M. shows the biasing effects of experience with words, while at the same time being unable to recall that experience. For example, H.M. is shown a word, such as "DEFINE," and asked to indicate how much he likes or dislikes it on a 1 to 5 scale. Next, he is given the stem "DEF" and asked to say the first word that comes to mind. Here he typically responds with the previously experienced word, even though it is not the most frequent completion of the stem "DEF" when biasing is absent. In contrast, he fails dramatically on subsequent recall and recognition testing with the same words (Gabrieli, Cohen, and Corkin, unpublished data).

In summary, H.M.'s impaired performance on traditional tests of delayed recall and recognition memory is in marked contrast to his normal performance on tests of motor, perceptual, and cognitive skill learning and on measures of biasing effects of experience with words. Among the various dichotomies that have been proposed to account for such findings, the distinction between procedural learning (knowing how) and declarative learning (knowing that) is perhaps the most appropriate to conceptualize the kind of knowledge that is spared in H.M. and the kind that is preserved.[57] Declarative knowledge appears to require medial temporal-lobe structures bilaterally for its expression; procedural knowledge is independent of that system.

REMOTE-MEMORY CAPACITIES

In an effort to explore some of H.M.'s premorbid memories in a natural environment, Dr. Neal Cohen and I accompanied H.M. to his 35th high school reunion in 1982. A number of his classmates remembered him and greeted him warmly; one woman even gave him a kiss. As far as we could determine, however, H.M. did not recognize anyone's face or name. But he was not alone in this respect. We met a woman who claimed that she too did not know anyone in the room. Clearly, she and H.M. were the exceptions in this regard, but her comment reminds us that as people age, they also forget. Thus, in evaluating H.M.'s remote memory function with objective tests, it has been important to compare his performance with that of age-matched control subjects.

In 1968, Milner, Corkin, and Teuber[30] reported that H.M.'s retrograde amnesia was restricted to about 2 years preceding the operation. This conclusion was based upon information from the neurosurgeon's office notes and on postoperative interviews with H.M. and his mother. Recently, objective tests have been used to probe the limits of H.M.'s remote memory for public and personal events.[58,59] The new data confirm the finding that H.M.'s remote memory impairment is temporally limited, but they extend the limits of the deficit back to 1942, 11 years before the medial temporal-lobe resection. The public events tests measure recall of famous tunes, verbal recognition of public events, and recall and recognition of famous scenes. In the famous tunes test (Marslen-Wilson, unpublished data), subjects hear samples of 48 tunes from the 1920s to the 1960s, and are asked to provide the titles. H.M.'s ability to name famous tunes is below the normal range for the 1930s, 1940s, and 1960s. A comparison of H.M.'s performance with that of two other amnesic patients suggests that the severity of the remote memory loss may be related to the severity of their anterograde amnesia. Errors in dating famous tunes were defined as the difference between the subject's dating and the actual date. Normal control subjects have an equal number of overshoots and undershoots, as does a patient with global amnesia secondary to encephalitis, although he is less accurate. H.M., in contrast, has a tendency to attribute most tunes to the 1940s so that he systematically overshoots in the 1920s and 1930s, and systematically undershoots in the 1950s and 1960s. On the verbal recognition test of public events,[60] there are 88 questions about events from the 1940s through the 1970s. On this test, H.M.'s performance is normal for the 1940s, borderline for the 1950s, and clearly impaired for the 1960s and 1970s. A comparison of these results with those for other amnesic patients suggests that the extent in time of the retrograde loss is related to the duration of the amnesic syndrome. The postencephalitic patient who had been amnesic for 26 years is impaired, whereas two other patients who had been amnesic for 10 years and 1 year, respectively, both performed normally. Items for the famous scenes test were selected because they depict an event that cannot be deduced from the picture itself. There are four pictures at each of five decades from the 1940s through the 1980s. In the recall test, subjects are first asked whether they have seen the picture before. They are then given one minute to describe the content and action in the picture, and what event it depicts. If the subject omits important details, they are probed for by specific questions. Finally, subjects are asked, "When was the picture taken?" A content score and a dating score are given for each picture. On the recall test, H.M.'s content scores are impaired for all decades except the 1940s, and his dating scores are impaired at all decades tested. The number of datings per decade is also noted, the actual number for each decade being four. Reminiscent of the famous tunes test, H.M. preferentially chooses the 1940s and 1950s at the expense of the 1960s through 1980s: His dating is shifted into his nonamnesic time period. It is striking that with this preference for the 1940s and 1950s, H.M. is still impaired in dating 1940s and 1950s items. Similar findings are obtained with the famous scenes recognition test.

The personal events test is a modified version of the Crovitz personal remote memory test.[58,59,61] Here, subjects are given eight concrete nouns, one at a time, and are asked to relate some personally experienced event cued by each noun, from any period of their life, and to state when the event took place. In order to establish the consistency of the memory, an attempt is made to invoke the same memory a day later, and to assess its content and dating. Day one and day two memories are scored from 0 to 3, according to their specificity. On this task, a perfect score is 30, and all subjects perform efficiently. A drop from day one to day two means either that the subject could not produce the day one memory on day two at all, or that the day two memory was less specific. H.M. and one other amnesic patient show a slight drop from day one to day two. Every time that a subject gives a memory that is specific enough to be scored 3, he is asked to date that memory. Normal control subjects and three amnesic patients who have been amnesic from 1 to 26 years produce memories across their life span up to their current age. In contrast, H.M's memories are all from age 16 years or younger, even though his operation took place at age 27. It is important to note that his major seizures began at age 16, however. This absence of memories over age 16 replicates our previous results (Cohen and Corkin, unpublished data). Consistent with this finding are the observations that H.M. does not remember the end of World War II, nor his high school graduation, both of which occurred after his 16th birthday and before his operation. The fact that H.M. produces no memories after age 16 is not evidence that he is unable to do so. He was therefore given the same words again and asked to relate memories only after the age of 16. Because the task becomes more difficult for everyone when responses are restricted to a particular time period, H.M.'s performance was compared with the performance of another amnesic patient whose responses were similarly constrained. The results indicate that H.M.'s total score is about half of what it was in the unconstrained condition, and poorer than the scores of the other amnesic patients in the constrained condition; that the memories that he does give are for ages 17 and 18 only, and when he is asked to redate these memories the same day and the next day, he dates three of the four below age 16; and that the consistency of memories from day one to day two is practically 0, again in contrast to his unconstrained performance and to the constrained performance of the other patient. These experiments, taken together, provide clear evidence that H.M.'s remote memory impairment extends from the present time back to age 16, 11 years before the operation that resulted in the severe anterograde amnesia. There are at least three factors that may account for this finding. First, there is likely to be a retrograde amnesia covering a period of years before the operation. This impairment would be a true loss of previously established memories. Second, there may also be an anterograde component due to the occurrence of seizures and the toxic doses of anticonvulsant medications prescribed to prevent them. This condition could have interfered with the acquisition of new information. Third, another factor may be a progressive deterioration of remote memories over the years due to impoverished rehearsal secondary to retrograde amnesia, anterograde amnesia, or both.

COMMENT

H.M.'s legacy to cognitive science and brain science has been to provide evidence relevant to distinctions between memory systems and among amnesias of different etiologies based upon the selective preservation or disturbance of specific capacities. H.M. shows a sparing of immediate but not lasting memory function, of skill learning and priming effects but not learning of facts and events, and of remote memories up to 11 years before operation but not after that. These findings suggest that processes in the storage of immediate memories are biologically independent of those underlying memories that endure, and that the acquisition of skills and priming effects is not supported by medial temporal-lobe structures, whereas the remembrance of people and episodes is. Further, H.M.'s preservation of immediate memory capacity and span, and his temporally limited remote memory loss distinguish him from patients with Korsakoff's syndrome and patients with Alzheimer's disease, who do show deficits in immediate memory, as well as in remote memory across all time periods examined.[24,62,63] The additional deficits seen in Korsakoff's syndrome and Alzheimer's disease are in part related to the more extensive pathologic changes in the brain. Results from patients with a variety of brain pathologies are needed to understand the neurology of memory.

In 1984, 31 years after H.M. underwent bilateral medial temporal lobectomy, research with this patient continues to provide new insights into the cognitive and biologic processes that constitute normal human learning and memory. Neuroscientists of present and future generations are indebted to H.M. for his ongoing contributions to our knowledge. We should also recognize the neurosurgeon Dr. Scoville for encouraging research with H.M., and for publicizing it himself in an effort to ensure that, in the patient group to which H.M. belongs, N = 1.

ACKNOWLEDGMENT

A great debt is owed Dr. Brenda Milner for permission to examine H.M. on repeated occasions, and for her incisive comments on this manuscript. My collaborators in this work included Neal J. Cohen, Howard Eichenbaum, John D.E. Gabrieli, Elizabeth Grove, Nancy Hebben, F. Jacob Huff, Thomas H. Morton, Mary Jo Nissen, Harry Potter, Harvey J. Sagar, and Edith V. Sullivan. Dr. Robert Ackerman of the Massachusetts General Hospital Department of Neuroradiology kindly interpreted H.M.'s CT scans. Valuable laboratory assistance was provided by Rae Ann Clegg, Karen Shedlack, Allison Feeley, Kathy Coffin, and Marguerite Randolph. The staff and facilities of the MIT Clinical Research Center provided the necessary environment for these studies. Much of the work described here was supported by USPHS grants MH24433, MH32724, MH06401, MH08280, NS19698, and RR00088, and by the Oxford Regional Health Authority.

REFERENCES

1. Scoville WB, Milner B: Loss of recent memory after bilateral hippocampal lesions. J Neurol Neurosurg Psychiatry 20:11–21, 1957
2. Scoville WB, Dunsmore RH, Liberson WT, Henry, CE, Pepe A: Observations of medial temporal lobotomy and uncotomy in the treatment of psychotic states. Proc Assoc Res Nerv Ment Dis 31:347–369, 1953
3. Scoville WB: Amnesia after bilateral mesial temporal-lobe excision: Introduction to Case H.M. Neuropsychologia 6:211–213, 1968
4. Toone BK, Wheeler M, Fenwick, PBC: Sex hormone changes in male epileptics. Clin Endocrinol 12:391–395, 1980
5. McEwen B: Glucocorticoids and hippocampus: Receptors in search of a function. In *Current Topics in Neuroendocrinology*, Vol 2. In Ganten D, Pfaff D (eds): Berlin: Springer, 1982, pp 23–43
6. Poletti CE, Sujatanond M: Evidence for a second hippocampal efferent pathway to hypothalamus and basal forebrain comparable to fornix system: A unit study in the awake monkey. J Neurophysiol 44:514–531, 1980
7. Aulhorn E, Harms H: Visual perimetry. In Jameson E, Hurvich LH (eds): *Handbook of Sensory Physiology*, VII. New York: Springer, 1972
8. Eichenbaum H, Morton TH, Potter H, Corkin S: Selective olfactory deficits in Case H.M. Brain 106:459–472, 1984
9. Corkin S, Milner B, Rasmussen T: Somatosensory thresholds: Contrasting effects of postcentral-gyrus and posterior parietal-lobe excisions. Arch Neurol 23:41–58, 1970
10. Hebben N, Corkin S, Eichenbaum H, Shedlack K: Diminished ability to interpret and report internal states after bilateral medial temporal resection: Case H.M. Submitted
11. Thurstone LL: *A Factorial Study of Perception.* Chicago: University Press, 1944
12. Corkin S, Growdon JH, Sullivan EV, Rosen TJ: Dissociation of sensorimotor functions in Alzheimer's disease. Submitted
13. Bucy PC: *Neurology*, 4th ed. Springfield, MA: Thomas, 1949
14. Brinkman J, Kuypers HGJM: Cerebral control of contralateral and ipsilateral arm, hand, and finger movements in the split-brain rhesus monkey. Brain 96:653–674, 1973
15. Milner B: Psychological defects produced by temporal-lobe excision. Res Public Assoc Res Nerv Ment Dis 36:244–257, 1958
16. Doppelt JE, Wallace WL: Standardization of the Wechsler adult intelligence scale for older persons. J Abnorm Soc Psychol 51:213–330, 1955
17. Torch WC, Hirano A, Solomon S: Anterograde transneuronal degeneration in the limbic system: Clinical-anatomical correlation. Neurology 27:1157–1163, 1977
18. Lackner JR: Observations on the speech processing capabilities of an amnesic patient: Several aspects of H.M.'s language function. Neuropsychologia 12:199–207, 1974

19. Kaplan E, Goodglass H, Weintraub S: *The Boston Naming Test,* experimental edition. Boston: Lea & Febinger, 1978
20. DeRenzi E, Vignolo LA: The token test: A sensitive test to detect receptive disturbances in aphasics. Brain 85:665–678, 1962
21. DeRenzi E, Ferrari C: The reporter's test: A sensitive test to detect expressive disturbances in aphasics. Cortex 14:279–293, 1978
22. Newcombe F: *Missile Wounds of the Brain.* London: Oxford University Press, 1969
23. Huff FJ, Corkin S, Growdon JH: Anomia in Alzheimer's disease: Associated cognitive deficits. Soc Neurosci Abstr 9:94, 1983
24. Corkin S: Some relationships between global amnesia and the memory impairments in Alzheimer's disease. In Corkin S, Davis KL, Growdon JH, Usdin E, Wurtman RJ (eds): *Alzheimer's Disease: a report of progress in research.* New York: Raven Press, 1982
25. O'Keefe J, Nadel L: *The Hippocampus as a Cognitive Map.* Oxford: Clarendon Press, 1978
26. Teuber H-L, Weinstein S: Ability to discover hidden figures after cerebral lesions. Arch Neurol Psychiatry 76:369–379, 1956
27. Corkin S: Hidden figures test performance: Lasting effects of unilateral penetrating head injury and transient effects of bilateral cingulotomy. Neuropsychologia 17:585–605, 1979
28. Semmes J, Weinstein S, Ghent L, Teuber H-L: Impaired orientation in personal and extrapersonal space. Brain 86:747–772, 1963
29. Hebb DO: *Organization of Behavior.* New York: John Wiley and Sons, 1949, p 278
30. Milner B, Corkin S, Teuber H-L: Further analysis of the hippocampal amnesic syndrome: 14-year follow-up study of H.M. Neuropsychologia 6:215–234, 1968
31. Milner B: Disorders of memory after brain lesions in man. Neuropsychologia 6:175–179, 1968
32. Lansdell HC: Effect of extent of temporal lobe ablations on two lateralized deficits. Physiol Behav 3:271–273, 1968
33. Cohen NJ, Corkin S: Chronic global amnesia after ruptured aneurysms of the anterior communicating artery. Soc Neurosci Abstr 8:25, 1982
34. Squire LR, Cohen NJ, Zola-Morgan S: Comparisons among forms of amnesia: Some deficits are unique to Korsakoff's syndrome. Soc Neurosci Abstr 8:24, 1982
35. Winocur G, Kinsbourne M, Moscovitch M: The effect of cueing on release from proactive interference in Korsakoff amnesic patients. J Exp Psychol [Hum Learn] 7:56–65, 1981
36. Milner B: Effects of different brain lesions on card sorting. Arch Neurol 9:90–100, 1963
37. Porteus SD: *Porteus Maze Test.* Palo Alto, CA: Pacific Books, 1965
38. Posner MI, Nissen MJ, Ogden WC: Attended and unattended processing modes: The role of set for spatial location. In Pick HL Jr, Saltzman E (eds): *Modes of Perceiving and Processing Information.* Hillsdale, NJ: Erlbaum, 1978
39. McCormick DA, Lavond DG, Clark GA, Kettner RE, et al: The engram found? Role of the cerebellum in classical conditioning of nictitating membrane and eyelid responses. Bull Psychonomic Soc 18:103–105, 1981
40. Solomon PR, Vander Shaaf ER, Nobre AC, Weisz DJ, Thompson RF: Hippocampus and trace conditioning of the rabbit's nictitating membrane response. Soc Neurosci Abstr 9:645, 1983
41. Corsi P: Human memory and the medial temporal region of the brain. Unpublished doctoral dissertation, McGill University, 1972
42. Wickelgren WA: Sparing of short-term memory in an amnesic patient: Implications for a strength theory of memory. Neuropsychologia 6:235–244, 1968
43. Drachman DA, Arbit J: Memory and the hippocampal complex. Arch Neurol 15:52–61, 1966
44. Prisko L: Short-term memory in focal cerebral damage. Unpublished doctoral dissertation, McGill University, 1963
45. Milner B: Memory and the medial temporal regions of the brain. In *Biology of Memory.* New York: Academic Press, 1970, pp 29–50
46. Smith ML, Milner B: The role of the right hippocampus in the recall of spatial location. Neuropsychologia 19:781–793, 1981
47. Jones MK: Imagery as a mnemonic aid after left temporal lobectomy: Contrast between material-specific and generalized memory disorders. Neuropsychologia 12:21–30, 1974
48. Milner, B: Visually guided maze learning in man: Effect of bilateral hippocampal, bilateral frontal, and unilateral cerebral lesions. Neuropsychologia 3:317–338, 1965
49. Corkin S: Tactually guided maze learning in man: Effects of unilateral cortical excisions and bilateral hippocampal lesions. Neuropsychologia 3:339–351, 1965
50. Penfield W, Milner B: Memory deficit produced by bilateral lesions in the hippocampal zone. Arch Neurol Psychiatry 79:475–497, 1958
51. Milner B, Kimura D: Dissociable visual learning defects after unilateral temporal lobectomy in man. Paper presented at the 35th annual meeting of the Eastern Psychological Association, Philadelphia, April, 1964
52. Milner B: Les troubles de la memoire accompagnant des lesions hippocampiques bilaterales. In *Physiologie de l'Hippocampe.* Paris: Centre National de la Recherche Scientifique, 1962, pp 257–272
53. Corkin S: Acquisition of motor skill after bilateral medial temporal-lobe excision. Neuropsychologia 6:255–264, 1968
54. Nissen MJ, Cohen NJ, Corkin S: The amnesic patient H.M.: Learning and retention of perceptual skills. Soc Neurosci Abstr 7:235, 1981
55. Cohen NJ, Corkin S: Normal learning of the Tower of Hanoi puzzle despite amnesia. Submitted
56. Cohen NJ, Corkin S: The amnesic patient H.M.: Learning and retention of a cognitive skill. Soc Neurosci Abstr 7:235, 1981
57. Cohen NJ, Squire L: Preserved learning and retention of pattern-analyzing skill in amnesia: Dissociation of knowing-how and knowing-that. Science, 210:207–210, 1980
58. Corkin S, Cohen NJ, Sagar HJ: Memory for remote personal and public events after bilateral medial temporal lobectomy. Soc Neurosci Abstr 9:28, 1983
59. Sagar HJ, Cohen NJ, Corkin S: Dissociations among processes in remote memory. To be presented at the Conference on Memory Dysfunctions, New York Academy of Sciences, June 1984
60. Squire LR: Remote memory as affected by aging. Neuropsychologia 12:429–435, 1974
61. Crovitz HF, Shiffman H: Frequency of episodic memories as a function of their age. Bull Psychonomic Soc 4:517–518, 1974
62. Butters N, Cermak LS: *Alcoholic Korsakoff's Syndrome.* New York: Academic Press, 1980
63. Cohen NJ, Squire LR: Retrograde amnesia and remote memory impairment. Neuropsychologia 19:337–356, 1981

42
D. L. Schacter
Implicit memory: History and current status

1987. *Journal of Experimental Psychology: Learning, Memory, and Cognition* 13: 501–518

Abstract
Memory for a recent event can be expressed *explicitly*, as conscious recollection, or *implicitly*, as a facilitation of test performance without conscious recollection. A growing number of recent studies have been concerned with implicit memory and its relation to explicit memory. This article presents an historical survey of observations concerning implicit memory, reviews the findings of contemporary experimental research, and delineates the strengths and weaknesses of alternative theoretical accounts of implicit memory. It is argued that dissociations between implicit and explicit memory have been documented across numerous tasks and subject populations, represent an important challenge for research and theory, and should be viewed in the context of other dissociations between implicit and explicit expressions of knowledge that have been documented in recent cognitive and neuropsychological research.

Psychological studies of memory have traditionally relied on tests such as free recall, cued recall, and recognition. A prominent feature of these tests is that they make explicit reference to, and require conscious recollection of, a specific learning episode. During the past several years, however, increasing attention has been paid to experimental situations in which information that was encoded during a particular episode is subsequently expressed without conscious or deliberate recollection. Instead of being asked to try to remember recently presented information, subjects are simply required to perform a task, such as completing a graphemic fragment of a word, indicating a preference for one of several stimuli, or reading mirror-inverted script; memory is revealed by a facilitation or change in task performance that is attributable to information acquired during a previous study episode. Graf and Schacter (1985, 1987; Schacter & Graf, 1986a, 1986b) have labeled this type of memory *implicit memory*, and have used the term *explicit memory* to refer to conscious recollection of recently presented information, as expressed on traditional tests of free recall, cued recall, and recognition.

Recent cognitive and neuropsychological research has demonstrated a variety of striking dissociations between implicit and explicit memory and has shown that under certain conditions, implicit and explicit memory can be entirely independent of one another. These observations have raised fundamental questions concerning the nature and composition of memory, questions that will have to be addressed by any satisfactory theory of memory. The purposes of this article are to present an historical survey of observations concerning implicit memory, to review modern experimental studies and theoretical analyses, with particular emphasis on recent work in cognitive psychology and neuropsychology, and to suggest directions for future research.

Before the historical survey is initiated, two points regarding the terms implicit and explicit memory should be clarified. First, I use these terms in the manner suggested by Graf and Schacter (1985). Implicit memory is revealed when previous experiences facilitate performance on a task that does not require conscious or intentional recollection of those experiences: explicit memory is revealed when performance on a task requires conscious recollection of previous experiences. Note that these are *descriptive* concepts that are primarily concerned with a person's psychological experience at the time of retrieval. Accordingly, the concepts of implicit and explicit memory neither refer to, nor imply the existence of, two independent or separate memory systems. The question of whether implicit and explicit memory depend on a single underlying system or on multiple underlying systems is not yet resolved, as will be discussed later in this article. Second, the term *implicit memory* resembles two more familiar terms from the psychological literature: unconscious memory (e.g., Freud & Breuer, 1966; Prince, 1914) and unaware memory or memory without awareness (e.g., Eriksen, 1960; Jacoby & Witherspoon, 1982). These two terms have been used to describe phenomena that will be referred to here with the term *implicit memory*. The main reason for adopting *implicit memory* in favor of either *unconscious memory* or *unaware memory* has to do with the conceptual ambiguity of the latter two terms. The terms *unconscious* and *unaware* have a large number of psychological meanings and implications (e.g., Bowers, 1984; Ellenberger, 1970; Eriksen, 1960), many of which do not apply to the phenomena of interest here. Although the term *implicit* is not entirely free of conceptual ambiguity, it is less saturated with multiple and possibly misleading meanings than are *unconscious* or *unaware*.

Implicit Memory: An Historical Survey

This section considers ideas and observations concerning implicit memory contributed by philosophers, psychologists, neurologists, psychiatrists, and others from the 17th century until the middle of the 20th century. Unless otherwise stated, these investigators did not actually use the term *implicit memory* in their writings. They did, however, describe and discuss situations in which memory for recent experiences was expressed in the absence of conscious recollection. I sometimes use the phrase *implicit memory phenomena* in reference to these observations. This is done purely for purposes of expositional clarity and should be seen as an attempt to put present concepts in the minds of past observers.

Philosophical Analysis: Descartes, Leibnitz, and Maine de Biran

It is widely recognized that both Plato and Aristotle commented extensively about the nature of memory, but both appear to have been concerned exclusively with explicit memory. During the Middle Ages, St. Augustine and St. Thomas Aquinas had a great deal to say about explicit retrieval and search processes, but I have not found any discussion of implicit memory in their writings.

The first clear reference to an implicit memory phenomenon appears to have been made by Descartes in his 1649 *The Passions of the Soul* (cited by Perry & Laurence, 1984), in which he observed that a frightening or aversive childhood experience may "remain imprinted on his [the child's] brain to the end of his life" without "any memory remaining of it afterwards" (Haldane & Ross, 1976, p. 391). Descartes did not, however, elaborate on the philosophical consequences of this phenomenon. In 1704, Gottfried Wilhelm Leibniz developed a systematic doctrine that both allowed for and made reference to implicit memory (Leibniz, 1916). He emphasized the importance of "insensible" or "unconscious" perceptions: ideas of which we are not consciously aware, but which do influence behavior. Leibniz explicitly claimed that people may have "remaining effects of former impressions without remembering them," and that "... often we have an extraordinary facility for conceiving certain things, because we formerly conceived them, without remembering them" (1916, p. 106). Although Leibniz's ideas concerning unconscious perceptions were later championed by several students and followers, they constituted a minority view during the 18th century, owing largely to the predominance of the British associationists. Locke, Hume, Mill, Brown, Hartley and others discussed memory at considerable length, but their analysis was restricted entirely to the domain of explicit memory; they had virtually nothing to say about implicit memory. Darwin (1974, p. 12) distinguished between *involuntary* and *voluntary* recollection, but both of these concepts were used in reference to explicit memory phenomena.

The first philosopher after Leibniz to systematically discuss phenomena of implicit memory was a French philosopher known by the surname Maine de Biran. Though virtually unknown today, he published an important treatise in 1804 entitled *The Influence of Habit on the Faculty of Thinking* (Maine de Biran, 1929). Like others before him, Maine de Biran believed that the analysis of habit was central to an understanding of hunman thought and behavior. Unlike others, however, Maine de Biran elucidated a feature of habit that had not been discussed previously in philosophical or scientific analyses: After sufficient repetition, a habit can eventually be executed *automatically* and *unconsciously* without awareness of the act itself or of the previous episodes in which the habit was learned. Thus, he observed that repeated actions are eventually executed with "such promptitude and facility that we no longer perceive the voluntary action which directs them and we are absolutely unaware of the source that they have" (p. 73). The most striking feature of Maine de Biran's system, however, was his delineation and detailed discussion of three different types of memory: mechanical, sensitive, and representative. The first two types are driven by habit and are involved in the largely unconscious or implicit expression of repeated movements (mechanical) and feelings (sensitive); the third type (representative) is involved in conscious recollection of ideas and events (pp. 156–157). Thus, according to Maine de Biran,

> If signs (in Maine de Biran's system, a *sign* is a motor response code) are absolutely empty of ideas or separated from every representative effect, from whatever cause this isolation may arise, recall is only a simple repetition of movements. I shall call this faculty for it *mechanical* memory. When the ... recall of the sign is accompanied or immediately followed by the clear appearance of a well circumscribed idea, I shall attribute to it *representative memory*. If the sign expresses an affective modification, a feeling or even a fantastic image whatsoever, a vague, uncertain concept, which cannot be brought back to sense impressions ... the recall of the sign ... will belong to *sensitive memory*. (p. 156)

Maine de Biran's scheme represents the first clear articulation of what we might now call a *multiple memory system* interpretation of differences between implicit and explicit memory. Although it is alleged that Maine de Biran influenced the thinking of both Pierre Janet and Henri Bergson (Ellenberger, 1970), his ideas went almost entirely unrecognized outside of France. Most subsequent 19th-century philosophers did not systematically discuss the implicit expressions of memory that were so central to Maine de Biran's view. One exception was Johann Friedrich Herbart, who in 1816 introduced the notion that "supressed ideas," which are unable to exceed the threshold of conscious awareness, can nevertheless influence conscious thinking (Herbart, 1896). The next systematic contributions were made by 19th-century scientists who approached the issue from the standpoint of biology and physiology.

Middle 19th Century: Unconscious Cerebration and Organic Memory

It is now widely recognized that various 19th-century thinkers were concerned with the general problem of unconscious mental processing (cf. Ellenberger, 1970; Perry & Laurence, 1984). One of the most prolific of them was the British physiologist William Carpenter, who invoked the term *unconscious cerebration* to refer to mental activity that occurs outside of awareness (Carpenter, 1874). To support this idea, Carpenter marshalled clinical and anecdotal observations which demonstrated that the effects of recent experiences could be expressed without conscious awareness of those experiences. For example, drawing on observations of automatic writing (writing that appears to occur involuntarily while a subject is in a hypnotic or similar state), he claimed that "It is a most remarkable confirmation of this view [unconscious cerebration], that ideas which have passed out of the *conscious* memory, sometimes express themselves in *involuntary muscular movements*, to the great surprise of the individuals executing them...." (1874, pp. 524–525). To Carpenter, the striking lack of autobiographical recognition or awareness that characterized implicit memory phenomena highlighted the critical role of such awareness in normal memory:

> Without this recognition, we should live in the present alone: for the reproduction of past states of consciousness would affect us only like the succession of fantasies presented to us in the play of the imagination... I am satisfied that I am the person to whom such and such experiences happened yesterday or a month, or a year, or twenty years ago; because I am not only conscious at the moment of the ideas which represent those experiences, but because I recognize them as the revived representations of my past experiences (1874, p. 455)

Carpenter's concept of unconscious cerebration and consequent interest in implicit memory derived from a more general attempt to relate physiology and psychology. A similar integrative effort was made by the Viennese physiologist Ewald Hering, who in 1870 introduced the idea of *organic* or *unconscious* memory (Hering, 1920). Hering criticized earlier writers for restricting their analyses to conscious or explicit memory: "The word 'memory' is often understood as though it meant nothing more than our faculty of intentionally reproducing ideas or series of ideas" (1920, p. 68). Hering argued that it is necessary to consider unconscious memory, which is involved in involuntary recall, the development of automatic and unconscious habitual actions, and even in the processes of ontogenetic development and heredity. Although this latter aspect of Hering's analysis clearly lies outside the domain of the present concerns, his psychological analyses of involuntary recall and the development of automaticity shared much in common with the earlier ideas of Maine de Biran. Following Hering's lead, a large number of psychologists, biologists, and others developed ideas concerning organic memory and its relation to what they referred to as conscious memory (see Schacter, 1982, chap. 7).

Late 19th and Early 20th Century: Systematic Empirical and Theoretical Developments

Toward the end of the 19th century, systematic empirical and theoretical analyses of implicit memory emerged in five different areas: "psychical" research, neurology, psychiatry, philosophy, and experimental psychology.

Psychical Research. Although modern practitioners might be reluctant to admit it, a good case can be made that 19th-century psychical researchers were the first to document implicit memory phenomena on the basis of controlled empirical observation. Two major "implicit memory tests" were used: crystal ball gazing and automatic writing. Both procedures were characterized by the main feature of an implicit memory test: When performing these tasks, subjects made no explicit reference to a specific past event: they either reported what they "saw" in the crystal or wrote whatever came to mind. Although the purpose of these procedures was to document phenomena such as telepathy and clairvoyance, several investigators reported that fragmentary representations of past experiences, devoid of any familiarity or autobiographical reference, frequently appeared during crystal gazing and automatic writing.

In an anonymously authored article in the *Journal of the Society for Psychical Research* (Miss X, 1889), it was reported that information that had been registered unconsciously (i.e., without attention) during the recent past often surfaced as an unfamiliar "vision" during crystal gazing. On the basis of this observation, the author questioned "spiritual" interpretations of crystal visions: "It is easy to see how visions of this kind, occurring in the age of supersition, almost irresistibly suggested the theory of spirit-visitation. The percipient, receiving information which he did not recognize as already in his own mind, would inevitably suppose it to be derived from some invisible and unknown source external to himself" (p. 513). In studies of automatic writing, several investigators described the emergence of knowledge acquired during past episodes which subjects were not aware that they possessed and that seemed foreign to their conscious personalities (Binet, 1890; Prince, 1914). On the basis of his own experiments with automatic writing, Barkworth (1891) concluded that "nothing is ever really forgotten, though the bygone memories evoked by pencil, or crystal, may appear so new and strange that we fail to recognize them as ever having been included in our experience" (p. 29).

Neurology. In 1845, the British physician Robert Dunn described the case of a woman who became amnesic after a near drowning and a long period of unconsciousness. During her amnesic state, the woman learned how to make dresses, even though she apparently did not explicitly remember that she had made any dresses: "She applied herself closely to her new occupation and abandoned altogether the old one. Still she had no recollection from day to day what she had done, and every morning began something new unless her unfinished work was placed before her" (1845, p. 588). Dunn did not discuss the theoretical implications of his observations.

Perhaps the first investigator to document implicit memory phenomena in neurological cases of amnesia and to delineate their theoretical implications was Sergei Korsakoff (1889). In one of his two classic papers describing the amnesic syndrome that now bears his name. Korsakoff observed that "... although the patient was not aware that he preserved traces of impressions that he received, those traces however probably existed and had an influence in one way or another on the course of ideas, at least in unconscious intellectual activity" (1889, p. 512). Korsakoff provided several insightful observations to support his notion. For example, he described a patient whom he had given an electrical shock. Though this patient did not explicitly remember being given any shocks, when Korsakoff showed him a case that contained the shock apparatus, "he told me that I probably came to electrify him, and meanwhile I knew well that he had only learned to know that machine during his illness" (p. 512). Korsakoff went on to argue that amnesic patients retained "weak" memory traces that could affect behavior unconsciously, but were not "strong" enough to enter conscious memory. He emphasized that his observations had important implications for psychologists:

> We notice that a whole series of traces which could in no way be restored to consciousness, neither actively nor passively, continue to exist in unconscious life, continue to direct the course of ideas of the patients, suggesting to him some or other inferences and decisions. That seems to me to be one of the most interesting peculiarities of the disturbance about which we are speaking. (p. 518)

Over 20 years later, Claparède (1911/1951) reported observations that were similar to Korsakoff's, although they are somewhat better known today. Claparède described the now famous example of an amnesic woman who refused to shake hands with him after he pricked her with a pin, even though she did not explicitly remember that Claparède had done so. Claparède interpreted this implicit expression of memory in terms of a disconnection between the ego and the memory trace. At about the same time, Schneider (1912, cited in Parkin, 1982) reported experiments in which he demonstrated that amnesic patients required progressively less information across learning trials to identify fragmented pictures, even though patients did not explicitly remember having seen the pictures before.

Psychiatry. Seminal observations concerning implicit memory were reported in the late 1880s and early 1890s by Pierre Janet and by Sigmund Freud, partly in collaboration with Joseph Breuer. For both Janet and Freud, the critical phenomena were observed in patients suffering hysterical amnesia as a result of emotional trauma. Although these patients could not explicitly remember the traumatic events, their memories of them were expressed indirectly (implicitly) in various ways. Janet (1893), for example, described a case in which a woman became amnesic after being mistakenly informed by a man who appeared suddenly in her doorway that her husband had died. Even though she subsequently could not consciously remember this incident, she "froze with terror" whenever she passed the door that the man had entered. In a later article, Janet (1904) described a woman who had become amnesic following the death of her mother. Though she could not consciously remember any of the events surrounding her mother's death, she experienced "hallucinations" that preserved the contents of those events. After describing numerous other cases of implicit memory in hysteric patients. Janet concluded that hysterical amnesia consists of two key factors: "1. the inability of the subject to evoke memories consciously and voluntarily, and 2. the automatic, compelling, and untimely activation of these same memories" (1904, p. 24). He theorized that hysteria was attributable to a pathological process of dissociation that interfered with the ability to synthesize memories into the "personal consciousness."

Freud's observations on hysteria were similar to Janet's insofar as he emphasized that traumatic memories, inacessible to consciousness, were expressed unconsciously by the patient as hysterical symptoms (see Freud & Breuer, 1966, for relevant cases). Although Freud later changed this view (Ellenberger, 1970), he never abandoned the idea that unconscious memories exert powerful influences on behavior.

Both Janet and Freud emphasized the role of unconscious or implicit memory in psychopathology. The

American psychiatrist Morton Prince clearly delineated the importance of implicit memory for normal cognitive function. In *The Unconscious* (1914), Prince drew together numerous observations of implicit memory from work with hysterical patients, hypnosis, dreams, and automatic writing, in which "... memories of the forgotten experiences [are expressed] without awareness therefore on the part of the personal consciousness" (p. 13). Noting that "... memories may be made to reveal themselves, without inducing recollection, at the very moment when the subject cannot voluntarily recall them" (p. 63), Prince concluded that "... a conscious experience that has passed out of mind may not only recur again as conscious memory, but may recur subconsciously below the threshold awareness" (p. 8). These observations, Prince argued, demonstrate that experiences that are not available to conscious or voluntary recall nevertheless influence cognition and behavior in everyday life:

> In normal life ideas of buried experiences of which we have no recollection intrude themselves from time to time and shape our judgments and the current of our thoughts without our realizing what has determined our mental processes. We have forgotten the source of our judgments, but this forgetfulness does not affect the mechanism of the process. (p. 68)

Philosophy. The major philosophical contribution to the analysis of implicit memory was made by Henri Bergson. In *Matter and Memory* (1911), he argued that "*The past survives under two distinct forms: first, in motor mechanisms; secondly, in independent recollections*" (p. 87). The first form of memory involves gradual learning of habits and skills and does not entail explicit reference to any specific past events; a learned habit "... bears upon it no mark which betrays its origin and classes it in the past: it is part of my present..." (p. 91). Bergson's second form of memory, recollection, entails explicit remembering of "memory-images" that represent specific events from one's past. Although this view is clearly reminiscent of Maine de Biran, Bergson did not actually discuss or even reference Maine de Biran's views anywhere in *Matter and Memory*.

Experimental Psychology. Experimental psychologists paid relatively little attention to implicit memory phenomena in the late 19th and early 20th centuries. Even though there was a large and thriving field in this post-Ebbinghausian era (cf. Schacter, 1982, chap. 8), most practitioners did not distinguish between explicit and implicit memory. Several exceptions, however, can be identified. Ebbinghaus (1885) himself acknowledged that not all effects of memory are expressed in conscious awareness (1885, p. 2). He also made a relevant empirical contribution, noting that savings was observed over a 24-hr retention interval for items that he did not consciously remember having studied before (pp. 58–59; see Slamecka, 1985a, 1985b; Tulving, 1985b). This intriguing observation was not systematically followed up by Ebbinghaus or others. Ebbinghaus' savings paradigm, in which memory is tested by relearning previously studied lists, can be viewed more generally as an implicit memory test: Explicit recollection of a prior episode or list is not called for during relearning (Slamecka, 1985b). Indeed, Ebbinghaus noted that one advantage of the savings method was that it could provide evidence for the existence in memory of information that could not be recollected consciously (1885, p. 8). Of course, numerous subsequent investigators used the savings method to analyze learning and transfer of training. Although there is a sense in which "the entire literature on transfer of training may be perceived as the study of implicit memory" (Slamecka, 1985b, p. 499), researchers did not view it as such and did not elaborate any distinctions like the one between implicit and explicit memory.

After Ebbinghaus, three lines of experimental investigation were concerned with certain aspects of implicit memory. First, Thorndike conducted a large number of experiments that, he claimed, demonstrated that subjects could learn various rules without conscious awareness of them or explicit memory for them (Thorndike & Rock, 1934; see Irwin, Kauffman, Prior, & Weaver, 1934, for methodological criticisms). Second, Poetzl reported in 1917 that unreported features of subliminally exposed pictures appeared in subjects' subsequent imagery and dreams, even though they did not remember these features and were allegedly unaware of them at the time of stimulus exposure (see Poetzl, 1960). Poetzl's experiments, however, were characterized by serious methodological deficiencies (Dixon, 1981; Erdelyi, 1970). Third, studies of hypnotic phenomena by Clark Hull (1933) and his students provided numerous demonstrations of implicit memory for skills, conditioned responses, and facts acquired during hypnosis. Hull's description of the quality of recall by hypnotic subjects resembled Claparède's and Korsakoff's earlier observations of organic amnesia: "In such cases they stated that the name seemed to come from 'nowhere' and was not accompanied by any recollection that the character or syllable had ever been encountered before" (1933, p. 134).

One further contribution from experimental psychology ought to be noted. In *Outline of Psychology* (1924), William McDougall became the first investigator to use the terms *implicit* and *explicit* with reference to the different ways in which memory can be expressed. He distinguished between explicit recognition, which involves conscious recollection of a past event, and implicit recognition, which involves a change in behavior that is attributable to a recent event yet contains no conscious recollection of it or explicit reference to it (1924, pp. 308–309).

Summary of Historical Survey

Four general points can be made regarding the historical survey. First, observations of implicit memory were reported across a broad range of tasks, subjects, and conditions. Perhaps the richest sources of implicit memory phenomena were the clinical observations made by Claparède. Freud, Janet, Korsakoff, Prince, and others. With the exception of Prince, these clinicians did not set out with the specific aim of distinguishing between forms of memory. Nevertheless, they were insightful observers who recognized clearly that the phenomena they described had important implications for theories of normal and abnormal mental function. Indeed, there were relatively few investigators who explicitly raised the issue of whether different forms of memory could be distinguished and then went on to report original empirical observations; Ebbinghaus and Prince should be counted prominently among them. A second, related point is that most empirical observations either were anecdotal, were made under relatively uncontrolled clinical conditions, or were reported in experiments that lacked methodological rigor. Thus, even though the early observers reported phenomena that are broadly similar to those of interest today, methodological inadequacies limit the degree to which they bear directly on contemporary theoretical concerns. Third, there were only a few attempts to develop theoretical accounts of the dissociations that had been observed. The most popular idea was that implicit memory phenomena were produced by memory traces that are too "weak" to exceed the threshold of strength or activation needed for explicit memory (Herbart, 1896; Leibniz, 1916; Korsakoff, 1889; Prince, 1914). As will be shown later, recent experimental work has provided grounds for rejecting this view. However, several other ideas were advanced, including the multiple-memories view of Maine de Biran and Bergson, and the notion of a dissociation between memory traces and the "self" articulated by Claparède and Janet. Fourth, the various investigators who were concerned with implicit memory phenomena exhibited little or no knowledge of each other's work. This circumstance is perhaps not surprising, because observations of implicit memory were made in disparate fields of study.

Modern Research on Implicit Memory

Let us now consider research concerning implicit memory from the 1950s to the present. Date from five different though partly overlapping research areas will first be reviewed: savings during relearning, effects of subliminally encoded stimuli, learning and conditioning without awareness, repetition priming, and preserved learning in amnesic patients. This review is followed by a consideration of contemporary theoretical approaches to implicit memory.

Savings During Relearning

As noted earlier, it is possible to view the phenomenon of savings during relearning as an index of implicit memory, in the sense that relearning a previously studied list does not require explicit reference to a prior learning episode, although the influence of the prior episode is revealed by savings (cf. Slamecka, 1985b). However, little of the voluminous research on savings has addressed the question of whether subjects do indeed rely on explicit memory for prior learning episodes when relearning a list, so it is not entirely clear what savings studies tell us about implicit memory. The most directly pertinent evidence has been provided by Nelson (1978), who has shown savings for items that are neither recalled nor recognized, which thereby suggests that savings can occur in an entirely implicit manner.

Effects of Subliminally Encoded Stimuli

The controversy concerning subliminal perception is well known to experimental psychologists (Dixon, 1971). Although early experiments purporting to demonstrate subliminal perception were severely criticized (Eriksen, 1960), recent studies using a variety of new experimental techniques have supplied more convincing evidence that stimuli that are not represented in subjective awareness (Cheesman & Merikle, 1986) are nevertheless processed to high levels by the perceptual system (e.g., Cheesman & Merikle, 1986; Dixon, 1981; Fowler, Wolford, Slade, & Tassinary, 1981; Marcel, 1983; see Holender, 1986, for a methodological critique). More relevant to the present concerns, several studies have purposed to show that stimuli that are not consciously perceived, and hence cannot be explicitly remembered, influence subsequent behavior and performance on tasks that do not require conscious recollection of the subliminal stimulus, such as free association (Haber & Erdelyi, 1967; Shevrin & Fritzler, 1968) and imaginative story and fantasy productions (Giddan, 1967; Pine, 1960). However, questions regarding interpretation of these results have been raised (Dixon, 1981; Erdelyi, 1970).

The foregoing experiments did not systematically examine the relation between implicit and explicit memory for subliminally exposed stimuli. However, recent studies have demonstrated implicit memory for subliminal or briefly exposed stimuli under conditions in which subjects exhibit little or no explicit memory. Kunst-Wilson and Zajonc (1980) showed subjects geometric shapes at exposure durations that they contended were too brief (1 ms) to permit conscious perception. Explicit memory for the shapes, as indexed by forced-choice recognition performance, was at chance. However, subjects demonstrated implicit memory by showing a reliable preference for the previously exposed shapes on a test in which they rated which of two shapes—one old, one new—they liked better. Similar results have been reported by Seamon, Brody, and Kauff (1983) and Wilson (1979). Mandler, Nakamura, and Van Zandt (in press) showed that brief stimulus exposures that yield chance levels of recognition memory can influence nonaffective stimulus judgments (i.e., brightness). Bargh and Pietromonaco (1982) examined the effects of subliminal exposures to "hostile" words (e.g., unkind, thoughtless) on a subsequent impression formation task. Subjects who had been given subliminal exposures to hostile words later rated a target person more negatively than did those who had not received such prior exposure, even though explicit recognition of the hostile words was at the change level. Bargh, Bond, Lombardi, and Tota (1986) observed similar implicit effects following subliminal exposure to various other types of words. Lewicki (1985) found that after subliminal exposure to adjective-noun pairs (e.g., *old–tree*) subjects tended to choose the previously exposed adjective in response to questions concerning how they "felt" about the noun (e.g., *Is a tree big or old*?)

A recent study by Eich (1984) that used a different method to attenuate conscious perception of target materials yielded data consistent with the foregoing results. Eich used an auditory divided attention task in which homophones were presented on the unattended channel together with words intended to bias the low frequency interpretation of the homophone (e.g., *taxi*–FARE). Subjects subsequently showed to explicit memory for the homophones on a *yes/no* recognition test. However, when required to spell the target words, subjects provided the low frequency spelling of the homophones more often than in baseline conditions, thereby demonstrating implicit memory for the unattended information.

Learning and Conditioning Without Awareness

In learning-without-awareness studies, subjects allegedly learn rules or contingencies without awareness of learning them and, hence, without explicit memory for them (cf. Greenspoon, 1955; Thorndike & Rock, 1934). The phenomenon was studied extensively during the 1950s in multitrial learning experiments in which subjects were reinforced for making specific responses or types of responses. Several investigators reported that subjects who were unaware of the reinforcement-response contingency provided the reinforced response with increasing frequency across trials, but others pointed to the lack of appropriate methods for determining subjects' awareness of the reinforcement-response contingency (for review, see Eriksen, 1960). Studies that used more rigorous methods for assessing awareness reported some positive evidence of learning without awareness (Giddan & Eriksen, 1959; Krieckhaus & Eriksen, 1960), as did research in which the reinforcement-response contingency was thoroughly disguised (Rosenfeld & Baer, 1969; see also Nisbett & Wilson, 1977). However, many negative observations were also reported (Brewer, 1974).

In related research, several investigators presented evidence that subjects could acquire various types of classically conditioned responses without awareness of conditioning contingencies (cf. Adams, 1957; Lacey & Smith, 1954), but assessment of awareness was often insufficient (Brewer, 1974). Along these same lines, research concerning the phenomenon of subception (Lazarus & McCleary, 1951) indicated that an experimentally acquired conditioned response, revealed by the galvanic skin response to nonsense syllables that had been accompanied by shock, could be subsequently elicited by brief exposures to the nonsense syllables, even though subjects did not detect the presence of the syllables. Although some questions and criticisms were raised about interpretations of the subception phenomenon, the finding that a conditioned response could sometimes be elicited by an unreported stimulus was not challenged (Eriksen, 1960, pp. 287–288).

Recent evidence concerning rule or contingency learning without awareness has been reported in a series of experiments by Reber and his colleagues concerning a phenomenon that they call *implicit learning* (e.g., Reber, 1976; Reber, Allen, & Regan, 1985; see also Brooks, 1978; Gordon & Holyoak, 1983; McAndrews & Moscovitch, 1985). In these studies, subjects were presented with letter strings that were organized according to various rules of a synthetic grammar. Reber and his associates reported that subjects learned to identify grammatically correct strings even when they were not consciously or explicitly aware of the appropriate rules (for critique and discussion, see Dulany, Carlson, & Dewey, 1984, 1985; Reber et al., 1985). Using a somewhat different procedure, Lewicki (1986) showed that contingencies between different features of stimulus information influenced latencies to respond to questions regarding the contingent features, even though none of the subjects could explicitly state the nature of the contingency.

Repetition Priming Effects

Most of the recent work in cognitive psychology that can be characterized as implicit memory research has been concerned with the phenomenon of direct or repetition priming (cf. Cofer, 1967): facilitation in the processing of a stimulus as a function of a recent encounter with the same stimulus. Repetition priming has been observed on a variety of tests that do not make explicit reference to a prior study episode. The tests most commonly used in priming research are *lexical decision*, *word indentification*, and *word stem* or *fragment completion*. On the lexical decision test (e.g., Forbach, Stanners, & Hochhaus, 1974; Scarborough, Gerard, & Cortese, 1979), subjects are required to state whether or not a particular letter string constitutes a legal word; priming is reflected by a decreased latency in the making of a lexical decision on the second presentation of a letter string relative to the first. On the word identification test (also referred to as *tachistoscopic identification* or *perceptual identification*: e.g., Feustel, Shiffrin, & Salasoo, 1983; Jacoby & Dallas, 1981; Neisser, 1954), subjects are given a brief exposure (e.g., 30 ms) to a stimulus and then attempt to identify it. Priming on this task is indicated by an increase in the accuracy of identifying recently exposed items relative to new items or by a decrease in the amount of exposure time necessary to identify recently exposed items. On word completion tests (e.g., Graf, Mandler, & Haden, 1982; Tulving, Schacter, & Stark, 1982; Warrington & Weiskrantz, 1974), subjects are either given a word *stem* (e.g., tab—for table) or *fragment* (e.g.,–ss–ss––for assassin) and are instructed to complete it with the first appropriate word that comes to mind. Here, priming is reflected by an enhanced tendency to complete test stems or fragments with words exposed on a prior study list. Other priming tests include reading of transformed script (Kolers, 1975, 1976; Masson, 1984), face identification (Bruce & Valentine, 1985; Young, McWeeny, Hay, & Ellis, 1986), and free association (Storms, 1958; Williamsen, Johnson, & Eriksen, 1965).

The current interest in repetition priming derives from two distinct and at times independent areas of investigation. The first area grew out of research on word recognition and lexcial organization. The general purpose of these studies was to use the pattern of priming effects observed on tasks such as word identification and lexical decision as a basis for making inferences about the nature of lexical access and representation (cf. Morton, 1979; Murrell & Morton, 1974; Scarborough et al., 1979). This line of research has yielded a number of useful findings about performance on implicit memory tests. Several investigators who attempted to distinguish between modality-specific and modality-nonspecific components of lexical organization by examining the effect of auditory–visual modality shifts on the magnitude of repetition priming reported little or no priming of tachistosopic identification (e.g., Kirsner & Smith, 1974; Kirsner, Milech, & Standen, 1983) and lexical decision performance (e.g., Kirsner et al., 1983; Scarborough et al., 1979) following an auditory study presentation. A number of studies have compared repetition priming of real words and nonwords, and have generally found that nonwords show either no priming or smaller amounts of priming than real words (Forbach et al., 1974; Forster & Daivs, 1984; Kirsner & Smith, 1974; Scarborough, Cortese, & Scarborough, 1977), although robust priming of nonwords has been observed under some experimental conditions (Feustel et al., 1983; Salasso, Shiffrin, & Feustel, 1985).

Several studies have demonstrated that priming of word identification performance occurs for morphologically similar words (e.g., exposure to *seen* facilitates identification of *sees*; Murrell & Morton, 1974), but not for visually similar words (*seen* does not facilitate *seed*; Murrell & Morton, 1974; see also Osgood & Hoosain, 1974) or phonologically similar words (*frays* does not facilitate *phrase*: Neisser, 1954). In an important study, Winnick and Daniel (1970) examined word identification performance following three types of study conditions: reading a familiar word from a visual presentation of it, generation of the word from a picture of it, or generation of the word from its definition. They observed significant priming on the word identification task following visual presentation but observed no priming in either of the generation conditions. By contrast, they found that free recall of words in both generation conditions was considerably higher than in the read condition. Although Winnick and Daniel did not set out to compare implicit and explicit memory, their results revealed a sharp dissociation between these two forms of memory (for similar results, see Jacoby, 1983b).

The second line of investigation concerned with priming effects was initiated in the context of research on episodic memory. It was stimulated largely by Warrington and Weiskrantz's (1968, 1974) work on amnesia, which will be reviewed in the next section. Their experiments demonstrated that amnesic patients showed excellent retention when required to complete three-letter stems of recently presented words, despite their inability to remember the prior occurrence of the words on a *yes/no* recognition test. Several investigators examined whether similar dissociations could be produced in normal subjects by manipulation of appropriate experimental variables (e.g., Graf et al., 1982; Jacoby & Dallas, 1981; Tulving et al., 1982), and thereby initiated systematic comparison of performance on implicit and explicit memory tests. Data generated by this line of investigation indicate that repetition priming effects on implicit memory tests can be experimentally dissociated from explicit recall and recognition in a number of ways.

First, several studies have demonstrated that variations in level or type of study processing have differential effects on priming and remembering, in conformity with the finding first reported by Winnick and Daniel (1970). For instance, Jacoby and Dallas (1981) showed subjects a list of familiar words and had them perform a study task that required elaborative processing (e.g., answering questions about the meaning of target words) or did not require elaborative processing (e.g., deciding whether or not a word contains a particular letter). Memory for the words was subsequently assessed with *yes/no* recognition and word identification tests. As expected on the basis of many previous experiments (cf. Craik & Tulving, 1975), explicit memory was influenced by type of study processing: Recognition performance was higher following elaborative study tasks than nonelaborative study tasks. Implicit memory, however, was unaffected by the study task manipulation; priming effects on word identification performance were about the same following the elaborative and nonelaborative processing tasks. Graf et al. (1982) reported a similar pattern of results by using free recall as an index of explicit memory and stem completion as an index of implicit memory. More recently, Grat and Mandler (1984) found dissociable effects of a study-task manipulation on implicit and explicit memory when test cues were identifical (i.e., three-letter word stems) and only instructions were varied. When subjects were told to use the stems to try to remember study-list words (explicit memory instructions), more items were recalled following elaborative study processing than following nonelaborative study processing. However, when subjects were instructed to write down the first word that came to mind in response to a test stem (implicit memory instructions), type of study task did not affect the amount of priming observed. Schacter and McGlynn (1987) assessed implicit memory for common idioms e.g., SOUR–GRAPES) with a free-association test (e.g., SOUR–?) in which subjects wrote down the first word that came to mind, and assessed explicit memory with a cued-recall test in which the same cue was provided and subjects were instructed to try to remember the appropriate study-list target. Implicit memory was invariant across several elaborative and nonelaborative study tasks that significantly influenced explicit memory.

A second type of dissociation between implicit and explicit memory involves the effect of study-test changes in modality of presentation and other types of surface information. As was noted earlier, priming effects on lexical decision and word identification tests are significantly reduced by study-test modality shifts (Clarke & Morton, 1983; Kirsner et al., 1983; Kirsner & Smith, 1974). Jacoby and Dallas (1981) compared the effects of modality shifts on implicit (word identification) and explicit (*yes/no* recognition) tasks. They found that changing modality of presentation from study (auditory) to test (visual) severely attenuated priming effects on word identification performance but had little or no effect on recognition performance. Graf, Shimamura, and Squire (1985) reported that priming effects on the stem-completion task were reduced by a study-test modality shift, whereas cued-recall performance was not significantly influenced by this manipulation, and Roediger and Blaxton (1987) found that priming of word-fragment completion performance was attenuated by modality shifts even though free-recall and recognition performance were largely unaffected. Along the same lines, several studies have shown that within the visual modality, priming effects on lexical decision, fragment completion, and reading tasks are highly sensitive to study-test changes of various types of surface information (Kolers, 1975, 1976; Roediger & Blaxton, 1987; Roediger & Weldon, 1987; Scarborough et al., 1979), whereas recall and recognition are either unaffected or slightly affected by such changes.

A third kind of evidence for implicit/explicit dissociations comes from studies that have manipulated retention interval. On both word-fragment completion (Komatsu & Ohta, 1984; Tulving et al., 1982) and word identification tests (Jacoby & Dallas, 1981), priming effects persist with little change across delays of days and weeks, whereas recognition memory declines across the same delays. In other situations, however, priming of word-stem completion (Graf & Mandler, 1984; Graf et al., 1984; Shimamura & Squire, 1984) and lexical decision (Forster & Davis, 1984) has proved to be a relatively transient phenomenon, decaying across delays of minutes and hours over which explicit remembering persists. Fourth, recent studies indicate that manipulations of retroactive and proactive interference that significantly impair explicit recall and recognition do not influence priming effects on either word-stem completion (Graf & Schacter, 1987) or word-fragment completion (Sloman, Hayman, Ohta, & Tulving, in press). A fifth and final type of evidence for dissociation between priming and remembering is the finding of statistical independence between performance on recognition tests and tests of word-fragment completion (Tulving et al., 1982), word-stem completion (Graf & Schacter, 1985), homophone spelling (Eich, 1984; Jacoby & Witherspoon, 1982), prototype identification (Metcalfe & Fisher, 1986), and reading of mirror inverted script (Kolers, 1976). In these experiments, successful performance on an implicit memory test was uncorrelated with success or failure on an explicit memory test.

Taken together, the foregoing studies provide impressive evidence that priming effects on implicit memory tests differ substantially from explicit recall and recognition. Other studies, however, have revealed several similarities between priming and remembering. First, under certain conditions manipulations of retention interval have parallel effects on priming effects and explicit memory (Jacoby, 1983a; Schacter & Graf, 1986a; Sloman et al., in press). Second, Jacoby (1983a) has shown that manipulating list context at the time of test, which is known to affect recognition memory, also affects performance on the word identification task: Identification performance was higher when 90% of tested words came from a previously studied list than when only 10% did. Third, both implicit and explicit memory are influenced by newly acquired associations between unrelated word pairs. On a variety of implicit memory tests, including word-stem completion (Graf & Schacter, 1985, 1987; Schacter & Graf, 1986a, 1986b), lexical decision (McKoon & Ratcliff, 1979, 1986), and reading of degraded word pairs (Moscovitch et al., 1986), more priming is observed when a target word is tested in the context of its study-list cue than when it is tested alone or in the presence of some other cue. Fourth, this phenomenon of *implicit memory for new associations* (cf. Graf & Schacter, 1985) resembles explicit remembering of new assoications insofar as it depends on some degree of elaborative processing at the time of study. For example, Schacter and Graf observed associative effects on word completion performance after subjects had performed study tasks that required them to elaborate semantic links between two unrelated words, such as generating sentences or reading meaningful sentences (e.g., *The injured* OFFICER *smelled the* FLOWER). When subjects engaged in study tasks that prevented elaboration of semantic relations, such as comparing the number of vowels and consonants in the target words or reading anomalous sentences (e.g., *The dusky* COW *multiplied the* EMPLOYER), implicit memory for new associations was not observed. Schacter and McGlynn (1987), using free-association and cued-recall tests, also found that both implicit and explicit memory for newly acquired associations depends on elaborative study processing. A fifth type of evidence showing a relation between implicit and explicit memory was reported by Johnston, Dark, & Jacoby (1985). They demonstrated that processes subserving implicit memory can affect performance on an explicit memory task: Recently studied words that were identified quickly on a word identification test were more likely to be given a recognition judgment of "old" than were more slowly identified words. These similarities between implicit and explicit memory have a number of implications that will be discussed later when alternative theoretical accounts of implicit memory are compared.

Implicit Memory in Amnesia

The amnesic syndrome, which is produced by lesions to the medial temporal and diencephalic regions of the brain (e.g., Moscovitch, 1982; Rozin, 1976; Squire, 1986; Weiskrantz, 1985), is characterized by normal perceptual, linguistic, and intellectual functioning together with an inability to remember explicitly recent events and new information. Amnesic patients are seriously impaired on standard tests of explicit recall and recognition, and they perform disastrously in real-life situations that require explicit remembering, such as recollecting actions and events during a round of golf (Schacter, 1983). Beginning with the previously discussed clinical observations of Korsakoff (1889) and Claparède (1911/1951), instances of implicit memory by amnesic patients have been documented widely. Most modern studies of implicit memory in amnesia can be classified into two broad categories: skill learning or repetition priming.

Research on skill learning in amnesia was initiated by Milner and Corkin and their colleagues in the 1960s. They demonstrated that the profoundly amnesic patient H. M. could acquire motor skills such as pursuit rotor and mirror tracing, even though he did not remember explicitly that he had previously performed the task (Milner, 1962; Milner, Corkin, & Teuber, 1968). Robust learning of motor skills has been observed in various other amnesic patients (e.g., Butters, 1987: Eslinger & Damasio, 1986; Starr & Phillips, 1970). Amnesic patients have also exhibited normal or near-normal learning of perceptual and cognitive skills, including skills, including reading of mirror-inverted script (Cohen & Squire, 1980; Moscovitch, 1982), puzzle solving (Brooks & Baddeley, 1976), rule learning (Kinsbourne & Wood, 1975), and serial pattern learning (Nissen & Bullemer, 1987), despite their failure to remember explicitly that they had previously performed the skills. Similar dissociations have been observed in drug-induced amnesia (Nissen, Knopman, & Schacter, in press) and multiple-personality amnesia (Nissen, Ross, Willingham, Mackenzie, & Schacter, in press).

The second major area of research on implicit memory in amnesia, concerned with repetition priming effects, was initiated by the important series of experiments conducted by Warrington and Weiskrantz (1968, 1970, 1974, 1978). They found that amnesic patients could show normal retention of a list of familiar words when tested with word-stem or fragment cues, whereas these same patients were profoundly impaired on free-recall and recognition tests. Indeed, Warrington and Weiskrantz (1968) noted that patients often did not remember that they had been shown any study-list items and treated the fragment test as a kind of "guessing game." In subsequent research using the fragment cuing procedure, amnesic patients' performance was sometimes impaired with respect to that of control subjects (e.g., Squire, Wetzel, & Slater, 1978).

It is now clear that whether or not amnesic patients show normal retention when tested with word fragments and various other cues depends critically on the implicit/explicit nature of the test. For example, Graf et al., (1984) demonstrated that when subjects were given explicit memory instructions—that is, they were told to use word stems as cues for *remembering* previously studied words—amnesics were impaired with respect to controls. By contrast, when subjects were given implicit memory instructions—that is, they were told to complete the stems with the first word that comes to mind—amnesics and controls showed comparable amounts of priming (see also Graf et al., 1985). In an early and often overlooked study, Gardner, Boller, Moreines, and Butters (1973) presented Korsakoff's syndrome amnesics and controls with a categorized word list. When subjects were subsequently given category cues and asked to respond with the first category member that came to mind, both amnesics and controls showed equivalent amounts of priming. When asked to remember list items in response to category cues, amnesics were impaired with respect to controls (see also Graf et al., 1985; see Kihlstrom, 1980, for priming of category production performance in hypnotic amnesia). Schacter (1985) found that amnesic patients showed normal priming effects after studying a list of common idioms (e.g., SOUR–GRAPES) and then writing down the first word that came to mind on a free-association test (e.g., SOUR–?). Amnesics were impaired, however, when instructed to try to use the same cues to remember study-list targets. Shimamura and Squire (1984) obtained a similar pattern of results with highly related paired associates (e.g., TABLE–CHAIR). On the basis of these studies, it seems reasonable to conclude that normal retention of a list of familiar items by amnesic patients occurs only when implicit tests are used. Consistent with this observation, amnesic patients have shown normal priming effects on various other implicit memory tests, including lexical decision (Moscovitch, 1982), perceptual identification (Cermak, Talbot, Chandler, & Wolbarst, 1985), and homophone spelling (Jacoby & Witherspoon, 1982; for more extensive review, see Schacter & Graf, 1986b; Shimamura, 1986).

In most of the priming experiments discussed thus far, study materials consisted of items with integrated or unitized preexisting memory representations, such as common words, linguistic idioms, or highly related paired associates. Recently, several investigators have examined whether amnesic patients show normal priming or implicit memory for novel information that does not have any preexisting representation as a unit in memory, such as nonwords or unrelated paired associates. The results thus far have been mixed. Cermak et al. (1985) found that amnesic patients do not show priming of nonwords on a perceptual identification task, and Diamond and Rozin (1984) obtained similar results when implicit memory was tested with three-letter stems. Using a word completion test, Graf and Schacter (1985) and Schacter and Graf (1986b) found that some amnesic patients—those with relatively mild memory disorders—showed normal implicit memory for a newly acquired association between unrelated words, whereas severely amnesic patients did not show implicit memory for new associations. Moscovitch et al. (1986) assessed implicit memory with a task that involved reading degraded pairs of unrelated words, and observed normal implicit memory for new associations in patients with severe memory disorders. McAndrews, Glisky, and Schacter (in press) investigated implicit memory for new information by presenting subjects with novel, difficult-to-comprehend sentences (e.g., *The haystack was important because the cloth ripped.*), and requiring them to generate cues that rendered the sentences comprehensible (e.g., *parachute*). They found that severely amnesic patients' ability to generate the correct cues was facilitated substantially by a single prior exposure to the cue-sentence pair, despite their complete lack of explicit memory for the sentences and cues.

The foregoing studies indicate that amnesic patients can show priming effects for newly acquired information, but they also suggest that such effects depend on the type of implicit memory test that is used and, in some instances, on the severity of amnesia. Another important issue concerning priming in amnesic patients concerns the duration of the phenomenon. Several investigators have reported that priming of word-completion performance in amnesic patients is a relatively transient phenomenon, lasting only a few hours (Diamond & Rozin, 1984; Graf et al., 1984; Rozin, 1976; Squire, Shimamura, & Graf, in press). By contrast, McAndrews et al. (in press) found that severely amnesic patients showed robust priming on their sentence puzzle task after a 1-week retention interval. These observations suggest that the duration of priming in amnesic patients may depend on the way that implicit memory is assessed and the nature of the target information.

In addition to skill learning and repetition priming phenomena, amnesic patients have also exhibited dissociations between implicit and explicit memory in various other situations. Schacter, Harbluk, and McLachlan (1984) demonstrated that amnesic patients could learn some fictitious information about people (e.g., *Bob Hope's father was a fireman*), but could not remember explicitly that they had just been told the information (see also Schacter & Tulving, 1982; Shimamura & Squire, 1987). Similarly, Luria (1976) observed that an amnesic patient produced bits and pieces of recently presented stories, even though he did not remember being told any stories. Glisky, Schacter, and Tulving (1986) showed that a densely amnesic patient could learn to program a microcomputer despite the patient's persistent failure to remember explicitly that he had ever worked on a microcomputer. Johnson, Kim, and Risse (1985) found that amnesics acquired preferences for previously exposed melodies, Crovitz, Harvey, and McClanahan (1979) demonstrated that amnesics could spot a hidden figure more quickly after a single exposure to it, and Weiskrantz and Warrington (1979) reported evidence of classical conditioning in amnesic patients—in all cases, with little or no explicit recollection of the experimental materials and of the learning episode itself.

Summary of Contemporary Studies

The research reviewed in the preceding five sections indicates that implicit memory has been documented across different tasks, materials, and subject populations. Although it is clear that a wide variety of phenomena can all be grouped together under the rather general heading of *implicit memory*, it is equally clear that there are differences among these diverse phenomena. One difference that may be significant theoretically concerns whether implicit memories are *accessible* or *inaccessible* explicitly—that is, whether or not information that is expressed implicitly can, under certain conditions, be remembered explicitly. Several studies have found substantial implicit memory when explicit recognition is at the chance level and explicit recall is at or close to the floor, thereby suggesting that the implicitly expressed information is inaccessible explicitly (e.g., Bargh & Pietromonaco, 1982; Eich, 1984; Graf et al., 1982, 1984; Kunst-Wilson & Zajonc, 1980; Lewicki, 1986; McAndrews et al., in press; Squire, Shimamura, & Graf, 1985). These findings come either from studies of amnesic patients or from experiments in which normal subjects are prevented from encoding target materials in a fully conscious or elaborative manner. By contrast, in studies of normal subjects that allow elaborative encoding of target materials, implicitly expressed information is generally accessible explicitly. For example, normal subjects who produce a previously studied word on a completion test following elaborative encoding are able to consciously remember having studied the word if an explicit recall test is given, whereas a densely amnesic patient who produces a recently studied word on a completion test cannot under any circumstances consciously or explicitly remember having studied the word.

The observation that many implicit memory phenomena in normal subjects fall into the category of "accessible explicitly" raises questions concerning the extent to which, and sense in which, such phenomena should be considered implicit. That is, if normal subjects *can* remember target information explicitly under appropriate test conditions, how can we be sure that they do not remember explicitly on a nominally implicit memory test? Some investigators have attempted to disguise the fact that previously presented items appear on a test by presenting an implicit memory task as one of several filler tasks during a retention interval, and by testing only a small proportion of previously studied items (e.g., Graf et al., 1984; Jacoby, 1983a; Schacter & Graf, 1986a). The point of these procedures is to prevent subjects from catching on concerning the nature of the test, or at least to discourage the use of explicit memory strategies. It seems quite likely, however, that subjects will "clue in" concerning the nature of the test once they have been exposed to, or have successfully produced, a number of list items. Nevertheless, the fact that several studies have shown differential effects of experimental variables on implicit and explicit memory tasks when identical test cues were provided, and only the implicit/explicit nature of test instructions were varied (e.g., Graf & Mandler, 1984; Schacter & Graf, 1986a), suggests that subjects do not deliberately use explicit memory strategies on implicit memory tasks. If subjects did use such strategies, we would expect to observe parallel effects of experimental variables when the same cues are provided on implicit and explicit tasks.

However, the foregoing considerations indicate only that it is possible to prevent intentional or *voluntary* explicit memory from influencing performance on implicit memory tests. It is possible that some instances of what appear to be implicit memory may be better described as *involuntary* explicit memory: cases in which a test cue leads to an unintentional but fully conscious and explicit "reminding" of the occurrence of a prior episode (cf. Ross, 1984). The possibility of confusing implicit memory with involuntary explicit memory would appear to be greatest in experiments with normal subjects that permit elaborative encoding of target materials. At present, we know little about the relation between implicit memory and involuntary explicit memory, but future research and theorizing should be directed toward this issue.

Another difference among the various implicit memory phenomena concerns whether or not target information acquired during a study episode is represented directly in consciousness at the time of test. For example, in repetition priming studies, the target material (i.e., *assassin*) is represented in consciousness at the time of test, such as when the subject completes a test fragment with a previously studied item. By contrast, in other situations target content is not represented in consciousness at the time of test, yet influences performance *indirectly*. For example, when subjects performing an impression-formation task rate a target person more negatively because of subliminal exposure to hostile words that cannot be recalled (e.g., Bargh & Pietromonaco, 1982), or when subjects make classification responses on the basis of rules that they cannot articulate (e.g., Lewicki, 1986; Reber, 1976), the influence of acquired information on implicit memory is indirect. Although we do not know whether direct and indirect expressions of implicit memory differ in theoretically significant ways, the issue has been previously overlooked and may be worth exploring in future studies.

The foregoing considerations also highlight the fact that we presently lack well-specified criteria for assessing whether subjects are explicitly aware of previous experiences at the time of test (Tulving, 1985c). Similar issues concerning criteria for determining awareness have been debated extensively in the literature on perception and learning without awareness (e.g., Chessman & Merikle, 1986; Eriksen, 1960; Nisbett & Wilson, 1977), and memory researchers would do well to attempt to incorporate some of the lessons from these investigations into research on implicit memory.

Theoretical Accounts of Implicit Memory

In view of the diversity of phenomena that can be grouped under the rubric of implicit memory, it is perhaps not surprising that no single theory has addressed, much less accounted for, all or even most of the observations discussed in this article. Rather, different theoretical views have been advanced to accommodate different subsets of the data. However, one general idea that can be rejected on the basis of recent research is the threshold view discussed in the historical section. The finding that implicit memory is unaffected by experimental variables that have large effects on explicit memory, and that performance on implicit tests is often statistically independent of performance on explicit tests, is inconsistent with a threshold model in which implicit and explicit tests differ only in their sensitivity to the strength of memory traces. In this section, three more viable theoretical approaches to implicit memory phenomena are considered, which are referred to, respectively, as *activation*, *processing*, and *multiple memory system* accounts. Each of these views has been concerned primarily with repetition priming effects and with dissociations observed in amnesic patients.

Activation views hold that priming effects on implicit memory tests are attributable to the temporary activation of preexisting representations, knowledge structures, or logogens (e.g., Graf & Mandler, 1984; Mandler, 1980; Morton, 1979; Rozin, 1976). Activation is assumed to occur automatically, independently of the elaborative processing that is necessary to establish new episodic memory traces. An activated representation readily "pops into mind" on an implicit memory test, but it contains no contextual information about an item's occurrence as part of a recent episode and therefore does not contribute to explicit remembering of the episode.

Processing views seek to understand differences between implicit and explicit memory by explicating the nature of and relations between encoding and retrieval process or procedures (e.g., Craik, 1983; Jacoby, 1983a, 1983b; Moscovitch et al., 1986; Roediger & Blaxton, 1987; Witherspoon & Moscovitch, 1986). Such views assume that both implicit and explicit memory rely on newly established episodic representations, and portray differences between them in terms of interactions between features of encoded representations and different demands posed by implicit and explicit tests. The best articulated version of this view relies on the distinction between *conceptually driven* processes and *data-driven* processes (Jacoby, 1983b; Roediger & Blaxton, 1987). Conceptually driven processes reflect subject-initiated activities such as elaborating, organizing, and reconstructing; data-driven processes are initiated and guided by the information or data that is presented in test materials. Although both explicit and implicit tests can have data-driven and conceptually driven components, it is argued that explicit memory tests typically draw primarily on conceptually driven processes, whereas implicit tests typically draw primarily on data-driven processes. Performance dissociations between implicit and explicit tests are thus attributed to differences between conceptually driven and data-driven processes.

Multiple memory system interpretations ascribe differences between implicit and explicit memory to the different properties of hypothesized underlying systems. For example, Squire and Cohen (1984) argued that conscious or explicit recollection is a property of, and supported by, a *declarative* memory system that is involved in the formation of new representations or data structures. By contrast, implicit memory phenomena such as learning of skills and repetition priming effects are attributed to a *procedural* system in which memory is expressed by on-line modification of procedures or processing operations. The distinction between episodic and semantic memory (Tulving, 1972, 1983) has also been invoked to account for dissociations on implicit and explicit tests (e.g., Cermak et al., 1985; Kinsbourne & Wood, 1975; Parkin, 1982; Schacter & Tulving, 1982; Tulving, 1983). The episodic memory system is viewed as the basis for explicit remembering of recent events, whereas semantic memory is seen as responsible for performance on tasks such as word completion, lexical decision, and word identification, which require subjects to make use of preexisting knowledge of words and concepts. A variety of other multiple memory system views have also been put forward (e.g., Johnson, 1983; O'Keefe & Nadel, 1978; Schacter & Moscovitch, 1984; Warrington & Weiskrantz, 1982).

Each of these three approaches is consistent with certain features of existing data and has difficulty accommodating others. Activation views account for the finding that priming of preexisting representations does not depend on elaborative processing (e.g., Graf et al., 1982; Jacoby & Dallas, 1981) and that under certain conditions, priming decays rapidly in both normals and amnesics (Cermak et al., 1985; Diamond & Rozin, 1984; Graf et al., 1984; Graf & Mandler, 1984; Shimamura & Squire, 1984; Squire et al., in press). Activation accounts are also consistent with the finding that some severely amnesic patients who show normal priming of items with preexisting memory representations (e.g., familiar words, idioms) do not show normal priming of nonwords or unrelated paired associates (Cermak et al., 1985; Diamond & Rozin, 1984; Schacter, 1985; Schacter & Graf, 1986b). However, an activation view does not readily accommodate those cases in which amnesic patients do show implicit memory for new information (Graf & Schacter, 1985; McAndrews et al., in press; Moscovitch et al., 1986), and has difficulty accounting for the effect of newly acquired associations on implicit memory tests in normal subjects (Graf & Schacter, 1985, 1987; McKoon & Ratcliff, 1979, 1986; Schacter & Graf, 1986a, 1986b; see Mandler in press, for discussion). The activation notion is also inconsistent with the persistence of facilitation on certain implicit memory tests over days, weeks, and months in normal subjects (Jacoby, 1983a; Jacoby & Dallas, 1981; Komatus & Ohta, 1984; Schacter & Graf, 1986a; Sloman et al., in press; Tulving et al., 1982) and amnesic patients (Crovitz et al., 1979; McAndrews et al., in press).

The strengths and weaknesses of the conceptual versus data-driven processing view are a virtual mirror image of those of the activation view. With its heavy emphasis on an episodic basis of implicit memory, this notion accounts well for observations of persistence, associative effects, contextual sensitivity, and study–test interactions (see Jacoby, 1983b; Roediger & Blaxton, 1987, for elaboration). However, it is less able to handle the findings on short-lived activation, dependence of some priming effects on preexisting representations in amnesic patients, and differences between priming of new and old representations in normals (cf. Feustel et al., 1983; Schacter & Graf, 1986a). This view also has difficulty accounting for the finding that implicit memory for newly acquired associations, as indexed by performance on the stem completion task, depends on some degree of elaborative study processing (e.g., Schacter & Graf, 1986a). Because it has been argued that elaborative study processing should not affect performance on data-driven implicit memory tasks such as stem completion (e.g., Roediger & Weldon, 1987), the finding that some aspects of performance on an implicit test are elaboration dependent is puzzling. It is also important to note that this view does not speak directly to the key feature of implicit memory phenomena: the absence of conscious recollection of a prior experience at the time of test. That is, it is not clear why data-driven processing should be associated with lack of explicit recollection of a prior experience, whereas conceptually driven processing is generally associated with conscious recollection of a prior experience (see Jacoby, 1984, for relevant discussion).

The strengths and weaknesses of multiple memory system views differ somewhat from the foregoing. The procedural/declarative view has been primarily applied to phenomena observed in amnesic patients. The strength of this view is that it provides a straightforward account of *normal* perceptual-motor skill learning in amnesics who lack conscious recollection of prior episodes: Skill learning is assumed to depend on a procedural memory system that is spared in amnesic patients, but does not provide a basis of explicit remembering. It has also been suggested that procedural memory is responsible for priming effects (Cohen, 1984; Squire, 1986). However, recent evidence indicates that priming and skill learning can be dissociated experimentally (Butters, 1987). This hypothesis also cannot readily account for amnesic patients' failure to show priming for nonwords: If priming reflects the modification of procedures used to encode target stimuli, it should occur for both old and new information. Moreover, amnesic patients show implicit memory in situations in which it is unlikely that performance is mediated by the procedural system. For example, amnesics can retrieve newly acquired facts and vocabulary even though they have no explicit recollection of having learned the information (Glisky et al., 1986; Schacter et al., 1984). It does not seem reasonable to attribute the implicit memory observed here to the procedural system, because learning of new facts is allegedly the responsibility of declarative memory (Squire & Cohen, 1984).

Proponents of the episodic-semantic distinction can account for some priming phenomena by postulating that performance on completion and identification tests depends upon activation of the semantic memory system, whereas explicit recall and recognition depend on episodic memory. This account would then be characterized by similar strengths and weaknesses as the activation view discussed earlier. Several other difficulties in applying the episodic–semantic distinction to implicit memory phenomena have been discussed elsewhere (McKoon, Ratcliff, & Dell, 1986; Roediger & Blaxton, 1987; Schacter & Tulving, 1982; Squire & Cohen, 1984; Tulving, 1983, 1986).

The foregoing considerations indicate that although each of the three main theoretical views accommodates certain aspects of the data, no single theoretical position accounts satisfactorily for all of the existing findings concerning implicit memory.

Implicit Memory: Future Directions

To conclude the article, I will first summarize key issues that need to be addressed in implicit memory research; I will then consider briefly a related domain of inquiry which may provide fruitful perspectives on implicit memory and suggest new directions for research.

Empirical and Theoretical Extensions of Implicit Memory Research

One of the most striking features of the historical survey and review of current research is the sheer diversity of implicit memory phenomena that have been observed. The fact that implicit memory has been observed across a wide variety of tasks and subject populations has both empirical and theoretical implications. On the empirical side, it seems clear that a critical task for future research is to delineate systematically the similarities and differences among the various implicit memory tests that have been used. Within the domain of repetition priming, for example, it would be desirable to further explore the relations among word-stem and fragment completion, word identification, lexical decision, free association, and other implicit memory tasks; each of these tests may be tapping different aspects of implicit memory (cf. Witherspoon & Moscovitch, 1986). Such research could help to clarify a number of unresolved issues. Consider, for example, the time course of repetition priming effects on implicit memory tests. It was noted earlier that activation views are consistent with findings of rapid decay of priming. However, the meaning of *rapid decay* varies widely, from seconds or minutes in some lexical decision paradigms (e.g., Forster & Davis, 1984) to several hours in stemcompletion paradigms (e.g., Diamond & Rozin, 1984; Graf & Mandler, 1984). Moreover, as discussed previously, priming in fragment completion, word identification, and other implicit memory paradigms can persist for days, weeks, and months (Jacoby, 1983a; McAndrews et al., in press; Schacter & Graf, 1986a; Sloman et al., in press; Tulving et al., 1982). To understand these differences in the time course of priming, researchers will need a better understanding of the nature of the information and processes tapped by different implicit memory tests.

It would also be desirable to attempt to relate the findings from priming studies to observations concerning implicit memory in other paradigms, such as implicit rule learning. One area that appears particularly promising concerns the role of implicit memory in affective and social phenomena such as mood states (Bowers, 1984), fears and phobias (Jacobs & Nadel, 1985), impression formation (Bargh & Pietromonaco, 1982), and self conceptions (Markus & Kunda, 1986). As revealed in the historical section, many striking implicit memory phenomena were reported by investigators concerned with the role of unconscious influences in affective states (e.g., Freud, Janet), and experimental studies of this issue could provide key insights into the functions of implicit memory. A second, related area that has not yet been fully exploited concerns the role of implicit memory in functional amnesias. A few investigators have examined implicit memory in hypnosis (Kihlstrom, 1980, 1984; Williamsen et al., 1965), multiple personality (Nissen, Ross, Willingham, Mackenzie, & Schacter, in press), and alcohol and drug intoxication (Hashtroudi, Parker, DeLisi, Wyatt, & Mutter, 1984; Nissen, Knopman, & Schacter, in press), but much work remains to be done. Third, research concerning the development of implicit memory in young and old populations is needed. Schacter and Moscovitch (1984) argued that infants and very young children may be capable of implicit memory only. However, there has been virtually no research that has explored the issue directly. Several studies have reported that older adults show intact repetition priming (Graf & Schacter, 1985; Light, Singh, & Capps, 1986) but little else is known about the relation between aging and implicit memory.

On the theoretical side, the diversity of implicit memory phenomena suggests that attempts to account for all relevant observations with a single construct or dichotomy will probably not be entirely successful. As was evident in the discussion of theoretical alternatives, no single position convincingly handles all relevant data. Accordingly, it is worth entertaining the idea that there are multiple sources of implicit memory phenomena. For example, Schacter and Graf (1986b) argued that automatic, relatively short-lived priming effects depend on activation of preexisting representations, whereas longer lasting, elaboration-dependent effects may be based on specific components of newly created episodic representations (see also Schacter & Graf, 1986a; Forster & Davis, 1984). Similarly, it is possible that some implicit memory phenomena, such as perceptual-motor skill learning in amnesic patients, reflect the operation of a memory system that is distinct from the system subserving explicit recall and recognition, whereas other implicit memory phenomena, such as associative effects on word-completion performance, depend on components of the same system that subserves recall and recognition. Unfortunately, firm criteria for distinguishing between multiple-system and single-system accounts do not exist, although some possibilities have been discussed (cf. Sherry & Schacter, in press; Tulving 1985a). Nevertheless, in view of the diversity of implicit memory phenomena, the activation, processing, and multiple-memory system views need not be mutually exclusive. Each may account well for certain aspects of the data, and may be useful in generating different questions and problems for future research.

The Generality of Implicit/Explicit Dissociations: A Theoretical Challenge

Recent research has revealed that implicit/explicit dissociations are not restricted to situations involving memory for recent events. These studies have produced dissociations that are remarkably similar to some of those discussed here in one crucial respect: Subjects demonstrate that they possess a particular kind of knowledge by their performance on a task, yet they are not consciously aware that they possess the knowledge and cannot gain access to it explicitly. In cognitive psychology, evidence of this kind, although somewhat controversial, has been provided by previously mentioned studies on perception without awareness (e.g., Cheesman & Merikle, 1986; Marcel, 1983).

Neuropsychological research has demonstrated that patients with various lesions and deficits show knowledge of stimuli that they cannot explicitly perceive, identify, or process semantically. First, patients with lesions to primary visual projection areas, who do not have conscious perceptual experiences within their hemianopic field, nevertheless perform at above-chance levels when given forced-choice discrimination tests concerning location, orientation, and other dimensions of a visual stimulus (e.g., Weiskrantz, 1986; see Champion, Latto, & Smith, 1983, for a critique). This phenomenon of "blind-sight" occurs in patients who claim that they are guessing the location and identity of the visual stimulus but do not "see" anything at all. A second, similar dissociation has been reported in patients with lesions of the right parieto-occipital cortex who have deficits orienting and attending to stimuli which are presented in their left visual fields. Such patients can make accurate same-different judgments regarding stimuli that are presented simultaneously in the left and right visual fields, despite the fact that they cannot state the identity of the stimulus in the left visual field and often deny the presence of any left-field stimulus (Volpe, LeDoux, & Gazzaniga, 1979). Third, patients with facial recognition deficits (prosopagnosia) show stronger galvanic skin responses to familiar than to unfamiliar faces, even though patients do not explicitly recognize any faces as familiar (Bauer, 1984; Tranel & Damasio, 1985). Fourth, alexic patients, who have serious problems reading common words, perform at above chance levels when required to make lexical decisions and semantic categorizations regarding words that they cannot explicitly or consciously identify (Coslett, 1986; Shallice & Saffran, 1986), or to point to objects corresponding to words that they deny seeing (Landis, Regard, & Serrant, 1980). Fifth, aphasic patients with severe comprehension deficits show semantic priming effects for related word pairs without conscious understanding of the semantic relation that links the words (Blumstein, Milberg, & Shrier, 1982; Milberg & Blumstein, 1981).

The foregoing phenomena differ from one another, and from the implicit memory phenomena discussed earlier, insofar as the performance of each type of patient reflects somewhat different residual or preserved capacities (for more detailed review, see Schacter, McAndrews, & Moscovitch, in press). The striking similarity, however, is that in all cases knowledge is expressed implicitly and does not give rise to a conscious experience of knowing, perceiving, or remembering. This observation suggests that conscious or explicit experiences of knowing, perceiving, or remembering are all in some way dependent upon the functioning of a common mechanism, a mechanism whose functioning is disrupted in various brain-damaged patients. Elsewhere, I have outlined a model that delineates some properties of this mechanism, describes how it is related to various memory structures, and suggests that it can be isolated or disconnected from specific memory and processing systems in different neuropsychological syndromes (Schacter, 1987). For the present purposes, the observation of implicit–explicit dissociations in multiple domains has several implications: It provides a possibly important clue for development of theories of implicit memory, it suggests that the study of implicit memory should be pursued in close conjunction with the study of related phenomena in normal and brain-damaged populations, and it highlights again the generality and pervasiveness of dissociations between implicit and explicit expressions of memory and knowledge.

Notes

This article was supported by a Special Research Program Grant from the Connaught Fund, University of Toronto, and by the Natural Sciences and Engineering Research Council of Canada Grant U0361.

I am indebted to numerous colleagues for comments on an earlier draft of the article, and I thank E. Eich, P. Gabel, E. Glisky, P. Graf, L. Jacoby, M. Johnson, J. Kihlstrom, G. Mandler, M. P. McAndrews, M. J. Nissen, A. Parkin, H. Roediger, T. Shallice, A. Shimamura, E. Tulving, A. Young, and the students in H. Roediger's graduate seminar for their helpful suggestions. I also thank C. Macdonald for excellent translations of material in French and for valuable aid with preparation of the manuscript.

Correspondence concerning this article should be addressed to Daniel L. Schacter, who is now at the Department of Psychology, University of Arizona, Tucson, Arizona 85721.

References

Adams, J. K. (1957). Laboratory studies of behavior without awareness. *Psychological Bulletin, 54*, 383–405.

Bargh, J. A., Bond, R. N., Lombardi, W. J., & Tota, M. E. (1986). The additive nature of chronic and temporary sources of construct accessibility. *Journal of Personality and Social Psychology, 50*, 869–878.

Bargh, J. A., & Pietromonaco, P. (1982). Automatic information processing and social perception: The influence of trait information presented outside of conscious awareness on impression formation. *Journal of Personality and Social Psychology, 43*, 437–449.

Barkworth, T. (1891). Some recent experiments in automatic writing. *Proceedings of the Society for Psychical Research, 7*, 23–29.

Bauer, R. M. (1984). Autonomic recognition of names and faces in prosopagnosia: A neuropsychological application of the guilty knowledge test. *Neuropsychologia, 22*, 457–469.

Bergson, H. (1911). *Matter and memory.* New York: Macmillan.

Binet, A. (1890). *On double consciousness.* Chicago: Open Court.

Blumstein, S. E., Milberg, W., & Shrier, R. (1982). Semantic processing in aphasia: Evidence from an auditory lexical decision task. *Brain and Language, 17*, 301–315.

Bowers, K. S. (1984). On being unconsciously influenced an informed. In K. S. Bowers & D. Meichenbaum (Eds.), *The unconscious reconsidered* (pp. 227–272). New York: Wiley.

Brewer, W. F. (1974). There is no convincing evidence for operant or classical conditioning in adult humans. In W. B. Weimer & D. S. Palermo (Eds.), *Cognition and the symbolic processes* (pp. 1–42). Hillsdale. NJ: Erlbaum.

Brooks, D. N., & Baddeley, A. D. (1976). What can amnesic patients learn? *Neuropsychologia, 14*, 111–122.

Brooks, L. (1978). Nonanalytic concept formation and memory for instances. In E. Rosch & B. B. Lloyd (Eds.), *Cognition and categorization* (pp. 169–211). Hillsdale, NJ: Erlbaum.

Bruce, V., & Valentine, T. (1985). Identity priming in the recognition of familiar faces. *British Journal of Psychology, 76*, 373–383.

Butters, N. (1987, February). *Procedural learning in dementia: A double dissociation between Alzheimer and Huntington's disease patients on verbal priming and motor skill learning.* Paper presented at the meeting of the International Neuropsychological Society, Washington, DC.

Campion, J., Latto, R., & Smith, Y. M. (1983). Is blindsight an effect of scattered light, spared cortex, and near-threshold vision? *The Behavioral and Brain Sciences, 6*, 423–486.

Carpenter, W. B. (1874). *Principles of mental physiology.* London: John Churchill.

Cermak, L. S., Talbot, N., Chandler, K., & Wolbarst, L. R. (1985). The perceptual priming phenomenon in amnesia. *Neuropsychologia, 23*, 615–622.

Cheesman, J., & Merikle, P. M. (1986). Word recognition and consciousness. In D. Besner, T. G. Waller, & G. E. Mackinnon (Eds.), *Reading research: Advances in theory and practice* (Vol. 5, pp. 311–352). New York: Academic Press.

Claparède, E. (1951). Recognition and 'me-ness.' In D. Rapaport (Ed.), *Organization and pathology of thought* (pp. 58–75). New York: Columbia University Press. (Reprinted from Archives de Psychologie, 1911, *11*, 79–90).

Clarke, R. G. B., & Morton, J. (1983). Cross modality facilitation in tachistoscopic word recognition. *Quarterly Journal of Experimental Psychology, 35A*, 79–96.

Cofer, C. C. (1967). Conditions for the use of verbal associations. *Psychological Bulletin, 68*, 1–12.

Cohen, N. J. (1984). Preserved learning capacity in amnesia: Evidence for multiple memory systems. In L. R. Squire & N. Butters (Eds.), *Neuropsychology of memory* (pp. 83–103). New York: Guilford Press.

Cohen, N. J., & Squire, L. R. (1980). Presented learning and retention of pattern-analyzing skill in amnesia: Dissociation of "knowing how" and "knowing that." *Science, 210*, 207–209.

Coslett, H. B. (1986, June). *Preservation of lexical access in alexia without agraphia.* Paper presented at the 9th European Conference of the International Neuropsychological Society, Veldhoven. The Netherlands.

Craik, F. I. M. (1983). On the transfer of information from temporary to permanent memory. *Philosophical Transactions of the Royal Society of London, 302*, 341–359.

Craik, F. I. M., & Tulving, E. (1975). Depth of processing and the retention of words in episodic memory. *Journal of Experimental Psychology: General, 104*, 268–294.

Crovitz, H. F., Harvey, M. T., & McClanahan, S. (1979). Hidden memory: A rapid method for the study of amnesia using perceptual learning. *Cortex, 17*, 273–278.

Darwin, E. (1794). *Zoonomia: or the laws of organic life.* (Vol. 1) London: J. Johnson.

Diamond, R., & Rozin, P. (1984). Activation of existing memories in the amnesic syndrome. *Journal of Abnormal Psychology, 93*, 98–105.

Dixon, N. F. (1971). *Subliminal perception: The nature of a controversy.* London: McGraw-Hill.

Dixon, N. F. (1981). *Preconscious processing.* New York: Wiley.

Dulany, D. E., Carlson, R. A., & Dewey, G. I. (1984). A case of syntactical learning and judgment: How conscious and how abstract? *Journal of Experimental Psychology: General, 113*, 541–555.

Dulany, D. E., Carlson, R. A., & Dewey, G. I. (1985). On consciousness in syntactic learning and judgment: A reply to Reber, Allen, and Regan. *Journal of Experimental Psychology: General, 114*, 25–32.

Dunn, R. (1845). Case of suspension of the mental faculties. *Lancet, 2*, 588–590.

Ebbinghaus, H. (1885). *Über das Gedächtnis* [Memory]. Leipzig: Duncker and Humblot.

Eich, E. (1984). Memory for unattended events: Remembering with and without awareness. *Memeory & Cognition, 12*, 105–111.

Ellenberger, H. F. (1970). *The discovery of the unconscious.* New York: Basic Books.

Erdelyi, M. H. (1970). Recovery of unavailable perceptual input. *Cognitive Psychology, 1*, 99–113.

Eriksen, C. W. (1960). Discrimination and learning without awareness: A methodological survey and evaluation. *Psychological Review, 67*, 279–300.

Eslinger, P. J., & Damasio, A. R. (1986). Preserved motor learning in Alzheimer's disease: Implications for anatomy and behavior. *The Journal of Neuroscience*, *6*, 3006–3009.

Feustel, T. C., Shiffrin, R. M., & Salasoo, A. (1983). Episodic and lexical contributions to the repetition effect in word identification. *Journal of Experimental Psychology: General*, *112*, 309–346.

Forbach, G. B., Stanners, R. F., & Hochhaus, L. (1974). Repetition and practice effects in a lexical decision task. *Memory & Cognition*, *2*, 337–339.

Forster, K. I., & Davis, C. (1984). Repetition priming and frequency attenuation in lexical access. *Journal of Experimental Psychology: Learning, Memory, and Cognition*, *10*, 680–698.

Fowler, C., Wolford, G., Slade, R., & Tassinary, L. (1981). Lexical access with and without awareness. *Journal of Experimental Psychology: General*, *110*, 341–362.

Freud, S., & Breuer, J. (1966). *Studies on hysteria*. (J. Strachey, Trans.). New York: Avon Books.

Gardner, H., Boller, F., Moreines, J., & Butters, N. (1973). Retrieving information from Korsakoff patients: Effects of categorical cues and reference to the task. *Cortex*, *9*, 165–175.

Giddan, N. S. (1967). Recovery through images of briefly flashed stimuli. *Journal of Personality*, *35*, 1–19.

Giddan, N. S., & Eriksen, C. W. (1959). Generalization of response biases acquired with and without verbal awareness. *Journal of Personality*, *27*, 104–115.

Glisky, E. L., Schacter, D. L., & Tulving, E. (1986). Computer learning by memory-impaired patients: Acquisition and retention of complex knowledge. *Neuropsychologia*, *24*, 313–328.

Gordon, P. C., & Holyoak, K. J. (1983). Implicit learning and generalization of the "mere exposure" effect. *Journal of Personality and Social Psychology*, *45*, 492–500.

Graf, P., & Mandler, G. (1984). Activation makes words more accessible, but not necessarily more retrievable. *Journal of Verbal Learning and Verbal Behavior*, *23*, 553–568.

Graf, P., Mandler, G., & Haden, P. (1982). Simulating amnesic symptoms in normal subjects. *Science*, *218*, 1243–1244.

Graf, P., & Schacter, D. L. (1985). Implicit and explicit memory for new associations in normal and amnesic subjects. *Journal of Experimental Psychology: Learning, Memory, and Cognition*, *11*, 501–518.

Graf, P., & Schacter, D. L. (1987). Selective effects of interference on implicit and explicit memory for new associations. *Journal of Experimental Psychology: Learning, Memory, and Cognition*, *13*, 45–53.

Graf, P., Shimamura, A. P., & Squire, L. R. (1985). Priming across modalities and priming across category levels: Extending the domain of preserved function in amnesia. *Journal of Experimental Psychology: Learning, Memory, and Cognition*, *11*, 385–395.

Graf, P., Squire, L. R., & Mandler, G. (1984). The information that amnesic patients do not forget. *Journal of Experimental Psychology: Learning, Memory, and Cognition*, *10*, 164–178.

Greenspoon, J. (1955). The reinforcing effect of two spoken sounds on the frequency of two responses. *American Journal of Psychology*, *68*, 409–416.

Haber, R. N., & Erdelyi, M. H. (1967). Emergence and recovery of initially unavailable perceptual material. *Journal of Verbal Learning and Verbal Behavior*, *6*, 618–628.

Haldane, E. S., & Ross, G. R. T. (Eds.). (1967). *The philosophical works of Descartes*. Cambridge: Cambridge University Press.

Hashtroudi, S., Parker, E. S., DeLisi, L. E., Wyatt, R. J., & Mutter, S. A. (1984). Intact retention in acute alcohol amnesia. *Journal of Experimental Psychology: Learning, Memory, and Cognition*, *10*, 156–163.

Herbart, J. F. (1896). *A text-book in psychology*. New York: D. Appleton.

Hering, E. (1920). Memory as a universal function of organized matter. In S. Butler (Ed.), *Unconscious memory* (pp. 63–86). London: Jonathan Cape.

Holender, D. (1986). Semantic activation without conscious identification in dichotic listening, parafoveal vision, and visual masking: A survey and appraisal. *The Behavioral and Brain Science*, *9*, 1–66.

Hull, C. L. (1933). *Hypnosis and suggestibility*. New York: Appleton Century.

Irwin, F. W., Kauffman, K., Prior, G., & Weaver, H. B. (1934). On 'learning without awareness of what is being learned.' *Journal of Experimental Psychology*, *17*, 823–827.

Jacobs, W. J., & Nadel, L. (1985). Stress-induced recovery of fears and phobias. *Psychological Review 92*, 512–531.

Jacoby, L. L. (1983a). Perceptual enhancement: Persistent effects of an experience. *Journal of Experimental Psychology: Learning, Memory, and Cognition*, *9*, 21–38.

Jacoby, L. L. (1983b). Remembering the data: Analyzing interactive process in reading. *Journal of Verbal Learning and Verbal Behavior*, *22*, 485–508.

Jacoby, L. L. (1984). Incidental versus intentional retrieval: Remembering and awareness as separate issues. In L. R. Squire & N. Butters (Eds.), *Neuropsychology of memory* (pp. 145–156). New York: Guilford Press.

Jacoby, L. L., & Dallas, M. (1981). On the relationship between autobiographical memory and perceptual learning. *Journal of Experimental Psychology: General*, *110*, 306–340.

Jacoby, L. L., & Witherspoon, D. (1982). Remembering without awareness. *Canadian Journal of Psychology*, *36*, 300–324.

Janet, P. (1893). L'amnésie continue [Continuous amnesia]. *Révue Générale Des Sciences*, *4*, 167–179.

Janet, P. (1904). L'amnésie et la dissociation des souvenirs par l'émotion [Amnesia and the dissociation of memories by emotion]. *Journal de Psychologie Normale et Pathologique*, *1*, 417–453.

Johnson, M. (1983). A multiple-entry, modular memory system. In G. H. Bower (Ed.), *The psychology of learning and motivation* (Vol. 17, pp. 81–123). New York: Academic Press.

Johnson, M. K., Kim, J. K., & Risse, G. (1985). Do alcoholic Korsakoff's syndrome patients acquire affective reactions? *Journal of Experimental Psychology: Learning, Memory, and Cognition*, *11*, 27–36.

Johnston, W. A., Dark, V. J., & Jacoby, L. L. (1985). Perceptual fluency and recognition judgments. *Journal of Experimental Psychology: Learning, Memory, and Cognition*, *11*, 3–11.

Kihlstrom, J. F. (1980). Posthypnotic amnesia for recently learned materials: Interactions with "episodic" and "semantic" memory. *Cognitive Psychology*, *12*, 227–251.

Kihlstrom, J. F. (1984). Conscious, subconscious, unconscious: A cognitive perspective. In K. S. Bowers & D. Meichenbaum (Eds.), *The unconscious reconsidered* (pp. 149–211). New York: Wiley.

Kinsbourne, M., & Wood, F. (1975). Short term memory and the amnesic syndrome. In D. D. Deutsch & J. A. Deutsch (Eds.), *Short-term memory* (pp. 258–291). New York: Academic Press.

Kirsner, K., Milech, D., & Standen, P. (1983). Common and modality-specific processes in the mental lexicon. *Memory & Cognition*, *11*, 621–630.

Kirsner, K., & Smith, M. C. (1974). Modality effects in word identification. *Memory & Cognition*, *2*, 637–640.

Kolers, P. A. (1975). Memorial consequences of automatized encoding. *Journal of Experimental Psychology: Human Learning and Memory*, *1*, 689–701.

Kolers, P. A. (1976). Reading a year later. *Journal of Experimental Psychology: Human Learning and Memory*, *2*, 554–565.

Komatsu, S.-I., & Ohta, N. (1984). Priming effects in word-fragment completion for short- and long-term retention intervals. *Japanese Psychological Research*, *26*, 194–200.

Korsakoff, S. S. (1898). Etude médico-psychologique sur une forme des maladies de la mémoire [Medical-psychological study of a form of diseases of memory]. *Révue Philosophique*, *28*, 501–530.

Krieckhaus, E. E., & Eriksen, C. W. (1960). A study of awareness and its effects on learning and generalization. *Journal of Personality*, *28*, 503–517.

Kunst-Wilson, W. R., & Zajonc, R. B. (1980). Affective discrimination of stimuli that cannot be recognized. *Science*, *207*, 557–558.

Lacey, J. L., & Smith, R. L. (1954). Conditioning and generalization of unconscious anxiety. *Science*, *120*, 1045–1052.

Landis, T., Regard, M., & Serrant, A. (1980). Iconic reading in a case of alexia without agraphia caused by a brain tumor: A tachistoscopic study. *Brain and Language*, *11*, 45–53.

Lazarus, R. S., & McCleary, R. (1951). Autonomic discrimination without awareness: A study of subception. *Psychological Review*, *58*, 113–122.

Leibniz, G. W. (1916). *New essays concerning human understanding*. Chicago: Open Court.

Lewicki, P. (1985). Nonconscious biasing effects of single instances on subsequent judgments. *Journal of Personality and Social Psychology*, *48*, 563–574.

Lewicki, P. (1986). Processing information about covariations that cannot be articulated. *Journal of Experimental Psychology: Learning, Memory, and Cognition*, *12*, 135–146.

Light, L. L., Singh, A., & Capps, J. L. (1986). Dissociation of memory and awareness in young and older adults. *Journal of Clinical and Experimental Neuropsychology*, *8*, 62–74.

Luria, A. R. (1976). *The neuropsychology of memory*. Washington, DC: V. H. Winston.

Maine de Biran. (1979). *The influence of habit on the faculty of thinking*. Baltimore: Williams & Wilkins.

Mandler, G. (1980). Recognizing: The judgment of previous occurrence. *Psychological Review*, *87*, 252–271.

Mandler, G. (in press). Memory: Conscious and unconscious. In P. R. Solomon, G. R. Goethals, C. M. Kelley, & B. R. Stephens (Eds.), *Memory—An interdisciplinary approach*. New York: Springer Verlag.

Mandler, G., Nakamura, Y., Van Zandt, B. J. S. (in press). Nonspecific effects of exposure on stimuli that cannot be recognized. *Journal of Experimental Psychology: Learning, Memory, and Cognition*.

Marcel, A. J. (1983). Conscious and unconscious perception: Experiments on visual masking and word recognition. *Cognitive Psychology*, *15*, 197–237.

Markus, H., & Kunda, Z. (1986). Stability and malleability of the self-concept. *Journal of Personality and Social Psychology*, *51*, 858–866.

Masson, M. E. J. (1984). Memory for the surface structure of sentences: Remembering with and without awareness. *Journal of Verbal Learning and Verbal Behavior*, *23*, 579–592.

McAndrews, M. P., Glisky, E. L., & Schacter, D. L. (in press). When priming persists: Long-lasting implicit memory for a single episode in amnesic patients. *Neuropsychologia*.

McAndrews, M. P., & Moscovitch, M. (1985). Rule-based and exemplar-based classification in artifical grammar learning. *Memory & Cognition*, *13*, 469–475.

McDougall, W. (1924). *Outline of psychology*. New York: Charles Scribner's Sons.

McKoon, G., & Ratcliff, R. (1979). Priming in episodic and semantic memory. *Journal of Verbal Learning and Verbal Behavior*, *18*, 463–480.

McKoon, G., & Ratcliff, R. (1986). Automatic activation of episodic information in a semantic memory task. *Journal of Experimental Psychology: Learning, Memory, and Cognition*, *12*, 108–115.

McKoon, G., Ratcliff, R., & Dell, G. (1986). A critical evaluation of the semantic-episodic distinction. *Journal of Experimental Psychology: Learning, Memory, and Cognition*, *12*, 295–306.

Metcalfe, J., & Fisher, R. P. (1986). The relation between recognition memory and classification learning. *Memory & Cognition*, *14*, 164–173.

Milberg, W., & Blumstein, S. E. (1981). Lexical decision and aphasia: Evidence for semantic processing. *Brain and Language*, *14*, 371–385.

Milner, B. (1962). Les troubles de la mémoire accompagnant des lésions hippocampiques bilatérales [Disorders of memory accompanying bilateral hippocampal lesions]. In *Physiologie de l'hippocampe*. Paris: Centre National de la Recherche Scientifique.

Milner, B., Corkin, S., & Teuber, H. L. (1968). Further analysis of the hippocampal amnesic syndrome: 14 year follow-up study of H. M. *Neuropsychologia*, *6*, 215–234.

Miss X. (1889). Recent experiments in crystal visions. *Proceedings of the Society for Psychical Research*, *5*, 486–521.

Morton, J. (1979). Facilitation in word recognition: Experiments causing change in the logogen models. In P. A. Kolers, M. E. Wrolstad, & H. Bouma (Eds.), *Processing of visible language* (Vol. 1, pp. 259–268). New York: Plenum.

Moscovitch. M. (1982). Multiple dissociations of function in amnesia. In L. S. Cermak (Ed.), *Human memory and amnesia* (pp. 337–370). Hillsdale, NJ: Erlbaum.

Moscovitch, M., Winocur, G., & McLachlan, D. (1986). Memory as assessed by recognition and reading time in normal and memory-impaired people with Alzheimer's disease and other neurological disorders. *Journal of Experimental Psychology: General*, *115*, 331–347.

Murrell, G. A., & Morton, J. (1974). Word recognition and morphemic structure. *Journal of Experimental Psychology*, *102*, 963–968.

Neisser, U. (1954). An experimental distinction between perceptual processes and verbal response. *Journal of Experimental Psychology*, *47*, 399–402.

Nelson, T. O. (1978). Detecting small amounts of information in memory: Savings for nonrecognized items. *Journal of Experimental Psychology: Human Learning and Memory*, *4*, 453–468.

Nisbett, R. E., & Wilson, T. D. (1977). Telling more than we can know: Verbal reports on mental processes. *Psychological Review*, *84*, 231–259.

Nissen, M. J., & Bullemer, P. (1987). Attentional requirements of learning: Evidence from performance measures. *Cognitive Psychology*, *19*, 1–32.

Nissen, M. J., Knopman, D., & Schacter, D. L. (in press). Neurochemical dissociation of memory systems. *Neurology*.

Nissen, M. J., Ross, J. L., Willingham, D. B., Mackenzie, T. B., & Schacter, D. L. (in press). Memory and awareness in a patient with multiple personality disorder. *Brain and Cognition.*

O'Keefe, J., & Nadel, L. (1978). *The hippocampus as a cognitive map.* Oxford: Clarendon Press.

Osgood, C. E., & Hoosain, R. (1974). Salience of the word as a unit in the perception of language. *Perception & Psychophysics, 15,* 168–192.

Parkin, A. (1982). Residual learning capability in organic amnesia. *Cortex, 18,* 417–440.

Perry, C., & Laurence, J. R. (1984). Mental processing outside of awareness: The contributors of Freud and Janet. In K. S. Bowers & D. Meichenbaum (Eds.), *The unconscious reconsidered* (pp. 9–48). New York: Wiley.

Pine, F. (1960). Incidental stimulation: A study of preconscious transformations. *Journal of Abnormal and Social Psychology, 60,* 68–75.

Poetzl, O. (1960). The relationship between experimentally induced dream images and indirect vision. Monograph No. 7. *Psychological Issues, 2,* 41–120.

Prince, M. (1914). *The unconscious.* New York: Macmillan.

Reber, A. S. (1976). Implicit learning of synthetic languages: The role of instructional set. *Journal of Experimental Psychology: Human Learning and Memory, 2,* 88–94.

Reber, A. S., Allen, A., & Regan, S. (1985). Syntactical learning and judgment, still unconscious and still abstract: Comment on Dulany, Carlson, and Dewey. *Journal of Experimental Psychology: General, 114,* 17–24.

Roediger, H. L. III, & Blaxton, T. A. (1987). Retrieval modes produce dissociations in memory for surface information. In D. S. Gorfein & R. R. Hoffman (Eds.), *Memory and cognitive processes: The Ebbinghaus centennial conference* (pp. 349–379). Hillsdale, NJ: Erlbaum.

Roediger, H. L. III, & Weldon, M. S. (1987). Reversing the picture superiority effect. In M. A. McDaniel & M. Pressley (Eds.), *Imagery and related mnemonic processes: theories, individual differences, and applications* (pp. 151–174.) New York: Springer-Verlag.

Rosenfeld, H. M., & Baer, D. M. (1969). Unnoticed verbal conditioning of an aware experimenter by a more aware subject: The double-agent effect. *Psychological Review, 76,* 425–432.

Ross, B. H. (1984). Remindings and their effects in learning a cognitive skill. *Cognitive Psychology, 16,* 371–416.

Rozin, P. (1976). The psychobiological approach to human memory. In M. R. Rosenzweig & E. L. Bennett (Eds.), *Neural mechanisms of learning and memory.* Cambridge, MA: MIT Press.

Salasoo, A., Shiffrin, R. M., & Feustel, T. (1985). Building permanent memory codes: Codification and repetition effects in word identification. *Journal of Experimental Psychology: General, 114,* 50–77.

Scarborough, D. L., Cortese, C., & Scarborough, H. S. (1977). Frequency and repetition effects in lexical memory. *Journal of Experimental Psychology: Human Perception and Performance, 3,* 1–17.

Scarborough, D. L., Gerard, L., & Cortese, C. (1979). Accessing lexical memory: The transfer of word repetition effects across task and modality. *Memory & Cognition, 7,* 3–12.

Schacter, D. L. (1982). *Stranger behind the engram: Theories of memory and the psychology of science.* Hillsdale. NJ: Erlbaum.

Schacter, D. L. (1983). Amnesia observed: Remembering and forgetting in a natural environment. *Journal of Abnormal Psychology, 92,* 236–242.

Schacter, D. L. (1985). Priming of old and new knowledge in amnesic patients and normal subjects. *Annals of the New York Academy of Sciences, 444,* 41–53.

Schacter, D. L. (1987, June). *On the relation between memory and consciousness: Dissociable interactions and conscious experience.* Paper presented at the Conference on Memory and Memory Dysfunction, Toronto, Ontario, Canada.

Schacter, D. L., & Graf, P. (1986a). Effects of elaborative processing on implicit and explicit memory for new associations. *Journal of Experimental Psychology: Learning, Memory, and Cognition, 12,* 432–444.

Schacter, D. L., & Graf, P. (1986b). Preserved learning in amnesic patients: Perspectives from research on direct priming. *Journal of Clinical and Experimental Neuropsychology, 8,* 727–743.

Schacter, D. L., Harbluk, J. L., & McLachlan, D. R. (1984). Retrieval without recollection: An experimental analysis of source amnesia. *Journal of Verbal Learning and Verbal Behavior, 23,* 593–611.

Schacter, D. L., McAndrews, M. P., & Moscovitch, M. (in press). Access to consciousness: Dissociations between implicit and explicit knowledge in neuropsychological syndromes. In L. Weiskrantz (Ed.), *Thought without language.* London: Oxford University Press.

Schacter, D. L., & Moscovitch, M. (1984). Infants, amnesics, and dissociable memory systems. In M. Moscovitch (Ed.), *Infant memory* (pp. 173–216). New York: Plenum.

Schacter, D. L., & Tulving, E. (1982). Memory, amnesia, and the episodic/semantic distinction. In R. L. Isaacson & N. E. Spear (Eds.), *The expression of knowledge* (pp. 33–65). New York: Plenum Press.

Schacter, D. L., & McGlynn, S. M. (1987). *Implicit memory: Effects of elaboration depend on unitization.* Manuscript submitted for publication.

Schneider, K. (1912). Über einige klinisch-pathologische Untersuchungsmethoden und ihre Ergebnisse. Zugleich ein Beitrag zur Psychopathologie der Korsakowschen Psychose [On certain clinical-pathological methods of research and their results. Together with a contribution to the psychopathology of Korsakoff's psychosis]. *Zeitschrift für Neurologie und Psychiatrie, 8,* 553–616.

Seamon, J. G., Brody, N., & Kauff, D. M. (1983). Affective discrimination of stimuli that are not recognized: Effects of shadowing, masking, and cerebral laterality. *Journal of Experimental Psychology: Learning, Memory, and Cognition, 9,* 544–555.

Shallice, T., & Saffran, E. (1986). Lexical processing in the absence of explicit word identification: Evidence from a letter-by-letter reader. *Cognitive Neuropsychology, 3,* 429–458.

Sherry, D. F., & Schacter, D. L. (in press). The evolution of multiple memory systems. *Psychological Review.*

Shevrin, H., & Fritzler, D. E. (1968). Visual evoked response correlates of unconscious mental processes. *Science, 161,* 295–298.

Shimamura, A. P. (1986). Priming effects in amnesia: Evidence for a dissociable memory function. *Quarterly Journal of Experimental Psychology, 38A,* 619–644.

Shimamura, A. P., & Squire, L. R. (1984). Paired-associate learning and priming effects in amnesia: A neuropsychological study. *Journal of Experimental Psychology: General, 113,* 556–570.

Shimamura, A. P., & Squire, L. R. (1987). A neuropsychological study of fact learning and source amnesia. *Journal of Experimental Psychology: Learning, Memory, and Cognition, 13,* 464–474.

Slamecka, N. J. (1985a). Ebbinghaus: Some associations. *Journal of Experimental Psychology: Learning, Memory, and Cognition, 11,* 414–435.

Slamecka, N. J. (1985b). Ebbinghaus: Some rejoinders. *Journal of Experimental Psychology: Learning, Memory, and Cognition, 11,* 496–500.

Sloman, S. A., Hayman, C. A. G., Ohta, N., & Tulving, E. (in press). Forgetting and interference in fragment completion. *Journal of Experimental Psychology: Learning, Memory, and Cognition.*

Squire, L. R. (1986). Mechanisms of memory. *Science, 232,* 1612–1619.

Squire, L. R., & Cohen, N. J. (1984). Human memory and amnesia. In J. McGaugh, G. Lynch, & N. Weinberger (Eds.), *Proceedings of the conference on the neurobiology of learning and memory* (pp. 3–64). New York: Guilford Press.

Squire, L. R., Shimamura, A. P., & Graf, P. (1985). Independence of recognition memory and priming effects: A neuropsychological analysis. *Journal of Experimental Psychology: Learning, Memory, and Cognition, 11,* 37–44.

Squire, L. R., Shimamura, A. P., & Graf, P. (in press). Strength and duration of priming effects in normal subjects and amnesic patients. *Neuropsychologia.*

Squire, L., Wetzel, C. D., & Slater, P. C. (1978). Anterograde amnesia following ECT: An analysis of beneficial effects of partial information. *Neuropsychologia, 16,* 339–348.

Starr, A., & Phillips, L. (1970). Verbal and motor memory in the amnesic syndrome. *Neuropsychologia, 8,* 75–88.

Storms, L. H. (1958). Apparent backward associations: A situational effect. *Journal of Experimental Psychology, 55,* 390–395.

Thorndike, E. L., & Rock, R. T., Jr. (1934). Learning without awareness of what is being learned or intent to learn it. *Journal of Experimental Psychology, 17,* 1–19.

Tranel, D., & Damasio, A. R. (1985). Knowledge without awareness: An autonomic index of facial recognition by prosopagnosics. *Science, 228,* 1453–1454.

Tulving, E. (1972). Episodic and semantic memory. In E. Tulving & W. Donaldson (Eds.), *Organization of memory* (pp. 381–403). New York: Academic Press.

Tulving, E. (1983). *Elements of episodic memory.* Oxford: The Clarendon Press.

Tulving, E. (1985a). On the classification problem in learning and memory. In L.-G. Nilsson & T. Archer (Eds.), *Perspectives in learning and memory* (pp. 67–94). Hillsdale, NJ: Erlbaum.

Tulving, E. (1985b). Ebbinghaus's memory: What did he learn and remember? *Journal of Experimental Psychology: Learning, Memory, and Cognition, 11,* 485–490.

Tulving, E. (1985c). Memory and consciousness. *Canadian Psychology, 25,* 1–12.

Tulving, E. (1986). What kind of a hypothesis is the distinction between episodic and semantic memory? *Journal of Experimental Psychology: Learning, Memory, and Cognition, 12,* 307–311.

Tulving, E., Schacter, D. L., & Stark, H. A. (1982). Priming effects in word-fragment completion are independent of recognition memory. *Journal of Experimental Psychology: Learning, Memory, and Cognition, 8,* 336–342.

Volpe, B, T., LeDoux, J. E., & Gazzaniga, M. S. (1979). Information processing of visual stimuli in an 'extinguished' field. *Nature, 282,* 722–724.

Warrington, E. K., & Weiskrantz, L. (1968). New method of testing long-term retention with special reference to amnesic patients. *Nature, 217,* 972–974.

Warrington, E. K., & Weiskrantz, L. (1970). Amnesia: Consolidation or retrieval? *Nature, 228,* 628–630.

Warrington, E. K., & Weiskrantz, L. (1974). The effect of prior learning on subsequent retention in amnesic patients. *Neuropsychologia, 12,* 419–428.

Warrington, E. K., & Weiskrantz, L. (1978). Further analysis of the prior learning effect in amnesic patients. *Neuropsychologia, 16,* 169–176.

Warrington, E. K., & Weiskrantz, L. (1982). Amnesia: A disconnection syndrome? *Neuropsychologia, 20,* 233–248.

Weiskrantz, L. (1985). On issues and theories of the human amnesic syndrome. In N. M. Weinberger, J. L. McGaugh, & G. Lynch (Eds.), *Memory systems of the brain* (pp. 380–415). New York: Guilford Press.

Weiskrantz, L. (1986). *Blindsight.* New York: Oxford University Press.

Weiskrantz, L., & Warrington, E. K. (1979). Conditioning in amnesic patients. *Neuropsychologia, 17,* 187–194.

Williamsen, J. A., Johnson, H. J., & Eriksen, C. W. (1965). Some characteristics of posthypnotic amnesia. *Journal of Abnormal Psychology, 70,* 123–131.

Wilson, W. R. (1979). Feeling more than we can know: Exposure effects without learning. *Journal of Personality and Social Psychology, 37,* 811–821.

Winnick, W. A., & Daniel, S. A. (1970). Two kinds of response priming in tachistoscopic recognition. *Journal of Experimental Psychology, 84,* 74–81.

Witherspoon, D., & Moscovitch, M. (1986). *Independence between word fragment completion perceptual identification.* Manuscript submitted for publication.

Young, A. W., McWenny, K. H., Hay, D. C., & Ellis, A. W. (1986). Access to identity-specific semantic codes from familiar faces. *Quarterly Journal of Experimental Psychology, 38A,* 271–295.

43

A. P. Shimamura, D. P. Salmon, L. R. Squire, and N. Butters

Memory dysfunction and word priming in dementia and amnesia

1987. *Behavioral Neuroscience* 101: 347–351

Alzheimer's disease is the most common form of dementing illness, affecting as many as 5% of persons over 65 years of age (Henderson, 1986; Huppert & Tym, 1986; Terry & Katzman, 1983). The disease is associated with progressive cortical, limbic, and subcortical brain damage (Arendt, Bigl, Arendt, & Tennstedt, 1983; Terry & Davies, 1980; Whitehouse, Price, Struble, Clark, & DeLong, 1982) and with a spectrum of cognitive changes including memory loss, deterioration of intellectual function, and personality change (Corkin, Davis, Growdon, Usdin, & Wurtman, 1982; Mohs, Greenwald, Dunn, & Davis, 1985; Weingartner et al., 1981). Because neuropathological information is obtained only at the end-stage of the disease process, little is known about the ordinary trajectory of the disease, that is, when specific brain regions become affected. Similarly, although memory impairment is recognized to be an early symptom of the disease, it is not known which aspects of memory are affected or at what point other cognitive functions become impaired.

Recent findings have shown that Alzheimer's disease prominently disrupts corticolimbic connections by damaging entorhinal and subicular cortices (Hyman, Van Hoesen, Damasio, & Barnes, 1984), thereby isolating the hippocampal formation from neocortex. This finding is critical, because damage to the hippocampal formation causes a selective amnesic disorder in humans (Scoville & Milner, 1957; Zola-Morgan, Amaral, & Squire, 1986). In such cases, amnesia occurs without impairment of other cognitive functions, such as language and intelligence. Patients with damage to the diencephalic midline (e.g., patients with Korsakoff's syndrome) also exhibit a selective memory disorder (Butters, 1984; Butters & Cermak, 1980; Mair, Warrington, & Weiskrantz, 1979; Squire & Shimamura, 1986; Talland, 1965). Although amnesic patients perform poorly when they are asked explicitly to recall or recognize material presented only a few minutes ago, they can exhibit sparing of certain memory functions, as indicated by normal performance on tests of digit span (Baddeley & Warrington, 1970; Drachman & Arbit, 1966), skill learning (Brooks & Baddeley, 1976; Cohen & Squire, 1980), and priming (Graf, Squire, & Mandler, 1984; Jacoby & Witherspoon, 1982; for review, see Shimamura, 1986).

These facts about amnesia have suggested that memory is organized in the brain as a set of dissociable processes or systems (Cohen, 1984; Mishkin, Malamut, & Bachevalier, 1984; Squire, 1986). The term *declarative memory* has been used to describe the memory system that is impaired in amnesia (Cohen, 1984; Squire, 1982). Declarative memory is available to conscious awareness and includes the facts and specific episodes learned in everyday experience. By contrast, *procedural memory* is implicit and is available only through performance. Skill learning, simple classical conditioning, and priming have been considered to be examples of procedural memory. Because procedural memory is spared in amnesic patients, it must depend on brain regions other than the medial temporal and diencephalic structures known to be affected in amnesia.

The relative status of procedural memory in Alzheimer's disease is not well understood. Alzheimer patients exhibited good performance on a perceptual-motor (pursuit rotor) skill task (Eslinger & Damasio, 1986); yet, in another study Alzheimer patients exhibited impaired performance on a cognitive (mirror-reading) skill task (Grober, 1985). Although loss of hippocampal function in Alzheimer's disease might explain deficits in declarative memory, this impairment alone could not explain deficits in procedural memory. Neuropathological studies have demonstrated damage to neocortex as well as damage to subcortical structures that provide cholinergic innervation to the forebrain (Pearson, Esiri, Hiorns, Wilcox, & Powell, 1985; Whitehouse et al., 1982), but it is not certain when this pathology occurs in the course of the disease. Thus it is not clear whether Alzheimer's disease *begins* as a selective impairment characteristic of amnesic syndromes or whether other kinds of memory processes are also affected at a relatively early stage of the disease.

This research was supported by the Medical Research Service of the Veterans Administration, National Institute of Aging Grant AG-05131, National Institute of Mental Health Grant MH24600, and the Office of Naval Research.

We thank Joyce Zouzounis, Lauren Lyon, Kim Rivero-Frink, and Deborah Rosenthal for research assistance.

Correspondence concerning this article should be addressed to Arthur P. Shimamura, Veterans Administration Medical Center, V-116A, 3350 La Jolla Village Drive, San Diego, California 92161.

In this study, we investigated the phenomenon of lexical priming in a group of mild to moderately impaired patients with Alzheimer's disease. Priming is the facilitation or modification of behavior by recently encountered stimuli, and it is intact even in severely amnesic patients. Lexical priming can be easily demonstrated in the word completion test (Graf et al., 1984; Squire, Shimamura, & Graf, in press). Subjects are presented a list of words (e.g., MOTEL, ABSTAIN) and then are asked simply to say the first word that comes to mind in response to three-letter word beginnings or stems (e.g., MOT, ABS). This test differs from standard tests of memory in that testing is conducted implicitly; that is, subjects are not told to use the stems as memory cues, and they apparently treat the task as a word puzzle. For amnesic patients, words appear to *pop* into mind in response to three-letter cues, yet the words are not recognized as familiar.

We tested both word completion priming and verbal memory ability in patients with Alzheimer's disease, patients with Korsakoff's syndrome, and patients with Huntington's disease. Patients with Korsakoff's syndrome have previously been found to exhibit intact priming ability (Graf et al., 1984; Shimamura & Squire, 1984; Squire et al., in press). Huntington's disease prominently affects the basal ganglia and impairs both motor and cognitive functions (Bruyn, Bots, & Dom, 1979; Butters, Sax, Montgomery, & Tarlow, 1978; Caine, Ebert, & Weingartner, 1977; Josiassen, Curry, & Mancall, 1983). Although patients with Huntington's disease exhibit impaired skill (mirror reading) learning (Martone, Butters, Payne, Becker, & Sax, 1984), nothing is known about their priming ability.

Method

Subjects

Patients with Alzheimer's disease. We tested a group of 8 patients with a clinical diagnosis of mild to moderate Alzheimer's disease (see Table 1). Because a definite diagnosis of Alzheimer's disease is not possible without neuropathologic evidence, we used the clinical criteria developed by the National Institute of Neurological and Communicative Disorders and Stroke and the Alzheimer's Disease and Related Disorders Association (McKann et al., 1984). Based on these criteria, a senior staff neurologist diagnosed five patients as probable Alzheimer's disease and three others as possible Alzheimer's disease. All patients scored at or above 104 out of a possible 144 points on the Dementia Rating Scale (DRS; average DRS = 118). The DRS is a test battery that assesses a spectrum of cognitive functions, including attention, memory, construction, and verbal fluency (Coblentz et al., 1973). In addition, the patients averaged 11.9 errors out of a possible 33 errors on the Blessed scale (Blessed, Tomlinson, & Roth, 1968), and they averaged 20.4 correct out of a possible 30 points on the Mini-Mental State (Folstein, Folstein, & McHugh, 1975). Testing occurred on the average 3.2 years after the appearance of the first symptoms (range = 1–5 years).

Patients with Huntington's disease. We tested a group of 8 patients with Huntington's disease (see Table 1). Diagnosis of Huntington's disease was made on the basis of a positive family history and the presence of choreiform movements. Their functional capacity was assessed with the Shoulson and Fahn (1979) scale, which rates functional disability on a 5-point scale (1 = *minimal*, 5 = *total*). One of the patients was rated at Functional Stage 1, two at Stage 2, four at Stage 3, and one at Stage 4.

Patients with Korsakoff's syndrome. We tested 7 patients with Korsakoff's syndrome (see Table 1) who have been studied in previous investigations (Shimamura & Squire, 1986a, 1986b). A detailed assessment of memory functions for 6 of these patients can be found in Squire and Shimamura (1986). Neuropsychological screening and independent neurological examination indicated that memory impairment was the only notable deficit of higher cortical functions.

Control subjects. Each of the three patient groups was matched to its own control group with respect to age and education level (see Table 1). The control group for patients with Alzheimer's disease consisted of 9 elderly individuals who averaged 69.6 years of age, and the control group for patients with Huntington's disease consisted of 8 younger individuals who averaged 50.1 years of age. We tested a group of 6 alcoholic individuals as control subjects for the patients with Korsakoff's syndrome. The alcoholic subjects were current or former participants in alcoholic treatment programs in San Diego County. All had abstained from alcohol for an average of 28.6 months prior to testing (range = 1–81 months).

Table 1
Description of Patient and Control Groups

Patient group	*N*	Age	ED	DRS
Alzheimer's disease	8	72.0	13.8	118
Older controls	9	69.6	13.9	140
Huntington's disease	8	48.9	13.6	128
Younger controls	8	50.1	13.5	141
Korsakoff's syndrome	7	53.9	11.7	128
Alcoholic controls	6	51.7	12.8	140

Note. DRS = Dementia Rating Scale; ED = education.

Procedure

We used a word completion test similar to those used in previous studies of word priming in amnesic patients (see Graf et al., 1984; Squire et al., in press). Subjects were asked to read 10 words (e.g., MOTEL, ABSTAIN) and to rate how much they liked each word on a 5-point scale (1 = *dislike extremely*, 5 = *like extremely*). Two additional filler words were placed at the beginning of the list and three at the end to reduce primacy and recency effects. In this way, words were presented for study without explicitly telling subjects to expect a memory test. Following a single presentation of the words, subjects were shown 20 three-letter word stems and were asked to complete each stem with the first word that came to mind (e.g., MOT, ABS). There were always at least 10 possible words that could be used to complete each target stem, only one of which was presented for the study. Ten of the stems could be completed using study words, and the other 10 stems were used to assess baseline guessing rates. The stems used to assess baseline rates were used as target stems for other subjects. The entire procedure was then repeated in exactly the same manner using a different list of 10 words. In this way, word completion was assessed twice, using two lists of 10 words.

In addition to the word completion test, we administered the Rey Auditory Verbal Learning Test (Lezak, 1983; Rey, 1964), which tests both recall and recognition memory. Subjects were given five study/test trials to learn a list of 15 words. In the recall version of the test, subjects were asked to recall as many words as possible immediately after each of the five word-list presentations. In the recognition test, we presented a different list of 15 words and tested subjects by presenting the 15 list words intermixed with 15 new words. After each of five list presentations, subjects were asked to say whether or not a word was just presented. Recognition performance was based on the percentage of correct responses out of 30 (i.e., correct hits + correct rejections).

Results

Figure 1 shows memory performance of patient and control groups on the Rey Auditory Verbal Learning Test. All three patient groups exhibited impaired verbal memory on both recall ($p < .01$) and recognition tests ($p < .01$). Patients with Alzheimer's disease and patients with Korsakoff's syndrome exhibited nearly the same level of impairment, $F(1, 12) < 1.0$, $p > .50$. Although patients with Huntington's disease exhibited impaired verbal memory, they performed significantly better than the other two patient groups on tests of both recall, $F(1, 13) = 5.6$, $p < .05$, and recognition, $F(1, 13) = 6.1$, $p < .05$).

In spite of the similarity in verbal memory performance between patients with Alzheimer's disease and patients with Korsakoff's syndrome, only patients with Alzheimer's disease exhibited impaired word completion priming (see Figure 2). In fact, the mean word completion score obtained by patients with Alzheimer's disease was significantly lower than the mean score obtained by any other group ($ps < .02$). By contrast, the mean completion scores obtained by patients with Korsakoff's syndrome and by patients with Huntington's disease were not significantly different from the mean scores obtained by their respective control groups: Korsakoff patients versus controls, $t(11) = 0.41$, $p = .69$; Huntington patients versus controls, $t(14) = 1.2$, $p = .25$. Thus all subject groups except patients with Alzheimer's disease increased their tendency to complete word stems to form previously presented words by 30% to 40% above baseline (baseline = 5–11%). Alzheimer patients, however, increased their tendency to use previously presented words only 10% above baseline (baseline = 6%).

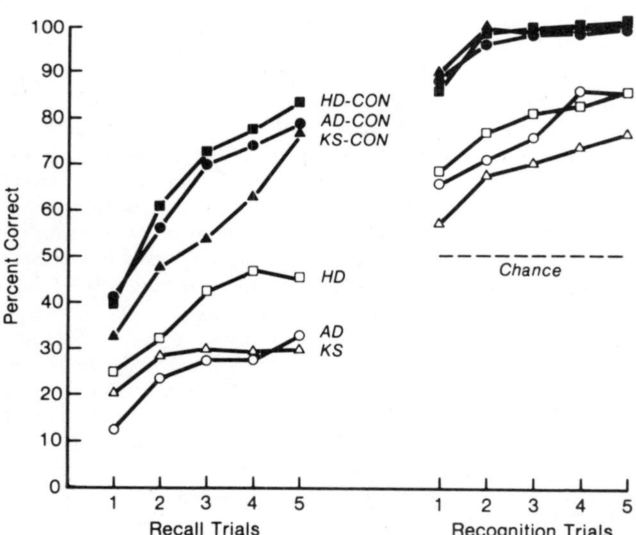

Figure 1. Recall (left) and recognition (right) memory performance across five study/test learning trials using the same 15 words on each trial. (A different set of 15 words was used for the recall and recognition trials. Figure shows performance by Alzheimer disease patients [AD; ○—○] and their controls [CON-AD; ●—●], Huntington disease patients [HD; □—□] and their controls [CON-HD; ■—■]; and Korsakoff syndrome patients [KS; △—△] and their alcoholic control subjects [CON-KS; ▲—▲].)

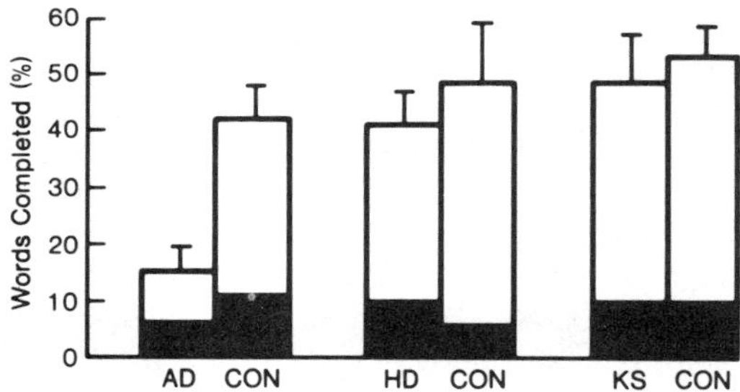

Figure 2. Lexical priming ability as measured by the word completion test. (Subjects were shown words [e.g., MOTEL] and later asked to complete three-letter word stems [e.g., MOT] with the first words that came to mind. Bars represent percentage of previously presented words that were used to complete word stems [total number of study words = 20]. Dark area represents baseline guessing performance, that is, the tendency to complete the same words under conditions when they had not been presented. Only Alzheimer disease patients [AD] exhibited impaired lexical priming. Figure shows AD patients, Huntington disease patients [HD], and Korsakoff syndrome patients [KS] adjacent to each of their respective control groups [CON].)

Although the ability to complete stems with previously presented words was impaired in Alzheimer patients, it is important to note that these patients were able to perform the basic task of completing word stems with words. Six patients with Alzheimer's disease completed all 20 stems with words, and the other 2 patients completed 18 of 20 stems. Thus these patients completed 98% of the stems with words—though usually not with a previously presented word.

The priming deficit seen in Alzheimer's disease was not simply related to overall dementia. Of the 8 patients with Huntington's disease, the 4 who obtained the lowest DRS scores had the same average DRS score as the Alzheimer patients (average DRS = 118 points). Yet, these 4 Huntington patients exhibited intact priming ability (44% completion, 10% baseline). Moreover, the 4 least-demented Alzheimer patients averaged 127.0 points on the DRS, which was only one point less than the average DRS scores of patients with Huntington's disease and Korsakoff's syndrome. Nevertheless, these 4 Alzheimer patients exhibited impaired priming ability (21% completion, 5% baseline).

Discussion

Explicit tests of verbal memory revealed a deficit in all three patient groups. In fact, patients with Alzheimer's disease and patients with Korsakoff's syndrome exhibited about the same level of verbal recall and recognition impairment. Nevertheless, only patients with Alzheimer's disease exhibited impaired priming ability. This is the first report of a deficit in word completion priming in any patient group. Because these findings were obtained in mild to moderately demented patients, they suggest that damage to brain regions in addition to those damaged in amnesia must occur at relatively early stages of the disease.

The deficit in priming may reflect an impairment in the ability to activate representations that store lexical memory. Accordingly, this deficit might account for problems in word finding and semantic memory that are prominent cognitive symptoms of Alzheimer's disease, particularly in later stages of the disease (Martin & Fedio, 1983; Ober, Dronkers, Koss, Delis, & Friedland, 1986; Schwartz, Marin, & Saffran, 1979; Warrington, 1974; Weingartner, Grafman, Boutelle, Kaye, & Martin, 1983). The finding of intact priming performance in patients with Huntington's disease suggests that the capacity for activation of representations in lexical memory does not depend on the brain areas damaged in this disease. The fact that a mirror reading skill was impaired in Huntington's disease (Martone et al., 1984) suggests that various forms of procedural memory can be dissociated from one another.

Several lines of evidence indicate that the word completion deficit in Alzheimer's disease reflects an impairment in memory activation rather than a global intellectual or cognitive impairment. First, patients with Alzheimer's disease were able to perform the task of completing word stems with words, so that poor performance could not be attributed simply to slowness or inability to comprehend instructions. Second, baseline guessing rates were normal in Alzheimer patients, which indicates that patients were not producing obscure or unusual words. Third, overall levels of dementia—within the range tested—were not related to impaired lexical priming. That is, even when subgroups of Huntington and Alzheimer patients were closely matched for degree of dementia, only the Alzheimer patients exhibited impaired priming.

The impairment in word priming exhibited by patients with Alzheimer's disease is robust. We have observed impaired lexical priming in a second independent sample of 13 other patients (Salmon, Shimamura, Butters, & Smith, 1987). In that study, instead of presenting words once, we presented words twice before testing for word completion. Nevertheless, the patients increased their tendency to use presented words only 15% above baseline (baseline = 11%), whereas control subjects increased their tendency to use presented words by 40% above baseline (baseline = 7%). Thus markedly impaired priming ability was observed altogether in 21 mild-to-moderately demented patients with Alzheimer's disease.

In summary, the most important finding was that patients with Alzheimer's disease exhibited impaired priming, whereas patients with Korsakoff's syndrome did not, despite the fact that these two patient groups exhibited a similar degree of impairment on explicit tests of recall and recognition memory. Patients with Korsakoff's syndrome, or patients with circumscribed medial temporal lobe damage, are impaired on explicit tests of memory, yet they exhibit intact priming. The impairment in priming must therefore reflect damage to regions other than the medial temporal and diencephalic brain structures affected in amnesia. Moreover, the finding of intact priming in patients with Huntington's disease suggests that the integrity of the neostriatum is not critical for normal priming effects. Impaired priming in Alzheimer's disease may be the result of damage to cortical representations that store lexical memory. If so, then involvement of neocortex must occur at a relatively early stage in the disease process, in conjunction with involvement of the structures responsible for the deficit in verbal or declarative memory. Further study of this and other aspects of memory impairment may help in determining the usual trajectory of the disease and in identifying which brain systems are first affected.

References

Arendt, T., Bigl, V., Arendt, A., & Tennstedt, A. (1983). Loss of neurons in the nucleus basalis of Meynert in Alzheimer's disease, paralysis agitans and Korsakoff's disease. *Acta Neuropathologica, 61,* 101–108.

Baddeley, A. D., & Warrington, E. K. (1970). Amnesia and the distinction between long- and short-term memory. *Journal of Verbal Learning and Verbal Behavior, 9,* 176–189.

Blessed, G., Tomlinson, B. E., & Roth, M. (1968). The association between quantitative measures of dementia and senile change in the cerebral gray matter of elderly subjects. *British Journal of Psychiatry, 114,* 797–811.

Brooks, D. N., & Baddeley, A. D. (1976). What can amnesic patients learn? *Neuropsychologia, 14,* 111–122.

Bruyn, G. W., Bots, G., & Dom, R. (1979). Huntington's chorea: Current neuropathological status. In T. Chase, N. Wexler, & A. Barbeau (Eds.), *Advances in neurology: Vol. 23. Huntington's disease.* Raven Press: New York.

Butters, N. (1984). Alcoholic Korsakoff's syndrome: An update. *Seminars in Neurology, 4,* 226–244.

Butters, N., & Cermak, L. S. (1980). *Alcoholic Korsakoff's syndrome: An information processing approach.* New York: Academic Press.

Butters, N., Sax, D. S., Montgomery, K., & Tarlow, S. (1978). Comparison of the neuropsychological deficits associated with early and advanced Huntington's disease. *Archives of Neurology, 35,* 585–589.

Caine, E., Ebert, M., & Weingartner, H. (1977). An outline for the analysis of dementia: The memory disorder of Huntington's disease. *Neurology, 27,* 1087–1092.

Coblentz, J. M., Mattis, S., Zingesser, L. H., Kasoff, S. S., Wisniewski, H. M., & Katzman, R. (1973). Presenile dementia: Clinical aspects and evaluation of cerebrospinal fluid dynamics. *Archives of Neurology, 29,* 299–308.

Cohen, N. J. (1984). Preserved learning capacity in amnesia: Evidence for multiple memory systems. In L. Squire & N. Butters (Eds.), *The neuropsychology of memory* (pp. 83–103). New York: Guilford Press.

Cohen, N. J., & Squire, L. R. (1980). Preserved learning and retention of pattern analyzing skill in amnesia: Dissociation of knowing how and knowing that. *Science, 210,* 207–209.

Corkin, S., Davis, K. L., Growdon, J. H., Usdin, E., & Wurtman, R. J. (Eds.). (1982). *Alzheimer's disease: A report of research in progress* (Vol. 19). New York: Raven Press.

Drachman, D. A., & Arbit, J. (1966). Memory and the hippocampal complex. *Archives of Neurology, 15,* 52–61.

Eslinger, P. J., & Damasio, A. R. (1986). Preserved motor learning in Alzheimer's disease: Implications for anatomy and behavior. *Journal of Neuroscience, 6,* 3006–3009.

Folstein, M. F., Folstein, S. E., & McHugh, P. R. (1975). Mini-mental state. A practical method for grading the cognitive state of patients for the clinician. *Journal of Psychiatric Research, 12,* 189–198.

Graf, P., Squire, L. R., & Mandler, G. (1984). The information that amnesic patients do not forget. *Journal of Experimental Psychology: Learning, Memory, and Cognition, 10,* 164–178.

Grober, E. (1985). Encoding of item-specific information in Alzheimer's disease. *Journal of Clinical and Experimental Neuropsychology, 7,* 614.

Henderson, A. S. (1986). The epidemiology of Alzheimer's disease. *British Medical Bulletin, 42,* 3–10.

Huppert, F. A., & Tym, E. (1986). Clinical and neuropsychological assessment of dementia. *British Medical Bulletin, 42,* 11–18.

Hyman, B. T., Van Hoesen, G. W., Damasio, A. R., & Barnes, C. L. (1984). Alzheimer's disease: Cell-specific pathology isolates the hippocampal formation. *Science, 225,* 1168–1170.

Jacoby, L. L., & Witherspoon, D. (1982). Remembering without awareness. *Canadian Journal of Psychology, 32,* 300–324.

Josiassen, R., Curry, L., & Mancall, E. (1983). Development of neuropsychological deficits in Huntington's disease. *Archives of Neurology, 40,* 791–796.

Lezak, M. D. (1983). *Neuropsychological assessment* (2nd ed.). New York: Oxford University Press.

Mair, W. G. P., Warrington, E. K., & Weiskrantz, L. (1979). Memory disorder in Korsakoff's psychosis: A neuropathological and neuropsychological investigation of two cases. *Brain, 102,* 749–783.

Martin, A., & Fedio, P. (1983). Word production and comprehension in Alzheimer's disease: The breakdown of semantic knowledge. *Brain and Language, 19,* 124–141.

Martone, M., Butters, N., Payne, M., Becker, J. T., & Sax, D. S. (1984). Dissociations between skill learning and verbal recognition in amnesia and dementia. *Archives of Neurology, 41,* 965–970.

McKann, G., Drachman, D., Folstein, M., Katzman, R., Price, D., & Stadlan, E. M. (1984). Clinical diagnosis of Alzheimer's disease: Report of the NINCDS-ADRDA Work Group under the auspicies of Department of Health and Human Services Task Force on Alzheimer's Disease. *Neurology, 34,* 939–944.

Mishkin, M., Malamut, B., & Bachevalier, J. (1984). Memories and habits: Two neural systems. In J. L. McGaugh, G. Lynch, & N. Weinberger (Eds.), *The neurobiology of learning and memory* (pp. 65–77). New York: Guilford Press.

Mohs, R. C., Greenwald, B. S., Dunn, D. D., & Davis, K. L. (1985). Assessment of cognition and affective symptoms in dementia. In J. Traber and W. H. Gispen (Eds.), *Senile dementia of the Alzheimer type.* Berlin: Springer-Verlag.

Ober, B. A., Dronkers, N. F., Koss, E., Delis, D. C., & Friedland, R. P. (1986). Retrieval from semantic memory in Alzheimer-type dementia. *Journal of Clinical and Experimental Neuropsychology, 8,* 75–92.

Pearson, R. C. A., Esiri, M. M., Hiorns, R. W., Wilcox, G. K., & Powell, T. P. S. (1985). Anatomical correlates of the distribution of the pathological changes in the neocortex in Alzheimer's disease. *Proceedings of the National Academy of Sciences, 82,* 4531–4534.

Rey, A. (1964). *L'examen clinique en psychologie.* [The clinical psychology examination]. Paris: Presses Universitaires de France.

Salmon, D. P., Shimamura, A. P., Butters, N., & Smith, S. (1987). *Lexical and semantic deficits in patients with Alzheimer's disease.* Manuscript submitted for publication.

Schwartz, M. F., Marin, O. S. M., & Saffran, E. M. (1979). Dissociations of language function in dementia: A case study. *Brain and Language, 7,* 277–306.

Scoville, W. B., & Milner, B. (1957). Loss of recent memory after bilateral hippocampal lesions. *Journal of Neurology, Neurosurgery, and Psychiatry, 20,* 11–21.

Shimamura, A. P. (1986). Priming effects in amnesia: Evidence for a dissociable memory function. *Quarterly Journal of Experimental Psychology, 38A,* 619–644.

Shimamura, A. P., & Squire, L. R. (1984). Paired-associate learning and priming effects in amnesia: A neuropsychological study. *Journal of Experimental Psychology: General, 113,* 556–570.

Shimamura, A. P., & Squire, L. R. (1986a). Memory and metamemory: A study of the feeling-of-knowing phenomenon in amnesic patients. *Journal of Experimental Psychology: Learning, Memory, and Cognition, 12,* 452–460.

Shimamura, A. P., & Squire, L. R. (1986b). Korsakoff's syndrome: The relation between anterograde amnesia and remote memory impairment. *Behavioral Neuroscience, 100,* 165–170.

Shoulson, I., & Fahn, S. (1979). Huntington's disease: Clinical care and evaluation. *Neurology, 29,* 1–3.

Squire, L. R. (1982). The neuropsychology of human memory. *Annual Review of Neuroscience, 5,* 241–273.

Squire, L. R. (1986). Mechanisms of memory. *Science, 232,* 1612–1619.

Squire, L. R., & Shimamura, A. P. (1986). Characterizing amnesic patients for neurobehavioral study. *Behavioral Neuroscience, 100,* 866–877.

Squire, L. R., Shimamura, A. P., & Graf, P. (in press). Strength and duration of priming effects in normal subjects and amnesic patients. *Neuropsychologia.*

Talland, G. A. (1965). *Deranged memory.* Academic Press: New York.

Terry, R. D., & Davies, P. (1980). Dementia of the Alzheimer type. *Annual Review of Neuroscience, 3,* 77–95.

Terry, R. D., & Katzman, R. (1983). *Annals of Neurology, 14,* 497.

Warrington, E. K. (1974). The selective impairment of semantic memory. *Quarterly Journal of Experimental Psychology, 27,* 635–657.

Weingartner, H., Grafman, J., Boutelle, W., Kaye, W., & Martin, P. R. (1983). Forms of memory failure. *Science, 221,* 380–382.

Weingartner, H., Kaye, W., Smallberg, S. A., Ebert, M. H., Gillin, J. C., & Staram, N. (1981). Memory failure in progressive idiopathic dementia. *Journal of Abnormal Psychology, 90,* 187–196.

Whitehouse, P. J., Price, D. L., Struble, R. G., Clark, A. W., & DeLong, M. R. (1982). Alzheimer's disease and senile dementia: Loss of neurons in the basal forebrain. *Science, 215,* 1237–1239.

Zola-Morgan, S., Amaral, D. G., & Squire, L. R. (1986). Human amnesia and the medial temporal region: Enduring memory impairment following a bilateral lesion limited to field CA1 of the hippocampus. *Journal of Neuroscience, 6,* 2950–2967.

V
Higher Cortical Functions

Introduction to Part V

One of the most exciting things about cognitive neuroscience is the promise that it can help us to understand two of the most "mental" activities, language and reasoning. The articles in this section illustrate two ways in which researchers gain leverage from considering how such functions are carried out in the brain. On the one hand, researchers have discovered important properties of the systems themselves. On the other, researchers use facts about allied perceptual and memory functions to place constraints on theories of how the brain accomplishes higher cognitive functions.

One of the themes that runs through this section is that higher cognitive functions are not unitary and undifferentiated but have a rich underlying structure—which is being revealed by cognitive neuroscience research. We have chosen articles that illustrate a number of different methods that have been used to this end, ranging from studies of behavioral deficits following brain damage, to studies of dissociations in the cerebral hemispheres, to studies of regional blood flow in the brain.

Reasoning

The goal of much of the work in the first section of this part is to decompose functions that we label with a single word or two and to examine the underlying structure of the processing systems. Farah shows that visual mental imagery is not accomplished by a single function and illustrates a method of fractionating a cognitive ability by examining the patterns of spared and impaired abilities following brain damage. Farah's work rests on the idea that individual functions are localized in different parts of the brain. It is likely that the functions she examines will themselves have a complex underlying structure. Thus, Farah's work shows that one need not have a complete theory in hand at the outset; rather, progress can be made even if only a few distinctions are used to guide an empirical investigation.

Roland and Friberg illustrate the power of another technique, Xe^{133} regional cerebral blood flow (rCBF) monitoring, to distinguish among distinct sets of cognitive processes. They find that different brain structures are active when subjects perform different kinds of mental activities; the dissociations among the activated brain areas provide good evidence that visual mental imagery is in fact distinct from auditory imagery. Furthermore, they find that mental imagery activates many areas that are also activated during like-modality perception. This is important because it implies that as we come to understand perception, we will gain leverage on understanding mental imagery. And as we understand mental imagery, we will gain leverage on understanding the types of reasoning in which it figures centrally.

Georgopoulos, Lurito, Petrides, Schwartz, and Massey show how this same imagery facet of reasoning can be studied profitably in nonhuman primates. Georgopoulos et al. studied the mechanisms that underlie one form of mental rotation, which was first reported by Roger Shepard and his colleagues. Humans require progressively more time to mentally rotate visualized objects through greater arcs; indeed, in some experiments response times increase linearly with the amount of rotation (see Shepard and Cooper, 1982). These findings suggested that a process was incrementing gradually through a set of intermediate positions. Georgopoulos et al. find that at least one form of mental rotation is related to motor planning; neurons in the primary motor area discharge systematically as a monkey is planning to reach to a rotated stimulus, with neurons tuned to intermediate positions firing in progression until neurons that are tuned to the appropriate orientation are activated.

Kosslyn uses a very different technique to provide evidence that there are two distinct ways to form visual mental images. This technique rests on demonstrating that some processes are more effective in the left cerebral hemisphere, whereas other processes are more effective in the right cerebral hemisphere. The fact that processes are relatively effective in different hemispheres is evidence that they are distinct; if only a single process were at work, it would generally be more effective in one hemisphere or would be equally effective in the two hemispheres.

At first glance, Kosslyn's findings may seem to contradict those of Farah, who reports that left-hemisphere damage selectively disrupts the ability to generate visual mental images. However, Kosslyn's findings may suggest that right-hemisphere-based imagery is more taxing than left-hemisphere-based imagery. Thus, Farah's results may reflect the fact that brain-damaged patients typically are generally slowed down and hence are more likely to fail at more challenging tasks. Thus even if the right-hemisphere mechanisms remain intact, these patients may not be able to use them effectively. Alternatively, it is possible that there is a critical subprocess used in all image generation that is implemented in the left hemisphere and that Kosslyn's findings reflect hemispheric differences in additional processes (such as those that arrange segments of objects in images, as he suggests). Given the differences in methodologies, there are many possible accounts for the different results (for further possible complications, see also Sergent 1990).

The power of examining differences between the cerebral hemispheres is brought home in force by Gazzaniga, Bogen, and Sperry, who study patients who (for medical reasons) have had their cerebral hemispheres surgically disconnected. In most cases, information presented to one hemisphere in these patients stays there; it does not cross over to the other side. Gazzaniga et al. show many previously unsuspected differences in the processing performed by the two hemispheres. Such dissociations provide strong hints about the architecture of the processing system that underlies much of cognition.

Finally, Milner and Petrides illustrate that the frontal lobes play a special role in reasoning. These structures presumably rely on much of the processing performed elsewhere in the brain, not only drawing inferences and deductions but also directing the course of attention, devising plans, and otherwise "managing" higher cortical functions. The frontal lobes have only recently begun to be studied in detail, which is not surprising: To a large extent, they direct and modulate other processes, and until we have some idea what those other processes do, it will be difficult to specify frontal lobe function in detail.

Language

This topic is much more difficult to investigate than visual cognition (let alone perception or memory), in large part because there are no good animal models of language. Hence we cannot gain the leverage from the kinds of neuroanatomical and neurophysiological studies that are helping us to understand other functions. Nevertheless, the theme of decomposing higher functions into more specific processes is also evident in this set of articles; in these studies, however, the evidence for distinct processing components rests in large part on patterns of dissociations and associations among behavioral deficits that follow brain damage.

A striking exception to the traditional method of studying behavioral deficits in patients with brain damage, however, is the work of Petersen, Fox, Posner, Mintun, and Raichle, who use PET to dissect the processing that underlies our ability to read single words. They show that at least two distinct sets of cortical areas are involved; the processes carried out by one set (in the occipital lobes) apparently are specifically involved in visually decoding written patterns into words, whereas the processes carried out by the other areas (in the frontal lobes) apparently access stored semantic information on the basis of these patterns. One reason these findings are important is that they implicate visual processes in reading, which often were neglected by researchers in experimental psychology. In addition, these findings add further insight into the functions of the frontal lobes.

At first glance, Petersen et al.'s findings may seem to be inconsistent with those reported in the paper by Ojemann, Ojemann, Lettich, and Berger. Whereas Petersen et al. find evidence that reading is accomplished in specific cortical areas, Ojemann et al. find that processes underlying spoken language may not be consistently localized to the same cortical areas in different people. These contrasting findings are intriguing in part because speech is a relatively late evolutionary development, whereas the perceptual processes that underlie reading presumably are not; furthermore, the semantic processing involved in reading also may have been present much earlier for use in identifying objects. Hence the processes used in reading may be more "hard wired" than those involved in other aspects of language. Depending on one's particular set of early experiences, it is possible that a number of alternative brain sites can be "initialized" to process language. But even so, these sites must receive the proper kinds of inputs and be connected to the brain areas that produce speech. Thus even language variability is restricted primarily to a specific zone of the brain.

We then reprint a paper by Geschwind, in which he describes his now-classic theory of language processing in the brain. Geschwind posits a logical progression of processing in a series of brain areas, which is inspired in large part by observations about neuroanatomy. In many ways, this project springs directly from the work of nineteenth-century researchers such as Wernicke, but is informed by additional neuroanatomical and neurophysiological findings. Geschwind's theory has a deep appeal: it is elegant and provides straightforward accounts for a raft of clinical findings. We now know enough to rule out this theory, however. Unfortunately, counter to his claims, words are not reflexively converted to auditory representations (see Petersen et al.), and much of language processing is not as tightly constrained by anatomical connections as he suggested (see Ojemann et al.). Nevertheless, the basic concept of using anatomical connections as one constraint on theorizing still stands, but this is not the only constraint—we must also think about the computational properties of neural networks and how networks are configured over the course of experience. It seems likely that some as-yet-unformulated network model will be required to illuminate the relation between anatomical and computational constraints in language processing.

McCarthy and Warrington find that brain damage can selectively disrupt meaningful information that is accessed in a specific sensory modality; these results suggest that different semantic information may be accessed when we see objects versus when we hear them. To many, this is a very surprising result, but it may not be so surprising from the perspective of Mishkin's and Squire's theories of memory. Recall that those theories emphasize the multiplicity of memories, and recall that perceptual systems serve double duty as memory systems. However McCarthy and Warrington's findings are interpreted, they will place strong constraints on theories of semantic representation.

The nature of the internal representation of meaning is further illuminated by Marshall and Newcombe, who discuss the syndrome of *deep dyslexia.* This syndrome is a collection of related disorders in reading, including the inability to sound out words properly and various problems in matching visual representations of words to the proper semantic representations in memory. By observing the patterns of errors made by these patients, researchers have gleaned important hints about how information is organized in semantic memory. In contrast, Coltheart, Masterson, Byng, Prior, and Riddoch illustrate another, in many ways complementary, syndrome, in which the "deep" aspects of meaning may be spared but the processes that access them may be awry; these patients may be forced to rely on the sounds that correspond to written words in order to interpret them. The two disorders together place strong constraints on theories of reading, which ultimately must address the pattern of results reported by Petersen et al.

The papers in this section span a wide range of topics, from mental imagery and reasoning to reading, speaking, and understanding language. Nevertheless, these papers all share a commitment toward carefully examining behaviors and relating aspects of the behaviors to neural function. Furthermore, although most of the papers do not use this terminology, all of these researchers aim to specify the underlying computations that must be performed to produce the behavior. Those who wish to build a system that behaves like the brain stand to gain numerous insights from the discoveries and inferences summarized here.

References

Sergent, J. 1990. The neuropsychology of visual image generation: Data, method, and theory. *Brain and Cognition* 13: 98–129.

Shepard, R. N., and L. A. Cooper. 1982. *Mental Images and Their Transformations.* Cambridge, MA: MIT Press.

44

M. J. Farah

The neurological basis of mental imagery: A componential analysis

1984. *Cognition* 18: 245–272

Abstract

The neurological literature contains numerous reports of loss of mental imagery following brain damage. This paper represents an attempt to interpret the patterns of deficits and preserved abilities in these reports in terms of a componential information-processing model of imagery. The principal result was a consistent pattern of deficit in a subset of patients, which could be attributed to a loss of the image generation component of imagery; examination of the lesion sites in this subset of patients implicated a region in the posterior left hemispheres as critical for the image generation process. The analysis also provided evidence that the long-term visual memories used in imagery are also used in recognition, and that dreaming and waking visual imagery share some underlying processes.

Cases of loss of visual imagery due to brain damage have been described in the neurological literature for decades. Despite the relatively long history of the study of this phenomenon, however, little progress has been made in understanding the neurological basis of visual imagery. This paper represents an attempt to synthesize what is now known about visual imagery in normal humans with the existing data on visual imagery deficits in brain-damaged humans, with the hope of shedding new light on both topics. In particular, the approach is to reinterpret the 'loss of imagery' literature in terms of a *theory* of imagery, making distinctions among the *components* of imagery ability that may be individually susceptible to brain damage. It will then be possible to look for the anatomical correlates of componentially-defined imagery deficits, as well as ways in which the breakdown of imagery ability after brain damage constrains our theories of imagery in normal individuals.

A search of the literature yielded 37 descriptions of cases of loss of imagery published in English. Where anatomical data are available, the areas of the brain that are implicated as relevant to visual imagery are varied: parietal lobe, occipital lobe and temporal lobe damage have all been associated with loss or severe deficit of visual imagery ability, and neither hemisphere can be excluded. Some authors have attempted to generalize about the critical lesion sites. For example, Nielsen (1946) has stated that a loss of imagery may be used as a diagnostic *localizing sign* of damage to the inferior convex portion of area 19 of the occipital lobes (p. 270). Arbuse (1947) has proposed a left parietal basis for imagery, and more recently Bisiach and his colleagues (Bisiach and Luzzati, 1978; Bisiach *et al.*, 1949) have demonstrated parietal involvement in the use of imagery. Humphrey and Zangwill's (1951) presentation of three cases of loss of dreaming and waking imagery is often cited as support for a right hemisphere locus for imagery, although the authors themselves asserted that "disorders of visual imagination appear liable to follow lesions on either side." Ehrlichman and Barrett (1983) cite many authors who assume that imagery is a function of the right hemisphere, but conclude that the evidence available does not support this assumption.

What are we to make of this lack of association between loss of imagery and damage to particular areas of the brain? Two possibilities suggest themselves. First, it is possible that imagery is not a 'faculty' of the brain, but merely a collection of epiphenomena which emerge when other memory and reasoning processes interact in particular ways, as has been argued by some psychologists (e.g. Pylyshyn, 1981). If this were the case, then damage to one or more of the interacting systems might or might not produce a manifest 'imagery deficit', depending upon the ability of the remaining systems to produce some of the alleged properties of imagery. This state of affairs would lead to just the complex and inconsistent pattern of data described in the last paragraph. An alternative possibility is that imagery is a faculty or, in Luria's (1973) terms, a "functional system" of the brain, and like language or perception it has an internal structure, the components of which have different physiological bases. If this were the case, then the inconsistencies would be only apparent, the result of our grouping together deficits in different components of visual imagery. A consistent picture would emerge if we were to look for the brain areas associated with these components individually. This second possibility may be thought of as a hypothesis: imagery is a faculty or system of the brain, made up of identifiable subsystems that each have a direct neurological instantiation.

In order to test this hypothesis using the published case reports of loss of visual imagery, and thereby to attempt to localize the components of the imagery system in the brain, two additional kinds of information are needed. First, we need a theory of visual imagery that specifies the components of the visual imagery system. Second, we need to know which of these components were destroyed in each of the case reports that form our data base.

A Theory of Visual Imagery

Kosslyn (1980) has provided a comprehensive and well-supported componential theory of visual imagery in normal adults. For present purposes, only the most general features of the theory will be used, corresponding to the highest level 'parse' of the imagery system into different kinds of information-bearing *structures* and information-manipulating *processes.* The long-term visual memory structures store information about the appearances of objects. Like other long-term memory structures, we are not conscious of this information except when it is being accessed or otherwise manipulated by one of the processes specified by the theory. A second kind of structure, the 'visual buffer', is not itself information-bearing but is the medium in which images occur. The visual buffer has been found to have certain invariant properties such as visual angle and grain which are independent of the image that is 'displayed' in it. The spatial, pictorial information-bearing structure that we consciously experience as an image consists of patterns of activation in the visual buffer.

The *processes* postulated by Kosslyn include those that 'generate', 'inspect' and 'transform' the image in the visual buffer. The generation process (actually decomposable into component processes, which are not relevant here) creates the image in the visual buffer from information stored in long-term visual memory. The inspection process converts the patterns of activation in the visual buffer into organized percepts, identifying parts and relations within the image. For example, when we image a Star of David by mentally combining two triangles, it is the inspection process that allows us to find the embedded hexagon in the center. This process has not been modeled in detail by Kosslyn but presumably resembles the elementary pattern recognition processes that Ullman (this issue) has called "visual routines". Finally, there are processes that transform (e.g., rotate, translate) the image.

Given this analysis of the imagery system, we might expect to find cases of loss of imagery that correspond to losses of different structural or processing components of imagery. That is, a patient would be expected to have no imagery on introspection, and be unable to perform tasks requiring the consulting of an image, if any of the following components were destroyed by brain damage: the long-term visual memories, the visual buffer, the generation process, or the inspect process. Loss of image transformation processes would be expected to give rise to distinct deficits in visual/spatial thought processes, but not to the loss of imagery altogether.

What remains to be done in order to carry out a componential analysis of the imagery deficits reported in the literature is to find a way to infer from the descriptions of patients' performances in various tasks *which* component or components of the imagery system must have been damaged. This was accomplished by the use of 'task analyses' of the tasks reported in each case study. A task analysis is a theory of the cognitive processing required to carry out a task. As such, task analyses are clearly dependent on a general theory of cognitive processing: the general theory specifies what components are available for performing a given task, how they will interact, and what their results will be.

There are six main kinds of task that are described in the case studies and are relevant to assessing imagery ability: question-answering tasks, introspection tasks, drawing and construction tasks, recognition tasks, and sensory and perceptual tasks. In order to write task analyses for these tasks, the processing components of the imagery model had to be augmented with some general (that is, non-imagery) components as described in the next section.

Additional Theoretical Assumptions

In order to model performance in all phases of the tasks included in the task analyses in this paper the following additional components were added to the basic Kosslyn model: a 'describe' component for question-answering tasks in which the contents of the visual buffer (either an internally generated image or a visually encoded percept) must be inspected and described, a 'copy' component for constructional tasks in which the contents of the visual buffer (either an internally generated image or a visually encoded percept) must be inspected and drawn or constructed, and a 'detect' component for simple visual perception tasks and imagery introspection tasks, in which the patterns of activation in the visual buffer need not be inspected (i.e., the structure or form of the pattern need not be processed) but the mere presence of activation must be detected. These additional components are obviously complex systems in their own right, and it may be misleading to refer to them as components. However, as will be seen shortly, care was taken to avoid making any inferences from the task analyses that could depend on the nature of these components; they function in the task analyses as place-holders for systems of non-imagery processing that are not directly relevant to assessing imagery ability.

In order to infer which component of imagery is damaged in each patient, it was also necessary to augment the imagery model with a visual encoding process that encodes stimuli into the visual buffer. Support for the claim that imagery and perception share a common visual buffer comes from findings of interactions between images and percepts in the visual buffer (Farah, In press; Finke and Schmidt, 1977, 1978; Finke and Shepard, In press) and from findings of many subtle, quantitative similarities between the visual buffer in imagery and in perception (Finke and Kosslyn, 1980;

Finke and Kurtzman, 1981; Podgorny and Shepard, 1978).

Finally, a recognition process was added to the framework of the Kosslyn imagery theory. The standard approach to modelling visual recognition (e.g. Marr, 1982; Selfridge and Neisser, 1960) was use: after a percept has been encoded into the visual buffer and inspected, it is translated into the format of the long-term visual memories and compared with those memories. Recognition consists of a match between the representation derived from the input and one of the long-term visual memories. In order to infer which component of imagery is damaged in each patient, it was necessary to assume initially that the long-term visual memories used in image generation are the same memories that are used in visual recognition. Although this assumption seems extremely reasonable on the grounds of parsimony, the only way to justify the assumption is by testing it. This was done by examining cases of *content-specific* imagery deficits, that is, cases in which the patient could visualize some kinds of objects but not others. If the long-term memories of the imagery system are also the basis for object recognition, then we would expect parallel content-specific recognition deficits in these patients. To anticipate the results of the analysis of the case reports, there were six cases of content-specific agnosia in which imagery ability was examined, and in four of these imagery for both recognizable and unrecognizable categories of stimuli was tested. All four of these cases displayed a parallel imagery deficit.

Figure 1 shows the complete theory from which the task analyses will be derived. From Kosslyn's theory come (1) the *long-term visual memories* of the appearance of objects, (2) the *visual buffer*, the short-term memory medium in which images occur, (3) the *generation* process, which takes the information about the

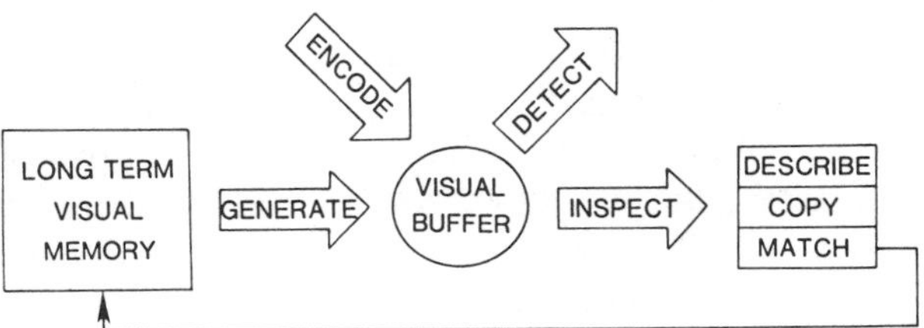

Figure 1. The general model of perception and imagery from which task analyses were derived. Patterns of activation are formed in the visual buffer either by an image generation process (from long term memories) or a perceptual encoding process. The presence of activation in the visual buffer may simply be detected, or an inspection process may read out structured patterns of activation for further processing: description (in the case of question-answering tasks), copying (in the case of drawing or construction tasks) or matching with long term visual memories (in the case of recognition tasks).

appearance of objects stored as deep images and creates a surface image, a spatial distribution of activation in the visual buffer, and (4) the *inspection* process, which organizes and transmits the information displayed in the visual buffer to other cognitive systems.

Added to the imagery structures and processes are (1) sensory processes that *encode* stimuli into the visual buffer and *detect* activation in the visual buffer, (2) recognition processes that *match* the inspected contents of the visual buffer with long-term visual memories, (3) visual to verbal translation processes that *describe* the inspected contents of the visual buffer, and (4) visual to motor translation processes that *copy* the inspected contents of the visual buffer.

Tasks and Task Analyses

Figures 2–8 show the task analyses for each of the relevant tasks described in the case reports. These include the tasks deemed by the authors of the case reports to require imagery, as well as other tasks that are useful as controls for possible non-imagery deficits.

The task most commonly used to infer a loss of imagery is to ask patients to describe or answer questions about the visual appearance of objects. Of course, it is always conceivable that a patient could perform adequately on such a task without consulting an image but instead by consulting explicitly encoded facts about the object's appearance; however, there is evidence from laboratory studies with normal humans that for retrieving information about aspects of appearance not often explicitly discussed (e.g. whether George Washington had a beard) and particularly spatial, relational information (e.g. whether the entrance to one's house is in the center or off to one side of the front) imagery is used (Eddy and Glass, 1981; Kosslyn and Jolicoeur, 1980). In most cases the authors of the case reports asked appropriately subtle questions. Some examples are: "Did George Washington have a beard?" (Brownell *et al.*, 1984), "What color are the stars on the American flag?" (Brownell *et al.*, 1984; Boyle and Nielsen, 1954), "Describe the exterior of your home." (Brain, 1954; Levine, 1978; Nielsen, 1946). In a few cases, the questions did not meet the criteria of requests for subtle relational and non-explicitly coded information, for example: "What are the colors of a canary? The sky? Gass?" (Levine, 1978; Nielsen, 1946). Similarly, the ability of an architect or builder to describe familiar buildings such as his own home was not taken as evidence for intact imagery because this information is likely to be explicitly encoded by such individuals (Brain, 1954, Case 1; Nielsen, 1946, p. 227). In these cases patients' answers were not used as evidence of imagery ability for the purpose of making inference to the damaged component. The task

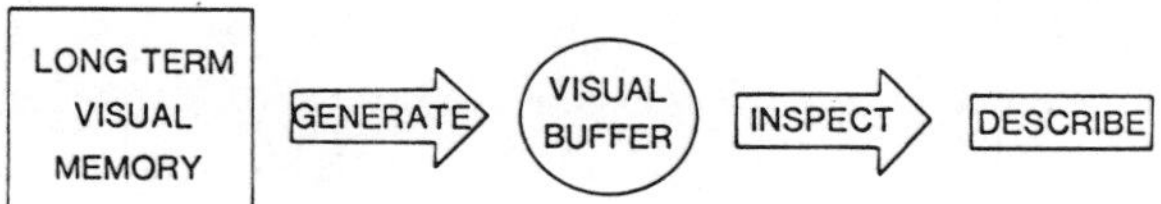

Figure 2. Task analysis for question-answering from memory.

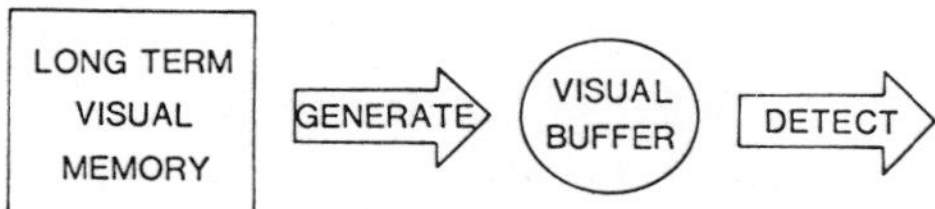

Figure 3. Task analysis for 'introspection': the detection of imagery.

analysis for the question-answering task is shown in Fig. 2. An image must be generated from long-term memory into the visual buffer, inspected and described.

Many patients spontaneously reported a loss of imagery based on their own introspection. In this context introspection does not involve the reporting of *how* a given thought process seems to the thinker to be proceeding, but rather a self-report about the existence of the thought process or, more accurately, the existence of a product of a thought process, a visual image. The task analysis for introspection is shown in Fig. 3. An image must be generated from long-term memory into the visual buffer, and its presence must be detected. Although the task analysis for introspection is very similar to the task analysis for question-answering, it should be noted that in introspection the patient is commenting more explicitly on his internal mental state than during question-answering, and there is therefore a greater chance of the patient's responses being affected by his or her naive theories about the mind. There are only three cases (Humphrey and Zangwill, 1955) in which any inferences rest on introspection alone.

Imagery deficits can also be detected in constructional tasks, either drawing a requested object or assembling it from parts such as sticks or blocks. As with question-answering and description from memory, not all drawing tasks require imagery; in particular, it is assumed that imagery is not needed to draw simple geometric shapes such as a circle or schematic cannonical forms such as a human stick figure. For constructional tasks, Fig. 4 shows the required structures and processes. An image must be generated from long-term memory into the visual buffer, inspected and copied.

Four further tasks are relevant to inferring the component of imagery ability that has been damaged. They are copying tasks, recognition tasks, perceptual tasks, and sensory tasks. In most cases in which a patient was asked to draw or construct something from memory,

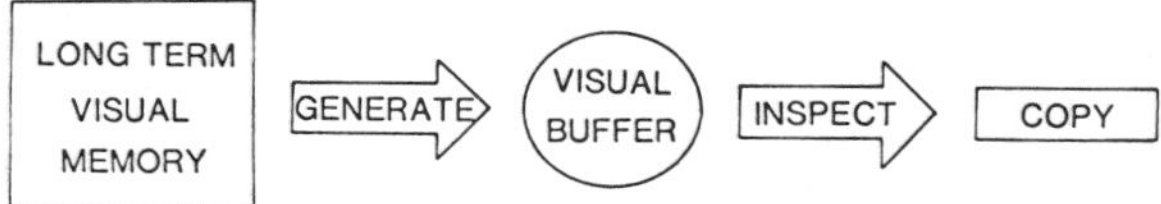

Figure 4. Task analysis for drawing or constructing from memory.

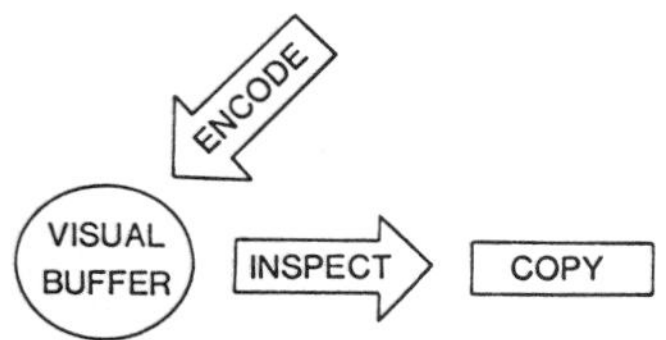

Figure 5. Task analysis for drawing or constructing from a visible model.

he or she was also asked to copy (from a visible model) either the same subject or a subject of comparable familiarity and complexity. Knowledge of a patient's performance in this task is clearly helpful in interpreting his or her performance at drawing or constructing from memory. The task analysis for copying a visible model is shown in Fig. 5 and consists of encoding the model into the visual buffer, inspecting it and copying it.

Finally, a patient's ability to perceive and recognize objects can be helpful in inferring which component of the visual imagery system has been damaged. Testing sensory, perceptual and object recognition ability is a standard part of any neurological examination following brain damage. Visual agnosia is the inability to recognize an object by sight alone, in the absence of any elementary perceptual or general intellectual impairment. To be diagnosed an 'associative visual agnosic', a patient must meet several requirements. He or she must have adequate sensory processes for encoding stimuli, and also have the ability to perceive stimuli as organized wholes (i.e., not have an 'apperceptive' visual agnosia, also called simultanagnosia or 'gestalt deficit'). The patient must be be generally alert, be able to identify objects by touch, sound, or other non-visual modalities, and yet be unable to identify the same objects by sight. The patient need not be able to name an object to demonstrate his or her recognition of it; simply indicating its function either verbally or motorically is adequate to rule out agnosia. Associative agnosia is thus a specific failure to associate a perceptual representation with a long-term memory representation. The task analyses for sensory, perceptual and recognition tasks are shown in Figs. 6–8. To demonstrate that he or she can see, a patient must be able to encode a stimulus into the visual buffer, and detect its presence (Fig. 6). To demonstrate complete perceptual abilities, a patient must be able to encode an object into

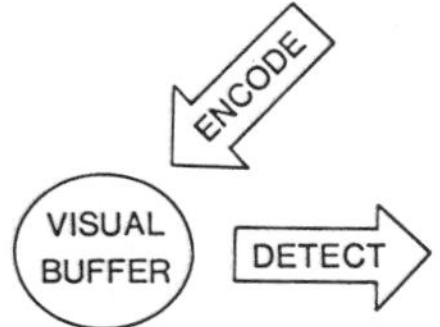

Figure 6. Task analysis for detection of visual stimuli.

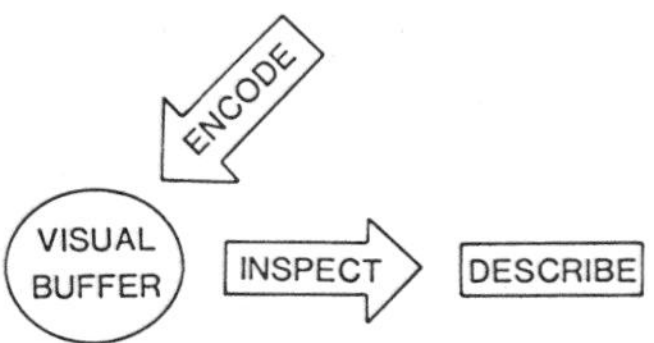

Figure 7. Task analysis for description of visual stimuli.

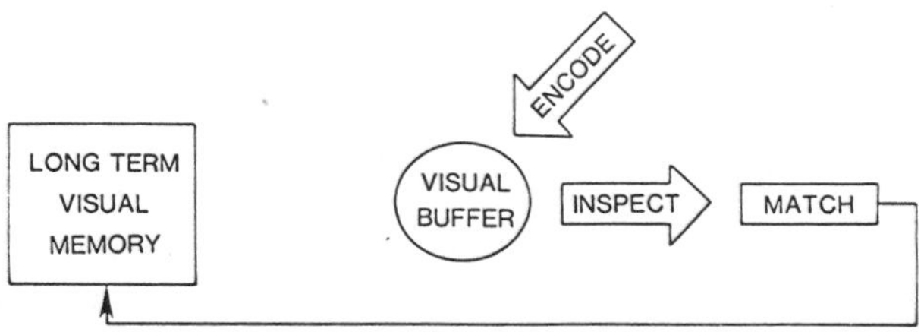

Figure 8. Task analysis for recognition of visual stimuli.

the visual buffer and produce a recognizable description of it (Fig. 7), for example by providing the colors, shapes, or names of objects or pictures. The ability to copy a stimulus from a model (Fig. 5) also is sometimes taken by neurologists as evidence for intact perceptual abilities. To demonstrate that he or she can recognize objects, a patient must be able to encode the object into the visual buffer, and match it with a long-term memory representation (Fig. 8).

The reliability with which the descriptions of tasks described in the case reports could be classified into the categories of tasks represented in Figs. 2–8 was tested by having a second reader perform the classifications independently. The second reader was shown the task analyses of Figs. 2–8 and given copies of the 37 case reports, with instructions to identify occurrences of the seven tasks in the case reports. The reader was an undergraduate psychology major who did not know the results of the original analysis. She also knew virtually nothing about neuroanatomy, ruling out the possibility of her grouping together tasks performed similarly by patients with similar lesions. The two readers' classifications were largely in agreement; specific differences are discussed in the next section.

Inferences Using Task Analyses

Once the task analyses have been constructed, the damaged imagery components can be inferred. If a patient cannot perform a task, then one or more of the cognitive components required for that task must be damaged. We can narrow down the candidate components by noting which of those same components are required by the tasks that the patient *can* perform. This is because if a patient can perform a task, then it is likely that all of the cognitive components required by that task are intact. Therefore, we can infer that a component is damaged if it is the only component in the task analysis of a failed task that does not also occur in the task analysis of a successfully performed task.

To summarize the differences between the second reader's classifications and my own original classifications, the second reader's were somewhat more inclusive than mine, resulting in more cases having been inferred to be cases of loss of imagery based on her classifications (27) than based on mine (25). For the 24 cases inferred to be cases of imagery deficit on the basis of both readers' task classifications, the inferences to the particular component of imagery that was damaged were always the same. Therefore, I will only report 'compromise' inferences, which resulted from a discussion between the two readers after the classifications were completed.

Cases classified as lacking evidence of imagery deficit are displayed in Table 1. The most common reason that cases were put into this category was that the original author of the report has simply stated that a patient had an imagery deficit without describing any of the behavioral evidence that presumably had led him to that conclusion.

Inferring the Damaged Component of Imagery

Among the 27 patients classified as having impaired imagery systems, there are three distinct patterns of abilities and deficits that emerge, from which we may infer damage to different components of the visual imagery system.

Generation Process Deficit

Eight patients display the following pattern of abilities and deficits, illustrated in Fig. 9. Figure 9a illustrates the performance of the patients of Brownell *et al.* (1984), Lyman, *et al.* (1938), and Nielsen (1946, pp. 200, 227), who were unable to answer questions requiring imagery, although they did possess the ability to answer similar questions about visible stimuli and could recognize visually presented stimuli. The patients of Brain (1954, Cases 1 and 2) displayed this same basic pattern of deficits, but with some unusual additional features. Whereas Case 1, a construction supervisor, was no longer able to visualize plans or elevations at work, Brain reports that the patient was able to give a satis-

Table 1. Cases for which an imagery deficit could not be inferred. For each case the primary topic of the case report, the etiology and the general anatomical area of cortical damage are listed

Case	Topic	Etiology	Lesion site
Arbuse (1947)	Gerstmann's syndrome	Neoplasm	Left parieto-occipital
Brown (1972) Case 11	Apperceptive visual agnosia	Anoxia	Bilateral posterior
Brown (1972) Case 12	Apperceptive visual agnosia	Cerebrovascular accident?	Bilateral posterior
Holmes (1945) p. 359 (cited as loss of imagery by Critchley, 1953)	Color agnosia	Cerebrovascular accident	Left occipital
Nielsen (1946) p. 203 (cited as loss of imagery, 1955)	Visual agnosia	Cerebrovascular accident	Right occipital
Nielsen (1946) p. 230 (cited as loss of imagery, 1955)	Gerstmann's syndrome	Cerebrovascular accident	Left parieto-occipital
Nielsen (1955) Case 7	Loss of imagery	Neoplasm	Left occipital
Nielsen (1955) postscript Case 1	Loss of imagery and dreaming	Neoplasm	Left occipital
Nielsen (1955) postscript Case 2	Loss of imagery and dreaming	Neoplasm	Left occipital
Wilbrand (1887) (described by Nielsen, 1955)	Loss of imagery	Cerebrovascular accident	Left posterior

factory description of "an object he could not visualize, e.g., his own house." Case 2 showed an inability to describe familiar objects or answer questions involving imagery only when his eyes were closed; with eyes open his performance inexplicably improved. Figure 9b illustrates the performance of the patients of Lyman *et al.* (1938) and Spalding and Zangwill (1950), who were unable to draw common objects from memory, although they were able to copy comparable or identical objects and recognize visually presented objects. Figure 9c illustrates the performance of the patients of Brain (1954, Cases 1 and 2), Humphrey and Zangwill (1951, Case 3), and Spalding and Zangwill (1951) who were unable to detect any imagery on introspection, although they were aware of being able to see. In each section of Fig. 9 the only component of the failed tasks that does not occur in the successful tasks is the image generation process. Therefore, in these patients the generation process is likely to be damaged.

When the eight cases inferred to have damage to the image generation process are considered as a separate group, a trend in lesion sites emerges, shown in Table 2. The two cases in the image generation process group that provide detailed anatomical data from surgery (Lyman *et al.*, 1938) or autopsy (Nielsen, 1946, p. 227) show tumors in the left parieto-occipital area, although in both cases signs of increased intracranial pressure were noted, implying possible pressure effects on the functioning of tissue distant from the tumors. Nielsen's case also had a left thalamic tumor. The remaining six cases provide varying amounts of information on lesion site. Spalding and Zangwill's (1950) patient was wounded by a penetrating missile, whose point of entry was between the left angular gyrus of the parietal lobe and area 19 of the occipital lobe. From skull X-rays and neurological signs, the authors assert that the left parieto-occipital area was the site of greatest damage. Of the remaining five cases of image generation process deficit shown in Table 2, there are two for which the available localizing signs indicate a left posterior focus of pathology (left parieto-occipital EEG abnormalities for Brain's (1954) head-injured Case 1 and clinical presentation indicating a left posterior cerebral artery stroke for Nielsen's (1946, p. 200) patient). In Brain's (1954) second case a physical examination provided no information on lesion site and further tests were not carried out. It was known that the patient had fallen and sustained a severe right fronto-vertical head injury, suggesting a probable right frontal lesion (coup) and, one might speculate, a possible left posterior lesion (contra-coup). Writing about this patient earlier, Brain (1950) proposed that the imagery deficit might be the result of contra-coup. The patient of Brownell *et al.* (1984) had extensive bilateral damage from several strokes, with a written description of a CT scan mentioning involvement of both parietal lobes (right more than left). The patient's records also included mention of possible left anterior damage on the basis of the patient's dysphasia. Finally, the third case of Humphrey and Zangwill (1951) had sustained a posterior right parietal lesion from a penetrating missile (shown in skull X-rays), but two factors suggest that this patient had reversed hemispheric dominance. He was a left-hander and, more importantly, his unilateral right-

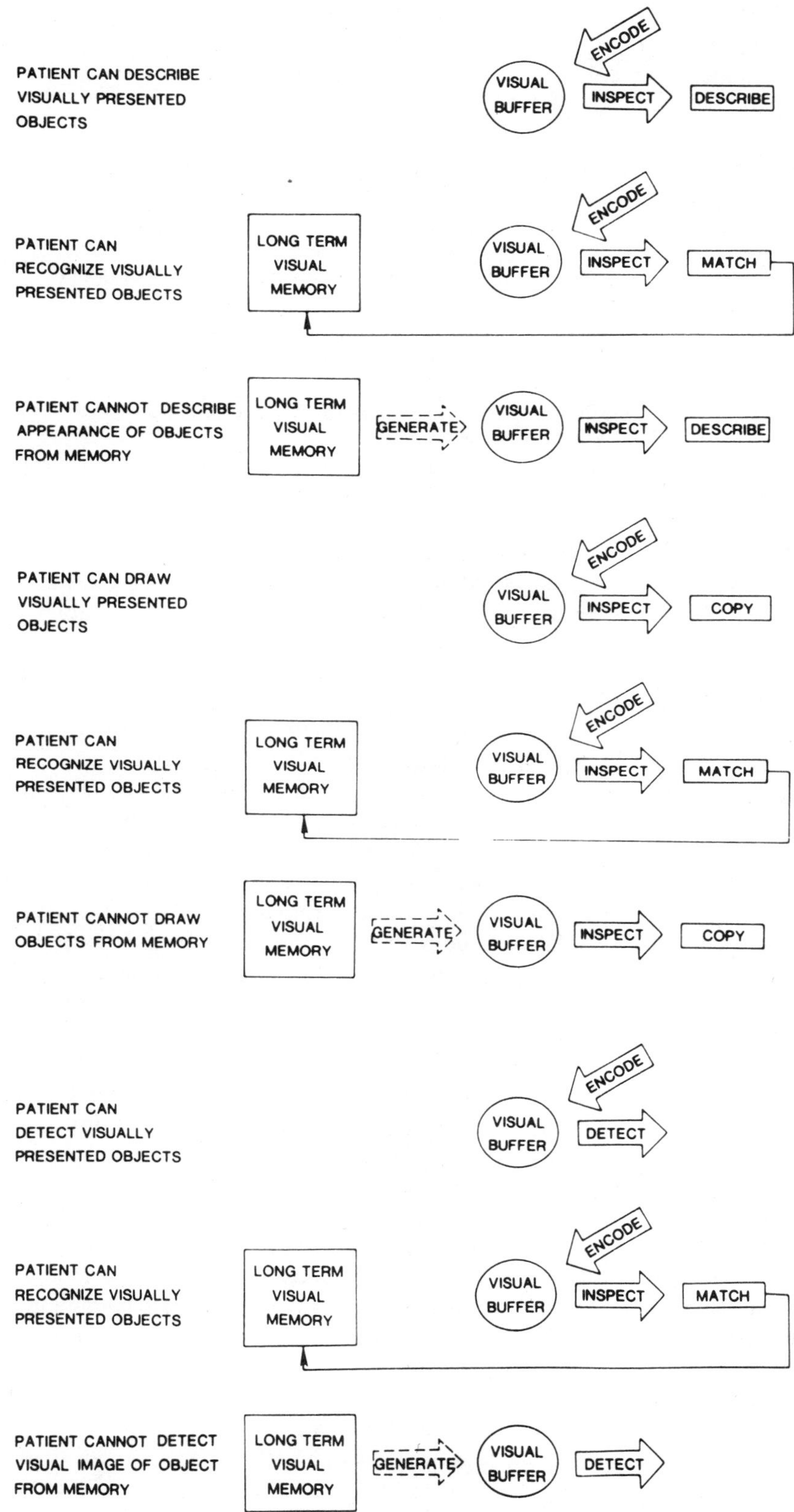

Figure 9. Inferring an image generation process deficit. Solid outline indicates that a component is ruled out as the reason for the patients' failure in the imagery tasks by virtue of appearing in the analysis of a successfully performed task.

Table 2. Cases inferred to have an image generation process deficit. For each case the primary topic of the case report, the etiology and the general anatomical area of cortical damage are listed

Case	Topic	Etiology	Lesion site
Brain (1951) Case 1	Loss of imagery	Head injury	Left poosterior
Brain (1951) Case 2	Loss of imagery	Head injury	?
Brownell *et al.* (1984)	Loss of imagery	Cerebrovascular accident	Bilateral parietal (greater on right), left frontal
Humphrey and Zangwill (1951) Case 3	Loss of dreaming	Penetrating head wound	Right posterior parietal (left handed)
Lyman *et al.* (1938)	Alexia and agraphia	Neoplasm	Left parieto-occipital
Nielsen (1946) p. 200	Topographic disorientation	Cerebrovascular accident	Left posterior
Nielsen (1946) p. 227	Gerstmann's syndrome	Neoplasm	Left parietal and occipital
Spalding and Zangwill (1950)	Loss of 'number form'	Penetrating head wound	Bilateral, greatest in left parieto-occipital

hemisphere damage left him dysphasic. Thus, this patient follows the trend for posterior dominant hemisphere damage.

It is clear that the quality of the localizing information and the nature of the lesions themselves (size and etiology) in these cases cannot support an inference to a critical lesion site in any individual case. The claim that the left posterior region contains critical structures for image generation is based on the trend observed across cases, *viz.*, in the seven cases with localizing information, six have predominantly or exclusively posterior dominant hemisphere damage.

For the sake of examining the trend towards left posterior damage found in these cases of image generation deficit, we can return to the *non-agnosic* cases of Table 1, in which the authors had claimed that the patients had lost imagery, but did not provide the information needed to infer a loss of imagery using task analyses. If these patients had indeed lost imagery, then their lack of an agnosia implies that they were cases of image generation process deficit (by the process of elimination depicted in Fig. 9). These patients all had left posterior damage: Arbuse's (1947) patient had a left parieto-occipital tumor (with increased intracranial pressure), Nielsen's (1946, p. 230) patient had a stroke with lesions in the left posterior parietal and occipital lobes as well as a small lesion in the motor strip, the case of Wilbrand described by Nielsen (1955) had a stroke with a right homonymous hemianopia as the only neurological sign, implying left posterior cerebral artery stroke, and Nielsen's (1955) Case 7 had what was described as a "small" tumor in the left occipital lobe. There are two additional cases of loss of imagery reported in a postscript to Nielsen's (1955) paper, with no mention of agnosia. Assuming that the presence of agnosia would have been mentioned, these patients are also likely to have had image generation deficits, and they, too, had left occipital tumors.

Long-Term Visual Memory Deficit

Thirteen patients display the following pattern, illustrated in Fig. 10. These patients are listed in Table 3. Figure 10a illustrates the performance of the patients of Albert, *et al.* (1975), Basso, *et al.* (1980), Beyn and Knyazeva (1962), Boyle and Nielsen (1954), Epstein (1979), Macrae and Trolle (1956), Nielsen (1946, p. 176), Ratcliff and Newcombe (1982), Shuttleworth *et al.* (1982, Case 2), Taylor and Warrington (1971), Wapner *et al.* (1978), and Wilbrand (1887, translated by Critchley, 1953) who were unable to recognize visual stimuli and also unable to answer questions requiring imagery, although they were able to describe and answer questions about the appearance of visual stimuli. In other words, in addition to their imagery deficit these patients had an associative visual agnosia. Figure 10b illustrates another aspect of the performance of the patients of Albert *et al.* (1975), Beyn and Knyazeva (1962), Macrae and Trolle (1956), Ratcliff and Newcombe (1982). Shuttleworth *et al.* (1982), Taylor and Warrington (1971) and Wapner *et al.* (1978), who, in addition to the disabilities already mentioned, were unable to draw objects from memory, although they were able to copy objects. Finally, Fig. 10c illustrates the performance of the patients of Basso *et al.* (1980), Humphrey and Zangwill (1951, Case 1), Macrae and Trolle (1956) and Shuttleworth *et al.* (1982), who, in addition to the above-mentioned recognition difficulties, were unable to detect their own imagery upon introspection, but were able to see.

From these patterns of performance we can conclude that either the long-term memories have been damaged or both the generation process and the matching process have been damaged. Several factors favor the inference that the long-term memories have been damaged. First, parsimony favors the interpretation that one component occurring in all and only failed tasks, is damaged, rather than the interpretation

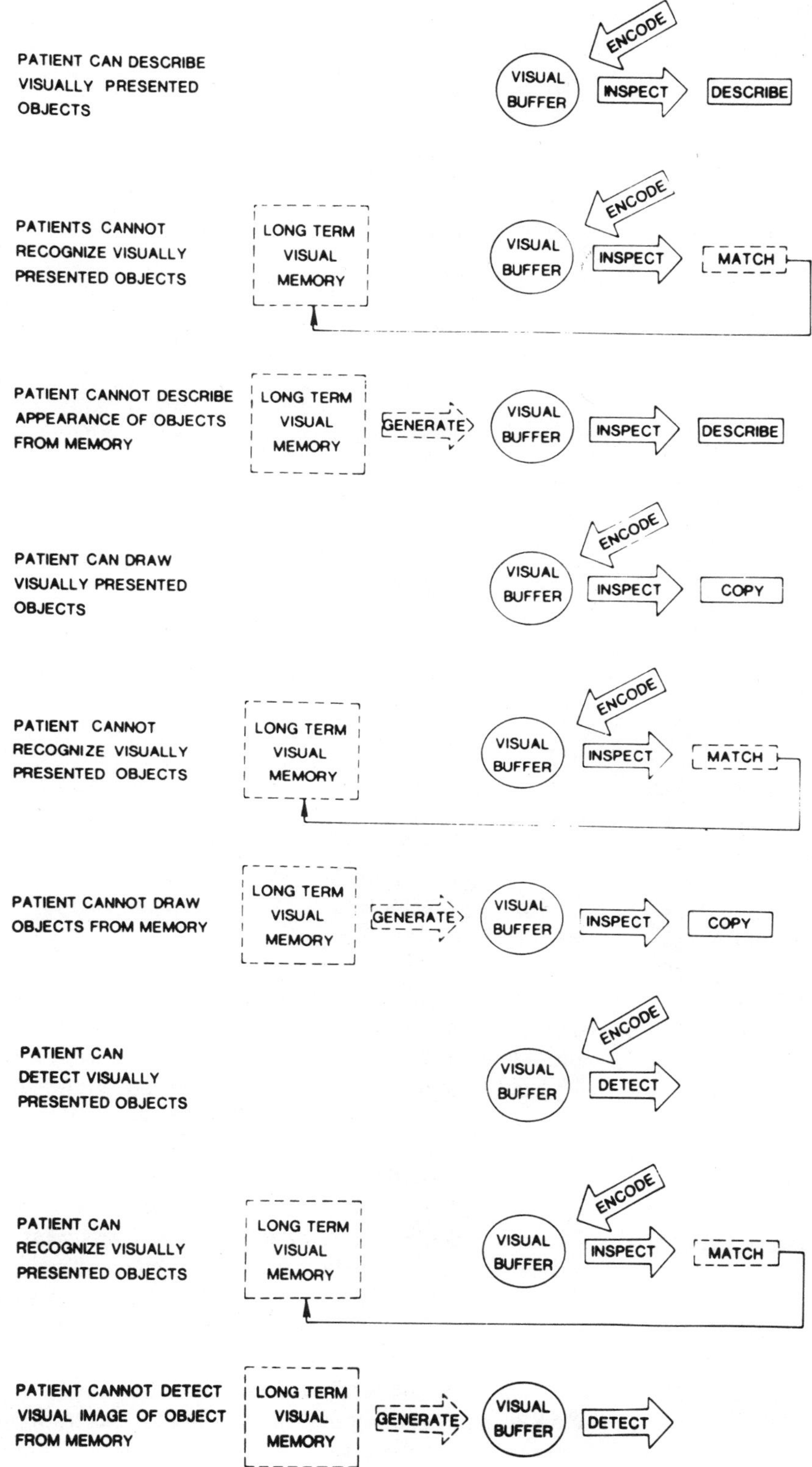

Figure 10. Inferring a long term visual memory deficit. Solid outline indicates that a component is ruled out as the reason for the patients' failure in the imagery tasks by virtue of appearing in the analysis of a successfully performed task.

Table 3. Cases inferred to have a long term visual memory deficit. For each case the primary topic of the case report, the etiology and the general anatomical area of cortical damage are listed

Case	Topic	Etiology	Lesion site
Albert *et al.* (1975)	Visual agnosia	Cerebrovascular accident?	Right anterior, bilateral posterior
Basso *et al.* (1980)	Loss of imagery	Cerebrovascular accident	Left temporal and occipital
Beyn and Kuyazeva (1962)	Prosopagnosia and visual object agnosia	Cerebrovascular accident	Bilateral posterior
Boyle and Nielsen (1954)	Visual agnosia	Neoplasm and surgical trauma	Bilateral occipital (greater on right)
Epstein (1979) Case 1	Loss of dreaming	Cerebrovascular accident	Left posterior (left handed)
Humphrey and Zangwill (1951) Case 1	Loss of dreaming	Penetrating head wound	Right parietal
Macrae and Trolle (1956)	Visual agnosia	Head injury	Bilateral temporal and parietal (greater on left)
Nielsen (1946) p. 176	Visual agnosia	Cerebrovascular accident	Right occipital, left temporal and parietal
Ratcliff and Newcombe (1982)	Visual agnosia	Cerebrovascular accident	Bilateral occipital, parietal, temporal (greater on right)
Shuttleworth, *et al.* (1982) Case 2	Prosopagnosia	Head injury	Bilateral posterior
Taylor and Warrington (1971)	Visual agnosia	Cortical atrophy	Diffuse (left more than right)
Wapner *et al.* (1978)	Visual agnosia	Cerebrovascular accident	Left temporal, bilateral occipital (greater on left) (left handed)
Wilbrand (1887, transl. Critchley, 1953)	Visual agnosia	Cerebrovascular accident	Bilateral posterior

that a pair of components, each of which occurs in one failed task are damaged. Second, a distinguishing feature of this group is that several of the cases showed content-specific imagery deficits, as well as content-specific agnosias. This suggests that damage has been done to one of the representational, or information-bearing, components of the imagery system. Third, when a content-specific imagery deficit exists, it is paralleled by a content-specific recognition deficit affecting the same class of stimuli, which suggests that the same component is responsible for both the imagery and recognition deficit: Beyn and Knyazeva's (1962) patient was able to recognize only 3 of 16 common objects that he could not reportedly image, but could recognize 13 out of 16 common objects that he could image. Wapner *et al.*'s (1978) patient was also better at imaging those objects he could recognize, as inferred from his drawing performance. Although Shuttleworth *et al.*'s (1982) second patient was not tested on imagery other than for faces, she introspected that she could image anything but faces, and her recognition difficulties were primarily encountered with faces. Despite his claims that he had lost all imagery, including auditory and olfactory imagery, Basso *et al.*'s (1980) patient could draw and describe from memory as well as recognize most common objects, but failed when these same tasks involved geographical locales and performed only mediocrely when they involved faces. For these three reasons I am classifying the patients discussed in this section as having damaged long-term visual memories rather than as having a combination of damaged generation and match processes. However, this classification is supported by a less direct inference than the preceding classification of image generation deficit.

In all but three of the cases of loss of long-term visual memories, the damage was known to involve one or both occipital lobes, as shown in Table 3. (Humphrey and Zangwill's (1951) Case 1 had sustained a penetrating head wound from a metal fragment that entered in the right posterior parietal region, which might or might not have caused occipital damage. Macrae and Trolle's, (1956) patient had a closed head injury causing abnormal EEG in the temporal and parietal regions. The anatomical information in this case is very weak, and so we cannot conclude much from a lack of positive evidence for occipital damage. Taylor and Warrington's (1971) patient had diffuse atrophy with no focal damage.)

There is less anatomical regularity within the long-term visual memory group than within the generation process group; there is no clear trend here either in laterality or in region within the posterior lobes. This greater heterogeneity could reflect the necessity for a further componential analysis of long-term visual memory deficit. That is, perhaps different cognitive components of the long-term visual memories, having different anatomical locations, have been disrupted in

Table 4. Case inferred to have either an image generation process deficit or a long-term visual memory deficit

Case	Topic	Etiology	Lesion site
Humphrey and Zangwill (1951) Case 2	Loss of dreaming	Penetrating head wound	Bilateral parieto-occipital (greater on left)

different cases. Unfortunately, there are not enough data available on the specific nature of the imagery and recognition deficits in these cases to suggest what the different components might be.

In one case (Humphrey and Zangwill, 1951, Case 2) there is not enough information to decide whether the imagery deficit was due to loss of the generation process or loss of long-term visual memories. This case is shown in Table 4. Although agnosia or recognition difficulties are not mentioned in this case, the report refers to "some topographic and related visual memory loss" (p. 323). On the one hand, if this "visual memory loss" refers to recognition memory then this patient has the pattern of deficits and abilities that would place him among the long-term visual memory cases. On the other hand, if it refers to his inability to recall visual information, then this patient belongs in the image generation process group. We are not aided in our decision by the following two quotes from the patient, one of which suggests a complete, across-the-board loss of imagery, and the other of which suggests a partial and possibly content-specific imagery deficit: "I think only in words, never in pictures," and, "If someone says: 'Can you visualize what your home is like?' Well I can do that, but I can't visualize a lot of things, such as faces sometimes or places I've been to." This patient's brain damage was in the parieto-occipital regions of both hemispheres, predominantly the left.

Inspection Process Deficit

Five patients showed a pattern of abilities and deficits indicative of damage to the inspection process. Four of these patients (Adler, 1944: Brain, 1941; Brown, 1972, Case 13, also described in Benson and Greenberg, 1969; Levine, 1978) showed the pattern of abilities and deficits illustrated in Fig. 11, and the fifth patient (Nielsen, 1946, p. 188) showed the same pattern except that his drawing ability was not tested. These patients were each the subjects of detailed examinations by their physicians, with the following results. These patients are not blind, but have difficulty describing complex stimuli. Their performance on imagery question-answering tasks is poor, and their descriptions of the appearances of objects from memory is reported to be vague, sparse, and inaccurate. For the four patients whose drawing ability was tested, both their copies and their drawings from memory were sketchy, inaccurate and disorganized. In view of their perceptual deficits, it is not surprising that these patients also had difficulty recognizing objects.

These patients are so impaired that there are very few components that can be ruled out by virtue of occurring in a successfully performed task. Therefore, an inference can only be made on the basis of parsimony. The only component that occurs in all and only the failed tasks is the inspection component. The simplest alternative account of these patients' deficits requires that three cognitive components be damaged: long-term visual memories, copy, and describe. The relevance of parsimony may be questioned here, however, in view of these patients' rather extensive bilateral damage, from carbon monoxide poisoning (Adler, 1944; Brown, 1972, Case 13), infection (Brain, 1941), surgical trauma (Levine, 1978), or multiple strokes (Nielsen, 1946, p. 188).

Associated Cognitive Deficits

Imagery has been hypothesized to play an essential role in many kinds of thinking and problem-solving. One might therefore expect loss of imagery to be accompanied by other cognitive deficits. Although most of the patients described here had some other cognitive deficits, none of these deficits appeared consistently, either across all patients or within a single group of patients. Indeed, Brain (1954) expressed surprise at the general sparing of intellectual ability in his patients who had lost imagery ability. This lack of consequence may reflect the flexibility of human cognition, and the availability of alternative means of performing what might normally be imagery-mediated tasks, such as route-finding, mental arithmetic, or spelling aloud.

The only consistent functional associate of loss of imagery in these cases was loss of dreaming. Of the 17 cases of loss of imagery which included information about dreaming, all but 3 reported either a total loss of dreaming (Basso *et al.*, 1980; Boyle and Nielsen. 1954; Humphrey and Zangwill, 1951, Cases 2 and 3; Lyman *et al.*, 1938; Nielsen, 1955, postscript Cases 1 and 2), a dramatic reduction in dreaming (described by the patient as, e.g., "almost no dreams": Epstein, 1979, Case 1; Humphrey and Zangwill, 1951, Case 1; Wilbrand, 1887, transl. Critchley, 1953), or a selective loss of the visual component of dreaming (Adler, 1944; Brain, 1954, Case 1; Brown, 1972, Case 13; Macrae and Trolle, 1956). The exceptions to this trend for impairment of dreaming were Shuttleworth *et al.*'s (1982, Case 2) prosopagnosic patient, who maintained that she did experience visual elements in her dreams, Brain's (1941) apperceptive agnosic child, who was able to relate a dream involving black and white dogs (which suggests that visual elements were present in the dream), and

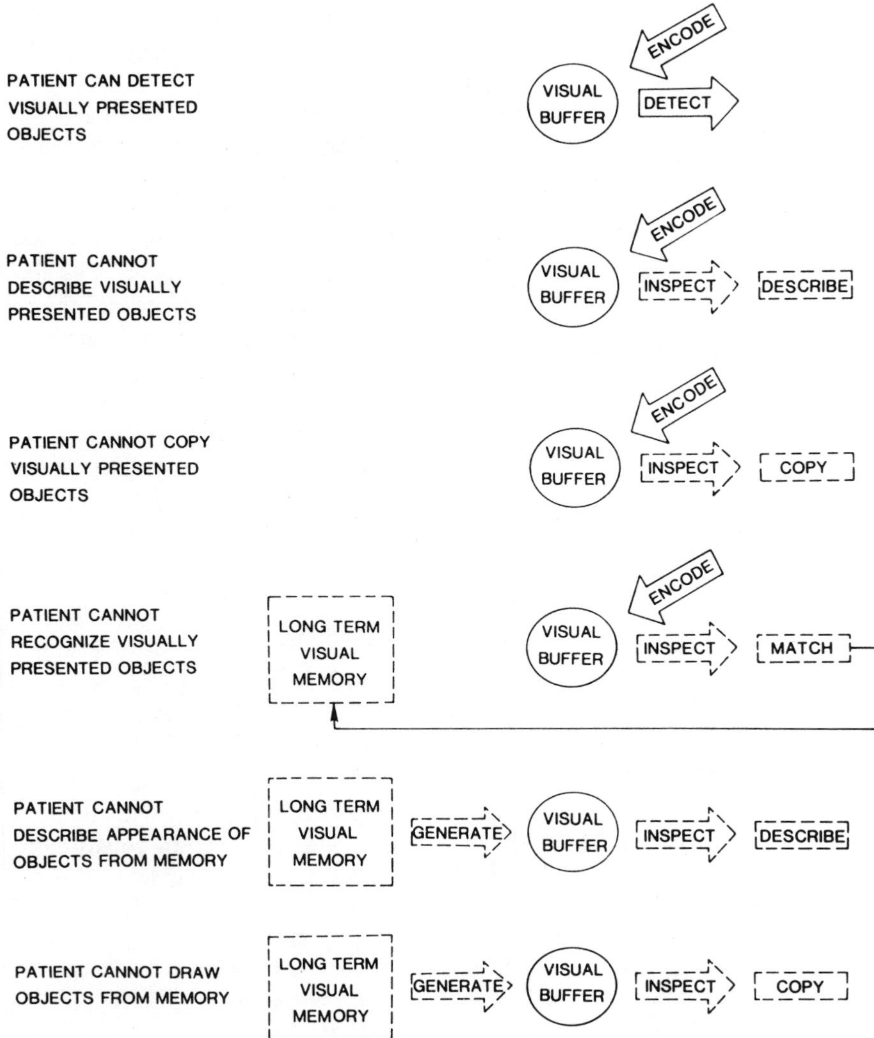

Figure 11. Inferring an inspection process deficit. Solid outline indicates that a component is ruled out as the reason for the patients' failure in the imagery tasks by virtue of appearing in the analysis of a successfully performed task.

Table 5. Cases inferred to have an inspection process deficit. For each case the primary topic of the case report, the etiology and the general anatomical area of cortical damage are listed

Case	Topic	Etiology	Lesion site
Adler (1944)	Visual agnosia	Anoxia	Diffuse (especially posterior)
Brain (1941)	Visual agnosia	Infection	Diffuse
Brown (1972) Case 13 (also described by Benson and Greenberg, 1969)	Visual agnosia	Anoxia	Diffuse (especially posterior)
Levine (1978)	Visual agnosia	Surgical trauma	Bilateral temporal, parietal and occipital (greater on right)
Nielsen (1946) p. 188	Simultanagnosia	Cerebrovascular accident	Bilateral parietal and occipital

Brown's (1972, Case 12) apperceptive agnosic who, while cortically blind, suffered from vivid nightmares. (The report of Brown's Case 12 did not make clear what the criteria were by which the patient was judged to have lost his imagery ability, leaving open the possibility that this patient had not actually lost imagery.) In order to decide whether these cases undermine the hypothesis that common structures and processes underlie dreaming and waking imagery we would want to know if the dreams of these patients, though present, have deficits that parallel the deficits of their waking imagery. For example, in the case of Shuttleworth *et al.*'s patient, the critical association or dissociation would not simply be between the presence of dreams and her waking imagery deficit, but between the presence of faces in her dreams and her waking imagery deficit, as this primarily involved faces. Although a selective deficit for dreaming of faces might seem a far-fetched idea, such a deficit has been described by Tzavaras (1967), in the context of prosopagnosia. Similarly, we would want to know whether Brain's patient could image a black dog as distinct from a white one while awake.

Cases of impaired dreaming with preserved waking imagery would naturally not be included in the present review of loss of imagery, but would nevertheless be relevant to assessing the strength of association between waking and dream imagery. Greenberg and Farah (1984) reviewed the loss of dreaming literature, including but not limited to the cases cited here, and found no cases of loss of dreaming in which loss of waking imagery was noted to be intact. Thus, there is a strong association between waking and dream imagery after brain damage, which suggests shared neural mechanisms for these two processes.

Summary and Discussion of Findings

Two general goals for this project were set out at the beginning of the paper: First, to use a componential analysis of imagery derived from studies of normal humans to understand the neurological phenomena of loss of imagery, and second, to use the results of this neurological study to illuminate the functioning of the intact imagery system. Most of the paper so far has focused on the first goal, by describing the componential model of imagery and the ways in which the different patterns of preserved abilities and deficits found in different cases can be interpreted in terms of the model: on the basis of the model we expected to find greater homogeneity within groups of patients sharing a deficit in the same underlying component than across different kinds of imagery deficits, and this expectation was borne out.

Patients with a deficit in the image generation process showed a consistent trend in lesion site, despite rather weak localizing information in many cases. Most of the patients had most or all of their damage in the posterior left quadrant of the brain. The quality of the localizing information makes a more precise localization impossible at present. However, the most obvious and perhaps the most striking aspect of this relatively coarse-grained localization is its laterality. As Ehrlichman and Barrett (1983) have documented, there exists a widespread assumption that imagery is a right hemisphere function. However, in reviewing the neuropsychology literature on the laterality of imagery, they found that the data supporting the 'right hemisphere' hypothesis do not actually apply to image generation *per se*, but rather to various forms of so-called 'spatial ability' and higher visual perceptual processing.

The laterality of the image generation process identified here is in agreement with the outcome of a recent case study of a split-brain patient (Farah *et al.*, In press). Whereas the disconnected left hemisphere could perform a task requiring image generation, the right hemisphere could not, despite its facility with all of the components of the imagery task except for image generation itself. Both hemispheres could classify briefly presented lower case letters as including or not including a long 'stem' (e.g. 't' and 'g' have long stems, 'a' and 'r' do not), and both could associate a briefly presented upper case letter with the corresponding lower case form. Their performances diverged sharply, however, in the corresponding imagery task: When given the upper case form of a letter as a cue to classify the lower case form as having or not having a long stem, the left hemisphere continued to perform essentially perfectly, and the right hemisphere dropped to chance levels of performance.

The present project provides inductive evidence that if a patient has lost the ability to generate images then he or she will have left posterior damage. We do not yet know what proportion of patients with damage in this area will also have an image generation deficit. Although published reports of loss of imagery are rare compared with reports of other cognitive disabilities (e.g. linguistic, attentional), this measure may greatly underestimate the incidence of imagery disorders for two reasons. First, the critical area for image generation may be close to the posterior language centers of the left hemisphere. Thus, many patients with lesions in this area may be unable to communicate their loss of imagery. Second, patients are not as likely to complain to their doctors about a loss of imagery as they are about a loss of language or vision. In this vein, it is interesting to note that of the seventeen cases of loss of imagery in which the patient's occupation or hobby was reported, eight patients worked in architecture, building, carpentry, painting or set design, activities that demand visualization.

Although an anatomical locus for long-term visual memories was not found, there was a trend for parallel content-specific deficits in imagery and recognition, implying that the imagery system shares representations with perceptual processes in the brain, an intuitively appealing idea (e.g. see Hebb, 1968) for which little evidence exists.

This analysis of loss of imagery also has implications for our understanding of the intact imagery system in normal humans. The most obvious implications have already been mentioned. Neuropsychological evidence for the existence of an image generation process, distinct from the long-term visual memories themselves and from other recall processes, and a functional localization for that process. Other relevant findings include the associations between waking imagery and dreaming, and between content-specific imagery and recognition deficits, which suggest the existence of shared components for these pairs of seemingly disparate processes in the functional architecture of the normal brain.

At a more general level, the results of this project support the existence of an imagery system distinct from other memory and reasoning processes, with an internal structure corresponding to the components outlined in this paper. On a 'single code' account of imagery, such as Pylyshyn (1981) has put forward, imagery consists of recalling and manipulating information about the appearances of objects in a way that is not fundamentally different from recalling and manipulating information about other memory contents, such as historical facts, philosophical arguments, etc. If this were true, then one would not expect to find cases of selective loss of imagery ability any more than of selective loss of history or philosophy ability, and one would certainly not expect to find a separate brain area dedicated to one of these abilities.

The ability of the componential analysis of imagery used in this paper to interpret the loss of imagery literature also provides support for that particular analysis. Despite an occasional stray datum, for example the effect of opening the eyes on Brain's (1954) second patient, there is a substantial match between the observed patterns of performance on different tasks under different conditions and the kinds of patterns that are allowed assuming the present componential model. The situation could have been otherwise: for example, patients might have been described who had content-specific imagery deficits but no recognition deficits, or an isolated imagery deficit for remote but not recent memories. By and large the deficits and abilities reported did divide up along the lines that the model can account for. Therefore, although the case reports were interpreted *assuming* the model to be true, it is not entirely circular to consider the ability of the model to interpret these cases as supporting the model.

The last 15 years in cognitive psychology have seen enormous growth in our understanding of mental imagery. This progress has been made almost entirely within the theoretical confines of the information-processing paradigm, which eschews all concerns with neural 'hardware'. This paper represents an initial attempt to make contact between the theoretical constructs of cognitive theories of imagery and neurological phenomena. The results presented here are preliminary, and limited by the quality of the cognitive and neurological information available in the case reports. Nevertheless, they are grounds for optimism for future studies of imagery in neurological patients, using the experimental methodologies as well as the theoretical framework of current cognitive psychology.

Note

Preparation of this paper was supported by PHS grant 1F32 MH 08876-01 and by the MIT Center for Cognitive Science under a grant from the Alfred P. Sloan Foundation. The author thanks Neal Cohen, Lee Cranberg, William Estes, Howard Gardner, Mark Greenberg, Stephen Kosslyn, David Levine, R. Duncan Luce and Steven Pinker for helpful comments and suggestions on earlier drafts of this paper. Reprint requests should be sent to Martha J. Farah, Department of Neurology, B.U. School of Medicine, Psychology Research, Mail Drop 116-B, B.V.A.M.C., 150 S. Huntington Ave., Boston, MA 02130, U.S.A.

References

Adler, A. (1944) Disintegration and restoration of optic recognition in visual agnosia. *Arch. Neurol. and Psychiat.*, *51*, 243–259.

Albert, M. L., Reches, A. and Silverberg, R. (1975) Associative visual agnosia without alexia. *Neurology*, *25*, 322–326.

Arbuse, D. I. (1947) The Gerstmann syndrome: Case report and review of the literature. *J. Nerv. Ment. Dis.*, *105*, 359–371.

Basso, A., Bisiach, E. and Luzzatti, C. (1980) Loss of mental imagery: A case study. *Neuropsychologia*, *8*, 435–442.

Benson, D. F. and Greenberg, J. P. (1969) Visual form agnosia. *Arch. Neurol.*, *20*, 82–89.

Beyn, E. S. and Knyazeva, G. R. (1962) The problem of prosopagnosia. *J. Neurol., Neurosurg. Psychiat.*, *25*, 154–158.

Bisiach, E. and Luzzatti, C. (1978) Unilateral neglect of representational space. *Cortex*, *14*, 129–133.

Bisiach, E., Luzzatti, C. and Persni, D. (1979) Unilateral neglect, representational schema and consciousness. *Brain*, *102*, 609–618.

Boyle, J. and Nielsen, J. M. (1954) Visual agnosia and loss of recall: Report of case. *Bull. Los Angeles Neurol. Soc.*, *19*, 39–43.

Brain, R. W. (1954) Loss of visualization. *Proc. R. Soc. Med.*, *47*, 288–290.

Brain, R. W. (1950) The cerebral basis of consciousness. *Brain*, *73*, 465–479.

Brain. R. W. (1941) Visual object agnosia with special reference to the Gestalt theory. *Brain, 64*, 43–62.

Brown, J. W. (1972) *Aphasia, Apraxia and Agnosia: Clinical and Theoretical Aspects.* Springfield, IL, Charles C. Thomas.

Brownell, H. H., Farah, M. J., Harley, J. P. and Kosslyn, S. M. (1984) Distinguishing imagistic and linguistic thought: A case report. Paper submitted for publication.

Critchley, M. (1953) *The Parietal Lobes.* London, Arnold.

Eddy, J. K. and Glass, A. L. (1981) Reading and listening to high and low imagery sentences. *J. verb. Learn. verb. Behav., 20*, 333–345.

Ehrlichman, H. and Barrett, J. (1983) Right hemispheric specialization for mental imagery: A review of the evidence. *Br. Cog., 2*, 39–52.

Epstein, A. W. (1979) Effect of certain cerebral diseases on dreaming. *Biol. Psychiat., 14*, 77–93.

Farah, M. J. (1984) Psychophysical evidence for a shared representational medium for visual images and percepts. *J. exp. Psychol: Gen.*, In press.

Farah, M. J., Gazzaniga, S. M., Holtzman, J. D. and Kosslyn, S. M. (1984) A left hemisphere basis for visual imagery. *Neuropsychologia*, In press.

Finke, R. A. and Kosslyn, S. M. (1980) Mental imagery acuity in the peripheral visual field. *J. exp. Psychol.: Hum. Percep. Perf., 6*, 126–139.

Finke, R. A. and Kurtzman, H. S. (1981) Area and contrast effects upon perceptual and imagery acuity. *J. exp. Psychol.: Hum. Percept. Perf., 7*, 825.

Finke, R. A. and Schmidt, M. J. (1977) Orientation-specific color aftereffects following imagination. *J. exp. Psychol.: Human. Percept. Perf., 3*, 599–606.

Finke, R. A. and Schmidt. M. J. (1978) The quantitative measurement of pattern representation in images using orientation-specific color aftereffects. *Percep. Psychophys., 23*, 515–520.

Finke, R. A. and Shepard, R. N. (In Press) Visual functions of mental imagery. In L. Kaufman and J. Thomas (eds.), *Handbook of Perception and Human Performance.* New York, John Wiley & Sons.

Greenberg, M. S. and Farah, M. J. (1984) The laterality of dreaming. Paper submitted for publication.

Hebb, D. O. (1968) Concerning imagery. *Psychol. Rev., 75*, 466–477.

Holmes, G. (1944) The organization of the visual cortex in man. *Proc. R. Soc. Lond., 132*, 348–361.

Humphrey, M. E. and Zangwill, O. L. (1981) Cessation of dreaming after brain injury. *J. neurol., Neurosurg. Psychiat., 14*, 322–325.

Kosslyn, S. M. and Jolicoeur, P. (1980) A theory-based approach to the study of individual differences in mental imagery. In R. E. Snow, P. A. Federico and W. E. Montague (eds.) *Aptitude, Learning and Instruction: Cognitive Processes Analysis of Aptitude*, Vol. 1. Hillsdale, NJ, Erlbaum.

Kosslyn, S. M. and Shwartz. S. P. (1977) A simulation of visual imagery. *Cog. Sci., 1*, 265–295.

Kosslyn, S. M. (1980) *Image and Mind.* Cambridge, MA, Harvard University Press.

Levine, D. N. (1978) Prosopagnosia and visual object agnosia: A behavioral study. *Br. Lang., 5*, 341–365.

Luria, A. R. (1973) *The Working Brain: An Introduction to Neuropsychology.* Baltimore, Penguin.

Lyman, R. S., Kwan, S. T. and Chao, W. H. (1938) Left occipito-parietal brain tumor with observations on alexia and agraphia in Chinese and English. *Chinese Med. J., 54*, 491–516.

Macrae and Trolle (1956).

Marr, D. (1982) *Vision.* San Francisco, W. H. Freemand & Co.

Nielsen, J. M. (1946) *Agnosia, Apraxia, Aphasia: Their Value in Cerebral Localization.* New York, Paul B. Hoeber.

Nielsen, J. M. (1955) Occipital lobes, dreams and psychosis. *J. nerv. ment. Dis., 121*, 30–32.

Podgorny, P. and Shepard, R. N. (1978) Functional representations common to visual perception and imagination. *J. exp. Psychol.: Hum. Percep. Perf., 4*, 21–35.

Pylyshyn, Z. W. (1981) The imagery debate: Analogue media versus tacit knowledge. *Psychol. Rev., 87*, 16–45.

Ratcliff, G. and Newcombe, F. (1982) Object recognition. In A. W. Ellis (ed.), *Normality and Pathology in Cognitive Functions.* New York, Academic Press.

Selfridge, O. G. and Neisser, U. (1960) Pattern recognition by machine. *Scient. Am, m 203*, 60–68.

Shulman, S. L., Remington, R. W. and McClean, M. C. (1979) Moving attention through visual space. *J. exp. Psychol.: Hum. Percep. Perf., 5*, 522–526.

Shuttleworth, E. C., Syring, V. and Allen, N. (1982) Further observations on the nature of prosopagnosia. *Br. Cog., 1*, 302–332.

Spalding, J. M. K. and Zangwill, O. L. (1950) Disturbance of number-form in a case of brain injury. *J. Neurol., Neurosurg. Psychiat., 13*, 24–29.

Taylor, A. and Warrington, E. K. (1971) Visual agnosia: A single case report. *Cortex, 7*, 152–161.

Triesman, A. M. and Gelade, G. (1980) A feature-integration theory of attention. *Cog. Psychol., 12*, 97–136.

Tzavaras, A. (1967) Contribution a l'etude de l'agnosie des physiognomies: Memoire pour le titre d'assistants etrangers. Paris, Faculte des Medicine de Paris, *1*.

Ullman, S. (1984) Visual Routines, *Cog., 18*, 97–159.

Wapner, W., Judd, T. and Gardner, H. (1978) Visual agnosia in an artist. *Cortex, 14*, 343–364.

45

P. E. Roland and L. Friberg

Localization of cortical areas activated by thinking

1985. *Journal of Neurophysiology* 53: 1219–1243

SUMMARY AND CONCLUSION

1. These experiments were undertaken to demonstrate that pure mental activity, thinking, increases the cerebral blood flow and that different types of thinking increase the regional cerebral blood flow (rCBF) in different cortical areas. As a first approach, thinking was defined as *brain work in the form of operations on internal information, done by an awake subject.*

2. The rCBF was measured in 254 cortical regions in 11 subjects with the intracarotid ^{133}Xe injection technique. In normal man, changes in the regional cortical metabolic rate of O_2 leads to proportional changes in rCBF. One control study was taken with the subjects at rest. Then the rCBF was measured during three different simple algorithm tasks, each consisting of retrieval of a specific memory followed by a simple operation on the retrieved information. Once started, the information processing went on in the brain without any communication with the outside world. In 50 − 3 thinking, the subjects started with 50 and then, in their minds only, continuously subtracted 3 from the result. In jingle thinking the subjects internally jumped every second word in a nine-word circular jingle. In route-finding thinking the subjects imagined that they started at their front door and then walked alternatively to the left or the right each time they reached a corner.

3. The rCBF increased only in homotypical cortical areas during thinking. The areas in the superior prefrontal cortex increased their rCBF equivalently during the three types of thinking. In the remaining parts of the prefrontal cortex there were multifocal increases of rCBF. The localizations and intensities of these rCBF increases depended on the type of internal operation occurring. The rCBF increased bilaterally in the angular cortex during 50 − 3 thinking. The rCBF increased in the right midtemporal cortex exclusively during jingle thinking. The intermediate and remote visual association areas, the superior occipital, posterior inferior temporal, and posterior superior parietal cortex, increased their rCBF exclusively during route-finding thinking. We observed no decreases in rCBF. All rCBF increases extended over a few square centimeters of the cortex.

4. The activation of the superior prefrontal cortex was attributed to the organization of thinking. The activation of the angular cortex in 50 − 3 thinking was attributed to the retrieval of the numerical memory and memory for subtractions. The activation of the right midtemporal cortex was attributed to the retrieval of the nonverbal auditory memory. The activation of the superior occipital, posterior inferior temporal, and posterior superior parietal cortex was attributed to the retrieval of the visual and spatial memory. Retrieval of different images gave rise to identical rCBF increases.

5. The main conclusions were as follows: Thinking was produced by activation of multiple cortical fields in the homotypical cortical zones outside the immediate sensory association areas. Different types of thinking activated different cortical fields. Thinking consumed cortical metabolic energy, reflected in multifield increases of rCBF. The estimated cortical energy consumption during thinking was equivalent or larger than the estimated cortical energy consumption during intense voluntary movements or intense processing of external sensory information. Retrieval of memory also consumed cortical metabolic energy. When a subject retrieved the visual and spatial memory or the nonverbal auditory memory to reevoke sensory events, the rCBF increased in the intermediate and remote sensory association areas belonging to the relevant modality. It was possible macroscopically to distinguish different types of thinking and to identify the kind of memory retrieved by the subjects, but it was not possible macroscopically to distinguish different images retrieved from a specific memory.

INTRODUCTION

Purely mental work, such as imagining a familiar face or the rain drumming against the window pane blocks the α-rhythm and augments the β-rhythm in the electroencephalogram (EEG) (12). If this desynchronization of the EEG is due to neurons increasing their excitation one would expect that mental work would increase the cerebral metabolism. If the presumed increase of neuronal excitation during mental work can be localized, one would expect to find localized increases of the neuronal metabolism during mental work. It has been shown many times (e.g., Refs. 2, 14) that there is a tight coupling between the regional cerebral metabolism and the regional cerebral blood flow in the normal brain. Measurements of one of these variables is thus an indicator of the metabolic work of the neurons and glia cells.

Sokoloff et al. (27) measured the cerebral blood flow and O_2 consumption in the brain while subjects did different complicated mental calculations. They could not find any changes of either the blood flow or the O_2 consumption of their subjects. They suggested that the efficiency of the neuronal work might increase during mental work. Or if this was not the case, then the energy consumption might increase in some regions of the brain while it decreased in other regions, such that the total metabolism and blood flow of the brain remained unchanged.

After Lassen and Ingvar (7, 8) introduced a method to measure the regional cerebral blood flow (rCBF) in the brain, Ingvar and Risberg (5) used this method to study changes in rCBF during psychological tasks. They found an increase of 6 $\text{ml} \cdot 100\ \text{g}^{-1} \cdot \text{min}^{-1}$ in the rCBF of the suprasylvian regions while subjects were repeating a sequence of digits presented backward to them. These subjects continually received instructions during the rCBF measurements. It could not be excluded, therefore, that the changes in rCBF were due to auditory stimulation. It was later shown that when subjects did a purely internal brain work in the form of programming but not executing a sequence of voluntary movements, the rCBF increased locally in the supplementary motor area and the superior prefrontal cortex (20, 21). Similarly, the pure anticipation of a very weak somatosensory stimulus increased the rCBF in the superior and middle prefrontal cortex and the somatotopically corresponding part of the contralateral somatosensory cortex (15). However, these two examples of purely mental work are too special to meet the general view of what thinking is. Thoughts are produced by retrieval of information from the brain itself. Thinking is the production of thoughts concatenated by internal operations. As a first operational approach, we define thinking as *brain work in the form of operations on internal information, done by an awake subject.* The subject should not prepare for voluntary movements or for the perception of sensory information, nor should he receive sensory information from the outside world or execute voluntary movements. The purpose of these experiments was to demonstrate that thinking increases the rCBF of the cerebral cortex and that different types of thinking give rise to rCBF increases in different cortical areas.

METHODS

Subjects

Eleven subjects who underwent carotid angiography participated. After informed consent from the subjects, the rCBF was determined in conjunction with the angiography. A patient was accepted for study if the angiogram, the rCBF measurement with the patient at rest, and the computerized axial tomography (CT-scan) of the brain were all normal. The brains of all participating subjects were thus anatomically intact. At the time of investigation none of the subjects had any neurological signs. Cases 454, 462, 493, and 500 received either diphenylhydantoin or carbamazepine for epilepsy; these drugs were within therapeutic blood levels. No clinical seizures or other ictal phenomena were observed in the EEG during the investigations. In addition, case 488 had one focal (psychomotor) seizure in his history. We compared the extents and localizations of the rCBF of these patients with epilepsy to the rCBFs of the remaining nonepileptics. As apparent from Figs. 7, 8, 10, and 11 we could not find any differences in extent and localization. When the intensities of the rCBF increases in the three types of thinking were compared, there were no statistical differences between the two groups ($P > 0.2$ and $P > 0.2$). All right hemispheres and all left hemispheres were therefore treated as two homogenous groups. Six dominant left hemispheres and five nondominant right hemispheres were infused with isotope. Hemisphere dominance (hemisphere in which language is located) was determined in all subjects who had their left hemisphere infused and in two of the right hemisphere cases (488, 493). The last three subjects were distinctly right handed. The determination was made by an intracarotid injection of the γ-aminobutyric acid agonist tetrahydroisoxazolopyridinol (THIP) as a preoperative evaluation before temporal lobe surgery (26).

Measurement of rCBF

The ^{133}Xe intracarotid injection method we used in the present experiments was a variant of the original Lassen and Ingvar method (8). This variant has been extensively described (15, 19). Briefly, the isotope was injected as a bolus through a catheter into the internal carotid artery. The washout of the isotope from 254 cortical regions was monitored by a 254-detector dynamic γ-camera (28). The rCBF in each of the 254 cortical regions was measured from the clearance curve segment between 12 and 60 s after the start of the injection

$$rCBF_i = 100\lambda|\alpha_i| \qquad (1)$$

in which α is the slope of the logarithmically transformed clearance curve, and λ is the blood cortex partition coefficient (ml/g). Measured this way $rCBF_i$ is the flow of the cerebral compartment with the highest blood flow, the gray matter. The clearance curve from each detector was examined for monoexponentiality. If there were deviations from monoexponentiality the subject was excluded. Arterial blood samples were taken during each rCBF measurement for determination of P_{CO_2}. Differences in rCBF due to differences in arterial P_{CO_2} between experiments were corrected by 4% per mmHg. All arterial P_{CO_2} values were between 37.0 and 46.9 mmHg. The intraarterial blood pressure and the pulse rate were measured.

Test procedures

Each subject went through at least four rCBF measurements according to a randomized schedule: one during rest; one during 50 − 3 thinking; one during jingle thinking; and one during route-finding thinking. All instructions were finished 15 s before the start of injection. For all rCBF measurements included, the status and behavior of the subjects were exactly the same in rest and during the three different types of thinking. The status of the surroundings was also exactly the same for all rCBF measurements included. Apart from the instructions, speech was prohibited in the examination room. All personnel wore rubber soles and cotton dresses. The room was darkened; only two small working lights far away from the subjects were lit.

The subjects started their thinking at the command *start,* which was given 5 s before the start of the isotope injection. All subjects spent between 80 and 90 min supine in the flow room. During each rCBF measurement the subjects were lying motionless, but between the measurements they were free to move and open their eyes. Every 5 min we asked the subjects about any discomfort they might have, itching, soreness from the catheter, etc. None of the subjects experienced any pain or discomfort, nervousness, or anxiety during the 1½ h testing period.

Each task was designed so that the subject had to retrieve information from a specific memory in the brain and then perform a simple operation on this information. The retrievals and operations could, once started, go on continuously without any communication between the subject and the surroundings. Another rationale behind the design was the formal similarity in the treatment of information during the three tasks; the flow of information was described by a simple loop with two intercalated operations (Figs. 1 and 2) or a cascade of two such loops (Fig. 3). Furthermore all operations were deterministic, and the algorithms were given beforehand.

Rest

This was the reference state. The subject was supine, relaxed, and awake. He did not receive any stimulation. The eyes were closed with cotton-wool pads that reduced eye movements, and the ears were plugged. The subjects were trained to avoid tensing the muscles, to relax, and to think of nothing. A pillow was placed under the neck; this helped the subjects to avoid tensing the neck muscles. The subjects were not allowed to make any movements, tense their muscles, speak, or change their respiratory rhythms. We did not record the EMG. Instead, two persons inspected the head, neck, and extremity muscles for contractions. Sometimes the subjects involuntarily wiggled their toes during the thinking. The thinking procedure was then repeated with a slight modification (i.e., 52 − 3 instead of 50 − 3) during a new measurement of rCBF. Subjects with even the slightest motor activity during this second

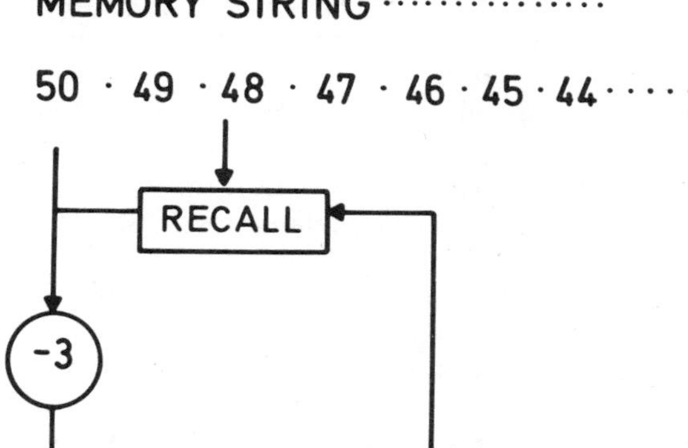

FIG. 1. Formal structure of the 50 − 3 task. Task is continuous, deterministic, and has the simplest algorithm of the three tasks. It consists of a recall from memory of ordered sequence of integers. From the integer 50 the subject continuously subtracts 3, or jumps 3 integers backward while the rCBF measurement was being taken.

attempt were excluded. In six subjects the EEG was recorded. These recordings were without motor artifacts.

In all subjects, with the exception of 462 and 488, we did two determinations of the rCBF during rest. In all cases of double-rest determination, the differences between the rCBF of the first rest and the second rest was <11% for any of the detector channels monitoring the brain. In all cases of double-rest determination the rCBF value that was used for the calculations was the mean of the two measurements. As in previous studies (15–22) we did several intracarotid sham injections of physiological saline to habituate the subjects to the examination. In all types of thinking the behavior of the subjects was as in rest.

Internal numerical operations: 50 − 3 thinking

All subjects were trained in a 100 − 7 task, in which they had to start with 100 and then continuously subtract 7, silently. When they performed the procedure perfectly, they received the instruction to start with 50 and then continuously subtract 3. They were told to go on even if they reached negative integers. They were not allowed to say anything or move until they were asked the control question *how far have you reached?*. The control question was asked 60–65 s after the start of the injection. If they made an error they were instructed in this task, as well as in the other tasks, to *just go on* and *not try to go back* and correct the error. The authors made sure that no movements occurred during the rCBF measurements. In four subjects an additional rCBF measurement was taken while they continuously subtracted 3 from 52. The structure of the task is shown in Fig. 1.

Jingle thinking

The jingle was the most well-known Danish jingle. It was known by heart by all the subjects. The structure of the task is shown in Fig. 2. The subjects were trained by jumping every third word of the closed-loop jingle. When they performed the procedure perfectly and were able to go on silently they received the test instruction. In the real task they were asked to jump every second word of the closed-loop jingle. Five to 10 seconds after the rCBF measurement was finished, subjects were asked how far they reached, and the number of jumps was calculated. The authors made sure that the status of the subjects included was exactly as in rest.

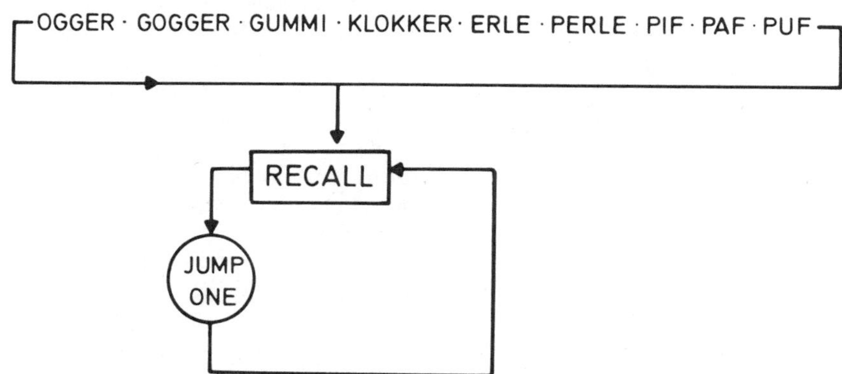

FIG. 2. Formal structure of the jingle task. Subjects recalled the ordered sequence of nonsense words from memory. Starting with *ogger* he continuously jumped over one word. The open sequence, however, initially had to be transformed into a closed loop consisting of the nine words. Thus when *puf* was reached the next jump would be to *gogger*.

Route finding

Also in this task the subjects were trained prior to the real task. They had to imagine that they were turning at every second corner, alternatively to the right and the left. As in the two other tasks, when the subjects were able to do the internal procedure perfectly, the instruction was given. In the real task the subjects *imagined* that they walked out their front door and then walked alternatively to the left and the right every time they reached a corner or a road on the appropriate side (Fig. 3). The subjects were told not to try to remember the names of the streets or surroundings they recalled, but to concentrate on the appearance of their familiar surroundings, i.e., to concentrate on what they saw with the mind's eye. Again, they did not try to correct errors if they made a wrong turn, but just continued as instructed, left-right. In five subjects, a second determination of rCBF was made while the subjects were imagining that they walked alternatively to the right and left.

Relation between rCBF pattern and functional anatomy of the cerebral cortex

The rCBF values from each of the 254 cortical regions were stored in an orthogonal matrix that could be displayed on a television screen (Figs. 5 and 6). This display is the image of the brain seen by the radially arranged detectors. The anatomic relations between the detector image and the brain surface were determined after a proportional stereotaxic system as described in earlier publications (15, 19, 21) (Fig. 5). The spatial resolution of the detector system was 1 cm, 3 cm from the surface of the collimators. The correlation of rCBF values between adjacent channels was <25% (17).

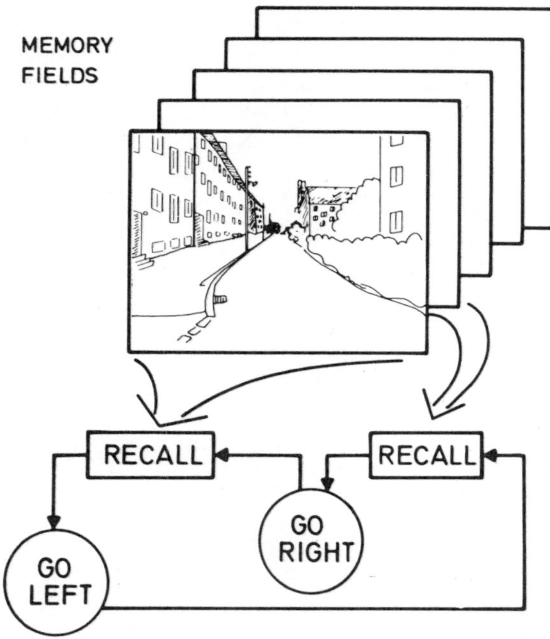

FIG. 3. Formal structure of the route-finding thinking. Subject *imagined* that he started at his front door and then walked alternatively left and right every time he reached a corner on the appropriate side. Thus the sequence of visual fields to be recalled next from the spatial-visual memory was contingent on content of visual field at the moment.

In Fig. 4 the cerebral cortex was subdivided into 31 regions based on earlier functional mapping and functional dissection studies of the human brain (5, 9, 13, 15–26). The subdivision was based on the results that different subsets of cortical fields were activated during different types of information processing by the brain (*functional mapping*). Moreover, when single steps of information processing of one type were altered the activation of some of the cortical fields belonging to the activated subset was also altered (*functional dissection;* Ref. 19). Activation means that the regional cerebral blood flow and the regional cerebral metabolism increased. Information processing means all sorts of generating, processing, storing, transferring, and using of information, which can be described with the terms and concepts of the theory of information and communication. The subdivision of the cerebral cortex in Fig. 4 is an abstraction and is preliminary. In principle, it would take an indefinite number of experiments to characterize the human cerebral cortex functionally and exactly. After the statistical analysis and proportional transformation of the matrix (Fig. 5) each activation or region without activation was assigned a name from Fig. 4 according to the subdivision in which most of the detector channels were localized.

A single cortical activation in an individual is a uniquely delimited field that does not necessarily respect the borders of the subdivisions in Fig. 4 (Figs. 6–8, 10, 11). In each subject the localization of an activated cortical field was determined in several independent ways (Fig. 5). First, the distances between the activated field and other well-defined smaller active fields was measured. All subjects participating in the present study had their motor mouth area, motor hand area, supplementary motor area, and auditory area activated during additional measurements of their rCBF. The activation procedures have been described elsewhere (21, 22, 26). Second, an activated field was localized by comparing the rCBF matrix with the matrix of the initial maximal counting rates. This matrix showed the passage of the radioactive bolus through the end part of the carotid artery, the anterior and middle cerebral arteries, and the insular portion of the ascending frontal vessels. Third, in each subject the same vessels were located on the carotid angiogram. The angiogram was taken with a picture magnification of 1:1.1

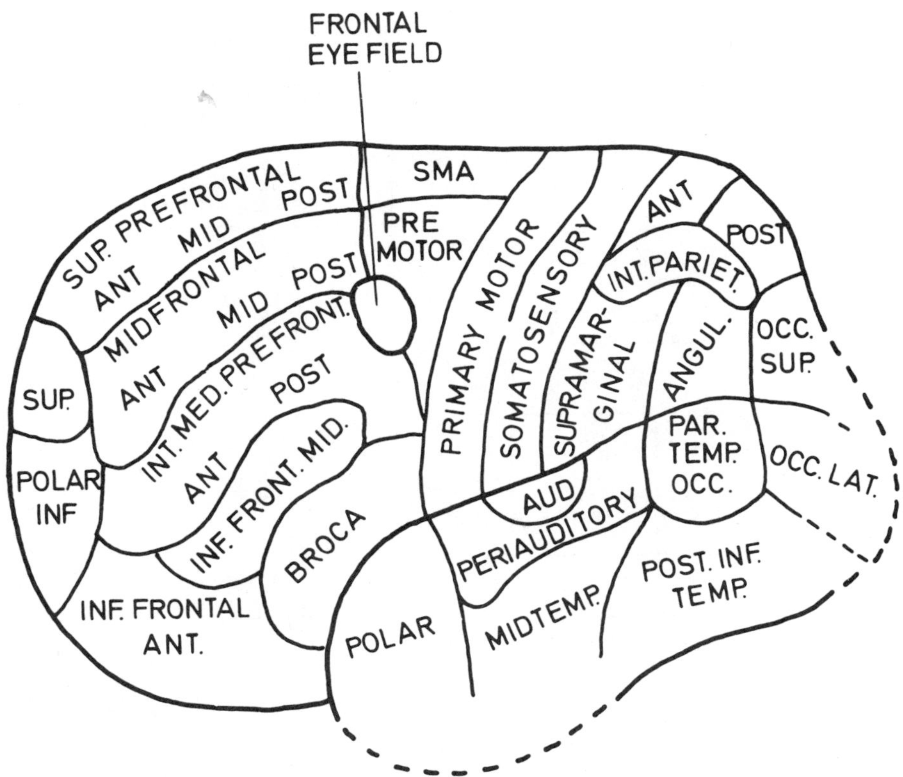

FIG. 4. The cerebral cortex is divided into the above regions for descriptive purposes. Figure is a standard view of the projection of the cerebral cortex obtained by 254 detectors. Upper part of mesial frontal cortical surface is projected as upper part of the superior prefrontal cortex. Superolateral border of brain runs through the middle of superior prefrontal region. Regions outside detector field or regions not provided by isotope with intracarotid method are shown with *broken lines*. Right homologue to the Broca area is called the posterior inferior frontal area.

with the two external acoustical meatus overprojected. Fourth, the display matrix of the distribution of the isotope 2–3 s after the injection showed the contour and size of the cerebral hemisphere. These four measures were all independent of the rCBF.

The relations between the display matrices, the X-ray pictures, and the cerebral hemisphere and the cerebral vessels were uniquely determined by the magnification factor and the radiation geometry obtained with the 254 collimators. The collimators were arranged perpendicular to the spherical collimator surface (19). The collimator surface facing the brain was shaped as a concave spherical segment with a curvature of 0.0666 cm^{-1}. This corresponded approximately to the curvature of the superolateral surface of the brain in the horizontal plane (29), whereas the minimum curvature in the frontal plane in an average brain was ~0.13 cm^{-1}. The display of the rCBF from the 254 cortical regions thus preserved the proportions of cortical areas better than scans with parallel ray paths. The axis of the collimator head was directed 15° posterior to the coronal plane of the head. The prefrontal cortex was consequently magnified and the parietal cortex minimized in the displays (Fig. 6). The mesiolateral border of the hemisphere and the upper part of the mesial surface were also visible due to this arrangement. In each subject the vertical and horizontal axes of the proportional stereotaxic system of Talairach et al. (29) were aligned to points of the brain contour and points of the course of the vessels (29). Each active cortical field for that particular subject was then localized in relation to these axes, and the subject's hemisphere was then proportionally subdivided (29). After the proportional subdivision each activated field was identified and named after one of the regions in Fig. 4. The uncertainty in determining the localization of a cortical focus in an individual brain with these methods was estimated to be 1.0 cm near the midfrontal plane and 1.9 cm near the poles (two-dimensional, 12% confidence intervals; or 88% confidence limits, 29). Since all activated fields were of the size of three detectors or larger, and since the smallest subdivision of the cortex, with the exception of the frontal eye fields, covered an area corresponding to a minimum of four detectors, the probability of mislocating an activated field with respect to

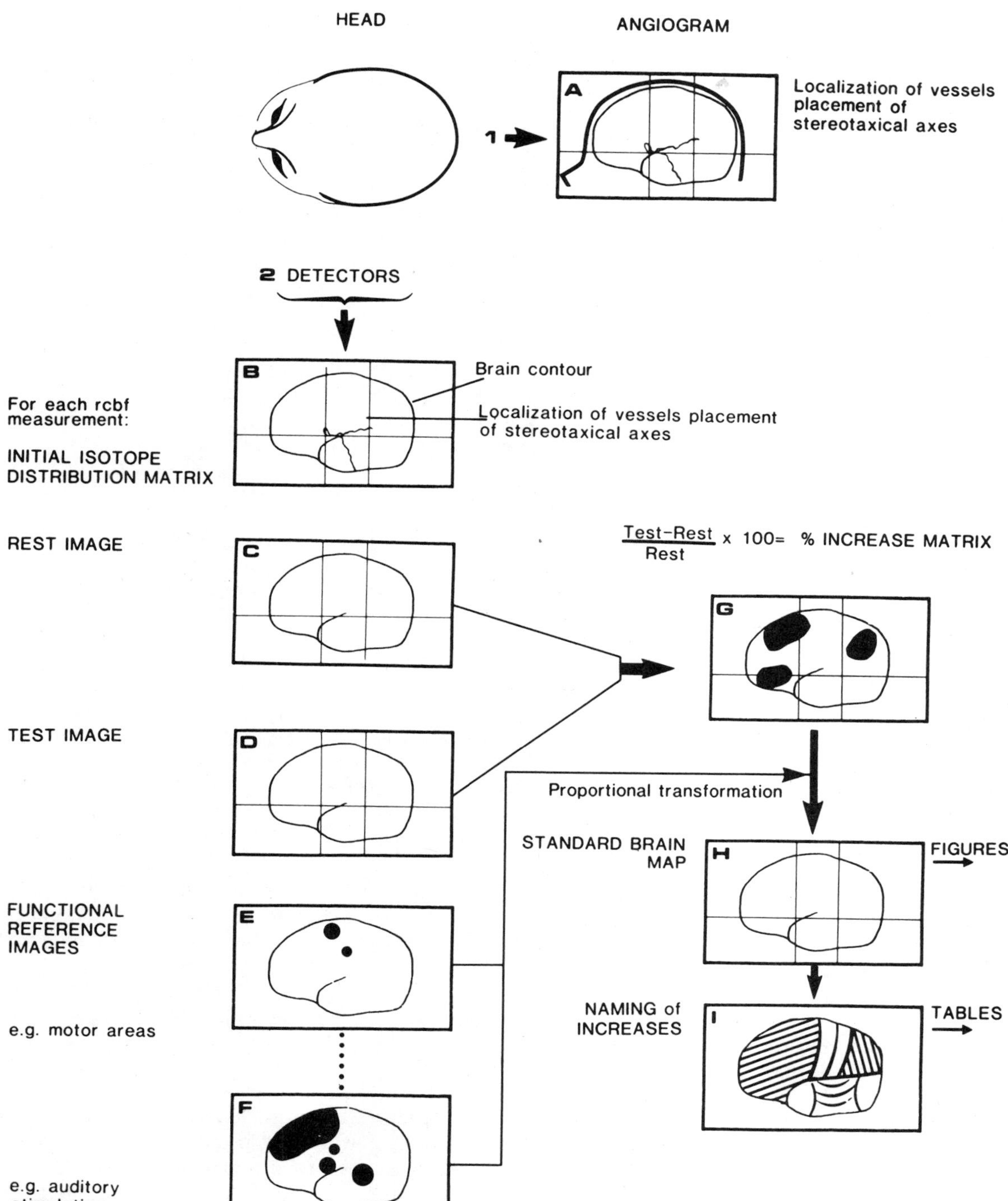

FIG. 5. Main steps in anatomic localization of changes in rCBF and data processing. The rCBF measurements are made in conjunction with carotid angiograms. *A*: in angiogram the stereotaxic axes are positioned in relation to skull anatomy and major vessels (29). *B*: in image of initial isotope distribution the brain contour and major vessels are reidentified and the stereotaxic axes positioned. *E* and *F*: by other activation procedures, e.g., finger movements (*E*) and auditory stimulation (*F*), motor areas, auditory areas, etc. are localized in the same subject and spatially correlated with the proportionally transformed matrix of percent changes in rCBF (*G*) on standard brain map (*H*). In each subject all activations are delimited on the % increase matrix (*G*). The percent increase matrix is then proportionally enlarged/reduced according to the proportional stereotaxic system and shown in Figs. 7, 8, 10, 11. Finally, the geometric mean of the proportionally transformed percent increase matrix, identical to the standard brain map *H* of all subjects is drawn (see Fig. 9). Statistical analysis of homogeneity of subareas within the matrix *C* and *D* is followed by a computation of mean rCBF (Tables 2 and 4) and mean increase in each statistically defined subarea. These statistically defined subareas are identical in rest and test and are named after areas in Fig. 4. Results of statistical analysis are shown in Tables 3 and 5.

A, B, E, F, matrices or images in Fig. 5 was considered insignificant. Especially because the location of the frontal polar region was obtained directly from the display of the initial isotope distribution.

For comparative and illustrative purposes only, the rCBF matrix with the activated fields delimited was transferred to a brain map of standard dimensions (29) by simple proportional enlargement/reduction (Figs. 7, 8, 10, 11). The geometric mean of the outline of each activation was then drawn for the whole group of subjects (Fig. 9). No attempt was made to correlate the localization of individual fields of activation with regional anatomic structures such as gyri and sulci. Consequently the 31 subdivisions in the tables of the cerebral cortex were given functional and descriptive names (Broca area, frontal eye field, angular area, etc.). In summary, the geometric means of individual activations and their average intensities are shown in the figures; the heuristic comparisons and the statistical analysis are shown in the tables.

Data treatment

The experimental design and data treatment were the same as described in earlier publications (15, 16, 25). The experimental statistical design was a paired comparison (3). Each subject served as his own control. For each subject (k) the state of physiological activation, thinking, was compared with the rest state. The changes in rCBF from rest to test were calculated by simple subtraction of the matrices

$$[\mathrm{DrCBF}_{i,k}] = [\mathrm{rCBF}_{i,k}\ \mathrm{test}] - [\mathrm{rCBF}_{i,k}\ \mathrm{rest}] \quad (2)$$

CALCULATION OF MEAN CHANGES OF rCBF IN PERCENT (FIG. 9). For each subject the percent change matrix was computed for each test (j) as

$$[\%\mathrm{DrCBF}_{i,k,j}] = \frac{[\mathrm{DrCBF}_{i,k,j}]}{[\mathrm{rCBF}_{i,k},\ \mathrm{rest}]} \cdot 100 \quad (3)$$

To each [$\%\mathrm{DrCBF}_{i,k,j}$] corresponded air image $I(\%\mathrm{DrCBF}_{i,k,j})$ as shown in Fig. 6, *C* and *D* $I(\%\mathrm{DrCBF}_{i,k,j})$ (Fig. 5*G*) was then proportionally enlarged or reduced (Fig. 5*H*) to $Ip(\%\mathrm{DrCBF}_{i,k,j})$. The corresponding matrix after proportional transformation was called $[\%\mathrm{DrCBF}_{i,k,j}]p$. The individual $Ip(\%\mathrm{DrCBF}_{i,k,j})$ images were then superimposed to give $SIp(\%\mathrm{DrCBF}_{i,\cdot,j})$. In this superimposed image from all subjects, $SIp(\%\mathrm{DrCBF}_{i,\cdot,j})$, the geometrical mean of each change in rCBF was drawn. These outlines are depicted in Fig. 9. The outline of each change in rCBF was then transferred to the matrix $[\%\mathrm{DrCBF}_{i,k,j}]p$ of each subject and a mean percent change of rCBF within the activated area consisting of (ak) channels was calculated.

$$E(a, k) = \frac{1}{ak} \sum_{i}^{ak} \%\mathrm{DrCBF}_{i,k,j} \quad (4)$$

and an overall mean was calculated and shown in Fig. 9

$$E(a) = \frac{1}{n} \sum_{k}^{n} E(a, k) \quad (5)$$

and an estimate of the variance $S^2(a)$

$$S^2(a) = \frac{1}{n-1} \sum [E(a) - E(a, k)]^2 \quad (6)$$

across subjects was calculated as well as a standard error of mean

$$SE = \frac{S}{\sqrt{n}} \quad (7)$$

The test statistic was a Student's t test with Dunnett's corrections for multiple comparisons with a control (1). In the computation of $E(a, k)$ it was neglected that the $\%\mathrm{DrCBF}_{k,j}$ of adjacent channels might be correlated up to a maximum of 25%.

THE FIGURES SHOWING INDIVIDUAL PERCENT CHANGES IN rCBF (FIGS. 7, 8, 10, 11). From earlier repeated measurements with the subjects at rest the coefficient of variation ($\mathrm{CV}_{i,k}$) of $\mathrm{rCBF}_{i,k,\ \mathrm{rest}}$ was 0.055 for i located in nonprefrontal regions and 0.076 for i located in prefrontal regions (19). In the present study the double determinations of $\mathrm{rCBF}_{i,k,\ \mathrm{rest}}$ gave similar results (the maximal difference in $\mathrm{rCBF}_{i,k,\ \mathrm{rest}}$ being 11%). If one assumes that $\mathrm{CV}(\mathrm{rCBF}_{i,k,\ \mathrm{rest}}) = \mathrm{CV}(\mathrm{rCBF}_{i,k,\ \mathrm{test}})$, then a reasonable criterion for determining whether a change in $\mathrm{rCBF}_{i,k}$ should be considered a significant change would be

$$1.64[\mathrm{SD}_{\mathrm{rest}}{}^2 + (\mathrm{SD}_{\mathrm{rest}} \cdot m)^2]^{1/2} < \mathrm{DrCBF}_{i,k} \quad (8)$$

in which SD is the standard deviation obtained from $\mathrm{CV}(\mathrm{rCBF}_{i,k,\ \mathrm{rest}})$ and $m = E(\mathrm{rCBF}_{i,k,\ \mathrm{test}})/E(\mathrm{rCBF}_{i,k,\ \mathrm{rest}})$, the ratio between the mean rCBF during test and during rest for channel i, in subject (k). The m ratio was estimated to be 1.1 because the increase of the mean cortical blood flow (Table 1) was close to 10% in all three tests. A usable single criterion then for the whole cortex (both prefrontal and nonprefrontal areas) would be to display all changes >15%. The changes depicted then would have 95% confidence limits. Figures 7, 8, 10, 11 show all changes >15.0%.

STATISTICAL ANALYSIS OF CORTICAL FIELDS IN REST AND DURING THINKING (TABLES 2, 3, 4, 5). Since the prejudgement for calculating a mean rCBF $E(\mathrm{rCBF}_{f,k})$ for a certain cortical field (f) was that all $\mathrm{rCBF}_{i,k}$, $i = (1, \ldots, f)$ belonged to the same distribution, the [$\mathrm{rCBF}_{i,k,\ \mathrm{test}}$] matrix and the [$\mathrm{rCBF}_{i,k,\ \mathrm{rest}}$] matrix was analyzed for homogeneity of the rCBF in smaller subdivisions of the matrices. We assumed that if the $\mathrm{rCBF}_{i,k,\ \mathrm{rest}}$ and the $\mathrm{rCBF}_{i,k,\ \mathrm{test}}$ were normally distributed and if the $\mathrm{CV}(\mathrm{rCBF}_{i,k,\ \mathrm{rest}}) = \mathrm{CV}(\mathrm{rCBF}_{i,k,\ \mathrm{test}}) = 0.055$,

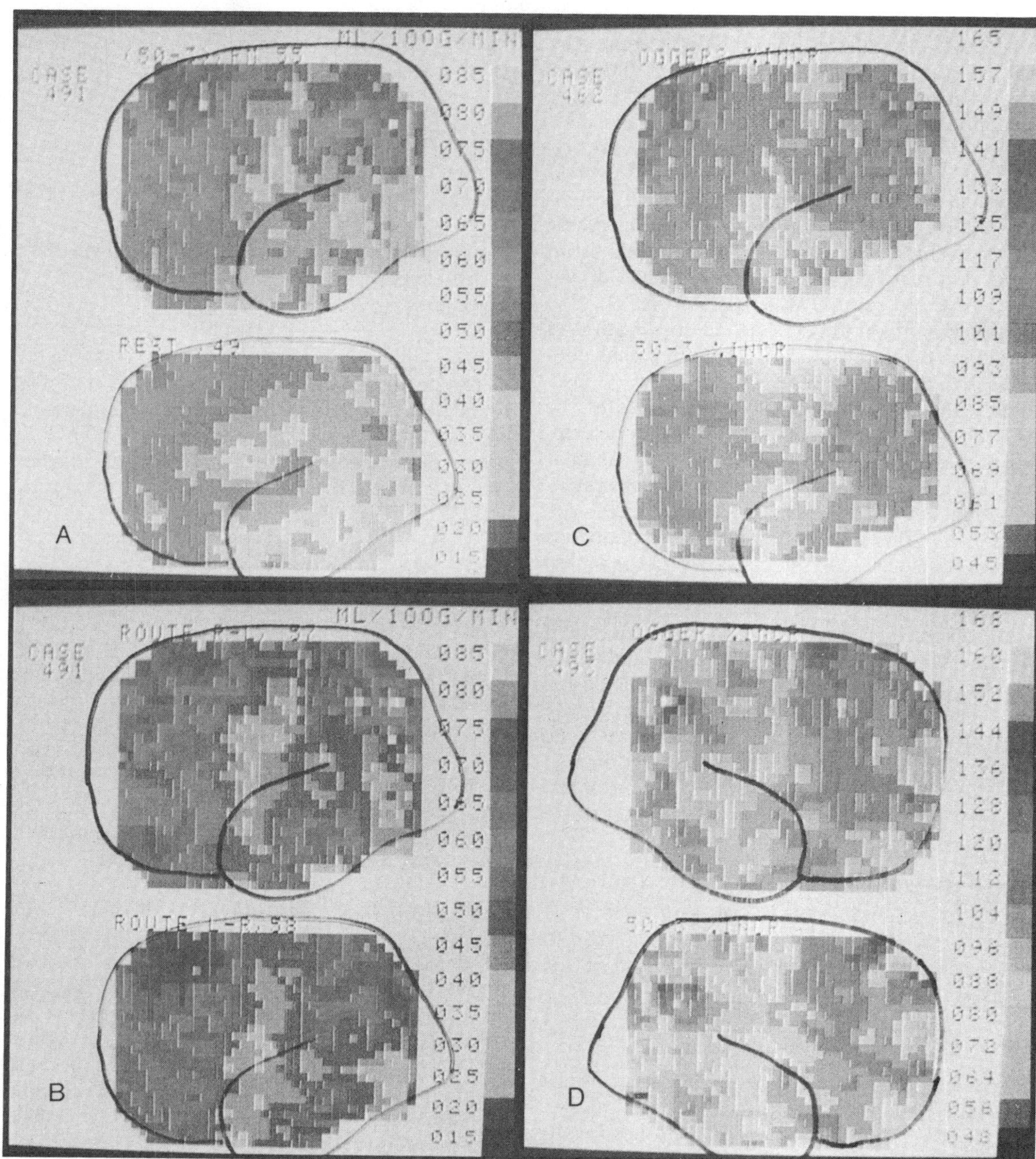

FIG. 6. The rCBF in three subjects during pure thinking. Subjects had closed eyes, plugged ears, showed no voluntary motor activity, and received no stimuli. No difference occurred in outside world between rest and three types of thinking. *A*: normal rest pattern (*lower*). Note increase in angular cortex and prefrontal cortex during 50 − 3 thinking (*top*). Scale rCBF in $\text{ml} \cdot 100\ \text{g}^{-1} \cdot \text{min}^{-1}$. *B*: route finding, same subject *imagining* he walked first right then left (*top*) and then during new measurement first left then right (*lower*). Note increases in visual association areas and reproducibility. *C*: percent increase of rCBF during jingle thinking, which preferentially activated supramarginal cortex (*top*), and percent increase in 50 − 3, which preferentially activated angular cortex (*lower*). *A, B, C*: left hemisphere. *D*: right hemisphere. Percent increase in jingle thinking (*top*) and 50 − 3 thinking (*lower*). *Scales* in *C* and *D*, percent increase + 100.

then a reasonable strategy was to subdivide the [$\text{rCBF}_{i,k,\text{test}}$] into fields ($f$) such that the CV-($\text{rCBF}_{i,k,\text{test}}$) within each field < 0.055. Within each field (f) delimited this way, the $\text{rCBF}_{i,k,\text{test}}$ would be very close and thus be likely to belong to the same distribution. We used this criterion to

TABLE 1. *Mean cortical blood flow, pulse rate, and blood pressure in rest and during thinking*

	Rest	50 − 3	Jingle	Route Finding
Mean cortical blood flow				
Left hemisphere	52.8	55.8	59.3	60.7 ml · 100 g^{-1} · min^{-1}
Right hemisphere	63.8	68.4	70.8	66.4 ml · 100 g^{-1} · min^{-1}
Mean % increase ± SE				
Left hemisphere		5.3 ± 1.6	12.2 ± 3.3	14.9 ± 1.6
Right hemisphere		7.7 ± 2.1	11.3 ± 1.8	8.6 ± 2.2
Mean arterial blood pressure	95.6	97.4	97.4	100.8 mmHg
Mean pulse rate	88.9	92.4*	92.0	93.8* min^{-1}

* $P < 0.05$; t test; two-sided significance limits.

subdivide the matrices [$rCBF_{i,k,\,50-3}$], [$rCBF_{i,k,\,jingle}$] and [$rCBF_{i,k,\,route}$] into the exact same fields. When this subdivision was applied on the [$rCBF_{i,k,\,rest}$] matrix it was apparent that the CV($rCBF_{i,k,\,rest}$) within each field in all cases is <0.080. That is, that the $rCBF_{i,k}$ within equally delimited fields in rest, 50 − 3 thinking, jingle thinking, and route finding was homogenous. Consequently, it was

TABLE 2. *rCBF in the left hemisphere during thinking*

Area	No. of Channels	50 − 3	Jingle	Route Finding
Superior prefrontal ant	5	68.4 ± 2.7	65.1 ± 2.5	69.0 ± 2.3
Superior prefrontal mid	5	75.4 ± 4.4	73.4 ± 4.2	73.4 ± 2.7
Superior prefrontal post	6	74.6 ± 3.7	76.2 ± 3.8	74.0 ± 2.8
Superior polar	4	65.5 ± 3.5	69.4 ± 3.9	66.7 ± 2.6
Inferior polar	6	60.3 ± 3.7	60.2 ± 3.2	62.1 ± 2.9
Midfrontal ant	5	64.3 ± 3.5	68.5 ± 3.8	71.2 ± 2.4
Midfrontal mid	5	57.5 ± 2.8	60.0 ± 2.6	66.1 ± 4.0
Midfrontal post	5	60.7 ± 2.8	66.0 ± 3.4	66.5 ± 3.2
Frontal eye field	2	60.7 ± 3.1	63.8 ± 3.2	64.5 ± 2.4
Intermediate prefrontal ant	5	60.2 ± 3.4	61.2 ± 3.9	61.7 ± 3.2
Intermediate prefrontal post	5	60.9 ± 3.3	64.0 ± 4.0	66.7 ± 3.7
Inferior frontal ant	9	62.3 ± 3.0	62.9 ± 3.7	68.4 ± 3.1
Inferior frontal mid	6	59.2 ± 2.8	63.0 ± 3.0	64.4 ± 2.7
Broca	7	62.6 ± 3.9	65.7 ± 3.4	63.3 ± 2.3
Orbitofrontal lat	8	62.1 ± 3.4	60.6 ± 2.7	63.6 ± 2.7
Premotor	5	53.4 ± 2.5	55.7 ± 3.4	56.2 ± 2.5
Supplementary motor	5	53.4 ± 3.6	51.3 ± 2.6	53.4 ± 1.1
Motor	10	49.1 ± 2.3	50.6 ± 2.0	50.7 ± 1.8
Somatosensory	10	48.8 ± 1.8	51.7 ± 1.6	50.5 ± 1.7
Superior parietal ant	5	50.7 ± 2.9	53.5 ± 2.6	54.8 ± 2.1
Superior parietal post	5	53.3 ± 3.4	55.6 ± 3.3	67.9 ± 4.2
Intraparietal	4	55.1 ± 2.9	58.8 ± 3.2	66.6 ± 4.0
Supramarginal	5	54.8 ± 2.0	64.1 ± 3.2	63.7 ± 3.6
Angular	5	63.0 ± 2.4	61.8 ± 3.3	55.8 ± 2.3
Parieto-temporo-occipital	5	44.3 ± 1.2	53.3 ± 2.3	51.8 ± 0.5
Auditory	4	50.6 ± 2.0	55.8 ± 3.1	53.8 ± 1.1
Periauditory	4	48.5 ± 1.8	52.3 ± 2.9	51.9 ± 1.6
Midtemporal	6	47.8 ± 2.8	52.2 ± 3.3	54.1 ± 3.3
Posterior inf temporal	6	49.7 ± 1.9	52.1 ± 3.8	59.6 ± 2.9
Temporal pole	7	45.2 ± 1.2	50.5 ± 1.7	47.6 ± 1.4
Occipital lat	5	44.6 ± 2.6	45.4 ± 1.9	46.7 ± 1.8
Occipital sup	6	50.6 ± 1.6	49.7 ± 1.6	60.6 ± 2.5

Values are means ± SE. rCBF in ml · 100 g^{-1} · min^{-1}.

possible to calculate a mean rCBF $E(\mathrm{rCBF}_{i,k,j})$ for each subject in rest as well as in test

$$E(\mathrm{rCBF}_{f,k,j}) = \frac{1}{i} \sum_{i}^{f} (\mathrm{rCBF}_{i,k,j}) \quad (9)$$

and an overall mean for the field (f)

$$E(\mathrm{rCBF}_{f,j}) = \frac{1}{n} \sum_{k}^{n} E(\mathrm{rCBF}_{f,k,j}) \quad (10)$$

and a standard deviation

$$\mathrm{SD} = \left(\frac{1}{n-1} \sum [E(\mathrm{rCBF}_{f,j}) - E(\mathrm{rCBF}_{f,k,j})^2]\right)^{1/2} \quad (11)$$

and a standard error

$$\mathrm{SE}_f = \frac{\mathrm{SD}}{\sqrt{n}} \quad (12)$$

Tables 2 and 4 show $E(\mathrm{rCBF}_{f,j}) \pm \mathrm{SE}_f$. Similarly it was possible to calculate

$$E(\mathrm{D\ rCBF}_{f,k,j}) = E(\mathrm{rCBF}_{f,k,\,\mathrm{test}}) - E(\mathrm{rCBF}_{f,k,\,\mathrm{test}}) \quad (13)$$

and

$$E(\mathrm{D\ rCBF}_{f,j}) = \frac{1}{n} \sum_{k}^{n} E\mathrm{D\ rCBF}_{f,k,j} \quad (14)$$

and the standard error $\mathrm{SE}_{\mathrm{D}f}$ of $E(\mathrm{DrCBF}_{f,j})$. Tables 3 and 5 show $E(\mathrm{DrCBF}_{f,j}) \pm \mathrm{SE}_{\mathrm{D}f}$.

The test statistic was a Student's t test with Dunnett's correction for multiple comparisons (1). Tables 3 and 5 also show the average number of detectors monitoring each field (f). The total number of channels listed in these tables is <254 because the channels that look outside the brain have been excluded, and because the channels monitoring cortex that received insufficient amount of isotope were also excluded from statistical analysis. Each field (f) was then assigned a name according to Fig. 4.

The probability of assigning a wrong name to an activated field in a subject cannot be assessed

TABLE 3. *Increases of rCBF in left hemisphere during thinking*

Area	No. of Channels	50 − 3	Jingle	Route Finding
Superior prefrontal ant	5	7.0 ± 2.0*	5.7 ± 1.6*	9.0 ± 1.1‡
Superior prefrontal mid	6	14.8 ± 3.2†	14.6 ± 2.8†	14.1 ± 1.1‡
Superior prefrontal post	6	12.9 ± 2.6†	16.1 ± 1.8‡	13.4 ± 0.8‡
Superior polar	4	5.6 ± 2.3	9.5 ± 2.6*	6.2 ± 2.5
Inferior polar	6	3.0 ± 1.8	2.9 ± 1.6	5.0 ± 1.9
Midfrontal ant	5	6.0 ± 0.9‡	10.2 ± 2.7*	13.1 ± 1.2‡
Midfrontal mid	5	1.4 ± 1.6	4.1 ± 2.4	9.6 ± 3.0
Midfrontal post	5	4.5 ± 3.0	10.2 ± 2.9*	11.1 ± 0.9‡
Frontal eye field	2	4.1 ± 2.7	7.0 ± 1.7*	8.9 ± 1.6†
Intermediate prefrontal ant	5	6.9 ± 1.7*	7.8 ± 2.1*	8.7 ± 1.5†
Intermediate prefrontal post	5	6.4 ± 1.9*	10.6 ± 2.8*	13.2 ± 1.4‡
Inferior frontal ant	9	2.9 ± 2.7	3.5 ± 2.2	9.2 ± 1.4‡
Inferior frontal mid	6	5.2 ± 2.0	8.9 ± 2.3*	9.8 ± 1.8‡
Broca	7	6.1 ± 1.3†	8.6 ± 1.2‡	7.1 ± 1.4†
Orbitofrontal lat	8	−5.0 ± 2.1	0.9 ± 3.7	3.0 ± 1.9
Premotor	5	−0.9 ± 0.6	1.2 ± 1.2	2.4 ± 1.2
Supplementary motor	5	0.3 ± 1.5	−0.1 ± 1.7	0.2 ± 1.8
Motor	10	−0.8 ± 0.7	0.7 ± 1.6	1.0 ± 0.8
Somatosensory	10	−1.2 ± 1.2	1.8 ± 2.4	1.5 ± 1.4
Superior parietal ant	5	0.0 ± 1.1	2.7 ± 1.1	3.7 ± 1.4
Superior parietal post	5	3.2 ± 2.4	5.4 ± 3.2	19.6 ± 2.6‡
Intraparietal	4	−0.3 ± 1.8	3.7 ± 5.3	13.3 ± 1.9‡
Supramarginal	5	2.8 ± 1.0	12.6 ± 2.5†	12.0 ± 2.3†
Angular	4	10.5 ± 1.6‡	7.8 ± 2.4*	4.3 ± 2.0
Parieto-temporo-occipital	5	−1.6 ± 1.4	4.5 ± 1.7	3.9 ± 1.8
Auditory	4	−4.8 ± 2.5	0.2 ± 2.8	−1.4 ± 1.7
Periauditory	4	−2.9 ± 1.1	0.2 ± 2.2	0.2 ± 0.5
Midtemporal	7	−1.1 ± 2.3	3.3 ± 3.8	5.9 ± 2.9
Posterior inf temporal	6	1.9 ± 2.3	4.3 ± 4.5	12.4 ± 3.6*
Temporal pole	7	−4.6 ± 2.2	0.6 ± 2.0	−1.9 ± 1.6
Occipital lat	5	−3.8 ± 0.9	3.0 ± 1.2	−0.9 ± 0.8
Occipital sup.	6	0.1 ± 2.8	0.3 ± 2.2	11.0 ± 3.2*

Values are means ± SE. rCBF, $\mathrm{ml \cdot 100\ g^{-1} \cdot mi^{-1}}$. * $P < 0.05$; † $P < 0.01$; ‡ $P < 0.005$. Two-tailed test (1).

TABLE 4. *rCBF in the right hemisphere during thinking*

Area	No. of Channels	50 − 3	Jingle	Route Finding
Superior prefrontal ant	5	77.8 ± 2.7	76.1 ± 1.9	89.3 ± 5.4
Superior prefrontal mid	6	83.4 ± 5.3	89.4 ± 4.4	81.3 ± 5.6
Superior prefrontal post	6	75.7 ± 5.2	74.7 ± 2.9	76.8 ± 4.2
Superior polar	4	83.6 ± 5.9	75.8 ± 4.7	79.4 ± 4.9
Inferior polar	6	76.6 ± 5.2	75.7 ± 5.8	71.7 ± 6.1
Midfrontal ant	5	76.4 ± 4.4	81.0 ± 4.4	75.9 ± 3.9
Midfrontal mid	5	71.7 ± 4.6	80.3 ± 6.5	75.7 ± 5.8
Midfrontal post	5	73.6 ± 4.5	77.9 ± 4.6	73.1 ± 5.4
Frontal eye field	2	73.3 ± 5.0	77.3 ± 5.4	75.1 ± 4.7
Intermedial prefrontal ant	5	77.3 ± 4.5	81.7 ± 8.3	75.5 ± 5.4
Intermedial prefrontal post	6	71.5 ± 6.9	74.9 ± 5.8	69.9 ± 5.8
Inferior frontal ant	9	80.4 ± 6.5	81.5 ± 6.5	78.4 ± 5.9
Inferior frontal mid	6	80.3 ± 5.3	84.7 ± 7.8	74.1 ± 5.3
Inferior frontal post	7	73.7 ± 5.3	73.6 ± 5.1	68.3 ± 4.7
Orbitofrontal lat	8	68.9 ± 3.6	70.4 ± 9.1	63.0 ± 6.3
Premotor	5	64.1 ± 3.0	68.6 ± 5.5	64.8 ± 5.1
Supplementary motor	5	65.3 ± 3.4	67.4 ± 3.5	66.6 ± 2.7
Motor	10	59.5 ± 4.1	64.4 ± 4.5	57.4 ± 3.8
Somatosensory	10	61.2 ± 4.4	63.9 ± 4.6	57.8 ± 3.2
Superior parietal ant	5	64.3 ± 5.7	65.4 ± 6.1	58.5 ± 4.1
Superior parietal post	5	64.6 ± 5.6	65.9 ± 4.9	70.2 ± 6.5
Intraparietal	4	66.2 ± 5.4	68.0 ± 6.1	62.4 ± 5.5
Supramarginal	5	70.1 ± 5.9	75.7 ± 7.2	67.3 ± 4.7
Angular	4	74.1 ± 4.2	71.8 ± 3.6	66.7 ± 4.6
Parieto-temporo-occipital	5	62.9 ± 5.0	61.8 ± 5.2	60.6 ± 3.7
Auditory	4	66.0 ± 3.9	67.6 ± 4.3	64.2 ± 3.3
Periauditory	4	64.3 ± 4.2	64.2 ± 3.8	61.4 ± 3.5
Midtemporal	6	65.8 ± 3.0	69.9 ± 4.1	57.8 ± 4.0
Posterior inf temporal	6	60.6 ± 3.9	59.2 ± 3.9	62.8 ± 3.8
Temporal pole	7	57.3 ± 4.1	59.9 ± 5.3	54.7 ± 3.9
Occipital lat	5	58.3 ± 3.6	58.4 ± 2.5	55.6 ± 2.1
Occipital sup	6	63.8 ± 5.9	61.6 ± 6.2	63.6 ± 4.2

Values are mean ± SE. rCBF in $ml \cdot 100\ g^{-1} \cdot min^{-1}$.

in general because it depends on the number of channels activated. From the data on the spatial resolution (19) and the uncertainty of localizing a channel with the Talairach stereotaxic system (29) a "worst case" can be calculated in which only one channel of activation determines whether an activation should be assigned to region x or y. With five channels activated in a field the probability of mislocating an activated field in a "worst case" is 0.40. Such worst cases occurred in 8% of all regions analyzed in all subjects. This uncertainty is therefore inherent in the construction of the Tables 2–6. With an increasing number of paired comparisons on normally distributed rCBF data there is a risk that some of the comparisons between rest and test might turn out to be statistically significant due to chance. With 62 regions compared, an average 3.1 regions will exceed a two-sided significance limit of 0.05. Since an analysis of variance is not appropriate to the present type of data, there is at present no standard procedure to compensate for the mass significance.

When the differences in rCBF increases between the different types of thinking were evaluated, we used a test for equality of three means (3).

RESULTS

All three types of thinking elicited marked increases of rCBF. These increases were always located outside the motor cortices and outside the primary sensory areas[1] and their immediate association areas. This was in accordance with the fact that the subjects did not make any voluntary movements nor did they receive any sensory stimulation. Each type of thinking provoked rCBF increases in different areas in the posterior part of the hemisphere. There were also differences in the localization of the rCBF increases in the prefrontal cortex (Fig. 6). Each of the

[1] Primary visual cortex could not be measured with this method.

TABLE 5. *Increase of rCBF in right hemisphere during thinking*

Area	No. of Channels	50 − 3	Jingle	Route Finding
Superior prefrontal ant	5	7.3 ± 2.6	5.6 ± 2.5	22.4 ± 4.5†
Superior prefrontal mid	6	15.6 ± 2.3‡	21.8 ± 2.8‡	15.1 ± 3.5†
Superior prefrontal post	6	8.3 ± 2.0*	7.5 ± 2.3	12.8 ± 1.4‡
Superior polar	4	13.7 ± 2.7†	5.9 ± 2.6	12.3 ± 2.8*
Inferior polar	6	6.8 ± 1.3†	5.8 ± 2.0	4.5 ± 3.4
Midfrontal ant	5	9.1 ± 1.5‡	13.9 ± 2.5†	11.6 ± 2.7*
Midfrontal mid	5	1.4 ± 1.6	10.0 ± 2.5*	13.4 ± 2.8*
Midfrontal post	5	4.9 ± 3.5	8.1 ± 1.4†	6.8 ± 2.3
Frontal eye field	2	3.2 ± 1.9	3.3 ± 3.3	7.5 ± 3.1
Intermediate prefrontal ant	5	11.9 ± 1.7‡	16.2 ± 4.0*	11.9 ± 2.8*
Intermediate prefrontal post	5	5.5 ± 2.4	8.9 ± 2.2*	8.9 ± 2.1*
Inferior frontal ant	9	10.1 ± 1.5‡	10.8 ± 2.9*	13.1 ± 1.8‡
Inferior frontal mid	6	10.3 ± 1.5‡	14.5 ± 3.7*	9.1 ± 2.6*
Inferior frontal post	7	3.6 ± 2.7	3.5 ± 1.7	2.1 ± 1.6
Orbitofrontal lat	8	2.0 ± 3.8	3.5 ± 2.8	2.1 ± 1.8
Premotor	5	−4.8 ± 3.0	0.0 ± 1.2	−2.6 ± 1.3
Supplementary motor	5	−0.3 ± 1.4	−0.2 ± 1.1	−1.2 ± 1.4
Motor	10	−2.2 ± 1.7	2.3 ± 1.4	−1.0 ± 1.5
Somatosensory	10	−0.3 ± 0.7	2.3 ± 1.0	−0.9 ± 0.7
Superior parietal ant	5	−2.4 ± 1.9	−1.3 ± 1.3	−1.3 ± 1.9
Superior parietal post	5	0.4 ± 1.7	1.6 ± 0.7	14.3 ± 3.0*
Intraparietal	4	1.8 ± 1.8	2.0 ± 1.2	4.0 ± 2.5
Supramarginal	5	8.1 ± 2.2*	13.7 ± 4.4	9.5 ± 2.6*
Angular	4	9.1 ± 1.4‡	6.8 ± 2.5	9.4 ± 1.3‡
Parieto-temporo-occipital	5	1.7 ± 2.4	1.2 ± 1.8	3.9 ± 1.7
Auditory	4	−0.8 ± 2.4	0.8 ± 1.8	−0.5 ± 0.7
Periauditory	4	0.1 ± 1.2	0.1 ± 1.7	1.8 ± 1.1
Midtemporal	7	5.3 ± 1.9	9.4 ± 2.4*	0.7 ± 1.7
Posterior inf temporal	6	0.0 ± 1.4	1.0 ± 0.7	8.3 ± 2.0*
Temporal pole	7	0.1 ± 2.6	2.7 ± 2.0	0.5 ± 1.6
Occipital lat	5	−1.0 ± 0.8	−1.4 ± 2.1	2.3 ± 2.8
Occipital sup	6	0.5 ± 0.6	−1.2 ± 1.9	6.2 ± 0.9‡

Values are means ± SE. rCBF in $ml \cdot 100\ g^{-1} \cdot min^{-1}$. * $P < 0.05$; † $P < 0.01$; ‡ $P < 0.005$. (1) Two tailed test.

rCBF increases usually occupied an area of 3–7 cm^2 of the cortex. Within each of the areas of increase the rCBF variance was small for the whole group of subjects (Tables 2 and 4). Sometimes the rCBF increases were confluent over larger areas of the cortex. The increases in rCBF were so intense that the mean cortical blood flow increased (Table 1). In 50 − 3 and route-finding thinking there was also an increase in the pulse rate. We did not find any areas of the cortex with significant decreases in rCBF during thinking. The changes of rCBF during thinking therefore cannot be due to any redistribution of rCBF.

We distinguished two different types of areas among the areas that raised their rCBF. The areas that were activated in every subject during one type of thinking were called *core regions.* The areas that were activated in some subjects with rCBF increases of more than 15%, but not in others, were called *facultative regions.*

The 50 − 3 thinking

This task had the most simple algorithm (Fig. 1). The greatest rCBFs in the left hemisphere were located in the superior prefrontal cortex, anterior midfrontal cortex, Broca area, and angular cortex (for nomenclature see Fig. 4). The greatest rCBF values indicate the cortical regions with the average greatest metabolism during the 48 s it took to measure the rCBF. Figure 6 shows that all subjects activated the left middle and posterior superior prefrontal cortex, the Broca area, and the angular cortex. The left anterior intermediate prefrontal cortex was also modestly

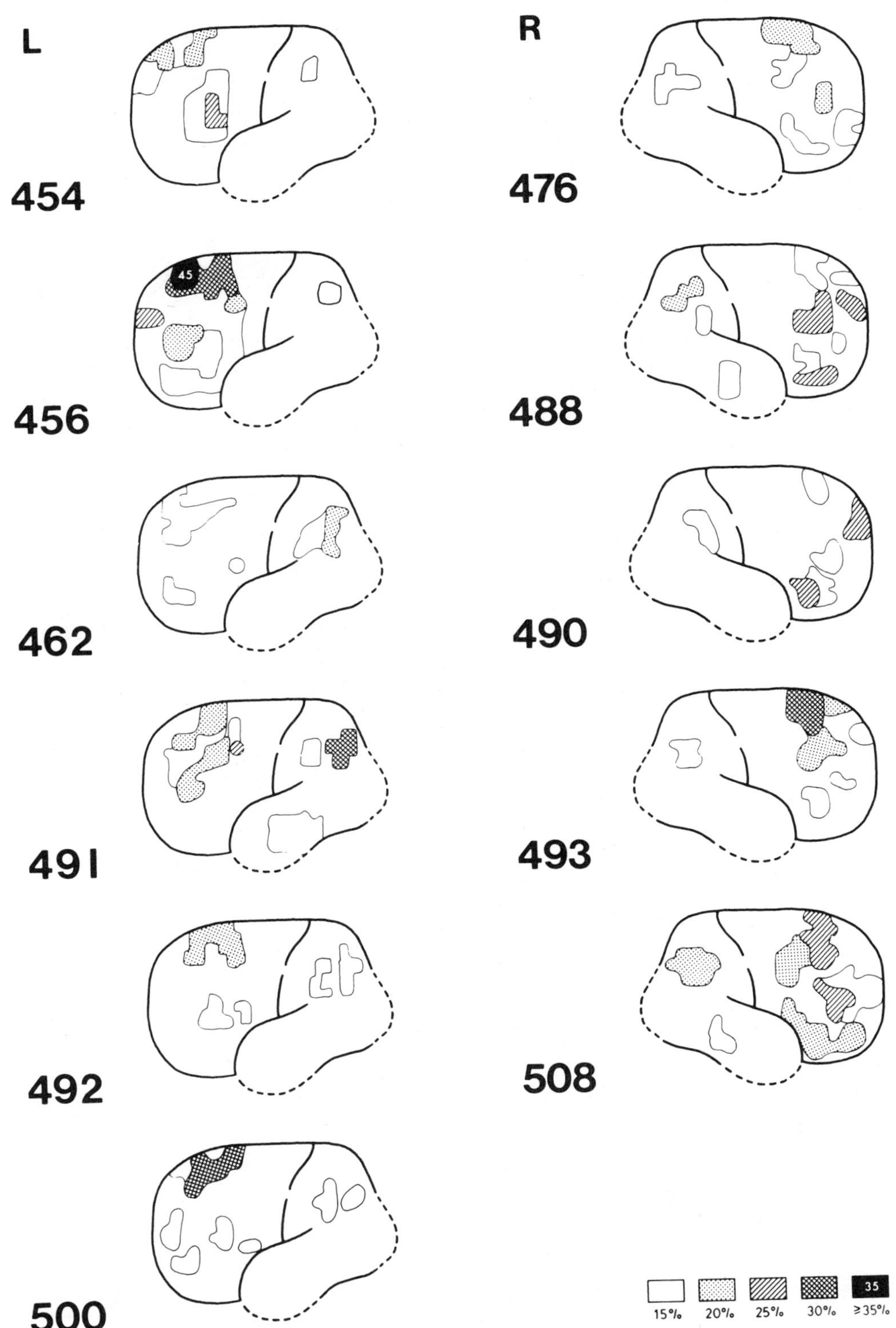

FIG. 7. Individual percent increases of rCBF during internal numerical operation, 50 − 3. All increases above 15% are shown. *Left,* left hemispheres; *Right,* right hemispheres. Note that all subjects had middle superior prefrontal cortex and angular cortex activated. In addition the left anterior intermediate prefrontal cortex was consistently activated in all subjects although the rCBF increases here were just below 15% in some subjects. In right hemisphere the anterior intermediate prefrontal cortex and anterior inferior prefrontal cortex was always activated in addition to the middle superior prefrontal cortex. In the left hemisphere the posterior superior prefrontal cortex and the Broca area were activated about 15% in all but one subject.

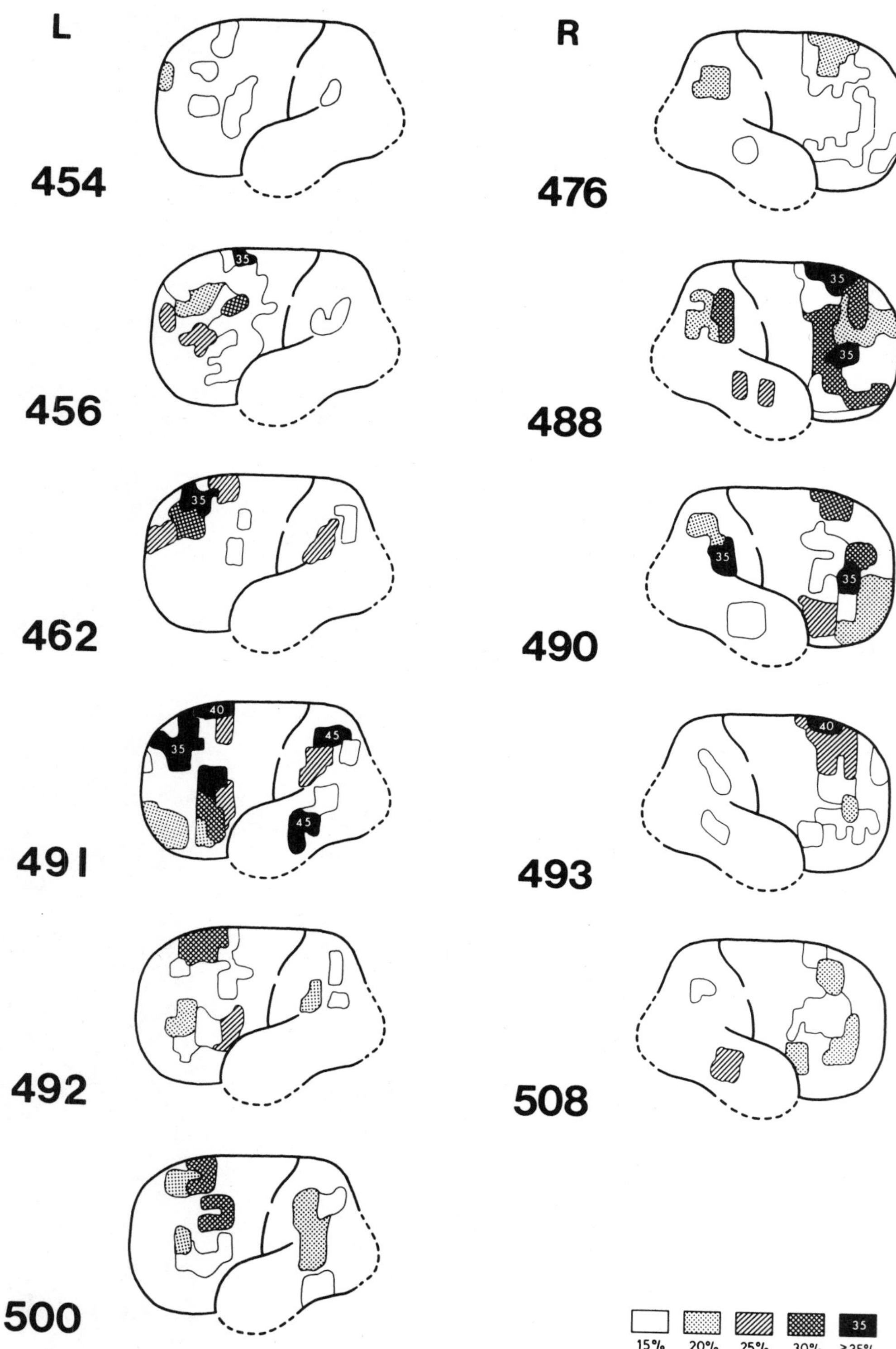

FIG. 8. Percent increases in rCBF in individuals while they did internal operations on the jingle. *Left*: left hemisphere, all subjects had the middle superior prefrontal cortex, the anterior and posterior midfrontal cortex, the Broca area, the middle inferior frontal cortex and the supramarginal cortex activated. All but one subject had the anterior and posterior intermediate prefrontal cortex activated. *Right*: right hemisphere. Here, core regions activated by all subjects were middle superior prefrontal cortex, anterior and middle midfrontal cortex, anterior intermediate prefrontal cortex, middle anterior frontal cortex, and supramarginal and midtemporal cortex.

activated in every subject (Fig. 9). This indicates that it either was repetitively activated for a shorter period during the 48 s it took to measure the rCBF, or that it was modestly activated continuously during the 48 s. These areas were the core areas in the left hemisphere for the 50 − 3 thinking. These core areas had the greatest rCBF values (Table 2) and the greatest increases of rCBF (Table 3). All subjects had at least two extra facultative areas activated. In addition to the core regions either the anterior and posterior midfrontal cortex or the middle inferior frontal cortex were activated in the left hemisphere (Fig. 7).

In the right hemisphere, the core regions were the middle superior prefrontal cortex, anterior midfrontal cortex, anterior intermediate prefrontal cortex, anterior and middle inferior frontal cortex, and the angular cortex (Figs. 7 and 9). These right-sided core regions together with the superior polar region had the greatest rCBF and the greatest rCBF increases (Tables 4 and 5). In addition either the superior or inferior polar region was activated as a facultative region.

The four subjects 490, 491, 492, and 508 did a repetition of the internal continuous subtraction in which they continuously subtracted 3 from 52. Neither the facultatively activated areas nor the core areas showed any decreases in rCBF during this repetition. In other words, the pattern and the intensities of the rCBF increases in each individual was unaltered ($P > 0.2$, multiple double comparison). The average extension of the cortical areas that had significant increases of rCBF are shown in Fig. 9. All core regions had a low interindividual variance of their rCBF increases. When the whole group was considered, not all facultative areas had statistically significant rCBF increases.

The subjects performed from 9 to 30 subtractions from the start of thinking until 5 s after the rCBF measurement was finished, when they were asked how far they had reached. It was not possible to find correlation between the rCBF increases in any of the areas activated in Fig. 7 or 9 and the number of subtractions made. Nor was it possible to find any correlations between the recruitment of facultative areas and correct versus incorrect subtractions. Since we knew the hemispheric dominance of our subjects, the activation patterns were analyzed for right-left differences. Table 6 shows the right regions that were more strongly activated than their left counterparts.

TABLE 6. *Differences in rCBF between the hemispheres during thinking*

50 − 3	
Superior polar	R > L
Intermediate prefrontal ant	R > L
Inferior frontal ant	R > L
Inferior frontal mid	R > L
Supramarginal	R > L
Jingle	
Superior prefrontal mid	R > L
Superior prefrontal post	L > R
Intermediate prefrontal ant	R > L
Inferior frontal ant	R > L
Route finding	
Superior prefrontal ant	R > L
Intraparietal	L > R
Angular	R > L

All differences statistically significant $P < 0.05$ (3). R, right; L, left.

Jingle thinking

This task required a more complicated operation on the retrieved information than the 50 − 3 thinking did. There were rCBF increases in more prefrontal cortical areas than during the 50 − 3 thinking (Fig. 6). The greatest rCBFs in the left hemisphere were localized to the core areas; the middle and posterior superior prefrontal cortex, anterior and posterior midfrontal cortex, Broca area, middle inferior frontal cortex, and supramarginal cortex (Table 2) (Fig. 8). The core regions also had the most intense increases of rCBF (Table 3).

In the right hemisphere, the core regions were the middle superior prefrontal cortex, anterior and middle inferior frontal cortex, supramarginal, and midtemporal cortex (Fig. 8). Of these regions, all except the midtemporal cortex had rCBF values among the nine greatest (Table 4). The most intense rCBF increases were located to these core regions (Table 5). It appeared that all subjects in addition had activation of either the posterior superior prefrontal cortex or the posterior intermediate prefrontal cortex (Fig. 8).

In Fig. 9 the average extensions of the cortical areas that had statistically significant increases are depicted. Many of the facultative areas had significant increases of rCBF, but usually with a greater variance of the mean percent increase (Fig. 8).

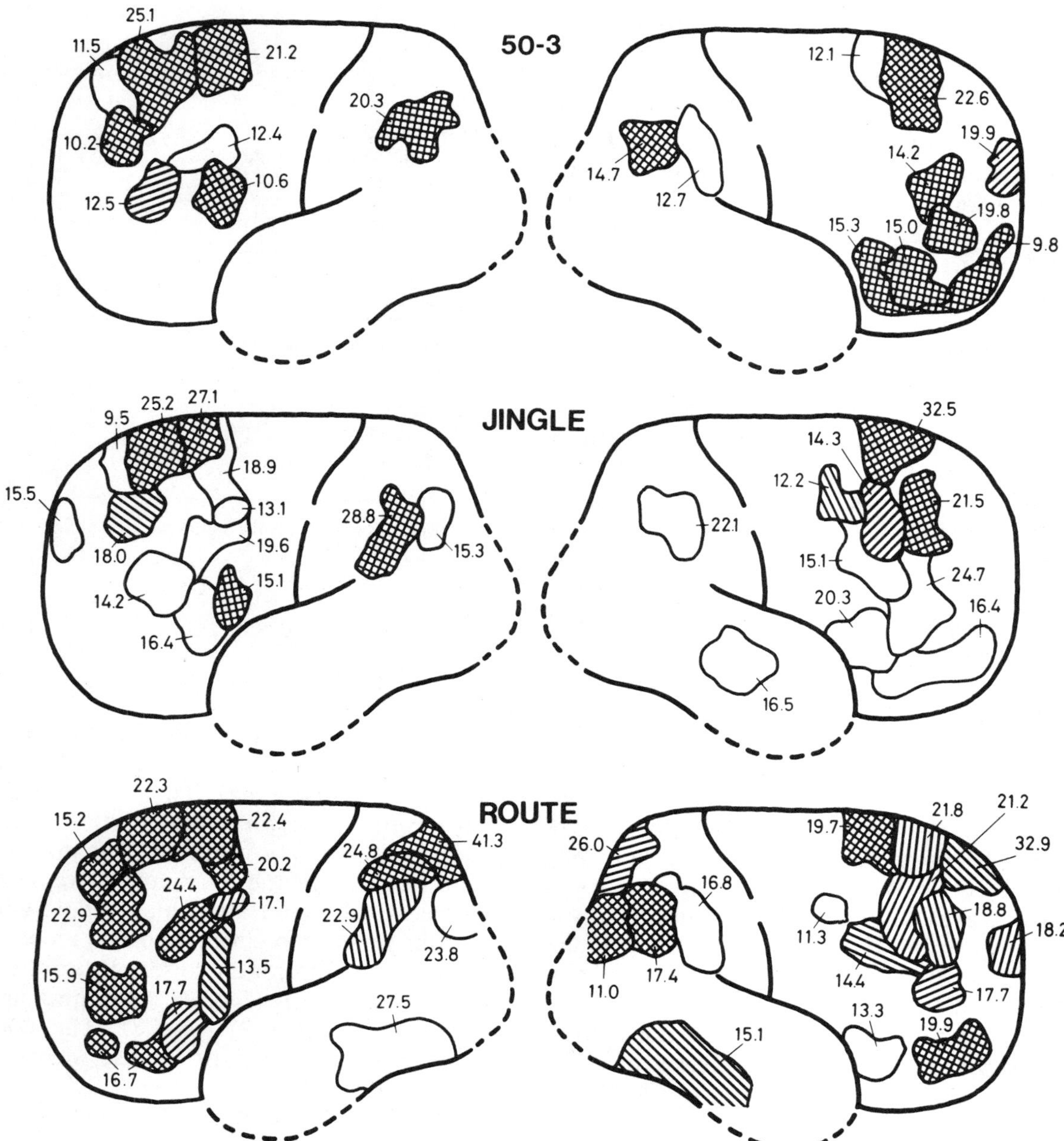

FIG. 9. Mean increases of rCBF in percent and their average distribution in cerebral cortex during three different types of thinking. *Left*: left hemisphere, six subjects. *Right*: right hemisphere, five subjects. *Crosshatched areas* have rCBF increases statistically significant at the 0.005 level (t test, two-sided comparison; Ref. 1) Hatched areas $P < 0.01$, other areas shown $P < 0.05$. Note that only the cortex outside the sensory and motor areas were activated and that no significant decreases in rCBF were observed.

During the 65 s the subjects were thinking about the jingle, they made from 8 to 26 jumps. Subjects 456, 500, 476, 488, and 508 had errors. It was impossible to correlate the sizes of the rCBF increases in any of the areas in Fig. 8 with the number of jumps or with erroneous performance. From Table 6 it is seen that there were right-left differences in the activation of four prefrontal areas.

Route-finding thinking

In contrast to the 50 − 3 thinking and the jingle thinking, in which the amount of information to be retrieved and operated upon was limited, route-finding thinking involved the retrieval of a considerable amount of information, i.e., memorized images of the outer world. The retrieved images then had to be analyzed for special features. Consequently, this analysis also covered a considerable amount of information (Fig. 3). As was the case during the two other types of thinking, the greatest rCBF values in the left dominant hemisphere were located in the middle and posterior superior prefrontal cortex (Fig. 6). However, the greatest increase in rCBF was located in the posterior superior parietal cortex (Figs. 10 and 11, Table 3). The (core) regions activated in all subjects were the middle and posterior superior prefrontal cortex, anterior and posterior midfrontal cortex, posterior intermediate prefrontal cortex, anterior inferior frontal cortex, intraparietal, supramarginal, posterior superior parietal cortex, and posterior inferior temporal cortex. The latter activation often occupied the lower part of the midtemporal cortex (Figs. 4, 10, 11). In addition to these core regions most of the subjects had activation of the superior occipital cortex. All subjects with activation of the superior occipital cortex also had their angular cortex activated. In addition to these activations all subjects had activation of either the anterior intermediate prefrontal cortex or the frontal eye field (Figs. 10, 11). The greatest increase of rCBF was seen in the core regions plus the intermediate visual association areas, the superior occipital area, and posterior inferior temporal area (Table 3).

The core regions in the right hemisphere were the whole superior prefrontal cortex, anterior and middle midfrontal cortex, and the angular and posterior superior parietal areas (Figs. 10 and 11). In case 476 the rCBF increase in the anterior superior prefrontal cortex was just below 15%. This region was therefore included in the core regions. All

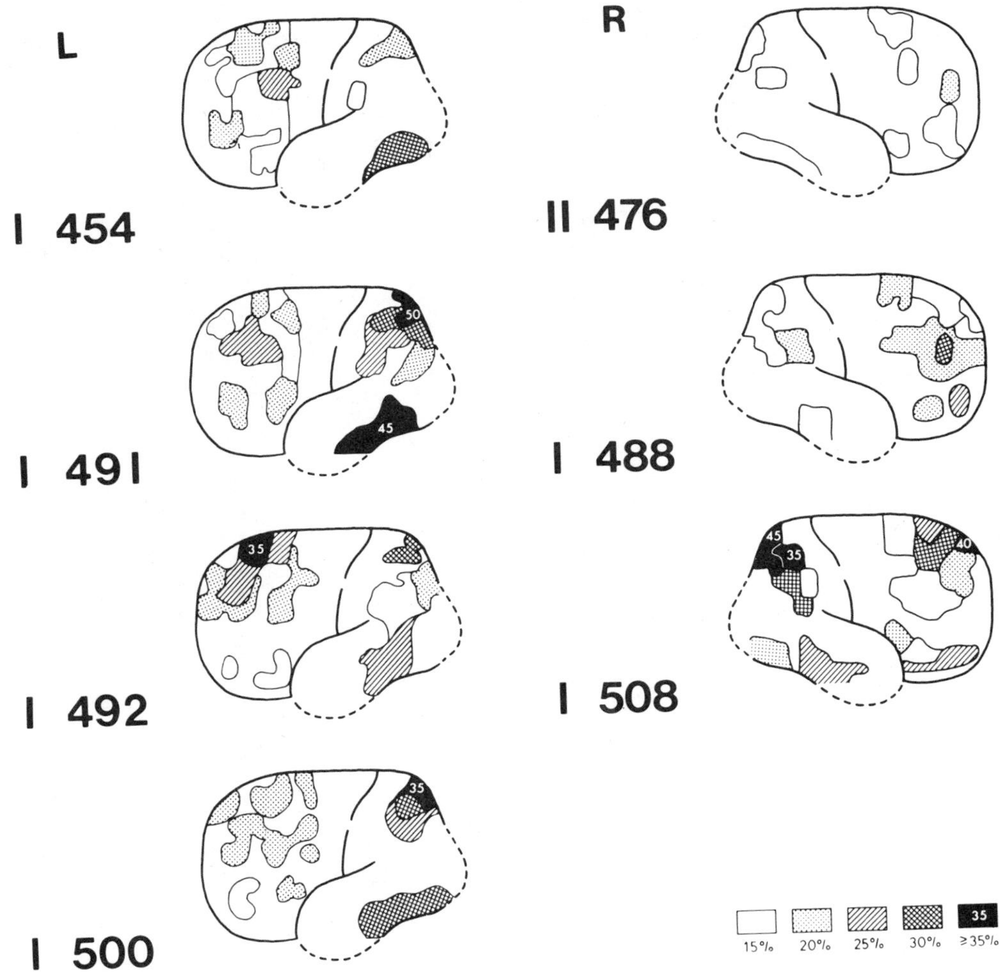

FIG. 10. Percent increase in subjects operating on visual images recalled from memory: route-finding thinking. Subjects were imagining that they were walking alternatively left and right. I, first measurement; II, second measurement. Left, left hemisphere; right, right hemisphere.

subjects had either the superior occipital cortex or the posterior inferior temporal cortex activated. These two regions plus the superior polar area and the anterior intermediate prefrontal area were activated in all but one subject (Figs. 10 and 11).

It was difficult to quantify the speed of information processing in the route-finding thinking. When the 62–65 s of thinking had passed we asked the subjects how far they had reached in their "internal walk." Their path was then located on a map of their home surroundings. The 11 subjects changed direction from 3 to 12 times. The distance covered varied from 300 to 8,300 m. It is probable that those measures were insufficient to reflect the rate of information transmission between the different cortical areas activated (Fig. 9), since it was impossible to find any correlation between the measures and the rCBF increases of these areas.

Five subjects, 491, 476, 488, 490, and 508,

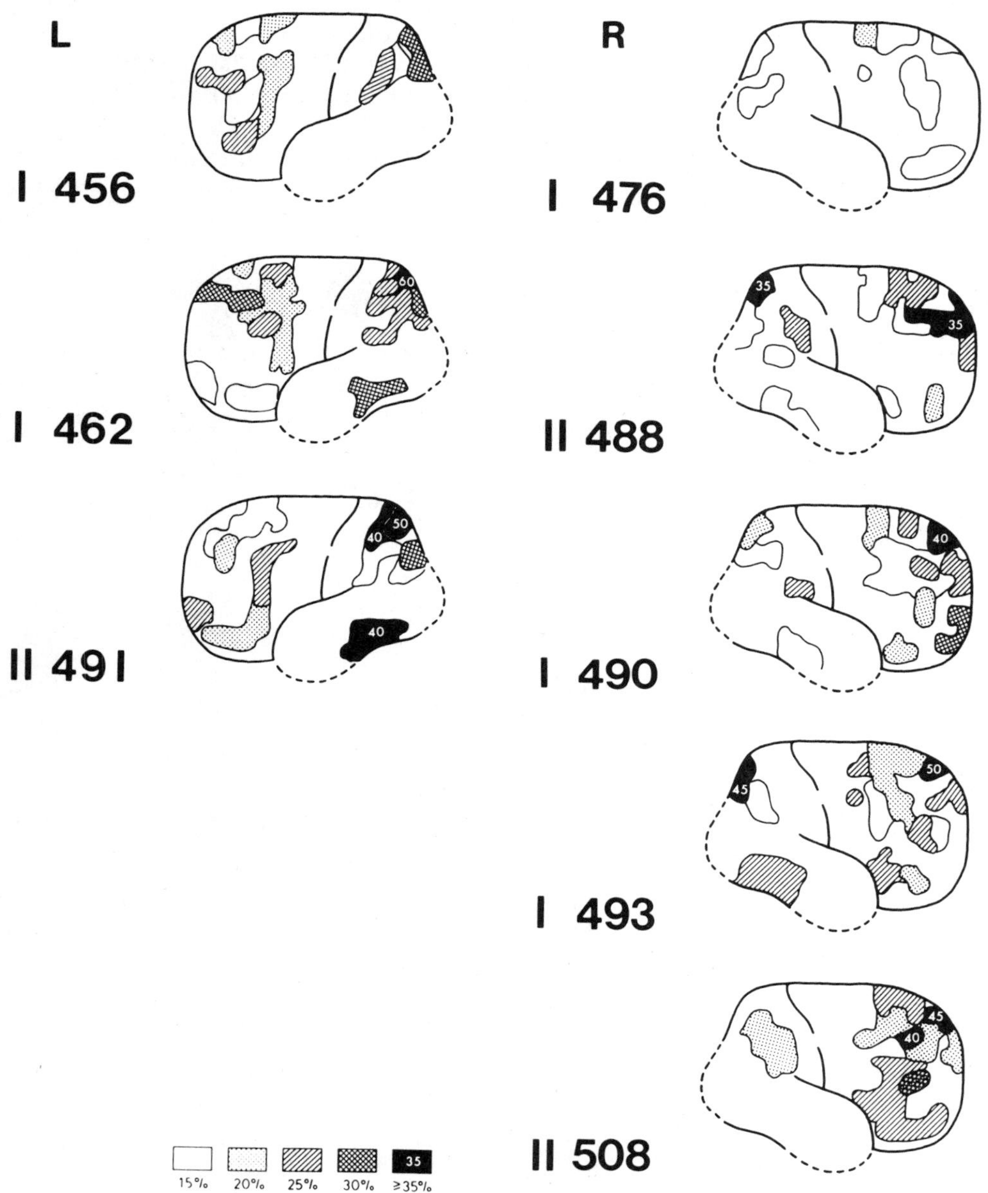

FIG. 11. Percent increase in subjects during route-finding thinking. Subjects were imagining that they were walking alternatively right and left. I, first measurement of route-finding thinking; II, second measurement. Left, left hemisphere; right, right hemisphere. In individuals, activations were of same shape and localization no matter whether subjects were asked to go right-left or left-right. Repetition of test in 490 is not shown since measurement was taken as a vertex view. Case 456 had insufficient isotope supply to the posterior inferior temporal cortex.

repeated the route-finding thinking. During the repetition the subjects imagined that they walked left-right-left, if they had previously walked right-left-right. The speed of information processing measured in the number of turns, and the distance covered was remarkably constant in each individual. There were no changes for the group of the five subjects ($P > 0.2$ for both walking distance and number of turns). The shape of the activated areas was reproducible for each subject (Fig. 6*B*, 10, 11). For the four subjects 476, 488, 490, and 508 in whom the right hemisphere was measured there were no changes in the sizes of the rCBF increases ($P > 0.1$ for all comparisons). In brief, there were no systematic changes in the rCBF with repetition of the route-finding thinking; the performance, pattern, and intensities of the rCBF increases were reproducible.

Similarities and differences in the activation patterns provoked by the three different types of thinking

The middle and posterior superior prefrontal cortex had high rCBF values no matter which type of thinking was occurring (Tables 2 and 4). In these areas the rCBF values and

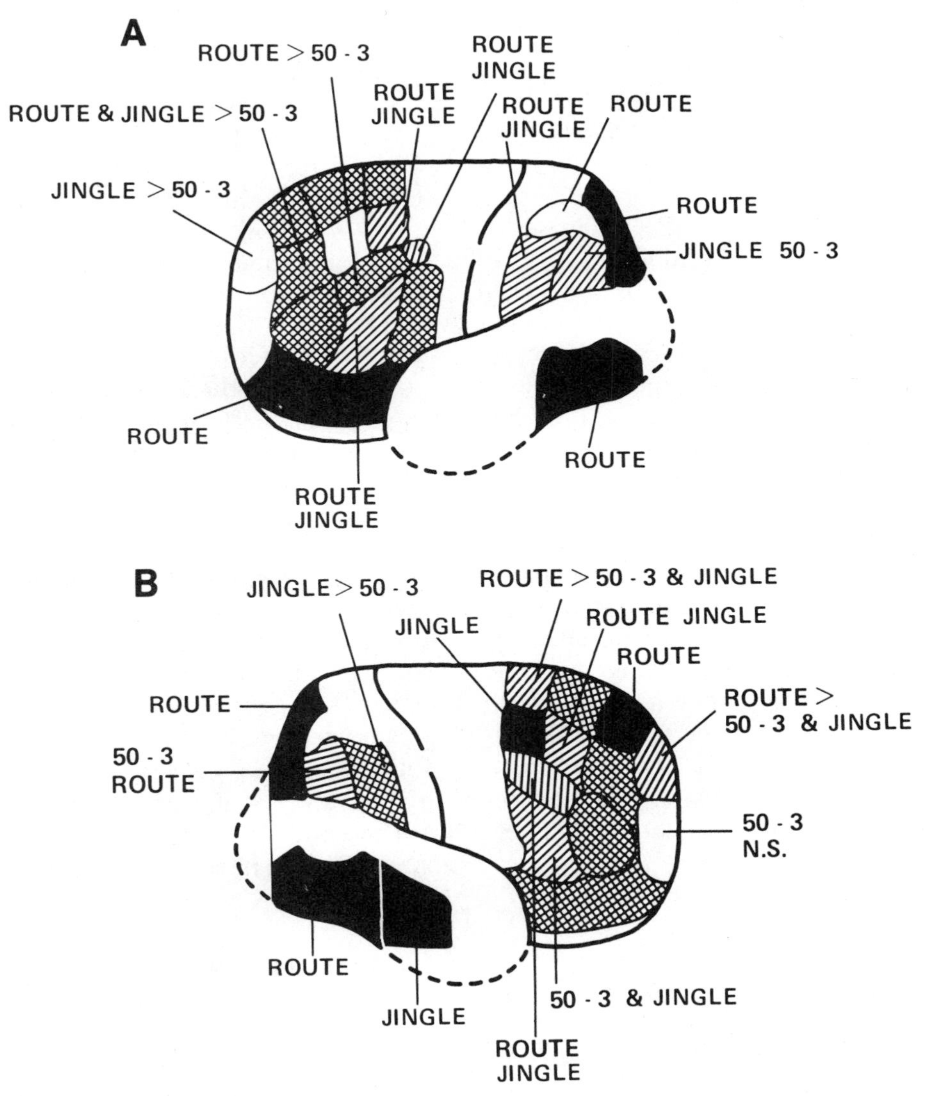

FIG. 12. Diagram of differences in cortical activations during three different types of thinking. Areas that were specifically and statistically significantly activated in one type of thinking only are shown *black*. Areas activated by two types of thinking only, are shown *hatched*. For example, the right superior polar region was activated in route-finding thinking and 50 − 3 task. The rCBF during these two tasks were significantly greater than rCBF during jingle thinking. In addition rCBF was greater during route-finding thinking than during the 50 − 3 thinking. *A*: left hemisphere; *B*: right hemisphere.

the increases of rCBF did not change significantly from one type of thinking to the next (Tables 3 and 5). The anterior parts of the midfrontal cortex and the intermediate prefrontal cortex were activated in both hemispheres during each type of thinking (Fig. 9). There were no statistically significant differences in the activations on the right side or in the left intermediate prefrontal cortex, whereas the route- and jingle thinking on average activated the left anterior midfrontal cortex more than 50 − 3 thinking did (Fig. 12). The Broca area and the right anterior inferior frontal cortex were also activated without any differences between the types of thinking. Not all these areas were core regions. The only cortical area activated in every subject in all three types of thinking was the middle superior prefrontal cortex.

The differences between the different types of thinking were most striking in the posterior parts of the hemispheres. This was evident by a comparison of the rCBF increases in each individual during the different types of thinking (compare Figs. 7, 8, 10, and 11). It is also evident from inspection of the average extensions of the statistically significant increases in Fig. 9 that some cortical areas were exclusively activated by one type of thinking. The right midtemporal cortex was exclusively activated during the jingle thinking (Fig. 12). This area is an intermediate auditory association area (13, 16, 17, 23). The intermediate visual association areas, superior occipital, posterior superior parietal, and posterior inferior temporal (16, 24), were exclusively activated during the route-finding thinking. Corresponding to the differences in rCBF increases in the posterior parts of the hemispheres, there were differences of the activation of the prefrontal cortex. Figure 12 summarizes the similarities and statistical differences.

DISCUSSION

Purely mental activity, thinking, was associated with increases of rCBF in multiple cortical fields. The rCBF increased only in homotypical cortical areas. Not all homotypical cortical areas were activated. The auditory, somatosensory, and visual immediate association areas were never activated. These results eliminated the possibility that the rCBF increases during thinking were diffuse increases in cortical blood flow due to general arousal or a state of grave apprehensiveness (6). Since different prefrontal, parietal, and temporal cortical areas were activated during the three types of thinking, and since many areas shared by the three types of thinking were activated with different intensities, the rCBF increases could not be due to a general activation of the homotypical zone. The modest increase in pulse rate during 50 − 3 thinking and route-finding thinking could not be taken as expressions of general arousal or anxiety, nor could these variables in any way be correlated with the patterns or the intensities of the rCBF. Neither would the results be compatible with activation of diffuse noradrenergic projections with regional preferences.

Since the subjects received three different verbal instructions, the different patterns of rCBF increases might have been due to the perception of three different verbal instructions. We think that this possibility could also be eliminated, because the increase in rCBF after a (verbal) stimulus lasts only 1–3 s (11), and the rCBF measurement was started 27 s after the instruction was finished. Furthermore, auditory perception and listening give rise to rCBF patterns very different from the present patterns (13, 23, 26).

The eye movements were suppressed, but the subjects could still have moved their eyes, which could be one of the explanations for the rCBF increases in the frontal eye fields. However, eye movements with the eyes closed do not give rise to rCBF increases elsewhere (10). For the subjects included we did not observe any signs of other muscular contractions or any rCBF increases in the primary motor area. Since the subjects did not receive any stimuli, nor in any way communicated with the outside world, the multifocal rCBF increases must have been evoked by internal brain work.

Cortical organization of the three types of thinking

The three different patterns of rCBF increases must have been evoked by different types of internal brain work. One of the explanations for the different patterns could have been that the subjects internally memorized the three different instructions. This could not be the full explanation since the subjects actually performed calculations, jingle jumping, and route finding. To assume that one kind of internal information processing (memorization of the instructions) gave rise to cortical rCBF increases, whereas another kind of internal information processing (operations on retrieved information) did not, would probably be untenable. Furthermore, the effect of memorizing an instruction has yet been limited to an activation of the left anterior superior prefrontal cortex. This area was activated in every task the subjects performed according to a prior given instruction (16, 17, 19–26). It was also unlikely that different degrees of difficulty of the three types of thinking could have produced these different cortical activations because the numbers of errors made by the subjects were roughly the same in the three tasks.

The middle superior prefrontal area and the left posterior superior prefrontal area were activated uniformly during all three types of thinking. Activation of these cortical areas was also observed in earlier investigations in which subjects had to operate in succession with two different sets of cortical areas (16, 17, 22). The greatest increases of rCBF in these areas were observed when the work of the second set was contingent on the work done by the first set (16, 17). The activations of these two cortical areas thus are not in any way specific for the present kinds of thinking. During all three types of thinking the subjects had to retrieve information from a memory and perform an operation on the retrieved information. In this two-step processing presumably two different sets of cortical areas would be activated.

In addition to these two areas only the right anterior midfrontal area was activated in all subjects. For the remaining homotypical cortical zone there were differences in the localization, intensity, and consistency (i.e., whether they were core areas or not) of the activated cortical fields during the three types of thinking.

To pursue further the interpretation of the results it is appropriate to answer two philosophical questions. First, are the three types of thinking really different? Second, do the differences in the formal communication theory description of the three types of information treatment correspond to similar differences in the biological information treatment? The algorithm of the three tasks was given in advance because it was part of the instruction to the subjects. The algorithm in each task consisted of a set of operations; these operations were exclusively defined on a specific information content. For example, it was not possible to subtract three from the appearance of one's home street or to turn alternatively to the right and left in the jingle. The outcome of the 50 − 3 operations could only be an integer less than 50. All subjects arrived at an integer less than 50, be it right or wrong. The outcome of the jingle operations could only be one of the nine nonsense words. All subjects arrived at one of these words. The outcome of the route-finding operations could only be a geographical point. All subjects arrived at a geographical point. In each of the subjects the end product was different from the start material. Each of the three products was also different for each subject. Since the subjects did not receive any outside information, the information they must have retrieved to arrive at the end products must have been internal. Furthermore, since the products could not have been achieved had the interval operations not been performed, we conclude that the subjects were thinking, i.e., producing a series of thoughts concatenated by internal operations, and that the three types of thinking were different.

Since the rCBF increases outside the frontal eye fields must be considered as due to internal brain work, we assume that at least part of the remaining rCBF increases are due to the three types of thinking. Since it was unlikely that non–task-related thinking, because of its expected randomness, would have produced consistent rCBF increases across subjects, we assume that at least the rCBF increases in the core areas were produced by the task-related thinking. Since the three different types of thinking elicited different rCBF increases and since these differences were consistent across subjects, one must assume that the differences in intensity and localization of the rCBF increases were produced by the differences in thinking. However, this does not imply that the information processing, transfer, and recall in the brain had a structure that could be described by the information-flow diagrams of Figs. 1, 2, and 3. On the contrary, during thinking as in other brain works (17, 18) multiple cortical fields were activated. Such activation patterns indicate that large populations of neurons are activated, and that the transmission between these populations is of another nature than the single-line transmission indicated in the information flow diagrams. Of course, the proper criterion for different types of thinking would be a biological one, i.e., that different cortical areas and subcortical structures were activated in an animal, for example, under the conditions listed in the introduction. So far, however, the knowledge about the way information operations and information recall is represented in the brain is too scant to apply such a criterion.

Although the algorithms and deterministic nature of the thinking tasks puts constraints on the thinking, there might nevertheless have been slightly different ways of treating the necessary retrieved information. For example, some subjects might have seen the integers, subtraction operations, or nonsense words with their mind's eye, and this could have given rise to rCBF increases in smaller remote visual association areas juxtaposed to the angular cortex without any possibility for us to distinguish such activations from an activation of the angular or intraparietal area. However, none of the larger visual association areas (posterior superior parietal, occipital superior, posterior inferior temporal) were activated in subjects during jingle thinking or 50 − 3 thinking. Moreover, all these types of thinking could to some extent have been embedded in more or less frequent internal verbal formulations, which in the former case could have activated the Broca area and maybe other areas facultatively.

Within the same type of thinking there were moderate differences in the activation of cortical areas between the subjects (Figs. 7, 8, 10, 11). In the 50 − 3 thinking and the route-finding thinking each subject had one or more facultative areas activated in addition to the core areas. When the 50 − 3 thinking and the route-finding thinking were repeated there was a remarkable reproducibility in the areas activated in each subject. This suggested that the influence of non-task-related thinking on the rCBF patterns was moderate. Each subject was recruiting and operating with the same cortical areas within each type of thinking. There were, consequently, slightly different individual ways of recruiting and operating with cortical areas during the same type of thinking. This kind of variability was also observed in sensory and motor tasks (16, 22–25). Still, each individual had clearly different rCBF activation patterns and activation intensities provoked by the three different types of thinking (Figs. 7, 8, 10, 11). Different types of thinking thus activate different cortical areas.

Retrieval of memory

The angular cortex, especially the left, was strongly activated in the 50 − 3 thinking. The angular cortex was activated in every subject only during the 50 − 3 thinking (Fig. 6). The left and right angular cortices were the only core areas in the posterior divisions of the hemispheres during 50 − 3 thinking. Lesions of the left or both angular gyri have been said to cause acalculia in its purest form: inability to perform the basic arithmetic operations and to perform stepwise computations (4). Only during the 50 − 3 thinking was the memory for subtraction operations and the numerical memory retrieved. It is likely then that the activation of the angular cortex during the 50 − 3 thinking was due to the retrieval of the memory for subtraction and integers that, at least partly, must have been located here.

The main difference in the three types of thinking was the type of memory to be retrieved. The right midtemporal cortex was activated exclusively during jingle thinking. This area was activated in all subjects. The midtemporal area has previously been activated in the nondominant hemisphere when subjects discriminated tone rhythms (16, 23). The area is a remote auditory association area (16). One of the most important characteristics of the jingle was its rhythmic structure. The retrieval of the specific memory for the rhythmic structure could then have activated the midtemporal cortex in the nondominant hemisphere.

The intermediate and remote visual association areas, superior occipital and posterior inferior temporal, plus the posterior superior parietal area and the left intraparietal cortex were activated exclusively during route-finding thinking. In other studies, exactly the same areas were activated when subjects discriminated the shape of ellipses (24) and when subjects were looking at familiar surroundings (9). The left posterior inferior temporal cortex was activated in every subject in whom there was sufficient isotope supply to this area. Also the left intraparietal cortex and the posterior superior parietal areas were activated in every subject. The retrieval of the memory of the home surroundings and their spatial relations most likely caused these activations during route-finding thinking. Since both the retrieval of memory for space directions and images of the home surroundings were linked together in the route-finding thinking, one cannot, on the basis of the present results, tell whether the images and the space directions were retrieved from different areas. However, it would agree with earlier results if the retrieval of space directions activated the posterior superior parietal cortex and the intraparietal cortex (22).

In the subjects in whom the route-finding thinking was repeated, the retrieved images during the second run must have been all different from the series of retrieved images during the first run. There were nevertheless no detectable differences in the shapes, localizations, or intensities of the rCBF increases in the superior occipital, posterior inferior temporal, intraparietal, and posterior superior parietal cortical areas. This meant that different retrieved images gave rise to rCBF increases of identical intensity, extension, and macroscopic localization.

A previous study (16) shows that when a subject simultaneously received visual, auditory, and somatosensory information from the external world, and the subject turned his attention toward the visual modality and discriminated the visual signals, the rCBF was further enhanced in the intermediate and remote visual association areas. This enhancement in the superior occipital, posterior inferior temporal, and the posterior superior parietal cortices occurred despite the fact that the stimulation of the three senses were unaltered (16). This means that the target areas for the retrieval of visual images from memory were the same as the target areas for the direction of attention toward visual spatial signals. The difference between reception and discrimination of external visual information and retrieval of internal stored visual information is that the primary visual area and the immediate visual association cortex is activated when the information comes from the external world but not when it is retrieved from visual-spatial memory. If the visual-spatial memory partly or fully was localized to the cerebral cortex, then apparently the same areas that finally reconstructed incoming visual and spatial information also stored this information.

Cortical energy consumption due to thinking and memory retrieval

Since there was a coupling between rCBF and the regional cortical O_2 consumption ($rCMRO_2$) the rCBF increases during thinking coupled to increases in $rCMRO_2$. Also, the cortical areas with the greatest rCBFs were those with the greatest regional cortical O_2 consumption ($rCMRO_2$). The greatest rCBFs appeared in the cortical areas that participated in thinking. These areas increased their rCBF from rest to thinking (Tables 2–5).

It has been shown that inhibition of the cerebral cortex induced by GABA agonists can reduce the cortical rCBF down to 25 $ml \cdot 100\ g^{-1} \cdot min^{-1}$ (26). On the other hand, physiological activations of the cerebral cortex during thinking as well as during sensory and motor tasks increased the rCBF multifocally in the cerebral cortex (13, 15–26). Provided that the rest was adequate, significant rCBF decreases were not observed either in the present study or in previous studies (13, 15–26). That is, physiological activations that were known to increase the net excitation of the cerebral cortex also increased the rCBF. None of the rCBF increases therefore could have been due to a net inhibition.

The total average increase in cortical blood flow (CBF) during programming and execution of a sequence of intense, fast, complicated voluntary movements (21) was 5.03 $ml \cdot 100\ g^{-1} \cdot min^{-1}$. Similarly, the cortical CBF increase during discrimination of tone rhythms (23) was 2.90 $ml \cdot 100\ g^{-1} \cdot min^{-1}$. From Table 1 it is evident, then, that for route-finding thinking and jingle thinking the cortical energy consumption was larger than for intense perceptual and motor tasks. There is, therefore, no reason to assume that the neuronal work underlying thoughts is any different from the neuronal work underlying voluntary movements or perceptions.

ACKNOWLEDGMENTS

We thank Chief Physician Dr. N. Lassen for his support and excellent working conditions, Professor H.

Hultborn, and Dr. P. Dyhre-Poulsen for their helpful suggestions on earlier versions of the manuscript.

Address for reprint requests: Dr. Rieland, Department of Clinical Neurophysiology, Karolinska Hospital, S10401, Stockholm, Sweden.

REFERENCES

1. DUNNETT, C. W. New tables for multiple comparison with a control. *Biometrics* 20: 482–491, 1964.
2. GREENBERG, F., HAND, P., SYLVESTRO, A., AND REIVICH, M. Localized metabolic flow couple during functional activity. *Acta Neurol. Scand. Suppl.* 72: 12–14, 1979.
3. HALD, A. *Statistical Theory With Engineering Applications.* New York: Wiley, 1952.
4. HÉCAEN, H., ANGELERGUES, R., AND HOUILLIER, S. Lés variétés cliniques des acalculies au cours des lésions rétrorolandiques: approche statistique du problème. *Rev. Neurol.* 105: 85–103, 1961.
5. INGVAR, D. H. AND RISBERG, J. Increase of regional cerebral blood flow during mental effort in normals and in patients with focal brain disorders. *Exp. Brain Res.* 3: 195–211, 1967.
6. KETY, S. S. Circulation and metabolism of the human brain in health and disease. *Am. J. Med.* 8: 205–217, 1950.
7. LASSEN, N. A. AND INGVAR, D. H. The blood flow of the cerebral cortex determined by radioactive Krypton-85. *Experientia* 17: 42–43, 1961.
8. LASSEN, N. A. AND INGVAR, D. H. Regional cerebral blood flow measurements in man. *Arch. Neurol. Psychiatry* 9: 615–622, 1963.
9. MAZZIOTTA, J. C., PHELPS, M. E., AND HALGREN, E. Local cerebral glucose metabolic response to audiovisual stimulation and deprivation: studies in human subjects with positron CT. *Human Neurobiol.* 2: 11–23, 1983.
10. MELAMED, E. AND LARSEN, B. Cortical activation pattern during saccadic eye movements in man: localization by focal cerebral blood flow increases. *Ann. Neurol.* 5: 79–88, 1979.
11. MOSKALENKO, Y. Y. Regional cerebral blood flow and its control at rest and during increased functional activity. In: *Brain Work,* edited by H. D. Ingvar and N. A. Lassen. Copenhagen: Munksgaard, 1975, p. 343–351.
12. MUNDY-CASTLE, A. C. The electroencephalogram and mental activity. *Electroencephalogr. Clin. Neurophysiol.* 9: 643–655, 1957.
13. NISHIZAWA, Y., OLSEN, T. S., LARSEN, B., AND LASSEN, N. A. Left-right cortical asymmetries of regional cerebral blood flow during listening to words. *J. Neurophysiol.* 48: 458–466, 1982.
14. RAICHLE, M. E., GRUBB, R. L., GADO, M. H., EICHLING, J. O., AND TER-POGOSSIAN, M. M. Correlation between regional cerebral blood flow and oxidative metabolism. *Arch. Neurol.* 33: 523–526, 1976.
15. ROLAND, P. E. Somatotopical tuning of postcentral gyrus during focal attention in man. A regional cerebral blood flow study. *J. Neurophysiol.* 46: 744–754, 1981.
16. ROLAND, P. E. Cortical regulation of selective attention in man. *J. Neurophysiol.* 48: 1059–1078, 1982.
17. ROLAND, P. E. Application of brain blood flow imaging in behavioral neurophysiology: the cortical field activation hypothesis. In: *Brain Imaging and Brain Function,* edited by L. Sokoloff. New York: Raven, 1985, p. 89–106.
18. ROLAND, P. E. Metabolic measurements of the working frontal cortex in man. *Trends Neurosci.* 7: 430–435, 1984.
19. ROLAND, P. E. AND LARSEN, B. Focal increase of cerebral blood flow during stereognostic testing in man. *Arch. Neurol.* 33: 557–558, 1976.
20. ROLAND, P. E., SKINHØJ, E., LARSEN, B., AND ENDO, H. Perception and voluntary action: localization of basic input and output functions as revealed by regional cerebral blood flow increases in the human brain. In: *Cerebral Vascular Disease,* edited by J. S. Meyer, H. Lechner, and M. Reivich. Amsterdam: Excerpta Medica, 1977, p. 40–44.
21. ROLAND, P. E., LARSEN, B., LASSEN, N. A., AND SKINHØJ, E. Supplementary motor area and other cortical areas in organization of voluntary movements in man. *J. Neurophysiol.* 43: 118–136, 1980.
22. ROLAND, P. E., SKINHØJ, E., LASSEN, N. A., AND LARSEN, B. Different cortical areas in man in organization of voluntary movements in extrapersonal space. *J. Neurophysiol.* 43: 137–150, 1980.
23. ROLAND, P. E., SKINHØJ, E., AND LASSEN, N. A. Focal activation of human cerebral cortex during auditory discrimination. *J. Neurophysiol.* 45: 1139–1151, 1981.
24. ROLAND, P. E. AND SKINHØJ, E. Focal activation of the cerebral cortex during visual discrimination in man. *Brain Res.* 222: 166–171, 1981.
25. ROLAND, P. E., MEYER, E., SHIBASAKI, T., YAMAMOTO, Y. L., AND THOMPSON, C. J. Regional cerebral blood flow changes in cortex and basal ganglia during voluntary movements in normal human volunteers. *J. Neurophysiol.* 48: 467–480, 1982.
26. ROLAND, P. E. AND FRIBERG, L. Are cortical rCBF increases during brain work in man due to synaptic excitation or inhibition? *J. Cereb. Blood Flow Metab.* 3 Suppl. 1: 244–254, 1983.
27. SOKOLOFF, L., MANGOLD, R., WECHSLER, R. L., KENNEDY, C., AND KETY, S. The effect of mental arithmetic on cerebral circulation and metabolism. *J. Clin. Invest.* 34: 1101–1108, 1955.
28. SVEINSDOTTIR, E., LARSEN, B., ROMMER, P., AND LASSEN, N. A. A multidetector scintillation camera with 254 channels. *J. Nucl. Med.* 18: 168–174, 1977.
29. TALAIRACH, J., SZIKLA, G., TOURNOUX, P., PROSSALENTIS, A., BORDAS-FERRER, M., COVELLO, L., IACOB, M., AND MEMPEL, E. *Atlas d'Anatomie Stéréotaxique du Téléncephale.* Paris: Masson, 1967.

46

A. P. Georgopoulos, J. T. Lurito, M. Petrides, A. B. Schwartz, and J. T. Massey

Mental rotation of the neuronal population vector

1989. *Science* 243: 234–236

Abstract

A rhesus monkey was trained to move its arm in a direction that was perpendicular to and counterclockwise from the direction of a target light that changed in position from trial to trial. Solution of this problem was hypothesized to involve the creation and mental rotation of an imagined movement vector from the direction of the light to the direction of the movement. This hypothesis was tested directly by recording the activity of cells in the motor cortex during performance of the task and computing the neuronal population vector in successive time intervals during the reaction time. The population vector rotated gradually counterclockwise from the direction of the light to the direction of the movement at an average rate of 732° per second. These results provide direct, neural evidence for the mental rotation hypothesis and indicate that the neuronal population vector is a useful tool for "reading out" and identifying cognitive operations of neuronal ensembles.

A fundamental problem in cognitive neuroscience is the identification and elucidation of brain events underlying cognitive operations (*1*). The technique of recording the activity of single cells in the brain of behaving animals (*2*) provides a direct tool for that purpose. Indeed, a wealth of knowledge has accumulated during the past 15 years concerning the activity of cells in several brain areas during performance by monkeys of complex tasks. A major finding of these studies has been that the activity of single cells in specific areas of the cerebral cortex changes during performance of particular tasks; these changes are thought to reflect the participation of the area under study in the cognitive function involved in the task (*3*). However, a direct visualization of a cognitive operation in terms of neuronal activation in the brain is lacking.

We chose as a test case for this problem the cognitive operation of mental rotation. Important work in experimental psychology during the past 20 years (*4*) has established the mental rotation paradigm as a standard in cognitive psychology and as a prime tool in investigating cognitive operations of the "analog" type. We adapted this procedure in a task that required movement of a handle in a direction that was at an angle with the direction of a stimulus. Under these conditions the reaction time increased with the angle, which suggests that the subject may solve this problem by a mental rotation of an imagined movement vector from the direction of the stimulus to the direction of the actual movement (*5*). Now, the direction of an upcoming movement in space seems to be represented in the motor cortex as the neuronal population vector (*6*), which is a weighted vector sum of contributions ("votes") of directionally tuned neurons: each neuron is assumed to vote in its own preferred direction with a strength that depends on how much the activity of the neuron changes for the movement under consideration. This vectorial analysis has proved useful in visualizing the directionality of the population in two- and three-dimensional space during the reaction time (*7*) and during an instructed delay period (*8*).

Given the mental rotation hypothesis above and the neuronal population vector as a neural representation of the movement direction, a strong test is as follows: if a monkey performs in the above-mentioned task and the neuronal activity in the motor cortex is recorded during performance, would the population vector rotate in time, as the hypothesis for a mental rotation of an imagined movement vector would predict? Because the appropriate movement direction can be arrived at by either a counterclockwise or a clockwise rotation, which of these two rotations would be realized by the population vector? Of course, there is no reason that the population vector should rotate at all, and if it rotates, there is no a priori reason that it should rotate in one or the other direction; for all we know, any of these alternatives is possible.

The activity of single cells in the motor cortex was recorded (*9*) while a rhesus monkey performed in the mental rotation task. In the beginning of a trial, a light appeared at the center of a plane in front of the animal, which moved its arm toward the light with a freely movable handle (*10*). After a variable period of time (0.75 to 2.25 s), the center light was turned off and turned on again, dim or bright, at one of eight positions on a circle of 2-cm radius (*11*). The monkey was trained to move the handle in the direction of the light when it came on dim (direct trials) or in a direction that was perpendicular (90°) to and counterclockwise from the direction of the light when it came on bright (rotation trials) (*12*). The movements of the animal were in the appropriate direction for both kinds of trials. The neuronal population vector was calculated every 10 ms starting from the onset of the peripheral light (that is, at the beginning of the reaction time). The preferred direction of each cell (n = 102 cells) was determined from the cell activity in the trials in which the animal moved toward the light (direct trials). For the calculation of the population vector, peristimulus time histograms (10-ms binwidth) were computed for each cell and each of the 16 combinations (classes) used [eight positions and two conditions (direct or rotation), see (*11*) above] with counts of fractional interspike intervals as a measure of the intensity of cell discharge. A square root transformation was applied to these counts to stabilize the variance (*13*). For a given time bin, each cell made a vectorial contribution in the direction of the cell's preferred direction and of magnitude equal to the change in cell activity from that observed during 0.5 s preceding the onset of the peripheral stimulus (control rate, that is, while the monkey was holding the handle at the center of the plane). The population vector **P** for the jth class and k^{th} time bin is

$$\mathbf{P}_{j,k} = \sum_{i}^{102} w_{i,j,k}\mathbf{C}_i$$

where $\mathbf{C}_i$ is the preferred direction of the ith cell and $w_{i,j,k}$ is a weighting function $w_{i,j,k} = (d_{i,j,k}) - a_{i,j}$ where $d_{i,j,k}$ is the square root–transformed (*13*) discharge rate of the ith cell for the jth class and k^{th} time bin, and $a_{i,j}$ is the similarly transformed control rate of the ith cell for the jth class.

Figure 1 illustrates the results obtained when the movement direction was the same (toward 9 o'clock) but the stimulus was either at 9 o'clock (direct trials, left panel) or at 12 o'clock (rotation trials, right panel). In the direct trials the population vector pointed in the direction of the movement (which coincided with the direction of the stimulus) (Fig. 1, left). However, in the rotation trials the population vector rotated in time counterclockwise from the direction of the stimulus to the direction of the movement (Fig. 1, right). Another example is shown in Fig. 2 and illustrated in the cover photograph. The working space is outlined in blue. The time axis is the white line directed upwards. The population vector is shown in green, as it rotates during the reaction time from the stimulus direction (between 1 and 2 o'clock) to the movement direction (between 10 and 11 o'clock). The population vector was calculated with a 20-ms bin sliding every 2 ms. The red lines are projections of the population vector onto the working space.

The rotation of the population vector was a linear function of time with an average slope (for the eight positions of the light used) of 732 ± 456°/s (mean ± SD). The population vector began to change in length 125 ± 28 ms (mean ± SD, $n = 8$) after the stimulus onset. At this point its direction was close to the direction of the stimulus; the average angle between the direction of the population vector and that of the stimulus was 17° counterclockwise (the average absolute angle was 29°). The population vector stabilized in direction at 225 ± 50 ms after stimulus onset. At this

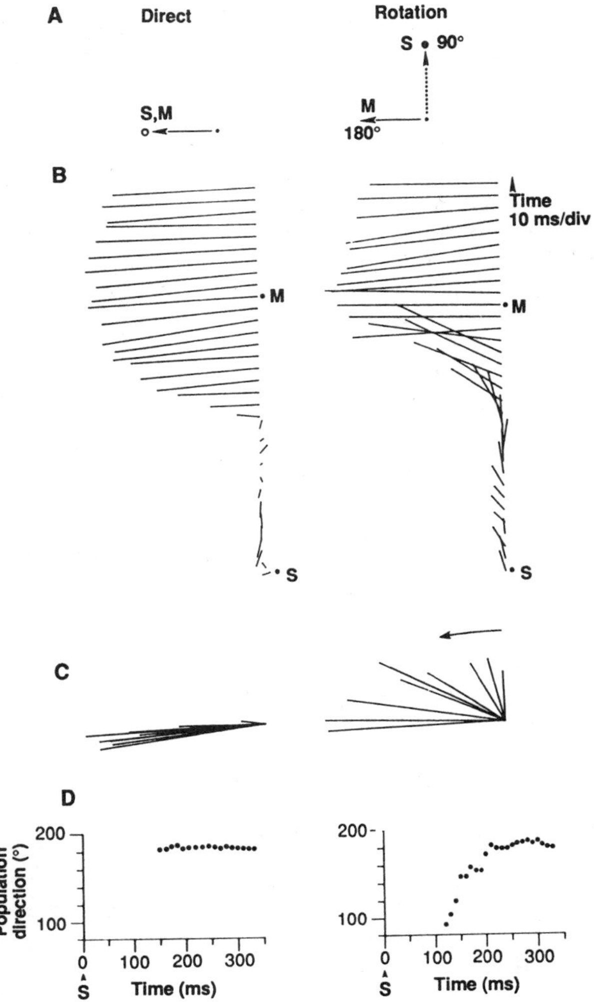

Figure 1. Results from a direct (left) and rotation (right) movement. (**A**) Task. Unfilled and filled circles indicate dim and bright light, respectively. Interrupted and continuous lines with arrows indicate stimulus (S) and movement (M) direction, respectively. (**B**) Neuronal population vectors calculated every 10 ms from the onset of the stimulus (S) at positions shown in (A) until after the onset of the movement (M). When the population vector lengthens, for the direct case (left) it points in the direction of the movement, whereas for the rotation case it points initially in the direction of the stimulus and then rotates counterclockwise (from 12 o'clock to 9 o'clock) and points in the direction of the movement. (**C**) Ten successive population vectors from (B) are shown in a spatial plot, starting from the first population vector that increased significantly in length. Notice the counterclockwise rotation of the population vector (right panel). (**D**) Scatter plots of the direction of the population vector as a function of time, starting from the first population vector that increased significantly in length after stimulus onset (S). For the direct case (left panel) the direction of the population vector is in the direction of the movement (~180°); for the rotation case (right panel) the direction of the population vector rotates counterclockwise from the direction of the stimulus (~90°) to the direction of the movement (~180°).

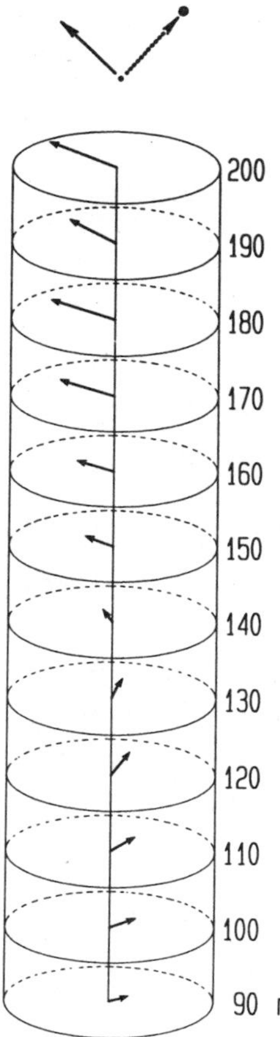

Figure 2. Rotation of the population vector for a different set of rotation trials. The stimulus and movement directions are indicated by the interrupted and continuous lines at the top. The population vector in the two-dimensional space is shown for successive time frames beginning 90 ms after stimulus onset. Notice its rotation counterclockwise from the direction of the stimulus to the direction of the movement.

point its direction was close to the direction of the movement; the average angle between the direction of the population vector and that of the movement was 0.5° clockwise (the average absolute angle was 8°). Finally, the movement began 260 ± 30 ms after stimulus onset, that is, 35 ms after the direction of the population vector became relatively stable; this difference was statistically significant ($P < 0.02$, paired t test).

These results support the hypothesis that the directional transformation required by the task was achieved by a counterclockwise rotation of an imagined movement vector. This process was reflected in the gradual change of activity of motor cortical cells, which led to the gradual rotation of the vectorial distribution of the neuronal ensemble and the population vector. The average slope of the rotation of the population vector (732°/s, see above) was comparable to but higher than that observed when human subjects performed a similar task (~400°/s) (*5*) and that observed in a task that involved mental rotation of two-dimensional images (~400°/s) (*14*). It is likely that all three experiments involved a process of mental rotation which, in the present case, was reflected in the motor cortical recordings of this study and identified by using the population vector analysis. Of course, other brain areas are probably involved in such complicated transformations; for example, recent experiments with measurements of regional cerebral blood flow (*15*) suggested that frontal and parietal areas seem to be involved in the mental rotation task of Shepard and Metzler (*16*), whereas frontal and central areas seem to be involved in a line orientation task (*15*); in both of these tasks there was a greater increase in blood flow in the right than in the left hemisphere.

The rotation of the neuronal population vector is of particular interest because there was no a priori reason for it to rotate at all. It is also interesting that the population vector rotated consistently in the counterclockwise direction: this suggests that the spatial-motor transformation imposed by the task was solved by a rotation through the shortest angular distance. Given that the mental rotation is time consuming, this solution was behaviorally meaningful, for it minimized both the time for the animal to get the reward and the computational effort which would have been longer if the rotation had been through 270° clockwise (*17*).

Finally, these results were obtained from one animal: because cognitive problems could be solved in different ways by different subjects, it is important that techniques for reading out brain operations be sensitive enough to be applied to single subjects. Indeed, the findings of our study indicate that the population vector is a sensitive tool by which an insight can be gained into the brain processes underlying cognitive operations in space.

References and Notes

1. See, for example, V. B. Mountcastle, *Trends Neurosci.* **9**, 505 (1986); M. A. Arbib and M. B. Hesse, *The Construction of Reality* (Cambridge Univ. Press, New York, 1986); J. Z. Young, *Philosophy and the Brain* (Oxford Univ. Press, New York, 1987).

2. R. N. Lemon, *Methods for Neuronal Recording in Conscious Animals* (Wiley, Chisester, 1984).

3. See, for example, *Handbook of Physiology*, Section 1, *The Nervous System, Higher Function of the Brain*, parts 1 and 2, V. B. Mountcastle, F. Plum, S. R. Geiger, Eds. (American Physiological Society, Bethesda, MD, 1987), vol. 5.

4. R. N. Shepard and J. Metzler, *Science* **171**, 701 (1971); R. N. Shepard and L. A. Cooper, *Mental Images and Their Transformations* (MIT Press, Cambridge, MA, 1982).

5. A. P. Georgopoulos and J. T. Massey, *Exp. Brain Res.* **65**, 361 (1987).

6. A. P. Georgopoulos, P. Caminiti, J. F. Kalaska, J. T. Massey, *ibid. Suppl.* 7, 327 (1983); A. P. Georgopoulos, A. B. Schwartz, R. E. Kettner, Science **233**, 1416 (1986); *J. Neurosci.* **8**, 2928 (1988).

7. A. P. Georgopoulos, J. F. Kalaska, M. D. Crutcher, R. Caminiti, J. T. Massey, in *Dynamic Aspects of Neocortical Function*, G. M. Edelman, W. E. Gall, W. M. Cowan, Eds. (Wiley, New York, 1984), pp. 501–524; A. P. Georgopoulos, A. B. Schwartz, R. E. Kettner, *J. Neurosci.* **8**, 2928 (1988).

8. A. P. Georgopoulos, M. D. Crutcher, A. B. Schwartz, *Exp. Brain Res.*, in press.

9. The electrical signs of activity of individual cells in the arm area of the motor cortex contralateral to the performing arm were recorded extracellularly [A. P. Georgopoulos, J. F. Kalaska, R. Caminiti, J. T. Massey, *J. Neurosci.* **2**, 1527 (1982)]. All surgical operations [A. P. Georgopoulos, J. F. Kalaska, R. Caminiti, J. T. Massey, *J. Neurosci.* **2**, 1527 (1982)] for the preparation of the animal for electrophysiological recordings were performed under general pentobarbital anesthesia. Behavioral control and data collection and analysis were performed with a laboratory minicomputer.

10. The apparatus was as described in A. P. Georgopoulos and J. T. Massey [*Exp. Brain Res.* **65**, 361 (1987)]. Briefly, it consisted of a 25 cm by 25 cm planar working surface made of frosted plexiglass onto which a He-Ne laser beam was back-projected with a system of mirrors and two galvanometers. The monkey (5 kg) sat comfortably on a primate chair and grasped a freely movable, articulated handle at its distal end, next to a 10-mm diameter transparent plexiglass circle within which the animal captured the center light.

11. The eight positions were equally spaced on the circle, that is, at angular intervals of 45°, and were the same throughout the experiment. The brightness condition (dim or bright) and the position of the light were mixed. The resulting 16 brightness-position combinations were randomized. Eight repetitions of these 16 combinations were presented in a randomized block design.

12. The term "counterclockwise" is simply descriptive; no counterclockwise or clockwise directions were indicated to the animal. The direction in which the animal was required to move can be described equivalently as either 90° counterclockwise or 270° clockwise. The animal received a liquid reward when its movement exceeded 3 cm and stayed within $\pm 25°$ of the direction required. The average direction of the actual movement trajectories was within $\pm 5°$ of the direction required. Performance was over 70% correct trials.

13. The square root transformation was used as a variance-stabilizing transformation for counts [G. W. Snedecor and W. G. Cochran, *Statistical Methods* (Iowa State Univ. Press, Ames, Iowa, ed. 7, 1980), pp. 288–290.] Although the results obtained without this transformation were similar, the transformation is more appropriate because of the small size of the time bins (10 ms), and, therefore, the small number of counts.

14. L. A. Cooper and R. N. Shepard, in *Visual Information Processing*, W. G. Chase, Ed. (Academic Press, New York, 1973), pp. 75–176; L. A. Cooper, *Cognitive Psychol.* **7**, 20 (1975).

15. G. Deutsch, W. T. Bourbon, A. C. Papanicolaou, H. M. Eisenberg *Neuropsychologia* **26**, 44 (1988).

16. R. N. Shepard and J. Metzler, *Science* **171**, 701 (1971).

17. The same principles of minimization of the time-to-reward and of reduction of computation load, even at the expense of mechanical work, were observed in strategies developed by human subjects and monkeys in a different task [J. T. Massey, A. P. Schwartz, A. P. Georgopoulos, *Exp. Brain Res. Suppl.* **15**, 242 (1986)].

18. We thank D. Brandt and N. Porter for help during some of the experiments. Supported by USPHS grants NS17413 and NS20868.

47

S. M. Kosslyn

Aspects of a cognitive neuroscience of mental imagery

1988. *Science* 240: 1621–1626

Although objects in visual mental images may seem to appear all of a piece, when the time to form images is measured this introspection is revealed to be incorrect; objects in images are constructed a part at a time. Studies with split-brain patients and normal subjects reveal that two classes of processes are used to form images—ones that activate stored memories of the appearances of parts and ones that arrange parts into the proper configuration. Some of the processes used to arrange parts are more effective in the left cerebral hemisphere and some are more effective in the right cerebral hemisphere; the notion that mental images are the product of right hemisphere activity is an oversimplification.

PERHAPS THE MOST FUNDAMENTAL INSIGHT OF CONTEMPOrary cognitive science is the discovery that mental faculties can be decomposed into multicomponent information-processing systems. Although mental faculties such as "memory," "thinking," "imagery," and so on intuitively may seem to be single abilities, they are not. How visual mental imagery is being analyzed into distinct processing components and how these functionally characterized components are coming to be identified with brain structures is the subject of this article. Only one facet of imagery is considered here, namely the way visual mental images are generated from stored information.

Mental imagery has played a key role in many theories of mental function, both historically and currently (*1–3*). Imagery consists of brain states like those that arise during perception but occurs in the absence of the appropriate immediate sensory input; such events are usually accompanied by the conscious experience of "seeing with the mind's eye," "hearing with the mind's ear," and so on. Visual imagery is a particularly useful place to begin in that it clearly draws on some of the mechanisms also used in visual perception (*2–5*), and the anatomy and physiology of vision is becoming relatively well understood (*6, 7*). Evidence for the use of common mechanisms in imagery and like-modality perception abounds. For example, visual perception is more difficult than auditory perception when one is simultaneously holding a visual mental image, and vice versa when one is holding an auditory mental image (*8*). In addition, some visual illusions also appear in visual imagery (*4*). Indeed, there is emerging evidence that visual areas of the brain are selectively activated during visual mental imagery (*5*).

Generating hypotheses about the processing that underlies imagery is aided by consideration of three kinds of factors. First, it is necessary to begin by characterizing the behavior of imagery mechanisms. Without such information, there is nothing to explain. Second, because a theory of human information processing is in fact a theory about how the brain functions, it is useful to have some knowledge of the underlying neural substrate. Given that imagery shares some modality-specific perceptual mechanisms, facts about the anatomy and physiology of the visual system can be used in generating hypotheses about the processing underlying imagery. Third, it is useful to perform an analysis of what would be required to build a system that would produce the observed behavior. The use of these three kinds of factors is illustrated in the following section.

Generating Visual Mental Images

Probably the most obvious behavioral property of the imagery system is that images are not present all the time, but only occur in specific circumstances. For example, if one is asked to decide whether the uppercase letters of the alphabet have only straight lines or contain any curved lines, images of the letters are likely to be used. These images come to mind only when one begins to perform the task. The question to be considered here is, what is the nature of the processing that produces mental images?

Behavioral characterization. When asked, most people report that images of simple objects, such as letters or line patterns, seem to pop into mind all at once. However, when the time course of image formation is charted, such introspections are revealed to be incorrect: imaged patterns are built up a part at a time. Consider the following task. First, observe the letter in the grid at the upper left of Fig. 1. If that letter were present in the grid at the upper right, would it cover the X mark? In these experiments, subjects first memorized a set of such block letters, which varied from two (L) to five segments (G). The subjects later were shown a blank grid with a lowercase letter beneath it, and were asked to decide whether the corresponding uppercase version of the letter—if drawn in the grid as previously seen—would fill the cells occupied by two such X marks. On half the trials the letter would have covered both X marks, whereas on the other half it would have covered only one (the other was in a cell that would have been adjacent to the letter). Subjects were told to respond as quickly as possible while being as accurate as possible; response time and accuracy were measured.

The key to this method is that the two probe marks appeared in the grid only 500 milliseconds after the lowercase cue letter was presented. Given that up to 250 ms are necessary to read a letter cue (*9*), and about 250 ms are required to move one's eyes up from the cue, there was not enough time to finish forming the image before the probes appeared. Hence the time to respond should in part reflect the time to form the image (*10*).

The author is professor of psychology at Harvard University, Cambridge, MA 02138.

The first result of interest was that the response times increased with the visual complexity (number of segments) of the queried letter (mean slope, 133 ms per segment; SE, 28 ms; $P < 0.0005$). Although this result suggests that more complex forms require more time to image, it could instead reflect the time to search for the probe marks. Thus, it is important that complexity had greatly reduced effects when these subjects evaluated probe marks with the figure actually present (mean slope, 10 ms; SE, 4 ms; $P < 0.05$); the results in the imagery task do not reflect only search and evaluation time. In addition, in another condition the probe marks were eliminated, and subjects now were asked simply to read the lowercase cue and form an image of the corresponding uppercase version in the grid; as soon as the image was fully formed, the subjects were to press a key. These times also increased for letters with more segments, and did so to a similar degree in this task and the image evaluation task (mean slope, 100 ms per segment; SE, 19 ms; $P < 0.0005$; $P > 0.1$ for the comparison of the two slopes). Thus, there is reason to infer that differences in response times in the experimental task reflect differences in image formation time (*11*).

In addition to varying the complexity of the stimuli, the positions of the probe marks were varied along the individual letters. If the image is being constructed a segment at a time, then some probes ought to require more time to reach than others. A separate group of 25 subjects was asked to copy the block letters into empty grids, and the order in which the segments were drawn was covertly observed; the order was highly consistent, with five of the letters being drawn in the same way by 100% of the subjects, and the remainder being drawn in the same way by at least 75% (when these letters were drawn differently it was always in the order of a single segment). As is illustrated in Fig. 2, more time was required in the image evaluation task when the "farthest" probe mark fell on a segment typically drawn later in the sequence (mean slope, 178 ms per segment; SE = 35 ms; $P < 0.0005$). This effect of probe position did not occur in the perception control task (mean slope, 2 ms per segment; SE, 7 ms; $P > 0.25$). Similar results were found for novel two-dimensional patterns (*11*) and three-dimensional shapes (*12*).

Thus, it appears that patterns in images are built up by activating parts individually and that parts are imaged in roughly the order in which they are typically drawn. These inferences were supported by a host of additional experiments controlling for various alternative accounts. For example, it was possible that the effect of probe position was due to scanning an imaged pattern in search of the probes (which might be different than inspecting a figure that is actually present). If so, then farther probes should require more time to evaluate than nearer ones, even when one has formed the image in advance of the probe; this did not occur. It was also possible that the effects reflect patterns of eye movements; nevertheless, they persisted even when subjects fixated on the center of the screen while performing the task (*11, 12*).

Additional research has been conducted to discover what factors determine the nature of the parts, and has shown that principles of perceptual organization also determine the part structure of images (*13*). That is, it has been known since the early part of this century that we see lines and regions as being organized into "perceptual units." For example, the pattern "------" is seen as a line (grouped by the "law of good continuation"), not six isolated dashes; "XXX XXX" is seen as two units (grouped by the "law of proximity"), not six solitary X's; and XXXooo is seen as two units (grouped by the "law of similarity"), not simply three X's and three o's. Similarly, lines that form a symmetrical pattern or that form enclosed areas tend to be grouped as units (*14*). In the block letter stimuli used in the image generation experiments, adjacent filled cells will form a unit (a bar) as per the law of good continuation. There is good evidence that these sorts of units are not only perceived, but also are stored in memory (*13*).

Thus, given that visual mental images are formed by activating previously stored perceptual information, it is easy to formulate a hypothesis about why images are constructed a part at a time: namely, when originally viewed the parts were stored individually and hence they are later activated into an image individually. But even so, the data suggest that parts are activated sequentially. Why are they not simply activated all at once to reconstruct the entire object in the image?

Neurological constraints. One possible reason why parts are imaged sequentially hinges on the way parts and spatial relations among them might be stored in memory. Ungerleider and Mishkin (*7*) summarize evidence for "two cortical visual systems" in primates (Fig. 3). The ventral system runs from area OC (primary visual cortex) through area TEO down to the inferior temporal lobe. This system has been identified with the analysis of shape ("what"). The dorsal system runs almost directly from circumstriate area OB to OA and then to PG (in the parietal lobe). This system has been identified with the analysis of location ("where").

Three sorts of data have been marshalled to support Ungerleider and Mishkin's claims. First, neuroanatomical investigations have documented the existence of the separate pathways. Indeed, each pathway has now been decomposed into connections among numerous distinct areas (*6, 7*).

Second, neurophysiological investigations of monkey brains have revealed that cells in both systems are sensitive to visual input, but have different functional properties. For example, cells in the inferior temporal lobe are sensitive to shape (often being highly tuned for specific shape properties), color, and have very large receptive fields that almost always include the fovea (*15, 16*). In contrast, cells in the parietal lobe are not particularly sensitive to shape or color, rarely include the fovea in their receptive fields, are sensitive to direction of motion, and some cells in this region respond selectively to an object's location (as gated by eye position) (*17*).

Third, behavioral data provide dramatic evidence of the distinct visual functions of the two systems. When the temporal lobes are ablated but the parietal lobes are spared, animals are severely impaired in learning to discriminate among patterns, but are relatively unimpaired in learning to discriminate among locations. In contrast, when the parietal lobes are ablated and the temporal lobes are spared, the animals are severely impaired in learning to discriminate locations, but are relatively unimpaired in learning to discriminate among patterns; corresponding results have also been reported in humans after stroke (*18*).

Information-processing analyses. The observation that "what" and "where" are processed separately during perception leads to an explanation of why parts are imaged sequentially if the shape of each part is stored separately, and a part's location is specified relative to another part. If so, then one needs to have the reference part already activated before one can know where a subsequent part belongs in an image. When generating an image of a block letter F, for example, one might have encoded that there is a vertical line on the left, a horizontal line connected at its left side to the top of the vertical line, and another horizontal line connected at its left side to the vertical line midway down (94% of the subjects we have observed print the segments in this order). When forming the image, then, the vertical line on the left is a prerequisite for the other two lines; the locations of the horizontal lines are specified relative to the vertical line. Thus, some parts should be imaged before others. Finally, because one needs to attend to a specific place on the reference part in order to place a new part, and focal attention is restricted to only a single region of space at a time (*19*), only one part can be imaged at a time.

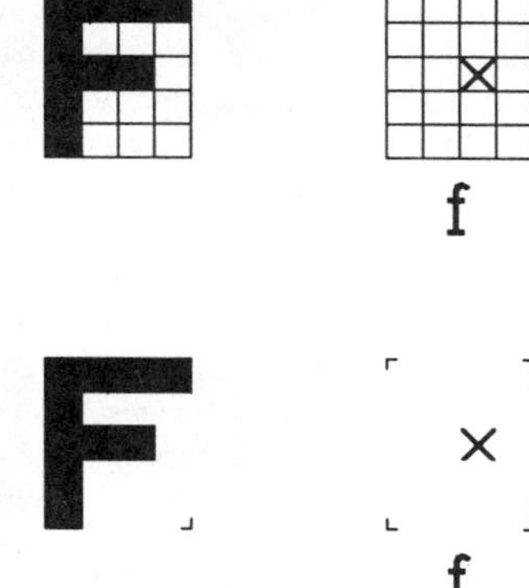

Fig. 1. (**Top left**) A letter formed by selectively filling in cells of a matrix. (**Top right**) Subjects were shown a lowercase cue and asked whether the corresponding uppercase block letter would occupy the cells containing one or two X marks. Because only 500 ms were allowed between presentation of the lowercase cue and the probe marks, which is not enough time to read the cue and finish forming the image, the decision times in part reflect the time to form the image in the matrix. (**Bottom**) An alternative way of presenting the stimuli, which was expected to induce a different method of arranging parts in the image.

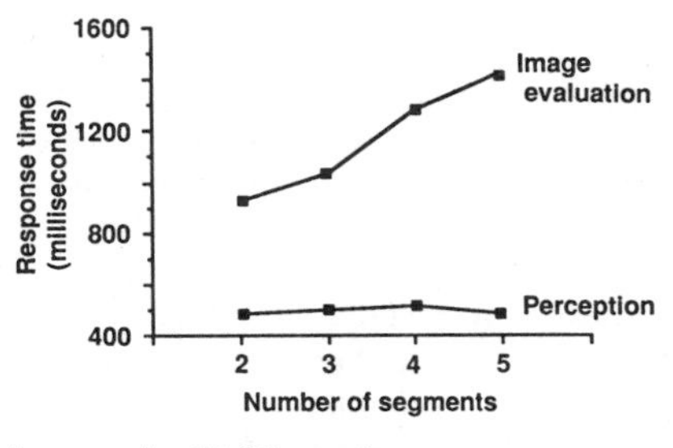

Fig. 2. The mean time to evaluate probe marks in the image evaluation and perception tasks when the farthest probe mark was on the first, second, third, or fourth segment typically drawn. The image evaluation task required deciding whether probes would have fallen on a letter, and the perception task required deciding whether probes actually did fall on a letter.

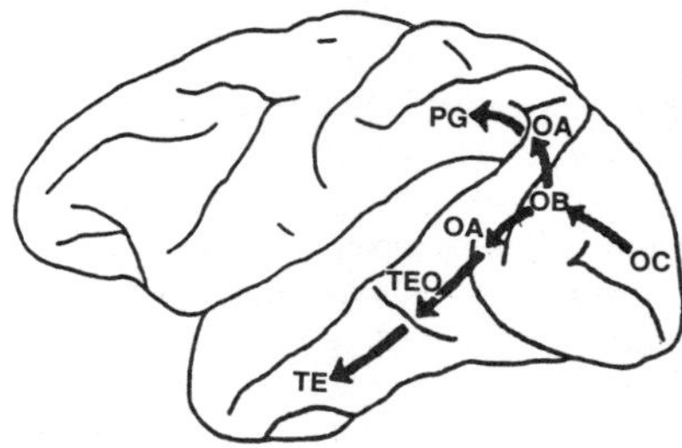

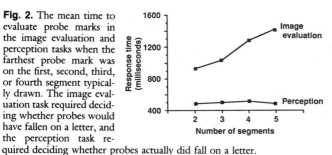

Fig. 3. The dorsal and ventral systems of the primate brain. [Adapted from (*32*)]

Consider first the assumption that individual parts of shapes are stored separately. When is this likely to occur? An important fact about the visual system is that it operates at multiple scales of analysis; it is sensitive to coarse overall features and to fine-grained features, and one can attend to a given scale. However, there appears to be a trade-off between scope and resolution (*20, 21*). For example, one can take in an entire human form, but not see much in the way of details about the face, or one can attend to individual features of the face at high resolution but lose the overall pattern. When one attends to details, the laws of perceptual organization serve to parse objects into parts, as was noted earlier (*13*). Attending to details is necessary to distinguish among similar objects that have different parts, such as letters; thus, parts should be encoded separately for such objects.

Consider next the assumption that part locations are stored relative to other parts. This assumption follows from an analysis of what would be required to build a machine that recognizes shape: for purposes of perceptual recognition, it is of limited use to store a single pattern to be matched against input as a template. Many objects (such as a dog, scissors, or a person) can assume a very large number of distinct shapes (as, for example, when a dog is scratching, sleeping, running, jumping, and so on). Similarly, many objects assume multiple variants on a shape, such as a letter of the alphabet (which comes in many fonts). In such cases, there are so many distinct shapes, and new ones occur all the time, that shapes may often arise that do not correspond to one previously seen and stored in memory. Thus, encoding a shape as a single pattern may not lead to a match with a previously stored shape.

A more effective way to represent such shapes is to extract specific properties that will not change when the object assumes a new configuration or a shape-variant appears. One such invariant is the type of spatial relation between parts. For example, no matter how a dog is contorted, the parts remain connected in the same way. I refer to this type of representation as categorical because equivalence classes of relations are specified. "Connected to" (or "above," "below," "inside," "next to," and so on) does not correspond to a particular topographic configuration, but rather specifies a large category of such configurations (for example, the foreleg remains "connected to" the upper leg no matter how the leg is bent or stretched. With such categorical representations, part locations are specified relative to other parts (*20*). If the appropriate categorical relations are used, a description of the arrangement of an object's parts will be the same across its various contortions and variations and, hence, will be useful for recognition.

Neuropsychological Hypothesis Testing

Images thus appear to be formed a part at a time because (i) shapes of individual parts of objects are stored separately, (ii) spatial relations among parts are stored separately from shapes, (iii) spatial relations specify location relative to other parts, (iv) stored parts and relations are used to form mental images, and (v) only a single reference point on a prior part can be located at a time. Hence, because parts can only be added when the reference part is present and the reference location on it has been found, parts will be imaged sequentially.

The separation of the storage of parts and spatial relations suggests a possible distinction between two classes of processes—ones that activate stored visual shapes and ones that gain access to and use stored spatial relations to arrange those shapes correctly. One way to garner evidence for this initial, rather coarse decomposition of the processing underlying image generation is to show that the two kinds of processing can be dissociated during image formation. Farah *et al.* and Kosslyn *et al.* have done just this in a series of experiments examining image generation in commissurotomy patients (*22, 23*).

One task we used required subjects to make judgments about letters. Letters were the initial stimuli of choice in part because of the evidence that they are imaged a segment at a time. The task was to decide from memory whether specific uppercase letters are composed only of straight lines (for example, A and H) or include at least one curved line (for example, B and D) (*24*); unless one has performed the task many times or intentionally memorized the responses, imagery is used to make this judgment (*23*). There were two critical assumptions in our experiments. First, we assumed that the shapes of letters are stored as segments and categorical spatial relations among them. Letters come in many different fonts, and one wants to recognize new instances; thus it is efficient to store categorical representations of the spatial relations among parts, which will apply to a wide range of different topographic positions. Second, we assumed that categorical relations are language-like (indeed, they almost always can be labeled by a word or two). This assumption was critical for our experiments because one uncontroversial fact about the functional specialization of the cerebral hemispheres is that for right-handed people the left hemisphere is superior to the right at producing and using language (*18*).

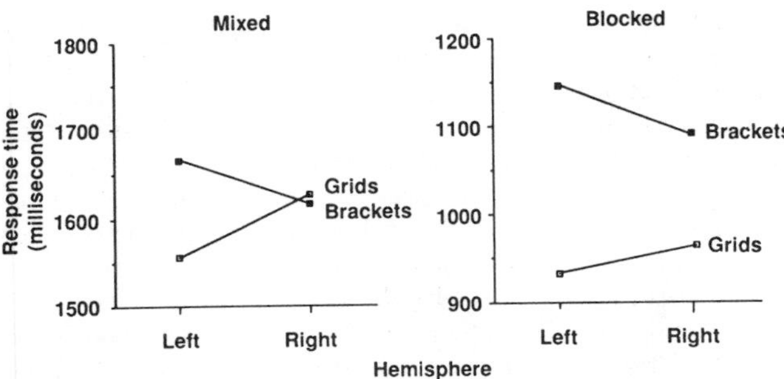

Fig. 4. The mean time required by normal right-handed people to evaluate single probe marks in lateralized grids. The grids were complete (grids) or reduced to four brackets at the corners (brackets) (see Fig. 1). (**Left**) Results when each letter was imaged only once before a new letter was presented (mixed trials). (**Right**) Results when the letter was imaged eight times in succession after the cue was presented (blocked trials). In mixed trials a lowercase cue was presented beneath the grid; in blocked trials the cue was presented at the central fixation point at the beginning of the trials.

Therefore, we expected that the left cerebral hemisphere would be better at generating images of letters, assuming that multiple parts would be composed by use of categorical spatial relations. In contrast, we expected no difference between the hemispheres in the ability to form images of single shapes, when separate representations of spatial relations would not be used; visual memories of shape should be equally available in both hemispheres. If we could document such a dissociation and implicate image generation differences as its cause, we would have evidence for a distinction between a mechanism that activates stored shapes and one that uses stored spatial relations to arrange them.

Documenting an Image-Generation Deficit

We tested these hypotheses by lateralizing lowercase letter cues. The lateralization procedure consisted of asking subjects to focus on a fixation point, and then to view stimuli presented 1.5° to the left or right of fixation. Because the cues were only presented for 150 ms, the subjects could not move their eyes to examine them, ensuring that the letter was projected onto only one half of the retina. Because the left half of each retina sends input only to the left cerebral hemisphere, and the right half of each retina sends input only to the right cerebral hemisphere, lateralizing stimuli in this way allowed us to provide input to the separate hemispheres (*25*).

The most detailed examination, which was conducted with patient J.W., will be summarized here (*23*). This patient had undergone surgery about 3 years before testing (for the treatment of otherwise intractable epilepsy), and magnetic resonance scanning revealed that his corpus callosum was fully sectioned. Because his corpus callosum was transected, information presented to one hemisphere was not available to the other hemisphere.

We began by lateralizing lowercase letters, and asking J.W. to judge whether the corresponding uppercase version had any curved lines. He pressed one key when he decided that the uppercase letter had at least one curved line and another if it had only straight lines. The results were striking: J.W.'s left hemisphere responded perfectly, whereas his right hemisphere was correct only 70% of the time; in a replication experiment, the left hemisphere again was perfect, whereas the right was correct only 65% of the time (*26*).

This finding is not enough to document an image generation deficit per se. A rather lengthy series of control experiments was required to eliminate various alternative accounts. The most simple control consisted of presenting J.W. with the uppercase letters themselves, and asking him to judge them as they appeared on the screen. Both hemispheres responded correctly on at least 97.5% of the trials. This result indicates that the right hemisphere deficit in the imagery task was not due to its being unable to perform the judgment, to encode letters, or produce appropriate key presses. In other control experiments we showed that both hemispheres could understand the correspondence between the lowercase cues and the uppercase letters, could retain images long enough to interpret their shapes, and could perform multipart tasks.

A selective deficit. We expected the right hemisphere to have difficulty generating images of letters if parts are activated sequentially and categorical representations of spatial relations are used to arrange the parts into the image. However, to argue that the difficulty lies in one class of processes and not others, it must be demonstrated that the right hemisphere can perform some imagery tasks, but not those in which the parts must be arranged with the use of categorical relations.

We reasoned that images should be constructed from parts whenever the task requires evaluation or comparison of parts; in these cases, high-resolution images of parts are necessary, and these representations were encoded and stored individually. In contrast, arranging parts should not be necessary to perform a task requiring imaging the overall shape of an object, if such a shape was encoded as a single perceptual unit. That is, even though such a template has little use in perceptual recognition for generalizing over variations in an object's shape, we expected relatively low-resolution patterns of overall shape to be encoded because they provide information about how an object is oriented in space, which is useful for navigation. If so, then we expected both hemispheres to be able to image such a pattern representing a single object. Although such a pattern would have a relatively low resolution, we reasoned that it should be sufficient to perform tasks that do not require comparing or evaluating parts (and hence high-resolution images of individual parts are not necessary).

In one task, J.W. was asked to decide which of two similar-sized animals (for example, a goat or a hog) was the larger, as seen from the side at the same distance; this task previously had been shown to require imagery (*27*). The name of one of the animals was lateralized, and hence only one hemisphere had the opportunity to perform the task. Only one error occurred during the entire testing session. This high level of performance is worrisome, however, in that it may reflect a "ceiling effect." The task may be so easy that it is insensitive to differences in hemispheric processing. Thus, we devised a second imagery task that did not require assembling parts, but which was considerably more difficult. J.W. was asked to decide whether named objects (book, nose, and buckle, for example) are taller than they are wide. This was a difficult task, given the stimuli we used, and resulted in overall worse performance. Nevertheless, both hemispheres could perform the task at better than chance levels of performance (50%), and did so equally well (70.8% versus 66.7% correct for the left and right hemispheres, respectively).

One could argue that all that has been shown is a difference for letters versus words. Thus, we conducted another task with the animal names presented in the size judgment experiment, but this task required comparing locations of parts, which we assumed required relatively high-resolution images of the parts—entailing the use of individually stored parts and spatial relations. We now asked J.W. to decide whether the named animal's ears protrude above the top of its skull (for example, an ape and a sheep versus a cat and a mouse). The left hemisphere performed correctly on 87.5% of the trials, whereas the right hemisphere performed correctly on only 45% of the trials. In short, the problem was not limited to letters, but apparently to tasks that involve juxtaposing parts.

Convergent evidence for the distinction between processes that activate images and that arrange parts is also available in the clinical literature. For example, Deleval *et al.* (*28*) describe a patient who experienced impaired imagery following left hemisphere damage. This patient claimed, "When I try to image a plant, an animal, an object, I can recall but one part, my inner vision is fleeting, fragmented; if I'm asked to imagine the head of a cow, I know that it has ears and horns, but I can't revisualize their respective places. In the same way, I cannot determine how many fingers a frog paw has, even though I have manipulated this animal each day in the laboratory. . . ."

Contrasting Left and Right Hemisphere Abilities

A second split-brain patient also provided evidence for a functional dissociation between processes that activate images and processes that arrange parts in images, with the left hemisphere being superior when the latter processes were required. However, only two subjects were tested, and these patients may have atypical cerebral organization due to years of severe epilepsy and the disconnection of the cerebral hemispheres at the time of testing. Thus it is important to show that the inferences about component processes and their neural realization generalize to normal people.

To obtain such converging evidence, a group of normal right-handed Harvard University students was tested in a variation of the grids imagery task described above (see the top panels of Fig. 1). After subjects memorized the block letters, they saw lateralized grids with a lowercase cue beneath them (64 trials, half presented in each visual field). The letters were presented in mixed order, with a letter not repeated in fewer than four trials. The grids now contained only a single "X" probe, as is illustrated in Fig. 1. Because the corpus callosa of these subjects is intact, information presented to one hemisphere will be transmitted to the other; thus, the primary measure of interest here was the time to respond: response times should be fastest when the hemisphere that receives the initial input is more effective in processing (*25*).

Consistent with the findings from the split-brain patients, these subjects evaluated the probes more quickly when the grid was presented to the right visual field (and hence was projected onto the left side of each retina and was seen first in the left cerebral hemisphere). However, it was possible that this result only reflected the left hemisphere's greater facility at reading the lowercase cues. Hence, as a control, an additional group of students was tested in a modified version of the task. The lowercase cue was now presented in the center (replacing the fixation point), not beneath the grid; after this, an empty grid with one probe mark was lateralized eight times (four in the left field, and four in the right, with no more than three trials appearing in the same field in a row and with the probe mark in a different location on each trial). Each new series of trials began with a different lowercase cue appearing in the center. As is evident in Fig. 4, although these subjects responded faster overall in this blocked design, a left hemisphere advantage was nevertheless obtained. Thus, the left hemisphere was shown to be better than the right hemisphere even in normal subjects at performing this multipart image generation task (*29*).

These experiments with normal subjects pushed the information-processing analyses one step further. The tests done with the split-brain patients hinged on the assumptions that categorical relations are used to arrange segments of letters and relative positions of animal parts in images, and that such relations are processed better in the left hemisphere. However, categorical representations cannot be the only method used by the brain to store spatial relations: what is a virtue for recognizing semirigid objects is a drawback for distinguishing among subtly different multipart shapes or for reaching or navigating. For these tasks, one needs to know the actual metric spatial relations among parts or objects. Knowing only that an object is "next to" the wall will not help one very much to find it and pick it up. For these sorts of tasks, the coordinates of an object must be internally represented. In short, information-processing considerations lead to the hypothesis that the brain can store spatial relations in two ways, either in terms of a category or in terms of more precise coordinates (*30*).

If this is so, then there should be two ways of forming images of a multipart object—by using either categorical or coordinate stored spatial relations to arrange parts. Given the evidence that the right hemisphere is more efficient at representing and processing metric spatial relations (*18*), the right hemisphere therefore should be better than the left when parts must be arranged in precise positions in an image. To test this idea, an additional group of students was tested in a modified version of the grids task; this task was the same as the grids task except that the internal lines were removed and only brackets at the four corners were depicted (as is illustrated in the bottom panels of Fig. 1). After subjects memorized the block letters as they appeared within the brackets, probe marks within the brackets were lateralized (lower right corner of Fig. 1), and the subjects were asked to decide whether the probe would fall on the letter were it within the brackets as previously shown. When grid lines are present, a categorical representation of how segments are connected is adequate; the grid lines are a crutch for placing segments properly in accordance with a description. In contrast, when only four corner brackets are present, more precise representations of segment location are necessary to determine whether an imaged letter would cover the X mark. Thus, it was expected that a process that uses coordinate representations to arrange parts would be recruited in this task, and that this process would be more effective in the right hemisphere.

The results from both the "grids" and "brackets" conditions are illustrated in Fig. 4. As expected, the subjects were faster when the brackets stimuli were presented to the left visual field, and hence were seen first in the right hemisphere. These results were obtained when lowercase cues were presented beneath the brackets ("mixed" presentation) or when an additional group saw them in the center before eight consecutive trials with that letter ("blocked" presentation); in both cases, these results are in sharp contrast to those obtained with grids, when categorical relations were presumably adequate.

In order to consider whether the results with the brackets were due to a right-hemisphere superiority at localizing the probe marks, and not due to image generation per se, a separate group of subjects was given an analog of the task that did not require image generation but did require encoding the probe location and comparing it to an uppercase letter. A probe X was lateralized within brackets (for 150 ms) and then replaced by an uppercase letter (as illustrated at the lower left of Fig. 1, for 100 ms). The task was to judge whether the X mark would have fallen on the letter, had they been superimposed. The letter served to mask the X, requiring subjects to encode its location into memory to be compared to the locations of the letter segments. As expected, the right hemisphere was superior when the metric location of the X had to be stored. However, this right hemisphere advantage was 3.2 times too small to account for the right hemisphere advantage for the brackets imagery task.

In short, both hemispheres can form images of the components, but the hemispheres apparently differ in the preferred way of arranging them. These results from normal subjects not only provide support for the inferences drawn from the split-brain subjects, but also provide evidence for a second means by which parts can be arranged in images (*31*).

Conclusions

In this article, I have illustrated how one can discover structure in mental abilities where none was obvious. After first examining behavior during task performance, facts about the brain and information-processing analyses can lead to relatively subtle hypotheses about processing. These hypotheses are testable in part by examining selective impairments in neuropathological populations. With this approach, it was found that the act of generating a visual mental image involves at least two classes of processes—ones that activate stored shapes and ones that use stored spatial relations to arrange shapes into an image. The discovery that the left hemisphere is better at arranging shapes when categorical information is appropriate, whereas the right hemisphere is better when coordinate information is necessary, suggests that the processes that arrange parts can be further decomposed into two classes that operate on different sorts of information.

The findings that under some circumstances the left cerebral hemisphere is better at mental imagery is counterintuitive to many. The left hemisphere has traditionally been identified with language, and the right with imagery *(22, 23, 28–30)*. However, neither hemisphere can be said to be the seat of mental imagery: imagery is carried out by multiple processes, not all of which are implemented equally effectively in the same part of the brain.

REFERENCES AND NOTES

1. A. Paivio, *Imagery and Verbal Processes* (Holt, Rinehart, & Winston, New York, 1971).
2. S. M. Kosslyn, *Image and Mind* (Harvard Univ. Press, Cambridge, 1980).
3. R. N. Shepard and L. A. Cooper, *Mental Images and Their Transformations* (MIT Press, Cambridge, 1982).
4. R. A. Finke and R. N. Shepard, in *Handbook of Perception and Human Performance*, K. R. Boff, L. Kaufman, J. P. Thomas, Eds. (Wiley, New York, 1986), vol. 37, p. 1.
5. M. J. Farah, *Psychol. Rev.*, in press.
6. D. C. Van Essen, in *Cerebral Cortex*, A. Peters and E. G. Jones, Eds. (Plenum, New York, 1985), vol. 3, p. 259.
7. L. G. Ungerleider and M. Mishkin, in *Analysis of Visual Behavior*, D. J. Ingle, M. A. Goodale, R. J. W. Mansfield, Eds. (MIT Press, Cambridge, 1982), p. 549.
8. S. J. Segal and V. Fusella, *J. Exp. Psychol.* **83**, 458 (1970).
9. C. W. Eriksen and B. A. Eriksen, *ibid.* **89**, 306 (1971).
10. This method was adapted from one developed to compare imagery and perception by P. Podgorny and R. N. Shepard, *J. Exp. Psychol.: Hum. Percept. Performance* **4**, 21 (1978).
11. S. M. Kosslyn, C. B. Cave, D. A. Provost, S. M. Von Gierke, *Cog. Psychol.*, in press.
12. J. D. Roth and S. M. Kosslyn, *Cog. Psychol.*, in press.
13. S. M. Kosslyn, B. J. Reiser, M. J. Farah, S. J. Fliegel, *J. Exp. Psychol. Gen.* **112**, 278 (1983); S. K. Reed and J. A. Johnsen, *Mem. Cog.* **3**, 569 (1975).
14. J. E. Hochberg, *Perception* (Prentice-Hall, New York, 1964); L. D. Kaufman, *Sight and Mind* (Oxford Univ. Press, New York, 1974); I. Biederman, *Psychol. Rev.* **94**, 115 (1987).
15. C. G. Gross, C. J. Bruce, R. Desimone, J. Fleming, R. Gattass, in *Cortical Sensory Organization II: Multiple Visual Areas*, C. N. Woolsey, Ed. (Humana, Clinton, NJ, 1984), p. 187.
16. R. Desimone, T. D. Albright, C. G. Gross, C. J. Bruce, *J. Neurosci.* **4**, 2051 (1984).
17. R. A. Andersen, G. K. Essick, R. M. Siegel, *Science* **230**, 456 (1985).
18. E. DeRenzi, *Disorders of Space Exploration and Cognition* (Wiley, New York, 1982); H. Hecaen and M. L. Albert, *Human Neuropsychology* (Wiley, New York, 1978).
19. C. J. Downing and S. Pinker, in *Attention and Performance XI*, M. I. Posner and O. S. I. Marin, Eds. (Erlbaum, Hillsdale, NJ, 1985), p. 177; D. LaBerge, *J. Exp. Psychol.: Hum. Percept. Performance* **9**, 371 (1983); M. I. Posner, C. R. R. Snyder, B. J. Davidson, *J. Exp. Psychol.: Gen.* **109**, 160 (1980); A. M. Treisman and G. Gelade, *Cog. Psychol.* **12**, 97 (1980).
20. D. Marr, *Vision* (Freeman, San Francisco, 1982).
21. H. Egeth in *The Psychology of Learning and Motivation*, G. H. Bower, Ed. (Academic Press, New York, 1977), p. 277; C. W. Eriksen and J. D. St. James, *Percept. Psychophys.* **40**, 225 (1986); J. Jonides, *Bull. Psychonomics Soc.* **21**, 247 (1983); G. L. Shulman and J. Wilson, *Perception* **16**, 89 (1987).
22. M. J. Farah, M. S. Gazzaniga, J. D. Holtzman, S. M. Kosslyn, *Neuropsychologia* **23**, 115 (1985).
23. S. M. Kosslyn, J. D. Holtzman, M. J. Farah, M. S. Gazzaniga, *J. Exp. Psychol. Gen.* **114**, 311 (1985).
24. This task is a variant of one developed by R. J. Weber and J. Castleman, *Percept. Psychophys.* **8**, 165 (1970).
25. J. G. Beaumont, Ed., *Divided Visual Field Studies of Cerebral Organization* (Academic Press, New York, 1982).
26. Both response time and accuracy were always measured in all of these experiments to ensure that errors were not made because of hurried decisions. Such possible speed-accuracy tradeoffs do not undermine the inferences drawn from any of the response time or accuracy results described here.
27. S. M. Kosslyn, G. L. Murphy, M. E. Bemesderfer, K. J. Feinstein, *J. Exp. Psychol.: Gen.* **106**, 341 (1977).
28. J. Deleval, J. De Mol, J. Noterman, *Acta Neurol. Belg.* **83**, 61 (1983) (M. J. Farah and O. Koenig, translators). See also M. J. Farah, D. N. Levine, R. Calvanio, *Brain Cog.*, in press; M. J. Farah, *Cognition* **18**, 245 (1984).
29. For additional converging results, see M. J. Farah, *Neuropsychologia* **24**, 541 (1986).
30. See S. M. Kosslyn [*Psychol. Rev.* **94**, 148 (1987)] for additional explication of, and evidence for, this distinction.
31. Only the results from the first set of trials are summarized here; additional trials were administered to assess possible changes in strategy with practice, as is describe by S. M. Kosslyn, J. R. Feldman, V. Maljkovic, S. Hamilton, unpublished manuscript.
32. M. Mishkin, L. G. Ungerleider, K. A. Macko, *Trends Neurosci.* **6**, 414 (1983).
33. Supported by NIMH grant MH 39478, ONR contract N00014-85-K-0291, and AFOSR contract 88-0012. Requests for reprints should be sent to S. M. Kosslyn, 1236 William James Hall, 33 Kirkland Street, Cambridge, MA 02138. I thank J. Gabrieli, O. Koenig and V. Maljkovic for critical readings, S. Hamilton and C. Moheban for technical assistance, and my collaborators and students cited herein for stimulating discussions and critical reviews of earlier works.

48

M. S. Gazzaniga, J. E. Bogen, and R. W. Sperry

Some functional effects of sectioning the cerebral commissures in man

1962. *Proceedings of the National Academy of Science* 48: 1765–1769

It has been possible in studies of callosum-sectioned cats and monkeys in recent years to obtain consistent demonstration of a variety of interhemispheric integrational functions mediated by the corpus callosum.[1,2] These animal findings stand in marked contrast to the apparent lack of corresponding functional deficits produced by similar surgery in human patients.[3–9] The general picture of callosal functions based on the animal studies tends to be supported in current early testing of a 48-year-old male war veteran with recent complete section of the corpus callosum, anterior and hippocampal commissures.

The patient (W. J.) had been having grand mal convulsions for fifteen years subsequent to war injuries suffered in 1944. The seizures were refractory to medical management with a frequency, at best, of about 1 per week and, at worst, of 7 to 10 per day culminating in status epilepticus every 2–3 months. The subject was right handed, had an I.Q. of 113, and showed no significant sensory, motor, or associative disturbances in a battery of visual, tactile, and motor tests applied prior to surgery, excepting a mild hypesthesia on the left side.

The commissures were sectioned in a single operation by exposure and retraction of right frontal and occipital lobes. The massa intermedia was judged by the surgeons[10] to be absent and some atrophy of the exposed right frontal pole was observed. Generalized weakness, akinesis, and mutism were evident immediately after surgery but had largely cleared when postoperative testing was started. Anticonvulsant medication was reinstated shortly after surgery. There have since been three brief attacks with loss of consciousness but as yet no major convulsions. Occasional brief episodes of clonic-like tremor confined to the distal portions of the right arm or leg have also been noted. The operation appears to have left no gross changes in temperament or intellect, and the patient has repeatedly remarked that he feels better generally than he has in many years.

The tests referred to below were carried out from the 6th to 20th weeks after surgery in weekly 3-hour sessions, mostly in the laboratory but on a few occasions in the patient's home, usually with the patient's physician and wife present. The general test repertoire included a considerable carry-over of items from previous clinical studies plus some new and revised test procedures designed on the basis of observed effects of brain bisection in animals.

Tests involving tactual function have revealed no significant impairments in the right side of the body connected to the dominant left hemisphere. Similar testing of the left hand, however, has indicated a severe agnosia, anomia, and agraphia. For example, in blindfold tests, the patient has regularly been able to manipulate and use correctly most familiar objects such as a pencil, cigarette, ring, pistol, hat, glasses, etc., but has been totally unable to name or to describe any of these. Prior to surgery he could write legibly with the left hand, but afterward has produced only a meaningless scribble.

Also, he locates accurately points of tactile stimulation on the fingers of either hand by touching with the thumb of the same hand, immediately or with a 5 sec delay imposed. He is quite unable, however, under similar conditions to cross-locate with either hand across to the other. Such cross localization is possible for points on the head, face, and upper neck. Taste and touch are both reported correctly from either side of the tongue. When tapped lightly one to four times on one foot or hand, the subject can accurately tap a corresponding number of times with the hand of the same side but is unable to tap the correct number with the opposite hand. Simple jigsaw cutouts could be put together correctly with either hand separately but not when cooperation between both hands was required. In general, when stimulus and response are confined to the same hemisphere in such tests, the performance goes well, but when cross-integration is required, the activity breaks down.

Visual tests were conducted with tachistoscopic presentation of stimuli at 1/10 and 1/100 sec. The results reveal no marked abnormality in response to stimulation of the right visual half-field, projected to the dominant hemisphere. In the left half-field, however, there is a profound agnosia for all stimuli presented. When very simple geometric designs, or single large numbers or letters are flashed to this half-field, the subject can retrieve the corresponding figure at a level 30 per cent above chance from among a series of five or more patterns on cards placed within easy reach of the left hand. He is unable to perform above chance, however, when colors are used, or when he is obliged to select the same cards with the opposite hand. Also, he has been unable to name, draw a rough semblance, or to otherwise describe the left field figures with either hand or verbally. More complicated written material is read easily in the right half-field but evokes only a blank response from the left field. In visuomotor studies with the right hand working a push button, he responds to the simple on-flash of a small light when it appears in the right half-field only, while with the left hand he is able to respond to the light signal in either field. When a choice between red and green lights was required, the reaction was correct only for responses of the right hand to stimuli in the right half field. In simple visual constructional tests, as in copying a sketch of a Necker cube, the drawings of the left hand were less defective than those of the right.

With respect to motor function no special coordinative difficulty has been observed in tests involving independent use of the right hand. The left hand also is capable of refined individuated finger movements and generally is adept and dextrous enough in the performance of familiar automatic activities such as handling and smoking a cigarette, lifting a coffee cup, putting on glasses, and the like. The left hand also works well along with the right in other habitual tasks such as tying a knot in the belt of his robe, folding towels, putting on and removing clothes. In other respects, however, the use of the left hand is obviously impaired. For example, if the patient is interrupted in any of the foregoing activities and asked to repeat on command with his left hand any of these motor performances or even to make much simpler movements, the left arm and hand may fail to respond at all or the response may be spasmodic and grossly inadequate. Much as in a stammerer's block, the more intense the effort, the more difficult to achieve the movement. In the early tests especially, a profound apraxia was apparent with respect to any independent movements of the left hand in response to a purely verbal command. Beginning with the 3rd month, however, if the test was presented with nonverbal aids, i.e., if the experimenter said. "Do this" and demonstrated the requested movement, then the patient with the left hand was usually able to follow very simple actions like writing a T or an L and lifting individual fingers as in a piano exercise.

Movements like lifting the left hand and placing it behind the head or using it to point to something, i.e., responses that could not be carried out by the left hand alone to a verbal command, were achieved readily when he was directed to use both hands to make the same or symmetrical movements. Frequently, when his left hand had been fumbling ineffectively at some task, he would become exasperated and reach across with the right hand to grab the left and place it in the proper position.

None of these apraxic difficulties was apparent in the use of the dominant right hand during the regular testing sessions. However, transient difficulty with the right hand was reportedly seen on a few occasions by the patient's wife. She has also noted antagonism between the actions of the right and left hands, e.g., the patient would pick up the evening paper with the right hand, but put it down abruptly with the left and then have to pick it up again with the right. Similar contradictory movements were observed occasionally in the course of dressing and undressing, and in other daily activities, at times on a scale sufficient to be distinctly bothersome. It was as if the control of the left hand were strongly centered in the minor hemisphere at such times and hence isolated from the main intent and prevailing directorship of the dominant hemisphere.

There were further indications that the separated hemispheres were each unaware of activity going on in the other in the case of those functions that are highly lateralized, e.g., visual perception within right or left half-field, language functions, or tactile and motor functions of the extremities. For example, the patient often retrieved a correct visual stimulus card with the left hand after exposure to the left visual half-field, but after the card had been turned over he was completely unable, on request, to describe or to otherwise use the major hemisphere to identify the figure he had chosen. Or, after responding intently with the correct count by the left hand to a series of tactile stimuli applied to the left leg or hand, it was often clear from his reply to question that in his literate hemisphere he had been totally unaware of having either felt the stimuli or made the response. In a few tests involving the learning of simple tactile discriminations with right or left hand, the learning did not carry over to the opposite hand.

The severe left apraxia following callosal section may have been exaggerated in this patient by an unnatural potentiation of cerebral dominance and the lateralization of volitional control as a result of the damage to the non-dominant cortex incurred in his injuries of 1944. On the other hand, since pre-operative studies suggested a focus in the left parietal lobe,[10] it is also possible that damage to the left hemisphere may have impaired its ipsilateral motor control thus leading to exaggeration of the left apraxia after commissurotomy. The extent to which visual perception is intact in the left half-field still remains something of a problem that it may be possible to settle with further tests that combine half-field presentation with non-verbal responses.

The question of how typical the findings in this case may be is complicated by the unknown amount and nature of the pre-existent cerebral damage. Nevertheless the marked differences between the pre- and post-operative results and most of the other impairments observed seem best ascribed to interruption of the commissural connections particularly those linking the sensory and motor areas of the right cerebral cortex with the speech and related centers of the dominant left hemisphere. The results are in line with the picture of callosal function obtained from recent animal studies and with certain minority interpretations of callosal lesions in man as reviewed by Sweet[11] and amplified recently by Geschwind.[12] They appear to favor the existence of a genuine callosal or cerebral deconnection syndrome in human adult subjects who have been free of childhood cerebral complications, and have the normal lateralization of language.

With regard to the discrepancy between the foregoing and the apparent absence of similar disconnection impairments is the majority of callosum-sectioned patients previously described, the following are of interest: Visual testing without tachistoscopic control in the present patient failed to demonstrate satisfactorily his left hemiagnosia. His depth perception and stereoscopic vision are preserved. Blindfold learning of part of a stylus maze of the same type used in the earlier studies[8] transferred at a high level in this patient also from either hand to the other. Further, the first author had earlier applied a number of the same visual and tactile tests to a nine-year-old boy of above-average intelligence with reported congenital agenesis of the corpus callosum complicated by postnatal hydrocephalus. This boy performed close to the level of normal control children with almost no indication of the disconnection effects observed in the adult surgical patient. Bilateralization of cortical speech centers and other compensatory developmental effects are presumed to be present in the boy with agenesis. On the other hand, the normal right-handedness of the surgical patient and correlated lateralization of speech, the development of which took a normal course to well beyond 30 years of age is considered important to the observed impairments. By contrast, many of the earlier cases studied had childhood neurological complications. Finally, it is entirely possible that a significant range of variability is normal in the development of callosal functions in different individuals, and that a corresponding spectrum is therefore to be expected in the syndrome of the corpus callosum. Even so, there remain some puzzling inconsistencies not satisfactorily resolved as yet. Testing is still in progress and more thorough detailed reports are contemplated.

Notes

The authors wish to express their regard and thanks to the patient and his wife for the invaluable cooperation throughout.

Aided by the F. P. Hixon Fund of the California Institute of Technology and by grants to the Institute, No. M3372 and No. 2G86, from the U.S. Public Health Service.

1. Sperry, R. W., *Fed. Proc.*, **20**, 609 (1961).

2. Sperry, R. W., *Science*, **133**, 1749 (1961).

3. Akelaitis, A. J., *Arch. Neurol. Psychiat.*, **45**, 788 (1941).

4. Akelaitis, A. J., *J. Neuropath. Exp. Neurol.*, **2**, 226 (1943).

5. Akelaitis, A. J., *J. Neurosurg.*, **1**, 94 (1944).

6. Bremer, F., J. Brihaye, and G. Andre-Balisaux, *Schweiz. Arch. Neurol. Psychiat.*, **78**, 31–87 (1956).

7. Bridgman, C. S., and K. U. Smith, *J. Comp. Neurol.*, **83**, 57–68 (1945).

8. Smith, K. U., *Science*, **114**, 117 (1951).

9. Smith, K. U., and A. J. Akelaitis, *Arch. Neurol. Psychiat.*, **47**, 519–543 (1942).

10. Bogen, J. E., and P. J. Vogel, *Bull. Los. Angeles Neurol. Soc.* (in press).

11. Sweet, W. H., *Arch. Neurol. Psychiat.*, **45**, 86–104 (1941).

12. Geschwind, N., *New Engl. J. Med.* (in press).

B. Milner and M. Petrides

Behavioural effects of frontal-lobe lesions in man

1984. *Trends in Neurosciences* 7: 403–407

Abstract

The study of patients with excisions from the frontal lobes has revealed specific cognitive deficits that appear against a background of normal functioning on a variety of perceptual and memory tasks, as well as on conventional intelligence tests. These deficits include a reduced output on fluency tasks, faulty regulation of behaviour of external cues, and impaired organization and monitoring of material to be remembered, and of the subject's own responses. Differential effects related to the side of the lesion are less consistently observed after frontal- than after temporal-lobe excisions. Such effects, when they do occur, may depend as much on the demands of the task as on the nature of the test material.

The part of the frontal lobe that lies anterior to the primary motor area reaches its maximum development in the human brain. The present article deals with the functions of this large expanse of cortex, excluding the speech area of Broca at the foot of the inferior frontal gyrus in the left hemisphere. The frontal cortex has major reciprocal connections with the posterior parietal, prestriate and temporal cortex[1,2]. It is thus in a position to influence as well as receive input from these posterior cortical regions, which are involved in the analysis and long-term storage of somatosensory, visual and auditory information. Its projections to structures such as the hypothalamus and amygdala allow for the regulation of emotional responses[3], whilst projections to the precentral cortex[4,5] and the neostriatum[6,7] provide direct routes to the motor systems[8].

Ideas concerning the functions of the frontal lobes have ranged widely over time. In sharp contrast to the claims of some early investigators who believed that the frontal lobes were 'the seat of intelligence', a number of studies have demonstrated that significant damage to this part of the brain is compatible with normal performance on conventional intelligence tests[9–12], as well as on various perceptual, linguistic, and memory tasks that can be sensitive indicators of damage to posterior cortex or to medial temporal-lobe structures[13,14]. Clinical observation, on the other hand, has suggested that many individuals with frontal-lobe lesions show poor adjustment to everyday life, not only because of changes in personality, but also because of inability to organize their everyday activities[15–17] and reduced flexibility and inventiveness in their approach to new problems[16]. During the past twenty years, several investigations have confirmed the existence of such cognitive deficits and have delineated them further by means of experimental procedures derived from the animal laboratory, as well as by a more extensive sampling of intellectual abilities than that provided by IQ tests[10–18].

Divergent Thinking

Traditional intelligence tests may be said to measure different aspects of convergent thinking[19], in the sense that there is usually just one correct answer to the question or problem set. Tests of divergent thinking, in contrast emphasize the number and variety of responses that can be produced to a single question; an example would be a task that required one to list different possible uses of a given object, such as a brick, within a prescribed time limit. Tasks of this kind are held to be better predictors of creative achievement than are standard intelligence tests[19], and Zangwill[20] has suggested that performance on such tasks may be particularly vulnerable to the effects of frontal-lobe injury. So far the strongest support for this notion comes from the domain of verbal fluency, where patients with left frontal-lobe lesions in the dominant hemisphere for speech have been repeatedly shown to be impaired on tasks such as the Thurstone Word Fluency Test, in which they are required to generate in a limited time as many four-letter words as possible beginning with a specified letter[10,20–23]. In addition, such patients, although not dysphasic, show a marked impoverishment of spontaneous speech and writing. The question of whether corresponding deficits on non-verbal fluency tasks might follow right non-dominant frontal-lobe lesions was explored by Jones-Gotman and Milner[24] in an experiment in which normal subjects and patients with various cortical excisions were asked to draw as many different, unnameable designs as they could invent in a given time. Patients with right frontal or right fronto-central lesions were the most severely impaired group, although a milder deficit followed lesions of the left frontal lobe. Thus, the evidence points to some complementary specialization of the left and right frontal lobes with respect to fluency, although laterality effects tend to be less easy to demonstrate in the case of the frontal than of the temporal lobes[13].

Temporal Organisation and Memory

Whether or not memory deficits can be demonstrated after frontal-lobe lesions depends more on how memory is tested than on the nature of the material to be retained, although there are minor material-specific effects that vary with the side of the lesion. Prisko[10] has shown that patients with frontal neocortical excisions do poorly on delayed-comparison tasks in which a few easily discriminable stimuli recur in different pairings throughout the test, and the subject must say on any given trial whether or not the second stimulus differed from the first (presented 60 seconds before). To succeed requires the suppression of the potentially interfering memory of previous trials; Prisko's results suggest that the frontal-lobe lesions affected the patients' ability to keep the various trials apart[25,26], and hence that in the absence of other contextual cues they were less able than normal subjects[27] to distinguish the immediately preceding stimulus from stimuli presented earlier.

Subsequent work by Corsi[26], using three tasks that embodied different kinds of stimulus material (concrete words, representational drawings and abstract paintings), has provided direct evidence that frontal-lobe lesions can impair the temporal ordering of recent events. On these recency-discrimination tasks, subjects were shown a long series of cards in fairly rapid succession, each card bearing two simulus-items; whenever a question-mark appeared between the items (as in Fig. 1), the subject had to indicate which of the two items had been seen more recently. Usually both items had been shown before (say, 8 cards ago as compared with 32), but in the limiting condition one of them was new, in which case the task reduced to a simple test of recognition memory. Patients with temporal-lobe lesions showed mild deficits on the recognition measures (verbal after left temporal lobectomy, non-verbal after right) but no impairment of recency discrimination as such. In contrast, patients with frontal-lobe lesions could distinguish normally between material that had been presented before and material that was new, but they were impaired in judging the relative recency of two previously seen items.

On such tasks, recency judgements are apt to be based on the relative salience of the items in memory, since the series are too long to permit rehearsal of the temporal order of the stimuli, and there is no scope for organization of the material by the subject. Under these conditions, we see a predominant role of the right frontal lobe in test performance, together with some interaction between the nature of the test material and the side of the lesion. Patients with left frontal-lobe lesions showed a moderate impairment on the verbal task, whereas the right frontal-lobe group performed at chance on the abstract paintings, as well as having a clear impairment on the representational drawings.

A somewhat different pattern of results emerged from another memory task, self-ordered pointing[28], in which subjects were presented with a small stack of cards (6, 8, 10 or 12), each bearing a regular array of stimulus-items, the relative position of which varied from card to card. The task was to go through the stack touching one item on each card, in any order, but never touching the same item twice. This meant that subjects had to keep track of their own past responses while actively planning the ones to come. As in the recency task, several kinds of material were used (concrete words, abstract words, representational drawings—cf. Fig. 2, and abstract designs), and this time the group with left frontal-lobe lesions was impaired on every version of the task, a deficit being evident on all but the six-item arrays. The right frontal-lobe group, in contrast, showed merely a mild impairment on the non-verbal tests.

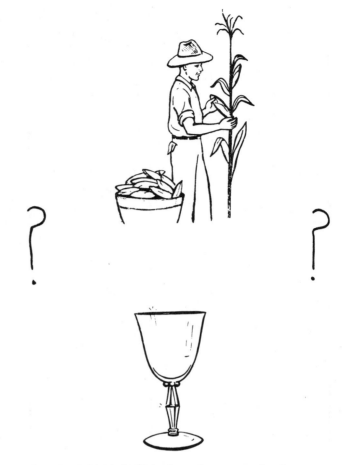

Figure 1. Recency-discrimination task: representational drawings. Sample test card. The subject must point to the item seen most recently.

Further evidence of a special contribution of the left frontal lobe to the organization and planning of responses comes from an experiment by Shallice and McCarthy[29] in which coloured beads threaded on rods in various configurations had to be transferred to specified target sites on these same rods in a minimum number of moves. Patients with right anterior lesions

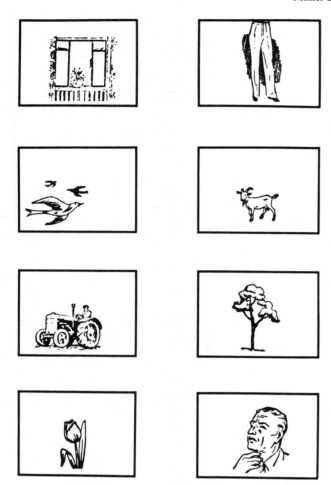

Figure 2. Self-ordered pointing task: stimuli used in the eight-item set of representational drawings.

were unimpaired, as were those with posterior lesions of either hemisphere, but patients with left anterior lesions were slower to develop the appropriate strategies and thus made more incorrect moves. Their failure did not seem to be attributable to verbal or spatial difficulties but rather to an inability to plan a few moves ahead. As we saw in the results for self-ordered pointing, such a planning deficit can impair performance on a memory task.

The poor performance of patients with unilateral excisions of dorsolateral frontal cortex on the memory tasks described above appears to result from a failure in the control processes of memory rather than from a deficit in retention as such. The next section deals with the question of generalized memory impairment following medial frontal-lobe lesions.

Amnesia after Aneurysms of the Anterior Communicating Artery

A global amnesic syndrome has been described in association with tumours invading the medial parts of the frontal lobes[30] or ruptured aneurysms of the anterior communicating artery[30,31], with presumed or demonstrated damage to the ventromedial frontal cortex. In such cases, the pathological changes have not been restricted to the frontal cortex but have extended to other basal forebrain regions, such as the septal nuclei and nucleus accumbens, as well as to related fibre systems (e.g. the columns of the fornix)[31,32]. It has, in fact, been suggested[31] that damage to these latter structures may have been responsible for the amnesic syndromes observed. A recent investigation by Mishkin and Bachevalier[33] has, however, provided some experimental evidence in favour of the notion that the ventromedial frontal cortex is directly involved in memory processes; this study demonstrated that monkeys with lesions of the ventromedial, but not of the dorsolateral frontal cortex, were impaired on a recognition-memory task.

Cues and the Regulation of Behaviour

Although patients with frontal-lobe lesions respond normally to environmental stimuli, they appear to have difficulty in using these stimuli to regulate their actions. A clear example of this is provided by the performance of such patients on a problem-solving task, the Wisconsin Card Sorting Test (illustrated in Fig. 3). In this task, the correct way of responding has first to be inferred from verbal feed-back provided by the examiner; then, once a particular mode of responding has been established, new sorting principles must be discovered, again on the basis of feed-back from the examiner. On tasks of this kind, the impairments observed after a frontal-lobe lesion appear to stem from the patient's inability to overcome previously established response tendencies, resulting in the generation of fewer hypotheses and, frequently, in a high incidence of errors involving perseveration[10,34,35]. No deficits are seen on the card-sorting test after unilateral orbital[10,34] or inferior[10] frontal-lobe lesions, whereas persistent impairment typically follows excisions from the superior frontal cortex[10,34]. The deficit may be seen after a frontal-lobe removal from either hemisphere but is more reliably associated with left-sided lesions than with right.

The inability of patients with frontal-lobe lesions to derive normal benefit from environmental signals elicited by their own responses is also evident in their performance on stylus-maze tasks (whether visual[10] or tactual[36]) in which the route cannot be figured out in advance but must be learned by trial-and-error on the basis of auditory feed-back from a bell or buzzer. The valence of the signals does not appear to be a relevant factor in the slowness of learning observed after frontal-lobe damage, since performance is impaired irre-

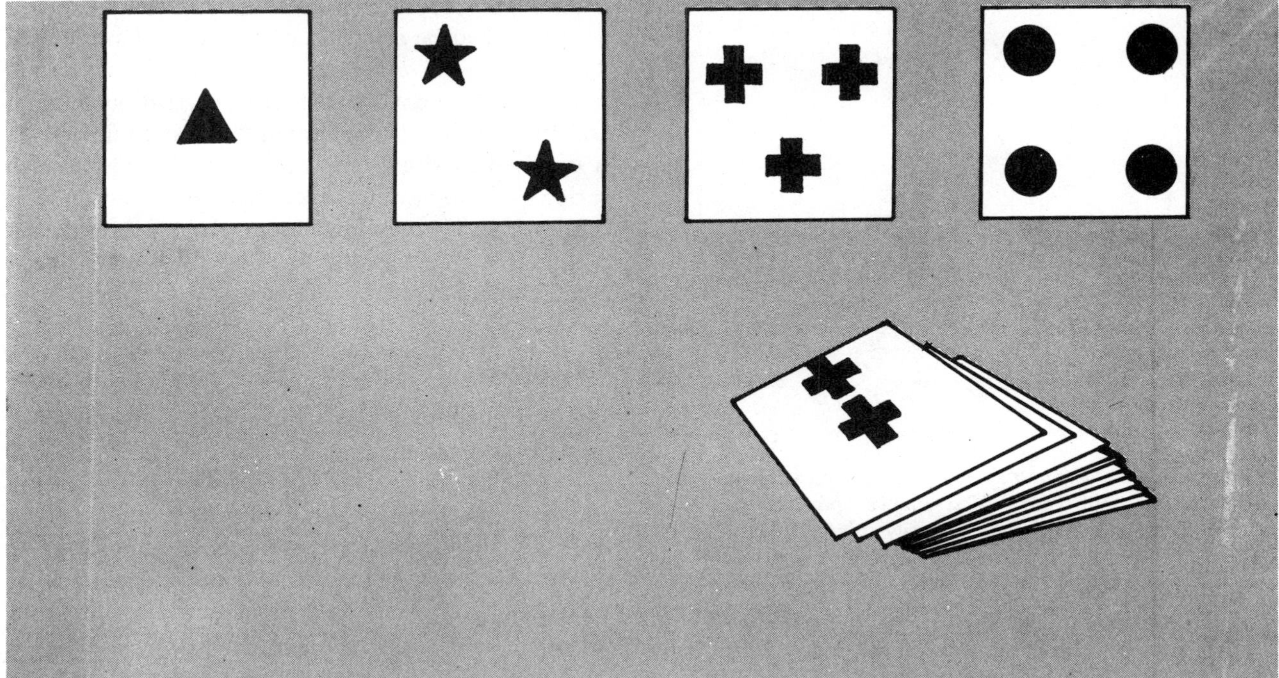

Figure 3. Wisconsin Card Sorting Test, showing the material as presented to the subject: stimulus cards above; response cards below. The instruction is to place each response card in front of one or other of the stimulus cards, wherever the subject thinks it should go; the examiner will then inform the subject whether the response was 'right' or 'wrong'. This information is to be used to get as many cards right as possible. Correction of mistakes is not allowed.

Colour is arbitrarily designated the first sorting category, all matches other than colour being called 'wrong': then, after 10 consecutive correct responses, the sorting principle shifts to form without warning, and subjects must modify their strategy accordingly. This procedure is repeated until six sorting categories (colour, form, number, colour, form, number) have been completed or until all the response cards have been placed. (*Reproduced from Ref 43 with permission of the publisher.*)

spective of whether the auditory signals follow correct or incorrect responses at a choice-point[37]. Luria[16] has argued that a disturbance in the verbal regulation of behaviour is a distinctive feature of frontal-lobe injury in man; these maze-learning results suggest that this formulation is too narrow, a similar disturbance being seen in the case of non-verbal signals. It is worth noting that the maze-learning deficits are more striking after right frontal-lobe lesions than after left, presumably reflecting the greater contribution of the right hemisphere to spatial processes.

In addition, patients with unilateral frontal-lobe excisions show a peculiarity of behaviour on maze-learning tasks that is rarely encountered in other subjects. This is a failure to comply with task instructions, the most noticeable example being to disregard the buzzer signalling an error, thereby continuing in the incorrect path and triggering further error signals[10]. This rule-breaking behaviour disappears spontaneously after a few trials[10,37], only to appear again on the next novel task. It seems reasonable to suppose that such behaviour is a special instance of the loss of inhibition that is often said to characterize the behaviour of such individuals in everyday life[16,17]. It also recalls the high incidence of impulsive errors observed on the Porteus mazes after frontal lobotomy[10], despite the fact that on those mazes the correct path is visible from the start.

An interesting example of lack of inhibition has recently been described by Lhermitte[38], who reported that patients with massive damage to the frontal lobes, unlike control subjects or patients with posterior cerebral lesions, would begin to use objects presented to them, such as a pen and a sheet of paper, without having been instructed to do so. Whether, however, such behaviour would occur after lesions restricted to the frontal cortex, without concomitant damage to the caudate nucleus or other subcortical structures, remains unclear.

Conditional Associative Learning

Following earlier work carried out with experimental animals[39–41], Petrides[26] has shown that patients who have sustained excisions from the frontal cortex are severely impaired in mastering conditional associative-learning tasks. In these tasks, the subjects have a set of responses available to them and must learn to produce the correct one when the appropriate stimulus is pre-

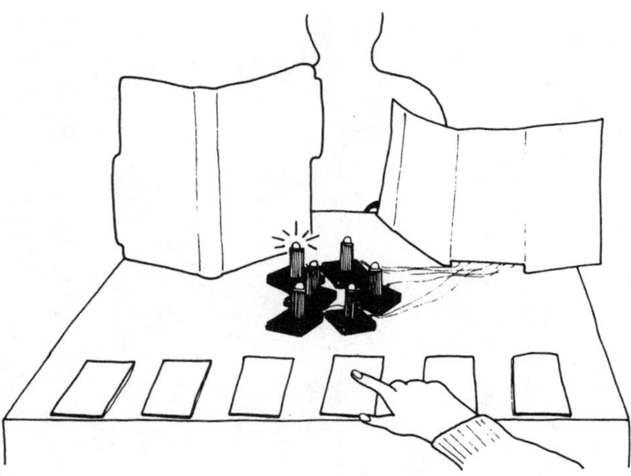

Figure 4. Sketch of apparatus used by Petrides to test spatial conditional associative-learning. The stimuli are presented by means of six identical blue lamps, randomly grouped together. When one of these lights up, the subject must respond by touching a particular one of the six identical response cards arranged horizontally in front of him. (*Reproduced from Ref. 26 with permission of the publisher.*)

sented. In one such task (see Fig. 4), the subject was faced with six white cards and six blue lamps. When one of these lamps was turned on, the subject had to respond by touching the cards one at a time until he found the correct one; after each response, the experimenter told the subject whether he was right or wrong. The lamp was turned off when the correct card had been touched, and a different lamp was lit to initiate the next trial. Patients with unilateral cortical excisions from the left or right frontal lobe exhibited marked impairments in learning this spatial conditional task, in contrast to patients with excisions of the left or right anterior temporal neocortex and amygdala who acquired it at a normal rate.

Deficits after unilateral frontal-lobe excisions were also observed on a non-spatial conditional task in which each of a set of six differently coloured stimuli was paired with one of six hand postures. The patients with frontal-lobe lesions could not learn to produce the correct responses to the stimuli, despite the fact that they had learned the hand postures before testing began and could reproduce them from memory throughout the test session.

In studies with patients, it is difficult to establish the critical regions within the frontal cortex involved in conditional learning because the excisions are rarely confined to anatomically distinct areas. In recent work with the monkey, the effect of selective lesions within the frontal cortex on the performance of analogous conditional tasks has been examined. It has been shown that lesions of the periarcuate cortex (areas 6 and 8) impair the acquisition of one such task[41]; in addition, postoperative retention of a similar task has been found to be deficient after lesions of area 6 (see Ref. 42).

The work on conditional tasks, carried out in man and monkey, has demonstrated that the frontal cortex is involved in situations where specific responses to various stimuli have to be learned and produced. The studies with monkeys, furthermore, have indicated that the posterior part of the dorsolateral frontal cortex may be the critical region.

Perspectives

The experimental work carried out in man and other primates has laid the groundwork for further exploration of the functions of the frontal cortex. It has become clear from both the behavioural and the anatomical work that the frontal cortex is neither functionally nor structurally homogeneous and that various subsystems can be identified. In the monkey, the investigation of the effects of restricted lesions, guided by the considerable anatomical knowledge now available, will undoubtedly continue to refine our understanding of these subsystems. The development of positron emission tomography, enabling the measurement of metabolic activity in relation to various psychological processes, opens up the possibility of identifying more precisely some of these subsystems in the human brain, as well as revealing functional relationships not only with other cortical areas but also with subcortical structures such as the basal ganglia, thalamus and brainstem, relationships clearly suggested by the anatomy and earlier behavioural work with nonhuman primates. In particular, it will be of interest to elucidate the interaction of frontal cortex with medial temporal-lobe structures in memory processes[30–33,44].

Acknowledgements

We thank the Linguaphone Institute for permission to reproduce the drawings illustrated in Fig. 2. The work of Brenda Milner was supported by the Medical Research Council of Canada.

Reading List

1. Jones, E. G. and Powell, T. P. S. (1970) *Brain* 93, 793–820.

2. Chavis, D. A. and Pandya, D. N. (1976) *Brain Res.* 117, 369–386.

3. Nauta, W. J. H. (1971) *J. Psychiatr. Res.* 8, 167–187.

4. Matsumura, M. and Kubota, K. (1979) *Neurosci. Lett.* 11, 241–246.

5. Muakkassa, K. F. and Strick, P. L. (1979) *Brain Res.* 177, 176–182.

6. Kemp, J. M. and Powell, T. P. S. (1970) *Brain* 93, 525–546.

7. Goldman, P. S. and Nauta. W. J. H. (1977) *J. Comp. Neurol.* 171, 369–385.

8. Kolb, B. and Milner, B. (1981) *Neuropsychologia* 19, 491–504.

9. Hebb, D. O. (1939) *J. Gen. Psychol.* 21, 73–87.

10. Milner, B. (1964) in *The Frontal Granular Cortex and Behavior* (Warren, J. M. and Akert, K., eds), pp. 313–334, McGraw-Hill, New York.

11. Teuber, H.-L. (1964) in *The Frontal Granular Cortex and Behavior* (Warren, J. M. and Akert, K.. eds), pp. 410–144, McGraw-Hill, New York.

12. Black, F. W. (1976) *J. Clin. Psychol.* 32, 366–372.

13. Milner, B. (1980) in *Nerve Cells, Transmitters and Behaviour* (Levi-Montalcini, R., ed.), pp. 601–625, Pont. Acad. Scientiarum, Vatican City.

14. Stuss, D. T., Kaplan, E. F., Benson, D. F., Weir, W. S., Chiulli, S. and Sarazin, F. F. (1982) *J. Comp. Physiol. Psychol.* 6, 913–925.

15. Penfield, W. and Evans, J. (1935) *Brain* 58, 115–133.

16. Luria, A. R. (1969) in *Handbook of Clinical Neurology* Vol. 2 (Vinken, P. J. and Bruyn, G. W., eds), pp. 725–757, North Holland, Amsterdam.

17. Fuster, J. M. (1980) *The Prefrontal Cortex: Anatomy, Physiology and Neurophyschology of the Frontal Lobe.* Raven Press, New York.

18. Shallice, T. and Evans, M. E. (1978) *Cortex* 14, 294–303.

19. Guilford, J. P. (1967) *The Nature of Human Intelligence*, McGraw-Hill, New York.

20. Zangwill, O. L. (1966) *Int. J. Neurol.* 5, 395–402.

21 Benton, A. L. (1968) *Neuropsychologia* 6, 53–60.

22. Ramier, A. M. and Hécaen, H. (1970) *Rev. Neurol.* 123, 17–22.

23. Perret, E. (1974) *Neuropsychologia* 12, 323–330.

24. Jones-Gotman, M. and Milner, B. (1977) *Neuropsychologia* 15, 653–674.

25. Pribram, K. H. and Tubbs, W. E. (1967) *Science*, 156, 1765–1767.

26. Milner, B. (1982) *Phil. Trans. R. Soc. London. Ser. B* 298, 211–226.

27. Yntema, D. B. and Trask, F. B. (1963) *J. Verb. Learn Verb. Behav.* 2, 65–74.

28. Petrides, M. and Milner, B. (1982) *Neuropsychologia* 20, 249–262.

29. Shallice, T. (1982) *Phil. Trans. R. Soc. London Ser. B* 298, 199–209.

30. Luria, A. R. (1976) *The Neuropsychology of Memory* John Wiley & Sons, New York.

31. Gade, A. (1982) *Surg. Neurol.* 18, 46–49.

32. Damasio, A. R., Graff-Radford, N. R., Eslinger, P. S. and Kassell, N. (1983) *Soc. Neurosci. Abstr.* 9, 29.

33. Mishkin, M. and Bachevalier, J. (1983) *Soc. Neurosci. Abstr.* 9, 29.

34. Drewe, E. A. (1974) *Cortex* 10, 159–170.

35. Cicerone, K. D., Lazar, R. M. and Shapiro, W. R. (1983) *Neuropsychologia* 21, 513–524.

36. Corkin, S. (1965) *Neuropsychologia* 3, 339–351.

37. Canavan, A. G. M. (1983) *Neuropsychologia* 21, 375–382.

38. Lhermitte, F. (1983) *Brain* 106, 237–256.

39. Konorski, J. (1972) *Acta Neurobiol. Exp.* 32, 595–613.

40. Goldman, P. S. and Rosvold, H. E. (1970) *Exp. Neurol.* 27, 291–304.

41. Petrides, M. (1982) *Behav. Brain. Res.* 5, 407–413.

42. Halsband, U. and Passingham, R. (1982) *Brain Res.* 240, 368–372.

43. Milner, B. (1963) *Arch. Neurol.* 9, 90–100.

44. Warrington, E. K. and Weiskrantz, L. (1982) *Neuropsychologia* 20, 233–248.

S. E. Petersen, P. T. Fox, M. I. Posner, M. Mintun, and M. E. Raichle

Positron emission tomographic studies of the cortical anatomy of single-word processing

1988. *Nature* 331: 585–589

The use of positron emission tomography to measure regional changes in average blood flow during processing of individual auditory and visual words provides support for multiple, parallel routes between localized sensory-specific, phonological, articulatory and semantic-coding areas.

LANGUAGE is an essential characteristic of the human species, and has been studied by disciplines ranging from philosophy to neurology. Because language is so complex, cognitive and neurological studies often focus on processing of individual words (lexical items). Cognitive models for lexical processing consider words perceived visually and auditorily to involve separate modality-specific codes, with access in parallel to shared output (articulatory) and meaning (semantic) codes[1-6]. In contrast, the model most widely accepted in the clinical neurological literature argues for serial processing, with an early recoding of visual input into an auditory-based code which is used in turn for semantic and articulatory access[7,8].

We have used recent advances in the precision of positron emission tomography (PET) for measuring activity-related changes in regional cerebral blood flow to identify brain regions active during three levels of single-word processing. Our results indicate localization of different codes in widely separated areas of the cerebral cortex. The results favour the idea of separate brain areas involved in separate visual and auditory coding of words, each with independent access to supramodal articulatory and semantic systems. These findings fit well with the parallel models, but argue against the obligatory visual-to-auditory recoding and serial nature of the clinical neurological models.

Methods

Brain blood flow was measured in 17 (11 female, 6 male) right-handed normal volunteers using a bolus intravenous injection of ^{15}O-labelled water (half-life, 123 s) and a 40-s data acquisition[9,10]. A series of 6–10 blood flow scans were obtained in each subject (10 m interscan interval). Within this series, conditions were designed as a hierarchy of paired comparisons to allow subtractive (task minus control) data analysis (see below).

Stimuli were presented throughout data acquisition. All stimuli were frequent English nouns presented at a rate of one per second. Visually presented words appeared on a colour monitor suspended 300 mm from the subject. Auditory words were presented through hearing-aid type speakers fitted within the ears and driven by a digital tape recorder.

Four behavioural conditions formed a three-level subtractive hierarchy (Table 1). Each task state was intended to add a small number of operations to those of its subordinate (control) state[11]. In the first-level comparison, the presentation of single words without a lexical task was compared to visual fixation without word presentation. Note that no motor output or volitional lexical processing was required in this task; rather, simple

Table 1 Paradigm design

Subtraction	Control state	Stimulated state	Task
Sensory task	Fixation point only	Passive words	Passive sensory processing Modality-specific word code
Output task	Passive words	Repeat words	Articulatory code Motor programming Motor output
Association Task	Repeat words	Generate uses	Semantic association Selection for action

The rationale of the three levels stepwise paradigm design is shown. At the second and third level, the control state is the stimulated state from the previous level. Some hypothesized cognitive operations are represented in the third column.

Table 2 Sensory tasks

Region	Coordinates (mm) Z	X	Y	Magnitude
Visual				
1. Striate cortex (L)	10	6	−72	2.28†
2. Striate cortex (R)	10	−12	−72	2.66†
3. Extrastriate cortex (L)	2	24	−58	3.82‡
4. Extrastriate cortex (R)	6	−26	−66	2.95‡
5. Inferior lateral occipital cortex (R)	−4	−34	−46	3.38‡
Auditory				
6. Posterior superior temporal cortex (L)	14	46	−10	2.46†
7. Temporal cortex (R)	12	−42	−16	2.76‡
8. Anterior superior temporal cortex (L)	−2	42	10	3.02†
9. Temporoparietal cortex (L)	14	54	−30	2.88‡
10. Lateral temporal cortex (R)	8	−62	−12	3.30‡
11. Inferior anterior cingulate cortex (L)	18	12	44	2.34†

Subtraction conditions: Passive words − Fixation point. For Tables 2-4, the following conventions are used: the region is given a mnemonic anatomical name associated with the coordinates. The coordinates and magnitudes of response are determined using a three-dimensional search algorithm on the averaged subtraction image. The coordinates are in mm from a 0, 0, 0 point that is at the level of a line drawn between the anterior and posterior commissures ($z = 0$), at the mid-line of the brain ($x = 0$), and located antero-posteriorly halfway between the commissures ($y = 0$). The magnitudes are the change in blood flow in ml/(100 g × min), and the statistical significance of the points is assessed with a two-stage testing procedure. The distribution of the magnitudes of local blood-flow change is tested for outliers using an omnibus gamma-2 test. For all averaged images presented here, there are statistically significant outliers. The foci with the largest magnitude of blood-flow change are then given a z-score with respect to the population of all local changes within an image. All foci of change with a P-value <0.03 are reported in the tables. † $P < 0.03$, ‡ $P < 0.01$.

In general, the passive presentation subtractions identify modality-specific foci of activation, whereas the higher level subtractions activate similar regions across modalities.

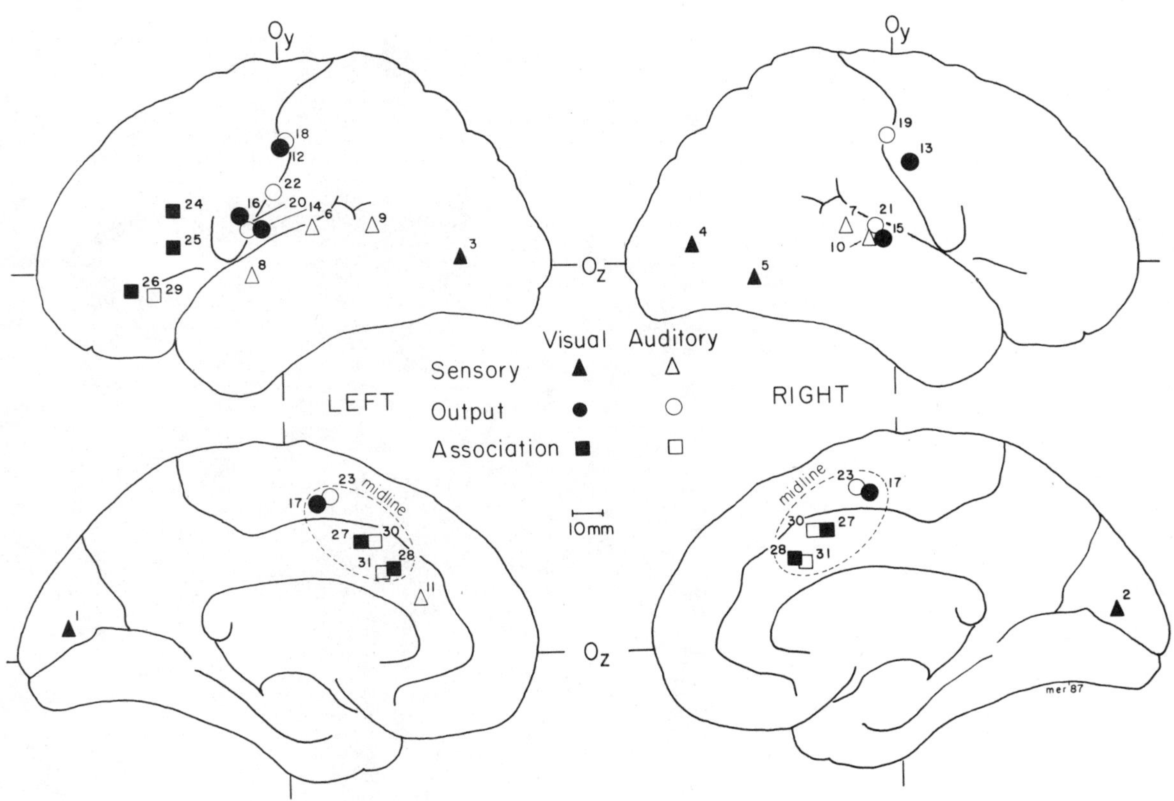

Fig. 1 Schematic lateral (upper) and medial (lower) surface views of the left and right hemispheres with superimposed cortical activation foci. O_y and O_z are 0 reference planes. Each numbered symbol represents a cortical focus of activation, the number referring to Focus number in Tables 2–4. The key to the activation conditions is in the figure. Notice that for passive subtractions, there is no overlap between visual (filled triangle) and auditory (open triangle) sensory tasks. There is considerable overlap, however, between presentation modality for the association and output foci.

sensory input and involuntary word-form processing were targeted by this subtraction (sensory task). In the second-level comparison, speaking each presented word was compared with word presentation without speech. Areas involved in output coding and motor control were targeted by this comparison. In the third-level comparison, saying a use for each presented word (for example, if 'cake' was presented, to say 'eat') was compared with speaking presented words. This comparison targeted areas involved in the task of semantic processing (verb-noun association), as distinct from speech, sensory input and involuntary word-form processing (association task).

Images were analysed by paired (intrasubject) subtraction. Task-state minus control-state subtractions created images of the regional blood flow changes associated with the operations of each cognitive level. Intersubject averaging was used to increase the signal-to-noise ratio of these subtracted images[12]. Averaging required anatomical standardization of all images; this was based on a previously described stereotactic method of anatomical localization for PET images[13,14].

Statistical significance was determined by distribution analysis of the entire population (both positive and negative) of independent regional changes within each averaged subtracted image. The location and magnitude of these changes were determined using a centre-of-mass computer search algorithm[15]. Each change distribution contained both noise and task-induced responses. During averaging, task-induced responses gained in magnitude relative to image noise, becoming 'outliers' in the distribution[12]. Significant responses, then, were defined using tests for outlier detection[16]. Statistical analysis was two-tiered: first, omnibus testing (gamma-2 statistic) determined whether an image (a distribution) contained any significant responses (any outliers); then, post-hoc analysis by Z-score ascribed significance levels to each response within the population. All distributions reported had a gamma-2 significance level of $P<0.05$. All cortical responses with a Z-score over 2.17 ($P<0.03$) are reported.

Lexical processing regions

Regions of activation are enumerated in Tables 2–4, and the cortical sites of activation are summarized in Fig. 1. The most striking aspect of Fig. 1 is that there are relatively few areas of activation added by each task and that these areas are clustered in a few critical parts of the cortex.

Modality-specific primary and non-primary sensory regions were activated by passive auditory or visual presentation of words (Table 2, Fig. 2*a* and *b*). No regions were activated for both auditory and visual presentation. The areas identified appear to support two different computational levels in each modality, one of passive sensory processing and a second level of modality-specific word-form processing.

For the visual modality, the main cortical activations are in the striate cortex and in a small set of prestriate areas reaching as far anterior as the temporal-occipital boundary. The primary striate responses were similar to those produced by other types of visual stimuli[17,18]. However, the regions of extrastriate occipital cortex in Table 2 have so far been activated only by the presentation of visual words. These regions may represent a network which codes for visual word form. Lesions near these regions sometimes cause pure alexia, that is, the inability to read words without other language deficits[19,20]. According to some cognitive models[1,3,21], a visual word form would be generated by a cooperative computational network including feature,

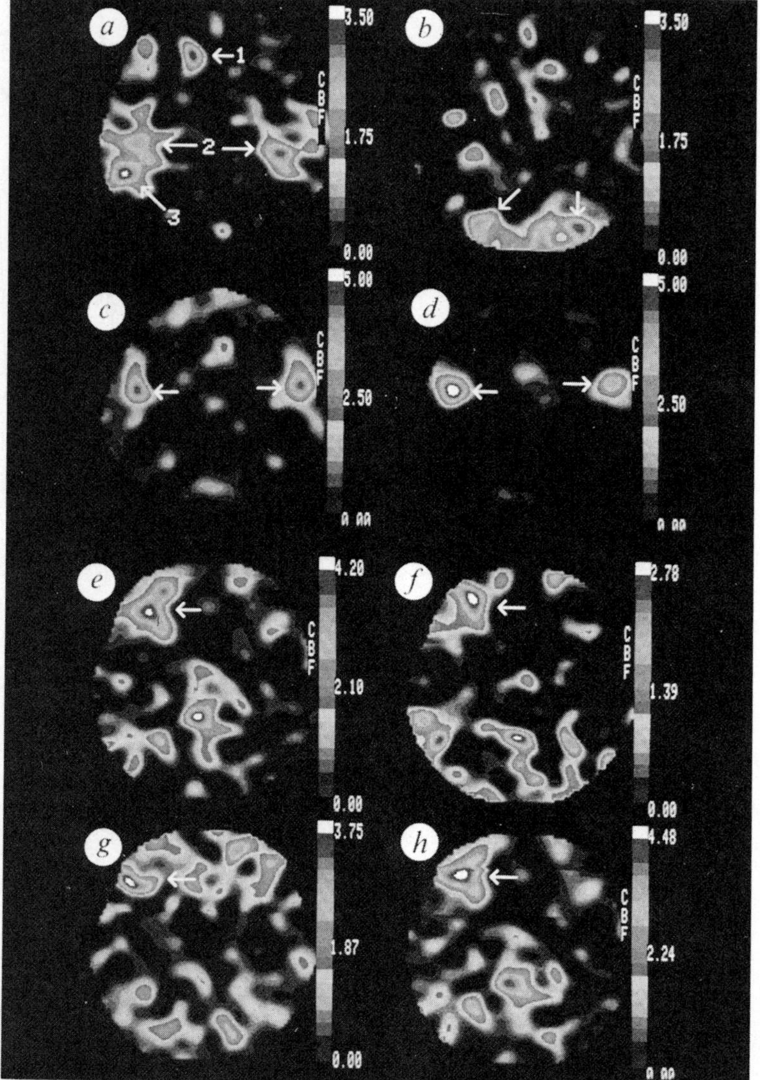

Fig. 2 *a* and *b*, Auditory versus visual comparison. A horizontal slice through averaged subtraction image represents blood-flow change when blood-flow during fixation is subtracted from blood flow present during presentation of word stimuli at 1 Hz (sensory task). Slice in *a* and *b* is taken 1.6 cm above AC–PC line. Foci of activity present at this level include temporoparietal cortex, bilateral superior posterior temporal cortex, inferior anterior cingulate for auditory presentation, and some occipital cortical activation for visual presentation. Note the non-overlapping distributions of activity for visual and auditory presentation in *a* and *b* during passive presentation. *c* and *d*, Auditory versus visual comparison. A horizontal slice through an averaged subtraction image representing blood-flow change when blood flow during passive presentation of words is subtracted from blood flow during vocal repetition of presented words (output task). Slice is taken 4.0 cm above AC–PC line. The foci present for both auditory and visual presentation are located on rolandic cortex, just anterior and superior to regions activated by somatosensory stimulation of the lips and probably represent the mouth representation of primary motor cortex. *e* and *f*, Auditory versus visual comparison. A horizontal slice through an averaged subtraction image representing blood-flow change when blood flow during repetition of presented words is subtracted from blood flow during vocalization of an appropriate use for the presented word (such as presentation of 'cake' ... output might be 'eat') (cognitive subtraction). Slice is taken 0.8 cm below AC–PC line. Foci for both presentation modalities occur in inferior anterior frontal cortex, probably area 47 of Brodmann. Those areas of activation are strongly left-lateralized. *g* and *h*, Comparison of activation in two semantic tasks. The slice on the right (*h*) is from the same condition as *e*; *g*, the blood-flow change when the blood flow during passive presentation of words at 2.5 Hz is subtracted from blood flow during a condition where the subject is asked to monitor this string of words for members of a specific semantic category. In the semantic monitoring task, there is no motor output during the scan. Subjects are asked after the scan for a gross estimate of the percentage of target words. The similar foci of activation in these two different semantic tasks implicate this region in semantic processing. Slice is taken 0.6 cm below AC–PC line.

letter, and word levels. The multiple areas activated could represent the different levels of such a network.

For auditory processing, areas of activity were found bilaterally in primary auditory cortex, and left-lateralized in temporoparietal cortex, anterior superior temporal cortex, and inferior anterior cingulate cortex. The temporoparietal and anterior superior temporal regions have not been activated by presentation of non-word auditory stimuli[22–24]. The temporoparietal region is near the angular and supramarginal gyri, areas that have been associated in lesion studies with the phonological deficits[25,26], and is a good candidate for a phonological coding region.

Areas related to motor output and articulatory coding are activated when words are repeated aloud (Table 3). In general, similar regions were activated for visual and auditory presentation. The activated regions included primary sensorimotor mouth cortex at a location corresponding to previous descriptions of sensorimotor topography[27]. Also activated were a set of premotor structures including a midline structure (supplementary motor area, SMA) and a set of activations around the sylvian fissure. The left sylvian regions are near Broca's area, a region often viewed as specifically serving language output[7,8]. But sylvian activation was also found in the right hemisphere, and this bilateral sylvian activation was also found when subjects were instructed to simply move their mouths and tongues, arguing against specialization of this region for speech output. Small lesions confined to classically defined Broca's area most frequently cause stuttering and oral apraxia rather than full-blown Broca's aphasia[28], adding further support to the view that these regions are related to general motor, rather than language-specific output programming.

The association tasks activated two areas of cerebral cortex for both auditory and visual presentation. A left inferior frontal area was identified that almost certainly participates in processing for semantic association. The second area, anterior cingulate gyrus, appears to be part of an anterior attentional system engaged in selection for action. This localization of function was suggested by the performance of a converging experiment in which subjects monitored lists of words for members of a semantic category (such as monitoring for dangerous animals). In the semantic monitoring condition, left-frontal activation was strong and was unaffected by the number of targets in the list, supporting a semantic-processing function. Anterior-cingulate activation, however, was much stronger for lists containing many targets than for those with few, suggesting activation only when target selection was frequent. Similarly, rapid uncued move-

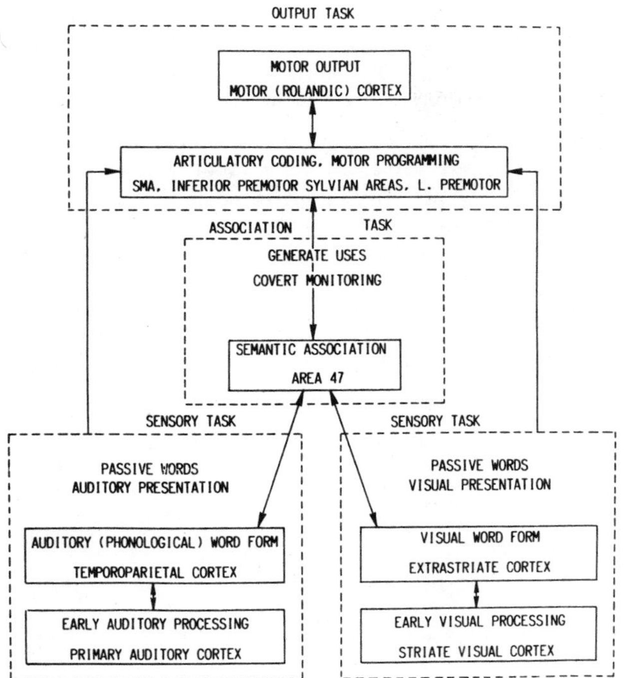

Fig. 3 A general network relating some of the areas of activation in this study to the different levels of lexical processing. There are many alternative networks consistent with the conditions under which the areas are activated, but this arrangement represents a simple design consistent with our results, and some convergent experiments from other types of studies. The dashed boxes outline the different subtractions. The solid boxes outline possible levels of coding and associated anatomical areas of activation.

ments and imagined movements activated anterior cingulate[29], whereas monitoring very low-frequency non-linguistic visual stimuli (J. V. Pardo, P.T.F., M.E.R., unpublished observations) activated neither cingulate nor left-frontal cortex. In accord with these observations, lesions of the anterior cingulate reduced the frequency of movements and speech (akinetic mutism)[30–32], whereas left-frontal lesions produced deficits in word-fluency tests[33], and in semantic-priming tasks[34,35].

Lexical processing models

What type of model do these results support? A serial single-route model has been widely accepted in clinical neurology[7,8]. In the serial model, access to semantics is by a phonological code, and access to output is by semantics. Thus, a visual word must be phonologically recoded (said to occur in the angular gyrus) and must establish semantic associations (Wernicke's area in the posterior temporal lobe) before output coding. Our results are more consistent with multiple-route models in concept[1–6,36–38], and are also quite inconsistent with the serial neurological model in detail.

First, there is no activation in any of our visual tasks near Wernicke's area or the angular gyrus in posterior temporal cortex. Visual information from occipital cortex appears to have access to output coding without undergoing phonological recoding in posterior temporal cortex. Second, tasks calling for semantic processing of single words activate frontal, rather than posterior, temporal regions. Third, sensory-specific information appears to have independent access to semantic codes and output codes; simple repetition (output tasks) of a presented word failed to activate the left-frontal semantic area (association tasks). A framework consistent with these results is presented in Fig. 3.

Table 3 Output tasks

Region	Coordinates (mm) Z	X	Y	Magnitude
Visual				
12. Mouth region, rolandic cortex (L)	40	46	0	4.34‡
13. Rolandic cortex (R)	32	−52	6	3.46‡
14. Buried sylvian cortex (L)	14	31	6	3.04†
15. Lateral sylvian cortex (R)	8	−63	−4	2.96†
16. Premotor cortex (L)	18	48	14	2.98†
17. Supplementary motor area (SMA)	50	−2	10	3.36†
Auditory				
18. Mouth region, rolandic cortex (L)	42	46	−2	3.64‡
19. Rolandic cortex (R)	40	−56	2	3.78‡
20. Buried sylvian cortex (L)	14	34	10	3.17†
21. Lateral sylvian cortex (R)	12	−62	−7	3.22‡
22. Premotor cortex (L)	26	52	2	3.06†
23. SMA	52	2	14	2.80†

Subtraction conditions: Repeat words − Passive visual words. See Table 2 legend for details of conventions used.

Table 4 Association tasks

Region	Coordinates (mm) Z	X	Y	Magnitude
Visual				
24. Dorsolateral prefrontal cortex (L)	20	44	36	2.98‡
25. Lateral prefrontal cortex (L)	8	38	36	2.96‡
26. Inferior prefrontal Cortex (L)	−6	−28	50	2.26†
27. Anterior cingulate	38	−6	24	3.12‡
28. Inferior anterior cingulate	28	−2	34	2.76‡
Auditory				
29. Inferior prefrontal cortex (L)	−6	33	43	3.10‡
30. Anterior cingulate	38	7	28	3.28‡
31. Inferior anterior cingulate	28	11	31	3.04‡

Subtraction conditions: Generate words − Repeat visual words. See Table 2 legend for details of conventions used.

The combination of cognitive and neurobiological approaches, of which this study is an example, has given us information about the functional anatomy of perception, attention, motor control, and language. As these endeavours proceed, solutions to the problem of mind-brain interaction that have intrigued us for so long should be illuminated.

This work was supported in part by the Office of Naval Research the National Institute of Health, and by the McDonnell Center for Higher Brain Function and the MacArthur Foundation.

1. LaBerge, D. & Samuels, J. *Cognitive Psychol.* **6,** 293-323 (1974).
2. Rumelhart, D. E. & McClelland, J. L. *Psychol. Rev.* **89,** 60-94 (1982).
3. Rumelhart, D. E. & McClelland, J. L. *Parallel Distributed Processing* Vols 1 and 2 (MIT, Cambridge, 1986).
4. Carr, T. H. & Pollatsek, A. *Reading Research* Vol. 5, 1-82 (Academic, New York, 1985).
5. Posner, M. I. in *Chronometric Explorations of Mind* (Posner, M. I. & Marin, O. S. M.) (Erlbaum, Englewood Height, N.J., 1978).
6. Coltheart, M. *Attention and Performance XI* (Erlbaum, Hilldale, N.J., 1985).

7. Geschwind, N. *Brain* **88,** 237-294, 585-644 (1965).
8. Geschwind, N. *Scient. Am.* **241,** 158-168 (1979).
9. Herscovitch, P., Markham, J. & Raichle, M. E. *J. Nucl. Med.* **24,** 782-789 (1983).
10. Raichle, M. E., Martin, W. R. W., Herscovitch, P., Mintun, M. A. & Markham, J. *J. Nucl. Med.* **24,** 790-798 (1983).
11. Sternberg, S. *Acta Psychol.* **30,** 276-315 (1969).
12. Fox, P. T., Mintun, M. A. & Raichle, M. E. *J. cerebral Blood Flow Metab.* (in the press).
13. Fox, P. T., Perlmutter, J. S. & Raichle, M. E. *J. Comp. Assist. Tomogr.* **9,** 141-153 (1985).
14. Tailarach, J. *et al. Atlas d'Anatomie Stereotaxique due Telencephale* (Masson, Cie., Park, 1967).
15. Mintun, M. A., Fox, P. T. & Raichle, M. E. *Soc. Neurosci. Abstr.* **13,** 850 (1987).
16. Snedecor, G. W. & Corcoran, W. G. *Statistical Methods* (Iowa University Press, Iowa City, 1980).
17. Fox, P. T. *et al. Nature* **323,** 806-809 (1986).
18. Fox, P. T., Miezin, F. M., Allman, J. M., Van Essen, D. C. & Raichle, M. E. *J. Neurosci.* **7,** 913-922 (1987).
19. Damasio, A. R. & Damasio, H. *Neurology* **33,** 1573-1583 (1983).
20. Henderson, V. W. *Brain Lang.* **29,** 119-133 (1986).
21. McClelland, J. L. & Rumelhart, D. E. *Psychol. Rev.* **88,** 375-407 (1981).
22. Lauter, J., Herscovitch, P., Formby, C. & Raichle, M. E. *Hearing Res.* **20,** 199-205 (1985).
23. Mazziota, J. C., Phelps, M. E., Carson, R. E. & Kuhl, D. E. *Neurology* **32,** 921-937 (1982).
24. Roland, P., Larson, B., Lassen, N. A. & Skinhoj, E. *J. Neurophysiol.* **43,** 118-136 (1980).
25. Roeltgen, D. P., Sevush, S. & Heilman, K. M. *Neurology* **33,** 755-765 (1983).
26. Shallice, T. *Brain* **104,** 413-429 (1981).
27. Fox, P. T. & Raichle, M. E. *Proc. natn. Acad. Sci. U.S.A.* **83,** 1140-1144 (1986).
28. Mohr, J. P. *et al. Neurology* **28,** 311-324 (1978).
29. Fox, P. T., Pardo, J. V., Petersen, S. E. & Raichle, M. E. *Soc. Neurosci. Abstr.* **13,** 1433 (1987).
30. Masdau, J. C., Schoene, W. C. & Funkenstein, H. *Neurology* **28,** 1220-1223 (1978).
31. Barris, R. W. & Schuman, H. R. *Neurology* **3,** 44-52 (1953).
32. Nielsen, J. M. & Jacobs, L. L. *Bull. L.A. Neurol. Soc.* **16,** 231-234 (1951).
33. Benton, A. L. *Neuropsychologia* **6,** 53-60 (1968).
34. Milberg, W. & Blumstein, S. E. *Brain Lang.* **14,** 371-385 (1981).
35. Milberg, W., Blumstein, S. E. & Dworetzky, B. *Brain Lang.* **31,** 138-150 (1987).
36. Humphreys, G. W. & Evett, E. J. *Behav. Brain Sci.* **8,** 689-740 (1985).
37. Shallice, T., McLeod, P. & Lewis, K. *Q. J. exp. Psychol.* **37A,** 507-532 (1985).
38. Coltheart, M., Davelaar, E., Jonasson, J. & Besner, D. in *Attention and Performance VI* (ed. Dornic, S.) (Academic, New York, 1977).

G. Ojemann, J. Ojemann, E. Lettich, and M. Berger

Cortical language localization in left, dominant hemisphere

1989. *Journal of Neurosurgery* 71: 316–326

The localization of cortical sites essential for language was assessed by stimulation mapping in the left, dominant hemispheres of 117 patients. Sites were related to language when stimulation at a current below the threshold for afterdischarge evoked repeated statistically significant errors in object naming. The language center was highly localized in many patients to form several mosaics of 1 to 2 sq cm, usually one in the frontal and one or more in the temporoparietal lobe. The area of individual mosaics, and the total area related to language was usually much smaller than the traditional Broca-Wernicke areas. There was substantial individual variability in the exact location of language function, some of which correlated with the patient's sex and verbal intelligence. These features were present for patients as young as 4 years and as old as 80 years, and for those with lesions acquired in early life or adulthood. These findings indicate a need for revision of the classical model of language localization. The combination of discrete localization in individual patients but substantial individual variability between patients also has major clinical implications for cortical resections of the dominant hemisphere, for it means that language cannot be reliably localized on anatomic criteria alone. A maximal resection with minimal risk of postoperative aphasia requires individual localization of language with a technique like stimulation mapping.

KEY WORDS • **language localization** • **cerebral cortex** • **stimulation mapping** • **epilepsy** • **dominant hemisphere**

THE generally accepted model of language localization in cortex, with a posterior inferior frontal Broca area and a temporoparietal Wernicke area, was developed over a century ago. Originally based on the location of strokes that altered language,[3,41] this approach has subsequently been supported by many but not all reports of aphasia with cortical lesions.[2,6,20] The investigation of language localization with electrical stimulation mapping during neurosurgical operations under local anesthesia provides a different perspective on this model. Devised by Penfield and Roberts,[33] stimulation mapping was based on the observation that applying a current to some cortical sites blocked ongoing object-naming, although no effect of stimulating these sites was reported by the quiet patient. Penfield and Roberts presented the results of stimulation mapping of the right or left hemispheres of a total of 110 patients; those authors reported that sites with evoked errors in naming were located in the rolandic cortex of both hemispheres and in the supplementary motor and classical Broca and Wernicke areas of the left hemisphere. However, a rather large number of left hemisphere sites outside those areas were associated with naming errors. Based on this work, stimulation mapping for language localization became an accepted part of the resective surgical technique for epilepsy[32] and has been the subject of a number of subsequent reports.[21,24,31,38]

The perspective on language localization provided by stimulation mapping differs from that derived from the effect of lesions. With the stimulation technique, language localization can be mapped in an individual subject, limited only by the surgical exposure; lesions generally damage only one cortical region in a patient, thus providing information on function of only a single area in that individual. The brief duration of stimulation makes any functional reorganization during the time it is applied unlikely; some degree of functional recovery usually occurs after lesions. Both stimulation mapping and lesions provide a different perspective on language localization from that derived from neuronal activity recording or blood flow or metabolic measurement techniques (such as positron emission tomography). The latter techniques indicate where neurons participate in language but not whether those neurons are essential for it. Stimulation and lesions indicate only areas essential for language, for the link with behavior is made only when the behavior fails.

In the present report, the cortical localization of language function as determined by stimulation mapping during naming was investigated in the left, dominant hemisphere of 117 patients. This is the largest experience with dominant hemisphere language localization with this technique reported to date. Several issues were investigated. Does the language area in an individual patient actually occupy all of the language cortex of the classical model? What is the variability in this localization between patients? Are there any demographic characteristics that correlate with the variability?

Clinical Material and Methods

Subjects

The study group included 117 patients undergoing left language-dominant frontal or frontotemporoparietal craniotomies. In two children, electrical stimulation mapping was accomplished through chronically implanted subdural electrode arrays.[15] In the remaining patients, stimulation mapping was performed during craniotomy under local anesthesia. The 117 patients were selected from a consecutive series of 129 patients undergoing stimulation mapping of the left language-dominant hemisphere as part of resective surgery for medically intractable epilepsy undertaken at the University of Washington Epilepsy Center through January, 1988. Twelve patients were excluded because of previous resections (four cases), inadequate data recording (two cases), preoperative aphasia (two cases), no statistically significant errors on stimulation (two cases), and congenital malformations of rolandic cortex that precluded use of the method for comparing cases (two cases). Thus, no subjects in the present study had previously experienced resection or a preoperative aphasia. All patients had evidence of left brain dominance for language. In 99 patients the evidence was based on language assessment with bilateral intracarotid amobarbital perfusion;[40,44] of these, 11 exhibited some language function in the right hemisphere as well. Patients for whom the amobarbital perfusion test showed exclusively or predominantly right language dominance were excluded.

The 117 patients included 56 males and 61 females, ranging in age from 4 to 80 years (mean 30.2 years). Preoperative verbal intelligence quotient (VIQ) data were available for 93 subjects (79%), and ranged from 70 to 126 (mean 99.1). There was no significant difference in VIQ between male and female subjects. In 37 patients the seizure disorder was related to adult-acquired lesions, 31 of which were tumors (most often a low-grade glioma). The sites of stimulation mapping were determined by the surgical exposure: this included both frontal and temporoparietal cortex in 90 subjects, only posterior frontal cortex in 11, and only temporoparietal cortex in 16.

Technique of Intraoperative Stimulation Mapping

Stimulation mapping is a technique for localizing language function within a hemisphere after lateralization has been determined preoperatively by the intracarotid amobarbital perfusion test. In order to insure that sites without evoked naming errors could be resected with a low risk of a postoperative language deficit, stimulation mapping must indicate both where language function is located and where it is not. In this series, the extent of the craniotomy was determined in part by this consideration, covering both the area of the proposed resection and also likely language locations.

Local anesthesia for the craniotomy was induced by a mixture of 0.5% lidocaine and 0.25% Marcaine (bupivacaine hydrochloride) given as a scalp field block and as an intradural injection on each side of the middle meningeal artery. Up to 1 cc of Innovar (droperidol and fentanyl citrate) neuroleptoanalgesia was administered shortly before the operation. No other medications were administered until after stimulation mapping, which was usually performed 3 to 4 hours after the operation was begun. Prior to language mapping, rolandic cortex was identified by stimulation and the threshold for afterdischarge in the electrocorticogram (ECoG) was established for the area of association cortex to be sampled with language mapping. Language mapping used the largest current that did not evoke afterdischarges. For the patients in this study, this ranged from 1.5 to 10 mA, measured between peaks of biphasic square-wave pulses with a total duration of 2.5 msec (1.25 msec for each phase). This was delivered from a constant-current stimulator in 4-second trains at 60 Hz across 1-mm bipolar electrodes separated by 5 mm. Sites for stimulation mapping were randomly selected to cover the exposed cortical surface, including areas where language function was likely to be located as well as the proposed resection. The stimulation sites, usually 10 to 20 per subject, were identified with sterile numbered tickets and the location of these tickets was recorded photographically.

Language function was measured by showing the patient slides of line drawings of objects with common names. These slides were projected at 4-second intervals, with the patient trained to name each one as it appeared. This is an easy task, and there were frequently no naming errors on slides presented in the absence of stimulation, with the highest error rate for the subjects of this study being 22%. While the patient named the slides, sites identified by the numbers were successively stimulated, with the current applied as the slide ap-

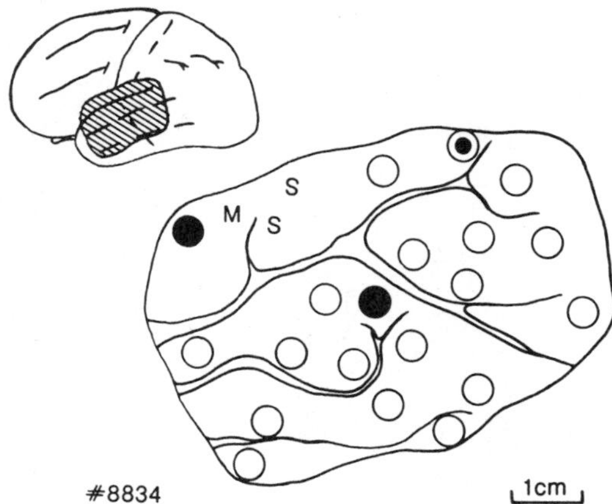

FIG. 1. Sites essential for naming *(filled circles)* in a 24-year-old woman with a verbal IQ of 81. Stimulation at 6 mA; control error rate in the absence of stimulation was 3.7%. *Open circles* indicate stimulation sites without evoked errors; single nonsignificant error shown by a *small dot.* M and S identify sites with motor (M) or sensory (S) responses. Note the localized posterior language area with closely spaced surrounding stimulation sites without errors.

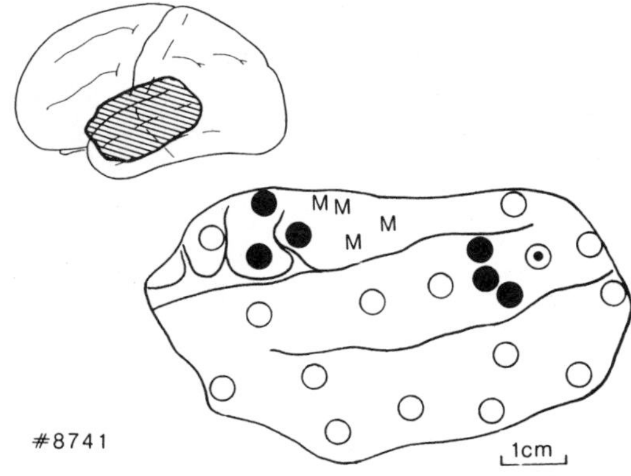

FIG. 2. Sites essential for naming *(filled circles)* in a 24-year-old woman with a verbal IQ of 94. Stimulation at 2 mA; control error rate in the absence of stimulation was 1.2%. *Open circles* indicate stimulation sites without evoked errors; single nonsignificant error shown by a *small dot.* The posterior language area (slightly larger than in the patient illustrated in Fig. 1) is oriented transversely to the superior temporal gyrus. Note also that the intensity of the stimulating current does not determine the size of language area (compare to Fig. 1). M indicates sites with motor response.

peared and continued until the appearance of the next slide. At least one slide without stimulation separated each stimulation, and no site was stimulated twice in succession; usually several slides intervened between each stimulation, and all sites were stimulated once before any site was stimulated a second time. Three samples of stimulation effect at each site were usually obtained. Intraoperative manual scoring of errors and their relation to stimulation provided immediate feedback to the surgeon. In addition, the patient's responses and markers indicating when and where stimulation had occurred were recorded on audio tape and used later to check the results before inclusion of the patient in this study.

Data Analysis

The accuracy of naming during the large number of slides presented in the absence of stimulation was compared to the accuracy of naming during stimulation of a given site, using the single sample binomial test.[36] A site was determined to be related to language function if the chance probability of errors evoked at that site was less than 0.05. With the low error rates in the absence of stimulation, evoking errors during two of the three stimulations at a site often achieved that level of statistical significance. The location of sites of stimulation in relation to rolandic cortex, the sylvian fissure, and sulci separating the major gyri was determined from the intraoperative photographs. Figures 1 to 7 and 9 to 11 are examples of the maps thus obtained for individual patients.

The variability in the location of sites with significant evoked changes in naming was determined by aligning the individual patient maps to rolandic cortex and sylvian fissure. Sites were then assigned to a zone defined by an arbitrary grid based on the same landmarks, as illustrated in Fig. 8. For frontal cortex, that grid included 1.5-cm segments in each of the inferior, middle and superior frontal gyri, beginning with the most anterior evoked motor response identifying the anterior limit of motor cortex. In addition, the inferior frontal gyrus was divided into superior and inferior zones by a line 1.5 cm above and parallel to the sylvian fissure. For temporoparietal cortex, that grid was based on a line extending from the posterior end of the sylvian fissure to the projection of the foot of the central sulcus onto that fissure. This line was subdivided into fourths,

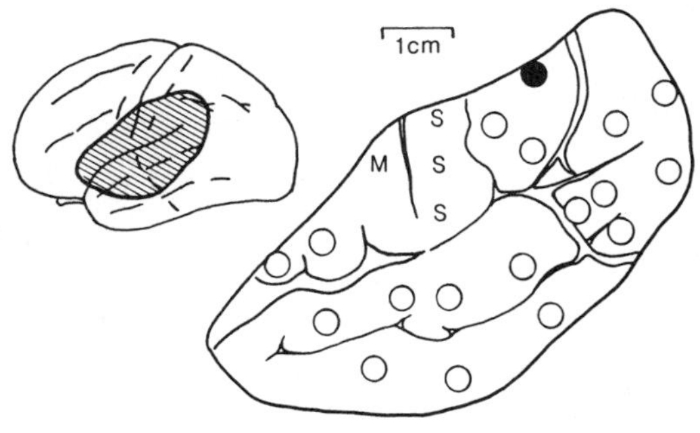

FIG. 3. Sites essential for naming *(filled circles)* in an 18-year-old woman with a verbal IQ of 95. Stimulation at 4 mA; control error rate in the absence of stimulation was 0%. *Open circles* indicate stimulation sites without evoked errors. This patient was left-handed, but had only left language according to the intracarotid amobarbital perfusion test. Language in this unusual parietal location imposes no limits on a temporal resection. M and S indicate sites with motor (M) or sensory (S) responses.

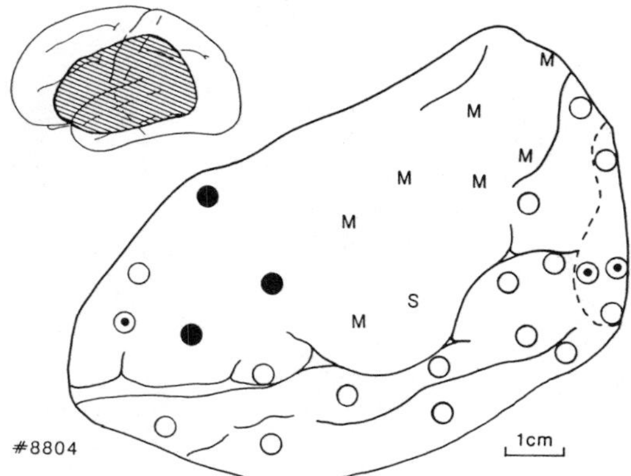

FIG. 4. Sites essential for naming *(filled circles)* in a 37-year-old woman with a verbal IQ of 99. Stimulation at 6 mA; control error rate in the absence of stimulation was 0%. *Open circles* indicate stimulation sites without evoked errors; single nonsignificant error shown by *small dots*. No posterior language sites were identified despite extensive mapping. A posterior temporal resection *(dashed line)* was associated with no language changes, even acutely. M and S indicate sites with motor (M) or sensory (S) responses.

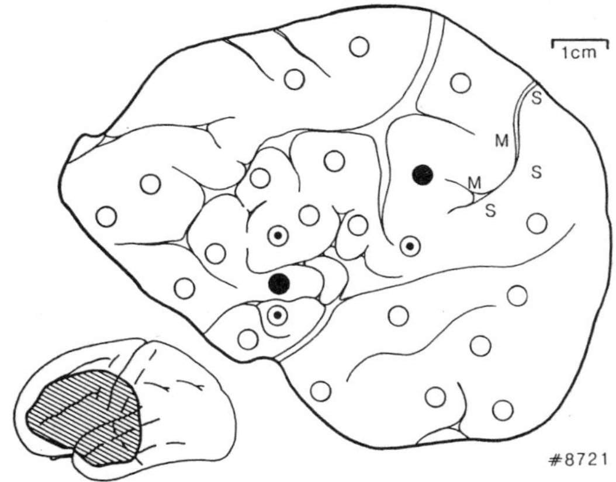

FIG. 6. Sites essential for naming *(filled circles)* in a 20-year-old man with a verbal IQ of 91. Stimulation at 5 mA; control error rate in the absence of stimulation was 0%. *Open circles* indicate stimulation sites without evoked errors; single nonsignificant error shown by *small dots*. Inferior frontal language sites extend nearly to the pterion. The frontal resection came within 1 cm of the anterior language area, and was followed by a significant expression aphasia lasting several weeks. M and S indicate sites with motor (M) or sensory (S) responses.

and zones were established in the superior, middle, and inferior temporal gyri and parietal operculum by these lines. Divisions of the retrosylvian portion of these gyri are also indicated in Fig. 8. The number of patients with sites within each of the zones was thus defined, and the percentage of those sites with significant evoked anomia was determined.

In order to compare patient characteristics with the variability in localization, zones were combined into five groups: superior or middle temporal gyri, inferior parietal lobe, inferior frontal gyrus, or elsewhere in frontal cortex. The proportion of patients with or without errors in each of these groups was compared in terms of age, preoperative VIQ, presence or absence of a lesion with adult onset, or presence of right hemisphere speech. Fisher's exact, chi-square, or Mann-Whitney U statistical tests were used.[36] A set of criteria to identify the extent of the cortical surface area with evoked anomia in each subject was also established. By these criteria, areas with evoked anomia were subdivided into: areas with clearly defined boundaries separated from sites without naming errors by 1 cm or less; areas that were of the same dimension but with mapping that did not absolutely define one boundary; and

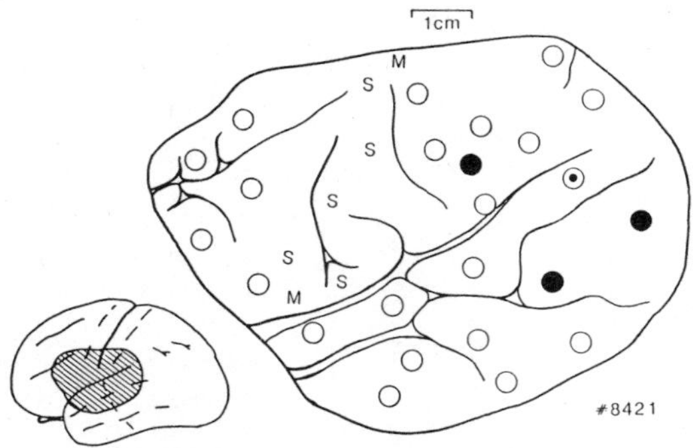

FIG. 5. Sites essential for naming *(filled circles)* in an 18-year-old man with a verbal IQ of 91. Stimulation at 5 mA; control error rate in the absence of stimulation was 1.7%. *Open circles* indicate stimulation sites without evoked errors; single nonsignificant error shown by a *small dot*. No changes in naming or counting were evoked at frontal sites. M and S indicate sites with motor (M) or sensory (S) responses.

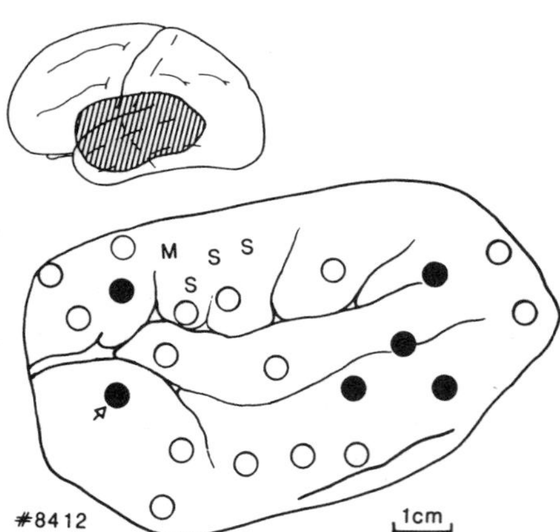

FIG. 7. Sites essential for naming *(filled circles)* in a 46-year-old woman with a verbal IQ of 91. Stimulation at 7 mA; control error rate in the absence of stimulation was 6%. *Open circles* indicate stimulation sites without evoked errors. Note the relatively large posterior language area, but very localized anterior language site, and a language site in the anterior superior temporal gyrus *(arrow)* in front of rolandic cortex, 4 cm from the temporal tip. M and S indicate sites with motor (M) or sensory (S) responses.

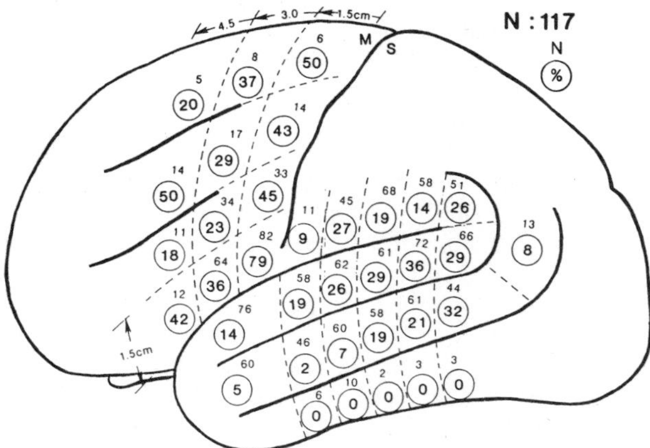

FIG. 8. Variability in language localization in 117 patients. Individual maps are aligned as described in the text, and cortex is divided into zones identified by *dashed lines*. *Upper number* in each zone is the number of patients with a site in that zone; *lower number in circle* is the percentage of those patients with sites of significant evoked naming errors in that zone. M and S indicate motor (M) or sensory (S) cortex.

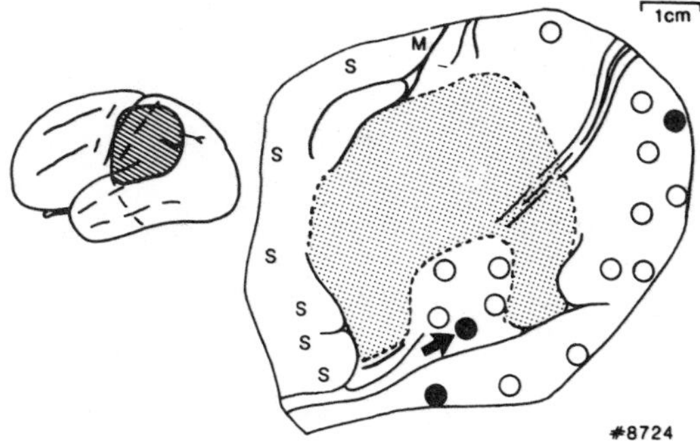

FIG. 10. Site of evoked naming errors *(filled circles)* in a 45-year-old man following removal of a parietal glioma *(shaded area)* that exposed the planum temporale. Note the localized site of evoked naming errors on the planum *(arrow)*, adjacent to a similar superior temporal gyrus surface site. Stimulation at 4 mA; control error rate in the absence of stimulation was 0.9%. *Open circles* indicate stimulation sites without evoked errors. No naming errors were evoked from stimulation of cortex overlying the tumor and no language disturbance followed the resection. M and S indicate sites with motor (M) or sensory (S) responses.

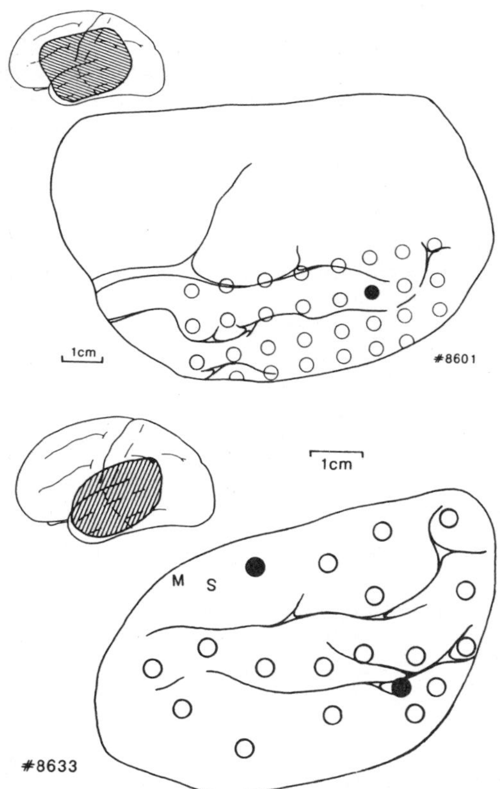

FIG. 9. Sites of significant evoked naming errors *(filled circles)* in a 4-year-old boy *(upper)* and a 70-year-old man *(lower)*, both with medial temporal lobe gliomas. *Open circles* indicate stimulation sites without evoked errors. The 4-year-old boy was stimulated through a chronic subdural grid. Note that both patients show very localized temporal language sites. M and S indicate sites with motor (M) or sensory (S) responses.

areas where contiguous sites with anomia extended over at least 2.5 cm. The study determined both the total area of mapping sites with evoked errors and areas of individual sites separated from others by sites with no stimulation effect on language.

Results

Language Localization in Individual Patients

In the most common pattern of individual localization encountered in the 117 patients, sites where stimulation evoked errors were separated by less than 1 cm in all directions from sites without errors. This discrete localization is shown for temporoparietal sites in Figs. 1 and 9, and for frontal sites in Fig. 7. Other examples have been presented elsewhere.[21,22] Within the limits of the surgical exposure and the number of sites sampled, in only 39% of the patients were errors evoked in any uninterrupted area of cortex larger than 1.5 cm in any dimension (approximately 2.25 sq cm). In only 14% was there an uninterrupted area of language cortex greater than 2.5 cm in the smallest dimension (but see Fig. 4). The populations with large or small extents of individual language areas could not be distinguished based on sex, preoperative VIQ, age, or levels of stimulation current. The margins of these areas were very sharp in many patients (Figs. 1, 3, 7, and 9); in others they were surrounded by cortex where single naming errors were evoked (Figs. 2, 5, and 6), suggesting a gradation between cortex with no role in naming to cortex that is essential for it. In an individual, then, essential areas for language were often organized in a mosaic pattern, 1 to 2 sq cm in extent.

In 67% of patients two or more such mosaics separated by "nonlanguage" cortex were identified (Figs. 5, 6, 7, 10, and 11); in 24% three or more were identified.

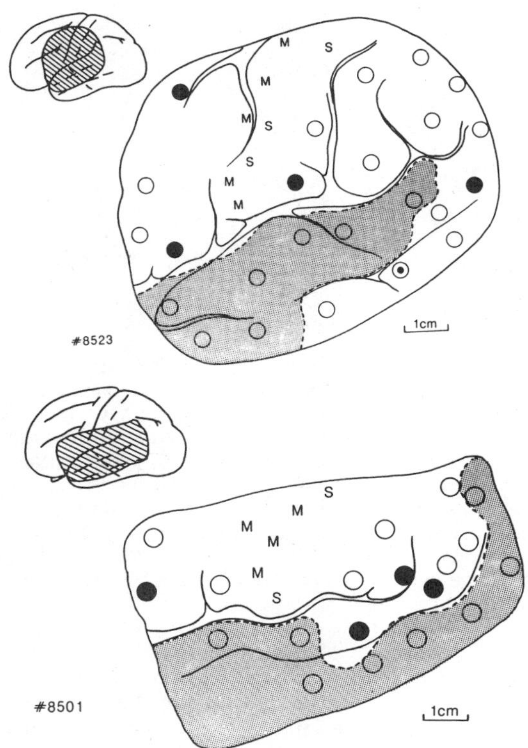

FIG. 11. Large dominant hemisphere temporoparietal resections of much of the classical Wernicke area in two patients, with no postoperative worsening of language function. The resections spared the sites of repeated evoked naming errors. Both patients had only left-sided speech areas based on preoperative intracarotid amobarbital perfusion testing. *Filled circles* indicate sites essential for naming; *open circles* indicate stimulation sites without evoked errors; single nonsignificant error shown by a *small dot.* M and S indicate sites with motor (M) or sensory (S) responses. *Upper:* This patient with superior temporal gyrus oligodendroglioma and intractable seizures experienced no language change after the resection delineated by the *shaded area.* The patient returned to teaching postoperatively. *Lower:* This patient with widespread lateral temporal epileptic focus had no language deficits preoperatively. Following the resection indicated by the *shaded area,* oral language returned to normal within a week, although reading remained slow for a longer period.

Almost all of the patients with multiple mosaics had at least one mosaic essential for language function in frontal cortex and another in temporoparietal cortex. Several separate mosaics in temporoparietal cortex were relatively common (Figs. 5, 7, 10, and 11); more rarely, several separate frontal mosaics were identified (Figs. 6 and 11).

When the total area of such mosaics in cortex available for mapping was estimated for each patient, 50% of the patients had total areas of 2.5 cm or less (Figs. 1, 3, and 9); only 16% had areas of 6 sq cm or larger (Fig. 7). Again, no statistically significant difference between patients with large or small total areas was identified, although patients with larger areas had lower average preoperative VIQ's than those with small areas (93.6 vs. 99.9).

Variability Between Patients

Although often highly localized in a given patient, sites essential for naming had exceedingly diverse anatomic locations throughout the population; these sites were not found uniformly in any given cortical region. Figure 4 illustrates mapping in a patient with a large frontal language area but no posterior sites. Neither extensive mapping nor resection of posterior temporal cortex in this patient had any effect on language. The reverse situation is seen in the patient whose responses are illustrated in Fig. 5, where naming changes were not evoked at frontal sites yet mapping at the same current evoked errors at multiple posterior sites. Figure 3 illustrates an even more unusual situation in which errors were evoked only in the parietal lobe, again in an area not exceeding 1 to 1.5 cm in any of the directions mapped; there were no errors in temporal or frontal sites, the areas where they would be expected given classical models of language localization. Naming sites were identified only in the frontal lobe in 17% and only in the temporoparietal lobe in 15% of the 90 patients with both frontal and temporoparietal mapping.

Figure 8 summarizes the variability in language localization in the 117 patients. Language sites were not uncommonly identified more anterior in the temporal or parietal lobe than might be predicted by the conventional extent of Wernicke's area. They were found far beyond the traditional boundaries of Broca's area. Equally variable was the presence of naming sites in the traditional language areas. No one zone in posterior cortex had errors evoked in more than 36% of patients with mapping there. Indeed, with the sole exception of inferior posterior frontal cortex, no zone exceeded 50% in the proportion of cases with significant naming sites. Even the 21% of patients with stimulation sites in posterior inferior frontal cortex did not have significant evoked naming errors. Thus, neither the location nor absence of language function at a given cortical site can be reliably predicted by anatomical considerations.

Patient Characteristics Correlating With Language Localization

Various characteristics of the population were somewhat predictive of language organization. Although the sex of the patient was not itself significant, preoperative VIQ and sex in some combinations corresponded to specific organizations of naming sites (Table 1). In the population of patients with a VIQ below the mean score, males were significantly more likely than females to have parietal language sites, an effect that was not evident in the half of the population with higher VIQ's. There was a suggestion of a similar effect for frontal zones outside the posterior inferior portion of the inferior frontal gyrus, but this difference did not reach statistical significance.

Significant differences in VIQ's for patients with or without evoked naming errors were present for males

TABLE 1
*Sex and VIQ differences in language localization**

Site	No. of Cases	% With Errors	Sex	Mean VIQ†	% Error Rate Low VIQ (≤ 99)	% Error Rate High VIQ (> 99)
parietal	102	40	M	96/101	59 } ‡	37
			F	100/98	25	27
superior temporal	104	65	M	97/105‡	78	56
			F	97/98	57	57
middle temporal	98	38	M	102/98§	33	50
			F	102/98	34	33
inferior frontal ‖	76	49	M	101/99 } §	53 } §	54
			F	102/98	27	55

* Data derived from stimulation-evoked errors in object naming. VIQ = verbal intelligence quotient. Significance of difference: ‡ = $p < 0.05$; § = $0.05 < p < 0.1$.

† Patients with errors/patients without errors.

‖ Outside posterior inferior zone.

with stimulation sites in the superior temporal gyrus (Table 1). In that group, patients with evoked errors had significantly lower VIQ's than those without errors. Suggestive differences showing higher VIQ's for patients of either sex with errors were present for stimulation at sites in inferior frontal cortex outside the posterior inferior frontal gyrus and at sites in the middle temporal gyrus. Comparing patterns of language localization in all patients with the highest VIQ's (≥ 110, 17 cases) to those with the lowest VIQ's (≤ 90, 21 cases) demonstrated a significantly greater proportion of superior temporal gyrus sites with errors in the low-VIQ group (81% errors in the low-VIQ group vs. 41% errors in the high-VIQ group, $p < 0.05$). Thus, the presence of evoked naming errors in the superior temporal gyrus seems to be associated with poor verbal abilities as measured by the VIQ, particularly in males. Sites in the middle temporal and frontal gyri may be associated with facile verbal abilities.

Several subgroups of language localization showed some correlation with sex and VIQ as well. Males with only temporoparietal and no frontal language sites had significantly lower VIQ's than males with both frontal and temporoparietal language sites (five males with only temporoparietal sites had a mean VIQ of 92; 13 males with both frontal and temporoparietal sites, both of which were mapped, had a mean VIQ of 101, $p < 0.05$). Females were suggestively but not significantly overrepresented among the patients with only frontal language sites (11 of 15 of that group were female, $0.05 < p < 0.1$).

The patterns of language localization in the 37 patients with lesions acquired in adulthood were compared to those in the 80 patients in whom the condition giving rise to epilepsy might have occurred perinatally. No significant differences were identified in the proportion of errors in frontal, parietal, superior, or middle temporal areas, even when the groups were matched by VIQ and sex. There was a single suggestive but not significant difference. Males with acquired lesions had more errors evoked by stimulation in the inferior frontal lobe outside the classical Broca's area (60% errors in 15 males with acquired lesions vs. 28% errors in 25 with possibly early-life lesions ($0.05 < p < 0.1$)).

Age was not a predictive factor with regard to language organization. No significant differences existed in location or extent of essential language areas between older and younger patients. Figure 9 illustrates this finding in a 4-year-old boy and a 70-year-old man, both showing highly localized temporal naming sites.

Discussion

Application of an electric current to the cortical surface has both excitatory and inhibitory effects on neuronal populations and *en passage* fibers, both locally and at a distance.[34] Empirically, language responses seem to represent a predominance of inhibitory effects, most likely from temporary inactivation of local populations of neurons by depolarizing blockade. The spatial extent of this blockade is not precisely known. One study using the extent of stimulation-evoked fluorescence with nicotinamide adenine dinucleotide, reduced form, suggested that the extent varied with repeated application of current to the same site.[39] However, the frequent uniform behavioral effect of repeated stimulation and the close proximity of sites with and without errors in many patients observed in the present study suggest that the evoked inactivation has little variation between stimulations and remains quite localized.

A second issue in interpreting stimulation effects is whether the behavioral change evoked by this local cortical inactivation represents an effect on the language process of naming, or on other processes such as perception or motor output system. Several observations suggest that usually the language process has been altered. Sites with evoked naming errors were not part of primary motor or sensory cortex, as indicated by the lack of evoked movements or sensations. Slides to be named carried a leader phrase, "this is a ——." Many patients successfully recited the phrase even when naming was incorrect, indicating that both perception and speech production were intact and implying that it was only the language process, naming, that was interrupted. In general, naming errors consisted of omission. Although nonsense words, jargon, and other errors occurred, they were rarely peculiar to one site. Thus, attempts at analyzing localization of different types of naming errors have generally proved to be nonproductive. When the patient did not produce the leader phrase, it was not possible to distinguish by means of naming tasks alone between failures in perception, naming, motor control, or even consciousness. However, in a subset of the present series, the stimulation effect on a memory measure was also assessed, and this was usually intact at sites where naming omissions occurred, indicating that consciousness, perception, and motor output were intact.[21] This procedure did not distinguish between an arrest of speech during naming and arrest of motor activity; indeed, at frontal premotor sites, such a distinction may be inappropriate. Lueders, *et al.*,[17] have suggested that posterior frontal premotor sites of speech arrest are really sites of "negative motor response," with arrest of hand movements as well as speech. Nevertheless, these sites are essential for language, and a motor aphasia often occurs if they are excised; this result is one of several lines of evidence for an intimate relationship between language and motor function in dominant hemisphere.[12,16,21]

There is evidence to support a correlation between sites with evoked naming errors and sites where lesions are likely to impair language. Penfield and Roberts[33] inferred this relationship. Direct evidence for anterior temporal resections was provided by Ojemann and Dodrill.[23] In that study a resection that came within 2 cm of a site of significant stimulation-evoked anomia was associated with a subtle but definite general language deficit observed on an aphasia battery administered 1 month after the operation. This deficit was not present when the resection avoided such sites by a wider margin, and could not be accounted for by the size of resection or other patient characteristics. Moreover, naming deficits are associated with all types of aphasias, suggesting that naming changes are likely to arise from manipulation of all cortex essential for language.[14] Thus, sites identified as essential for naming by stimulation mapping probably represent essential areas for language, even when assessed by lesion criteria.

In addition to defining the extent of cortical inactivation and the meaning of the naming errors, interpretation of these data requires addressing the type of population examined — one that was necessarily (by virtue of requiring craniotomies) neurologically abnormal. One might expect cortical reorganization or malformation to be related to lesions appearing in early life. However, no differences were identified between patients with lesions of early or adult onset. Thus, the variations seen in this study do not seem to be related to abnormal early development.

The pattern of organization of language in association cortex derived from this study includes localized essential areas (often as small as 1 sq cm), in some cases with very sharp boundaries and in others with a small area of surrounding cortex where single errors were evoked suggesting a more graded border to the area of repeated errors.[42] This type of organization would seem most compatible with modules or mosaics of association cortex devoted to language. Each patient usually has several of these, most often at least one frontally and one or more temporoparietally. A minority of patients, however, seem to have only frontal or only temporoparietal language modules. The more common pattern with distributed module-mosaics has become a standard model of cortical organization in animals.[9] Based on the finding here, human association cortex is also organized in distributed modules, but on an expanded scale compared to the primate. This localized mosaic pattern was present in the youngest patient investigated (a 4-year-old boy) at a time when language was being acquired.

In some patients the language function mosaics seemed to be oriented transversely to the axis of the gyrus (Fig. 2). Such an alignment suggests that areas essential for language reflect the pattern of connections of these cortical areas; in animals, efferent fibers to temporal association cortex are often oriented in bands perpendicular to the gyral axis (O Creutzfeldt, personal communication). How far the mosaics essential for language extend into the sulci is not entirely known, but several observations suggest that any extension is rather limited. If mosaics essential for language occurred exclusively in buried cortex or extended far from surface sites, then the surface sites would not be the good markers that they are for planning resections extending along a gyrus to avoid language deficits. Moreover, on a few occasions the extent of essential areas for language has been mapped in sulci. In one case (illustrated in Fig. 10), an essential area in the planum temporale, buried in the sylvian fissure, was an extension of a superior temporal surface site. Similarly, in another case, a posterior inferior frontal language area extension into buried frontal opercular cortex was identified.[31] No language changes were evoked from the sulcus immediately adjacent to a frontal language site in a third patient (G Ojemann, unpublished observation, Case 8844). To date, no buried sites not represented by adjacent surface sites have been identified.

The mosaics essential for language can also be distinguished from surrounding cortex by physiological changes identified during naming. However, changes in neuronal activity *per se* do not provide this distinction: recordings of neuronal activity in the human temporal lobe during language have identified changes in activity correlated with naming at sites clearly not essential for that function, based on both stimulation mapping and the effects of excision.[5,27] The patterns of those changes in neuronal activity related to language were usually tonic shifts in the level of neuronal firing, most suggestive of mechanisms of selective attention. Because of the invasive nature of microelectrode recording, neuronal activity in essential areas for language has not been investigated. The physiological changes that distinguish essential areas for language from surrounding cortex during naming were identified in the ECoG. During naming, temporoparietal sites essential for language were differentiated from surrounding cortex by local desynchronization,[7,29] and frontal sites essential for language were distinguished from surrounding cortex by a slow evoked potential.[7] The ECoG changes that differentiate frontal and temporoparietal sites essential for language from surrounding cortex during naming occur simultaneously.[7] Thus, frontal and posterior language sites function at least partly in parallel. Physiological evidence for serial processing from posterior to anterior language areas has yet to be obtained. Parallel processing of the separated mosaics has also been a feature of the organization of animal association cortex.[9] One mechanism for both a local cortical desynchronization and a frontal slow potential in animals is activity of the thalamocortical activating system,[11,37] producing selective attention. A lateral thalamic role in language, also thought to be related to mechanisms of activation-attention, has been described in studies of left thalamic stimulation.[25] During language, the mosaics essential for language are likely selected in parallel by a thalamocortical activating system producing intense local selective attention.

What has not been appreciated previously is the marked individual variability in the location of the mosaics essential for language. However, previous investigations of language localization with intraoperative stimulation mapping have shown sites in unexpected locations: for example, in midfrontal or midparietal,[33] and posterior temporoparietal locations.[38] In addition, stimulation mapping of language sites through chronic subdural electrode arrays has also demonstrated variation in the exact location of language.[15,18] Substantial variability has been evident in the University of Washington series, even when it consisted of only eight cases.[24,31] This variability is quite marked in all areas related to language except the most posterior portion of the inferior frontal gyrus. Even there, enough variability is present so that the classical Broca's area is occasionally not involved in language. This variability is probably the explanation for the difficulty in determining the exact location of the Wernicke language area from the extent of temporoparietal lesions producing aphasia.[2] Indeed, in each zone within the classical Wernicke area, sites related to language were present in less than 40% of the patients who had language assessed there. Moreover, this variability in location of posterior language areas is also evident when sites are combined over larger areas: only 65% of patients with sites anywhere in the superior temporal gyrus showed evoked naming errors, with lower percentages for those with middle temporal gyrus or parietal lobe sites (Table 1). The Wernicke language area of the classical model is clearly an artifact of combining the locations of these essential areas in different patients, for rarely if ever are essential language areas covering the entire classical Wernicke area found in an individual patient. Indeed, the entire extent of the classical Broca and Wernicke language areas is seldom essential for language in an individual patient. In the maps presented by Penfield and Roberts,[33] those combined areas cover over 8 sq cm — an extent encountered in less than one-sixth of our patients. In over half of our patients the identified extent of essential language cortex was less than one-quarter of the area delineated by Penfield and Roberts.

This variability in language localization outside the inferior frontal gyrus exceeds even the considerable variability in gross anatomy of the human perisylvian gyri.[35,43] Considered over the entire population, essential areas for language do not correspond to any described cytoarchitectonic areas of cortex. The individual variability in cytoarchitectonic areas has been little investigated, although one study of the "TP" area in the planum temporale suggested a moderate degree of variability in extent;[8] however, this degree of variation is also not nearly enough to account for the observed variability in language localization. Individual variability in gross localization of functions in animal cortex has received little attention, but considerable variability in the extent of monkey rolandic cortex, some of which was related to previous sensorimotor experiences, has been reported.[19]

There is little evidence in the present study to suggest that experience changes the localization of areas essential for language. The pattern in the patient with the least experience with language, at the age of 4 years, was similar to that in patients with the longest experience, at the ages of 70 and 80 years. In all of these cases the essential areas were localized to mosaics of 1 sq cm. In an earlier study in which the extent of areas essential for naming in different languages was investigated in bilingual patients, the areas essential for the language in which the subjects were least competent were larger than those for the language in which they had greater competence, although the actual items named had similar error rates in the two languages.[30] This suggested that essential areas might become smaller with increasing facility with a language. That suggestion received only slight corroboration in the present study, from the lower VIQ's in patients with larger total language area.

Some of the variation in language localization reflects differences based on language ability and sex. Differences between males and females in proportion of naming errors evoked from parietal and frontal sites (outside Broca's area) were noted in an analysis of the first 21 cases of the present series.[21] In the present much larger series, the parietal lobe seems to be the location of the major difference based on sex, with effects evident only in the low-VIQ group; males were more likely to have naming errors evoked from that area. In addition, there was suggestive evidence that females were overrepresented in the small subgroup of patients with only frontal language sites. Kimura[13] suggested that language deficits after temporoparietal strokes were less likely in females. From this hypothesis, she suggested that the posterior language area differed according to sex, with those language functions located in the left parietal lobe of males subserved by left frontal lobe in females. The data from the present study provide some support for that view.

Differences in language organization based on VIQ seemed to involve primarily the temporal lobe. In the present study, naming errors evoked from the superior temporal gyrus were significantly more likely in subjects with low VIQ's. Subjects with high VIQ's were suggestively more likely to have errors evoked from the middle temporal gyrus. An even clearer relationship between patterns of temporal lobe language organization and

VIQ was evident in an investigation of stimulation effects on both naming and simple-sentence reading in the 55 patients in the present series in whom both had been tested.[26] In that study, the presence of superior temporal sites where *only* naming errors were evoked and middle temporal sites with *only* reading errors was significantly associated with low VIQ's, while the reverse pattern (sites with *only* reading errors in the superior gyrus and sites with *only* naming errors in the middle gyrus) was associated with high VIQ's. Sites where both naming and reading errors were evoked did not differ based on VIQ. This probably explains why the present study showed a somewhat less robust relationship between language location and VIQ for, when only naming was mapped, sites with errors included those related to naming alone (related to VIQ) and to more general language function including reading (not related to VIQ). Stimulation mapping studies, then, clearly indicate that the biological substrate for language differs in patients with differing verbal abilities.

The clinical implications of the present study derive from the combination of discrete localization of essential areas for language in individual patients, and the marked variability between patients. Figure 8 indicates the probability of encountering essential areas for language in various portions of perisylvian cortex. As is evident from that figure, no anatomic landmark reliably indicates the presence or absence of language, outside the posterior inferior frontal lobe. Anterior temporal resections in front of rolandic cortex and sparing superior temporal gyrus are only relatively safe: 5% of our sample had essential areas for language in that cortex. The probability of encroaching on such essential areas increases substantially if the superior temporal gyrus anterior to rolandic cortex is included in the resection. Figure 7 illustrates a case with language function in this area. Damage to those language areas probably accounts for cases of persisting aphasia after anterior temporal lobectomy.[10] In the frontal lobe, sites essential for language occasionally extend forward to the pterion (Fig. 6). On the other hand, the marked individual variability means that in some patients cortex that is considered essential for language based on anatomic criteria can be safely resected without risk of aphasia: for example, in the patients whose language areas are illustrated in Figs. 3, 4, 10, and 11. These findings indicate that, if the maximum resections are to be undertaken with maximum safety to language areas, then the location of language function should be established in that individual patient with a technique like stimulation mapping.

The question for the surgeon becomes whether lateral cortical surface stimulation mapping with naming is reliable in indicating cortical areas that are and are not essential for language. The evidence that sites of stimulation-evoked errors identify the cortex that must be preserved to prevent aphasia after an anterior temporal resection has already been presented. However, to provide this type of information, stimulation mapping must indicate both where language is located and where it is not. Only when both are known can cortex without evoked naming errors be safely resected. Entirely negative stimulation mapping does not provide the information needed to plan a resection. The choice of stimulation currents is particularly important in this regard, for too low a current may not adequately block local cortical function, while too large a current is likely to evoke seizures. Thus, determining the afterdischarge threshold on ECoG and using a current just below that threshold are important parts of accurately identifying language cortex with stimulation mapping.

Although lateral cortical surface stimulation seems to provide the information needed to plan a resection, there is some evidence that it does not identify all of the cortex essential for language even in the temporal lobe. Sites of repeated stimulation-evoked language errors have been identified in the fusiform gyrus on the undersurface of the temporal lobe.[18] Stimulation mapping during reading of simple sentences and naming in second languages has provided some evidence that sites essential for naming in the primary language do not define all cortex essential for all language functions.[21,26,30] Nor does the location of sites essential for naming indicate cortex important for recent verbal memory function.[28] Thus, when resections are planned very close to language areas, particularly in patients dependent on facile function in these other language-related functions, additional stimulation mapping with reading or memory assessment may be desirable.

For most patients however, localizing language with lateral cortical surface stimulation mapping during naming provides the information needed to plan a cortical resection, providing that there is a margin of about 2 cm around identified sites, at least along a contiguous gyrus. Even with this margin, knowing where essential areas for naming are located often allowed for resections in classical language areas of the dominant hemisphere without postoperative aphasias (Figs. 4, 10, and 11). Although originally developed to allow maximum resection of epileptic foci in the dominant hemisphere with a minimum risk of subsequent language disturbance, the technique is equally useful for safely maximizing the extent of other cortical resections near language cortex, especially those for low-grade gliomas[1] and arteriovenous malformations.[4]

Acknowledgments

Dr. Carl Dodrill provided intracarotid amobarbital and VIQ data. Drs. H. Whitaker, C. Mateer, I. Fried, T. Sandquist, and D. Cawthon assisted in patient testing. The operations on 18 patients seen early in the study were performed by Dr. A. A. Ward, Jr., or Dr. A. Wyler.

References

1. Berger MS, Ojemann GA: Cortical mapping techniques used to maximize tumor resection and safety in children with brain tumors. **Ann Neurol 24:**361, 1988 (Abstract)
2. Bogen J, Bogen G: Wernicke's region — where is it? **Ann**

NY Acad Sci **280**:834–843, 1975
3. Broca P: Remarques sur le siège de la faculté du language articulé, suivies d'une observation d'aphémie (perte de la parole). **Bull Soc Anat 36**:330–357, 1861
4. Burchiel KJ, Clark H, Ojemann GA, et al: Use of stimulation mapping and corticography in the excision of arteriovenous malformations in sensorimotor and language-related neocortex. **Neurosurgery 24**:323–327, 1989
5. Cawthon D, Lettich E, Ojemann G: Human temporal lobe neuronal activity: inhibition during naming in only one of two languages. **Soc Neurosci Abst 13**:839, 1987
6. Damasio A: Concluding remarks: neuroscience and cognitive science in the study of language and the brain, in Plum F (ed): **Language, Communication and the Brain.** New York: Raven Press, 1988, pp 275–282
7. Fried I, Ojemann GA, Fetz EE: Language-related potentials specific to human language cortex. **Science 212**: 353–356, 1981
8. Galaburda AM, Sanides F, Geschwind N: Human brain. Cytoarchitectonic left-right asymmetries in the temporal speech region. **Arch Neurol 35**:812–817, 1978
9. Goldman-Rakic PS: Topography of cognition: parallel distributed networks in primate association cortex. **Annu Rev Neurosci 11**:137–156, 1988
10. Heilman KM, Wilder BJ, Malzone WF: Anomic aphasia following anterior temporal lobectomy. **Trans Am Neurol Assoc 97**:291–293, 1972
11. Jasper HH: Unspecific thalamocortical relations, in Field J, Magoun HW (eds): **Handbook of Physiology. Neurophysiology.** Washington, DC: American Physiology Society, Vol 2, Part 2, 1960, pp 1307–1321
12. Kimura D: Left-hemisphere control of oral and brachial movements and their relation to communication. **Philos Trans R Soc Lond (Biol) 298**:135–149, 1982
13. Kimura D: Sex differences in cerebral organization for speech and praxic functions. **Can J Psychol 37**:19–35, 1983
14. Kohn SE, Goodglass H: Picture-naming in aphasia. **Brain Lang 24**:266–283, 1985
15. Lesser RP, Lueders H, Dinner DS, et al: The location of speech and writing functions in the frontal language area. Results of extraoperative cortical stimulation. **Brain 107**: 275–291, 1984
16. Liberman AM, Cooper FS, Shankweiler DP, et al: Perception of the speech code. **Psychol Rev 74**:431–461, 1967
17. Lueders H, Lesser RP, Dinner DS, et al: Inhibition of motor activity by elicited electrical stimulation of the human cortex. **Epilepsia 24**:519, 1983 (Abstract)
18. Lueders H, Lesser RP, Hahn J, et al: Basal temporal language area demonstrated by electrical stimulation. **Neurology 36**:505–510, 1986
19. Merzenich MM, Nelson RJ, Kaas JH, et al: Variability in hand surface representations in areas 3b and 1 in adult owl and squirrel monkeys. **J Comp Neurol 258**:281–296, 1987
20. Mohr JP: Broca's area and Broca's aphasia, in Whitaker H, Whitaker HA (eds): **Studies in Neurolinguistics.** New York: Academic Press, 1976, Vol 1, pp 201–236
21. Ojemann GA: Brain organization for language from the perspective of electrical stimulation mapping. **Behav Brain Sci 6**:189–206, 1983
22. Ojemann GA: Effect of cortical and subcortical stimulation in human language and verbal memory, in Plum F (ed): **Language Communication and the Brain.** New York: Raven Press, 1988, pp 101–115
23. Ojemann GA: Electrical stimulation and the neurobiology of language. **Behav Brain Sci 6**:221–230, 1983
24. Ojemann GA: Individual variability in cortical localization of language. **J Neurosurg 50**:164–169, 1979
25. Ojemann GA: Language and the thalamus: object naming and recall during and after thalamic stimulation. **Brain Lang 2**:101–120, 1975
26. Ojemann GA: Some brain mechanisms for reading, in von Euler C (ed): **Brain and Reading.** New York: Macmillan, 1989, pp 47–59
27. Ojemann GA, Creutzfeldt O, Lettich E, et al: Neuronal activity in human lateral temporal cortex related to short-term verbal memory, naming and reading. **Brain 111**: 1383–1403, 1988
28. Ojemann GA, Dodrill CB: Verbal memory deficits after left temporal lobectomy for epilepsy. Mechanism and intraoperative prediction. **J Neurosurg 62**:101–107, 1985
29. Ojemann GA, Fried I, Lettich E: Electrocorticographic (ECoG) correlates of language: I. Desynchronization in temporal language cortex during object naming. **EEG Clin Neurophysiol** (In press, 1989)
30. Ojemann GA, Whitaker HA: The bilingual brain. **Arch Neurol 35**:409–412, 1978
31. Ojemann GA, Whitaker HA: Language localization and variability. **Brain Lang 6**:239–260, 1978
32. Penfield W, Jasper HH: **Epilepsy and the Functional Anatomy of the Human Brain.** Boston: Little, Brown & Co, 1954
33. Penfield W, Roberts L: **Speech and Brain Mechanisms.** Princeton, NJ: Princeton University Press, 1959
34. Ranck JB Jr: Which elements are excited in electrical stimulation of mammalian central nervous system: a review. **Brain Res 98**:417–440, 1975
35. Rubens AB, Mahowald MW, Hutton JT: Asymmetry of the lateral (sylvian) fissures in man. **Neurology 26**: 620–624, 1976
36. Siegel S: **Nonparametric Statistics for the Behavioral Sciences.** New York: McGraw-Hill, 1956
37. Skinner J, Yingling C: Central grating mechanisms that regulate event-related potentials and behavior: a neural model for attention. **Prog Clin Neurophysiol 1**:30–69, 1977
38. Van Buren JM, Fedio P, Frederick GC: Mechanism and localization of speech in the parietotemporal cortex. **Neurosurgery 2**:233–239, 1978
39. Van Buren JM, Lewis DV, Schuette WH, et al: Fluorometric monitoring of NADH levels in cerebral cortex: preliminary observations in human epilepsy. **Neurosurgery 2**:114–121, 1978
40. Wada J, Rasmussen T: Intracarotid injections of sodium amytal for the lateralization of cerebral speech dominance. **J Neurosurg 17**:266–282, 1960
41. Wernicke C: **Der Aphasische Symptomen Komplex.** Breslau: Cohn & Weigart, 1874
42. Whitaker H, Selnes O: Anatomic variations in the cortex: individual differences and the problem of the localization of language functions. **Ann NY Acad Sci 280**:844–854, 1975
43. Whitaker HA, Ojemann GA: Graded localisation of naming from electrical stimulation mapping of left cerebral cortex. **Nature 270**:50–51, 1978
44. Woods RP, Dodrill CB, Ojemann GA: Brain injury, handedness, and speech lateralization in a series of amobarbital studies. **Ann Neurol 23**:510–518, 1988

Manuscript received November 14, 1988.
This work was supported by National Institutes of Health Grants NS17111, 21724, and 20482.
Address reprint requests to: George Ojemann, M.D., Department of Neurological Surgery, University of Washington, RI-20, Seattle, Washington 98195.

52
N. Geschwind
The organization of language and the brain
1965. *Science* 170: 940–944

Many problems relating to the functions of the nervous system can effectively be studied by investigation in animals, which permits controlled and repeatable experiments on large groups of subjects. When we come, however, to consider the relationship of the brain to language, we must recognize that our knowledge is based entirely on findings in man. Some authors would even argue that language is exclusively a human attribute, so that no experiments on animals could ever be relevant. Although I believe that forerunners of language do exist in lower forms (*1*), the direct contributions to this area of experimentation on the brains of animals still lie in the future.

Brain Lesions in Man

Information in this area has come from several sources. Cases of brain tumor are of limited value, since tumors distort the brain and produce effects at a distance. Cases of penetrating brain wounds (*2*) have been of considerable use but are not the best source of anatomical data, since postmortem information is usually lacking. Analysis of the sites at which the skull was penetrated is of use statistically, but, because of variations in the paths taken by missiles, cannot provide precise data concerning the location of lesions producing language disorders. Stimulation during surgery (*3*) has been another most important source of information but, because of limitation of time at operation and the accessibility of only certain structures, has not covered the full range of phenomena observed clinically.

The elegant studies of Milner and her co-workers on patients undergoing excision of cortical regions for epilepsy represent the largest corpus of truly experimental studies of the higher brain functions in man (*4*). They are limited, however, with respect to the range of phenomena observed. Furthermore, since most of these patients were undergoing removal of areas of brain which had been the site of epileptic discharges since childhood, there is reason to believe that the effects seen after surgery may not represent the full range of phenomena seen after damage to the adult brain. The Wada test (*5*), in which sodium amytal is injected into one carotid artery, has been a major source of knowledge concerning the lateralization of language functions in the brain.

Although important information has been obtained by the above methods, it is still true that the bulk of our knowledge concerning the relationship of the brain to language has been derived from the study of adults in whom delimited areas of brain have been damaged as the result of occlusion of blood vessels, who have been studied carefully over long periods, and whose brains have been subjected to careful postmortem examination. Although fully suitable cases of this type are not common, the experience of nearly 100 years of study has built up a large body of reliable knowledge.

Aphasic Disorders

The generic term *aphasia* is used to describe the disorders of language resulting from damage to the brain. Early in the history of the study of aphasia the distinction between language and speech was stressed. In disorders of speech the verbal output was impaired because of weakness or incoordination of the muscles of articulation. The criterion of a disorder of language was that the verbal output be *linguistically* incorrect. The muscles of articulation might be used normally in nonlinguistic activities. Similarly, in aphasic disorders of comprehension the patient might lose the ability to comprehend spoken or written language and yet show normal hearing or vision when tested nonverbally. Furthermore, these disorders could occur without impairment of other intellectual abilities. The aphasias were thus the first demonstrations of the fact that selective damage to the brain could affect one class of learned behavior while sparing other classes, and thus gave origin to the field of study of brain-behavior relationships. The discovery of these phenomena was one of the greatest achievements of the last half of the 19th century.

Some cases of aphasia had been described before the mid-1800's, but it was Paul Broca who in 1861 began the study of the relationship of aphasia to the brain, with two major contributions (*6*). He was the first to prove that aphasia was linked to specific lesions, and to show that these lesions were predominantly in the left half of the brain. The man who was, however, most responsible for initiating the modern study of this field was Carl Wernicke (Fig. 1), who in 1874, at the age of 26, published his classic work, *The Symptom Complex of Aphasia*, which carried the appropriate subtitle, "A

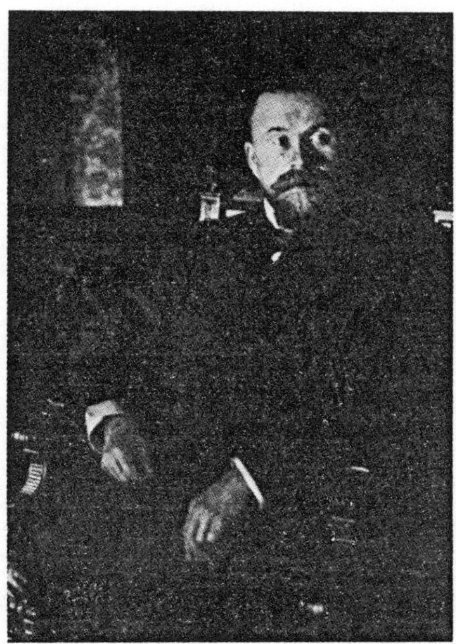

Figure 1. Carl Wernicke (1848–1904), who, at the age of 26, published the monograph *Der aphasische Symptomencomplex*, which was to be the major influence on the anatomical study of aphasia in the period preceding World War I. During his tenure as professor at Breslau, his assistants and students included many of the later leaders of German neurology, such as Otfrid Foerster, Hugo Liepmann, Karl Bonhoeffer, and Kurt Goldstein.

Psychological Study on an Anatomical Basis" (*7*). Wernicke established clearly the fact that there were linguistic differences between the aphasias produced by damage in the left temporal lobe, in what is now called Wernicke's area, and those produced by lesions in the frontal lobe in Broca's area (Fig. 2) (*8*).

Linguistic Changes in Aphasia

The aphasic of the Broca's type characteristically produces little speech, which is emitted slowly, with great effort, and with poor articulation. It is not, however, only at the phonemic level that the speech of these patients is abnormal, since the patient clearly fails to produce correct English sentences. Characteristically the small grammatical words and endings are omitted. This failure persists despite urging by the examiner, and even when the patient attempts to repeat the correct sentence as produced by the examiner. These patients may show a surprising capacity to find single words. Thus, asked about the weather, the patient might say, "Overcast." Urged to produce a sentence he may say, "Weather . . . overcast." These patients invariably show a comparable disorder in their written output, but they may comprehend spoken and written language normally. In striking contrast to these performances, the patient may retain his musical capacities.

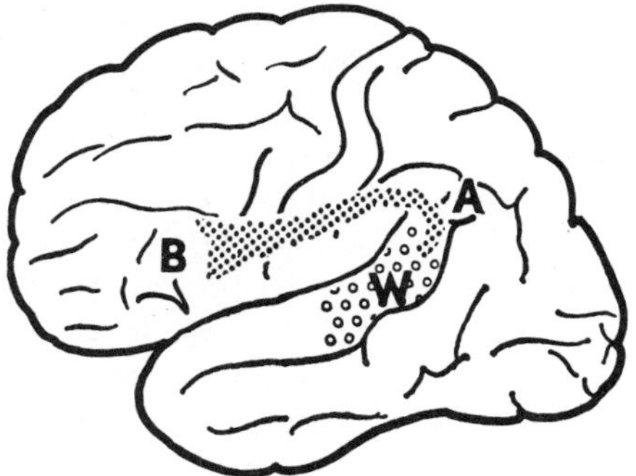

Figure 2. Lateral surface of the left hemisphere of the human brain. *B*, Broca's area, which lies anterior to the lower end of the motor cortex; *W* (open circles), Wernicke's area; *A* (closed circles), arcuate fasciculus, which connects Wernicke's to Broca's area. (See text.)

It is a common but most dramatic finding to observe a patient who produces single substantive words with great effort and poor articulation and yet sings a melody correctly and even elegantly. Because Broca's area lies so close to the motor cortex (Fig. 2), this latter region is often damaged simultaneously, so that these patients frequently suffer from paralysis of the right side of the body.

The Wernicke's aphasic contrasts sharply with the Broca's type. The patient usually has no paralysis of the opposite side, a fact which reflects the difference in the anatomical localization of his lesion. The speech output can be rapid and effortless, and in many cases the rate of production of words exceeds the normal. The output has the rhythm and melody of normal speech, but it is remarkably empty and conveys little or no information. The patient uses many filler words, and the speech is filled with circumlocutions. There may be many errors in word usage, which are called paraphasias. These may take the form of the well-articulated replacement of single sounds (so-called literal or phonemic paraphasias), such as "spoot" for "spoon," or the replacement of one word for another (verbal paraphasias), such as "fork" for "spoon." A typical production might be, "I was over in the other one, and then after they had been in the department, I was in this one." The grammatical skeleton appears to be preserved, but there is a remarkable lack of words with specific denotation.

The Wernicke's aphasic may, in writing, produce well-formed letters, but the output exhibits the same linguistic defects which are observed in the patient's speech. He shows a profound failure to understand both spoken and written language, although he suffers from no elementary impairment of hearing or sight.

The localization of these forms of aphasia has been confirmed repeatedly. It is important to stress this point, since there is a common misconception that the classical localizations were rejected because powerful arguments were raised against their validity. The two authors whose names are most frequently quoted as critics are Kurt Goldstein and Henry Head. As I have pointed out in greater detail elsewhere (*9*), Goldstein, who had been a student under Wernicke at the University of Breslau, despite the holistic views which he expressed in his philosophical discussions, actually explicitly stated his support of the classical localizations throughout his career. Head did indeed violently attack these views early in the first volume of his famous work on aphasia (*10*). His argument was, however, vitiated by the fact that, later in the same volume, the localizations which he himself supported turned out to be essentially identical to the ones he had previously dismissed as invalid.

Wernicke's Theory

Wernicke's contribution lay not only in establishing the syndrome patterns and their localizations but also in providing a theoretical analysis of the mechanisms of aphasia (Fig. 2). He pointed out that Broca's area was located just in front of the cortical region in which lay the motor representation for the face, tongue, lips, palate, and vocal cords—that is, the organs of speech. It seemed reasonable to assume that Broca's area contained the rules by which heard language could be coded into articulatory form. This formulation still appears reasonable. There is no need to assume that this coding need be a simple one. By contrast, Wernicke's area lies next to the cortical representation of hearing, and it was reasonable to assume that this area was somehow involved in the recognition of the patterns of spoken language. There is also no need to assume that this coding is a simple one.

Wernicke then added the natural assumption that these two areas must be connected. The general pattern was now clear. Destruction of Wernicke's area would lead to failure to comprehend spoken language. Wernicke pointed out that, for most people, written language was learned by reference to the spoken form and that therefore a lesion of this region would abolish comprehension of printed and written language. The act of speaking would consist in arousing in some way the auditory form of words, which would then be relayed forward to Broca's area to be transduced into the complex programming of the speech organs, and therefore, with damage to Wernicke's area, language output would also be disordered.

The model could readily be complicated further. Wernicke himself and those who followed him filled in further details. The comprehension of written language would require connections from the visual to the speech regions, and destruction of these connections should be able to cause isolated difficulties in reading comprehension. Since the language abilities were localized in the left hemisphere, language performances by the right hemisphere would depend on information transmission over the corpus callosum.

Clearly the validation of a theory is not a function of its surface plausibility but is dependent on other factors. It is important to remember that Wernicke's theory has been the only one in the history of aphasia which could in a real sense be put to experimental test. It was possible, on the basis of the theory, to predict that certain lesions should produce syndromes not previously described. Furthermore, it was possible, on being confronted with previously undescribed syndromes, to predict the site of the anatomical lesion. The most dramatic examples of this appear in the writings of Hugo Liepmann (*11*) on the syndromes of the corpus callosum. On the basis of his clinical examination he predicted the presence of callosal lesions, which were later confirmed at postmortem examination.

Several remarkable disorders of language have been described which fit readily into the Wernicke theory. In pure word deafness, the patient, with intact hearing as measured by ordinary nonverbal tests, fails to comprehend spoken language although he has essentially normal ability to express himself verbally and in writing and to comprehend written language. In this syndrome the area of damage generally lies deep in the left temporal lobe, sparing Wernicke's area but destroying both the direct auditory pathway to the left hemisphere and the callosal connections from the opposite auditory region. Although elementary hearing is intact because the right auditory region is spared, there is no means for auditory stimulation to reach Wernicke's area, and therefore the patient does not understand spoken language, although his ability to express himself in spoken and written language and his comprehension of the written language are essentially intact (*12*).

In conduction aphasia, there is fluent paraphasic speech, and writing, while comprehension of spoken and written language remains intact. Despite the good comprehension of spoken language there is a gross defect in repetition. The lesion for this disorder typically lies in the lower parietal lobe (Fig. 2), and is so placed as to disconnect Wernicke's area from Broca's area. Because Broca's area is preserved, speech is fluent, but abnormal. The preservation of Wernicke's area insures normal comprehension, but the gross defect in repetition is the result of disruption of the connection between this region and Broca's area. The disorder in repetition exhibits some remarkable linguistic features which are not yet explained. The disorder is greatest for the small grammatical words such as *the*, *if*, and *is*;

thus, a patient who may successfully repeat "big dog" or even "presidential succession" may fail totally on "He is here." The most difficult phrase for these patients to repeat is "No ifs, ands, or buts." In many of these patients the ability to repeat numbers may be preserved best of all, so that, given a phrase such as "seventy-five percent," the patient may repeat the "seventy-five" rapidly and effortlessly but may fail on "percent" (*12*).

Pure Alexia without Agraphia

Many examples of pure alexia without agraphia were described in the 1880's, but the first postmortem study of this syndrome was described in 1892, by Dejerine (*13*). His patient suddenly developed a right visual field defect and lost the ability to read. He could, however, copy the words that he could not understand. He was able, moreover, to write spontaneously, although he could not read later the sentences he had written. All other aspects of his use and comprehension of language were normal. At postmortem Dejerine found that the left visual cortex had been destroyed. In addition, the posterior portion of the corpus callosum was destroyed, the part of this structure which connects the visual regions of the two hemispheres (Fig. 3). Dejerine advanced a simple explanation. Because of the destruction of the left visual cortex, written language could reach only the right hemisphere. In order to be dealt with as language it had to be transmitted to the speech regions in the left hemisphere, but the portion of the corpus callosum necessary for this was destroyed. Thus, written language, although seen clearly, was without meaning. This was the first demonstration of the effects of a lesion of the corpus callosum in preventing transfer of information between the hemispheres.

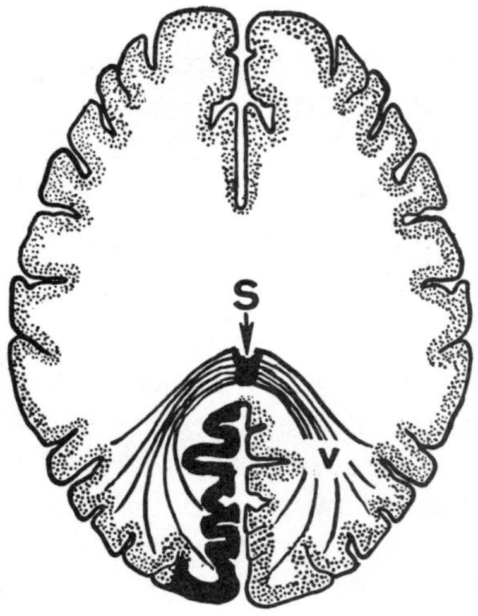

Figure 3. Horizontal section of the human brain, illustrating the mechanism of pure alexia without agraphia; *V*, visual region. The visual cortex on the left is destroyed (heavy black line). As a result, the patient can perceive written material only in the intact right visual region. For this material to be appreciated as language it must be relayed to the speech areas on the left side through the splenium, which is the posterior portion of the corpus callosum. As a result of damage to the splenium (*S*), this transfer cannot take place, and therefore the patient cannot comprehend the written words whose form he perceives clearly.

Dejerine's thesis has received striking confirmation. In 1925 Foix and Hillemand (*14*) showed that destruction of the left visual cortex in the absence of a callosal lesion does not produce this syndrome. In 1937 Trescher and Ford (*15*) described the first case in which a surgical lesion of the corpus callosum was shown to have a definite effect. Their patient had sustained section of the posterior end of the corpus callosum for removal of a tumor from the third ventricle. The patient could not read in the left visual field, but could read normally on the right side. This result is implied by the Dejerine theory and was confirmed by Maspes in 1948 (*16*) and more recently by Gazzaniga, Bogen, and Sperry (*17*). Many authors have confirmed Dejerine's anatomical findings. Michael Fusillo and I studied a patient with alexia without agraphia who demonstrated another intriguing disorder (*18, 19*). For approximately 3 months after his stroke he suffered from a disorder of verbal memory, which then cleared, leaving him with the reading difficulty, which remained unchanged until his death several months later. At postmortem, in addition to the anatomical findings of destruction of the left visual cortex and of the posterior end of the corpus callosum, the brain showed destruction of the left hippocampal region. It is now generally accepted that bilateral destruction of the hippocampal region leads to a permanent memory disorder. The transient memory disorder in our patient appeared to be the result of the destruction of the left hippocampal region—that is, the one located in the same hemisphere as the speech areas. Presumably it is the left hippocampal region which is necessary for the memory functions of speech cortex. After a period, the brain manages to compensate, presumably by making use of the opposite hippocampal region. Since publication of our paper (*18*), I have seem several other cases of this syndrome in which memory disorder was present at the onset. It is well known that the posterior cerebral artery supplies not only the visual cortex and the posterior end of the corpus callosum but also the hippocampal region. In a certain number of cases of occlusion of the left posterior cerebral artery, all of these structures are damaged. In other cases, however, the hippocampal region is spared. Meyer and Yates (*20*) and Milner (*4*) have demonstrated that, after removal of the left anterior temporal region for epilepsy, a verbal memory disorder is observed, which is, however, generally much milder than that found in the case

Fusillo and I reported, and which is not present after right anterior temporal ablation. The mildness of the disorder after left temporal ablation is probably the result of the fact that these patients had suffered from left temporal epilepsy for years and had therefore already begun to use the right hippocampal region to a considerable degree.

Isolation of the Speech Area

Another syndrome, called "isolation of the speech area," is explained readily by the Wernicke theory. This syndrome was described first by Kurt Goldstein (*21*) and has been described more recently by Geschwind, Quadfasel, and Segarra (*22*). We studied our patient for nearly 9 years after an episode of carbon monoxide poisoning. During this period she showed no evidence of language comprehension in the ordinary sense, and never uttered a sentence of propositional speech. She was totally helpless and required complete nursing care. In striking contrast to this state were her language performances in certain special areas. She would repeat perfectly, with normal articulation, sentences said to her by the examiner. She would, however, go beyond mere repetition, since she would complete phrases spoken by the examiner. For example, if he said, "Roses are red," she would say, "violets are blue, sugar is sweet, and so are you." Even more surprising, it was found that she was still capable of verbal learning. Songs which did not exist before her illness were played to her several times. Eventually, when the record player was started she would begin to sing. If the record player was then turned off she would continue singing the words and music correctly to the end, despite the lack of a model. Postmortem examination by Segarra showed a remarkable lesion, which was essentially symmetrical. The classical speech area, including Wernicke's area, Broca's area, and the connections between them, was intact, as were the auditory inflow pathways and the motor outflow pathways for the speech organs. In the regions surrounding the speech area either the cortex or the underlying white matter was destroyed. The speech area was indeed isolated. The patient's failure to comprehend presumably resulted from the fact that the language inputs could arouse no associations elsewhere in the brain, and since information from other portions of the brain could not reach the speech areas, there was no propositional speech. On the other hand the intactness of the speech region and its internal connections insured correct repetition. The preservation of verbal learning is particularly interesting. In addition to the speech area, the hippocampal region, which is involved in learning, was also preserved, and this probably accounts for her remarkable ability to carry on the memorizing of verbal material.

Callosal Syndromes

Although pure alexia without agraphia (*13*) was the first syndrome in which damage to the corpus callosum was shown to play a role by interrupting transfer of information between the hemispheres, it was a group of Wernicke's students, including Hugo Liepmann, Kurt Goldstein, and Karl Bonhoeffer, who elucidated the full syndrome of callosal disconnection in cases in which eventually there was careful postmortem confirmation of the predicted sites of the lesions (*11*, *12*). While the callosal syndromes continued to be recognized by German authors (*23*), their existence was either forgotten or indeed totally denied in the English-language literature. In November 1961, Edith Kaplan and I presented a patient to the Boston Society of Psychiatry and Neurology who was, we believed, suffering from a callosal disconnection syndrome—a diagnosis which was later confirmed at postmortem examination by Segarra. [Since that time several cases of confirmed callosal disconnection have been described (*24*).] I will mention here briefly only a few of the aspects of our patient's condition which fit into the Wernicke theory. When writing with the right hand the patient produced linguistically correct words and sentences and carried out calculations correctly. When writing with the left hand he produced incorrect words (for example, "run" for "go") and performed calculations incorrectly. The theory outlined above implies that, for writing to be carried out correctly with the left hand, the information must be transmitted from the speech areas across the corpus callosum, whose interruption in our patient explained his failures. Similarly, the patient could correctly name objects (concealed from vision) which he palpated with the right hand. On the other hand he would misname objects palpated with the left hand, although it could be shown by nonverbal means that his right hemisphere recognized the object. Thus, if a pencil was placed in his left hand the patient could draw the object previously held in that hand. Again, the Wernicke theory implies that, for an individual to correctly name an object held in the left hand, the information must be transmitted from the sensory regions in the right hemisphere to the speech regions via the corpus callosum, which had been destroyed in this patient. On the other hand, the patient could read in the left as well as the right visual field. This led us to conclude that the destruction of the corpus callosum had spared the posterior end, a prediction also confirmed at post-mortem.

Cerebral Dominance

Let me turn to another bit of knowledge which fits very well into the scheme presented above. One of the most remarkable features of man is cerebral dominance—that is, the fact that in the adult the capacities for speech are overwhelmingly controlled by the left hemisphere. Out of 100 adult aphasics, at least 96 percent have damage to the left side of the brain (*25*). We do not know of any example in any other mammal of a class of learning which is predominantly controlled by one half of the brain (*26*). What underlies human speech dominance? It is widely stated in the literature that the human brain is symmetrical, and this had led either to the assumption that speech dominance must reflect some subtle physiological difference between the hemispheres, or indeed even to the assumption that speech dominance is somehow acquired as the result of postnatal experience. My colleague Walter Levitsky and I (*27*) decided to reinvestigate this problem, particularly since we found that some earlier authors had claimed that there were in fact anatomical differences between the hemispheres. We demonstrated that such differences exist and are indeed readily visible to the naked eye. The area that lies behind the primary auditory cortex in the upper surface of the temporal lobe is larger on the left side in 65 percent of brains, and larger on the right in only 11 percent. This region on the left side is, on the average, nearly a centimeter longer than its fellow on the opposite side—that is, larger by one-third than the corresponding area on the right. More recently Wada (*28*) has confirmed our results. He has, in addition, studied this region in the brains of infants and has found that these differences are present at birth. This region which is larger in the left hemisphere is, in fact, a portion of Wernicke's area, whose major importance for speech was first shown nearly 100 years ago. It is reasonable to assume that there are other anatomical asymmetries in the hemispheres of the human brain, reflecting other aspects of dominance.

The study of the organization of the brain for language has been based of necessity on investigations in man. The bulk of our information in this area has come from careful studies of patients suffering from isolated damage as a result of vascular disease, whose brains have, after death, been subjected to careful anatomical examination. Disorders of language resulting from brain damage, almost always on the left side, are called aphasias. Carl Wernicke, nearly 100 years ago, described the linguistic differences between aphasias resulting from damage in different anatomical locations and outlined a theory of the organization of language in the brain. Not only have Wernicke's localizations stood up under repeated examination but his theory has been the only one which has permitted the prediction of new phenomena, or has been able to account for new observations. Several remarkable disorders, such as isolated disturbances of reading and the symptomatology of the corpus callosum, are examples of the explanatory power of this theory.

The phenomenon of cerebral dominance—that is, the predominant importance of one side of the brain for a class of learned behavior—occurs, as far as we know, in no mammal other than man. The dominance of the left side of the brain for speech is the most striking example of this phenomenon. Contrary to generally accepted views, there is a striking anatomical asymmetry between the temporal speech region on the left side and the corresponding region of the right hemisphere.

References and Notes

1. I have argued elsewhere that language is based on the striking development of the angular gyrus region in man, a region which receives inputs from all cortical sensory areas [see N. Geschwind, in *Monograph Series on Languages and Linguistics, No. 17* (Georgetown Univ. Press, Washington, D.C., 1964), pp, 155–169, *Brain* **88**, 237 (1965); *ibid.*, p. 585]. D. Pandya and H. Kuypers [*Brain Res.* **13**, 13 (1969)] have shown that a forerunner of this region exists in the macaque. R. A. Gardner and B. T. Gardner [*Science* **165**, 664 (1969)] and D. Premack (in a paper presented at the Symposium on Cognitive Processes of Nonhuman Primates, Pittsburgh, March 1970) have described what appears to be a definite degree of linguistic behavior in chimpanzees.

2. A R. Luria, *Traumatic Aphasia* (Mouton, The Hague, 1969).

3. O. Foerster, in *Handbuch der Neurologie*, O. Bumke and O. Foerster, Eds. (Springer, Berlin, 1936), vol. 6, pp. 1–448; W. Penfield and L. Roberts, *Speech and Brain-Mechanisms* (Princeton Univ. Press, Princeton, N.J., 1959).

4. See for example, B. Milner, in *Interhemispheric Relations and Cerebral Dominance*, V. B. Mountcastle, Ed. (Johns Hopkins Press, Baltimore, 1962), pp. 177–195.

5. J. Wada and T. Rasmussen, *J. Neurosurg.* **17**, 266 (1960); C. Branch, B, Milner, T. Rasmussen, *ibid.* **21**, 399 (1964).

6. A. L. Benton [*Cortex* **1**, 314 (1964)] summarizes the earlier literature; R. J. Joynt (*ibid.*, p. 206) gives an account of Broca's contributions.

7. C. Wernicke, *Der aphasische Symptomen-complex* (Franck and Weigert, Breslau, 1874). An English translation has recently appeared in *Boston Studies in the Philosophy of Science*, R. S. Cohen and M. W. Wartofsky, Eds. (Reidel, Dordrecht, 1969), vol. 4, pp. 34–97. For a more complete evaluation of Wernicke's work, see N. Geschwind, *ibid.*, pp. 1–33.

8. R. Jakobson [in *Brain Function*, E. C. Carterette, Ed. (Univ. of California Press, Berkeley, 1966), vol. 3, pp. 67–92] has given a vivid description of these linguistic differences.

9. N. Geschwind, *Cortex* **1**, 214 (1964).

10. H. Head, *Aphasia and Kindred Disorders of Speech* (Cambridge Univ. Press, London, 1926).

11. H. Liepmann, *Drei Aufsatze aus dem Apraxiegebiet* (Karger, Berlin, 1908).

12. N. Geschwind, *Brain* **88**, 237 (1965); *ibid.*, p. 585. There is another, less readily understood, lesion in some cases of pure word deafness which is discussed in these two communications.

13. J. Dejerine, *Mem. Soc. Biol.* **4**, 61 (1892).

14. C. Foix and P. Hillemand, *Bull. Mem. Soc. Med. Hop. Paris* **49**, 393 (1925).

15. J. H. Trescher and F. R. Ford, *Arch. Neurol. Psychiat.* **37**, 959 (1937).

16. P. E. Maspes, *Rev. Neurol.* **80**, 100 (1948).

17. M. S. Gazzaniga, J. E. Bogen, R. W. Sperry, Brain **88**, 221 (1965).

18. N. Geschwind and M. Fusillo, *Arch. Neural* **15**, 137 (1966).

19. For a review of the different varieties of alexia, see D. F. Benson and N. Geschwind, in *Handbook of Clinical Neurology*, P. J. Vinken and G. W. Bruyn, Eds. (North-Holland, Amsterdam, 1969), vol. 4, pp. 112–140.

20. V. Meyer and H. J. Yates, *J. Neurol. Neurosurg. Psychiat.* **18**, 44 (1955).

21. K. Goldstein, *Die transkortikalen Aphasien* (Fischer, Jena, 1917).

22. N. Geschwind, F. A. Quadfasel, J. M. Segarra, *Neuropsychologia* **4**, 327 (1968).

23. J. Lange, in *Handbuch der Neurologie*, O. Bumke and O. Foerster, Eds. (Springer, Berlin, 1936), vol. 6, pp. 885–960; O. Sittig, *Über Apraxie* (Karger, Berlin, 1931).

24. N. Geschwind and B. Kaplan, *Neurology* **12**, 675 (1962); M. S. Gazzaniga, J. E. Bogen, R. W. Sperry, *Proc. Nat. Acad. Sci. U.S.* **48**, 1765 (1962).

25. For a review, see O. Zangwill, *Cerebral Dominance and Its Relation to Psychological Function* (Thomas, Springfield, Ill., 1960).

26. In *submammalian* forms there are examples of behaviors whose neural control appears to be predominantly unilateral—for example, bird song [see F. Nottebohm, *Science* **167**, 950 (1970)]. These may represent, not an earlier stage of dominance, but rather a separate development.

27. N. Geschwind and W. Levitsky, *Science* **161**, 186 (1968).

28. J. Wada, paper presented at the 9th International Congress of Neurology, New York, 1969.

29. The work discussed has been supported in part by grant NS 06209 from the National Institutes of Health to the Boston University School of Medicine.

R. A. McCarthy and E. K. Warrington

Evidence for modality-specific meaning systems in the brain

1988. *Nature* 334: 428–430

Abstract

Patients with cerebral lesions offer a unique opportunity to investigate the organization of meaning systems in the brain. Clinical neurologists have long been aware that knowledge of particular classes or categories of information may be selectively impaired in some cases and selectively spared in others. For example, knowledge of letters, colours, objects, or people may be lost as a consequence of damage to the left hemisphere of the brain[1–4]. Recently there has been quantitative evidence for even more specific impairment and preservation of particular classes of knowledge[5–8]. More recently the evidence for knowledge of living things as compared with inanimate objects is particularly striking[9–12]. Such observations have suggested that our semantic knowledge base is categorical in its organization. In this preliminary report, we describe a patient whose semantic knowledge deficit was not only category specific, but also modality specific. Although his knowledge of the visual world was almost entirely normal, his knowledge of living things (but not objects!) was gravely impaired when assessed in the verbal domain. These findings call into question the widely accepted view that the brain has a single all-purpose meaning store[13].

Category-specific effects are most plausibly considered as arising from a deficit within the central meaning system itself. The alternative possibilities, namely failure at an earlier stage of processing, or disruption of the links between earlier (presemantic) processes and the meaning system can be discounted. For a category-specific deficit to arise in the first place it is necessary that the information should have already been categorized along a semantic dimension. Evidence for a degradation of categories of semantic knowledge, rather than failure to access an intact set of meaning representations, is based on two further converging sources of evidence. Firstly, patients may be highly consistent over testing sessions with regard to the specific items that they can or cannot comprehend. Such a pattern of response would be unlikely to arise simply as a product of 'random noise' in the meaning system, or in access to it. This evidence is more plausibly considered as reflecting the loss of particular items of information[11]. Secondly, the loss of certain items is not absolute. The errors made by such patients indicate partial knowledge of the target, so that broad category information is preserved (that is, a type of bird, vegetable, object and so on), but at the same time more detailed knowledge is lost (such as colour, size, type of material). Thus a patient would know that a canary was a bird, but not know that it was yellow[5]. This invariant hierarchy of partial knowledge is difficult to account for in terms of a deficit at a presemantic level of processing, but is entirely compatible with a degradation of the meaning representations themselves.

The question remains as to whether these findings can be explained in terms of a disorder to an all-purpose meaning system, or whether there are a number of dissociable meaning systems corresponding to different sensory modalities (auditory or visual for example). The majority of cases with category-specific disorders have shown some impairment in comprehending both the spoken word and in demonstrating knowledge of the same class of material when it is presented in pictorial form[13]. However, there may be a less than perfect concordance between the two sensory modalities, both in terms of the severity of deficit and the specific items that are affected[11]. The best-documented modality-specific disorder is the syndrome of visual associative agnosia, in which the patient is unable to assign meaning to objects or pictures presented visually, but may be able to perform normally when asked to define their appropriate verbal labels. For example, the patient may be unable to recognize a hammer, but have no difficulty in giving an adequate definition of the spoken word 'hammer'[14]. This single dissociation, although it is suggestive of there being modality-specific meaning systems, could be incorporated into a model postulating a single all-purpose meaning system, by postulating a disconnection syndrome[11]. However, a modality-specific impairment in which there was not only clear evidence of category specificity, but which also showed the hallmarks of a degradation of the meaning representations, would be strong evidence for multiple modality-specific meaning systems.

The patient we have investigated (T.O.B.) was a 63-year-old senior civil servant who complained of progressive deterioration in his use of language and comprehension of the spoken word. There was no other abnormality on neurological examination. PET (positron emission tomography) scanning demonstrated a relatively well circumscribed abnormality in the left temporal lobe (P. J. Tyrell, D. Perani and M. N. Rossor, personal communication). He spoke freely and fluently, using a somewhat repetitive and limited vocabulary. He frequently resorted to stereotyped phrases in his attempts to circumvent his obvious word-finding difficulties. Very occasional minor errors of syntax were also noted. He was tested on the Wechsler Adult Intelligence Scale and obtained an average verbal IQ of 95 and a high average performance IQ of 116. The only feature of note was his total failure to define a number of relatively common words which must have once been well within his vocabulary. This deficit accounted for the relative depression of his verbal IQ. His reading and writing were also somewhat impaired. His performance was also very weak on formal tests of naming: for example, he failed to score at all on a Graded Difficulty Naming Test. He had equal difficulty in matching a spoken name to a picture. Clinical observation suggested that his difficulty was not simply one of word retrieval, but that in addition certain spoken names appeared to be almost totally meaningless to him. This contrasted with an excellent ability to derive meaning from a picture. For example, when asked to define the word 'rhinoceros', he responded, "Animal, can't give you any functions." But when shown a picture of a rhinoceros he responded, "Enormous, weighs over one ton, lives in Africa". Asked to define 'dolphin', he replied, "A fish or a bird"; but when shown a picture he responded, "Dolphin lives in water ... they are trained to jump up and come out ... In America during the war years they started to get this particular animal to go through to look into ships." It was further observed that he appeared to have much greater difficulty in comprehending the names of animate things as compared with inanimate objects. For example, when asked to define 'pig', he responded, "Animal", and when asked to define 'lighthouse', he replied, "Round the coast, built up, tall building, lights revolve to warn ships." His definition of the word 'wheelbarrow' was, "The item we have here in the gardens for carrying bits and pieces; wheelbarrows are used by people doing maintenance here on your buildings. They can put their cement and all sorts of things in it to carry it around." By contrast, for peacock he replied, "Common name, can't place it." These observations were formally tested using a matched set of items divided into two categories, namely living things (36 animals and 12 plants) and objects[11]. T.O.B. was asked either to define a spoken word, or to explain what was represented in a picture. His responses were recorded on video and scored by independent raters using a lenient criterion that only the core concept need be conveyed. The percentage correct in each condition for the two categories is shown in Table 1. He was clearly impaired in only one of the four conditions, namely the definition of the spoken names of living things.

Although they are among the first words in a child's vocabulary, the names of animals tend to be of lower frequency in adult language than the names of objects.

Table 1. Picture and word identification†

	Pictures	Words
Living things	94%	33%
Objects	98%	89%

† % Correct. $n = 48$.

Table 2. Word definitions†

	Animals	Objects
1st attempt	30%	64%
2nd attempt	36%	70%

† % Correct. $n = 56$.

T.O.B. was given a second, purely verbal version of the definition task, using new stimuli in which the material from animate and inanimate categories was precisely matched for their frequency in the language. He was tested on two separate occasions to establish the degree of consistency in his responses. The percentage correct for each category for each condition is shown in Table 2. These findings replicate those from the previous test in showing a selective impairment in T.O.B.'s knowledge of the spoken names of animals. Furthermore, when re-tested he showed a highly consistent pattern of performance, failing the same items on each occasion. Indeed, his responses were only discrepant on 5 of the 56 object stimuli and 3 of the 56 animal stimuli.

In summary, we report evidence that T.O.B. has a category-specific impairment that affects in particular his knowledge of spoken names of living things, and that this impairment is consistent across time. These effects are prominent in the verbal domain, but at the same time his visual knowledge of the same items appears relatively unaffected. The view that the brain has a single 'all-purpose' meaning store is inadequate as an account of this pattern of results[13]. Firstly, the fact that it is one semantic category rather than another that is affected places this deficit within the domain of meaning. Secondly, the fact that T.O.B.'s impairment is consistent from one occasion to another clearly indicates that he shows degradation within the meaning representations themselves, rather than a failure of access to them. Therefore the observation that T.O.B.'s degradation deficit is confined to one modality and to one category within that modality (namely, living things) not only refutes the notion of an 'all-purpose' meaning store, but also provides positive evidence for multiple meaning representations.

T.O.B.'s knowledge of the visual world appears to be relatively intact, whereas his verbal knowledge is gravely impaired within one semantic category. We have argued that this pattern of performance indicates that there are dissociable modality-specific meaning systems in the brain. It has previously been suggested that the differential salience of information from different sensory and motor channels in the acquisition of knowledge is at the basis of the categorical organization of meaning[10]. The modality-specific organization of meaning can plausibly be viewed as having a similar developmental basis to that of category specificity. We would further speculate that this basic categorical organization of meaning provides a blueprint, which is to some extent duplicated in functionally independent modality-specific meaning systems. Indeed, the basic facts of phylogeny and ontogeny make such an organization eminently reasonable, if not inevitable.

We are grateful to Drs J. E. Rees and M. N. Rossor for permission to investigate T.O.B., a patient under their care. We wish to acknowledge the MRC Cyclotron Unit, Hammersmith Hospital and the staff of the Psychology Department, National Hospital. R.A.M.'s research was funded by Cambridge University.

Notes

1. Lissauer, H. *Cognitive Neuropsychol.* **5**, 153–192 (1988).

2. Nielson, J. M. in *Memory and Amnesia* (San Lucas, Los Angeles, 1958).

3. Konorski, J. in *Integrative activity of the brain: An interdisciplinary approach* (University of Chicago Press, 1967).

4. Coughlan, A. K. & Warrington, E. K. *Brain* **101**, 163–185 (1978).

5. Warrington, E. K. *Quart. J. exp. Psychol.* **27**, 635–657 (1975).

6. Goodglass, H. & Budin, C. *Neuropsychologia* **26**, 67–78 (1988).

7. McCarthy, R. A. & Warrington, E. K. *Neuropsychologia* **23**, 709–727 (1985).

8. Hart, J., Berndt, R. S. & Caramazza, A. *Nature* **316**, 439–440 (1985).

9. Warrington, E. K. & McCarthy, R. A. *Brain* **106**, 859–878 (1983).

10. Warrington, E. K. & McCarthy, R. A. *Brain* **110**, 1273–1296 (1987).

11. Warrington, E. K. & Shallice, T. *Brain* **107**, 829–853 (1984).

12. Sartori, G. & Job, R. *Cognitive Neuropsychol.* **5**, 105–132 (1988).

13. Riddoch, M. J., Humphreys, G. W., Coltheart, M. & Funnell, E. *Cognitive Neuropsychol.* **5**, 3–25 (1988).

14. McCarthy R. A. & Warrington, E. K. *J. Neurol. Neurosurg. Psychiat.* **49**, 1233–1240 (1986).

54

J. C. Marshall and F. Newcombe

The conceptual status of deep dyslexia: An historical perspective

1980. In *Deep Dyslexia*, edited by M. Coltheart, K. Patterson, and J. C. Marshall. London: Routledge & Kegan Paul

In our paper for the 1971 meeting of the International Neuropsychology Society at Engelberg we insinuated the existence of a symptom-complex that we called deep dyslexia (Marshall and Newcombe, 1973). We say 'insinuated' rather than 'argued for' because our efforts there were restricted to bringing together a set of brain-injured patients under a common label which was really no more than a promissory note for the syndrome we were conjecturing. The most striking aspect of the behaviour of the patient that we studied (Marshall and Newcombe, 1966) was that he would produce surprising numbers of frank semantic errors when attempting to read aloud individual words (without context, time pressure, or stimulus degradation). Table 1 shows a representative sample of such errors from our subject, G.R., an intelligent and, prior to sustaining a left hemisphere injury, literate adult.

In addition, G.R. would sometimes make derivational errors, misreading, for example, an adjective or verb as its related nominal (or vice versa). Errors of this nature (discussed in Marshall, Newcombe, and Marshall, 1970) are displayed in Table 2.

Errors in which there was a clear visual (shape) similarity between stimulus and (the written form of) his (oral) response were also common (Table 3).

A syntactic hierarchy could also be observed such that concrete nouns stood the best chance of being read correctly. Adjectives, verbs and abstract nouns were of intermediate difficulty, and function words were very rarely read correctly. G.R.'s most frequent response to presentation of a function word was 'Don't know!' Occasionally, however, his response would be rather more informative; a sample of his 'better' attempts at coping with the 'little words' (his phrase) is given in Table 4.

Finally, we note that G.R. can never read aloud a non-word–an orthographically legal character string which happens not to have found a semantic niche in the English language. Once more, G.R.'s typical response upon being presented with a pronounceable non-word is to indicate that he simply cannot perform the task. Table 5, however, also includes some responses where the non-word has been read as if it were a visually similar real word.

Let us surmise, then, that this particular cluster of error-types and differential difficulty in response to lexical formatives, grammatical formatives, and legal non-words does indeed constitute a symptom-complex in, at least, the minimal sense that if substantial numbers of semantic errors are present then the other four features will reliably co-occur. The logic of any more profound analysis of deep dyslexia as a symptom-complex would seem to presuppose some basic statistical regularity in the error-types which do (and do not) appear together. Thus, to pick a well known example of this kind of argumentation, the first line of attack upon the Gerstmann syndrome (Gerstmann, 1930) is to suggest that the four defining characteristics (finger agnosia, right–left confusion, agraphia, and acalculia) do not co-occur with any greater strength than any other collection of, in this case, parietal signs (Benton, 1961). Similarly for deep dyslexia: the notion would be considerably weakened if different numbers (from zero to *n*!) of error-types co-occurred with semantic errors in different patients. It is with the above 'null hypothesis' in mind that we now turn to review the (putative) cases of deep dyslexia (in alphabetically written languages) that were reported prior to our 1966 paper.

1. Franz (1930)

In his presidential address to the Western Psychological Association in July 1928, Shepherd Ivory Franz reported a patient who made frequent semantic errors to individual words and continued to do so despite intensive remedial practice and training in reading. The subject was a professional man (an architect), presumably middle-aged (he seems from Franz's description to have occupied a position of some seniority), and presumably right-handed (no indication is given to the contrary). He sustained a closed head injury, having 'been hit on the head by a brick which had fallen from the tenth storey of a building the construction of which he was supervising'. The man had a right-sided hemiplegia, but no information is given concerning visual functions (e.g. visual fields).

His spontaneous speech was very severely impaired: 'For a relatively long time he could use only two affirmative, one negative, and two affective expressions.' Although some improvement took place over the two years that Franz followed his progress, his (spontaneous) vocabulary remained very restricted: 'Under the older neurological classification, he would have been classed as a complete motor aphasic.' His comprehension of speech, however, seems to have been remarkably good, extending to the appreciation of jokes. He seems to have had no difficulty in repeating individual words; no information is given concerning memory span, object-naming or colour-naming. Some general ability was preserved, at least to the extent that the

Table 1. (G.R.) Semantic errors

act	→ 'play'
close	→ 'shut'
dinner	→ 'food'
afternoon	→ 'tonight'
uncle	→ 'cousin'
tall	→ 'long'

Table 2. (G.R.) Derivational errors

wise	→ 'wisdom'
strange	→ 'stranger'
entertain	→ 'entertainment'
pray	→ 'prayers'
truth	→ 'true'
birth	→ 'born'

Table 3. (G.R.) Visual errors

stock	→ 'shock'
quiz	→ 'queue'
deuce	→ 'duel'
saucer	→ 'sausage'
crowd	→ 'crown'
crocus	→ 'crocodile'

Table 4. (G.R.) Function words

for	→ 'and'
his	→ 'she'
the	→ 'yes'
in	→ 'those'
be	→ 'Smali words are the worst'
some	→ 'One of them horrid words again'

Table 5. (G.R.) Non-words

wux	→ 'don't know'
nol	→ 'no idea'
zul	→ 'zulu'
wep	→ 'wet'
dup	→ 'damp'
tud	→ 'omo ... tide'[a]

[a] Both responses are the names of common detergents. *Tud* is visually similar to *tide*; in addition, it is possible that *tud* was 'misread' as *sud*, an 'internal' response that was followed by an overt semantic error.

patient could play dominoes (both fairly and with cheating).

When asked to read individually presented words, the subject made such responses as *hen* → 'egg' or *cat* → 'mice'. Errors of this nature persisted despite Franz's showing the card, pronouncing the correct response himself, and having the patient repeat it thirty or forty times. Little or no improvement took place over a period of two years post-injury. Sometimes quite long sequences of semantic errors (single words) were given to a particular stimulus, and Franz had the impression that the patient recognized (in some cases at least) that his response was wrong, and that he was attempting to correct himself. Very occasionally the patient would produce a neologistic response but in all cases they could plausibly be interpreted as inaccurate vocalizations of a real word, e.g. *lost* → 'sol' (= soul), or *hand* → 'chiff' (= handkerchief). There was one such instance that Franz regarded as a derivational error, *push* → 'pudden' (= pushing, or pulling). No other error-types were mentioned, although it is reported that the patient would sometimes recognize and call attention to familiar names in the newspaper. Writing ability (with the left hand) was essentially non-existent; the patient could write his signature, albeit very badly. The ability to produce complex architectural drawings and plans was, however, extremely well preserved. When Franz thought he detected an error in such sketches it always turned out finally that the patient was right and Franz wrong.

Franz interpreted the semantic errors in reading as a disorder of association—'a dissociation of ideas and reactions'. He emphasized the fluctuations in performance and drew a partial analogy with semantic errors in second language learning. Franz conducted a number of 'free-association' tests (orally) with the patient, and although his responses were sometimes rather bizarre ('blind' → 'good', 'cellar' → 'sweet'), Franz emphasized that under these conditions the patient's expressive vocabulary was much larger than was apparent during spontaneous speech. Verbs, adjectives, adverbs, and abstract nouns were all elicited in association tests. Many of the patient's associations appear to be 'mediate', and Franz seemed to think that the reading problem arose from a similar disorder of selection; too many responses are potentially available and the subject cannot 'pick' the correct one when reading. Although some of the patient's associations are 'fixed' (e.g. 'up' → 'down', 'east' → 'west', 'cup' → 'saucer'), it is the variation in response from trial to trial (in both reading and association) that Franz stressed.

While the paradigm for interpretation that Franz used is perfectly clear, he emphasized that he had not provided an *explanation* for the phenomena:

> Brain destruction may be an important incident in making speech associations difficult, but at the present time the brain destruction is neither explanatory of the associative losses nor can it be definitely classificatory until we further investigate speech from the standpoint of abilities and disabilities of association.

Franz's challenge still stands.

2. Beringer and Stein (1930)

Our next putative example was reported by Kurt Beringer and Johannes Stein at a joint conference of the Swiss Association for Psychiatry and the South West German Psychiatrists' Group in Basle in October 1929. Their patient was a woman, aged 64, educational level unspecified, and (presumably) right-handed. She had sustained an embolism of one branch of the left posterior cerebral artery. She had a right homonymous hemianopia, and 'a tendency to tire abnormally quickly in the apparently intact field of vision'. No information is given concerning the state of the motor system.

Beringer and Stein report the case as an example of 'pure alexia', for it would seem that her spontaneous speech, comprehension of speech, and repetition ability were unimpaired, as was her spontaneous writing. Kleist, Goldstein, and Minkowski were in the audience and joined in the discussion which followed the lecture. Minkowski, for one, was clearly absolutely amazed that a patient could make outright semantic errors in reading without the presence of associated language deficit: he asked, in an obviously rhetorical tone of voice, whether

> a patient who was observed and examined in such detail was really totally free from aphasic disturbances, whether she did not suffer some damage, in part at least, in vocabulary or in grammatical constructions with respect to the smaller language units, as is often the case not only with the restitution of motor aphasia but also with other aphasic types.

We have been unable to locate any published answer to Minkowski's question.

Beringer and Stein described the woman's alexia as 'characterized by agnosia for letters and words', and as uninfluenced by the form of the input (handwriting, Gothic, or Roman type). Errors on word-reading were, however, frequently drawn from the same 'sphere of meaning' as the stimulus item; examples include *Reichstag* (Parliament) → 'Berlin' (Berlin), *Indien* (India) → 'Elefant' (elephant), and *Fuchs* (fox) → 'Hase' (hare). Her performance was dramatically improved by being given (semantic) cues to the sense of the stimuli: 'She was completely puzzled by the word "sixteen", and was unable to recognize either the whole word or the individual letters, but she read it at once on being told that it was a number.' She was asked to read out the animals, or the musical instruments from a (semantically) mixed list of fifteen words—'she succeeded, although she had previously been alectic for these very words, such as cello, and horse.' Similarly, if presented with a list of words all drawn from the same category, she was initially quite unable to read any of them. But told that they were all, for example, tools, she succeeded in reading eleven out of twelve correctly. Similar results are reported for lists of virtues, crimes, and temporal expressions, although occasional derivational errors were made (e.g. *mercy* → 'merciful'). Beringer and Stein report that she could cope with abstract words just as well (or as badly) as with concrete words, but there does seem to be a syntactic hierarchy in her performance. She continued to try to read the newspaper following her embolism, and would sometimes succeed in reading out correctly a whole series of words, 'especially *nouns*'. In all conditions of testing, however, function words (*is, and, although, would,* etc.) were read particularly badly. She would sometimes attempt to spell out the sequence of letter names in the stimulus, either before or after trying to read the word as a whole, but numerous errors were made. The patient was quite uncertain as to the correct spelling, and even in cases where she had got it right she 'would abandon her own correct spelling when a false one was suggested to her'.

The patient made numerous mistakes when copying letters and geometric designs. However, she 'succeeded readily with spontaneous writing' although she could not (after a delay) read back what she herself had written.

Beringer and Stein provide two inter-related explanations for the nature of the reading deficit. In the first place they draw attention to the restricted, labile, fluctuating, and easily fatigued state of the patient's visual performance. Perimetric investigation showed various departures from normality in the apparently 'intact' visual field. The limits of the field seemed to vary more than in normal subjects as a function of size, intensity, and duration of stimulation. Likewise, the discrepancy between perception of moving versus static stimuli was outside the normal range. The just noticeable difference for a light-stimulus that gradually increased in intensity was also abnormal. Furthermore, the perception of movement was disturbed:

> very rapid movements were not recognised. When watching a cartoon film she did not notice, for instance, the leap of an animal from one side of the picture to the other when this happened very quickly. The patient was aware only that the animal was suddenly there, or that it had been at one side and was now at the other. On one occasion she deduced from this that the animal had jumped. On another she drew from the false perception the conclusion that there were two animals.

Other investigations are reported from which it appears that the subject's ability to recognize 'poorly illuminated geometrical shapes in a darkened room' was weaker than normal. The relevance of 'visual fatigue' to reading performance was pointed out by the subject herself who stated: 'If I want to read the paper, I must often wait for a moment and look away, then I can read again.' Beringer and Stein attempt to check this by getting the patient to relax in a darkened room and then putting the light on:

She was asked to read immediately after this relaxation, and at once read the first three words correctly, then her performance became uncertain and incorrect. After another period of darkness she again read correctly at first then wrongly, and she repeated this several times.

Now, this 'instability' of vision does not, of course, in itself serve to explain the occurrence of semantic errors in reading. Accordingly, Beringer and Stein suggest that although the fluctuating visual image of the word is not sufficient to determine directly and uniquely a (correct) vocal output it does suffice to evoke the appropriate 'sphere of meaning'. This notion is reminiscent of the two-threshold logogen model that Morton (1968) proposed in explanation of our own early results (Marshall and Newcombe, 1966), with the following difference: the *form* of representation that Beringer and Stein implied for the 'sphere of meaning' was in part at least, imagistic. They seem to be suggesting (or more accurately their patient suggests) that the word conjures up an appropriate visual image, which is in turn responded to as in an object- or scene-naming task. Thus the patient read *Reichstag* as 'Berlin' and then explained: 'I had the impression of somewhere I had been, where there was so much to see and to look at, you just had to sit down on a park bench and then look at it all, the whole picture.' Although such commentaries are interesting, it is, of course, not required that one takes them as veridical accounts of the actual process that was involved in the production of the overt response 'Berlin'. (Pylyshyn, 1973, and Nisbett and Wilson, 1977, discuss some of the more general theoretical issues that are at stake.) As Minkowski remarks: 'the associative connection is obvious and intelligible without any further consideration'. None the less, the notion needs airing for the idea of 'picturability' will turn up again in the later history of our topic (e.g. in Faust, 1955).

3. Low (1931)

The next case was seen by A. A. Low in Chicago in 1929. The patient, a man of 38, education and handedness unspecified, was admitted to hospital following, we presume, a left-hemisphere stroke. His vision appears to have been normal, but there was a complete right-sided hemiplegia and 'the tongue protruded toward the right side and showed a slight tremor'.

When the patient was admitted in July he seems to have suffered a total loss of speech; by September he had 'a partial motor aphasia and expressed himself with difficulty. He could name objects and was able to carry out simple commands but was unable to carry out complicated orders or to name the use of objects.' Further restitution of function is observed and by the middle of November

the patient had a fair ability to use spontaneous speech. He spoke in well-formed sentences, though with some difficulty in finding words. No agrammatism was noted in spontaneous speech. He was well able to point to objects named verbally or in print, to name the objects indicated by the examiner and to designate the use of objects.

Immediate repetition was essentially without error for both words and nonsense words, irrespective of number of syllables. The patient had thus made a remarkably good recovery in his oral language abilities (albeit with some residual aphasic signs) by the time that the investigations of visual language processing were launched. In contrast, writing to dictation was very poorly performed, although copying (with the left hand) of both print and cursive handwriting was quite good.

At this time the patient's 'reading aloud was fair for most words.' However, 'when given a sentence or paragraph to read, he left out many words and combinations of words, giving a distinct impression of agrammatical reading.' As Low writes, 'The agrammatical disturbance being confined to reading aloud only, the case represented a rare instance of an agrammatical disturbance in an isolated faculty of speech and called for detailed study.' Over the next few months Low devised and administered an astonishing number and variety of reading (and other) tests to his patient. Although Low's taxonomy of errors differs from our own it is clear from his examples that *all* the features we discussed in relation to G.R. are to be found in the performance of Low's patient. The patient makes semantic errors (*dad* → 'father', *child* → 'girl', *vice* → 'wicked'), derivational errors (*goes* → 'go', *reinstatement* → 'instate', *fleeing* → 'flee'), and visual errors (*life* → 'wife', *sword* → 'words', *shirt* → 'skirt'). Of all parts of speech the patient experienced the greatest difficulty when attempting to read (short) 'particles' (pronouns, articles, prepositions, conjunctions, adverbs, and auxiliary verbs). The patient also conspicuously failed to read pronounceable nonsense syllables, and would frequently 'infuse meaning into the material' (*sto* → 'story', *jun* → 'jump', *lom* → 'lemon'). A similar 'tendency toward supplementing meaning was again in evidence' when the patient was asked to read isolated letters or abbreviations (*J* → 'John', *A. A. Low, M.D.* → 'Low, doctor medicine').

Low is particularly careful in his attempts to isolate the exact nature of the patient's errors. The following quotation illustrates the type of argument that Low uses to support the claim that some errors are indeed visual:

> Mistakes like 'wife' for 'life', 'space' for 'pace' referred to a substitution of words which both look and sound alike. From such errors it is impossible to infer whether the patient read primarily with the aid of visual or of auditory images. But if he misread 'words' for 'sword', it was obvious that what he substituted was two words that merely looked alike. This mistake was obviously made because of a misapprehension of the visual images. A mistake which would have pointed definitely to a misapprehension of the auditory image, like 'tree' for 'key' was never made, although the tests provided ample opportunity for such errors.

With respect to the distinction between grammatical and lexical formatives, Low notes that while the patient 'simplified' complex words by dropping prefixes and suffixes (re-, de-, -ment, -s, -ing), he did *not* typically simplify compound nouns (e.g. armchair, doghouse, songbird, farmhand) in which both elements have full semantic value. Such compounds are read as easily as 'their isolated components'. Some of the derivational errors can be eliminated by context. Low tested the patient three times on sixty 'determined plurals' (e.g. *many houses, much money*) where 'after the patient reads "many" no choice is left him but to follow up with a plural formation. Similarly, after the pronunciation of the word "much" no room is left but for a succeeding singular.' Low continues:

> The fact that in three separate performances not one confusion of plural and singular occurred was taken as undisputable evidence that the patient had a considerable facility for handling singular and plural, and that the mistakes observed in the preceding tests referred to a tendency to leave out affixes, not to an ignorance of 'grammar'.

Low is careful, wherever possible, to check that his syntactic interpretations of error rates are valid. Thus having observed that the patient is particularly poor at reading 'short' particles (*at, from, to, as,* etc.) he rules out the possibility that 'shortness' (rather than grammatical function) is responsible for the deficit by noting that the patient is good at reading short (three-letter) nouns and adjectives.

Low concludes:

> All the defects of the various functions were reduced to a relative inefficiency to analyse parts out of a whole, on the one hand, and to a relative preference for synthesizing parts into a whole, on the other hand. All the symptoms were thus traced to one unifying lesion.

This vague theoretical account does not, of course, specify a psychological mechanism responsible for the 'analytic' impairment. None the less, Low's strategy is obviously sensible; one should consider the strongest possible claim—a unitary source for the observed symptoms—in order to facilitate its refutation. (We have not discussed here the many other psycholinguistic tests—including sentence and paragraph reading—that were administered. We would simply urge anyone interested in the psychology of language to read Low's descriptive masterpiece for themselves.)

4. Goldstein (1948)

We have previously mentioned that Kurt Goldstein was in the audience for Beringer and Stein's presentation in 1929. Finally, with Marianne Simmel, he observed a similar case of his own.* The patient (case 23) was a young man of 26, who had sustained a gunshot injury leading to 'occlusion of left carotid artery with cerebral infarction.' The bullet, it seems, 'went out at the base of the skull without apparently injuring actual brain matter.' The man was left-handed and his 'formal' education was rather limited. He was, however, an avid reader and had an extensive knowledge of Shakespeare and of Voltaire and Rousseau (the latter two in translation). He had also picked up 'a not inconsiderable amount of Greek' whilst in reformatory or jail. Visual functions seem to have been normal (although no formal testing is reported) as were motor functions with the exception of 'tactile agnosia' in the right hand.

The man had a severe expressive aphasia, and indeed 'spoke very little spontaneously'. What he did say was restricted to nouns and verbs (with very clear pronunciation). Speech in response to questions was somewhat better in terms of vocabulary size although here too he would produce one-word sentences and 'occasionally a noun and verb or adjective together, but never the article'. Some stock phrases might also be uttered ('pretty good', 'I know', 'I'm lost', 'I don't mind'). His comprehension was not good. Simple commands (sit down) would be understood but 'he failed whenever such a request contained more than one concrete item, e.g. "stand up and close your eyes".' Immediate repetition was good for single words, with the exception of function words, but very poor for short sentences. Digit span was restricted to one or two items. Spontaneous writing was poor and writing to dictation very bad, although copying was unimpaired.

When attempting to read aloud individual words numerous semantic errors were made (e.g. *era* → 'time',

* Some of the data reported in this section were very kindly supplied by Professor Simmel.

tide → 'water', *down* → 'up', *low* → 'small', *big* → 'little', *draw* → 'paint'). Similar semantic errors were found in tests of object-naming (*pipe* → 'cigar', *toaster* → 'eat', *lamp* → 'table'). Derivational (*lived* → 'live') and visual (*puddle* → 'puppy') errors also occurred in reading. Function words (*in*, *on*, *of*, *the*) were never read correctly; the most frequent response to them was no response, although sometimes they were misread as content words (e.g. *but* → 'button'). Goldstein checked that the function word phenomenon was not a purely output deficit. The patient could read *inn* but not *in*, *four* but not *for*, *two* but not *to*.

Reading of nonsense syllables was not investigated, although a (perhaps) related condition of testing is reported, namely the reading of 'mutilated words'. The patient would, for example, read *hsptl* as 'hospital' or *gradn* as 'garden'. Presented with mixed lists of correctly spelt words and their respective 'mutilated' forms he could pick out the correct form; this could be regarded as a forerunner of the lexical decision paradigm.

In his discussion of the case, Goldstein naturally stresses the role of comprehension in determining the patient's reading performance: 'Whenever the patient was able to read a word . . . there was never *any question as to his understanding* of the word. He *never*, as far as could be determined, *was able to read a word which he did not understand*, while at the same time he seemed to recognize a number of words and understand them without being able to read them correctly.'

The patient could 'recognize instantly' (both in free vision and with very short tachistoscopic exposure) '*a great number of words*, mostly nouns and verbs, but also a few adjectives, especially color names.' However, if the patient '*did not recognize a word instantly, no matter how much time he was given, he could not read it*.'

Goldstein accordingly regards the patient as reading by a holistic rather than a sequential strategy: '*Reading as a process starting from left to right was something completely alien to him*.' He could not, in other words, 'read by reading syllable after syllable.' Goldstein explains whatever success the patient did have in reading by invoking his '*extraordinary capacity of visual memory and imagery*.' Thus 'his visual memory made it possible for him to "read" a great number of words by simple recognition of the visual form.'

Given the patient's performance with stimuli such as *gradn* one might wonder exactly what is the form of this visual form. And one might also note that such an explanation of *correct* responses does not help us to understand the source of the *semantic* errors. Goldstein refers to the deficit as an 'impairment of abstraction and abnormal concreteness' but it is hard to see how one could cast these notions in the shape of an explicit information-processing model.

5. Simmel and Goldschmidt (1953)

A few years later, in 1950, Marianne Simmel was to observe another case whose reading disability was quite similar to that shown by the patient she investigated with Goldstein. The new patient was a left-handed woman of 24 who left school in order to get married after three years of high school. She is reported to have been an intelligent girl who did well in school. Seven years prior to the investigation, she had a child. 'A day or so before the baby's birth the patient began to have convulsions . . . she had 14 more convulsions after delivery by forceps, and was in a coma for several days.' For some time after she came out of coma the patient appears to have been severely agnostic, aphasic, and amnesic.

Seven years later the patient had made substantial recovery although numerous residual deficits were still in evidence. Ophthalmological and neurological findings, however, were within normal limits, with the exception of a marked reduction in visual flicker fusion frequency. No motor deficits were observed, including no 'primary dysarthria'.

The patient's spontaneous speech was 'on the whole very good', although some word-finding difficulties were noted. Verbal paraphasias did occur, albeit infrequently; literal paraphasias occurred very infrequently. Mistakes were occasionally made with function words (paragrammatism) but it is stressed that the patient did *not* speak in telegram style. 'Reactive' speech was much poorer: there were difficulties in remembering the question, and verbal paraphasias were frequent. In general, comprehension was only fair. Simple sentences were understood and simple instructions followed, but 'more complicated instructions or explanations which involved the simultaneous presentation of several factors seemed to present almost insurmountable obstacles to her.'

Oral repetition was well preserved for sentences, words, and nonsense syllables, but object-naming was grossly impaired. Numerous semantic paraphasias and considerable circumlocution were observed.

Writing, either spontaneously or to dictation was impossible, with the exception of the alphabet, the number series, and the patient's own name. Copying was 'generally poor and very laborious'. Although the patient could eventually copy letters and words 'the unit of her procedure was not the letter, but the single stroke, which gave rise to occasional constructive malformations.'

Reading 'consisted only of the recognition of individual words, primarily nouns, adjectives, and verbs. There was no reading of sentences, although she would occasionally read a "phrase"—a response similar to her spontaneous use of such automatic phrases.' Both visual (*chairman* → 'airmail', *shell* → 'tell') and semantic errors (*cents* → 'pennies', *blades* → 'razor') were frequently observed in single word reading. Function words were almost never read correctly (*not* → 'stop'); short (three-letter) nouns and verbs also occasioned great difficulty. Errors often had 'a similar letter configuration' to the correct response, e.g. *on* → 'no', *of* → 'for', *and* → 'can', *that* → 'plant', *but* → 'put', *shall* → 'tell'. Derivational errors are not reported and it seems that the reading of nonsense syllables was not tested.

Simmel and Goldschmidt discuss the patient's level of awareness of her errors. On some trials there was 'real "guessing", of which she was perfectly conscious.' On the majority of trials which produced 'verbal paraphasias', however, 'she seemed satisfied with her performance; but when asked whether she was sure of the correctness of her productions, she usually said, "I don't know" or "You tell me".' (It is not reported whether the patient's confidence in her responses differed as a consequence of whether the error was visual or semantic.) When the patient failed to recognize a word, she occasionally 'started spelling the word, i.e. reading the single letters, more or less correctly. This procedure did not, however, help her in finding the word.'

No general interpretation of the patient's pattern of loss and preservation is given, although an impairment of the 'abstract attitude' is implied: 'on the Goldstein Block Design test, the Weigl test and object-sorting tests the patient's performance was extremely "concrete".'

6. Faust (1955)

It is not really clear that we should include Faust's patient (W.E.) in our survey, but for the sake of completeness we will give a brief description of the case. The patient was a partially left-handed man (age and education unspecified) who sustained a left parietal gunshot injury in the Second World War. A bullet was removed at operation two days later. He had a right-sided spastic paralysis and initially was totally unable to speak.

Capacity for speech slowly returned although there were considerable residual aphasic signs. Spontaneous speech was poorly articulated with long pauses and occasional word-finding difficulties. He did, however, have 'enough circumlocutions at his disposal to make himself understood'. Repetition of number and letter series was also impaired and the patient would often stop halfway through a series and after some time return to the beginning. No information is given about the patient's comprehension or ability to repeat. Colour-naming was severely impaired; the deficit was associated with perceptual disturbance—the patient's discrimination and sorting of colours was quite poor.

The patient's writing to dictation was fair and he was hesitant with longer words. Performance was improved when the examiner articulated the syllables of multisyllabic words separately, and this strategy was employed with some success by the patient himself. When asked to write isolated nouns he would often add the article. In copying written material, the patient would 'draw a copy of the shape of the letter, without any understanding of it'.

Reading performance was very poor, even for material that the patient had himself written earlier: 'Single words were very seldom read correctly. If a word was not grasped at once, further reading was impossible.'

It is not entirely clear from Faust's report whether or not the patient made *outright* semantic errors that he thought were (or might have been) correct responses. The patient did, however, show by description and circumlocution that he had at least partial comprehension of the words that he could not read aloud. Thus given *table*, *chair*, and *cupboard*, the patient, although unable to read the words individually, remarked 'I know that, those are all furniture.' Similarly, given *Hans*, *Andreas*, and *Martin*, the patient could indicate that the words were all forenames (although again he could not read them aloud). The patient was quite unable to cope with reading function words such as articles or prepositions.

When he could not read a word the patient essayed the strategy of reading the initial letters:

> He only succeeded in doing this when the rest of the word was covered up. He could not analyse the whole word (into its letters). If he covered up a part of the word, then he could read the initial letter correctly. However, it was impossible for him to combine with this the letter which followed and so read the first and second letters together.

No information is given concerning the other error-types that are pertinent to our proposed symptom-complex.

Faust stresses the role of an unfolding 'sphere of meaning' in determining the patient's performance, and he refers back to Beringer and Stein's case as showing a similar impairment. He notes that the patient did sometimes understand words with a 'concrete meaning' and that 'the further the meaning of a word is from the concrete, the more strongly marked is the impairment to recognition.' Words with an 'abstract meaning' (such as articles, prepositions, and some verbs) are thus 'the most difficult to read'. Faust summarizes this point by remarking that 'it is not the length of the word which is crucial for recognition of it, but rather its relation to concrete objects and to what is visually-picturable.' Faust's interpretation is thus related both to the *imageability hypothesis* and to the *operativity hypothesis* of Gardner (1973).

Preliminary Discussion

A summary of the six cases is given in Table 6. This table cites examples of the pattern of reading impairment of these subjects as it relates to the initial conjecture: that deep dyslexia is indeed a symptom-complex. On the whole, there is some support for our suggestion that semantic errors occur in the context of derivational and visual errors, and that impairment is maximal when attempting to read function words or nonsense syllables. At very least, there are no counterexamples in the cases we have reviewed. The table, however, contains too many question marks (where information is simply not available) to permit the making of very strong claims.

It would seem that the syndrome (if such it be) is specific to reading performance in the following sense: although the majority of the patients reported do have additional aphasic symptoms neither the nature nor the severity of the associated impairment is (even approximately) constant. Spontaneous speech may be grossly non-fluent (and agrammatic) or fluent paraphasic, or anomic. If we are to believe Beringer and Stein's claim, speech may be quite unimpaired. Comprehension deficits are usually in evidence, but again they may range from severe to quite mild. The nature (and perhaps even the primary locus) of the brain injury (and the associated neurological disturbances) is likewise variable. The patient population is itself heterogenous—men and women, old and young, left-handed and right-handed. The patients, prior to sustaining brain injury, were neither unintelligent nor poor readers. Indeed, if anything they appear to have had an above average interest and competence in reading. We have no information about how they were taught to read or what strategies they adopted as mature readers prior to injury. A reasonable guess would be that they had been 'chinese' rather than 'phoenician' readers (Baron and Strawson, 1976). The reading problem does seem to co-occur with a writing deficit, which is often more severe than the disturbance of reading. (In some cases spontaneous and dictated writing is abolished.) Even this deficit does not, however, seem to be an invariant concomitant of deep dyslexia. Spontaneous writing seems to have been preserved in Beringer and Stein's case (and in Faust's patient writing performance was far superior to reading).

The evidence so far assembled does not, then, enable us (yet) to reject the hypothesis that deep dyslexia is indeed a functional, dynamic deficit of the *reading* system (or at least of one sub-type of possible reading systems). Despite the involvement of semantic and syntactic variables in determining performance the condition does not seem to be secondary to a more widespread (multi- or supra-modal) disturbance of linguistic ability. That is, theoretical interpretations of the condition may not need to make specific reference to the associated aphasic deficits that are found in the majority of the patients who have thus far been studied. It may be that no particular constellation of aphasic signs constitute necessary and sufficient conditions for the emergence of deep dyslexia. But all of this leaves us more or less where we started—in search of a psychological explanation (an information-processing model consistent with linguistic descriptions of the condition, and with available neurological constraints) for a uniquely perplexing disorder.

Three very general questions thus arise. First, to what extent can we interpret deep dyslexia as a structured breakdown in the (or a) primary reading mechanism employed by the normal, fluent adult reader (Ellis and Marshall, 1978; Holmes, Marshall and Newcombe, 1971)? Second, if real insight is not forthcoming by adoption of the first viewpoint, can we achieve a new synthesis by conjecturing that the responsible lesions have uncovered and allowed to emerge overtly an intact but subsidiary reading system, the neurological substrate for which is perhaps to be found in the right hemisphere (Coltheart, 1977)? Third, can we begin to discover universal and specific constraints upon reading mechanisms by comparing dyslexic breakdown across a variety of script-types, in particular by

Table 6

Study	Semantic errors	Derivational errors	Visual errors	Function words	Nonsense syllables
Franz (1930)	*cat* → 'mice'	*push* → 'pudden'	?	?	?
Beringer & Stein (1930)	*Reichstag* → 'Berlin'	*mercy* → 'merciful'	?	very poor	?
Low (1931)	*child* → 'girl'	*goes* → 'go'	*sword* → 'words'	very poor	*jun* → 'jump'
Goldstein (1948)	*draw* → 'paint'	*lived* → 'live'	*puddle* → 'puppy'	very poor	*gradn* → 'garden'
Simmel & Goldschmidt (1953)	*cents* → 'pennies'	?	*top* → 'put'	very poor	?
Faust (1955)	semantic descriptions	?	?	very poor	?

investigating languages written in non-alphabetic orthographies (Marshall, 1976)?

Finally, we wish to emphasize yet again the importance of attempts to falsify the claim that deep dyslexia is a real syndrome. Any valid taxonomic classification presupposes a functional unity in the pattern of impaired and preserved abilities within and between classes. The effects of a chance constellation of lesions, however often observed, or even of a single lesion that for purely topological reasons (Brain, 1964) impairs a variety of independent systems, are unlikely to be theoretically revealing. Our own preference is that there is indeed a disruption of a single underlying mechanism which shows itself in a meaningful cluster of surface manifestations. But we must not ignore the possibility that we are studying an accident of anatomy or sampling, whose consequences have misled us by their tantalizing appearance of order. In short, deep dyslexia will not exist unless or until it finds a place within a credible neurolinguistic theory.

References

Baron, J. and Strawson, C. (1976) Use of orthographic and word-specific knowledge in reading words aloud. *Journal of Experimental Psychology, Human Perception and Performance*, *2*, 386–93.

Benton, A. L. (1961) The fiction of the 'Gerstmann Syndrome'. *Journal of Neurology, Neurosurgery and Psychiatry*, *24*, 176–81.

Beringer, K. and Stein, J. (1930) Analyse eines Falles von 'Reiner' Alexie. *Zeitschrift für die Gesamte Neurologie und Psychiatrie*, *123*, 473–8.

Brain, Lord (1964) Statement of the problem. In A. V. D. de Reuck and M. O'Connor (eds), *Disorders of Language*. London: Churchill.

Coltheart, M. (1977) Phonemic dyslexia: some comments on its interpretation and its implications for the study of normal reading. Paper presented at the International Neuropsychology Society Meeting, Oxford.

Ellis, A. W. and Marshall, J. C. (1978) Semantic errors or statistical flukes? A note on Allport's 'On knowing the meaning of words we are unable to report'. *Quarterly Journal of Experimental Psychology*, *30*, 569–75.

Faust, C. (1955) *Die zerebralen Herdstörungen bei Hinterhauptsverletzungen und ihr Beurteilung*. Stuttgart: Thieme.

Franz, S. I. (1930) The relations of aphasia. *Journal of General Psychology*, *3*, 401–11.

Gardner, H. (1973) The contribution of operativity to naming capacity in aphasic patients. *Neuropsychologia*, *11*, 213–20.

Gerstmann, J. (1930) Zur Symptomatologie der Hirnläsionen im Übergangsgebiet der unteren Parietal—und mittleren Occipitalwindung. *Nervenartzt*, *3*, 691–5.

Goldstein, K. (1948) *Language and Language Disturbances*. New York: Grune & Stratton.

Holmes, J. M., Marshall, J. C. and Newcombe, F. (1971) Syntactic class as a determinant of word-retrieval in normal and dyslexic subjects. *Nature*, *234*, 416.

Low, A. A. (1931) A case of agrammatism in the English language. *Archives of Neurology and Psychiatry*, *25*, 556–97.

Marshall, J. C. (1976) Neuropsychological aspects of orthographic representation. In R. J. Wales and E. Walker (eds), *New Approaches to Language Mechanisms*. Amsterdam: North Holland.

Marshall, J. C. and Newcombe, F. (1966) Syntactic and semantic errors in paralexia. *Neuropsychologia*, *4*, 169–76.

Marshall, J. C. and Newcombe, F. (1973) Patterns of paralexia. *Journal of Psycholinguistic Research*, *2*, 175–99.

Marshall, M., Newcombe, F. and Marshall, J. C. (1970) The microstructure of word-finding difficulties in a dysphasic subject. In G. B. Flores d'Arcais and W. J. M. Levelt (eds), *Advances in Psycholinguistics*. Amsterdam: North Holland.

Morton, J. (1968) Grammar and computation in language behavior. *Progress Report No. 6*, Center for Research in Language and Language Behavior, University of Michigan.

Nisbett, R. E. and Wilson, T. D. (1977) Telling more than we can know: verbal reports on mental processes. *Psychological Review*, *84*, 231–59.

Pylyshyn, Z. W. (1973) What the mind's eye tells the mind's brain: a critique of mental imagery. *Psychological Bulletin*, *80*, 1–24.

Simmel, M. L. and Goldschmidt, K. H. (1953) Prolonged post-eclamptic aphasia: report of a case. *A.M.A. Archives of Neurology and Psychiatry*, *69*, 80–3.

M. Coltheart, J. Masterson, S. Byng, M. Prior, and J. Riddoch

Surface dyslexia

1983. *Quarterly Journal of Experimental Psychology* 35A: 469–495

Abstract

Two cases of surface dyslexia are described. In this disorder, irregular words such as *broad* or *steak* are less likely to be read aloud correctly than regularly-spelled words like *breed* or *steam*; and when irregular words are misread the incorrect response is often a regularisation (reading *broad* as "brode" and *steak* as "steek", for example). When reading comprehension was tested, homophones were often confused with each other: for example, *soar* was understood as an instrument for cutting, and *route* was understood as being part of a tree. Spelling was also impaired, with the majority of spelling errors being phonologically correct: for example, "search" was spelled *surch*. "Orthographic" errors in reading aloud (omitting, altering, adding or transposing letters) were also noted. These errors were not due to defects at elementary levels of visual processing.

One of our cases was a developmental dyslexic, and the other was an acquired dyslexic. The close similarity of their reading and spelling performance supports the view that surface dyslexia can occur both as a developmental and as an acquired dyslexia.

A theoretical interpretation of surface dyslexia within the framework of the logogen model (including a grapheme–phoneme correspondence system for reading non-words) was offered: defects within the input logogen system, and in communication from that system to semantics, were postulated as responsible for most of the symptoms of surface dyslexia.

Introduction

Consider the word *gauge*. In this word, the vowel digraph *au* is given the pronunciation /eɪ/. There are no other words of English in which this particular orthographic–phonological correspondence occurs. The usual pronunciation for *au* is /ɔ/. Since the pronunciation of *au* in *gauge* is unique to that word, the word could only be read aloud correctly by accessing stored information which is specifically about the word gauge.

In contrast, for words like *gaunt*, in which *au* is given its usual pronunciation, correct reading aloud could be accomplished by using general information of the form *g* → /g/, *au* → /ɔ/, *n* → /n/ and *t* → /t/, information which applies to a large variety of different words. Information specifically about the word *gaunt* is not mandatory for correct reading aloud.

Words containing the digraph *au* with the pronunciation /ɔ/ may be termed *regular* words (assuming their other orthographic-phonological correspondences are also the usual ones); those words in which *au* is given some other pronunciation may be termed *irregular* words.

A reader who relied solely on general information about orthographic–phonological correspondences to read aloud, and did not consult sources of word-specific information, would read regular words correctly but would misread irregular words, and the misreadings of irregular words would take the form of regularisations: reading *gauge* as /gɔdʒ/, for example.

If, as a consequence of brain damage, a person lacks adequate access to word-specific information about pronunciation, or if a person has not developed this in the course of learning to read, whilst relatively good access to general information about orthographic–phonological correspondences is possible, it follows that a prominent symptom of this form of disordered reading would be difficulty in reading irregular words aloud, with the erroneous readings consisting of regularisation errors. Precisely this variety of dyslexia has been described by Marshall and Newcombe (1973): they named it *surface dyslexia*, and described two cases, J.C. and S.T.

Both cases had suffered penetrating missile wounds to the left temporo-parietal region of the brain, 20 or more years before the investigations of their reading capabilities. The writing and oral spelling of both patients was severely impaired, as well as their reading. Spontaneous speech was unimpaired (in the case of J.C.) or reasonably fluent (in the case of S.T.). Regularisation errors such as broad → /broʊd/ and route → /raʊt/ were present in their attempts at reading aloud. Evidently, one way to detect surface dyslexia is to compare the accuracy of reading aloud of regular and irregular words. A convenient matched set of 39 irregular and 39 regular words was published by Coltheart, Besner, Jonasson and Davelaar (1979) and used by Shallice and Warrington (1980) in their investigations of a case of surface dyslexia (they used the term "semantic dyslexia" to refer to this syndrome). Their patient, R.O.G., was correct in reading aloud for 36 out of 39 regular words and 25 out of 39 irregular words. She had fluent expressive speech with occasional word-finding difficulties, and poor spelling as well as poor reading. Her reading error included regularisations: for example, she read *broad* as "brode".

To judge from four recent general reviews of acquired dyslexia (Patterson, 1981; Shallice, 1981; Coltheart, 1981; Newcombe and Marshall, 1981), there is a consensus in favour of the view that an essential symptom of surface dyslexia is the kind of difficulty with irregular words that we have just been discussing.

There is by no means agreement, however, as to the procedure by which regularisation errors are produced when irregular words are misread. When a patient reads *broad* as "brode", for example, it is evident that he has failed to access word-specific information about the irregular word *broad*. His choice of "brode" as a response, however, could be explained in at least four different ways. These explanations are considered later in the paper: briefly, the possibilities which have been proposed are that a system of grapheme–phoneme correspondences are used, that correspondences for orthographic units larger than the grapheme (e.g. *br* and *oad*) are used, that correspondences between *morphemes* and phonology are used (the relevant morpheme here being *road*), and that analogies with orthographically similar words (here, for example, *road*, *goad*, *load*) are used.

The main aim of our paper is not to attempt to adjudicate between these views of surface dyslexic reading, since we consider that this may not yet be possible. Instead, we wish to provide further information about the nature of surface dyslexia. In particular, we concentrate upon three topics: reading comprehension, error types in surface dyslexic reading, and the nature of the spelling disorder which accompanies surface dyslexia.

Reading comprehension in surface dyslexia has not yet been systematically investigated, though a number of pertinent observations were made by Marshall and Newcombe (1973). Their patient, J.C., for example, not only read *listen* as "Liston", but added the gloss "... that's the boxer", indicating that his view about what this word meant was obtained via the use of his (incorrect) phonological recoding, rather than being based directly upon an orthographic code for the word. We investigate how frequent this phenomenon is—that is, how often the surface dyslexic's comprehension of a printed word depends upon his phonological recoding of that word with neglect of the word's orthographic code, as in the Liston example. We also investigate what additional kinds of errors (other than the regularisation error) can be observed in surface dyslexic reading; and whether there are systematic kinds of error in spelling to dictation and spontaneous writing.

Finally, our paper also considers the relationship between developmental and acquired surface dyslexia. So far in this paper we have considered cases of acquired dyslexia—that is, of reading disorder produced by brain damage in a previously competent reader. Some poor readers, of course, have never attained competence in reading, and the term "developmental dys lexia" may be used here. An interesting but little-explored question concerns what relationships (if any) exist between the forms of acquired dyslexia and developmental dyslexia. This question is dealt with in unpublished work by Holmes (1973; see also Holmes, 1978) which reports investigations of J.C. and S.T., who exhibited *acquired* surface dyslexia, and of four *developmental* dyslexic. Holmes contended that the pattern of reading errors exhibited by these developmental dyslexics corresponded to the pattern exhibited by the acquired dyslexics and examinations of the corpus of errors she provided support her view. Holmes therefore concluded that surface dyslexia exists not only as an acquired dyslexia but also as a developmental dyslexia. This conclusion is consistent with the work of Boder (1973), in that one of the forms of developmental dyslexia Boder postulated—her term for it was "dyseidetic dyslexia"—appears to be equivalent to surface dyslexia.

We report investigations of the reading, writing and spelling performance of two individuals: C.D. and A.B. We will argue that C.D. is a developmental dyslexic, that A.B. is an acquired dyslexic, and that both are surface dyslexics. We hope, then, not only to provide further information about the nature of surface dyslexia itself, but also further evidence for the view that surface dyslexia occurs both as a developmental dyslexia and as an acquired dyslexia.

Developmental Surface Dyslexia

Case History

C.D., a right-handed girl, was born in February 1964. She has one sibling, a left-handed brother; her father is left-handed and her mother is right-handed. Neither her parents nor her brother are said to have had difficulties in reading or any other aspect of language, but C.D. was always slow at reading, and dyslexic difficulties were suspected as early as the age of 7 years. She has lived for periods in Switzerland, where she attended a French school and spoke and wrote in French, but English is her native language. There is no history or current evidence of any form of neurological abnormality. Her speech production and comprehension appear to be entirely normal.

At the age of 9, she was administered the WISC and obtained a Full Scale IQ of 104. The WISC was administered again on 26 April 1979: she obtained a Full Scale IQ of 104 again (Verbal IQ, 105; Performance IQ, 101). At this time, she performed at the Bright Normal level on two sub-tests and at the Average level on all remaining sub-tests (including a Digit Span scale score of 10). In more extensive testing of digit span in February 1980 she was given four spoken five-digit sequences to repeat: three were repeated correctly and one with an order error of two adjacent digits. Of four six-digit sequences, three were repeated correctly and one with an order error or two adjacent digits. Sequences of

Table I. Performance of C.D. on standardised tests of reading and spelling

	Date	Age score	Chronological age
Schonell reading test	26 April 1979	11:0	15:2
Schonell spelling test	26 April 1979	9:0	15:2
Schonell reading test	28 January 1980	10:1	15:11
Schonell spelling test A (written responses)	4 February 1980	9:4	16:0
Schonell spelling test B (oral responses)	25 February 1980	7:5	16:0
English picture vocabulary test (printed words to be matched to pictures)	29 September 1980	13:2	16:7

fewer than four digits were repeated without error. When the task was to repeat the digits back in reverse order, four-digit and shorter sequences were repeated correctly; one of two five-digit sequences was correct, the other produced an omission. These results indicate that C.D. exhibits a somewhat reduced digit span (an estimated age score of 12:6).

Her reading and spelling abilities have been tested on several occasions, with the results shown in Table I. These results indicate severe backwardness in reading aloud, silent reading comprehension, written spelling and oral spelling. These difficulties in dealing with written language occur in the context of normal intelligence and normal ability in dealing with spoken language: not only do C.D.'s spoken language and speech comprehension appear entirely normal, but when her word comprehension was tested using the English Picture Vocabulary Test with each word *spoken* (rather than *written*, as in Table 1), on 7 July 1980, her age score was 17:5. Further evidence indicating that her ability to comprehend single printed words is very much inferior to her ability to comprehend comparable single spoken words is given later in the paper.

This pattern of performance (normal intelligence and normal ability to deal with spoken language plus severe difficulties in dealing with printed language, in the absence of neurological abnormalities and emotional problems) is usually taken as justifying the description "developmental dyslexia". We next wish to indicate why we consider that the particular form of dyslexia exhibited by C.D. is surface dyslexia as defined by Marshall and Newcombe (1973) and Holmes (1973).

Evidence for Surface Dyslexia in C.D.

Reading Aloud Regular and Irregular Words On 28 November 1979 C.D. was asked to read aloud the 39 regular and 39 matched irregular words listed in Coltheart *et al.* (1979). Her responses were correct for 35 out of 39 regular words and for 26 out of 39 irregular words ($\chi^2 = 6.08, P < 0.02$).[1] These value may be compared with those produced by R.O.G. (Shallice and Warrington, 1980), who was suffering from an acquired surface dyslexia produced by a left-hemisphere haemorrhage; R.O.G. scored 36 out of 39 and 25 out of 39 on the regular and irregular words. For reasons described above, reading aloud which is significantly worse for irregular words than for regular words is one of the cardinal symptoms of surface dyslexia.

Homophone Matching We pursued this regularity effect further by investigating whether it could be obtained in a task which, whilst requiring the subject to convert printed letter strings into phonological codes, did not require a spoken response. The task we used was judging whether two different letter strings had identical or different pronunciations—"homophone matching". Three different forms of the test were devised: one using only regular words, another using irregular words, and a third using only non-words.

Consider the homophone pair *hair/hare.* A subject who was poor at phonological recoding might nevertheless judge that these two words were homophones by using an orthographic strategy: that is, judging word pairs to be homophonous when there is considerable orthographic overlap between them, as in the case *hair/hare.* On this strategy, however, if *hair* and *hare* are considered to be homophonous, then *hair* and *hard* would also be considered homophonous, since the orthographic overlap between *hair* and *hare* is the same as the overlap between *hair* and *hard.* With such stringent matching of orthographic overlap between "Same" (homophonic) stimulus pairs and "Different" (non-homophonic) stimulus pairs, it is impossible for the task to be performed using any code except a phonological one. We therefore selected 25 pairs of homophones (all 50 of these words being regularly spelled) and 25 orthographically-matched non-homophonic word pairs (all 50 of these words being regularly spelled also). This constituted the "regular homophone matching" task.

An "irregular homophone matching" task was constructed in exactly the same way (25 homophonic pairs plus 25 orthographically matched non-homophonic pairs). Here, of the four words making up a homophonic pair and its orthographically-matched non-homophonic pair, one word was irregular. This ensured that a person who always generated an incorrect phonological code (a regularisation) for an irregular word would score at chance on the irregular-words version of the homophone matching task. For example, with the matched pairs *so/sew* and *no/new*, there would be a correct "Different" response to the second pair and an *incorrect* "Different" response to the first pair (since the irregular word *sew* would not be given the same phonological code as *so*); whilst with the matched pairs *ale/ail* and *are/air*, there would be a correct "Same" response to the first pair and *incorrect* "Same" response to the second pair (since the irregular word *are* would be regularised and hence given the same phonological code as *air*).

Finally a "non-word homophone matching" task was constructed using only non-words, with orthographic matching as before: there were 25 pairs of non-word homophones and 25 matched pairs of non-word non-homophones (e.g. *fid/phid* vs. *fid/prid*).

These three homophone-matching tasks were administered to C.D. In each case, the 50 item pairs were typed in lower case letters on cards, one pair per card, and these were given to C.D. one card at a time. Her task was to sort the cards into two piles (one for pairs with identical pronunciations and one for pairs with different pronunciations) without reading the items aloud.

The results were as follows: regular words, 44 out of 50 (four false alarms, two misses); non-words, 39 out of 50 (four false alarms, six misses; irregular words, 34 out of 50 (10 false alarms, six misses). The three conditions differed significantly ($\chi^2_{(2)} = 8.73$, $P < 0.02$) and performance was significantly worse with irregular words than with regular words ($\chi^2_{(1)} = 5.82$, $P < 0.02$).

Thus, whether a phonological code is required overtly (as in reading aloud) or only covertly (as in silent homophone matching), C.D. performs worse with irregular words than with regular words.

Error Types As we discussed earlier in this paper, a failure to use word-specific information when attempting to read words aloud would result not only in worse performance with irregular words as compared to irregular words, but would also result in regularisation errors. Furthermore, since English has no perfectly applicable general system for specifying correct stress in polysyllabic words, word-specific information will often be needed if words are to be pronounced with correct stress. Inadequate access to such information should therefore lead to stress errors in reading aloud, and indeed Marshall and Newcombe (1973) reported such errors in their patients: for example, the words *omit* and *imply* were read with stress on the first syllable and an unstressed second syllable.

In reading aloud, C.D. produced examples of both regularisation errors and stress errors. Some of these are shown in Table II. All six surface dyslexics discussed by Holmes (1973) made regularisation errors and stress errors, as examination of her error corpus shows.

Table II. Regularisations and stress errors in surface-dyslexic reading (C.D.)

bear	→ "beer"	shove	→ /ʃoɷv/
gauge	→ "gorge"	apex	→ /ə'pɛks/
duet	→ /djut/	oboe	→ /ɛ'boɷ/
pint	→ /pɪnt/	break	→ /brik/
billed	→ /'bɪlə:d/	are	→ "air"
quay	→ /kweɪ/	surplus	→ /sə'plus/
angel	→ /'æŋgɷ/	come	→ /koɷm/
subtle	→ /'sʌbtaɪl/	bury	→ /bjuri/

Other aspects of surface dyslexia as it was discussed by Marshall and Newcombe (1973)—for example, "visual" errors—are discussed later in this paper. For the moment, we conclude that the regularity effects, regularisation errors and stress errors displayed by C.D. justify classifying her as a surface dyslexic; and we turn now to a consideration of reading comprehension in this case of surface dyslexia.

Reading Comprehension Given that C.D. read *bear* as "beer", for example, it is clearly important to know how she would have responded if her task had been to *understand* this printed word rather than to read it aloud. Would she have understood it as an animal (the way it is spelled) or as a drink (the way she read it aloud)?

We decided to study reading comprehension by asking C.D. to say what printed words meant as well as reading them aloud. She was shown single printed words, asked to define each word, and only after having done this to read the word aloud (to avoid, as far as possible, any contamination of the comprehension response by a previous oral reading response). She was also asked to spell each word aloud (with the word remaining in view) after she had first indicated what it meant and secondly read it aloud. We used this spelling aloud task because it might be argued that a response such as *bear* → "beer" is not a regularisation at all, but instead is due to a letter misperception: the *a* of *bear* is misperceived as *e*. If letter misperceptions at any *elementary* level are a significant factor in C.D.'s reading errors, they should be evident when she spells aloud words which she is looking at.

We selected a set of 95 words which in previous testing C.D. had read wrongly. Each word was presented singly on an index card, and she was asked first to say what the word meant, then to read it aloud, and then to spell it aloud, while the card was still being viewed.

It was overwhelmingly the case that the definition she gave corresponded to the subsequent oral reading response, *irrespective of whether the word was read aloud correctly or not.* Of the 95 words, 49 were read correctly and 46 were not.[2] Of the 46 misread words, 44 were defined in accordance with the subsequent oral reading response: some examples are: *bear*, "a drink ...

beer" and *enigma*, "a picture ... image". There were only four examples where the definition and the subsequent reading aloud did not match:

debt → "when you owe something ... depth"
quay → "quiver ... to move ... /kweɪ/" (?quake)
throng → "pained ... throng" (?throb)
surplus → "some news, a surplus which goes round ... surplus"

These results indicate that, when the surface dyslexic's oral reading response differs from the word presented for reading, the comprehension of the word is determined via the incorrect pronunciation, even if the comprehension test precedes the oral reading. Thus C.D. understands a word in terms of the way she would read it aloud, not the way it is spelled.

This dominance of comprehension by phonology is not a consequence of requiring subsequent oral reading, because it occurs when no reading aloud is required. C.D. was presented with a four-alternative forced-choice test, in which a spoken definition was given to her and she was asked then to choose from a set of four printed words that word which fitted the definition. The four words included the correct response, a homophone of the correct response, a foil which was at least as orthographically similar to the correct response as the homophone was, and a fourth foil which was orthographically similar to the homophonic foil (example: "It means to complain": *moat*, *mown*, *moan*, *morn*).

The test consisted on 100 such items. C.D.'s choice was correct for 74 items. Of the 26 errors, 24 consisted of choosing the homophonic foil; the two other foil types were chosen once each.

In the definitions and oral readings given by C.D., there were many errors which involved the regularisation of irregular words, but there are also others (such as the response to *enigma*) which cannot be interpreted as regularisations. We take this point up later; for the moment, we will consider the possible role of letter misperceptions and misperceptions of letter order in surface-dyslexic reading.

One might argue that the response *bear* → "a drink" occurs because of a misperception of the *a* as an *e*, that *plain* → "to make preparations for" involves a failure to percieve the *i* at all, and that *spare* → "a weapon" and *enigma* → "a picture" involve misperceptions of the relative spatial locations of letters. If this were so, these elementary perceptual errors should occur when C.D. spells these words aloud after having just defined them and read them aloud. This did not happen. There was only a single instance in which the spelling-aloud response did not match the word presented: *debt* was spelled aloud as "D,E,P ... D,E,D,T". Thus we observed responses such as *bowl* → "wind ... blow ... B,O,W,L", and *enigma* → "a picture ... image ... E,N,I,G,M,A".

We conclude that the reading-aloud errors and comprehension errors of the surface dyslexic do not arise at some *elementary* perceptual level at which individual letters are misidentified or their relative positions misperceived, since C.D. was essentially perfect at reading out the correct letters in their correct positions in the spelling-aloud task. This has implications for some traditional findings on developmental dyslexia: responses such as *bowl* → "blow" or *spare* → "spear" have in the past sometimes been offered as evidence for a deficiency in sequential visual perception but it is difficult to accept this if we know that immediately after these incorrect responses the letters in words will be correctly read aloud in their correct sequence, as happens on virtually every occasion. This spelling-aloud control task has not always been used in studies of "sequential disorders" in dyslexia. Of course, it is quite possible that *some* dyslexic readers *would* err in the spelling-aloud task.

In this tripartite task requiring comprehension, pronunciation and spelling, then, the surface dyslexic's comprehension is governed by the way the word would be said, whilst the spelling-aloud performance is governed by the way the word is seen. Hence comprehension errors occur (because pronunciation errors occur), whilst spelling-aloud errors do not occur.

Asking C.D. to comprehend then read aloud then spell printed words thus proved very useful in elucidating a number of aspects of surface dyslexia. What is more, it revealed an interesting and frequent form of error which has not previously been reported in studies of surface dyslexia, since it could only be discovered when comprehension is tested—the homophone confusion, in which reading aloud is correct but comprehension is incorrect; examples are *pane*, "something which hurts" and *bowled*, "fierce, big".

We suggest below that these homophone confusions in comprehension are of considerable theoretical significance.

Latency of Reading C.D.'s, reading, even when incorrect, was usually prompt, and multiple attempts at reading a single word were rare. In a session when she read aloud eight lists of words, each consisting of a column of 25 words, time to read the lists ranged from 25 to 30 seconds per list, and error rate ranged from 12 to 32% across lists. Of these 200 responses, only two involved multiple attempts at reading.

Auditory Comprehension In order to compare C.D.'s auditory comprehension with her reading comprehension, the 95 words used for testing reading comprehension were subsequently (2.5 months later) given in spo-

Table III. Comprehension of spoken words compared to comprehension of printed words (C.D.)

Visual	Auditory: Comprehended	Auditory: Not comprehended	Total
Read correctly and comprehended correctly	38	0	38
Read as another word and comprehended as that word	21	3	24
Read as a non-word; "don't know" given as comprehension response	5	6	11
Read as a word; "don't know" given as comprehension response	0	1	1
Other	0	2	2
	64	12	76

ken form, and she was asked to say what the word spoken to her meant.

As mentioned above, it happened that some of these 95 words (19, to be exact) were homophones. Asking for a definition of a spoken homophone is clearly an unsatisfactory request, so we consider for the moment only the 76 non-homophones. These results are shown in Table III. Correct comprehension occurred for 84% of the words when they were heard and for 50% of the words when they were read ($\chi^2_{(1)} = 20.14$, $P < 0.01$). Furthermore, every word which had been comprehended correctly when presented visually was comprehended when presented in speech, whilst there were 25 words which were comprehended correctly in speech but not in print. The 12 words which were not comprehended in speech were *satirical, sepulchre, oblivion, pinnacle, surplus, beguile, throng, enigma, billet, gawky, mode* and *siege*: all relatively infrequent words.

Thus single words were comprehended much better when they were heard than when they were read. Furthermore, those words which were not comprehended when they were heard were all sufficiently rare for these results to be consistent with the suggestion made earlier that C.D.'s speech comprehension is normal.

What of the 19 homophones? In the speech comprehension test, these were disambiguated by spelling each one aloud to C.D. after it had been spoken as a whole word. In spite of the disambiguation, 11 of these spoken homophones were wrongly defined; and in every case the definition corresponded to the other sense of the homophone (e.g. *tacks* defined as "money", *quay* as "main figure"). As Table I shows, C.D. has a very marked deficit in spelling as well as in reading, and this failure to use heard spelling to disambiguate spoken homophones is presumably another reflection of her spelling deficit, a point to which we return later.

Table IV. Phonologically correct errors in spelling to dictation by C.D.

Written spelling		Oral spelling	
worry	→ worrey	view	→ vew
else	→ elce	mortgage	→ morgage
search	→ surch	health	→ helth
description	→ discription	familiar	→ fermillyer
mechanical	→ macanical	cemetery	→ cemertery
capacity	→ capasaty	sufficient	→ surfichent
coarse	→ cource	equally	→ equaly
definite	→ defenat	bargain	→ bargan
anniversary	→ anerversery	account	→ acount

Spelling Administration of two parallel forms of the Schonell spelling test, with written spelling required for form A and oral spelling for form B, indicated that C.D.'s spelling, whether written or oral, is at least as markedly impaired as her reading (see Table 1).

The majority (about 60%) of her spelling errors in these two tests were phonologically correct, and examples of these are shown in Table IV. However, there were some examples which were not phonologically correct, such as "colonel" → *curanly*, "signature" → *signaation*, "cough" → *coulg*, "appreciate" → *aperatch*, "institution" → *intertune* and "exaggerate" → *exadert*. Misspellings, again mainly phonologically correct, were also fairly common in her spontaneous writing of prose.

Some Experiments with French

C.D.'s parents and grandparents speak French, though English is the usual language of her parents; she herself speaks French too, and spent some time in a French-speaking school in Switzerland.

She was asked to write down the English equivalents of 30 single spoken French words (all cooking terms). She omitted three items, not recognising the French words (poivre. épice. agneau) and made one translation error ("poire" → *pepper*). Of the remaining 26 correctly understood words, the English spellings were incorrect for 10 (most misspellings being phonologically correct or almost correct). Three months later, she was given this task in reverse, i.e. the English words were spoken and she was asked to write down their French equivalents. Five were not attempted; of the remaining 25, the French spellings were incorrect for 14, and phonologically correct misspellings occurred here too ("snail" → *escargo*, "wine" → *du vain*, "vinegar" → *vineigre*).

The occurrence of phonologically correct misspellings in these translation tasks is of some importance. When such misspellings occur in a monolingual task, it is possible to argue that the spoken word is not recognised and hence is treated as a non-word: if so, a phonologically correct spelling error is not a spelling error. If one does not recognise "search" as a word, then *surch* is a correct spelling.[3] Since our contention is that C.D.'s speech recognition is normal, we would not wish to entertain this explanation of her phonological spelling errors; and the explanation may be dismissed because of the occurrence of these errors in translation tasks. If she spells "légumes" as *vegterbales* and "wine" as *vain*, as she did, she must have recognised the spoken words, since she translated them correctly into another language. Thus the phonological spelling errors here actually are *spelling* errors.

Types of Error in Reading Aloud

So far we have discussed two of the forms of oral reading error—the regularisation error and the stress error. However, there are many errors in C.D.'s oral reading which cannot be assigned to either of these categories: *bowl* → "blow", *check* → "cheek" and *enigma* → "image", for example.

When Marshall and Newcombe (1973) considered this issue, they mentioned several categories of error which could not arise simply through phonological reading. Some of their categories were purely descriptive (difficulties with consonant clusters, difficulties with vowel clusters) and others were theoretically based (visual errors, partial failure of grapheme–phoneme conversions). We will propose a somewhat different approach to the classification of these sorts of errors.

Because C.D. produced numerous errors which involved omission of letters but which could not be described as "partial failure of grapheme–phoneme rules" (e.g. *frog* → "fog", *varnish* → "vanish", *saucer* → "sauce"), it becomes unclear whether an error such as *bike* → "bik" explained by Marshall and Newcombe as a partial failure of grapheme–phoneme rules, requires such an explanation. This error might instead be an example of a more general error type (letter omission). Analogously, since their patient, J.C., read *cable* as "able", his reading of *niece* as "nice" might not be due to a specific difficulty with vowel clusters (as they proposed) but instead to a more general tendency to omit letters.

"Difficulties with consonant clusters" were illustrated by Marshall and Newcombe (1973) with examples such as *pigsty* → "pigisti", but could instead be due to a more general tendency to add letters; and C.D. exhibited such a tendency (*topic* → "tropic", *utter* → "butter", *stake* → "/streɪk/").

Marshall and Newcombe (1973) also referred to "occasional visual errors" such as *spy* → "shy" or *polite* → "police". Given that *t* is not visually similar to *c*, we take it that they meant by "visual error" a response where a letter has not been omitted or added, but merely changed: and C.D. produced such responses (*shrug* → "/strʌg/", *flight* → "fright", *tacks* → "/plæks/"). Visual similarity between letters appeared to be unimportant here: when stimulus and response differed by a single letter, the mismatching letters were frequently not visually similar to each other.

In addition to letter omissions, additions and changes, errors of letter position also occurred in C.D.'s responses (*enigma* → "image", *board* → "broad", *gaol* → "/gæloʊ/", *dare* → "dear", for example).

We should emphasise that the errors we describe as letter omissions, additions, changes and position errors are not unique to C.D. When the error corpus provided by Holmes (1973) is scrutinised, examples of all four error types can be found in all six of the cases she describes.

To describe reading errors in terms of these four labels is, of course, theoretically arid, and scarcely amounts even to a classification, since, if an error is made and the response has any similarity to the stimulus, all conceivable errors would represent one of the four error types, or some combination of them. Our aim has been to show, however, that the theoretically fertile classification proposed by Marshall and Newcombe may be inadequate, since the error examples they offered can be subsumed under the error typology we propose whilst, we have argued, the error examples we have offered cannot be subsumed under their categorisation scheme. Further work will be needed if it is to be shown that, for example, an error like *bike* → "bik" is not simply another example of an error like *frog* → "fog".

Reading Non-Words Aloud We have shown that C.D.'s ability to read words aloud is impaired. What of her ability to read non-words?

She was given 30 three-letter non-words to read aloud. Of these, 15 were pseudohomophones (i.e. were pronounced exactly like some English word) and 15 were not. She pronounced 21 out of 30 correctly; three of her nine errors were with pseudohomophones.

With a set of 50 monosyllabic non-words three to five letters long she scored 12 out of 50 correct; with a set of 120 non-words one to three syllables and four to six letters long she scored 28 out of 120 correct.

Evaluating these results is not entirely straightforward, since one cannot take normal performance in reading non-words as 100% correct performance. First of all, there is not universal agreement amongst normal readers as to what is the correct pronunciation of all non-words. Secondly, pronunciations which scarcely anyone would regard as possibly correct can be found in non-word reading by skilled readers: examples we have observed with university undergraduate subjects reading non-words aloud include *crom* → "/krʌm/", *glond* → "/blɒnd/", *brilmit* → "/brɪmlɪt/", *taid* → "/taɪd/" and *gebe* → "/gibə/". Consequently, it would be desirable to have normative data against which to evaluate C.D.'s reading of non-words. However, we consider it very unlikely indeed that any normal reader would produce scores as low as 12 out of 50 and 28 out of 120 when reading aloud our lists of non-words.

It is worth pointing out that amongst C.D.'s non-word reading errors were letter omissions (*nade* → /næd/, *girter* → /gɪtə/), letter changes (*pleck* → /plæck/, *drig* → /drɪd/), letter additions (*coab* → /koɷbə/, *drace* → /dræns/, and letter position errors (*syphet* → /saɪpɛθ/, *civid* → /ˈsaɪdɪv/). Thus all the "orthographic" or "visual" errors evident in reading words aloud are also present when non-words are read aloud.

A second feature of her non-word reading was that incorrect responses were sometimes non-words and sometimes real words. For example, in the set of 120 non-words mentioned above, where 92 were misread, 59.8% of error responses were real words; of the 38 incorrect responses to the 50 non-words mentioned above, 42.1% were real words. In these tests, all the items in the test were non-words and C.D. was informed of this; the tendency to produced word responses to non-word stimuli might well be higher in lists consisting of randomly intermixed words and non-words, where prior information as to whether an item is a word or not would not be available.

The tendency to "lexicalise" (to read a non-word as a word) has been discussed, in relation to surface dyslexia, by Marcel (1980). Although C.D. produces numerous lexicalisations, we do not regard this kind of behaviour as characteristic of surface dyslexia in general, because it is not shown by other surface dyslexics we have studied and are studying. For example, the acquired surface dyslexic E.E, who misread 71 of the 120 non-words referred to in the previous paragraph, produced only six word responses. Furthermore, even when all stimuli are *words*, non-word responses are common: when the set of 78 regular and irregular words were given to six surface dyslexics (three acquired, three developmental) the percentage of errors where the response was *not* a word ranged from 41 to 84%.

Acquired Surface Dyslexia

Case History

A.B., born in 1963, is left-handed except that he has always written with his right hand, and his father is left-handed. His school reported that he has a mature attitude to his work but would not be likely to pass higher CSE examinations; he was very good at metal design and mathematics, but "found English very hard". (We have no further information about this.) He took a job as an apprentice fitter.

On 31 July 1979 he had a motorcycle accident on a wet road, and suffered a compound comminuted depressed fracture of the right frontal area of the skull and a fractured right arm. He was unconscious for approximately 1 month. Bone fragments were excised from the right frontal area of the brain. The only brain damage noted was contusion in the right frontal area. We presume that he was right-hemisphere lateralised for language; all other reported cases of acquired surface dyslexia had left-hemisphere damage. Residual problems included occasional minor epileptic fits, often involving only an aura, some mild difficulties in balance and co-ordination, and difficulty in logical thinking, reasoning and higher language functions.

Evidence for Surface Dyslexia in A.B.

Regular vs. Irregular Words. On 26 June 1980, A.B. was asked to read aloud the 39 regular and 39 irregular words referred to earlier. He was correct with 30 out of 39 regular words and 18 out of 39 irregular words ($\chi^2_{(1)} = 7.8$, $P < 0.01$).[4] He was also given the three silent homophone-matching tasks described above. The results were as follows: regular, 39 out of 50 (three false alarms, eight misses); non-words, 35 out of 50 (three false alarms, 16 misses); irregular words, 30 out of 50 (10 false alarms, six misses). The effect of word type approached significance ($\chi^2_{(2)} = 5.22$, $0.1 > P > 0.05$), as did the difference between regular and irregular ($\chi^2_{(1)} = 3.79$, $0.1 > P > 0.05$).

On 14 July 1980, A.B. was given the Schonell reading and spelling tests. He scored 46 out of 100 on the reading test (reading age = 9:3), and 38 out of 100 on the spelling test (spelling age = 8:8). His oral reading responses included unambiguous examples of all the kinds of errors discussed earlier in connection with C.D. (that is, regularisations, stress errors, letter omissions, letter additions, letter changes and position errors).

His spelling errors on the Schonell spelling test included a number which were phonologically correct, and such errors were also made when he wrote a half-page paragraph describing his job. Examples of these errors are given in Table V.

Thus A.B.'s reading and spelling demonstrates all the abnormalities which we have described in connection with C.D.: (a) better oral reading of regular than irregular words; (b) silent homophone matching which is best for regular words, next best for non-words, and worst for regular words; (c) regularisations and stress errors in reading aloud; (d) frequent phonologically correct misspellings; and (e) letter omissions, changes, additions and position errors in reading aloud.

Comprehending, Pronouncing and Spelling We performed with A.B. the tripartite comprehension test

Table V. Phonologically-correct misspellings A.B.

Writing single words to dictation			
son → sun		method → methered	
seem → seam		freeze → frise	
four → for		assist → asist	
dancing → danceing		readily → redaly	
search → surch		various → veryuse	
concert → consert		genuine → jenuwen	
domestic → damesteck		signature → signiture	
topic → Top-pick			
Spontaneous prose writing			
firm → phurm		bigger → biger	
firm → furm		cranes → crain's	
trial → tryal		compressors → compresers	
an apprentice → anaprentis		hour → ouwer	
trucks → trucs		two → to	

described earlier: that is, he was given single printed words and asked first to say what the word meant, then to read it aloud, then to spell it. This test was performed with a set of 107 words (these were *not* all words which had previously been misread).

Of these, there were 36 which were not comprehended correctly. In two cases, it was not clear what word the patient was attempting to define; in all the other cases, the definition corresponded to the subsequent pronunciation of a word. These correspondences included "don't know" responses to a word subsequently read as a neologism, such as *shove* → "don't know . . . /ʃoωv/" and *gang* → "don't know . . . /gændʒ/". There were also homophone confusions such as *soul* → "shoe" and *route* → "what holds the apple tree in the ground and makes it grow". In addition, there were instances where the response was a word phonologically different from the stimulus—here there were letter omissions, letter changes, letter additions and position errors, as in these examples:

scarce → "fairly serious cut . . . scar"
thyme → "certain part of the orchestra, music that the orchestra's playing, sort of meaning of what they are playing . . . theme"
debt → "to have a long discussion on something . . . debate"
subtle → "to stand firm . . . stable"

The spelling-aloud task (that is, naming all the letters of a word while looking at the word) was performed incorrectly with five of the 107 words. All of these words had been defined and read aloud correctly.

In this test, then, A.B. behaved exactly like C.D. If his oral reading response is erroneous, his prior comprehension of the word matches the subsequent incorrect oral reading response, not the stimulus, whilst at the same time his spelling-aloud response virtually always matches the stimulus, and not the oral reading response. This can lead to gross discrepancies between the reading and spelling responses, such as *build* → "bull . . . B,U,I,L,D" and *subtle* → "stable . . . S,U,B,T,L,E". In the comprehension test, A.B. also exhibited the kinds of homophone confusions which C.D. showed.

Auditory Comprehension A set of 48 short words was presented to A.B. Each word was spoken, then spelled aloud. His task was to say what each word meant. He made no errors to the 27 of these words which were not homophones. Of the 21 homophones, eight were wrongly defined: in every case the definition was of the other member of the homophone pair. Thus A.B. again behaves like C.D.: both are very poor at using heard spelling to disambiguate spoken homophones, but otherwise good at comprehending spoken words, at least for the sets of words we used.

Response to Spelled-Aloud Words When the 78 regular and irregular words were spelled aloud to P.M. (another surface dyslexic we have studied), his task being to respond by saying each word aloud, performance was better with the regular words (33 out of 39 vs. 24 out of 39), and the incorrect responses included regularisations (C,O,M,E, → /koωm/, M,O,V,E, → /moωv/). Another acquired surface dyslexic (E.E.) responded similarly (28 out of 39 regular words correct vs. 20 out of 39 irregular words) with regularisations such as S,E,W, → /su/). Thus features of surface dyslexia (homophone confusions, regularisations, poorer performance with irregular words) occur even when the stimulus is spelled aloud to the patient rather than being presented visually.

Premorbid and Familial Spelling No standardised test results were available here, but a school workbook completed prior to A.B.'s injury was, and in it spelling is imperfect, and there are examples of phonologically correct misspellings such as separately → *seperatly*, breaks → *brakes*, differences → diffrances. However, scrutiny of this workbook indicates that A.B.'s spelling was certainly far better before his accident than after it.

Some written communications from his mother (who works as a nurse) to his speech therapist were also studied. These included numerous spelling errors, many of which were phonologically correct (e.g. sure → *shore*).

In the absence of adequate information about the educational level and general language abilities of A.B.'s mother and (premorbidly) of A.B., it is difficult to evaluate these data. An extreme possibility is that both A.B. and his mother were developmental surface dyslexics, and that A.B.'s head injury simply exacerbated an already present condition. We consider this unlikely and in any case are confident that such an analysis cannot be offered for all cases of surface dyslexia, since we have studied one case of acquired dyslexia where the symptoms corresponded very closely to those of A.B. and C.D. and where a high degree of premorbid literacy was certainly present (the patient had written books on architectural history). Furthermore, it is already known that phonological spelling of the kind displayed by A.B. can occur as part of an acquired dysgraphia in a patient whose premorbid spelling was excellent: this is shown by case T.P., studied by Patterson and Kay (1982).

Symptoms of Surface Dyslexia: An Interim List

The symptoms shown by A.B. and C.D. (and by the four other surface dyslexics, two acquired and two developmental, whom we have studied) are as follows:

(1) Regular words are more likely to be read aloud correctly than irregular words.

(2) Incorrect readings of irregular words are often regularisations.

(3) Incorrect readings of polysyllabic words are sometimes correct except for being wrongly stressed.

(4) Silent homophone matching is more accurate with regular words, next best with non-words, and worst with irregular words.

(5) Silent reading comprehension is often mediated by prior phonological recoding; this is always the case when the phonological recoding is incorrect.

(6) Homophone confusions occur in silent reading comprehension.[5]

(7) Even when speech comprehension is otherwise intact, when a word is spelled aloud to the surface dyslexic (the task being to say or understand the word) the same errors occur as are seen in reading aloud. Thus one can observe homophone confusions and regularisations in response to spelled-aloud words.

(8) "Orthographic" errors (letter additions, alterations, omissions or transpositions) occur in reading aloud, and impair the reading of non-words as well as the reading of words.[6]

(9) Spelling is defective, with the majority of spelling errors being phonologically correct.

We suggest that the first of these symptoms may be considered necessary and sufficient for the diagnosis of surface dyslexia—i.e. we suggest that this symptom does not occur in any dyslexia except surface dyslexia, and that it occurs in all cases of surface dyslexia. We assume that whenever the first symptom is observed symptoms (2), (3) and (4) will also occur, since we argue below that these symptoms have a single common cause.

Although all of the surface dyslexics we have studied have exhibited comprehension defects due to the use of a phonological code for comprehension (symptoms (5) and (6)), we do not think such defects will invariably occur in surface dyslexia. There are two reasons for this. The first is that, on the theoretical account of surface dyslexia we offer below, symptoms (1) to (4) could occur without symptoms (5) and (6). The second is that there are already some suggestions of the occurrence of surface dyslexia without phonologically-based comprehension errors (Sasanuma, 1980; Goldblum, 1982). Sasanuma's case, K.K., was poor at reading aloud the Japanese ideographic script *kanji* whilst good at reading the syllabic script *kana*. If this corresponds to being poorer at reading irregular than regular words, then case K.K. represents the Japanese form of surface dyslexia. However, K.K. was not worse at *comprehending* kanji than at comprehending kana. Goldblum's case (who was French) regularised (and hence mispronounced) irregular words but appeared to be able to understand them correctly.

Whether the last three symptoms invariably occur in surface dyslexia can only be determined by studies of other cases of the disorder. Certainly the ninth symptom — phonologically correct misspellings — is not *confined* to surface dyslexia, since it has been reported as accompanying at least one case of a different dyslexia, phonological dyslexia (Beauvois and Dérouesné, 1979, Case R.G.)

Regularisation Errors as Normal Responses

There are irregular words so infrequent that they would not be known to the normal skilled reader of English: *fleury*, for example. When confronted with such words, and asked to read them aloud, the normal skilled reader produces regularisation errors, of course. It is therefore imprecise to state that the occurrence of regularisation errors is *sufficient* for the diagnosis of surface dyslexia; the sufficient condition is the occurrence of regularisation errors with common words (words, that is, which should have been known to the patient premorbidly) and the demonstration of an abnormal tendency to regularise may thus sometimes require comparisons between a patient and a control group, or between a patient's postmorbid and premorbid reading of irregular words. This is unlikely to be a difficulty with respect to acquired surface dyslexia, since the irregular words in the lists of regular and irregular words we referred to early are mostly common words. However, this characteristic of surface dyslexia sets it aside from other acquired dyslexias: under normal conditions, normal readers never make semantic errors in reading isolated words (as the deep dyslexic does) or fail drastically at reading non-words (as the phonological dyslexic does) or identify words letter by letter (as the pure alexic does).

The fact that regularisation errors cannot in themselves be regarded as abnormal responses has somewhat more complicated consequences for the interpretation of developmental surface dyslexia. There will be many quite common irregular words which will be unfamiliar to the young normal reader, and since young normal readers will have a good knowledge of the orthographic–phonological correspondences of English (see, for example, Doctor and Coltheart, 1980), regularisation errors will be frequent when young normal readers are reading irregular words aloud. Indeed, a good knowledge of the relationships between orthography and phonology (in both directions) should produce not only regularisations but also homophone confusions in reading comprehension, and phonological spelling errors, in young normal readers. It would not be at all surprising, then, if most or all of the symptoms of surface dyslexia could be demonstrated in young normal readers—a possibility raised by Marcel (1980). It follows that, if we compared the performance of our developmental surface dyslexic C.D. to the performance of normal readers having her reading age, her reading might be shown to be qualitatively and quantitatively indistinguishable from theirs.

Our view here is that one must distinguish between two issues: whether a putative developmental dyslexic's reading is abnormal, on the one hand, and whether his or her reading pattern is qualitatively distinct from young normal reading, on the other. The first issue is investigated by using controls matched for chronological age; the second by using controls matched for reading age. The first type of control establishes whether a reader should be regarded as developmentally dyslexic; the second type of control establishes whether the form of developmental dyslexia present corresponds to "delay" or to "deviance"—that is, whether the abnormality consists of failing to progress beyond normal early stages of reading or to the occurrence of abnormal patterns of reading not characteristic of any stage of learning to read. If varieties of developmental dyslexia exist, some may correspond to the former type of abnormality (for example, developmental surface dyslexia, corresponding to the "dyseidetic dyslexia" of Boder, 1973) and others to the latter kind of abnormality (for example, developmental deep dyslexia, if it exists: this would correspond to the "dysphonetic dyslexia" of Boder, 1973).

The Theoretical Interpretation of Surface Dyslexia

Suggestions as to the theoretical interpretation of surface dyslexia—that is, as to how it might be explained within the context of an explicit model of the processes involved in *normal* reading—have been made by a number of authors (for example, Marshall and Newcombe, 1973; Coltheart, 1978, 1981; Shallice and Warrington, 1980; Shallice, 1981; Marcel, 1980; Patterson, 1981; Henderson, 1982). We discuss below differences between views expressed by these authors: for the moment, however, we will discuss what they have in common. It is uniformly considered that when the surface dyslexic reads *broad* as "brode", this occurs because of a failure to access some previously stored representation of the whole word *broad*, a failure which leads to the word being treated as a novel unfamiliar letter string—that is, as a non-word. Thus the processing system used by the surface dyslexic to read *broad* here is the processing system we all use when reading a non-word aloud.

It follows that the form of one's explanation of reading in surface dyslexia will be largely governed by one's model of how non-words are read aloud; and it is because various models of non-word reading have been proposed that various explanations of surface dyslexia have been suggested.

A non-word is a novel stimulus, and so cannot be read aloud by accessing, from the *orthographic* form of the non-word as a whole, the *phonological* from of the non-word as a whole, because there has been no way of acquiring from experience such a specific one-to-one mapping. A non-word therefore must be read aloud by recourse to previously acquired information about mappings between *orthographic components* of the non-word's spelling and *phonological components* of its pronunciation; and the various views of how we read non-words differ according to the size and nature of the orthographic components which are mapped onto phonological components. The following views as to how this piecemeal mapping process might proceed have been proposed (we use the pronunciation of the non-word *bink* to illustrate these views):

(1) The orthographic unit used is the *grapheme* (where "grapheme" refers to any letter or letter group which represents a single phoneme:[7] thus *sprint* consists of six graphemes whilst *sheath* consists of only three). The reader has learned a system of correspondences between grapheme and phonemes, and uses the correspondences *b* → /b/, *i* → /ɪ/, *n* → /ŋ/ and *k* → /k/ to convert *bink* to /bɪŋk/. The conversion of *n* to /ŋ/, rather than to /n/, could be accomplished either by having a context-sensitive grapheme–phoneme correspondence or by the operation of phonotactic constraints at some output stage.

(2) Correspondences between multiple graphemes and multiple phonemes, such as *bi* → /bɪ/ or *nk* → /ŋk/, can be used. Here units larger than the grapheme are involved.

(3) The conversion of *ink* to /ɪŋk/ when reading *bink* as /bɪŋk/ occurs because *ink* is a morpheme, and a system of morpheme-to-phonology correspondences plays a part in reading non-words. Subsequently, in some way, the phoneme /b/ is added to /ɪŋk/ to yield /bɪŋk/ as a pronunciation for *bink*.

(4) The non-word *bink* activates those words which are its "orthographic neighbours"—pink, mink, sink, etc.,—and from this set of neighbours the common phonological termination /ɪŋk/ is abstracted. Subsequently, in some way, the phoneme /b/ is added to /ɪŋk/ to yield /bɪŋk/ as a pronunciation for *bink*.

Theorists have not always confined themselves to just one of these four possibilities. For example, on the account proposed by Shallice and Warrington (1980) and Shallice (1981) both the morpheme and the multigraphemic letter sequence can be used in mapping orthography onto phonology; and in the account of reading aloud offered by Glushko (1979) it would seem, as noted by Coltheart (1981), that both the multigraphemic letter sequence and the orthographic neighbourhood can be involved. Furthermore, *any* account of the processes involved in reading aloud non-words must include the use of orthographic units no larger than the grapheme, because one can devise non-words which could not be read aloud in any other way. For example, *zwuk* contains no morphemes, has no orthographic neighbours (since no words of English end *uk*) and contains some consecutive letters which do not exist as consecutive letters in any English words (so that there are no multiple graphemes for which multiple phoneme correspondences can have been learned through prior experience with words of English). Therefore, the grapheme must be the unit used when *zwuk* is read aloud. This is not to say, of course, that grapheme–phoneme correspondences are not simply one part of a broader system of orthographic–phonological correspondences.

It follows that any theory about how non-words are read aloud must include correspondences at the grapheme–phoneme level: disputes as to which is the correct account of how non-words are read aloud will be disputes as to what other levels, if any, are used. As far as surface dyslexia is concerned, then, the question is whether one can find examples of reading responses which appear to require that some unit other than the grapheme is being used, when reading via the whole word has failed. There are various ways in which one might set about doing this: one might try, for example, to show that a regular word like *sink* (which contains the morpheme *ink*) is more likely to be read correctly than a regular word like *sick* (which contains no morphemes). If such effects were to be demonstrable in surface dyslexia, then this would suggest that the morpheme is sometimes used as a unit to mediate translation from print to phonology when translation via a whole-word representation fails. Alternatively, one could sift through the responses made by surface dyslexics, collecting those which appear to be inexplicable in terms of the use solely of grapheme–phoneme correspondences. Such responses can be found: for example, C.D. read *borough* as /brʌf/ and *thorough* as /θərʌf/, and this, as Marcel (personal communication) has pointed out, suggests that the morphemic correspondence *rough* → /rʌf/ is being used.

As yet, however, there is no substantial evidence to indicate that any unit larger than the grapheme is used by the surface dyslexic to read those words for which the whole-word level fails. We will therefore offer an interpretation of surface dyslexia in which no units intermediate between the whole word and the grapheme are used for converting print to phonology, and leave it to future work on surface dyslexia to compel one to adopt the view that such intermediate units do in fact play a part. We do not wish at all to claim that, if an interpretation based upon the grapheme–phoneme correspondence mechanism appears to offer an acceptable explanation of what is currently known about surface dyslexia, this should be regarded as evidence counting against other kinds of interpretation, since other interpretations might produce equally acceptable explanations.

The model we will use to offer an interpretation of surface dyslexia is a revised version of the logogen model, adapted from Morton and Patterson (1980). The relevant components of this model are (a) *visual input logogens*; devices for the visual recognition of printed words; (b) *ouput logogens*; devices for generating the spoken forms of words; (c) *the cognitive system*; which deals with the processing of semantic information; (d) *grapheme–phoneme conversion* (GPC), which is used to account for our ability to read non-words aloud.

On this model, one can read aloud via the output logogens or via grapheme–phoneme conversion. Since non-words do not have logogens, however, only words can be read aloud via the output logogens; and since irregular words are incorrectly processed via the GPC system, only regular words and non-words can be read aloud correctly via this system.

What kind of damage to this system for reading might produce the symptoms of surface dyslexia? We will assume the cognitive system is intact (since C.D., a typical surface dyslexic, showed no impairment of speech comprehension, and we assume that the cognitive system is used both for comprehending print and for comprehending speech). We will also assume that the output logogen system, and its communication from the cognitive system, are intact, since this indicated by the intactness of C.D.'s spontaneous speech. These assumptions hold for nearly all of the surface dyslexics we have studied.

Suppose that a word has no accessible representation in the visual input logogen system. When this is so, and the task is to read aloud the word, it will be necessary to use the grapheme–phoneme conversion system to accomplish this task. This system correctly translates regular words from print to phonology, but produces incorrect translations for irregular words. Thus, if there are failures of access within the visual input logogen level, this will lead to errors in the reading aloud of irregular words but not to errors in the reading aloud of regular words. Hence the first of the nine symptoms we listed earlier will arise: an advantage for regular over irregular words in reading aloud. The second symptom, the regularisation error, will also arise, because on those occasions when the grapheme–phoneme correspondence system is used to read an irregular word, the resulting incorrect phonological code will, of course, be a regularisation. The third symptom, the stress error, will arise in the same way: even for regular words, whose individual phonemes are correctly obtained via the grapheme–phoneme system, it will not always be possible to decide, when these words are polysyllabic, where stress should fall. For example, if *apron* is treated as a non-word how could one decide whether it should be stressed like *April*, like *upon* or like *aptly*? Hence J.C. read *apron* as /a|prɒn/ (Holmes 1973).

Homophone Matching

We are not suggesting that, in surface dyslexia, words *never* access their representations in the visual input logogen system: if this were so, irregular words would *never* be read aloud correctly by the surface dyslexic, and yet they often are. We are suggesting that, in any testing session, some input logogens are correctly accessed and others are not.[8] Those occasions on which an input logogen is accessed are responsible for the above-chance performance on homophone matching with irregular words, and for the better performance with regular words than non-words in homophone matching. Because there are occasions when a word's visual input logogen is not accessible, however, so that a phonological code yielded by the grapheme–phoneme system must be used for the homophone-matching task, regular words will produce better performance than irregular words in this task; and non-words will yield above-chance performance because homophone matching can be achieved using the grapheme–phoneme system. Thus a partial defect at the level of the visual input logogens would produce the pattern of homophone-matching performance we observed with C.D. and A.B.: irregular word performance is above chance, so is non-word performance, and regular word performance is superior both to non-word performance and regular word performance. In other words, the fourth of the symptoms we listed finds an explanation.

Comprehension

So far in this section of the paper we have discussed reading aloud. Suppose, however, that on one of those occasions when the appropriate visual input logogen is inaccessible, the surface dyslexic has been asked to *understand* the printed word. The normal route from print to semantics is via the visual input logogen system, but this route is not available on this occasion. What *is* available, however, is a phonological representation of the word, obtained by using the grapheme–phoneme system. We suggest that in these circumstances all that the surface dyslexic can do is use this representation to access the cognitive system—to behave, that is, as if he or she were understanding a spoken, not a printed, word. A plausible route for this procedure, in the context of the logogen model proposed by Morton and Patterson (1980), is: visual analysis → grapheme–phoneme conversion → response buffer → auditory input logogens → cognitive system. It is the use of this route which is responsible for our finding that, when access to a visual input logogen fails, comprehension is based entirely upon mediation by a phonological code.

This mediation can still produce correct comprehension, but only if the printed word is both (a) regular and also (b) not a homophone. If the word is irregular, the phonological code produced by the grapheme–phoneme system will be incorrect, and hence comprehension cannot be correct: in this way responses such as pint → "don't know", and *gauge* → "a big dip" occur. If the word is a homophone, the phonological code produced by the grapheme–phoneme system will be ambiguous. This ambiguity could only be resolved by using orthographic information; use of such information would require the correct functioning of the visual input logogen system or a spelling system, and neither system functions normally in surface dyslexia. In this way homophone confusions such as *soar* → "to cut" or *pane* → "something which hurts" will occur.

Thus the fifth and sixth symptoms of surface dyslexia that were listed earlier, as well as the first four symptoms, can be explained in terms of failure of access within the visual input logogen level, with use of a phonological code (obtained from the grapheme–phoneme system) for comprehension. Shallice and Warrington (1980) characterised surface dyslexia as "phonological reading" and one interpretation of this term is the one we have offered: reading via the grapheme–phoneme system (whereas reading via the visual input logogens would be "visual reading").

We have shown that when words are spelled aloud to a surface dyslexic, and a comprehension or pronunciation response is requested, the errors characteristic of surface dyslexic *reading* occur, even though speech comprehension is otherwise intact. If, as suggested by Coltheart (1981), the input to the visual input logogen system is a set of abstract letter identities, one might argue that such identities are evoked not only by print but also by spoken letter names, so that the task of understanding a word when it has been spelled aloud depends upon the visual input logogen system, and hence is akin to reading rather than to speech perception. If so, the surface dyslexic should be surface dyslexic not only in response to a printed stimulus, but also in response to spelled-aloud stimuli. In this way, the seventh of our list of symptoms might be explained.

Homophone Confusions with Irregularly-Spelled Homophones

Some of the homophone confusions produced by C.D. and A.B. in the tripartite comprehension task occurred with irregularly-spelled homophones; for example, *bury* → "a fruit on a tree", and *bowled* → "fierce, big".

Irregular homophone confusions are important because they show that an explanation of surface dyslexia as arising solely from the inaccessibility of visual input logogens in insufficient, for the following reason. Since the above words were misunderstood, they could not have reached their appropriate entries in the cognitive system. However, since the definitions offered indicated that each word was confused with its homophone, the correct phonological representations of the words were obtained. These cannot have been obtained via the grapheme–phoneme system, because this system yields *incorrect* phonological codes for irregular words; *correct* phonological codes for such words are provided only by the output logogen system. Therefore these words must have reached their correct entries in the output logogen system. In terms of the theoretical framework we have adopted), such correct access cannot occur unless there is correct access within the visual input logogen system: but if the correct visual input logogen was accessed, why were these words misunderstood?

Our suggestion is that in these cases there is correct access within the visual input logogen system, but a failure of communication between this system and the cognitive system, whilst at the same time communication from the visual input logogen system to the output logogen system is achieved; and a phonological code can thus be obtained in this way. If comprehension is required, this phonological code can access the semantic system, perhaps via the auditory input logogens. This represents a second form of phonological reading: here "phonological reading" means reading via the output logogen system. This differs from the first kind of phonological reading we mentioned, which consisted of reading via the grapheme–phoneme system.

One reason for the theoretical importance of these irregular-homophone confusions is that they would appear to require, for their explanation, the existence of a direct (non-semantic) route from visual input logogens to output logogens. Such a route was included in the version of the logogen model proposed by Morton and Patterson (1980), but it is not required by any data collected from studies of normal reading, even though the logogen model was developed originally solely from studies of normal language behaviour. The evidence that this direct route exists comes only from studies of acquired dyslexia. The existence of the route is, we have argued, implied by the occurrence of irregular-homophone confusions in surface dyslexia; and a completely independent piece of evidence for this route comes from a different kind of acquired dyslexia, that studied by Schwartz, Saffran and Marin (1980). Their patient could read aloud irregular words which she could not comprehend. This reading aloud could not have been mediated by the grapheme–phoneme system (since the words were irregular) nor via semantics (since the words could not be understood); hence a third route would seem to be required.

Spelling

We have nothing further to say about the phonological spelling errors characteristic of surface dyslexia, since the logogen model as we have employed it contains no machinery for performing spelling tasks (though see Morton, 1980, for discussion of the extension of the model to spelling). We merely ask whether it can be simply a coincidence that phonological reading and phonological spelling have co-occurred in all those cases of the disorder where both reading and spelling have been studied. This conjunction may perhaps be due to some *general* loss of information about the orthographic forms of words, a loss affecting some system used equally for accepting orthographic input (reading) and producing orthographic output (spelling).

Unresolved Problems

A major problem for explanations of surface dyslexia based upon dual-route models in which the reading of irregular words and the reading of non-words depend upon two independent systems is that surface dyslexics should be observed in whom impairment of the "lexical" or "direct" reading route is accompanied by intactness of the "non-lexical" reading route (i.e. the grapheme–phoneme correspondence system, according to the theoretical framework we have adopted). Intactness of the grapheme–phoneme system can be assessed by ability to read non-words. As we have argued, one cannot require 100% performance in non-word reading as the criterion for claiming intactness of the grapheme–phoneme correspondence system. Furthermore, success in non-word reading depends on type of non-word: if there is a one-to-one and context-insensitive relationship of letter to phoneme (*stup*) the task of reading non-words may be simpler than when context-sensitivity is required (*cimy*) or when a one-to-one relationship does not hold (*choe*). Such issues complicate the question of whether non-word reading can be unimparied in cases of surface dyslexia, but, as we have said, it is clear that C.D.'s ability to read non-words was abnormally poor. If future work on surface dyslexia fails to demonstrate cases where non-word reading is within the normal range, models with independent lexical and non-lexical procedures for reading aloud will be compromised.

In terms of the theoretical framework we have been using, a selective deficit for irregular words, with regularisation and stress errors, could arise in more than one way [as Shallice and Warrington (1980) pointed out, in relation to a rather different model]. A loss of entries for words in the *output* logogen system, accompanied by relative sparing of the grapheme–phoneme correspondence system, would produce the first four symptoms of our symptom list and hence would, for us, count as surface dyslexia. However, a patient with this defect would have normal access to the semantic system and hence would not show surface-dyslexic effects in *comprehension.* As we have noted, the Japanese patient K.K (Sasanuma, 1980) could be an example of this kind of surface dyslexic, but no examples in English have been reported. The interpretation of surface dyslexia we offer makes strong predictions about this output-logogen form of surface dyslexia. Since the output logogens are necessary not only for reading irregular words but also for picture-naming and spontaneous speech, any surface dyslexic who has intact reading comprehension (and hence by inference has an output-logogen defect) must show anomic defects in spontaneous speech and in picture-naming. The patient K.K showed these symptoms (fluent paraphasic speech and very impaired object naming).

The French patient described by Goldblum (1982), however, who was surface dyslexic in oral reading but appeared to have access to semantics for misread words (as tested by requiring her to give semantic associates to the printed stimulus), seemed not to have an output logogen defect; word-finding difficulties in spontaneous speech or object-naming were not evident. Goldblum (1982) suggests that the lexical route was intact in this patient and was used when reading comprehension was required, but not when reading aloud was required. The results we refer to in the footnote on p. 7 might be taken to indicate something similar, namely that defects of the lexical route are not absolute, and that the requirement to comprehend induces the surface dyslexic to use this route (even for reading aloud) more than the route would be used when the task is simply to read aloud. If effects of this sort can be documented in sufficient detail, it will be necessary to think again about what we mean when we say that word representations in the lexical system are "inaccessible".

Notes

We thank Karalyn Patterson, Tony Marcel, Leslie Henderson, Tim Shallice, John Morton and an anonymous reviewer for criticisms of previous versions of this paper. Work reported here was supported by grant G979/827/N from the Medical Research Council.

1. See Appendix for error corpus.

2. C.D.'s incorrect readings are sufficiently consistent from occasion to occasion, with re-presentation of the same set of words, for us to be surprised at this success rate (52% correct when on previous presentation no words had been read correctly). One possibility is that the requirement to comprehend before reading aloud increases the accuracy of reading aloud. The same effect occurred with our second case, A.B., described later. He scored 46 out of 78 correct on the regular and irregular words when simply asked to read them aloud. On a subsequent occasion, when asked to define then read aloud, he scored 58 out of 78. Fourteen words read wrongly on the first occasion were read correctly on the second, when a prior definition was required. Further investigation of this issue is needed.

3. One could, of course, rule out this possibility by using a monolingual task in which heard words are defined and then spelled and showing that phonological spelling errors accompany correct definitions.

4. See Appendix for error corpus.

5. Given that both A.B. and C.D. made various kinds of "orthographic" errors, one might argue that *steak* → "fencing post" was not a homophone confusion but a letter position error (like *stale* → "slate"). We think this is unlikely, because there are homophone confusions where the stimulus and response are orthographically rather dissimilar. For example, E.E., a surface dyslexic we are currently studying, defined the word *I* as to do with the organs of sight (pointing to his eyes); other examples are *soar* defined as saw, *build* as billed and *paced* as paste.

6. We have not provided information as to the proportions of incorrect responses which fall into the various error categories (regularisations, stress errors and the various kinds of orthographic error) because such information can often be misleading. For example, the proportion of regularisations will depend upon the proportion of stimulus words which are irregular, and the proportion of stress errors will depend upon the proportion of stimulus words which are polysyllabic. Thus error proportions for these two error types will at least to some extent be arbitrary since they depend upon the (arbitrary) choice of the proportion of irregular words and polysyllabic words to be included in the stimuli presented to the surface dyslexic.

7. Venezky (1970) distinguishes between "grapheme" (an abstract letter) and "functional spelling unit" (any grapheme or sequence of graphemes which map onto a single phoneme). Because we do not consider his reason for rejecting the term "letter" compelling, because of the widespread use of the term "grapheme–phoneme correspondence" and because of the clumsiness of the term "functional spelling unit" we follow Coltheart (1978) in using "letter" where Venezky (1970) uses "grapheme", and using "grapheme" where he uses "functional spelling unit".

8. The question of consistency across testing occasions is clearly of relevance here. If the surface dyslexic is repeatedly tested on the same set of irregular words, will there be any consistency across occasions in those words he fails to read? Preliminary studies suggest that there is a great deal of such consistency.

References

Beauvois, M. F. and Dérouesné J. (1979). Phonological alexia: three dissociations. *Journal of Neurology, Neurosurgery and Psychiatry*, **42**, 1115–24.

Boder, E. (1973). Developmental dyslexia: a diagnostic approach based on three atypical reading–spelling patterns. *Developmental Medicine and Child Neurology*, **15**, 663–87.

Coltheart, M. (1978). Lexical access in simple reading tasks. In Underwood, G. (Ed.), *Strategies of Information Processing*. London: Academic Press.

Coltheart, M. (1980). Deep dyslexia: a right-hemisphere hypothesis. In Coltheart, M., Patterson, K. E. and Marshall, J. C. (Eds), *Deep Dyslexia*. London: Routledge and Kegan Paul.

Coltheart, M. (1981) Disorders of reading and their implications for models of normal reading. *Visible Language*, **15**, 245–86.

Coltheart, M., Patterson, K. E. and Marshall, J. C. (Eds) (1980). *Deep Dyslexia*. London: Routledge and Kegan Paul.

Coltheart, M., Besner, D., Jonasson, J. T. and Davelaar, E. (1979). Phonological recoding in the lexical decision task. *Quarterly Journal of Experimental Psychology*, **31**, 489–508.

Doctor, E. A. and Coltheart, M. (1980). Children's use of phonological encoding when reading for meaning. *Memory and Cognition*, **8**, 195–209.

Glushko, R. J. (1979). The organisation and activation of orthographic knowledge in reading aloud. *Journal of Experimental Psychology* (*Human Perception and Performance*), **5**, 674–91.

Goldblum, M. C. (1982). Comprehension in surface dyslexia Paper presented at the International Neuropsychological Society Meeting, Deauville.

Henderson, L. (1982). *Orthography and Word Recognition in Reading*. London: Academic Press.

Holmes, J. M. (1973). Dyslexia: a neurolinguistic study of traumatic and developmental disorders of reading. PhD thesis, University of Edinburgh.

Holmes, J. M. (1978). "Regression" and reading breakdown. In Caramazza, A. and Zurif, E. B. (Eds.) *Language Acquisition and Language Breakdown: Parallels and Divergencies*. Baltimore: Johns Hopkins Press.

Marcel, A. J. (1980). Surface dyslexia and beginning reading: a revised hypothesis of the pronunciation of print and its impairments. In Coltheart, M., Patterson, K. E. and Marshall, J. C. (Eds.), *Deep Dyslexia*. London: Routledge and Kegan Paul.

Marshall, J. C. and Newcombe, F. (1973). Patterns of paralexia: a psycholinguistic approach. *Journal of Psycholinguistic Research*, **2**, 175–99.

Morton, J. (1980). The logogen model and orthographic structure. In Frith, U. (Ed.), *Cognitive Processes in Spelling*. London: Academic Press.

Morton, J. and Patterson, K. E. (1980). A new attempt at an interpretation, or an attempt at a new interpretation. In Coltheart, M., Patterson, K. E. and Marshall, J. C. (Eds), *Deep Dyslexia*. London: Routledge and Kegan Paul.

Newcombe, F. and Marshall, J. C. (1981). On psycholinguistic classifications of the acquired dyslexias. *Bulletin of the Orton Society*, **31**, 29–46.

Patterson, K. E. (1978). Phonemic dyslexia: errors of meaning and the meaning of errors. *Quarterly Journal of Experimental Psychology*, **30**, 387–601.

Patterson, K. E. (1981). Neuropsychological approaches to the study of reading. *British Journal of Psychology*, **72**, 151–74.

Patterson, K. E. and Kay, J. (1982). Letter-by-letter reading: psychological descriptions of a neurological syndrome. *Quarterly Journal of Experimental Psychology*, In press.

Sasanuma, S. (1980). Acquired dyslexia in Japanese: clinical features and underlying mechanisms. In Coltheart, M., Patterson, K. E. and Marshall, J. C. (Eds), *Deep Dyslexia*. London: Routledge and Kegan Paul.

Schwartz, M. F., Saffran, E. M. and Marin, O. S. M. (1980). Fractionating the reading process in dementia: evidence for word-specific print-to-sound associations. In Coltheart, M., Patterson, K. E. and Marshall, J. C. (Eds), *Deep Dyslexia*. London: Routledge and Kegan Paul.

Shallice, T. (1981). Neurological impairment of cognitive processes. *British Medical Bulletin*, **37**, 187–92.

Shallice, T. and Warrington, E. K. (1977). The possible role of selective attention in acquired dyslexia. *Neuropsychologia*, **15**, 31–41.

Shallice, T. and Warrington, E. K. (1980). Single and multiple component central dyslexic syndromes. In Coltheart, M., Patterson, K. E., and Marshall, J. C. (Eds), *Deep Dyslexia*. London: Routledge and Kegan Paul.

Venezky, R. L. (1970). *The Structure of English Orthography*. The Hague: Mouton.

Appendix

Errors by C.D. and A.B. in reading the 78 regular and irregular words of Coltheart et al (1979)

C.D.

Regular	*Irregular*
pine → /peɪn/	gauge → /gruəl/ . . . /grʌdʒ/
spade → /spid/	debt → /dɛp/
duel → /diəl/	pint → /peɪnt/
barge → /bræg/	mortgage → /mɔteɪdʒ/
	come → /koɷm/
	shove → /ʃoɷv/
	bury → /bjuri/
	thorough → /θərʌf/
	trough → /θrɒŋ/
	bowl → /bloɷ/
	subtle → /sʌbtaɪl/
	broad → /bɔd/
	borough → /brʌf/

A.B.

Regular		*Irregular*	
quick	→ /rɪk/	gauge	→ (no response)
strewn	→ /straɪn/	sure	→ /ʃru/
spade	→ (no response)	trough	→ /θru/
sherry	→ /ʃɛərɪ/	cough	→ (no response)
shampoo	→ (no response)	yacht	→ (no response)
check	→ /tʃik/	sword	→ /swɔd/
base	→ /pas/	sew	→ /dʒu/
pine	→ /pɛni/	lose	→ /lɒs/
cult	→ /kʌoɷlt/	circuit	→ /sɘ:kjut/
gang	→ /gæg/	biscuit	→ /baɪsɪkjut/
dance	→ (no response)	castle	→ /kæsəl/
capsule	→ /kæpsəl/	soul	→ /sɒlt/
		scarce	→ /ska/
		debt	→ (no response)
		thorough	→ /θru/
		borough	→ /bɒroɷ/
		bury	→ (no response)
		gross	→ /krɒs/
		broad	→ /bɒroɷd/
		subtle	→ (no response)

Name Index

Italicized page numbers indicate papers appearing in this volume.

Subject Index